SURFACE CHEMISTRY AND ELECTROCHEMISTRY OF MEMBRANES

SURFACTANT SCIENCE SERIES

ADDITIONAL VOLUMES IN PREPARATION

Silicone Surfactants, *edited by Randal M. Hill*

Surface Characterization Methods: Principles, Techniques, and Applications, *edited by Andrew J. Milling*

SURFACE CHEMISTRY AND ELECTROCHEMISTRY OF MEMBRANES

edited by

Torben Smith Sørensen

Physical Chemistry, Modelling & Thermodynamics/DTH
Vanløse (Copenhagen), Denmark

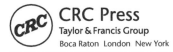

CRC Press
Taylor & Francis Group
Boca Raton London New York

CRC Press is an imprint of the
Taylor & Francis Group, an **informa** business

CRC Press
Taylor & Francis Group
6000 Broken Sound Parkway NW, Suite 300
Boca Raton, FL 33487-2742

First issued in paperback 2019

© 1999 by Taylor Francis Group, LLC
CRC Press is an imprint of Taylor & Francis Group, an Informa business

No claim to original U.S. Government works

ISBN-13: 978-0-8247-1922-7 (hbk)
ISBN-13: 978-0-367-39993-1 (pbk)

**Visit the Taylor & Francis Web site at
http://www.taylorandfrancis.com**

**and the CRC Press Web site at
http://www.crcpress.com**

Preface

Interest in the functioning of membranes is growing continuously, as is reflected in the overwhelming output of scientific papers in the field every year. There is increasing awareness of the crucial role played by the membrane surface—not only in synthetic membranes for reverse osmosis, desalination, purification, hemodialysis, and so on, but also in the biological membranes. The surface properties may be of a general physical nature (as in static or dynamic electric double layers) of a physicochemical nature (as the frozen-in two-phase structure of membranes with phase inversion during casting), or of a more specific chemical nature.

On the other hand, membrane transport takes place in a complicated interplay between the membrane surface, the membrane interior and the surrounding fluid phases, and many disciplines are called for in order to fully understand and describe the behavior: colloid and interface science, irreversible and statistical thermodynamics, electrochemistry, various forms of spectroscopy, and modern forms of microscopy to mention just a few.

The objective of this volume is to present a multiauthored and multidisciplinary book inside the general areas delineated above. It is hoped that such a book will attract the interest of physical chemists; surface scientists; inorganic, organic, and polymer chemists; physicists; chemical engineers; biophysicists; biologists; or anyone interested in gaining new inspiration for further research in a complex, rich, and useful scientific field of investigation.

In a monograph of limited size some important topics may necessarily be left out or be superficially treated. However, there is enough material here to make the book highly interesting in providing a unique constellation of the present state of the art. For this, I have to thank the many authors from so many different countries and cultures for their inventiveness and for their cooperation in making the changes necessary to promote the clarity of presentation.

The volume is divided into five main sections. In Part I, the topic of chemical and physical structure of synthetic membranes and membrane surfaces is discussed. The chapters in this section are concerned with atomic force microscopy of membrane surfaces, methods for the evaluation of pore sizes, the organic chemistry of surface functionalization of polymer membranes, and the fractal formation process of silica polymers and membranes.

In Part II, chapters are concerned with the phenomenology of transport and separation phenomena in synthetic membranes. Topics include solution–diffusion description and irreversible thermodynamics models of pervaporation and ultrafiltration, the treatment of protein fouling of ultrafiltration membranes, the diffusion of dyes in porous membranes, and the osmotic properties of membranes of polyelectrolyte gels.

In Part III, electrochemical processes are highlighted. The chapters in this section essentially deal with the theory and measurements of ion transport numbers in the bulk and on the surface of membranes, the transfer of water, ions, and entropy in ion exchange membranes, surface irreversible thermodynamics in an electrochemical fuel cell, electroosmotic phenomena, photoirradiation-controlled anion exchange membranes, and electroconvective mechanisms in membranes for electrodialysis.

Part IV is a "book within the book" concerning the important and useful techniques of impedance or dielectric spectroscopy in synthetic and biological membranes and in polymer films containing ion impurities. The—relatively little known—theoretical background for these techniques is advanced to such a state for the three chapters in this section, and so many experimental examples are given, that further use of impedance and dielectric spectroscopy in membrane science will surely be provoked.

Finally, Part V contains chapters on biological or biology-related membranes and on biomembrane surfaces. Chapter topics include the role of water in shaping transport in lipid bilayers, the role of surface electrostatics in ion binding in biological membranes, models of ion transport through "soft" polar interfaces (models of biomembranes), and the nonlinear instability of biological membrane surfaces of importance for bioadhesion.

All the authors have put special emphasis on the didactic side to make the presentations comprehensible and motivating for the well-informed nonspecialist of the topic in focus.

I would like to give my special thanks to Professor Arthur T. Hubbard, Director of The Surface Center at the University of Cincinnati, Ohio, and Senior Advisor to the Marcel Dekker, Inc., Surfactant Science series, for his suggestion to create this monograph and entrusting me to be the editor. I am the one to blame, however, if the result is less perfect than it could have been.

Torben Smith Sørensen

Contents

Contributors

Vicente Aguilella Departament de Ciències Experimentals, Universitat "Jaume I," de Castelló, Castelló, Spain

V. M. Barragán García Department of Applied Physics I, University Complutense of Madrid, Madrid, Spain

Dick Bedeaux Leiden Institute of Chemistry, Gorlaeus Laboratory, Leiden University, Leiden, The Netherlands

Marina Belaya Institute of Plant Physiology, Russian Academy of Sciences, Moscow, Russia

W. Richard Bowen Centre for Complex Fluids Processing, Department of Chemical and Biological Process Engineering, University of Wales Swansea, Swansea, United Kingdom

José Ignacio Calvo Department of Thermodynamics and Applied Physics, University of Valladolid, Valladolid, Spain

Terry C. Chilcott UNESCO Centre for Membrane Science and Technology, and Department of Biophysics, School of Physics, University of New South Wales, Sydney, New South Wales, Australia

Hans G. L. Coster UNESCO Centre for Membrane Science and Technology, and Department of Biophysics, School of Physics, University of New South Wales, Sydney, New South Wales, Australia

E. Anibal Disalvo   Laboratory of Physical Chemistry of Lipid Membranes, University of Buenos Aires, Buenos Aires, Argentina

Dominique Gallez   Service de Chimie Physique, Université Libre de Bruxelles, Brussels, Belgium

Antonio Hernández   Department of Thermodynamics and Applied Physics, University of Valladolid, Valladolid, Spain

Nidal Hilal   Centre for Complex Fluids Processing, Department of Chemical and Biological Process Engineering, University of Wales Swansea, Swansea, United Kingdom

Klaas Keizer   Department of Chemistry, Potchefstroom University for Christian Higher Education, Potchefstroom, Republic of South Africa

Signe Kjelstrup   Department of Physical Chemistry, Norwegian University of Science and Technology, Trondheim, Norway

Kyösti Kontturi   Department of Chemical Engineering, Helsinki University of Technology, Espoo, Finland

Victor Levadny   The Scientific Council for Cybernetics, Russian Academy of Sciences, Moscow, Russia

Robert W. Lovitt   Centre for Complex Fluids Processing, Department of Chemical and Biological Process Engineering, University of Wales Swansea, Swansea, United Kingdom

Masako Maekawa   Division of Life Science and Human Technology, Nara Women's University, Nara, Japan

Norbert Maene   VITO, Mol, Belgium

Salvador Mafé   Department of Thermodynamics, University of Valencia, Burjasot, Spain

José A. Manzanares   Department of Thermodynamics, University of Valencia, Burjasot, Spain

Jacqueline Marchand-Brynaert   Département de Chimie, Université catholique de Louvain, Louvain-la-Neuve, Belgium

Balagopal N. Nair Japan Chemical Innovation Institute, Tokyo, Japan

Shin-Ichi Nakao Department of Chemical System Engineering, University of Tokyo, Tokyo, Japan

Tatsuhiro Okada Department of Polymer Physics, National Institute of Materials and Chemical Research, Ibaraki, Japan

Tatsuya Okubo Department of Chemical System Engineering, University of Tokyo, Tokyo, Japan

Magnar Ottøy The Membrane Research Group, Telemark Technical Research and Development Center, Porsgrunn, Norway

Laura Palacio Department of Thermodynamics and Applied Physics, University of Valladolid, Valladolid, Spain

K. G. Papadokostaki Physical Chemistry Institute, Democritos National Research Centre, Athens, Greece

J. H. Petropoulos Physical Chemistry Institute, Democritos National Research Centre, Athens, Greece

Pedro Prádanos Department of Thermodynamics and Applied Physics, University of Valladolid, Valladolid, Spain

Patricio Ramírez Departament de Ciències Experimentals, Universitat "Jaume I" de Castelló, Castelló, Spain

Sergio Roberto Rivera* Departamento de Físico-Química, Universidad de Concepción, Concepción, Chile

V. G. J. Rodgers Department of Chemical and Biochemical Engineering, The University of Iowa, Iowa City, Iowa

I. Rubinstein Department of Environmental Physics and Energy Research, Blaustein Institute for Desert Research, Ben-Gurion University of the Negev, Sede Boqer Campus, Israel

---

* *Current affiliation*: SQM-Salar, Atacama Desert, Antofagasta, Chile.

C. Ruíz Bauzá   Department of Applied Physics I, University Complutense of Madrid, Madrid, Spain

M. Sanopoulou   Physical Chemistry Institute, Democritos National Research Centre, Athens, Greece

Toshikatsu Sata   Department of Applied Chemistry and Chemical Engineering, Yamaguchi University, Yamaguchi, Japan

Torben Smith Sørensen*   Physical Chemistry, Modelling & Thermodynamics/DTH, Nørager Plads 3, DK 2720 Vanløse (Copenhagen), Denmark

A. Steinchen   Université d'Aix-Marseille, Marseille, France

Suren A. Tatulian   Department of Molecular Physiology and Biological Physics, University of Virginia Health Sciences Center, Charlottesville, Virginia

Preben J. S. Vie   Department of Physical Chemistry, Norwegian University of Science and Technology, Trondheim, Norway

Dietrich Woermann   Institute of Physical Chemistry, University of Köln, Köln, Germany

Chris J. Wright   Centre for Complex Fluids Processing, Department of Chemical and Biological Process Engineering, University of Wales Swansea, Swansea, United Kingdom

B. Zaltzman   Department of Environmental Physics and Energy Research, Blaustein Institute for Desert Research, Ben-Gurion University of the Negev, Sede Boqer Campus, Israel

Emilij K. Zholkovskij   Institute of Bio-Colloid Chemistry of Ukrainian Academy of Sciences, Kiev, Ukraine

---

* Also affiliated with The Danish National Museum, Department of Conservation, Brede, Denmark, as a senior scientist.

SURFACE CHEMISTRY AND ELECTROCHEMISTRY OF MEMBRANES

1

Atomic Force Microscope Studies of Membrane Surfaces

**W. RICHARD BOWEN,* NIDAL HILAL, ROBERT W. LOVITT and
CHRIS J. WRIGHT** Centre for Complex Fluids Processing, Department of
Chemical and Biological Process Engineering, University of Wales Swansea,
Swansea, United Kingdom

---

* Corresponding author.

Abstract

Atomic force microscopy (AFM) is an extremely versatile tool for the membrane technologist. This powerful imaging device allows the topographical study of membrane surfaces both in air and process relevant aqueous environments. This chapter presents systematic studies of microfiltration, ultrafiltration and nanofiltration membranes in air and liquid. The chapter describes how accurate images of membrane surfaces are produced and how these can provide quantitative data on pore size distributions and surface morphology. However, AFM is not only an imaging technique. Measurements in electrolyte solutions can provide quantitative information on the surface charge properties of membranes. Furthermore, the instrument can directly quantify the forces of interaction between a membrane surface and a pertinent colloidal particle. Such a colloid probe AFM technique allows direct quantification of surface adhesion. Hence, AFM may be used to quantify the three parameters that most influence membrane separation performance: pore size distribution, membrane surface electrical properties and membrane adhesion (fouling). In each case AFM has substantial advantages over competing methods. AFM is a new technology and the range of its applications is growing rapidly. The chapter ends with a discussion of the future prospects of AFM and some of the potential applications within membrane science. AFM is fast becoming essential for the research and development of membrane separation processes.

I.   INTRODUCTION

Since its invention in 1986, atomic force microscopy (AFM) [1] has evolved as a valuable imaging technique with resolution in the micrometer to sub-nanometer range. The ability of AFM to image both insulating and conducting surfaces in a variety of environments has facilitated molecular resolution images of a wide range of materials, including proteins [2], lipids [3] and DNA [4]. In addition to its imaging abilities, AFM can also be employed to probe spatial variations in surface properties, such as adhesiveness [5] and elasticity [6].

In this chapter we start with a basic introduction to the technology of AFM and then demonstrate how we have found AFM to be an essential tool for our study of membrane surfaces. As the reader progresses through the chapter we hope that he or she will pick up on the excitement we have for this new technology in that it is not only a powerful imaging tool, but also an analytical device for quantitative measurement of the forces controlling membrane separation processes. We end the chapter exploring the future prospects of AFM and what this holds for the membrane technologist.

II. PRINCIPLES OF ATOMIC FORCE MICROSCOPY

The underlying concept of Atomic Force Microscopy is beautifully simple, a contrast to the complex, intricate insights this new technology has given. A tip that is located at the free end of a cantilever systematically probes a surface of interest in order to generate a topographical image. The analogy of a stylus tracking the grooves of a vinyl record is often used. However, the atomic force microscope probes the surface of a sample with a sharp tip, only a couple of microns long and often less than 10 nm in diameter at the end. The cantilever is 100–200 μm long. As the tip scans the sample the forces between the tip and the surface cause the cantilever to bend. A detector such as an optical lever measures this deflection and allows a computer to generate a map of the surface topography. A consequence of the straightforward nature of AFM has been that both conducting and nonconducting materials have been studied, including biological surfaces, with relatively little sample preparation and within environments pertinent to the surface under study.

The atomic force microscope used in our laboratory measures the deflection of the cantilever using optical techniques. Figure 1 is a schematic representation of the optical beam detection method used in our instrument. A laser beam is focused on the reflective gold-plated back of a cantilever and the position of the reflected beam is registered by a position-sensitive photodetector (PSPD). As the cantilever bends, the position of the incident laser beam on the detector shifts. The PSPD can measure displacements of light as small as 1 nm. The ratio of the path length between the cantilever and the detector to the length of the cantilever itself produces a mechanical amplification. As a result, the system can detect sub-nanometer vertical movements of the cantilever tip.

As the AFM cantilever is rastered across (actually the sample is moved by a piezo) a surface several forces contribute to its deflection. The dependence of the total interatomic force upon the distance between the tip and the sample, in air, is shown in Fig. 2 [7]. Two distinct regions of this curve are exploited by AFM methods. In contact mode the cantilever is less than a nanometer from the surface, the interatomic force between the cantilever and the sample

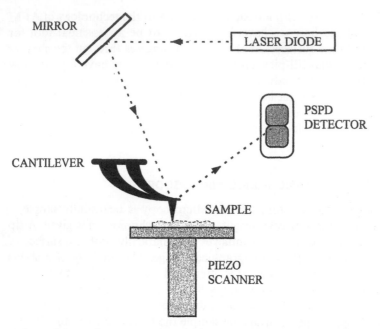

FIG. 1 Schematic representation of the beam-bounce detection scheme.

is repulsive, and the dominant force component is Born repulsion. In the non-contact mode, the cantilever is held in the order of several nanometers from the sample surface, and the interatomic force between the cantilever and the sample is dominated by long-range attractive van der Waals interactions.

When imaging new membranes and surfaces we adopt a systematic procedure using different imaging modes to optimize the image production. The discussion below introduces the different imaging techniques we have used in imaging membranes. A more detailed account of the AFM imaging modes is given in [8].

A. Contact Mode

Conceptually, contact mode is the most straightforward AFM imaging mode. As described above, the cantilever tip is held close to the sample surface and the sample surface rastered underneath the tip. As the sample surface is moved, the change in topography results in a change in tip–sample interaction. Thus, the force incident on the cantilever tip is altered (Fig. 2) and the equilibrium between the elastic force of the deflected cantilever and the applied force changed. The AFM operates in either of two ways. In constant height mode the cantilever is held in a fixed position with respect to the piezo so that the change in the cantilever deflection is used directly to generate a topo-

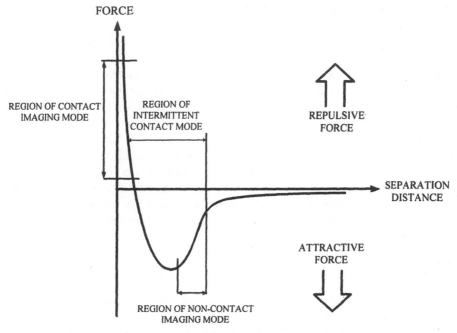

FIG. 2 Force vs. distance curve showing the tip–sample separation of different AFM operating modes.

graphic image. In constant force mode the total force between the cantilever tip and the sample is held constant by means of a feedback loop. The scanner moves up and down to keep the cantilever deflection constant as the topography changes under the cantilever.

Constant force mode is generally the preferred mode of operation. The total force exerted by the tip on the sample being within controlled limits. However, the response time of the feedback circuit and the movement of the scanner limits the effective scanning speed. The advantage of constant height mode is that it can have high scan speeds allowing the recording of real-time images of changing surfaces. Constant height mode is often used for taking atomic scale images of atomically flat surfaces where the variation of force and thus cantilever deflection is small.

When imaging a new membrane surface in contact mode the choice of cantilever is important. We have found it useful to choose from a range of cantilevers in order to optimize the production of images of different membranes. A soft cantilever which is sensitive to changes in applied force will resolve greater surface detail than a stiffer cantilever. However, there is a danger that the cantilever may crash into the surface, potentially damaging the sample surface or cantilever tip but definitely compromising the image quality. A stiff cantilever may reduce the danger of the tip crashing but the sensitivity of the system is reduced. A compromise must be reached.

The deflected cantilever pushes the tip in contact with the surface, this exerts a force which can damage the surface structure. The typical operating range of forces that are exerted on the surface by the tip are in the range 10^{-7} to 10^{-6} N. If the surface cannot withstand these forces then another imaging technique should be considered. Thus, contact mode is not the chosen method for the AFM imaging of soft samples.

We have found that contact mode is inadequate [9] when imaging membranes with small pores such as ultrafiltration and nanofiltration membranes. The reason for this is that diameter of the cantilever tip apex is greater than the pore diameter. When the tip is passed over the small pore the tip cannot penetrate into the pore and there is not a great change in cantilever deflection. To image soft samples or small pores the next imaging mode that should be considered is that of noncontact.

B. Noncontact Mode

Noncontact AFM (NC-AFM) is one of several vibrating cantilever techniques in which an AFM cantilever is vibrated near the surface of the sample. The cantilever is held at 5–10 nm distance away from the surface, within a region of the force distance curve where the long-range van der Waals forces are dominant (Fig. 2).

In simple terms, an applied force serves to change the vibrational amplitude and resonant frequency of a vibrating cantilever. Thus, as the sample is rastered under the vibrating cantilever tip the topography gives a change in the tip–sample interaction. This gives a resultant change in the vibrational parameters measured by the NC-AFM. A feedback system is employed in the AFM hardware to keep the monitored resonant frequency or the vibrational amplitude of the cantilever constant. The scanner moves the sample up and down maintaining the average tip to sample distance. As with contact AFM (in constant-force mode), the motion of the scanner is used to generate the data set.

The NC-AFM operating mode requires an AC detection scheme that is more sensitive than that of contact operation. The force between the tip and the sample in NC-AFM can be several orders of magnitude lower than the forces in contact mode. In addition, stiff cantilevers are used in NC-AFM because soft cantilevers can be pulled into contact with the sample surface. The use of stiffer cantilevers reduces the change in cantilever deflection and vibrational amplitude, giving a need for a sensitive detection scheme.

A principle advantage of NC-AFM is that the surface is imaged with no contact between the tip and the sample, which is desirable when studying soft surfaces. The total force between the tip and the sample is generally about

10^{-12} N. Samples are not damaged or contaminated through contact with the tip. In contrast, after repeated scanning in contact mode, samples are sometimes observed to be degraded. In general, we have found that NC-AFM is more effective than other modes for imaging ultrafiltration and nanofiltration membranes [9,10].

One potential disadvantage of NC-AFM is that in humid conditions the layer of condensed water lying on the sample surface may be too thick and will obscure features of interest. The AFM will image the surface of the liquid. Contact imaging mode, however, will penetrate the liquid layer to image the underlying surface.

C. Intermittent-Contact AFM

A further AFM imaging mode is that of intermittent contact (IC-AFM) and is a hybrid of contact and noncontact systems. As in NC-AFM a cantilever is vibrated, but the cantilever is held at a tip–sample distance closer to the region of contact imaging (Fig. 2) so that at the lower limit of the cantilever movement it just touches or taps the sample surface. Hence, the name intermittent contact or tapping mode. As for NC-AFM an image is produced by monitoring the changes in the cantilever oscillation amplitude as the tip to sample distance changes with surface topography.

The intermittent contact of the tip with the sample surface means that lateral forces (friction or drag) are reduced so that IC-AFM is less likely than contact mode to damage the sample surface. This is extremely useful when imaging soft samples. IC-AFM has become an important AFM technique since it overcomes some of the limitations of both contact and noncontact AFM.

D. Surface and Line Analysis

Once the AFM has taken an image the instrument software stores the picture as a data matrix of co-ordinates. Modern instruments have extensive image analysis capabilities that have proven essential for the effective study of surfaces. Surface statistics such as surface roughness, average height, and maximum peak-to-valley distance may be collected. These surface statistics are very useful for comparison of surfaces. For example, we have used such comparison to confirm that protein has adsorbed onto a surface when studying protein–protein interactions [11] and also in silica adhesion studies to ensure a range of silica surfaces with different roughness [12]. A line can also be selected in an image to study desirable features on the surface in terms of height, spacing and angle.

The ability to measure the size of pores is obviously useful when studying membranes once a good image has been produced. AFM is not a push of a button technique, however, and there are protocols that can be adopted to alter parameters within imaging modes and to switch to different techniques and ensure that the best image of the surface is achieved. We will discuss later in this chapter the best methods we have found to produce images of membrane surfaces. As the series of images are produced, surface and line analysis assess these images, identifying surface landmarks and differentiating imaging or preparation artefacts. We have found that when surface analysis is combined with an approximate prior knowledge of membrane pore size or molecular weight cut off as determined by indirect measurements, the production of good images of ultrafiltration and nanofiltration membranes is greatly facilitated.

E. Force Measurement

When AFM was first developed it was essentially an imaging technique that complemented and was added to the arsenal of imaging devices. Recently, however, the power of a further AFM capability has been realized, that of force measurement. The AFM can measure the forces of interaction found at surfaces such as membranes with obvious implications for membrane separation science. To generate a force–distance curve the change in deflection of a cantilever is recorded as a function of separation distance as the piezo scanner of the AFM raises and retracts the sample surface. As in imaging mode, the cantilever deflection is measured by the change in position of a laser beam bounced off the back of the cantilever and incident on the PSPD.

Figure 3 shows an experimental force–distance curve measured between an AFM tip and silica surface in electrolyte solution with schematic annotation of the tip and surface positioning. To the left of the curve the scanner is at maximum retraction and the cantilever is assumed to be undeflected. As the sample is raised, the separation distance between the tip and the sample decreases and the tip interacts with the sample surface inducing the cantilever to deflect. On further extension of the scanner a point is reached where the tip and the surface are in contact and on subsequent scanner extension the tip and the sample move in unison. Hence, the straight line to the right of the curve is called the region of constant compliance. The scanner reaches a maximum extension and then starts to retract. The retraction force curve does not lie on top of that of the approach because of the hysteresis of the piezo scanner movement.

The force–distance curve in Fig. 3 has an important feature on the retraction trace. This is due to tip–sample adhesion and is sometimes termed the snap-back point. As the scanner retracts away from the region of constant compliance the tip and sample adhere until a threshold is reached where the adhesive force is equalled by the force of a bent cantilever and the tip snaps away from the surface. Force–distance curves are characteristic of the system under study. In the case of Fig. 3, an adhesive force was observed between a

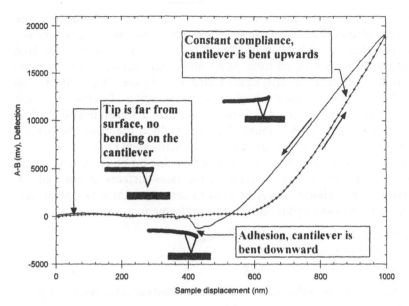

FIG. 3 Force (in terms of cantilever deflection) vs. sample displacement curve measured between an AFM silica tip and silica surface in electrolyte solution. The curve is annotated to show the positioning of the AFM tip and the surface when the sample is raised and retracted.

silica tip and a silica surface studied in an aqueous environment. However, other features can be seen on force curves. In air a snap-in point is often observed where the tip–sample separation reaches a certain value as the scanner extends and the tip experiences an attractive force causing the cantilever to be pulled towards the sample surface. Snap-back points are often observed with force curves measured in air due to the capillary force and adhesion of the tip to the water layer condensed on the surface of the sample. If other layers of liquid are present, such as oil films, multiple snap-back points will be observed. The positions and amplitudes of the snap-back points depend upon the viscosity and thickness of the layers present on the surface.

The slope of the constant compliance region is related to the elastic modulii of the surface material and cantilever. When the cantilever is more flexible than the sample surface the slope of the constant compliance region mostly reflects the spring constant of the cantilever. When a stiffer cantilever is used the elastic properties of the surfaces can be investigated.

To convert the cantilever deflection vs. sample displacement data to a force vs. tip–sample separation curve, it is necessary to know the spring constant of the cantilever and to define zeros of both force and separation. A number of different methods for the determination of spring constant have been reported

[13]. The zero of force is chosen where the tip and surface of sample are far apart and the zero of distance is chosen when the tip and sample start moving together. For this, the deflection of the cantilever from its position at large distances has to be subtracted from piezo movement values, point by point. The plot of this difference (x-axis) against force (y-axis) becomes vertical at the point of contact. This defines the beginning of the region of constant compliance where the output of the photodiode becomes a linear function of the sample displacement. We have found that this method identifies the onset of this region more effectively than the method normally used [14].

The atomic force microscope is a valuable machine for imaging virgin membrane surfaces and measuring interactions on these surfaces in both air and liquid environments. Hence, it may be used to determine three key parameters that influence membrane separation process performance:

Pore size distribution and surface morphology
Surface electrical properties
Surface adhesion—membrane fouling.

In each case the AFM technique has substantial advantages over competing techniques.

III. IMAGING MEMBRANE SURFACES IN AIR

The techniques which have been most widely used for the study of membrane morphology and pore characteristics are electron microscopy, mercury intrusion, extended bubble point, gas adsorption–desorption, thermoporometry, solvent permeability, and solute challenge [15]. Of these, only electron microscopy can provide direct and detailed information on the size distribution, shape and topography of the pores. However, electron microscopy has a number of disadvantages in the examination of porous polymeric structures. These include the fact that it is a high vacuum technique (which results in extensive drying of the sample), the requirement for extensive preparation such as metal coating or formation of a replica (both of which can produce artefacts with finely porous materials), and the possibility of damage by the electron beam. Electron microscopy gives images of only dry membrane surfaces. It is for reasons such as this that the use of AFM is so tantalizing to membrane technologists, since it produces images of membrane surfaces in both air and in solution.

A. Microfiltration Membranes

Atomic force microscopy has been used to investigate microfiltration and ultrafiltration membrane surface structure [16–24]. AFM has also been used to elucidate the mechanisms giving rise to inefficiencies (fouling) in membranes processing [25]. However, with one exception [23], membranes have been studied in "contact mode." The recent development of "noncontact mode" of operation described earlier in Sec. II.B, where the tip responds to attractive van der Waals interactions with the sample, is proving useful for the study of membranes. This mode of operation is especially suitable for materials which are soft or liable to mechanical damage as the forces used for imaging are also lower. Polymeric membranes are one such class of material. Further, it has been reported [23] that the use of noncontact mode can in some cases allow imaging of membrane surfaces which cannot be imaged in contact mode. However, there has been little systematic use of noncontact AFM for quantifying the surface pore structure of membranes.

We have used noncontact AFM to investigate the surface pore structure of different types of microfiltration membrane, both polymeric and inorganic [26]. The only preparation of the membranes for AFM was their attachment to steel disks with double-sided-scotch tape. In the next section we show results for Cyclopore track-etched polycarbonate microfiltration membranes. The measurements were made directly in air operating in noncontact mode.

1. Cyclopore Membranes

Three Cyclopore membranes (Whatman International Ltd). C01, C02 and C04 of different nominal pore size, 0.1, 0.2 and 0.4 μm, respectively, were examined. Figures 4a–c show AFM micrographs of the surfaces of these membranes. All images are given over areas of 3×3 μm, with the light regions being the highest points, and the dark regions the depressions (pores). The figures show that the overall surface structure is similar for the three membranes, but they have very different numbers of pores distributed nonuniformly over the scanned area. Comparing these membranes at higher magnification shows the approximately circular shape of the pore entrances and the increase in pore size from C01 to C04.

The AFM software allows quantitative determination of the diameter of pores by use of the images in conjunction with digitally stored line profiles

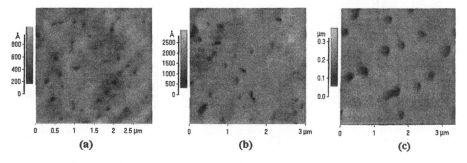

FIG. 4 2D images of C01, C02, and C04 Cyclopore membranes.

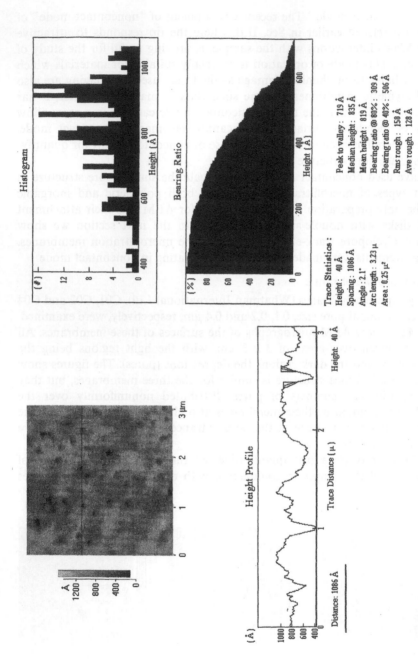

FIG. 5 Measurement of pore size of a Cyclopore membrane using line analysis mode. The figure is divided into five regions. (Top left) Actual image to be analyzed. (Bottom left) A plot which displays an individual cross-section (height profile) shown as a line on the image. (Bottom right) Line measurements. On the right there are two plots that display the height distribution along the line shown on the image and the bearing ratio, essentially an integral of the height histogram.

[25]. The simultaneous use of images and profiles greatly facilitates identification of the entrance of individual pores. Figure 5 shows measurement of a 0.109 μm pore entrance of a Cyclopore membrane in the line analysis mode of the AFM. In this mode the operator can work with 2D image or height profiles of the data where an arbitrary line on the image, including a short segment, can be selected and quantitative measurements of surface features such as pores on the membrane surface can be made by moving cursors along the line. Surface statistics can be collected as shown in Fig. 5. For capillary pore membranes, such as those used in the present work, there is very good agreement between pore diameters obtained by AFM and pore diameters calculated from hydraulic permeabilities [25]. (However, the diameter deep in the membrane may not be determined directly by surface AFM due to convolution between the tip shape and the pore). Pore diameters were determined in this way for 64 pores for the C01 membrane, 89 pores for the C02 membrane and 60 pores for the C04 membrane. The resulting pore size distributions are found to be: for the C01 membrane the range of pore sizes was 0.0824–0.165 μm with a mean of 0.109 μm and a standard deviation of 0.017 μm; for the C02 membrane the range was 0.117–0.273 μm with a mean of 0.184 μm and a standard deviation of 0.033 μm; for the C04 membrane the range was 0.312–0.546 μm with a mean of 0.412 μm and a standard deviation of 0.056 μm. These data show that the membranes have a narrow size distribution with a mean corresponding well to the manufacturer's specification.

We have also conducted a detailed study of Anopore microfiltration membranes [26].

2. Comparison of Results of Noncontact and Contact AFM

It is also possible to image microfiltration membranes using the AFM in contact mode. This posed some additional practical problems compared to the use of noncontact mode. For instance images obtained in contact mode for the Anopore membrane were less sharp, probably a result of the roughness of the surface, while in the case of the Cyclopore membranes there was a tendency for the membrane to tear due to the intimate contact between the tip and the membrane surface. However, successful images showed the same features in both modes. Pore dimensions obtained by both techniques were also in very good agreement. For example, the mean pore diameter obtained for the C02 membrane imaged in contact mode was 0.196 μm (standard deviation 0.047 μm) compared to 0.184 μm (standard deviation 0.033 μm) in noncontact mode.

3. Assessment

Atomic force microscopy is an effective means of investigating the surface structure and morphology of microfiltration membranes. Samples can be examined by AFM without preparative procedures that may alter the membrane structure. The value of atomic force microscopy is enhanced by the capability to operate in the noncontact mode. The surface topography of

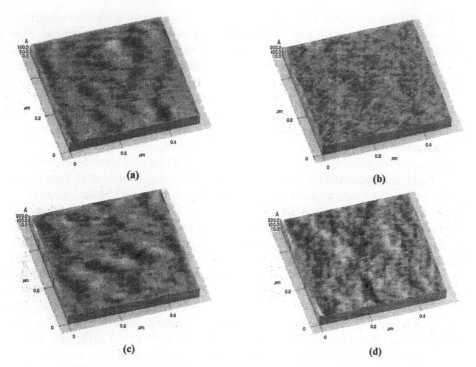

FIG. 6 3D images of YM Diaflo membranes, (a) YM3, (b) YM10, (c) YM30, (d) YM100. Courtesy University of Wales Swansea.

membranes can then be explored without distortion when the membrane is in the dry state. The noncontact AFM mode is able to image the original, unprepared surface of microfiltration membranes in air with single pore resolution. Image analysis can provide detailed information on the surface pore structure and allows quantitative determination of the pore size distribution. These benefits, combined with the ease of use of the technique, suggest that AFM should be considered as the method of first choice for determination of the surface pore characteristics of microfiltration membranes.

B. Ultrafiltration Membranes

Atomic Force Microscopy was used to image ultrafiltration membrane surfaces directly in air using the noncontact mode. We describe the protocol and present a study of the surfaces of four Diaflo (Amicon Inc. USA) YM series as an example of ultrafiltration membranes—YM3, YM10, YM30 and YM100, with molecular weight cut-off (MWCO) of 3000, 10,000, 30,000 and 100,000 daltons, respectively, made from regenerated cellulose. These membranes, were chosen due to their wide availability and application and as they cover a wide range of MWCO [27]. A full study on other ultrafiltration membranes of different polymers such as PM and XM Diaflo has been described elsewhere [9]. The only preparation of the membranes required, as in the case of the microfiltration membranes (Sec. III.A), was their attachment to steel discs with double-sided scotch tape.

Figures 6a–d show AFM images of the YM3, YM10, YM30 and YM100 membranes. The images are shown in three-dimensional form over areas of 0.5 × 0.5 μm. The pores are clearly visible as small well-defined dark areas on the images. In some cases they appear to occur in clusters, and for the higher MWCO membranes there is an increasing tendency for the pores to occur at the bottom of depressions in the membrane surface. The increase in pore diameter with increasing MWCO of the membranes is immediately apparent on comparing the images. There is also a visually apparent increase in surface roughness as the MWCO increases.

Table 1 presents statistical information on the mean size, standard deviation and size range. It may be seen that the mean pore diameter increases systematically as the specified MWCO of the membranes increases with a relatively small standard deviation in all cases. The root mean square roughness also increases as the nominal molecular weight cut off increases, though the magnitude is in all cases relatively low.

1. Comparison with other data

In previous investigations of membranes using AFM, there have been few systematic measurements of pore size distribution, though none using noncontact AFM. So the first point of comparison of the present data is with pore size distributions determined by contact AFM. The most systematic previous investigation [19] included data for three membranes with specified MWCO 10,000, one with MWCO 40,000 (polyethersulfone) and three of MWCO 100,000 (one polysulfone and two polyethersulfone). These membranes were from different manufacturers to those of the present work. For the 10,000 MWCO membranes, mean pore sizes of 14.1 nm, 12.6 nm, and 18.8 nm were reported. Comparison with the data for YM10 shows that such results are

TABLE 1 Statistical Characterization of Diaflo Membranes

Diaflo membrane	YM3	YM10	YM30	YM100
MWCO (Da)	3000	10,000	30,000	100,000
Mean pore diameter (nm)	8.7	11.3	13.2	19.4
Standard deviation (nm)	1.3	2.4	2.8	4.2
Size range (nm)	6.2–12.3	6.1–18.0	8.2–22.6	10.1–32.4
Number of counted pores	96	90	80	78
Rms[a] roughness (nm)	0.36	0.53	0.6	0.77

[a] Rms = root mean square.

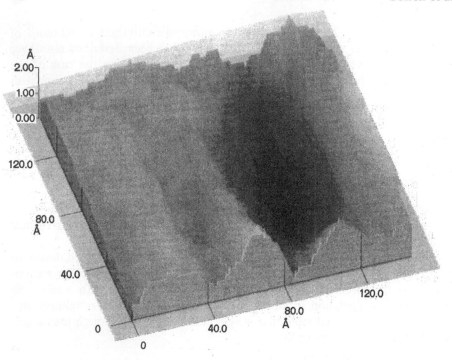

FIG. 7   3D image of a 5 nm single pore in ES625 membrane (MWCO 25,000). Courtesy University of Wales Swansea.

consistent with the present data. For the 40,000 MWCO membrane, a mean pore diameter of 11.6 nm was reported which is comparable to the present results for YM30. For the 100,000 MWCO membranes, mean pore sizes of 22.1 nm, 25.2 nm and 26.2 nm, were reported, which are comparable to but greater than the value obtained for YM100 in the present work. The width of pore size ranges reported previously are comparable to those in Table 1.

Other published pore size data from AFM has been sparse, though these include a range of 15–25 nm and 50–60 nm for polyethersulfone membranes of MWCO 30,000 and 100,000, respectively [20], 7–9 nm for a 10,000 MWCO polyethersulfone membrane [21] and 12–20 nm for a 30,000 MWCO polyacrylonitrile membrane [23]. Comparison with the data of Table 1 again shows that previous AFM studies are broadly consistent with the present work.

The second important type of comparison which can be carried out is with the results from electron microscopy. Electron microscopy data for membranes can require careful interpretation due to the extensive sample preparation required. An example of such studies using a high resolution field emission scanning electron microscope (FESEM) can be seen elsewhere [28].

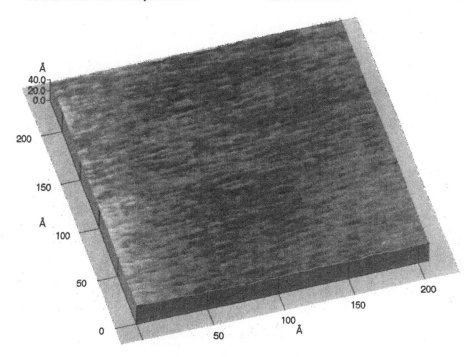

FIG. 8 3D image of ETNA01A nanofiltration membrane. Courtesy University of Wales Swansea.

Even operating the FESEM with the lowest energy electron beam (2 kV), it was found that the YM membranes were damaged.

The noncontact AFM data of the above ultrafiltration membranes is internally consistent and is in good agreement with previous contact AFM studies of membranes. SEM tends to give somewhat lower values for pore sizes. The discrepancies between pore sizes determined by AFM and EM are not easily resolved. SEM requires deposition of a conducting coating on the sample and TEM requires the preparation of a replica. The lengthy preparation techniques used in both cases can produce artefacts. Both coatings and replica formation are likely to lead to underestimation of pore sizes. Structural change may also arise due to damage by the electron beam or the requirement to operate in high vacuum.

Noncontact AFM has the tremendous advantage of operation in air with no sample preparation. Generally, care has to be taken in the use of AFM for detemination of pore sizes as the measured pore dimensions are a result of the convolution between tip and pore shape, which can become complex if the tip and surface pore sizes are comparable. However, this effect is expected to be much less significant for noncontact AFM than contact AFM as in the former case the tip is held at a significant distance from the surface and responding to

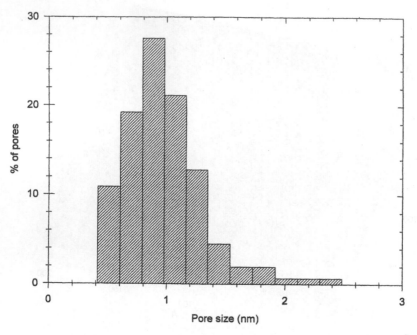

FIG. 9 Histogram of pore size distribution of ETNA01A nanofiltration membrane.

a variation in attractive forces in scanning. In favorable circumstances it is possible to image single pores in ultrafiltration membranes at very high resolution [10]. Figure 7 shows such an image for an ES625 membrane of MWCO 25,000 (PCI Membrane Systems Ltd). The pore diameter is ~5 nm.

2. Assessment

We have successfully used the AFM to image ultrafiltration membranes and to produce accurate surface statistics. This was achieved without pretreatment of the membranes and the risk of damaging the sample. This is in contrast to SEM techniques where even very low energy electron beams may damage the sensitive membrane material. As with microfiltration membranes we recommend that AFM is the first choice method for the determination of surface pore characteristics of ultrafiltration membranes. Both microfiltration and ultrafiltration membranes were imaged in a dry condition in air. We will see later that imaging in liquids opens the exciting prospect of visualization of such membrane surfaces under their conditions of use.

C. Nanofiltration Membranes

Nanofiltration membranes have a pore size of the order of 1 nm diameter and are made from a variety of polymers. As a consequence of differences in their manufacturer nanofiltration membranes have different surface roughness.

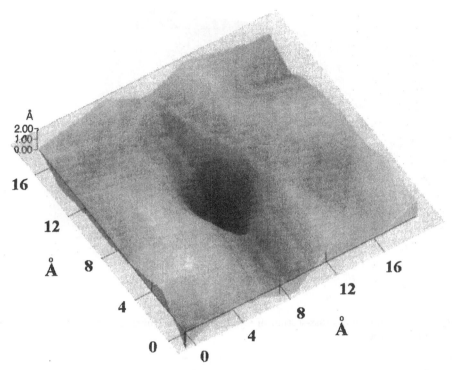

FIG. 10 3D image of a 0.5 nm single pore in XP117 membrane (MWCO 4000). Courtesy University of Wales Swansea.

We have studied a number of nanofiltration membranes in both air and liquid environments and have found greater success when imaging in air using noncontact mode [29]. Figure 8 shows a three-dimensional image of an ETNA01A membrane (DDS Filtration) imaged in air using the noncontact mode. The pores in the figure are readily distinguishable and the pore size distribution compared favorably with the MWCO quoted for this membrane. Figure 9 shows a histogram of pore size distribution of this membrane.

In some cases, ultrafiltration membranes may also have pores of subnanometer dimensions. Figure 10 shows a high resolution image of a single pore of ~0.5 nm dimensions in a XP117 membrane (MWCO 4000, PCI Membrane Systems Ltd).

D. Imaging Cross-Sections of Membranes

The AFM study of membrane surface topography yields much useful data. However, further information can be gained by imaging a cross-section of a membrane. Figures 11 and 12 show three-dimensional cross-section images of Cyclopore and Anopore microfiltration membranes. Both figures demonstrate

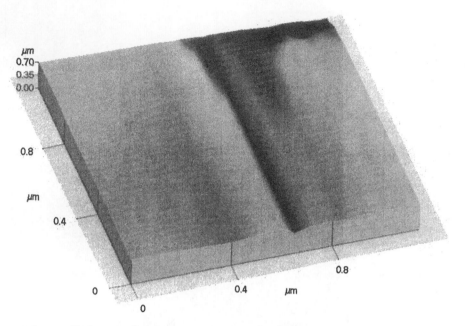

FIG. 11   3D image of cross-section of Cyclopore C02 membrane. Courtesy University of Wales Swansea.

clearly that the pores are straight and run from one side of the membrane surface to the other.

To produce a cross-section of a polymeric membrane we found freeze fracturing of the membrane to be the most effective method. The membrane was fractured after being frozen in liquid nitrogen for 5 min. When microtone and ultratone machines were used to slice the membrane the cross-sections of the pores were damaged. This was the case when both untreated membranes and membranes soaked in resin were sectioned. The fractured membrane sections were held in place on top of the AFM scanner by a clamping device especially fabricated for the purpose. This clamp held the membrane section in a vertical position so that the very thin area could be rastered underneath the AFM tip.

IV.   IMAGING MEMBRANE SURFACES IN LIQUID (DOUBLE LAYER MODE)

As outlined in Sec. II, the most widely used imaging method is "contact mode" in which the tip is responding to very short range repulsive (Born) forces. A second mode of operation is "noncontact mode" in which the tip responds to attractive van der Waals interactions with the sample. These have

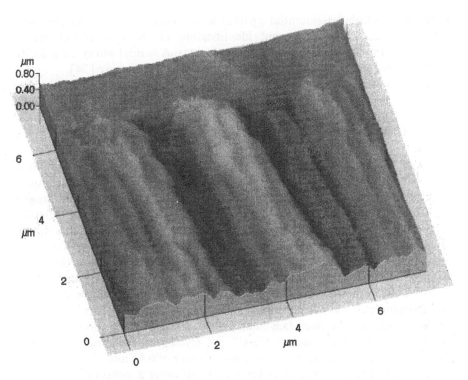

FIG. 12 3D image of cross-section of 0.02 μm Anophore membrane. The clamp holding the membrane cross-section can be seen at the top of the image. Courtesy University of Wales Swansea.

been the most widely used modes and virtually all AFM membrane studies have been carried out in these modes. However, in electrolyte solutions it is possible to image surfaces in "electrical double layer mode" [30] in which the tip responds to the electrical double layer interactions between itself and the surface. This mode may, however, be especially useful for membrane studies as it allows imaging under the processing conditions used for aqueous process streams—all membranes used under such conditions acquire a surface charge [31].

An important prior step to electrical double layer mode imaging is the determination of force–distance curves for the approach of the AFM tip to the sample surface [14,32,33]. Hence, we discuss here such data for a nominally 0.1 μm Cyclopore microfiltration membrane. AFM images for this membrane are then presented, produced at a range of forces in NaCl solutions at four ionic strengths. Image analysis allows the determination of pore size distributions—see Sec. III.A.1. The variation in image quality of membranes with imaging conditions is discussed in terms of the force–distance curves and numerically calculated potential profiles at the entrance to a charged pore. This allows an explanation and identification of the best conditions for imaging such membranes in electrolyte solutions. A similar study on a 25,000 MWCO ultrafiltration membrane has been presented elsewhere [34].

The Cyclopore membrane is a track etched polycarbonate microfiltration (Whatman International Ltd). All force and image measurements were made in a closed, unsealed liquid cell. Tubes allowed the exchange of the solution in the cell. These membranes were also studied using AFM in air (Sec. III.A.1) [10,26].

The AFM allows measurement of the force between the tip and a sample as a function of the displacement of the sample (see Sec. II.E). The deflection of the cantilever obtained with the membranes in the constant compliance region did not depend on the ionic strength of the solution. However, the deflection differed slightly from that obtained with a silicon dioxide surface in solution, indicating that some deformation of the membrane surface may have been taking place. It should be noted that the bending of the cantilever has to be taken into account in calculating the tip–sample separation distance as described earlier in Sec. II.E. Further, specification of a tip–sample distance is only meaningful if the sample surface roughness is small compared to the distances measured. For pore free areas of 16×16 nm it was found that the root-mean-square roughness of the 0.1 μm Cyclopore membrane in air was 0.077 nm with a maximum peak-to-valley distance of 0.43 nm.

The membrane was imaged in the liquid cell using a constant force in the electrical double layer mode. Before taking any image, a force–distance curve was measured. This allowed conversion of the arbitrary readings of the imaging force slider bar into real force values [34]. The membrane was then imaged at the selected force using a scan rate of 1 Hz with 256×256 pixel resolution. In all cases, 50 pores were measured to determine the size distribution. Measurements presented here were made in aqueous solutions of sodium chloride at concentrations in the range 10^{-1} to 10^{-4} M at pH 6.5 at room temperature ($18.5 \pm 1.2°C$).

A. Force Measurements Between AFM Tip and Membrane Surface

The forces between the cantilever tip and the membranes as a function of separation distance in NaCl solution at four ionic strengths are shown in Fig. 13. The force vs. distance curves were measured on pore free areas of the membranes. In each case the force is repulsive at all separations. This shows that the double layer electrostatic interaction between the silicon oxide surface of the tip and the membrane surface is dominant in all cases. Silicon oxide surfaces are known to have a negative potential under such conditions [35] as is also expected for the membranes [36]. At very small distances it may be that

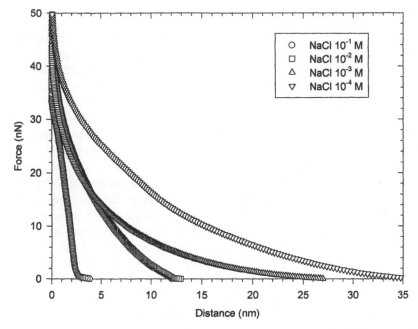

FIG. 13 Force vs. distance curves for the approach of an AFM tip to a Cyclopore membrane in NaCl solutions of various ionic strengths at pH 6.5.

the Born repulsion becomes significant. There is no indication of attractive dispersion (London-van-der-Waals) forces at short distances. Such dominant electrostatic behavior has also been observed in an AFM for the mutual interaction of silicon oxide surfaces [14]. The magnitude of the forces measured indicates that the effective area of interaction between the tip and the membrane surface may have been increased by some deformation of the membrane surface. Similar force measurements for an ultrafiltration membrane have been reported for an ES625 membrane of 25,000 MWCO [34].

The range of the measurable interaction increases as the ionic strength decreases, up to a maximum of ~ 35 nm, as is expected from electrical double layer theory [37]. The maximum interaction close to the membrane surface is of comparable magnitude at the different ionic strengths. The curves showed good reproducibility, including those regions where the curves at differing ionic strengths show some overlap—such overlap has also been reported in AFM force measurements between other types of surfaces [14,32]. The force vs. distance curves shown in the figure are for the approach of the tip to the membrane surface as is the usual practice for such work in electrolyte solutions.

B. Electrical Double Layer Mode Imaging of Membranes

Having carried out force vs. distance measurements it is possible to image the membrane at specified forces and so study the best means of imaging membranes in solution. Figure 14 shows images of the Cyclopore membrane produced at three different forces in 10^{-1} M NaCl solution (a–c) and at approximately constant force in 10^{-1}, 10^{-2}, 10^{-3} and 10^{-4} M NaCl solution (c, d–f). The images cover an area of 2.5 × 2.5 μm. The color intensity shows the vertical profile of the membrane surfaces, with light regions being the highest points and the dark regions being the depressions and pores.

Considering first the images obtained in 10^{-1} M solution at different forces. The image obtained with a force of 33.8 nN, and hence by reference to Fig. 13 with the tip very close to the membrane surface, gives the sharpest image containing the greatest detail. The pores are clearly visible as well-defined dark areas on the images. As the imaging force is reduced to 12.9 nN and then 4.35 nN, so the tip–membrane distance increases to 1.7 nm and 2.2 nm, respectively, and the image quality deteriorates with a significant loss of sharpness and detail. Variation of ionic strength with essentially constant force also gives variation in image quality. Images in 10^{-2} and 10^{-3} M solution (tip–sample distances 0.7 and 0.5 nm, respectively) are similar in quality to those in 10^{-1}

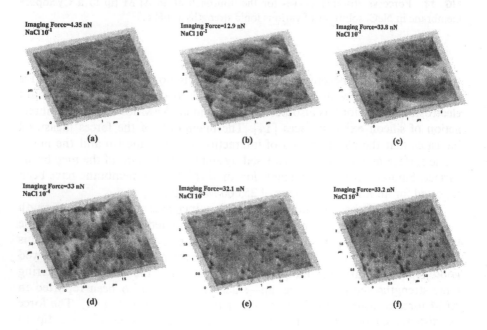

FIG. 14 3D images of a Cyclopore membrane at different imaging forces and different ionic strengths of NaCl solutions. Courtesy University of Wales Swansea.

M solution. However, the image in 10^{-4} M solution is significantly less good. For the latter image the tip–membrane distance has increased to 1.9 nm (see Fig. 13).

Pore size distributions for the imaging conditions shown in Fig. 14 are shown with statistical information summarized in Table 2. A number of trends are apparent. Firstly, for the three highest ionic strengths the mean pore diameter decreases with decreasing imaging force, but the values of the mean at the highest imaging force are comparable. These "high force" means are also comparable to that obtained for such a membrane by AFM in air, 0.109 μm with a standard deviation of 0.017 μm [26]. Secondly, in 10^{-4} M solution the size distribution and mean size show a tendency to move to higher values. Both of these trends will be discussed further in Sec. IV.C.

C. Potential Distribution at the Entrance to a Charged Pore

An exact interpretation of the force vs. distance curves measured in electrolyte solutions and of the images obtained in electrical double layer mode requires a calculation of the force of interaction between the tip and the membrane surface at any position of the tip above the surface. Important requirements for such a calculation are a knowledge of the exact shape of the AFM tip, a knowledge of the surface potential or surface charge (or better still the surface chemistry giving rise to the surface electrostatic properties) of the tip, a comparable knowledge of the surface properties of the membrane, and a solution of the nonlinear Poisson–Boltzmann equation for the appropriate geometry. The force at any distance can then be obtained by integrating the electric

TABLE 2 Pore Size Statistics for Cyclopore Membrane in NaCl Solutions Imaged at Different Forces

Ionic strength (M)	Imaging force (nN)	Mean size (μm)	Standard deviation (μm)	Size range (μm)
10^{-1}	33.8	0.111	0.020	0.078–0.132
	12.9	0.098	0.013	0.077–0.119
	4.4	0.098	0.020	0.067–0.131
10^{-2}	33.2	0.101	0.025	0.070–0.128
	23.4	0.095	0.025	0.054–0.134
	15.0	0.086	0.039	0.052–0.105
10^{-3}	33.1	0.103	0.022	0.076–0.136
	25.7	0.102	0.030	0.058–0.128
	21.4	0.094	0.018	0.066–0.125
10^{-4}	33.0	0.130	0.029	0.084–0.177
	30.0	0.135	0.029	0.094–0.177
	25.7	0.130	0.030	0.090–0.182

tensor on the tip surface. Such a complete calculation is very challenging and beyond the scope of the present work. In particular, the solution of the nonlinear Poisson–Boltzmann equation for the tip scanning across and interacting with a pore in a membrane surface requires a full three-dimensional numerical calculation by a technique such as the finite element method.

Fortunately, the main features of electrical double layer imaging of pores can be interpreted using a simpler approach. We have recently used the finite element technique to calculate the electrical potential distribution at the entrance to cylindrical charged pores [38]. This also requires a solution of the nonlinear Poisson–Boltzmann equation, but in two dimensions rather than three due to the axis of symmetry in the pore. Results of such calculations are presented in the present section.

Figure 15 shows the results of such calculations for a pore of diameter 0.1 μm, which is representative of the Cyclopore membrane under study. Both parts of the figure show a half section through the pore. In both cases the membrane surface (front surface and pore wall) is assumed to have a dimensionless potential of 1.0, corresponding to ~ 25 mV. This is typical of the zeta-potential of polymeric membranes [31,36]. The figures are for the extremes of ionic strength used in the present work, 10^{-1} M in Fig. 15a and 10^{-4} M in Fig. 15b. Isopotential lines in the solution are shown. It may be seen that the potential falls off much faster with distance at the higher ionic strength. To a first approximation, and for the purpose of elucidating the experimental results previously presented, a tip scanning at constant force in electrical double layer mode may be thought of as moving along one such isopotential line. In scanning at high force it could be thought of as moving along a high value isopotential line in solution close to the surface. At lower scanning force the tip could be thought of as moving along a lower value isopotential line, at a greater distance from the surface.

Comparison of Figs. 15a and 15b helps elucidate a number of the observations and trends apparent in Fig. 14 and Table 2. Firstly, it was found that the image obtained in 10^{-1} solution gave a sharper definition of the pores than that in 10^{-4} M solution. This may be understood from Fig. 15, for at the high ionic strength the isopotential lines follow the pore entrance more closely than at the low ionic strength. Secondly, it was found that statistical analysis of pore diameters gave a decrease in the measured pore diameter as the imaging force was decreased. In our approximation, imaging at low force corresponds to tracking a low value isopotential line. These occur some distance from the actual membrane surface and so the lower measured diameter may be understood. Thirdly, not only was the image obtained in 10^{-4} M solution less sharp, but the mean pore size determined was greater than at the higher ionic strengths and also greater than the value obtained in air. This is most probably an error in measurement induced by the difficulty in identifying the pore entrance when, in our approximation, tracking an isopotential line which

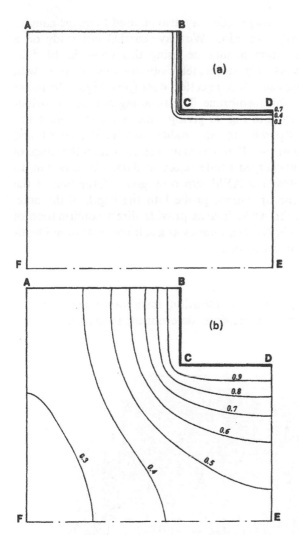

FIG. 15 Solution of the nonlinear Poisson–Boltzmann equation for a pore of 0.1 μm diameter, which represents the Cyclopore membrane under study. A half-section of a single pore is shown. BC represents the front surface of the membrane and CD the pore wall.

at this ionic strength will have appreciable curvature, even with the assumption of a sharp right-angle entrance to the pore. The real pore entrance will itself be somewhat rounded, so compounding the difficulty in practice. Data about the surface electrical properties of the membranes may also be obtained from this type of study.

Electrostatic double layer imaging mode may also be used to image nanofiltration membranes in electrolyte solution. We have carried out study on a PES5 (Hoechst AG) nanofiltration membrane using this mode in 10^{-2} M NaCl and compared the results of pore diameter obtained using AFM with that obtained from salt/uncharged solute rejection data [39]. Figure 16 shows a three-dimensional image of this membrane. The resulting pore size distribution based on 116 pores is shown in Fig. 17 giving a mean surface pore diameter of ~1.18 nm. This is comparable to but smaller than the diameter found by analysis of salt-rejection data ~1.86 nm. It is also smaller than the range of values found by analysis of uncharged solute rejection data, 2.24–2.64 nm. In this context it should be noted that AFM can only give information of the surface pore dimensions as the tip cannot probe into the depth of the pore. However, most importantly, the AFM images provide direct confirmation of the existence of discrete pores in NF membranes at a salt concentration identical to that used in the rejection experiments.

D. Assessment

Microfiltration, ultrafiltration and nanofiltration membranes may be successfully imaged, and their pore dimensions determined, in electrolyte solu-

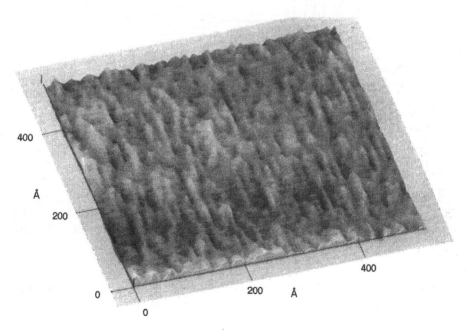

FIG. 16   3D image of PES5 nanofiltration membrane in 10^{-2} NaCl solution. Courtesy University of Wales Swansea.

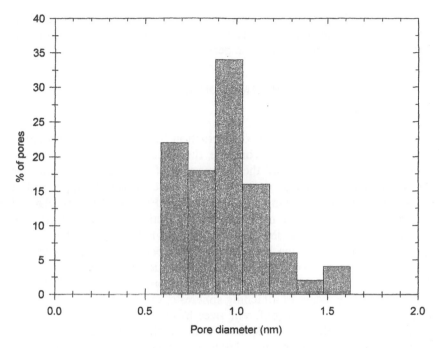

FIG. 17 Histogram of pore size distribution of PES5 nanofiltration membrane.

tions by atomic force microscopy (AFM). Such imaging may be carried out due to the long-range electrostatic interactions between the tip and the membrane surface—the electrical double layer mode of imaging.

An important requirement for the success of this technique is the prior determination of the force vs. distance curve for the interaction between the tip and the membrane surface. Commercial AFM equipment allows the user to specify the imaging force. For successful imaging it is important that a force sufficient to bring the tip quite close to the membrane surface is used. High electrolyte concentrations give the sharpest images with the best definitions of the pores. Use of a force sufficient to bring the tip close to the surface at high electrolyte concentration gives pore sizes and size distributions in good agreement with those obtained by AFM in air. The choice of such optimum conditions is especially important for ultrafiltration membranes where the decay length of the potential from a charged membrane in solution is comparable to the pore dimensions. The interpretation of these experimental findings is aided and confirmed by comparison with numerically calculated potential distributions at pore entrances.

AFM imaging of membranes in electrolyte solutions also provides information on the surface electrical properties of membranes, which can have an important influence on their separation performance.

V. ADHESION MEASUREMENT AND FOULING OF MEMBRANES

A. Colloid Probes

In Sec. IV.4 we discussed the forces of interaction between an AFM tip and a surface in solution. However, to compare the force curves with theoretical predictions it is important that the geometries of the interacting surfaces should be defined. The geometry of the AFM probe tip is not simple and in some cases not known. Attaching a sphere to the AFM cantilever, in place of the tip, makes it possible to measure the interaction between surfaces of known geometry. Such a "colloid probe" is shown in Fig. 18. This is an extremely interesting technique because the forces between colloidal particles dominate their behavior, and the forces between such particles and a membrane surface have a great influence on separation performance. We have developed innovative means of attaching spheres of different materials, such as silica and polystyrene, and of different sizes from 0.75 μm to 15 μm to the AFM cantilever. In addition the spheres held on the end of the tip can be coated with different polymers in order to investigate the interaction of the polymer with relevant surface. For example, we have immobilized protein onto

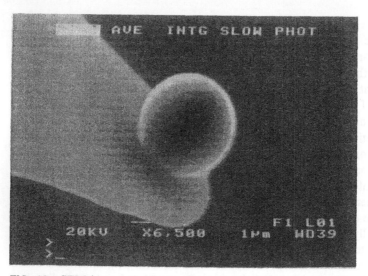

FIG. 18 SEM image of a 5 μm silicon dioxide sphere attached to an AFM cantilever (colloid probe).

a silica sphere and studied the interaction between protein layers adsorbed on the sphere probe and on a silica surface [11].

The colloid probes were prepared by attaching a sphere to a standard V-shaped AFM tipless cantilever. The colloid particles were glued to the cantilever with proprietary glues suitable for the colloid material. For example, Loctite Glass Bond (Loctite UK Ltd) was used to attach silica spheres to the silicon nitride cantilever. The fabrication of the "colloid probes" was achieved by using the optical microscope and the step-motor of the AFM apparatus. A "cell probe" was produced in a similar way by immobilizing a single living cell at the end of the cantilever [40].

The "colloid probes" and the "cell probes" can be used in the study of colloidal particle interactions with membranes. The approach of the probe to a membrane allows the measurement of colloid–membrane interaction forces. The separation of the probe from the membrane surface allows the measurement of adhesion forces. Quantification of these colloid–membrane interaction forces is important in the development of theoretical prediction and thus optimization and control of membrane separation processes. Adhesion of different materials to membranes is an important determinant of the membranes' fouling properties. Process testing of new membranes can be time consuming and costly. Thus, the development of an AFM method that quantifies the adhesion of different materials to a membrane may prove very useful to the membrane technologist.

B. Membrane Adhesion

Of the many well-established means of membrane characterization [14], none allows the direct measurement of the force of adhesion of fine particles and colloids to a membrane surface. The AFM colloid probe technique allows such measurement. The membrane technologist can now measure the force of adhesion of colloids to membrane surfaces and thus predict the membrane fouling properties of the colloidal material.

The AFM colloid probe technique allows the direct measurement of the force of adhesion of a single particle in a direction normal to the surface at which interaction is taking place. Measurements can be made in liquid environments matching those occurring in practice. A few such measurements have been reported for inorganic systems [41,42]. In our research laboratory we have demonstrated the potential of the AFM colloid probe technique to differentiate membranes on the grounds of their different adhesion properties. We studied two commercially available membranes both of nominal MWCO 4000 Da manufactured by PCI Membrane Systems Ltd (UK). The first, ES 404, is made from polyethersulfone, a relatively conventional polymer. The second, XP 117, is made from a mixture of polymers chosen with the aim of achieving low membrane fouling.

Colloid probes were prepared by attaching polystyrene spheres approximately 11 μm in diameter (Sigma, catalogue number LB-120) with epoxy resin (DP 105, Scotch-Weld) to a standard V-shaped AFM tipless cantilever. The measurements were made in aqueous solutions of sodium chloride at a concentration of 10^{-2} at pH 8 at room temperature with the membrane mounted in a closed, unsealed liquid cell.

Table 3 details the analysis of the surface morphology of the two membranes. The surface pore properties for both membranes are in the range expected from the nominal MWCO. All the parameters listed infer that the ES 404 membrane has a greater surface roughness than the XP 117 membrane. Surface roughness is an important physical parameter that needs to be considered in studies of adhesion [12]. Another important parameter of the measured adhesive force is that of loading force [12,41]. Loading force is the force that is applied by the deflected cantilever on the surface. This force was kept constant (222 nN $\pm$ 0.7%) when the adhesion of the colloid probe to the two different membranes was measured.

Figure 19 shows plots of normalized force (force/particle radius) vs. piezo-displacement as a colloid probe was retracted from the membrane surfaces. The colloid probe was in momentary contact with the membrane surfaces. From A to A' the colloid probe and membrane move together with no displacement relative to the piezo. From A' to B there is a stretching of the probe and/or membrane which gives them a relative movement with respect to the piezo. From B to C the stretching continues and the contact between the colloid probe and membrane is finally broken at C. From C to D the probe and membrane move further apart. The difference in force between B and C is a direct measurement of the adhesive interaction, in this case 1.98 mN/m for the ES404 membrane and 0.38 mN/m for the XP117 membrane. The XP117 membrane adhesive interaction is 5 times less than that of the ES404 membrane. The results show that the manufacturer has genuinely produced a membrane to which the test polystyrene particle attaches only weakly. That is, the membrane has the potential for being genuinely low fouling in process applications.

TABLE 3 Surface Morphology Analysis of Membranes Over an Area of 20 nm × 20 nm

Membrane	MWCO (Da)	Mean height (nm)	Peak to valley (nm)	Av. roughness (nm)	Rms[a] roughness (nm)
ES 404	4000	0.92	1.70	0.15	0.20
XP 117	4000	0.55	1.10	0.09	0.11

[a] Rms = root mean square.

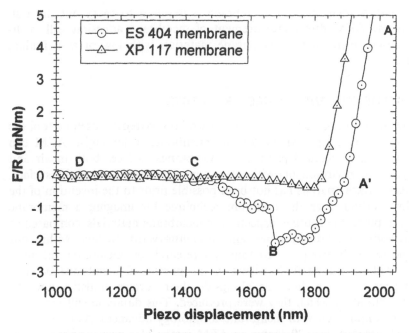

FIG. 19 Normalized force vs. piezo displacement plot (retraction) for a polystyrene colloid probe at an ES404 and a XP 117 membrane (10^{-2} M NaCl, pH 8).

The shape of the force–distance curves which show adhesion is also interesting (Fig. 19). In the case of the membrane adhesion measured with the polystyrene "colloid probe" the adhesive interaction took place over a distance of 400 nm. When we studied the adhesion of a "cell probe" to a silica surface we also found the adhesive interaction to take place over a large distance [40]. The cell probe and the polystyrene are both soft materials. Thus, the distance of the adhesive interaction in both cases is probably due to the stretching of the surfaces in contact. When adhesion is studied in a system of hard inorganic surfaces the adhesive interaction takes place over a very short distance, a couple of nanometers [12,41,42]. This is a consideration for the membrane technologist when studying such a heterogeneous range of materials.

We have studied the adhesion of silica and the protein bovine serum albumin (BSA) to the same membranes. In the case of silica there was no adhesion whereas BSA exhibited significant adhesion to both membranes. This further demonstrates the versatility of the "colloid probe" technique. The development of the colloid probe as a sensor for quantifying the adhesive force at membrane surfaces allows a relatively fast procedure for assessing the potential fouling of membrane surfaces by particles of different materials. In addition only a small piece of membrane is required to carry out the test. Utimately the AFM direct measurement of membrane adhesion will facilitate the development of new membrane materials with low or zero fouling properties.

VI. CONCLUSIONS AND FUTURE PROSPECTS

In conclusion, we hope this chapter has shown how extremely useful a tool the atomic force microscope can be for the membrane technologist. AFM can generate extremely detailed pictures of membranes surfaces both in air and process relevant environments without any invasive treatment of the surface. Such direct surface analysis has not been possible prior to the invention of the AFM. In addition once the optimum technique for imaging a membrane surface is in place, the routine inspection of membrane materials, compared to other methods, is relatively quick and straightforward. In fact, within our membrane research group we combine all research on membrane filtration processes with a routine AFM check of the purchased membrane batches. These images are in a database alongside their surface statistics and the optimum method by which they were produced. This database will grow and improve in conjunction with membrane technology advances. As an example of a recent advance, Fig. 20 shows an AFM image of a new membrane type called a micro sieve (Microfiltration B.V) where the pores in a silicon nitride surface were laser etched. This method of production has produced a membrane with extremely uniform pore size, shape and distribution.

Further advantages of AFM that need to be highlighted are that only a small piece of membrane is required to assess the surface morphology in both air and liquid. In addition the AFM functions both as an imaging tool and also a powerful force measuring device. This has meant that specific areas on a membrane surface can be located and probed in a desired environment. All of these are useful experimental options for the membrane technologist.

AFM is a new technology with much focused scientific endeavour and consequently the possibilities offered by AFM to the membrane technologist are constantly increasing in number. This is not only in terms of image production refinement but also as an analytical tool for the quantification of forces. In our research group we have exploited the colloid probe technique and initiated the cell probe technique in order to study the interaction of colloids with membranes and other process relevant surfaces. This direction of study has only just begun and we continue to increase the number of surfaces we have studied. The AFM has provided our research group with an experimental means to measure the interaction forces and compare them with those predicted by our theoretical studies of membrane separation processes. In the near future it will be possible to quantify the forces that are incident on a colloid particle as it enters a membrane pore, a concept that has obvious implications

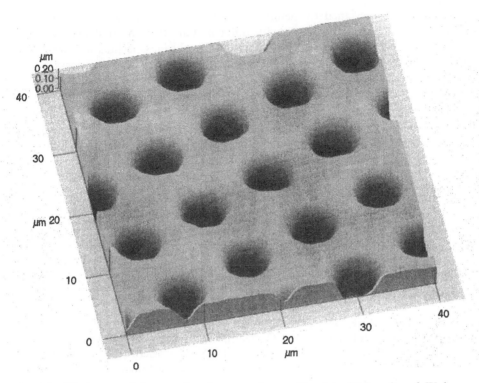

FIG. 20 3D image of 6 μm microsieve membrane. Courtesy University of Wales Swansea.

in membrane separation research and that has already been considered in theoretical terms [38].

Another promise offered by the colloid probe to the study of membrane surfaces is the quantification of zeta potentials of membrane surfaces by comparing the forces of interaction with theoretical predictions based on fitted potential values. An important advantage of this approach compared to electrokinetic methods is that it allows examination of differences in potential across the surface.

The colloid probe technique may prove very useful to membrane manufacture. The quantification of interaction forces between membranes and a range of materials may guide the production of novel membrane materials. For example, the adhesion of proteins to different materials as quantified by the colloid probe technique will aid the choice of materials when designing a membrane for the purification of proteins. This will serve to reduce the need for expensive pilot plant studies of new membranes. In addition the interaction of different colloid probes with different membranes may lead to further specifications assigned to membranes. For example, alongside porosity data, interaction of the membrane with different relevant materials such as silica, proteins or cells may be included in the membrane specification sheet. This will facilitate the choice of membranes when a new separation process is being designed.

AFM technology is at a stage of development where it is still defining its place as a scientific tool. The widespread utility of AFM, only invented in 1986, to the scientific community is only just being realized. The AFM has a lot more to offer the membrane technologist.

ACKNOWLEDGMENTS

This work was supported by the UK Engineering and Physical Sciences Research Council and the UK Biotechnology and Biological Sciences Research Council.

REFERENCES

1. G. Binnig, C. F. Quate, and C. Gerber, Phys. Rev. Lett. 56:930 (1986).
2. H. X. You and C. R. Lowe, J. Colloid Interface Sci. 182:586 (1996).
3. J. Yang, L. K. Tamm, A. P. Somlyo, and Z. Shao, J. Microscopy 171:183 (1993).
4. M. Benzanilla, S. Manne, D. E. Laney, Y. L. Lyubchenko, and H. G. Hansma, Langmuir 11:655 (1995).
5. W. R. Bowen, N. Hilal, R. W. Lovitt, and C. J. Wright, J. Membrane Sci. 139:269 (1998).
6. N. A. Burnham and R. J. Colton, J. Vac. Sci. Technol. A7:2906 (1989).
7. J. Israelachvili, Intermolecular and Surfaces Forces, 2nd ed., Academic Press, London, 1991.
8. D. Sarid, Scanning Force Microscopy, Oxford University Press, 1994.
9. W. R. Bowen, N. Hilal, R. W. Lovitt, and P. M. Williams, J. Colloid Interface. Sci. 180:350 (1996).
10. W. R. Bowen, N. Hilal, R. W. Lovitt, and P. M. Williams, J. Membrane Sci. 110:229 (1996).
11. W. R. Bowen, N. Hilal, R. W. Lovitt, and C. J. Wright, J. Colloid Interface. Sci. 197:348 (1997).
12. W. R. Bowen, N. Hilal, R. W. Lovitt, and C. J. Wright, Colloids and Surfaces A: Physicochemical and Engineering Aspects (1998), submitted for publication.
13. J. P. Cleveland, S. Manne, D. Bocek, and P. K. Hansma, Rev. Sci. Instruments 64:403 (1993).
14. W. A. Ducker, T. J. Senden, and P. M. Pashley, Langmuir 8:1831 (1992).
15. M. Mulder, Basic Principles of Membrane Technology, Kluwer Academic Publishers, Dordrecht, 1991.
16. A Chahboun, R. Coratger, F. Ajustron, J. Beauvillain, P. Aimar, and V. Sanchez, Ultramicroscopy 41:235 (1992).

17. A. Bessières, M. Meireles, P. Aimar, V. Sanchez, R. Coratgar, and J. Beauvillain. *Récent progrès en génie des procédés—Membrane preparation fouling-emerging processes* (P. Aimar and P. Aptel, eds), Vol. 6, CPIC, Nancy, 1992, pp. 111–116.

18. T. Miwa, M. Yamaki, H. Yoshimusa, S. Ebina, and K. Nagayama, Jpn. J. Appl. Phys. *31*: L1495 (1992).

19. P. Dietz, P. K. Hansma, O. Inacker, H. D. Lehmann, and K. H. Herrmann, J. Membrane Sci. *65*: 101 (1992).

20. A. K. Fritzsche, A. R. Arevalo, A. F. Connolly, M. D. Moore, V. B. Elings, K. Kjoller, and C. M. Wu, J. Appl. Polym. Sci. *45*: 1945 (1992).

21. A. K. Fritzsche, A. R. Arevalo, M. D. Moore, C. J. Weber, V. B. Elings, K. Kjoller, and C. M. Wu, J. Appl. Polym. Sci. *46*: 167 (1992).

22. A. K. Fritzsche, A. R. Arevalo, and M. D. Moore, in *Récent progrès en génie des procédés* (P. Aimar and P. Aptel, eds), Vol. 6, CPIC, Nancy, 1992, pp. 59–64.

23. A. K. Fritzsche, A. R. Arevalo, M. D. Moore, and C. O'Hara, J. Membrane Sci. *81*: 109 (1993).

24. A. Bottino, G. Capannelli, A. Grosso, O. Monticelli, O. Cavalleri, R. Rolandi, and R. Soria, J. Membrane Sci. *95*: (1994) 289.

25. W. R. Bowen and N. J. Hall, Biotech. Bioeng. *46*: 28 (1995).

26. W. R. Bowen, N. Hilal, R. W. Lovitt, and P. M. Williams, J. Membrane Sci. *110*: 233 (1996).

27. *Membrane Filtration/Chromatography Catalogue*, Amicon Inc., USA, 1993.

28. K. J. Kim, A. G. Fane, C. J. D. Fell, T. Suzuki, and M. R. Dickinson, J. Membrane Sci. *54*: 89 (1990).

29. W. R. Bowen, N. Hilal, R. W. Lovitt, and P. M. Williams, *Proceedings of Euromembrane '95*, Vol. 1 (W. R. Bowen, R. W. Field, and J. A. Howell, eds), ESMST, Bath, UK, 1995, pp. 136–139.

30. T. J. Senden, C. J. Drummond, and P. Kékicheff, Langmuir *10*: 358 (1994).

31. W. R. Bowen, in *Membranes in Bioprocessing* (J. A. Howell, V. Sanchez, and R. W. Field, eds), Blackie, London, 1993, pp. 265–291.

32. T. J. Senden and C. J. Drummond, Colloids and Surfaces A: Physicochemical and Engineering Aspects. *94*: 29 (1995).

33. H-J. Butt, M. Jaschke and W. Ducker, Bioelectrochemistry and Bioenergetics, *38*: 191 (1995).

34. W. R. Bowen, N. Hilal, R. W. Lovitt, A. O. Sharif and P. M. Williams, J. Membrane Sci. *126*: 77 (1997).

35. A. Grabbe and R. G. Horn, J. J. Colloid Interface. Sci. *157*: 375 (1993).

36. W. R. Bowen and R. J. Cooke, J. Colloid Interface. Sci. *141*: 280 (1991).

37. R. J. Hunter, *Foundations of Colloid Science*, Oxford University Press, Oxford, 1993.

38. W. R. Bowen and A. O. Sharif, Proc. Roy. Soc. Lond, Series A, *A452*: 2121 (1996).

39. W. R. Bowen, A. W. Mohammed, and N. Hilal, J. Membrane Sci. *126*: 91 (1997).

40. W. R. Bowen, N. Hilal, R. W. Lovitt, and C. J. Wright, Colloids and Surfaces A: Physicochemical and Engineering Aspects *136*: 231 (1998).

41. G. Toikka, R. A. Hayes, and J. Ralston, J. Colloid Interface. Sci. *180*: 239 (1996).

42. S. Veeramasunei, M. R. Yalamanchili, and J. D. Miller, J. Colloid Interface. Sci. *184*: 594 (1996).

2

A Multidisciplinary Approach Towards Pore Size Distributions of Microporous and Mesoporous Membranes

ANTONIO HERNÁNDEZ, JOSÉ IGNACIO CALVO, PEDRO PRÁDANOS, and LAURA PALACIO Department of Thermodynamics and Applied Physics, University of Valladolid, Valladolid, Spain

Abstract

There are several independent methods for determining pore statistics or pore size distributions. The most useful and common are presented here. In particular: Electron and atomic force microscopy techniques and computerized image analysis, gas–liquid and liquid–liquid displacement methods, mercury porosimetry, adsorption–desorption techniques, perm-porometry, thermoporometry and solute retention methods. For all these methods some examples are shown in this chapter. The different methods are described and the physical principles, operative conditions and mathematical procedures shown in some detail here. While other less developed methods are also mentioned. These methods are shown to cover complementary ranges and different characteristics linked with structure and permeation in porous membranes used in micro-, ultra- and nanofiltration as well as other porous materials. The value and drawbacks of each method are discussed and compared for very regular track-etched membranes. The effect of pore size distribution on electro-kinetic parameters, focusing on streaming potential, is also shown.

I. INTRODUCTION

Membranes can be classified according to their material components and structure as being porous or dense. What can be understood as dense membranes is depending on the scale to which they are studied. In this type of membrane, the performance (permeability and selectivity) is determined by the intrinsic properties of the material by solution–diffusion through the molecular interstices in the membrane material. When this is not the main mechanism, the membranes can be called porous. In this case, the selectivity is mainly determined by the dimension of the pores and the material has only an effect through phenomena such as adsorption and chemical stability under the conditions of actual application and membrane cleaning [1].

Some liquid or gas membranes are embedded into solid matrices whose porous structure may play a role in actual transport. On the other hand, solid dense membranes are usually fixed on a porous support whose structure can penetrate into the dense layer leading to defects in the dense material and corrections to the expected flow. Even if these defects are not present, the transport through the support material can play a significative role in process features.

The processes where porous membranes find their main application are pressure driven ones such as: microfiltration, ultrafiltration, and nanofiltration. These processes are also especially interesting attending to their wide range of practical applications. They can be used for the processing of fine particles, colloids, and biological materials such as protein precipitates and microorganisms [2]. Membranes used are commonly polymeric materials but innovative development has been made in the fields of ceramic and inorganic membranes. The prediction of the process performances of these membranes for industrially relevant separations ultimately rests on the development and application of effective procedures for membrane characterization.

Most membrane manufacturers characterize their products by a single pore size or a molecular weight cut-off value. These data are usually obtained by measuring the rejection of various macromolecules or particles of increasing hydrodynamic diameter or molecular weight. Nevertheless, it is clear that this single value does not allow to know neither the separation properties of the membrane nor its structure. In any case, the molecular weight cut-off can be accepted as a datum only useful for preliminary selection. However, all membranes must be assumed as containing size-distributed pores.

There are several independent methods for determining pore statistics [1,3–6]. The major ones are presented below [7]:

1. Electron microscopy. This method uses several electronic microscopy techniques which are available to view the top or cross-sections of membranes, as SEM (scanning electron microscopy), TEM (transmission electron microscopy), FESEM (field effect scanning electron microscopy), etc. Computerized image analysis of the corresponding micrographs is frequently used to obtain pore size distributions [8].
2. Atomic force microscopy. This technique allows the surface study of nonconducting materials, down to the scale of nanometers. It was developed by Binnig et al. [9], and its main advantage over the electron microscopy techniques is that no previous preparation of the sample is needed [8]. Although it is a relatively novel technique, application to membranes, both biological and synthetic ones, is growing rapidly [10,11].
3. Bubble pressure breakthrough. This method, introduced by Bechhold [12], is based on the measurement of the pressure necessary to make a fluid pass through a liquid-filled porous membrane. Bubble point and related methods (both liquid–liquid and gas–liquid displacement techniques) have been frequently used for estimation of mean pore size and pore size distributions of many commercial membranes [13–15], and have reached the status of recommended standards [16,17].
4. Mercury porosimetry. The method is based on the same principles as the bubble pressure method; but now mercury (a nonwetting fluid) is used to fill a dry membrane [18].
5. Adsorption–desorption methods [19]. An analysis of pore size distribution can also be accomplished by gas adsorption–desorption devices. The technique is based on the Kelvin equation, which relates the reduced vapor pressure of a liquid with a curved surface to the equilibrium vapor pres-

sure of the same liquid in a plane [20]. Also, application of BET adsorption theory to gas adsorption isotherms is commonly used to obtain specific surface areas.

6. Permporometry. The technique is based on the controlled blocking of pores by condensation of vapor, present as a component of a gas mixture, and the simultaneous measurement of the gas flux through the membrane [21]. If the Kelvin equation is used, the pore size distribution is obtained.

7. Thermoporometry. Another method suggested by Brun et al. [22], based on the fact that the solidification point of the vapor condensed in the pores is a function of the interface curvature. By using a differential scanning calorimeter (DSC), the phase transition can be easily monitored and the pore size distribution calculated.

8. Solute retention test. Rejection is measured, under more or less standardized conditions, for various solutes of increasing molecular weights or hydrodynamic sizes, thus pore sizes can be evaluated [23,24].

These techniques will be described in some detail here. Of course they are clearly not the only methods that can be used, but certainly are the most useful and widespread. The pore size ranges covered are summarized in Fig. 1. It is clear that they can be included in two main groups, some of these methods (the ones developed for the characterization of general porous materials) directly give morphological properties, while others give parameters related with the membrane permeation (those designed specifically to characterize membrane materials) [25]. Once we discuss them in some detail we will come back to their classification.

Other techniques can also be used for determining pores and pore sizes in filters as, for example, NMR measurements, wide angle X-ray diffraction, small angle X-ray scattering, electrical conductance, etc. Glaves and Smith [26] have demonstrated the determination of pore size in water-saturated membranes using nuclear magnetic resonance (NMR), spin-lattice relaxation measurements. The NMR measurements must be calibrated using a known pore population material, but nevertheless no specific pore geometry has to be assumed. Wide angle X-ray diffraction allows to determine the degree of crystallinity of the membrane material, which can be related to the pore sizes [27]. Otherwise, small angle X-ray scattering gives important structural information on pores producing the distinct heterogeneities of the electronic density [28]. Finally, electrical conductance measurements have been used to find pore sizes of mica sheets by Bean et al. [29].

Other techniques can give important physical and chemical parameters, other than pore size distributions, of porous materials as: ESCA (Electron Spectroscopy for Chemical Analysis), FTIR (Fourier Transform InfraRed spectroscopy) or contact angle determinations.

It is clearly interesting to know which are the principal features of each technique, in order to be able to adequately choose the more interesting tech-

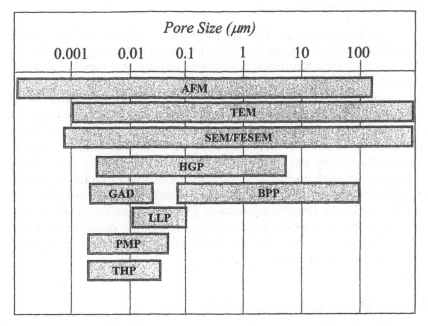

FIG. 1 Ranges of the main methods to analyze pore size distributions: AFM, atomic force microscopy; TEM, transmission electron microscopy; SEM/FESEM, scanning electron microscopy/field emission scanning electron microscopy; HGP, mercury porosimetry; GAD, gas adsorption–desorption; BPP, bubble point porometry (gas–liquid displacement porometry); LLP, liquid–liquid displacement porometry; PMP, permporometry and THP, thermoporometry.

nique for a given membrane and purpose. An initial factor of decision could be the range of pore sizes that each technique covers. Another important factor is the number of samples required to perform a characterization experience. While bubble point extended methods, solute retention challenge and microscopic methods need only a small quantity of membrane; the techniques of gas adsorption and mercury porosimetry require a considerable amount of sample area, depending on the porosity of the membrane. Moreover SEM, solute retention and mercury intrusion can destroy (or at least lead to a change in performance of) most of the membrane materials (especially mercury intrusion which adds the highly contaminant character of mercury).

Appropriate elucidation of structure is not only relevant to describe sieving effects but also to study solute–material interactions, as far as the corresponding interfaces are placed inside the pores. Thus, electrically determined membrane properties act on the solutes inside the pores and transport is affected by these properties (zeta potential, surface charges, etc.) in such a way that makes necessary a detailed knowledge of pore geometry to adequately correlate interactions with their effects on flux.

II. MICROSCOPIC TECHNIQUES

In this section, we will consider the characterization methods based on microscopic techniques that in conjunction with the appropriate image analysis lead to the evaluation of the membrane parameters without any previous assumption about the pore geometry.

Microscopic techniques were used very early in the characterization of membrane filters. Visual inspection of pore structure is an invaluable tool for a deep knowledge of the filters themselves. Nevertheless, as the developed filters entered the range of submicronic pores, i.e., pores with sizes under a micrometer, optical microscopy was not useful to achieve a real picture of the membrane structure, given that resolution is limited by the light diffraction pattern. Only the development of nonoptical microscopic techniques allowed us to skip this problem. First the electron microscopy [30], and now the probe microscopy [9], have given a gentle push to the microscopic characterization of membranes, so that we can now have information of membrane surfaces covering the full range of membrane filters.

A. Electron Microscopy: SEM and TEM

When a solid is bombarded with high energy electrons, there is a number of interactions between the solid material and the electron beam, that can be used to identify the specimen and the elements present in it, but also to characterize physically the holes and pores present at the surfaces.

Transmission electron microscopy (TEM) operates by flooding the sample with an electron beam, most commonly at 100–200 keV and detecting the image generated by both elastically and inelastically scattered electrons passing through the sample. TEM operates in the magnification range from $600 \times$ to $10^6 \times$.

Similarly, a fine beam of medium energy electrons (5–50 keV) causes several interactions with the material, being secondary electrons used in the SEM technique. SEM equipments are able to achieve magnifications ranging from $20 \times$ to $10^5 \times$, giving images marked by a great depth of field, thus leading to considerable information about the surface texture of the particles.

The main problems and difficulties of the microscopic observation by both transmission and scanning electron microscopy are how to prepare a membrane sample without any artefacts. The first step of the preparation is a careful drying of the sample, and in order to avoid collapse of the original structure, the freeze-dry technique using liquid nitrogen or the critical-point drying method with carbon dioxide is usually employed.

In order to observe cross-sections by SEM the dried membrane is first fractured at liquid nitrogen temperature, and then fixed perpendicularly to the sample holder. Usually, samples are afterwards covered by a thin metallic layer (normally a gold film of some hundreds of angstroms), increasing the production of secondary electrons and improving therefore image contrast, [31]. For TEM observation, a more complicated procedure is required. The dried sample is first embedded, if necessary, and then cut by a microtome. An embedding media which has no influence on the membrane must be chosen. The section must be thin enough for electrons to penetrate, i.e., less than 50 nm. If only surface is to be analyzed, a replica technique can be used by coating the membrane with a carbon film and then removing the membrane material, by dissolving it for example, and analyzing this replica [32].

The maximum resolution of TEM is ~0.3–0.5 nm, while SEM has 10 times greater resolution and in both cases a high electron beam energy is applied. Therefore the sample surface can be seriously damaged, especially for polymeric membranes, which makes observation difficult. In the early 1980s the Field Emission Scanning Electron Microscopy (FESEM), which nowadays achieves very high resolution (up to 0.7 nm) even at low beam energy: accelerating voltage of 1.5–4 kV, was developed and used to observe surface pores of ultrafiltration membranes [33].

As an example, a SEM picture is shown in Fig. 2 for a C04 membrane (track etched filter with a nominal pore size of 0.4 μm made by Cyclopore) SEM picture is shown. It has been made with a JEOL microscope (JSM-820) with potentials of 20 kV on a sample coated with a layer of gold by ion sputtering on a JEOL (SCD-004) [34].

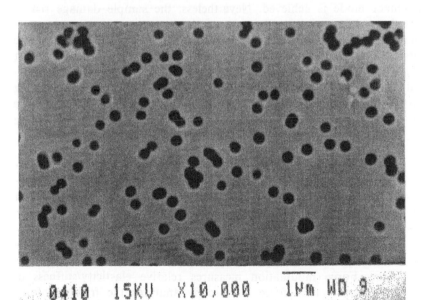

0410 15KV X10,000 1μm WD 9

FIG. 2 SEM picture of the C04 membrane.

B.   Probe Microscopy: STM and AFM

Atomic force microscopy (AFM), is a newly developed characterization technique which presents very high possibilities of development and application in
the field of microscopic observation and characterization of various surfaces.
A very small tip scans the surface and moves vertically according to its interaction with the sample, similarly to what is done in scanning tunneling microscopy (STM).

Both the techniques differ in the method used to detect interactions. In
STM the tip is so close to the sample (both being electrically conducting) to
allow a current to flow by tunnel effect and the sample or tip moves to keep
this current constant. While in AFM the tip is placed on a cantilever whose
deflection can be detected by the reflection of a laser beam appropriately
focused. This allows analysis of nonconducting materials, and makes the
method more convenient for the study of membrane materials [35–37].

Several operation procedures can be used in AFM.

1. Contact mode AFM. Measures the sample topography by sliding the
    probe tip across the sample surface. The tip–sample distance is maintained
    in the repulsive range of the van der Waals forces.
2. Noncontact mode AFM. Similarly, the topography of the sample is mea-
    sured by sensing the van der Waals attractive forces between the surface
    and the probe tip held above the surface. Of course, lower resolution than
    by contact mode is achieved. Nevertheless, the sample damage risk is
    avoided or minimized.
3. Tapping or intermittent contact mode AFM. It is a variation of the
    contact mode and operationally it is similar to noncontact mode, then it
    features the best characteristics of both methods. The cantilever is oscil-
    lated at its resonant frequency with high amplitude (over 100 nm) allowing
    it to touch the sample during the oscillation. This method maintains the
    high resolutions achieved in the contact mode, but minimizes the surface
    damage, as far as it eliminates the lateral friction forces.

These previously commented techniques give account of the sample topography. Moreover, other properties of the surfaces can be obtained, by analyzing different forces between sample and tip. For example, the phase contrast
provides information about differences in surface adhesion and viscoelasticity.
Magnetic and electric force microscopy (MFM and EFM) both measure magnetic (or electric) force gradient distribution above the sample surface. Surface
potential microscopy measures differences in local surface potential across the
sample surface. Force modulation measures relative elasticity/stiffness of
surface features and lateral force microscopy analyzes the frictional force
between the probe top and the sample surface. Finally, electrochemical
microscopy measures the surface structure and properties of conducting

materials immersed in electrolyte solutions with or without potential control. In many of these techniques, appropriate treatment of the measured forces is necessary to eliminate the contribution of the topographical images.

In Fig. 3 an AFM tapping mode image of C04 membrane is shown. It was obtained with a Nanoscope IIIA from Digital Instruments.

C. Computerized Image Analysis

Image analysis can be carried out by means of a plethora of software packages, some of which are supplied by the main optical or electronic microscopic manufacturers (Jeol, Leica, Karl Zeiss, Nikon, etc.) as a complement of their devices.

In all cases each photograph is first of all digitalized by assigning to each pixel a grey level ranging from 0 (black) to 255 (white). Then, a clearfield equalization is made to each image field to eliminate parasite changes in grey

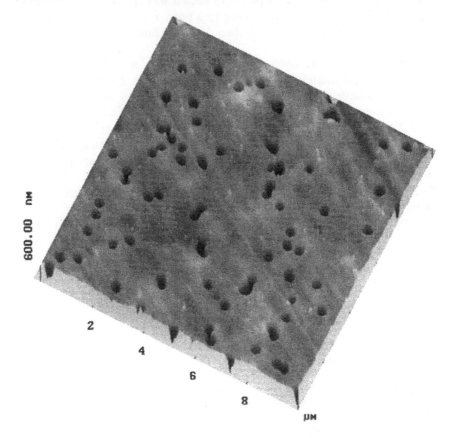

FIG. 3 AFM picture of the C04 membrane in a 3D projection.

levels due to uneven illumination. Obviously, a perfect clearfield equalization should require a blank image with a perfect flat sample of the same material equally treated and acquired in the same way. In fact this is impossible and even unconvenient, since far as uneven illumination can be due to the roughness of the sample itself. What can be done is to use what is called pseudoclearfield equalization by dividing the original image into a convenient number of rectangles. Then we can assign to all pixels the intensity such that a 95% of the original pixels have a lower intensity. Finally these rectangles are placed together by linear interpolation from rectangle to rectangle and subtracted from the original picture.

Once illumination effects are eliminated, the image grey spectrum is spanned to get the maximum contrast and definition. Then the images are redefined according to an assigned grey threshold level under which every pixel is assigned to 1 and the rest to 0. The resulting binary picture is improved by scrapping isolated pixels, in such a way that all the remaining 1's in the matrix are assumed as belonging to a pore. Finally the pore borders are smoothed in order to reduce the influence of the finite size of pixels and low definition.

Of course a correct selection of threshold grey level is fundamental to perform a correct analysis of accurate assigned pores. Customarily the grey spectrum is analyzed and the threshold placed centered in the valley of the almost bimodal distributions obtained. Unfortunately sometimes the spectra are so flat that this technique is only of relative help to make a correct threshold election [38]. In any case, eye inspection facilitates the process of selection of several reasonable threshold candidates whose outcomes are conveniently averaged.

Some parameters can be obtained directly from the SEM pictures, [34,39,40], for example: the surface pore density or number of pores per surface unit, N_T, and the porosity or porous surface fraction, Θ. In order to get the pore size distribution other parameters can be selected to study their statistical distributions, namely: pore area A_p and pore perimeter P_p along with two indirect parameters that can be defined as follows [34,41].

The equivalent or Feret pore diameter

$$d_p = 2\sqrt{\frac{A_p}{\pi}} \tag{1}$$

and the pore shape factor

$$s_p = 4\pi \frac{A_p}{P_p^2} \tag{2}$$

According to these definitions, the equivalent pore diameter is the diameter that a pore of area A_p should have if it had a circular section in the surface, while the pore shape factor is the ratio between the actual pore area and the corresponding area of a circle with the same perimeter. Actually s_p should be unity if the pore sections on the membrane surface were perfectly circular.

Consequently, the area and perimeter of each pore are measured immediately from the microphotographs, while diameter and shape factor are calculated by using Eqs. (1) and (2). Then we obtain, for each membrane, four size distributions: pore area, perimeter, diameter, and shape factor.

In the case of AFM pictures, we have also information on height which permits the study of pore entrances in greater detail. In this case, it is possible to use flat projections of the surface at different heights along with the level profiles at differently randomly chosen lines [42]. The simultaneous use of images and profiles greatly facilitates identification of the entrance of individual pores (however, the diameter deep in the membrane may not be determined directly by surface AFM due to convolution between the tip shape and the pore).

In Fig. 4, the pore size distribution for the C04 membrane is shown as obtained from their SEM pictures. Some other parameters are specific for AFM and are usually implemented by the on and/or offline analysis software included with the apparatus. In particular, roughness can be analyzed. This

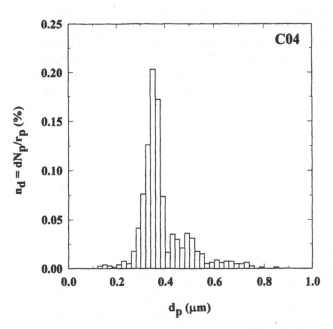

FIG. 4 Differential distribution for the number of pores of a given diameter for the C04 membrane from SEM pictures.

analysis is based on determining the heights of the tip over a baseline or reference level, Z. A statistical treatment of such heights leads to definition of the median value, Z_{med}, the mean, Z_m, or the maximum peak to valley height in the profile, R_t.

Moreover, some typical roughness parameters are defined, as the average roughness, R_a,

$$R_a = \frac{1}{n} \sum_{i=0}^{n} |Z_i - Z_m| \tag{3}$$

where n is the total number of points in the image matrix. Also the mean square roughness, R_{ms}, is usually evaluated from the Fourier transform of the surface profile. The corresponding values for the image of the C04 membrane shown in Fig. 3 are $R_a = 7.428$ nm and $R_{ms} = 10.974$ nm.

III. FLUID PENETRATION TECHNIQUES

It is well known that, when a liquid drop freely falls into a gas (for example water into air) or into another immiscible liquid phase, the drop tends to decrease its surface. If the drop size and density are so small that gravitational effects can be neglected, the drop acquires a spherical shape. The equilibrium is reached when the work done by the surface to decrease the area equals the liquid compression work. The mathematical description of this phenomenon leads to the Young–Laplace equation (1805) [43,44], which establishes that the pressure difference between both phases, Δp, is directly proportional to the surface tension of the interface, γ, and inversely proportional to the drop radius, R_d.

$$\Delta p = \frac{2\gamma}{R_d} \tag{4}$$

This equation can be expressed in a more general form, for whatever surface,

$$\Delta p = \gamma \left(\frac{1}{R_1} + \frac{1}{R_2} \right) \tag{5}$$

being R_1 and R_2 the principal radii of curvature that define this surface. When $R_1 = R_2$, the spherical surface equation is then recovered.

When the gas–liquid or liquid–liquid interface is confined to move inside a capillary tube, the surface behavior is also conditioned by the liquid–solid interface. But taking into account that the solid cannot change its shape and size, it will be only the liquid which shall change. The meniscus in the liquid–gas or liquid–liquid interface will be convex or concave depending on the liquid–solid interaction. In effect, it will be determined by the Young–Laplace equation. If the tube diameter is small enough (as it is in a capillary tube), we can consider this meniscus as an spherical segment of radius R_d. According to Fig. 5, the radius of the sphere is related with the capillary radius r_p by: $r_p = R_d | \cos \theta |$, being θ the so-called contact angle. According to this, the pressure necessary to intrude or expel the fluid from the capillary is given by the Young–Laplace equation as follows

$$\Delta p = \frac{2\gamma \cos \theta}{r_p} \qquad (6)$$

Note that for nonwetting liquids $\theta > 90°$ thus Δp is also negative. This equation is referred to as Washburn equation [45]. Moreover, if we have a zero contact angle, $\cos \theta = 1$, we arrive at what is usually called the Cantor equation [46].

Bechhold in 1908 [47] was the first using the Cantor's equation to evaluate pore sizes by measuring the pressure necessary to blow air through a water-filled membrane. The method so developed has been thoroughly used to characterize membranes and it is called the bubble point method. This method is only able to obtain the maximum pore size present in the pore distribution, corresponding to the minimum pressure necessary to blow the firstly observed air bubble. Furthermore, using water as wetting fluid, the pressure necessary to evaluate pore sizes as, for example 0.01 μm, can be as high as 145 bar.

To avoid having to use very high pressures, Bechhold et al. and Erbe [12,48], used two different liquids instead of an air–liquid interface, reducing appreciably the surface tension. For example, using isobutyl alcohol–water

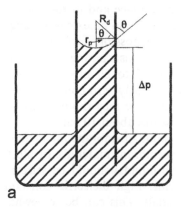
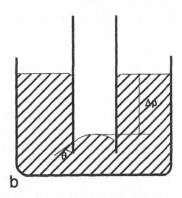

a   b

FIG. 5 Contact angle of a wetting (a) and nonwetting (b) liquid inside a capillary. Underpressure and overpressure are shown here in terms of ascents and depression under a gravitatory field.

interface, the measurement of pore sizes 40 times lower is achieved, as compared with the air–water interface.

Bechhold and co-workers [12] found that the observed pore size depends on the rate of pressure increase

$$r_p = \frac{2\gamma}{\Delta p} \left\{ 1 + \frac{2\,\Delta x}{\gamma} \left[\frac{d(\Delta p)}{dt} \, \bar{\eta} \right]^{1/2} \right\} \tag{7}$$

where $\bar{\eta}$ is the mean velocity of the permanent and soaking fluids and Δx is the thickness of the membrane.

A. Liquid Displacement

The bubble point and solvent permeability methods can be combined to yield a measure of the pore size distribution [49]. Stepwise increments of the pressure applied allows one to calculate [50] the number of pores corresponding to each diameter present in the pore distribution. The method has been recently improved for both liquid–gas interfaces [51,52], and liquid–liquid ones [53,54], allowing the evaluation of pore sizes corresponding to a wide range of porous materials.

1. Gas–Liquid Interface

The wetted sample is subjected to increasing pressure applied to a gas source. As the pressure of gas increases, it will reach a point where it can overcome the surface tension of the liquid in the largest pores and will push the liquid out. Increasing the pressure still further allows the gas to flow through smaller pores, according to the Washburn equation. The range of applicability of this method depends on the characteristics of the liquid soaking the membrane, due to both the surface tension of the gas–liquid interface and to the contact angle between liquid and membrane material. So, to obtain an extensive range of applicability, the liquid needs to have the lowest possible surface tension and a contact angle as near as possible to zero. There exists a range of organic liquids having low surface tensions ranging from 15 to 20 mN/m at temperatures between 293 and 313 K. They have also nearly zero contact angles with the most common membrane materials. In this case they should allow to analyze pore sizes below 0.1 μm, with applied pressures about 10 bar.

Given that the contact angle depends on the liquid–membrane interaction, different liquids should be preferred for different membrane materials. In effect, liquids with low dielectric constant (hydrophobic liquids) should be selected when dealing with hydrophobic membranes, while high dielectric constant liquids should be preferred for hydrophilic materials. This can be somewhat inconvenient when having different materials whose hydrophilicities differ or are unknown. In this case, a single liquid should be selected as a standard. Normally those exhibiting both radicals hydrophilic and hydrophobic (as, for example, hydrocarbonated compounds having a polar functional group) should be elected. This is the case, for instance, of alcohols or halogenated compounds.

Other interesting features that should be demanded are high chemical compatibility with most of the polymeric materials used in membrane manufacturing (it is well known that inorganic membranes do not have critical chemical compatibility problems) and a low vapor pressure at the working conditions of temperature and pressure. The last aspect being specially important, since liquid evaporation during the measurements can lead to erroneous results. Finally it is worth mentioning that, given that this kind of measurement is dynamically performed, it is convenient to choose liquids having viscosities as low as possible to avoid the influence of the measurement speed on the results.

A good candidate as wetting liquid, very frequently used in this kind of porometric analysis, is the iso-propyl alcohol, that has a surface tension (air–alcohol) of 20.86 mN/m and a vapor pressure of 5.8 kPa at 298 K. There exist, of course, commercial liquids specially designed for these kinds of determinations, having very optimized properties. For example, the Porofil (patented by Coulter) has a surface tension of 16 mN/m with a vapor pressure of 400 Pa at 298 K.

When different pores of diverse sizes are opened, the volume flow of gas, J_V, increases accordingly until all the pores are emptied. By monitoring the applied pressure and the flow of gas through the sample when liquid is being expelled, a wet run is obtained. If the sample is then tested dry (without liquid in its pores), a dry run follows. Computer-controlled instruments with software-driven experiment execution, data acquisition, processing, storage, and plotting are now commercially available. These are, for example, the Porometer series instruments manufactured by Coulter Electronics, the complete filter analyzer available from Porous Materials Inc., etc.

Figure 6 shows an example of the porometric results for a C08 membrane (which is a polycarbonate track-etched filter made by Cyclopore whose nominal pore size is 0.8 μm). Thus, the volume flow for the wet run, J_V^w, and for the dry one, J_V^d, vs. the applied pressure, allows to evaluate several statistical parameters, [55–57]. In effect, the cumulative flow for the pores with diameters below $d_p(j)$ is, [58],

$$f_a(j) = \frac{J_V^w(j)}{J_V^d(j)} \tag{8}$$

and the differential flow through pores in class jth ($j = 1, \ldots, n$); i.e., with a pore size $d_p(j)$, is

$$f_d(j) = \frac{f_a(j+1) - f_a(j-1)}{2} \tag{9}$$

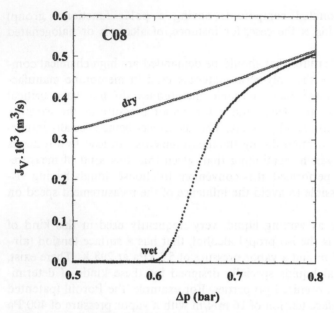

FIG. 6 Wet and dry runs obtained by air–liquid displacement technique on membrane C08.

While taking into account that flow is proportional to pore area, the fraction of pores with size $d_p(j)$ is

$$n_d(j) = K \frac{f_d(j)}{d_p(j)^2} \tag{10}$$

where K is a normalization factor that can be evaluated as

$$K = \frac{f_a(n)}{n'_a(n)} \tag{11}$$

n being the last class of sizes and

$$n'_a(n) = \sum_{j=0}^{n} n'_d(j) \tag{12}$$

with

$$n'_d(j) = \frac{f_d(j)}{d_p(j)^2} \tag{13}$$

Finally, the cumulative distribution of number of pores is

$$n_a(j) = \sum_{k=1}^{j} n_d(k) \tag{14}$$

In this way, the cumulative and differential distributions of relative number of pores and flow, n_a, n_d, f_a, and f_d, can be obtained. Nevertheless, if the absolute number of pores and porosity are to be evaluated, a model for the gas flow through the pores must be assumed.

The model for gas flow should be determined by the relation between the mean free path of the gas molecules and the pore size. In a first view, three simple models can be proposed to describe gas flow: the Hagen–Poiseuille viscous flow, the Knudsen molecular one and some transitional regimes between both.

(a) *Hagen–Poiseuille Model.* The volume flow for each pore diameter in the distribution should be given by the so-called Hagen–Poiseuille equation, [1]

$$J_V(d_p) = \frac{\pi N(d_p)}{128} \frac{d_p^4}{\eta \psi} \frac{\Delta p}{\Delta x} \tag{15}$$

where $N(d_p)$ is the density of pores of diameter d_p, ψ is a constriction-tortuosity factor, η is the gas viscosity. By assuming that all the pores have straight circular sections, Eq. (15) is

$$J_V(d_p) = \frac{\Theta(d_p)}{32} \frac{d_p^2}{\eta \psi} \frac{\Delta p}{\Delta x} \tag{16}$$

$\Theta(d_p)$ being the porosity for which pores of diameter d_p are responsible.

Some, mainly ultrafiltration membranes, have a granular structure. According to this model, an ultrafiltration membrane should be made out of granules of diameter d_g with a volume flow given by [1,59]

$$J_V = \frac{\Theta_V^3}{72(1 - \Theta_V)^2} \left(\frac{d_g^2}{\eta \psi}\right) \frac{\Delta p}{\Delta x} \tag{17}$$

where Θ_V is the volume or overall porosity, according to the Carman–Kozeny equation. This model leads to the same results as the Hagen–Poiseuille equation for equal pores if an equivalent pore diameter is defined as

$$d_p = \frac{2}{3} \left(\frac{\Theta_V}{1 - \Theta_V}\right) d_g \tag{18}$$

(b) *Knudsen Model.* The Hagen–Poiseuille formula strictly apply only if the mean free path of the gas molecules, λ, is much lower than the capillary diameter, because only in this limit can one properly assume that gas velocity at the capillary walls is equal to zero. If this condition is not fulfilled the basic equations for viscous flow cannot be applied. The mean free path for an ideal gas can be written as

$$\lambda = \frac{1}{\pi\sqrt{2}} \left(\frac{kT}{p'}\right) \frac{1}{d_m^2} \tag{19}$$

where p' is the pressure, d_m the molecular diameter, k the Boltzmann constant and T is temperature.

When pressure and/or pore size are so low that the mean free path greatly exceeds the tube diameter, the flow also becomes amenable to simple theoretical treatment. The flow in this limit is commonly referred to as free-molecule diffusion or Knudsen flow. In this case the flow of the gas is determined almost entirely by the collisions with the wall that can be considered highly irregular, at a molecular level, giving diffuse reflection of the gas molecules after collisions. In this way the volume flow is [1,60,61]

$$J_V(d_p) = \frac{2\pi N(d_p)}{3} \left(\frac{RT}{8\pi M_w}\right)^{1/2} \frac{d_p^3}{p_d \psi} \frac{\Delta p}{\Delta x} \tag{20}$$

where R is the gas constant, M_w is the molecular weight of the gas and p_d is the downstream pressure [51].

(c) *Knudsen–Poisseuille Transition Regime.* No quantitative kinetic-theory treatment of the flow in the transition region where λ and d_p are comparable exists. For a given gas, the question of the limit radii to pass from one to the other of these regimes has been frequently discussed [62–64]. This problem can be bridged if we look for the limit pore size where the representation of $[J_V \psi \Delta x/\Delta p]$ for both the regimes intersect. For air ($M_w = 29 \times 10^{-3}$ kg/mol, $\eta = 1.904 \times 10^{-5}$ Pa·s) at $T = 313$ K with a downstream pressure $p = 1$ bar, this happens at a pore diameter of 0.96 μm [65]. Of course, in a more or less wide zone around this limit diameter, the flow should be better described by a smooth curve. Given that there is not an easy way to establish this transitional regime, a reasonably good approximation should be reached by using Knudsen flow for pores below the limit diameter and Hagen–Poiseuille one for those over it.

If it is assumed that for pores until those in the mth class, $d_p(m) = 0.96$ μm, the transport is of the Knudsen type while for diameters over $d_p(m)$ there exists a viscous flow, the total number of pores per surface unit, $N_T(j)$, is

$$N_T(j) = \frac{L_p(j)}{l_p} \tag{21}$$

where $L_p(j)$ is the air permeability of the porous matrix at the jth pressure, while l_p is

$$l_p = \frac{\pi}{\Delta x} \left[\frac{2}{3p} \left(\frac{RT}{8\pi M_w}\right)^{1/2} \sum_{j=1}^{m} n_d(j) d_p^3(j) + \frac{1}{128\eta} \sum_{j=m}^{n} n_d(j) d_p^4(j)\right] \tag{22}$$

Due to some nonidealities, the air permeability of the dry membrane is not constant. Thus when calculating N_T, different values are obtained for each pressure leading to $N_T(j)$. Finally, the absolute differential distribution of pores per surface unit can be obtained as

$$N_d(j) = n_d(j)N_T(j) \tag{23}$$

While the absolute cumulative distribution is

$$N_a(j) = \sum_{k=1}^{j} N_d(k) \tag{24}$$

in such a way that the total surface density of pores should be $N_a(n)$.

Figure 7 show the distributions of pore number as a function of the pore size for two membranes (C08 and C10, Cyclopore filters with nominal pore sizes of 0.8 μm and 1.0 μm, respectively) where flux should be mainly of the Knudsen type and of the Hagen–Poiseuille type, respectively.

2. Liquid–Liquid Interface

The pore size distribution can also be estimated by using two immiscible liquids, one of them soaking the membrane structure and the other permeating liquid, which expels the wetting one [53,66]. This technique allows to determine pore sizes from 5 to 140 nm by using immiscible liquids with appropriately low surface tensions. This permits us to characterize typical

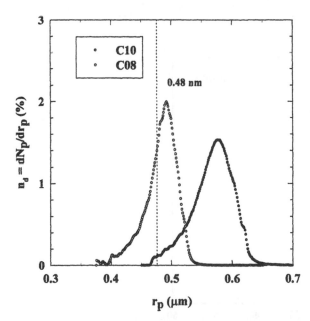

FIG. 7 Differential distribution for the number of pores for both C08 and C10 obtained by the air–liquid displacement technique. The radius corresponding to a change from Knudsen to Hagen–Poiseuille regime is shown by a dashed arrow. Note that only C10 is totally within the Hagen–Poiseuille range.

ultrafiltration membranes. The main advantage of this technique is the absence of high applied pressures (always below 10 bar). Examples of typical used pairs of liquids are: Distilled water–water saturated isobutanol ($\gamma = 1.7$ mN/m), distilled water–mixture of isobutanol, methanol and water (5:1:4 v/v) ($\gamma = 0.8$ mN/m) or distilled water–mixture of isobutanol, methanol and water (1:7:25 v/v) ($\gamma = 0.35$ mN/m) [53].

Evidently, here the question of the flow regime does not apply as far as the permeating fluid is a liquid, thus pore numbers require a viscous flux model. If usual assumptions on the pore geometry are done, Hagen–Poiseuille or Carman–Kozeny models should be applied.

In the case of hydrophilic membranes, when using liquids as those already mentioned, it is reasonable to suppose zero contact angle (or nearly) and to use the Cantor equation to relate the applied pressures and the pore sizes. Finally, the same calculation procedure described for gas–liquid interface should be used to calculate the differential flux and pore number distributions.

The technique has been successfully applied to symmetric as well as asymmetric membranes in the ultrafiltration range. An example is shown in Fig. 8, where the pore size distribution of a Nuclepore membrane with a nominal size of 30 nm (N003) has been obtained by reelaboration of results of Munari et al. [54].

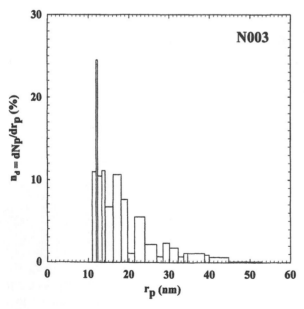

FIG. 8 Differential distribution for the number of pores for N003 membrane obtained by liquid–liquid displacement technique. Data adapted from [54].

B. Mercury Porosimetry

Another characterization method that can be included with those based on the Laplace equation is the mercury intrusion porosimetry. The method (also firstly proposed by Washburn [67]) was developed by Ritter and Drake [6], and applied for the first time to characterize membrane filters by Honold and Skau [68]. It has been shown to be a reliable method for the characterization of pore size distributions, pore structure and specific surface areas. Here, a Hg–air interface appears inside each pore. Thus the Washburn formula, Eq. (6), is also followed. However, in this case, mercury does not wet practically any kind of sample (the corresponding contact angles ranging from 112° to 150°) [6,67].

Plots of intruded and/or extruded volumes vs. pressure, usually called porograms, can show a great variety of shapes depending on the characteristics and distribution of pores and voids, if present in the sample. But two common features are always present in porograms [6].

1. Hysteresis is always obtained, i.e. the extrusion path does not follow the intrusion curve.
2. Moreover, after completion of an intrusion–extrusion cycle some portion of mercury is always retained by the sample (pore entrapment) avoiding loop closing. This phenomenon usually ceases after the second pressurization–depressurization run.

Both phenomena have been frequently attributed to "ink-bottle-pores" [69]. This explanation should indicate a very spread distribution of "ink-bottle" pores. A possibly more realistic point to explain hysteresis and entrapment is the assumption of a network of differently sized intersecting pores. Androutsopoulous and Mann [70], have calculated the consequences of assuming a bi-dimensional square network of cylindrical intersecting pores. Their predictions fairly agree with the actual hysteresis and entrapment behavior of catalytic materials where pelleted structure can be assumed. Lowell and Shields [71] have shown that coincidence between intrusion and extrusion curves is possible, at least in the second and subsequent cycles, if the contact angle θ is adjusted to distinguish between advancing (θ_i) and receding (θ_e) contact angles. Nevertheless, the first cycle in the porogram cannot be totally closed due to the mercury entrapment which varies greatly (from nearly zero to almost 100%) [70].

The mercury intrusion porosimetry has been used for a long time, as commented before, as an experimental standard technique for the characterization of pore and void structure. The usual application range goes from 0.002 to 1000 μm pore size. Nevertheless, to achieve the lower range, really high pressures are necessary, up to 4500 bar, which increases dangerously the risk of distorting the porous structure.

Some manufacturers of Mercury Porosimeters are Carlo Erba, Fisons, Micromeritics and Quantachrome Co. In almost all porosimeters, the amount of mercury intruded is determined by the fall in the level of the interface between the mercury and the compressing fluid. All porosimeters include certain common features. First, the sample is evacuated and then the penetrometer is backfilled with Hg in the low pressure port. The second step of the low pressure analysis is the collection of the data at pressures up to the last low pressure point specified. When the low pressure analysis is complete, the high pressure measurement is carried out up to the maximum pressure. Pore volume data are calculated by determining the volume of Hg remaining in the penetrometer stem. When the maximum pressure is achieved, the extrusion curve starts by reducing slowly the applied pressure. Commercial instruments can work in one or both modes: incremental and continuous. In the former the pressure, or amount of Hg introduced, is increased step by step and the system allowed to stabilize before the next step. In the continuous mode the pressure is increased continually at a predetermined rate [72].

From the data on intruded volume vs. applied pressures the pore size distributions can be obtained according to the following outlined procedure. The differential pore size distribution corresponding to specific volumes, $D_V(d_p)$

$$D_V(d_p) = \frac{p}{d_p} \frac{dV}{dp} \tag{25}$$

being p the applied pressure, d_p the diameter corresponding to that pressure according to Washburn equation, V the specific volume (volume of mercury intruded divided by the sample weight) and dV/dp the derivative of the intruded specific volume vs. pressure. Normally, the data acquisition software allows us to use appropriate derivation algorithms to smooth the resulting curves. The relative population of pores in each class is obtained from

$$n_d(j) = \frac{\dfrac{D_V(d_p)[d_p(j) - d_p(j-1)]}{\{[d_p(j) + d_p(j-1)]/2\}^2}}{\displaystyle\sum_{i=1}^{n} \frac{D_V(d_p)[d_p(i) - d_p(i-1)]}{\{[d_p(i) + d_p(i-1)]/2\}^2}} \tag{26}$$

The question of which contact angle should be used in the Washburn equation remains open, and it should be taken into account that errors of one degree out of 140 should lead to errors in all pore radii of a 1.4% [6]. A contact angle of $\theta = 130°$ seems to be valid for a wide range of materials and it is normally set as default value in most of the commercial equipment [6], along with a Hg–air surface tension, $\gamma = 0.474$ N/m [73]. Nevertheless, some authors calibrate porosimetric results in order to reproduce previous independent calculations on the pore size distributions. This approach has been followed by Liabastre and Orr [67], for Nuclepore membranes, comparing with

Computerized Image Analysis of Scanning Electron Microscopy (SEM-CIA) pictures leading to a contact angle of 126.3°. This method can induce very inexact estimations of pore size distributions if the reference method is not adequately chosen. In this way, SEM photographs seem an unfortunate selection as far as they refer to surface characteristics of the membrane that should be necessarily different from those referring to bulk structure [34]. For polymeric membranes, a value of $\theta = 140°$ seems to work reasonably well, giving good accordance with other characterization methods [74].

A typical pattern for the directly measured intrusion and extrusion curves is shown in Fig. 9 for a C04 membrane (Cyclopore membrane with 0.4 μm nominal pore size) from an Autoscan 33 10X manufactured by Quantachrome Co. Note the common features previously commented: hysteresis and entrapment. In our case entrapment was always low, as corresponding to very cylindrical pores [70,75]. The resulting pore size distribution for the C04 membrane is shown in Fig. 10.

IV. TECHNIQUES BASED ON GAS ADSORPTION–DESORPTION

Adsorption phenomena have been long known. In 1777, Scheele demonstrated that air makes carbon to increase its volume several times; this phenomenon being reversible, thus when heating the carbon, the air was evacuated from the solid. He dealt with adsorption of a gas (called adsorbate) onto a solid sub-

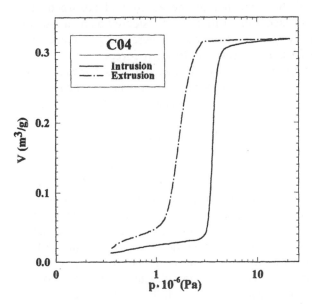

FIG. 9 Intrusion and extrusion Hg porograms for membrane C04.

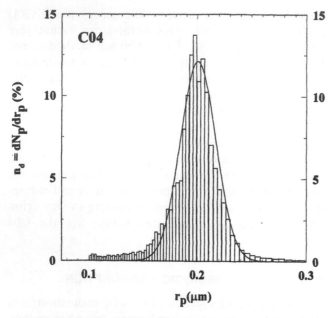

FIG. 10 Differential distribution for the number of pores obtained from Hg porosimetry for the C04 membrane.

strate (the adsorbent). Nevertheless, the complete phenomenon is much more general. Experimental work has shown that the amount of adsorbed gas is proportional to the solid surface, thus it must be considered as a surface phenomenon, taking place at the gas–solid interface, where the gas molecules fix themselves to the solid surface, due to several attractive forces.

The nature of these forces can be very diverse, but it is conventional to speak of physisorption or chemisorption, depending on whether the forces are of a physical (van der Waals forces) or a chemical (bonding forces) nature, respectively.

The study of this kind of systems it is fulfilled by determining the so-called adsorption isotherm. An adsorption isotherm consists in the evaluation of the amount of adsorbed gas as a function of the equilibrium pressure at a constant temperature. The physical adsorption is the predominant process for inert gases at temperatures below their critical point. Normally, in the adsorption isotherm, the pressure is expressed by the relative pressure $p_r = p/p_0$ where p_0 is the saturation pressure at a given temperature) and the amount may be expressed by the mass of gas or its volume at standard temperature and pressure (STP).

When dealing with porous solids, it is usual to classify the pores according to their size in three main categories. This classification lacks precision and universality but a tentative one, usually accepted, follows. Namely: micropores are those having sizes below 2 nm, mesopores range from 2 nm to 50 nm, and

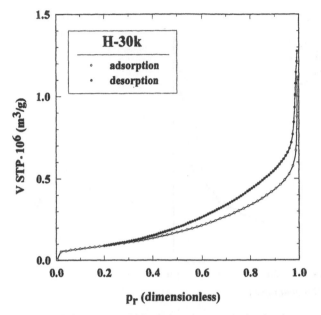

FIG. 11 Adsorption desorption isotherm for membrane H-30k. It is of the type I for low p_r and type IV according to the hysteresis loop.

finally macropores have sizes bigger than 50 nm. The reason for this classification is the applicability of the Kelvin equation (which will be conveniently analyzed below) with N_2 at 77 K as adsorbate.

The shape of the adsorption isotherm is related with the inner structure of the adsorbate in such a way that, according to the IUPAC recommendations, six main groups can be distinguished:

Type I: It corresponds to the usual Langmuir isotherm [76], and it is found when only micropores are present in the analyzed material.

Types II and III: They correspond to non-porous solids or solids containing only macropores. The type III isotherm differs from the type II on the relatively weakness of the solid–gas interaction present when type III isotherms are obtained.

Types IV and V: They correspond to processes presenting a hysteresis loop between adsorption and desorption paths. They are found in solid having only mesopores, to whom the Kelvin equation is fully applicable. Type IV differs from type V also in the weaker interaction present in the last case.

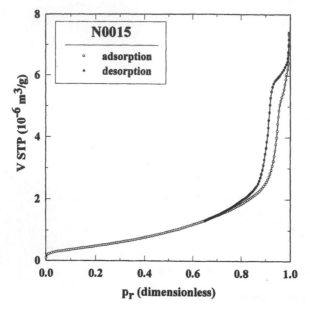

FIG. 12 Adsorption desorption isotherm for membrane N0015. It is type IV.

Type VI: It is the stepped adsorption isotherm which comes
                      from phase transition of the adsorbed molecular layer
                      or adsorption on the different faces of the crystalline
                      solids.

From the point of view of porous materials whose distribution of pores are
to be determined with this technique, we will only consider the isotherms of
types: I (micropores), IV and V (mesopores). In Figs. 11 and 12, corresponding
to results of N_2 adsorption–desorption on ultrafiltration membranes made by
Hoechst AG (Nadir UF-PES-30H/PP100) that here will be called H-30k [37],
and Nuclepore (N0015) [36], respectively, the typical shape of these isotherms
it is depicted. Both present type IV adsorption while Nadir membrane presents also a type I (micropores) at low relative pressures.

A. Gas Adsorption–Desorption Porosimetry

There exists a range of commercially available apparatus that allow determination of the adsorption isotherms of solids with gases or vapors. Taking into
account the measurement method, they can be divided into three groups:

those which measure the volume and the gas pressure in the equilibrium (static or continuous), those measuring in a continuous manner based on chromatographic methods and, finally, those determining the variation of the solid mass with a microbalance.

Some equipments measuring statically are: Belsorp 28 from Bel Co.; Sorpty 1750 from Carlo Erba; Fisons Sorptomatic 1900 Series; Horiba SA6200 Series; ASAP 2000, Accusorb 2100E, Digisorb 2600 and Gemini from Micromeritics; Nova 1000 and Nova 1200 from Quantachrome; Omnisorp series from Coulter Ltd., etc. Some based on continuous flow gas chromatography methods are: Series 4200, 4201, and 4203 from Beta Scientific; Model 4200 from Leeds & Northrup; Rapid Surface Area Analyzer 2300 and Flowsorb II2300 from Micromeritics; Monosorb, Quantasorb and Quantasorb Jr. from Quantachrome, etc. Finally we can mention some gravimetric apparatus as, for example: DVS analyzer from Surface Measurement Systems; Gravimat from Netzch, etc. [72].

When these methods are used to determine pore size distributions (physisorption), mainly N_2 and sometimes argon are chosen as adsorbate. Nevertheless, some other gases can be used when special characteristics of the materials are to be studied. For example, it can be interesting to study its hydrophilic/hydrophobic character or the dependence of the material accessible for adsorption on the molecular size of the gas. In these cases vapors from water, hydrocarbon compounds, alcohols, etc. can be used.

The following paragraphs will be devoted to describing the methods for determining of the pore size distributions of membranes and other porous materials, according to the scope of this chapter. As previously mentioned, these materials can be divided into two groups (presence of micropores or mesopores). However, as a first step we will consider the determination of the total adsorption surface of these materials by gas adsorption—not only because this parameter is an important structural characteristic but also due to the relevance of the models used in its determination as the basis of some of the usual methods for calculating pore size distributions.

1. Surface Area

The total surface area of a membrane where adsorption can occur may be determined by using the Brunauer–Emmett–Teller (BET) method, which is generally regarded as the standard procedure. This method relies on a kinetic model for adsorption [77], whose main assumptions are briefly summarized:

1. In all layers, except the first one, the molar adsorption enthalpy corresponds to the condensation enthalpy, L.
2. In all layers, except the first one, the condensation–evaporation conditions are equal.
3. At the saturation pressure (i.e., when $p_r = 1$), all the gas condenses onto the solid surface leading to an infinite number of adsorbed layers.

Accordingly a relatively simple expression is obtained

$$\frac{p}{V(p_0 - p)} = \frac{1}{V_m C} + \frac{C - 1}{V_m C} \frac{p}{p_0}$$ (27)

where V_m is the total volume adsorbed in a monolayer per mass unit of sample, V is the volume adsorbed per mass unit of the sample, and C is a parameter related to the molar adsorption enthalpy [36], as follows

$$C = \frac{A_1 \omega_i}{A_i \omega_1} \exp \frac{E_1 - L}{RT}$$ (28)

A_i is the fraction of adsorbate molecules that condense in the ith layer and ω_i is the frequency of vibration of the molecules perpendicular to the solid surface in ith layer ($i = 1, 2, \ldots, \infty$). Both these coefficients should be equal for $i > 1$. E_1 is the molar adsorption enthalpy for the first layer, while L corresponds to the rest of layers, as previously assumed.

Accordingly, a plot of $p/[V(p_0 - p)]$ against p_r should give a straight line, allowing evaluation of both C and V_m from the slope and ordinate intercept of the plot. In practice, such a simple model accurately serves only for relative pressures in the range from 0.05 to 0.3. In fact, what ought be done is to check the linear range to be used; in most cases, p_r from 0.05 to 0.1 should lead to correlation coefficients over 0.9999. Finally, by taking into account the molecular size of the adsorbate A_m (16.2 Å² for a nitrogen molecule), the specific adsorption area of the membrane should be

$$S = \left(\frac{V_m}{v_g} \right) N_A A_m$$ (29)

where v_g is the molar volume of the gas at standard temperature and pressure and N_A is Avogadro's number.

2. Pore Size Distribution

As already mentioned, the pore size ranges that define micro, meso and macro porosity are far from being clearly and sharply defined. In any case, ultrafiltration or nanofiltration membranes could present all of them, when they are composite and/or asymmetric.

Thus, it seems useful to perform both micropore and mesopore analysis for the N_2 adsorption–desorption isotherms. In the following sections features and differences of both analysis are envisaged. Although the adsorption isotherm near the condensation pressure ($p_r = 1$) gives important information on macropores, such an analysis is not practical for accurate measurements, because serious condensation on the apparatus walls begins near the saturated vapor pressure.

(a) *Mesopore Analysis.* Capillary condensation of the adsorbate molecules into the adsorbant pores is the key mechanism of adsorption in mesopores. In this case, the molecules adsorbed on a solid surface behave as being in the liquid state. This is true for all adsorption layers except the first ones (strictly the first one within the frame of the BET model). Thus, the interface between the gas and the already adsorbed molecules is a vapor–liquid equilibrium. This equilibrium is determined by the surface curvature which, when referring to a porous material, depends mainly on the geometry and size of the pores. This dependency is accounted for by the Kelvin equation.

$$\ln\left(\frac{p}{p_0}\right) = \left(-\frac{\gamma_l}{RT}\right)\cos\theta\left(\frac{1}{r_{k1}} + \frac{1}{r_{k2}}\right) \tag{30}$$

where γ is the surface tension, v_l is the molar volume of the liquid, θ is the contact angle of the liquid on the solar surface, and r_{k1} and r_{k2} are the Kelvin principal radii which are related with the principal curvature radii of the interface [19], according to $r_{ki} = R_{di}\cos\theta$ (see Fig. 5).

The Kelvin equation can easily be deduced from thermodynamic considerations along with the Young–Laplace equation. Given that a vapor–liquid equilibrium exists in capillar condensation, both their chemical potentials should be equal: $\mu_l = \mu_v$. Moreover, by taking into account the Gibbs–Duhem equation for each phase

$$s_l\,dT - v_l\,dp_l + d\mu_l = 0$$
$$s_v\,dT - v_v\,dp_v + d\mu_v = 0 \tag{31}$$

where s and v are the molar entropy and volume. Thus, at constant temperature

$$v_l\,dp_l = v_v\,dp_v \tag{32}$$

or

$$dp_l = \frac{v_v}{v_l}\,dp_v \tag{33}$$

But according to the Young–Laplace equation

$$p_v - p_l = \gamma\left(\frac{1}{r_{k2}} + \frac{1}{r_{k1}}\right)\cos\theta \tag{34}$$

and after derivation and substitution we have

$$d\left[\gamma\left(\frac{1}{r_{k2}} + \frac{1}{r_{k1}}\right)\cos\theta\right] = \frac{v_l - v_v}{v_l}\,dp_v \tag{35}$$

It can be assumed that $v_l - v_v \approx -v_v$ and that the gas behaves ideally

$$d\left[\gamma\left(\frac{1}{r_{k2}} + \frac{1}{r_{k1}}\right)\cos\theta\right] = -\frac{RT}{v_l}\,d(\ln p_v) \tag{36}$$

which after integration leads to the Kelvin equation.

The Kelvin equation can be simplified if the pores are supposed to be open capillaries and the liquid perfectly wets the solid ($\cos \theta = 1$)

$$\ln\left(\frac{p}{p_0}\right) = \left(-\frac{a\gamma v_1}{RT r_k}\right) \tag{37}$$

were $a = 2$ for the desorption process given that $r_{k1} = r_{k2} \equiv r_k$ while $a = 1$ for the adsorption process as far as $r_{k1} \equiv r_k$ and $r_{k2} = \infty$. See Fig. 13 for details, where it can also see that r_k (which is called Kelvin radius) is the pore radius, r_p, minus the thickness of the adsorbed layer, t, that appears before condensation and remains after vaporization; i.e.

$$r_p = r_k + t \tag{38}$$

The appropriate evaluation of this thickness t is a critical point to correctly relate relative pressures to pore sizes as far as, rigorously speaking, it should be measured for a totally flat surface of the same material. This is frequently impracticable, thus what is usually done is to apply a phenomenological correlation as did Halsey [78]. His correlation is based on a high number of measurements on flat materials to give t in angstroms as

$$t = 0.354\left[\frac{5}{\ln\left(\dfrac{p_0}{p}\right)}\right]^{(1/3)} \tag{39}$$

Once p_r data are converted to the corresponding values of r_p, the differential distribution of specific volume of the pores with r_p radius, dV_p/dr_p, can be obtained by the method of Dollimore and Heal assuming cylindrical pores [19,20]. This can be done both for adsorption and desorption results. Never-

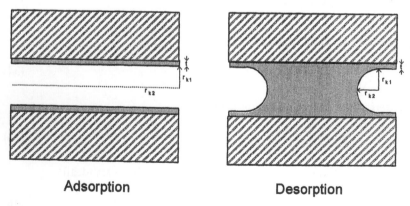

Adsorption   Desorption

FIG. 13 Sketch of the adsorption and desorption processes.

theless, it should be noted that the adsorption isotherm can only be used if the total specific area of the sample is known. We may use that obtained from the BET method. An example of the volume differential distribution obtained from both adsorption and desorption is shown in Fig. 14 for membrane N0015 (Nuclepore membrane of a nominal pore size of 15 nm).

The differential distribution of specific surface area, dS_p/dr_p, can be easily calculated given that

$$S_p = \frac{2V_p}{r_p} \tag{40}$$

Finally, if we know the pore length (that can be taken as equal to the membrane thickness for membranes with mean pore bending angle close to zero), the pore number differential distribution can be obtained by taking into account that for each pore radius

$$N(r_p) = \frac{V_p}{\pi r_p^2 \Delta x} \tag{41}$$

The corresponding number distribution for membrane N0015 is shown in Fig. 15.

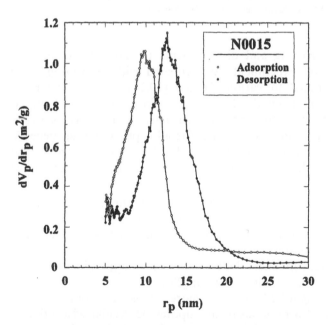

FIG. 14 Differential distribution for the volume per mass unit of the sample obtained from both N_2 adsorption and desorption runs for membrane N0015. The mesopores method has been used.

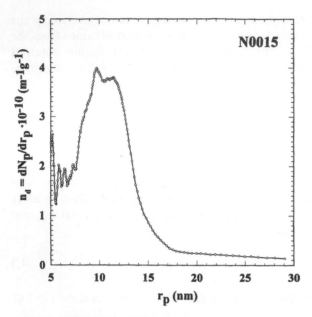

FIG. 15 Differential distribution for the number of pores obtained from N_2 desorption for membrane N0015. The mesopores method has been used.

Slight distribution widening and displacements to the right are usually obtained from adsorption experiments as compared with desorption ones; which have been attributed to various factors [19,28], such as the pore-network effect or a tensile strength phenomenon. However, for track-etched membranes, a left shift was observed and attributed to the existence of a portion of dead end pores [36]. In any case, the adsorption analysis depends on the BET area and a great dependency on the chosen lower edge for the pore size analysis can be shown. This makes adsorption analysis uncertain for practical purposes.

(b) *Micropore Analysis.* In the microporous range, the Kelvin equation loses its validity. Several approximations for adsorption isotherm analysis in the micropores range have been used. The simplest ones are based on reformulations of the Kelvin equation to take into account the thickness of the adsorbed layer in different manners. Nevertheless, these approximations lead to inconsistent results mainly at low pore radii [28].

Further refinements might be based on a more sophisticated description of the thermodynamics of adsorption inside micropores. Molecular adsorption in micropores can be well described by the Dubinin–Radushkevich equation [79], with the assumption of a Gaussian distribution for the pores. Also a calculation of the potential functions of Lennard–Jones, using the Horváth–

Kawazoe method [80], should lead to an evaluation of the pore size distribution corresponding to micropores.

Both analysis methods give reasonable accuracy but they need considerable mathematical calculations and previous knowledge about the details of the adsorbent–adsorbate interaction. Moreover, the results should be considered with some caution and the distributions obtained should only be considered as effective ones. Here we will consider a calculation method for micropore analysis, that gives reasonably good result for microporous membranes. The model, called micropores method (or MP-method) by the authors [81] is based on the De Boer t-plot. De Boer and coworkers developed a method suitable for analysis of micropores structure, by plotting the adsorption isotherm in terms of the statistical adsorbate film thickness instead of the reduced pressure [82].

Mikhail and coworkers considered that the t-plot starts to deviate from the initial slope (which should give the total BET surface area) due to the presence of micropores. Then, the subsequent slopes can be converted into microporous surface areas or the equivalent micropore volumes corresponding to each increment in the abscissa (Δt).

So, the volume of the micropores comprised between two adjacent values of the adsorbate thickness (t_i and t_{i+1}) can be evaluated from the slopes (S_i and S_{i+1}) of the t-plot corresponding to these thicknesses, as follows

$$V_i = (S_i - S_{i+1})\left(\frac{t_i + t_{i+1}}{2}\right) \tag{42}$$

Here t_i is identified with the pore radius given that the micropores adsorption is based on a pore filling mechanism.

As with the mesopores analysis, a major point in having reasonable results is the use of an adequate t-plot for the given adsorbate. In this case, values of t can be evaluated from an empirical relation given by Harkin and Jura

$$t = \left[\frac{13.99}{0.034 + \ln\left(\frac{p_0}{p}\right)}\right]^{(1/2)} \tag{43}$$

which gives better results in the analysis of micropores than that of Halsey [83]. The adequacy of the Harkin and Jura correlation is confirmed by noting the fair agreement of the surface as obtained from the initial slope of the so obtained t-plot and the independently calculated BET one.

Finally, the pore volume distributions may be calculated. However, it is worth noting that slope calculation imprecisions may even lead to negative volumes. This is why signal should be conveniently filtered and smoothed prior to the calculation of the pore size distribution. Absolute distributions of number of pores are not obtained because of the difficulty in assessing a determinate pore geometry to micropores.

As an example, Fig. 16 shows the results obtained for the H-30k. The differential pore volume distributions can be fitted to a log-normal distributions as usually found for ultrafiltration membranes; i.e.

$$f(x) = f_{max}(\mu)\exp\left\{-\left[\frac{\log\left(\dfrac{x}{\mu}\right)}{\log\sigma}\right]^2\right\} \tag{44}$$

where μ is the mean x and σ its standard deviation. Here r_p plays the role of the x variable, leading to fitted means and standard deviations with confidence levels over 99.5%. The values of μ and σ thus obtained for the volume distributions are shown in the figure along with the pore volume distribution in the microporous range.

B. Permporometry

Permporometry is a technique based on the principles of the capillary condensation of a vapor inside the membrane pores and the permeability of another noncondensable gas through these pores. As we saw above, capillary conden-

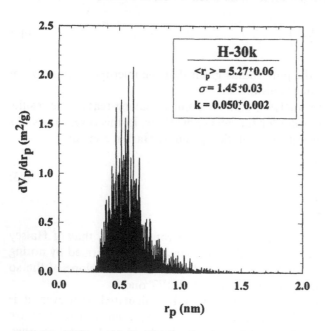

FIG. 16 Differential distribution for the volume per mass unit of the sample obtained from N_2 adsorption for membrane H-30k. The micropores method has been used.

sation is a process which can be modeled with Kelvin equation, in such a way that a control of the relative vapor pressure of the condensable gas allows to determine the size of the pores open to flow of the noncondensable gas.

If flux measurements are started when the relative vapor pressure of the condensable gas equals to one, all the pores in the membrane should be closed (i.e., filled with condensed liquid), avoiding any diffusive flux of the noncondensable gas through the membrane. When relative vapor pressure is slightly below 1 the liquid contained in the biggest pores start to vaporize opening these pores. Kelvin equation allows to correlate pressure with the size of the pores already opened to flux (Kelvin radius, r_k). The measured flow of the noncondensable gas can be easily translated in terms of pore number once the appropriate gas transport model is taken into account. By decreasing steadily the relative pressure until all the pores are already open, both the differential and integral pore size distributions can be obtained.

In this kind of determinations, as occurs in the case of the mesopores analysis through adsorption–desorption measurements, it must be taken into account that the size available to flux is not the real size of the pore. So it is necessary to add the thickness of the adsorbate layer, t, which is a function of pressure, as shown above. A good approximation to determine t is again the Halsey correlation.

Once a geometric model for the pore and a model for the gas transport through the pores are supposed, this method (as the liquid displacement technique) allows to determine the absolute distribution (differential or integral) of number of pores active to flux for the membrane. The model to be used should depend on the working conditions (type of gas, temperature, pore sizes, etc.). However, in most of the experiments where this technique was used, a diffusive Knudsen model seems to be adequate.

Cuperus [25], uses counterdiffusion of two gases (N_2 and O_2) that at operative conditions of pressure and temperature are inert and nonadsorbent and water vapor (or some organic vapors) plays the role of the adsorbate. In any case no pressure gradient is established across the membrane. Thus, the driving force for the mass transport is the concentration difference of both noncondensable gases between both sides of the membrane. Then, by measuring the concentration of one gas (the ith one) at one side of the membrane (with, for example, a selective electrode), we can determine the flux of such a gas, which can be calculated as follows

$$J_{k,i} = \frac{\pi N_T r_p^2 D_{k,i} \Delta p_i}{RT \psi \Delta x} \tag{45}$$

being $J_{k,i}$ the diffusional flux, $D_{k,i}$ the Knudsen diffusion coeficient, r_p the pore radius, Δx the membrane thickness, N_T the number of pores per surface unit, Δp_i the gradient of partial pressure and ψ the tortuosity. The diffusion coeficient can be calculated as

$$D_{k,i} = 0.66 r_p \left(\frac{8RT}{\pi M_{w,i}} \right)^{1/2}$$ (46)

being $M_{w,i}$ the molecular weight for the diffusing gas. These measurements should be done for different overall pressures; i.e., for different relative pressures of the condensable gas.

Since this technique is based on the Kelvin equation, it is applicable only to mesopores, whose strict limits are conditioned by the gas and working pressure. However, these limits can be considered, as previously commented, as ranging from 2 to 50 nm.

The method has been used and compared with other ultrafiltration membranes characterization methods, with very good results [21,25,84,85]. As an example we can compare results obtained by Cuperus, for the N0015 membrane. He obtained a value of about 10 nm from permporometric methods. This gives very good accordance with the mean value of 10–11.4 nm obtained by the present authors from adsorption–desorption data. Evidently the accordance shown in this case is related to the fact that the membrane can be considered as having cylindrically shaped pores, with a very narrow distribution and almost no tortuosity.

V. TECHNIQUES BASED ON CAPILLARY SOLIDIFICATION: THERMOPOROMETRY

This method is based on the dependence of the melting or solidification point of a substance with its surface curvature. Thus, when a fluid is introduced inside a porous material, since the pores change the surface curvature of the fluid, the determination of the resulting distribution of melting or solidification temperatures, can give us information about the size distribution present in the analyzed sample. As a first approximation, pore size can be related with freezing and melting temperatures empirically; such a phenomenological correlation should be obtained by using well known porous substances as test substances. However, it is also possible to obtain equations based on equilibrium thermodynamics, relating those parameters.

When a liquid totally saturates a porous material and it reaches an equilibrium with the solid phase, the thermodynamics of phase equilibria (based on Laplace and Gibbs–Duhem equations) shows that the solid–liquid interface curvature (determined by the pore size) can be related with the temperature of phase change [86]

$$T = T_0 - \int_T^{T_0} \frac{v_l}{\Delta s_F} d(\gamma_{sl} C_{sl})$$ (47)

being T the temperature for the phase change at a given curvature radius, T_0 is this temperature for a flat surface, v_l is the molar volume of the liquid, Δs_F is the molar entropy change, γ_{sl} is the surface tension at the solid–liquid interface and C_{sl} is the interfacial curvature. This curvature parameter is given by

$$C_{sl} = \frac{a}{r_p - t} \tag{48}$$

where $(r_p - t)$ is the radius of curvature of the solid–liquid interface, with r_p the geometrical radius of the pore and t being the thickness of the condensation layer on the wall that doesnot change its state of aggregation. The parameter a is 2 for an approximately spherical surface (for both melting and solidification), while for a cylindrical pore $a = 1$ when melting and $a = 2$ for solidification. These differences are due to the way solidification and melting take place. Solidification can proceed by either a classical mechanism of nucleation or a progressive penetration of the liquid–solid meniscus formed previously at the inlet of the pores. Melting, on the other hand, proceeds always from the center of the pores as shown in Fig. 17.

According to both these equations the decrease in phase equilibrium temperature, $\Delta T = T - T_0$, can be related with pore radius. It is worth mentioning that differences in melting and solidification processes appear in the same way as in the adsorption–desorption processes. Brun et al. [87] found that for water these relationships are

$$r_p(\text{nm}) = -\frac{64.67}{\Delta T} + 0.57 \quad \text{(solidification)}$$

$$r_p(\text{nm}) = -\frac{32.33}{\Delta T} + 0.68 \quad \text{(melting)} \tag{49}$$

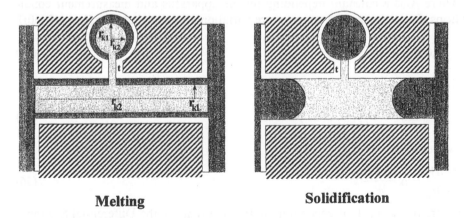

Melting   **Solidification**

FIG. 17 Sketch of the melting and solidification processes. Note that cylindrical pores melt and solidify differently. □, liquid, ■, solid.

with a ΔT from 0 to -40 K and assuming $t = 0.8$ nm. For benzene, [87]

$$r_p(nm) = -\frac{131.6}{\Delta T} + 0.54 \quad \text{(solidification)}$$

$$r_p(nm) = -\frac{65.8}{\Delta T} + 0.92 \quad \text{(melting)} \tag{50}$$

with ΔT ranging from 0 to -60 K, assuming $t = 1.33$ nm. Water should be used for hydrophilic materials while benzene should be preferred for hydrophobous membranes.

The latent heat of phase change depends on the decrease of phase equilibrium temperature along with γ_{sl} and the pore wall curvature, leading to apparent energies of phase change given in J/g^{-1} as [87]

$$W_a = -5.56 \times 10^{-2} \Delta T^2 - 7.43 \Delta T - 332 \quad \text{(solidification)}$$
$$W_a = -0.155 \times 10^{-2} \Delta T^2 - 11.39 \Delta T - 332 \quad \text{(melting)} \tag{51}$$

for water, and

$$W_a = -8.87 \times 10^{-3} \Delta T^2 - 1.76 \Delta T - 127 \quad \text{(solidification)}$$
$$W_a = -2.73 \times 10^{-2} \Delta T^2 - 2.94 \Delta T \quad \text{(melting)} \tag{52}$$

for benzene.

To change the temperature of a given porous material–soaking liquid system in ΔT we spend a power y. Then the differential volume of liquid changing its phase when temperature changes in $d(\Delta T)$ is

$$dV = \Lambda' \frac{y}{W_a} d(\Delta T) \tag{53}$$

where Λ' is a constant depending on the apparatus and measurement conditions. But pore size and temperature variation are related as [see Eqs. (49–50)]

$$r_p(nm) = -\frac{A}{\Delta T} + B \tag{54}$$

the differential of which is

$$dr_p(nm) = -\frac{A}{(\Delta T)^2} d(\Delta T) \tag{55}$$

We arrive at

$$\frac{dV}{dr_p} = \Lambda \frac{(\Delta T)^2}{W_a} y \tag{56}$$

where Λ is a constant depending on the sensitivity of the Differential Scanning Calorimeter (DSC) used along with the speed of temperature variation, the mass of the sample, the density of the liquid and the constant A.

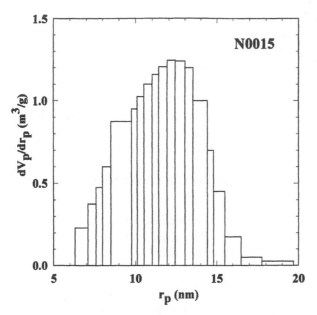

FIG. 18 Differential distribution for the volume per mass unit of the sample for N0015 membrane obtained by water thermoporometry. Data adapted from [91].

It is worth noting that the cooling or melting speed must be low enough ($\sim$1–6 K/h) for the three phases to remain in constant equilibrium and the temperature to be the same throughout the sample.

This method has been used to characterize porous materials and specifically ultrafiltration membranes, giving good results for pore size distributions in the range of 2–30 nm [84,88–90]. As an example, results of Quinson et al. [91], for N0015 membrane have been reelaborated in Fig. 18. The results are comparable to those, already mentioned, of Cuperus [25] and the present authors [36].

VI. TECHNIQUES BASED ON FUNCTIONAL PERFORMANCE: SOLUTE RETENTION TEST

The methods based on solute retention are extraordinarily interesting from the application point of view, as far as the factors to be considered to translate actual geometrical or structural characteristics into solute retention performances are especially complex (friction, elasticity, electrical or chemical interaction, hydrophilicity or hydrophobicity, diffusion into the solid matrix, etc.). A first approximation should consider sieve factors as the only or the most relevant phenomena by avoiding to consider friction or elasticity (mechanically or chemically determined) appearing in the hydrodynamical interaction of solute molecules and membrane material. In any case this is equivalent to consider an equivalent pore size including such factors. In this way, if a polydisperse solution is filtered through a membrane and its molecular weight and/or size distributions are analyzed up and downstream, an equivalent pore size distribution should be determined by sieving effects. On the other hand, the correlation of molecular weight and sizes depends on both the solute–solute and solute–solvent interactions. These, say, colloidal properties make necessary to fix standard conditions of concentration, solvent type, pH, ionic strength, etc.

On the other hand the process of mass transfer on the membrane is determined by several factors:

1. Adsorption and fouling on the membrane surfaces during the process [92].
2. Formation of a concentration polarization layer due to solute accumulation on the high pressures side of the membrane with retrodiffusion and possible gel formation, [93].
3. Other limiting factors such as osmotic pressure may appear [94].

Among these factors the most difficult to quantify and thus to be taken into account are both adsorption and fouling. In order to approximate ourselves as much as possible to the actual structural characterization of the membrane, low interacting solutions should be used under conditions leading to low fouling levels. Nevertheless, since it is impossible in practice to avoid fouling absolutely, its influence on the porous structure should be evaluated. This can be accomplished by measuring the flow vs. time decay and the pure water permeability both before and after operation [95]. Appropriate models can then be used to take into account the modifications induced on the porous matrix. In order to have reproducible conditions we should place ourselves in conditions of stationary flux after fouling.

The concentration polarization layer can be analyzed by using several different models but none of them gives good results, neither for all membranes (reverse osmosis, nanofiltration, ultrafiltration or microfiltration ones) nor under all hydrodynamic conditions on the retentate surface. Nevertheless the so called film model gives good results in spite of its simplicity for membranes in the reverse osmosis to ultrafiltration ranges [96]. Some precautions should be followed as well to ensure its applicability, namely: mass transfer through the membrane system is limited by the concentration polarization layer more than by the whole membrane; cross flow (tangential flow) filtration devices should be used; and the retentate should be recirculated onto the membrane at a high speed.

As a consequence of all these factors, the solute should be chosen to have low concentrations and to be accessible at a broad molecular weight range without significant changes in their physico-chemical properties.

In order to study nano- and ultrafiltration membranes some linear polymers could be chosen as polyethylene glycols or dextranes. Nevertheless their linearity makes difficult to assign a clearly defined size, what is not the case with globular macromolecules as proteins for instance. In the case of microfiltration membranes: latex, silica, alumina particles, etc. could be used.

A. Film Model

As mentioned, due to accumulation of the solute on the membrane, a concentration polarization layer appears that can be studied under simple conditions within the frame of the film model which can be outlined as follows.

The output or permeate concentration, c_p, can be given in terms of the feed concentration, c_0, through the so called observed or apparent retention coefficient

$$R_0 = 1 - \frac{c_p}{c_0} \tag{57}$$

This retention coefficient is a function of pressure, recirculation speed and molecular weight [97].

Actually, there is a concentration $c_m(>c_0)$ in contact with the membrane due to the accumulation resulting from the balance of convection through the membrane and back diffusion (concentration–polarization). Then a true retention coefficient can be defined as

$$R = 1 - \frac{c_p}{c_m} \tag{58}$$

which relates the actual concentrations on both faces of the membrane.

In the film model, a zone is assumed where the concentration decreases from c_m on the membrane to c_0 at a distance δ inside the retentate phase. This hypothesis leads to a permeate volume flow per unit of exposed area of the membrane, J_V, given by [98],

$$J_V = K_m \ln \frac{c_m - c_p}{c_0 - c_p} \tag{59}$$

where $K_m = D/\delta$ is the so-called mass transfer coefficient and D is the diffusion coefficient.

In order to evaluate the mass transfer coefficient without using highly concentrated solutions, whose high viscosities and very important solute–solute interactions and formation of aggregates should be inconvenient, we can rearrange Eq. (59) by taking into account Eq. (58), to

$$\ln \frac{1 - R_0}{R_0} = \ln \frac{1 - R}{R} + \frac{J_V}{K_m} \tag{60}$$

According to the traditional film model, when there is almost gelation on the retentate face of the membrane, c_m increases very slowly and the volume flow is approximately independent of Δp. Then the transport through the membrane can be assumed to be mainly convective, leading to a virtually constant ratio c_p/c_m and a maximum true retention coefficient, R_{max}. Thus the first term of the right-hand side of Eq. (60) can be taken as constant and a plot of $\ln[(1 - R_0)/R_0]$ against J_V would be a straight with $1/K_m$ as slope, and R_{max} can be obtained from the ordinate intercept.

On the other hand, the mass transfer coefficient can be calculated on the basis of heat transfer analogies by some kind of combination of the dimensionless Sherwood, Reynolds and Schmidt numbers [99]

$$Sh = A(Re)^\alpha (Sc)^\beta \tag{61}$$

where $Sh = K_m \, d_h/D$, $Re = v\rho \, d_h/\eta$ and $Sc = \eta/(D\rho)$; d_h being of diameter of the hydraulic channel, ρ is the solution density, η the solution viscosity and v is the mean recirculation velocity. The constants A, α and β depend on the flow regime and channel geometry. In any case, equation (61) implies

$$K_m = \Phi v^\alpha \tag{62}$$

where Φ depends on the solute diffusivity and the channel dimensions.

Then Eq. (60) can be written as

$$\ln \frac{1 - R_0}{R_0} = \ln \frac{1 - R}{R} + \frac{J_V}{\Phi v^\alpha} \tag{63}$$

Thus, the slope of a representation of $\ln[(1 - R_0)/R_0]$ against J_V/V^α would be $1/\Phi$ and the ordiate intercept would give R_{max}. Once Φ is known, R can be calculated for any condition.

Several values have been proposed for the coefficients A, α and β. These exponents [100,101] seem to depend on the flow regime in such a way that values of $\alpha = 1/3$ or $1/2$ can be used for the laminar regime and $\alpha = 0.8$ in the case of turbulence.

B. Pore Size Distributions

In order to evaluate the pore size distributions of a partially retaining membrane, it can be assumed that the retention is due to a sieving mechanism, in such a way that for each molecular weight there is a fraction of totally retaining pores while the rest of them allow a free pass of the molecules [102]. Then we can write the mass balance for each molecular weight as

$$J_V c_p = J_{V,t} c_m \tag{64}$$

where $J_{V,t}$ is the volume flow transmitted through the nonrejection fraction of pores. On the other hand the ratio of the transmitted volume and water ($J_{w,t}$)

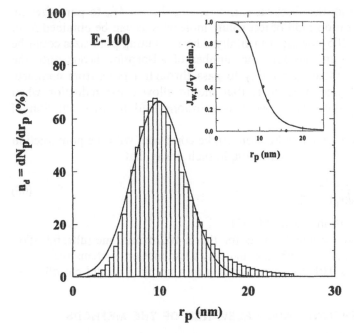

FIG. 19 Differential distribution for the number of pores obtained by solute retention of several proteins for E-100 membrane. The $J_{w,t}/J_V$ ratios are also shown.

fluxes is

$$\frac{J_{V,t}}{J_{w,t}} = \frac{\eta(c_m)}{\eta(0)} \tag{65}$$

being $\eta(c_m)$ and $\eta(0)$ the solution and solvent viscosities. But for low c_m this ratio can be approximated by 1 in such a way that according to Eq. (58), (64) and (65) we have, [24]

$$\left.\begin{array}{l} J_{w,t} = J_V(1 - R) \\ J_{w,r} = J_V R \end{array}\right\} \tag{66}$$

Therefore $J_{w,t}$ and $J_{w,r}$ (retented) can be evaluated once J_V for each R is known. Then, by using again the mass balance

$$\left.\begin{array}{l} J_V c_p = J_s \\ J_V - J_s = J_w \end{array}\right\} \tag{67}$$

J_w can be obtained. Thus, $J_{w,t}/J_w$ vs. the molecular weight gives the accumulated fraction of flow passing through the nonrejecting pores. The derivative of this function should thus provide the flux carrying molecules of a given molecular weight.

On the other hand, the abscissas can be changed from M_w to pore sizes by considering the gyration radii of test solute molecules as can be obtained from literature, [23,103–105], or experimentally. These resulting pore sizes could be modified by taking into account the number of adsorption layers onto the pore walls and the molecular ability to pass through a pore, from complete rigidity to some degree of elasticity that should allow a size reduction when crossing the membrane. Thus, these assumptions lead to an evaluation of $d(J_{w,t}/J_w)/d(r_p)$.

Finally, the differential flow fraction can be correlated with the pore fraction through the Hagen–Poiseuille equation, in such a way that

$$\frac{d(N_p/N_T)}{d(r_p)} = \frac{d(J_{w,t}/J_w)}{d(r_p)} \frac{K}{r_p^4} \tag{68}$$

K being a normalization constant [106].

In Fig. 19 the so obtained results for the E-100 membrane (ultrafiltration asymmetric polysulfonic membrane made by Desalination Systems Inc. whose nominal pore size is 0.01 μm corresponding to a nominal weight cut off of 35 kDa) are shown.

VII. COMPLEMENTARITY AND RELEVANCE OF THE METHODS

When dealing with porous membranes, porosity or pore size distribution analysis is a key factor in all operative characterization of permeation and selectivity. However, this characterization of the structure of porous materials can be achieved, as shown above, by using several different and independent methods. Some of these techniques elucidate the aspects of the structure of the membrane that influence permeation (open pores, etc.) while others refer to purely structural characteristics. Among them some yield information only or mainly about surface structures while others focus on the bulk organization of the porous material. A classification, along these lines, of the techniques outlined here are shown in Table 1.

The techniques related with permeation parameters (liquid displacement methods, solute retention test, permporometry, etc.) allow for the determination of the pore size distributions for the pores open to flux, obtaining a

TABLE 1 Character of the Methods Exposed

	Structure	Permeation
Bulk	Adsorption–desorption	
	Hg-porosimetry	Gas–liquid displacement
	Thermoporometry	Liquid–liquid displacement
Surface	Electronic microscopy	Permporometry
	AFM	Solute retention

pore radius value close to that of the lowest cross-section present along the whole pore. These techniques are useful to characterize the thin layer in asymmetric membranes but they don't give any insight into the remaining membrane structure.

On the other hand, the morphology related techniques (electron microscopy, atomic force microscopy, mercury porosimetry, gas adsorption–desorption, thermoporometry, etc.) give a complete information of the porous structure. Nevertheless, in the case of thermoporometry, gas adsorption and mercury intrusion techniques, it is necessary to suppose a structural model for the pores, and the interpretation of the obtained results is quite complex, especially in the case of asymmetric membranes. In contrast, the microscopical techniques, using surface and cross-sectional images, allow to obtain a complete knowledge of the actual membrane structure. Since the cross-sectional imaging of membrane filters presents considerable difficulties (for example, the risk of distorting the pore structure in the cutting process), only surface studies are commonly used (see, however, chap. 1, Sec. III.D).

It is worth noting that for most of the membranes actually in use, the features revealed by permeation methods are determined by the surface structure more than by the bulk one. In fact when permeation is mainly determined by narrow pores, the membrane should be as thin as possible. This along with mechanical requirements makes necessary to work with asymmetrical or composite membranes including a thin active layer that mainly determines the flow and retention. This active layer layer should be placed on the top of the membrane to avoid internal fouling. In contrast, microfiltration membranes are usually symmetrical.

All techniques are useful, as far as structure elucidating techniques both focusing on surface and bulk can be compared with the permeation ones. This comparison can give an indication of the thickness of the retentive layer (sometimes it can include part of the a priori support or porous layer). On the other hand, internal adsorption appears frequently and thus it is useful to know where it takes place. The divergences between actual and effective pore size distribution should be explained, as already mentioned, by taking into account all solute–solute and solute–membrane interactions along the flow path.

On the other hand, all techniques may be used with new or used membranes, or with membranes cleaned according to different procedures. This helps to establish where and how adsorption and/or fouling takes place under different operative conditions [95,107].

Thus, discerning which characterization technique is the most useful for a complete knowledge of microporous membranes is counter productive; as far as they are complementary rather than competitive.

Of course, when dealing with asymmetrical or composite membranes, or even other types of membranes which are not very regular, differences are sometimes high, especially between bulk and surface characterizing methods. However, very regular membranes, as for example filters that can be assumed to consist in a parallel bunch of cylindrical capillaries perpendicular to the membrane surface, give an almost exact accordance for all methods. In Fig. 20 the mean pore size is shown against the nominal pore sizes of several track-etched membranes. These membranes are known to have pores whose shape is actually very close to cylindrical with a tortuosity factor very close to one. A regression of all results is also shown which reproduces fairly the nominal pore sizes. The small dispersion of results coming from different techniques is also shown as far as all data are within the 95% confidence interval. Even for these highly regular membranes that in fact cannot be perfectly symmetric, small differences between permeation and surface methods applied to both sides of the membrane can be used to deduce the thickness of the actual active layer [40].

A correct characterization of the structure of membranes is also needed in order to deduce electrical properties of membrane materials (surface charge density, zeta potential, etc.). This can be shown for electrokinetic phenomena, for example.

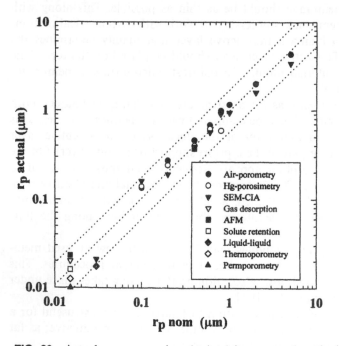

FIG. 20 Actual mean pore size obtained from several methods vs. the nominal ones. Only results for polycarbonate track-etched membranes with pore diameters ranging from 15 nm to 5000 nm are shown.

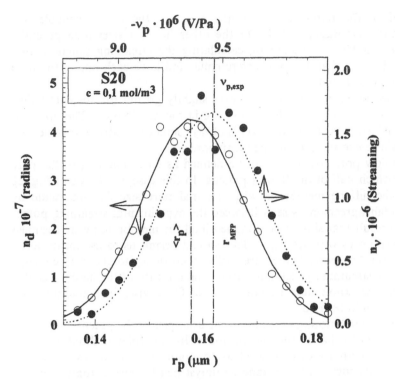

FIG. 21 Pore size distribution compared to the corresponding streaming potential distribution for S20 and a NaCl concentration of 0.1 mol/m³.

It is known that when an electrolytic solution is pushed through the membrane some socalled electrokinetic effects appear. All of them can be analyzed in terms of the fine capillary method, which needs to assume, in its first formulations, pores of equal radii to solve numerically the transport equations (Nernst–Planck, Navier–Stokes, Poisson, and charge and mass conservation) with the adequate boundary conditions. Such models are used to obtain the electrokinetic coefficients for an assumed pore charge. But, when one of them is measured, the streaming potential for instance, the surface charge density can be fitted to get the experimental result for each concentration. Thus, the adsorption isotherm or adsorbed surface charge density vs. concentration can be obtained [108–110], and extrapolated to get the actual surface charge density of the membrane material.

In fact this can be done by using a measured pore size distribution. The results so obtained are seen to deviate only slightly from those that should be obtained if all the pores were assumed equal to the most probable one (homoporous membrane), [111]. On the other hand, a streaming potential distribution can be constructed by calculating the streaming potential that should be obtained if all the pores were equal and have each one of the pore sizes in the real distribution.

Actual streaming potentials are always slightly greater (in absolute value) than those corresponding to the mean pore in the distribution. The obtained zeta potential (surface charge density) is always smaller (in absolute value too) than the value corresponding to the mean pore size.

A mean flow pore size, r_{MFP}, can be defined as corresponding to the pore size below which half of the flow is passing. In this case, as shown in Fig. 21 (S20 polyethersulfone membrane with nominal pore size 0.2 μm, made by Gelman), a fair agreement is seen between the experimental streaming potential and the result that should be obtained if all the membranes were assumed to have equal pores with size r_{MFP}. This should permit us to use mean pores, or better mean flow pores (which are easily measurable), to get surface charge densities from streaming potentials without taking care of the actual size distribution once we know they are not too wide. Otherwise, the actual pore size distribution should be used.

Finally it is worth noting that only some examples of the potential utility of the methods studied have been shown above. In particular it should be clear that all these methods can be applied to nonmembrane or even nonfilm porous materials such as, for instance, catalyst pellets, chromatographic supports, mineral samples, powders, etc.

REFERENCES

1. M. Mulder, *Basic Principles of Membrane Technology*, Kluwer, Dordrecht, The Netherlands, 1991.
2. W. S. W. Ho and K. K. Sirkar, *Membrane Handbook*, Van Nostrand Reinhold, New York, USA, 1992.
3. K. Kamide and S. Manabe, in *Ultrafiltration Membranes and Applications*, A. R. Cooper (ed.), Plenum Press, New York, NY, USA, 1980.
4. B. Rasneur, *Porosimetry (Characterization of Porous Membranes)*, Summer School on Membr. and Tech., Cadarache, France, 1984.
5. R. E. Kesting, *Synthetic Polymeric Membranes, A Structural Perspective*, 2nd. ed., John Wiley and Sons, New York, NY, USA, 1985.
6. S. Lowell and J. E. Shields, *Powder Surface Area and Porosity*, Powder Technology Series, B. Scarlett (ed.), J. Wiley and Sons Inc., New York, NY, USA, 1987.
7. S. S. Kulkarni, E. W. Funk and N. N. Li, in *Membrane Handbook*, W. S. W. Ho and K. K. Sirkar (eds), Van Nostrand Reinhold, New York, USA, 1992.
8. S. Nakao, J. Membr. Sci, 96: 131 (1994).

9. G. Binnig, C. F. Quate, and Ch. Gerber, Phys. Rev. Lett. *56*:930 (1986).
10. A. K.Fritzsche, A. R. Arevalo, M. D. Moore, C. J. Weber, V. B. Elings, K. Kjoller, and C. M. Wu, J. Membr. Sci. *68*:65 (1992).
11. P. Dietz, P. K. Hansma, O. Inacker, H. D. Lehmann, and K. H. Herrmann, J. Membr. Sci. *65*:101 (1992).
12. H. Bechhold, M. Schlesinger, K. Silbereisen, L. Maier, and W. Nurnberger, Kolloid, Z. *55*:172 (1931).
13. K. Schneider, W. Hölz, R. Wollbeck, and S. Ripperger, J. Membr. Sci. *39*:25 (1988).
14. G. Reichelt, J. Membr. Sci. *60*:253 (1991).
15. L. Zeman, J. Membr. Sci. *71*:233 (1992).
16. ASTM F316, *Standard Test Method for Pore Size Characteristics of Membrane Filters by Bubble Point and Mean Flow Pore Test.*
17. ASTM E1294, *Standard Test Methods for Pore Size Characteristics of Membrane Filters Using Automated Liquid Porosimeter.*
18. E. Honold and E. L. Skau, Science *120*:805 (1954).
19. S. J. Gregg and K. S. W. Sing, *Adsorption, Surface Area and Porosity*, Academic Press, London, UK, 1982.
20. D. Dollimore and G. R. Heal, J. Appl. Chem. *14*:109 (1964).
21. A. Mey-Marom and M. G. Katz, J. Membr. Sci. *27*:119 (1986).
22. M. Brun, A. Lallemand, J. F. Quinson, and C. Eyraud, J. Chim. Phys. *6*:973 (1973).
23. M. Sarbolouki, Sep. Sci. and Technol. *17*:381 (1982).
24. R. Nobrega, H. de Balmann, P. Aimar, and V. Sánchez, J. Membr. Sci. *45*:17 (1989).
25. F. P. Cuperus, *Characterization of Ultrafiltration Membranes*, Ph.D. Thesis, Twente, The Netherlands, 1990.
26. C. L. Glaves and D. M. Smith, J. Membr. Sci. *46*:167 (1989).
27. K. Sakai, J. Membr. Sci. *96*:91 (1994).
28. K. Kaneko, J. Membr. Sci. *96*:59 (1994).
29. C. P. Bean, M. V. Doyle, and G. Entine, J. Appl. Phys. *41*:1454 (1970).
30. R. L. Riley, J. O. Gardner, and U. Merten, Science *143*:801 (1964).
31. C. Riedel and R. Spohr, J. Membr. Sci. *7*:225 (1980).
32. T. Allen, *Particle Size Measurement*, Vol. 1, Chapman and Hall, London, 1997.
33. K. J. Kim, A. G. Fane, C. J. D. Fell, T. Suzuki, and M. R. Dickson, J. Membr. Sci. *54*:89 (1990).
34. J. I. Calvo, A. Hernández, G. Caruana, and L. Martínez, J. Colloid Interface Sci. *175*:138 (1995).
35. A. K. Fritzsche, A. R. Arevalo, M. D. Moore, V. B. Elings, K. Kjoller, and C. M. Wu, J. Membr. Sci. *68*:65 (1992).
36. P. Prádanos, M. L. Rodriguez, J. I. Calvo, A. Hernández, F. Tejerina, and J. A. de Saja, J. Membr. Sci. *117*:291 (1996).
37. J. I. Calvo, P. Prádanos, A. Hernández, W. R. Bowen, N. Hilal, R. W. Lovitt, and P. M. Williams, J. Member. Sci. *128*:7 (1997).
38. L. Zeman and L. Denault, J. Membr. Sci. *71*:221 (1992).
39. R. Swenson and J. R. Attle, Amer. Lab. *11*:50 (1979).

40. A. Hernández, J. I. Calvo, P. Prádanos, L. Palacio, M. L. Rodríguez, and J. A. de Saja, J, Membr. Sci. *137*: 89 (1997).

41. F. Martínez Villa, *Contribución a la Caracterización Morfológico-Estructural y Funcional de Membranas Poliméricas Microporosas. Estudio y Modelización de Flujos y Permeabilidades*, PhD Thesis, Valladolid, 1987.

42. A. Hernánez, J. I. Calvo, P. Prádanos, and F. Tejerina, Colloids and Surfaces A, *133*: 391 (1998).

43. T. Young, in *Miscellaneous Works*, (G. Peacock, ed.) J. Murray, London, 1855.

44. P. S. Laplace, *Mechanique Celeste*, Supplement to Book 10, 1806.

45. E. W. Washburn, Phys. Rev. *17*: 273 (1921).

46. M. Cantor, Ann. Phys. *47*: 399 (1892).

47. H. Bechhold, Z. Phys. Chem. *64*: 328 (1908).

48. F. Erbe, Kolloid Z. *59*: 195 (1932).

49. F. Erbe, Kolloid Z. *63*: 277 (1933).

50. P. Grabar and S. Niktine, J. Chim. Phys. *33*: 50 (1936).

51. H. Steinhauser, H. Scholz, A. Hübner, and C. Hellinghorst, in *Proc. ICOM'90*, Chicago, USA, 1990.

52. S. Pereira-Nunes and K. V. Peinemann, J. Membr. Sci. *77*: 25 (1992).

53. G. Capannelli, F. Vigo, and S. Munari, J. Membr. Sci. *15*: 289 (1983).

54. S. Munari, A. Bottino, P. Moretti, G. Capannelli, and I. Becchi, J. Membr. Sci. *41*: 69 (1989).

55. R. A. Wenman and B. V. Miller, in *Particle Size Analysis 1985* (P. J. Lloyd ed.), J. Wiley & Sons, NY, USA, 1987.

56. K. Venkataraman, W. T. Choate, E. R. Torre, R. D. Husung, and H. R. Batchu, J. Membr. Sci. *39*: 259 (1988).

57. H. Batchu, J. G. Harfield, and R. A. Wenman, *Fluid/particle Sep. J.*, *2*: 5 (1989).

58. *Coulter Porometer II, Reference Manual*, Coulter Electronics Ltd., Luton, UK, 1991.

59. R. F. Probstein, *Physicochemical Hydrodynamics: An Introduction*, Butterworth-Heinemann, Boston, USA, 1989.

60 R. D. Present, *Kinetic Theory of Gases*, McGraw-Hill, New York, USA, 1958.

61. S. Hwang and K. Kammermeyer, *Membranes in Separations*, R. Krieger, Malabar, USA, 1984.

62. R. W. Schofield, A. G. Fane, and C. J. D. Fell, J. Membr. Sci. *53*: 159 (1990).

63. K. K. Sirkar, in *Membrane Handbook* (W. S. W. Ho and K. K. Sirkar eds), Van Nostrand Reinhold, New York, USA, 1992.

64. H. Kreulen, G. F. Versteeg, C. A. Smolders, and W. P. M. van Swaaij, in *Proc. ICOM'90*, Chicago, USA, 1990.

65. A. Hernández, J. I. Calvo, P. Prádanos, and F. Tejerina, J. Membr. Sci. *112*: 1 (1996).

66. G. Capanelli, I. Becchi, A. Bottino, P. Moretti, and S. Munari, in *Characterization of Porous Solids* (K. K. Unger, J. Rouquesol, K. S. W. Sing and K. Kral eds), Elsevier, Amsterdam, The Netherlands, 1988.

67. A. A. Liabastre and C. Orr, J. Colloid Interface Sci. *64*: 1 (1978).

68. E. Honold and E. L. Skau, Science *120*: 805 (1954).

69. H. M. Rootare and C. F. Prenzlow, J. Phys. Chem. *71*: 2733 (1967).

70. G. P. Andreoutsopoulos and R. Mann, Chem. Eng. Sci. *34*: 1203 (1979).
71. S. Lowell and J. E. Shields, J. Colloid Interface Sci. *83*: 273 (1981).
72. T. Allen, *Particle Size Measurement*, Vol. 2, Chapman and Hall, London, 1997.
73. H. M. Rootare, Aminco Laboratory News 24, No. 3. Fall, 1968.
74. J. I. Calvo, A. Hernández, P. Prádanos, L. Martínez, and R. Bowen, J. Colloid Interface Sci. *176*: 476 (1995).
75. A. W. Adamson, *Physical Chemistry of Surfaces*, 4th. ed., Wiley-Interscience, New York, USA, 1982.
76. I. Langmuir, J. Am. Chem. Soc. *40*: 1368 (1918).
77. S. Brunauer, P. H. Emmett, and E. Teller, J. Am. Chem. Soc. *60*: 309 (1938).
78. J. Seifert and G. Emig, Chem. Eng. Tech. *59*: 475 (1987).
79. M. M. Dubinin, Carbon *27*: 457 (1989).
80. G. Horváth and K. Kawazoe, J. Chem. Eng. Jpn. *16*: 470 (1983).
81. R. Sh. Mikhail, S. Brunauer, and E. E. Bodor, J. Colloid Interface Sci. *26*: 45 (1968).
82. B. C. Lippen and H. H. de Boer, J. Catal. *4*: 319 (1965).
83. Coulter Electronics Ltd., *Omnisorp 100/360 Series Manual*, USA, 1991.
84. Ch. Eyraud, M. Bontemps, J. F. Quinson, F. Chatelut, M. Brun, and B. Rasneur, Bull. Soc. Chim. France *9–10*: I-237 (1984).
85. M. Katz and G. Baruch, Desalination *58*: 199 (1986).
86. M. Brun, A. Lallemand, J. F. Quinson, and Ch. Eyraud, J. Chim. Phys. *6*: 973 (1973).
87. M. Brun, A. Lallemand, J. F. Quinson, and Ch. Eyraud, Thermochim. Acta *21*: 59 (1977).
88. F. P. Cuperus, D. Bargeman, and C. A. Smolders, J. Membr. Sci. *66*: 45 (1992).
89. C. A. Smolders and E. Vugteveen, Polym. Mater. Sci. Eng. *50*: 177 (1984).
90. A. P. Broek, H. A. Tennis, D. Bergeman, E. D. Sprengers, and C. A. Smolders, J. Membr. Sci. *73*: 143 (1992).
91. J. F. Quinson, N. Maneri, L. Guihard, and B. Bariou, J. Membr. Sci. *58*: 191 (1991).
92. E. Mathlason, J. Membr. Sci. *16*: 23 (1983).
93. V. Gekas and B. Hallström, J. Membr. Sci. *30*: 153 (1987).
94. P. Prádanos, J. De Abajo, J. G. de la Campa, and A. Hernández, J. Membr. Sci. *108*: 129 (1995).
95. G. Jonsson, P. Prádanos, and A. Hernández, J. Membr. Sci. *112*: 171 (1996).
96. S. Nakao, T. Nomura, and S. Kimura, AIChE J. *25*: 615 (1979).
97. S. Nakao and S. Kimura, J. Chem. Eng. Jpn. *14*: 32 (1981).
98. G. Jonsson and C. E. Boessen, Desalination *21*: 1 (1977).
99. V. L. Vilker, C. K. Colton, and K. A. Smith, AIChE J. *27*: 632 (1981).
100. V. Gekas, G. Trägårth and B. Hallström, *Ultrafiltration Membrane Performance Fundamentals*, Swedish Foundation for Membrane Technology, Lund, Sweden, 1993.
101. G. B. Van der Berg, I. G. Rácz, and C. A. Smolders, J. Membr. Sci. *47*: 25 (1989).
102. M. Le and J. A. Howell, Chem. Eng. Res. Des. *62*: 373 (1984).
103. M. Bodzek and K. Konieczny, J. Membr. Sci. *61*: 131 (1991).
104. D. R. Lu, S. J. Lee, and K. Park, J. Biomater. Sci., Polym. End. *3*: 127 (1991).

105. S. Nakatsuka and A. S. Michaels, J. Memb. Sci. *69*:189 (1992).
106. P. Prádanos and A. Hernández, Biotechnol. Bioeng. *47*:617 (1995).
107. C. Herrero, P. Prádanos, J. I. Calvo, F. Tejerina, and A. Hernández, J. Colloid Interface Sci. 187:334 (1997).
108. G. B. Westerman-Clark and L. Anderson, J. Electrochem. Soc. *130*:839 (1983).
109. L. Martínez, M. Gigosos, A. Hernández, and F. Tejerina, J. Member. Sci. *35*:1 (1987).
110. J. I. Calvo, A. Hernández, P. Prádanos, and F. Tejerina, J. Colloid Interface Sci. *181*:399 (1996).
111. R. Pastor, J. I. Calvo, P. Prádanos, and A. Hernández, J. Membr. Sci. *137*:109 (1997).

3

Surface Functionalization of Polymer Membranes

JACQUELINE MARCHAND-BRYNAERT Département de Chimie, Université catholique de Louvain, Louvain-la-Neuve, Belgium

Abstract

The surface functionalization of polymer membranes and some surface chemical and physical characterization techniques are reviewed in order to give an impression of the current research trend toward "intelligent" membrane materials for highly specific purposes: development of nano-materials, template synthesis of conductive polymers, hemo-compatibilization of synthetic membranes, tissue engineering, controlled drug delivery systems. Surface functionalization and tagging techniques are discussed for membranes of different polymers, made by the phase-inversion process (tortuous-pore membranes) or by the track-etching technique (capillary-pore membranes). Especially fluorine tagging for X-ray photoelectron spectroscopy (XPS) analysis, and radiochemical tagging for liquid scintillation counting (LSC) analysis are treated, but other methods of surface characterization are also surveyed (SIMS, AFM, FTIR).

I. INTRODUCTION

A. Classification of Membranes

A membrane is a thin barrier (10 μm to 50 μm) which separates two phases and permits the selective transport of various (chemical) species. Membranes can be made of inorganic or organic, synthetic or biological products [1–4].

Several classifications of membranes exist, based on their *configurations* (sheets, tubes, hollow fibers, capsules ...), *morphologies* (symmetric membranes having the same chemical and physical structure throughout the hole, and asymmetric membranes in which the pores are much larger on one side than on the other), *chemical natures* (ceramic, metal and glass membranes, polymer, thermoplastic and composite membranes, biological membranes), and *applications* (microfiltration (MF), ultrafiltration (UF), reverse osmosis (RO), dialysis (D), ion exchange (IE) or electrodialysis, hemodialysis, pervaporation and gas separation).

Membranes are usually characterized by their *pore sizes*; when the holes are smaller than 0.001 μm in diameter, the membrane is called nonporous. Membranes with holes of about 0.001 to 0.005 μm and 0.005 to 10 μm in diameters are called, respectively, microporous and porous. The microfiltration membranes allow the separation of particles of about 0.03–10 μm in diameter; their industrial development in the 1940s originates from the need for the bacterial analysis of water (*Pseudomonas diminuta* = 0.28 μm; *Staphylococcus* bacteria = 1 μm). The commercial polymer membranes for microfiltration applications are made of cellulose derivatives, aromatic polyamide and polyimide, polyacrylonitrile copolymers, polysulfone, polycarbonate and polyester, polytetrafluoroethylene, polypropylene, poly(vinylidene difluoride) and polyethylene. Microfiltration membranes are currently used in medical care, food industry, and electronics.

The ultrafiltration membranes aim to separate particles of about 0.005–0.01 μm. Since they can retain virus (influenza virus = 1.000 Å), such membranes are extensively utilized in the medical and pharmaceutical field (sterilization), but also in the bio-industries (bioreactors), and for the manufacture of super-pure water (electronics industry). The commercial polymer membranes for ultrafiltration applications are made of cellulose derivatives, aromatic polyamide and polyimide, polyacrylonitrile, polyethersulfone, poly(dimethylphenylene oxide), poly(vinylidene difluoride), poly(methyl methacrylate), and polyelectrolyte complexes.

The earliest application of reverse osmosis membranes was for sea water desalination. Dialysis membranes cover two domains of application: the recovery of metals and other impurities in the industrial field, and the blood purification of uremia patients (removal of low molecular weight metabolic waste) in the medical field (hemodialysis, artificial kidney). Reverse osmosis and dialysis membranes are made of cellulose derivatives, aromatic polyamide, polyacrylonitrile copolymers, polysulfone and poly(methyl methacrylate).

Ion-exchange membranes are mainly utilized by the manufacturer of salts and in the desalination processes. They are made of styrene–divinylbenzene copolymers subsequently functionalized by sulfonation (cation-exchange) or amination (anion-exchange).

Finally, the gas separation membranes are nonporous membranes allowing selective gas dissolution and diffusion. They are made of cellulose acetate, polysulfone, poly(dimethylphenylene oxide), and polydimethylsiloxane.

B. Preparation of Membranes

In this paper, we focus on the membranes prepared from synthetic polymers. All the currently used microfiltration and ultrafiltration membranes may be classified into two categories, the "tortuous-pore" and the "capillary-pore" membranes [3].

1. The "Tortuous-Pore" Membranes

These membranes are prepared by the classical phase inversion process (casting process). Briefly, the polymers (or blends) are dissolved in a solvent and then precipitated by the addition of a nonsolvent. The tortuous-pore structure resembles a sponge with a network of interconnecting nonregular holes. Therefore, the surface pore openings, that can be examined with a scanning electron microscope (SEM), do not correspond to the limiting pore size within the depth of the membrane. Polymers not soluble at room temperature are dissolved at elevated temperature in the selected solvent. The membrane is then formed by controlled cooling of the solution (thermal-phase-inversion process). For chemically resistant polymers (PTFE), a stretching process has been developed for making porous membranes.

Normally, the casting and stretching processes do not change the chemical nature of the native polymer during the membrane manufacture.

2. The "Capillary-Pore" Membranes

The track-etching process allows the preparation of capillary microporous membranes [5–9] with very uniform, nearly perfectly round cylindrical pores.

These membranes are made in two steps, from homogeneous 10–20 μm thick polymer film precursors. The usual precursors are bisphenol-A polycarbonate, poly(ethylene terephthalate), and poly(vinylidene difluoride).

The film is first bombarded by heavy ions (Ar^{+9}), accelerated with a cyclotron. When passing through the polymer, the particles leave "damage tracks" where chemical bonds of the backbone are broken, and reactive termini (ions, radicals) are formed. The irradiated film is then immersed into an appropriate solution of reagents which preferentially etches the tracks, leading to the creation of pores. In some cases, UV irradiation, before etching, can improve the diffusion of the solution along the tracks [6].

The pore density of a track-etched membrane is determined by the residence time in the irradiator (10^5–10^9 pores/cm^2), while the pore diameter is controlled by the residence time in the etching bath (0.01–10 μm). However, there is an upper limit to the pore size, because the polymer dissolution occurs, not only along the sensitized tracks, but also on both surfaces of the thin film.

The mean pore diameter and the pore density are easily measured by scanning electron microscopy (SEM) [10]. Air porometry (extended bubble point method) and mercury intrusion porometry are also used for the characterization of track-etched filters [11].

From a chemical point of view, the manufacture of membranes by track-etching appears totally different from the previous process (Sec. I.B.1). Indeed, new functionalities (chain-endings) are created by the chemical treatment, onto the pore walls and the apparent surface. The nature of the surface-displayed functions can be determined from the study of model compounds (small molecules) submitted to the track-etching conditions [12]. Another approach toward the chemical characterization of track-etched membranes is based on the open-surface labeling with selective derivatization reagents (see Sec. III.C and III.D).

C. Surface Modifications

The standard membranes for (ultra)filtration purposes are generally made from chemically resistant, themostable, hydrophobic polymers. As a result of this chemical nature, undesired adsorption phenomena and fouling can occur [13–17]. For instance, protein fouling is a major problem within many industrial applications [18]. Strong experimental evidences have demonstrated that hydrophilic membranes are less accessible to fouling [3]. Accordingly, the main surface modification processes actually developed aim at rendering the surfaces more hydrophilic. On the other hand, highly hydrophobic surfaces are also required for specific applications (gas separation [19] and reverse osmosis membranes [20], hemocompatible materials [21]).

The modification of surface properties often results from polymer bulk modifications [22,23]; for instance, (i) membranes are prepared from acrylonitrile (co)polymers on which chemical transformations have been carried out in bulk [24]; (ii) ultrafiltration membranes are prepared by casting blends of poly(vinylidene difluoride) and poly(methyl methacrylate) or poly(ethylene glycol) [25]; (iii) membrane precursors are obtained by the copolymerization of traditional monomers with functionalized monomers [26]. These approaches will not be considered in the present paper. We are interested here in selective surface modifications, i.e., modifications that affect only the outermost layers of the membranes, and leave the bulk properties unchanged (thermal stability, physical and mechanical properties, permeability and selectivity).

The most relevant reasons for surface modifications are (i) to improve, in a controlled manner, the surface wettability properties responsible for the interactions with the surrounding media; (ii) to introduce specific functional groups susceptible to render the surface somewhat charged at physiological pH ($-SO_3^-$, $-NH_3^+$) and to direct the adhesion of proteins and cells; (iii) to offer potential anchorage points for the covalent coupling of various molecular architectures responsible for designed interactions (intelligent materials).

II. SURFACE FUNCTIONALIZATION BY WET CHEMISTRY

A. Surface Modification Strategies

New interfacial properties of polymer membrancs can be achieved using different methods [14]. *Preadsorption* (*coating*) of more or less hydrophilic compounds (β-lactoglobuline, methyl cellulose, poly(vinyl methyl ether ...)) decreases the susceptibility of the membranes to protein fouling [27]. The stable *physical entrapment of poly(ethylene oxide)* [28] within the surface network of poly(ethylene terephthalate) gives an intcresting biorcpclling material.

Discharges in oxygen atmosphcre (*plasma treatments*) [29] can be used to enhance the wettability of polymer surfaces, whilst CF_4 plasma treatments render the sufaces more hydrophobic [30]. Such treatments are nonselective and various chemical functions are created on the polymer surfaces. *Photo-oxidative treatments* are also described to improve the selectivity of polymide membranes [31].

In the *surface grafting* technique, the surface modification is achieved by the covalent bonding of new macromolecules on top of the substrate. The great majority of graft-polymerization processes involves the creation of reactive species (anchoring sites) on the substrate surface, followed by the polymerization via a radical mechanism, of hydrophilic vinyl monomers such as acrylic or methacrylic acid, acrylamide, 2-hydroxyethyl methacrylate (HEMA) and poly(ethylene glycol) (PEG) methacrylates. The surface activation is acomplished by different methods: γ-irradiation [32,33], UV photoirradiation [34–

36], plasma treatments [37–40], or thermal decomposition of peroxides [41]. Recently, nonthrombogenic membranes of polyurethane have been prepared by surface graft-polymerization of an acrylamide derivative of a thrombin inhibitor [42]. Similarly, grafting of poly(ethyleneimine) (PEI) on the polyurethane surface by using ozone induced or photoinduced activation, followed by immobilization of heparin via the reducive coupling with glutaraldehyde, also furnishes a blood compatible material [43].

Lastly, *wet treatments* [44], i.e., chemical reactions carried out at the solid–liquid interface, have been performed for modifying polymer surface properties. The goal of this mild approach is to create well defined functional groups on the surface, by using the arsenal of chemoselective transformations offered by organic chemistry.

There are important differences between standard organic chemistry (conducted in homogeneous solutions) and surface wet chemistry. Polymer surface modifications are necessarily heterogeneous; such reactions are often characterized by lower rates and yields, as a result of the reduction of dimensionality (constrained functional groups). The reactions are carried out at the interface between the membrane substrate and a solvent containing appropriate reagents. Depending on the choice of solvent (wetting and diffusion properties), and reaction temperature, the thickness of the modified layer can vary from a few Å to several microns. Also, the modified polymer surface (i.e., the product of the reaction) may interact with the solvent to a different extent than does the native polymer; this can lead to some surface solubilization and etching. When a polymer surface displays amorphous and crystalline domains, the effect of a wet treatment is not homogeneous, the amorphous domains being more rapidly attacked. Another problem concerns the final desorption of the excess of reagents and low-molecular weight materials; repeated washings can lead to some interface erosion.

Finally, the isolated modified surface can further change when exposed to air atmosphere (hydrophobic medium), by the reorientation and diffusion of polar groups away from the outermost surface and into the polymer bulk. This physical process, called "surface reconstruction" tends to diminish the surface free energy by leaving the most hydrophobic segments exposed. Surface reconstruction is usually followed by contact angle measurements.

Thus, the polymer wet chemistry is a complex phenomenon that requires appropriate analytical tools for characterizing the modified surfaces (see Sec. III).

In the following subsections, we will describe typical surface treatments, recently published. Our aim is not to present an exhaustive revue on the subject, but rather to illustrate the scope of the wet chemistry approach for modifying membranes. We have considered three categories of polymers: the chemically resistant polymers on which reactive sites have to be created to further develop surface functionalization, the polymers that naturally offer reactive pendant functional groups and, therefore, can be easily derivatized without chain breaking, and the polymers that exhibit reactive chain-endings, naturally occurring or created by hydrolysis of main-chain functionalities (esters, carbonates ...).

B. Chemical Attack on Poorly Reactive Polymers

1. Polypropylene (PP)

Two examples have been selected that involve the chemical attack of polypropylene membranes under strong oxidizing conditions. Most probably, the surface modifications were initiated by the creation of radical intermediates at the tertiary carbon atoms of the polyolefinic chains.

The surface wettability of PP membranes has been increased by insertion of acid, ester, and amide functionalities [45]. The process involves photooxidation followed by photosubstitution. Polypropylene films were soaked in various alcohols or amines, then the surfaces were exposed to UV irradiation at 185–253 nm under air atmosphere. Reflectance FTIR analysis of the samples clearly showed the presence of acid, ester, and amide groups. The surface modified PP membranes are useful for the separation of extraction solvents, such as furfural and N-methyl-pyrimidone, from diesel fuel extract or refine.

Extracoporal membrane oxygenation (ECMO) support has been improved by the covalent bonding of heparin [46]. The process involves ozone oxidation, grafting of a polyethyleneimine (PEI) spacer, coupling of heparin with glutaraldehyde and reduction of the Schiff's base intermediate (Scheme 1). The heparin bonded surface was able to maintain high levels of heparin bioactivity, suppressing platelet adhesion/activation and complement activation.

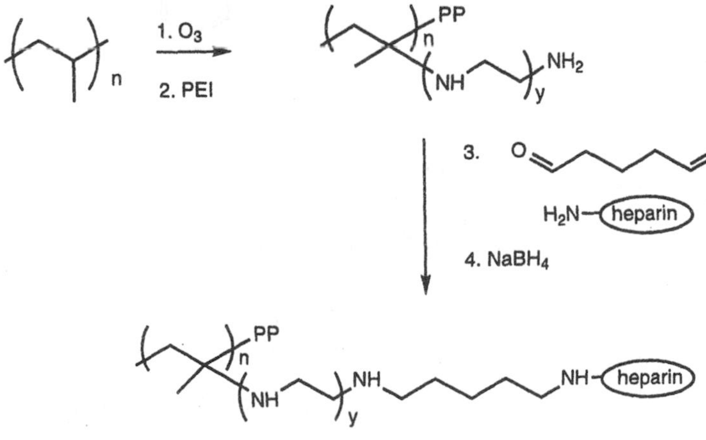

SCHEME 1 Covalent binding of heparin to ECMO support.

2. Poly(vinylidene difluoride) (PVDF)

Surface modifications of PVDF membranes generally result from initial HF elimination under strong basic conditions [47–50]. The insaturations created on the main chains allowed subsequent reactions, like halogenation, hydroboration, oxidation and nucleophilic addition. Water addition followed by reduction gave surfaces displaying hydroxyl functions [51]. Tracked PVDF membranes were etched in an aqueous solution of potassium hydroxide, potassium permanganate and potassium periodate [52]; this oxidative treatment should create carboxyl functions.

Polyallylamine has been attached on PVDF membrane by nucleophilic addition on the KOH etched support (Scheme 2). Reaction of the amino groups with 1,4-phenylene diisothiocyanate, followed by immobilization of

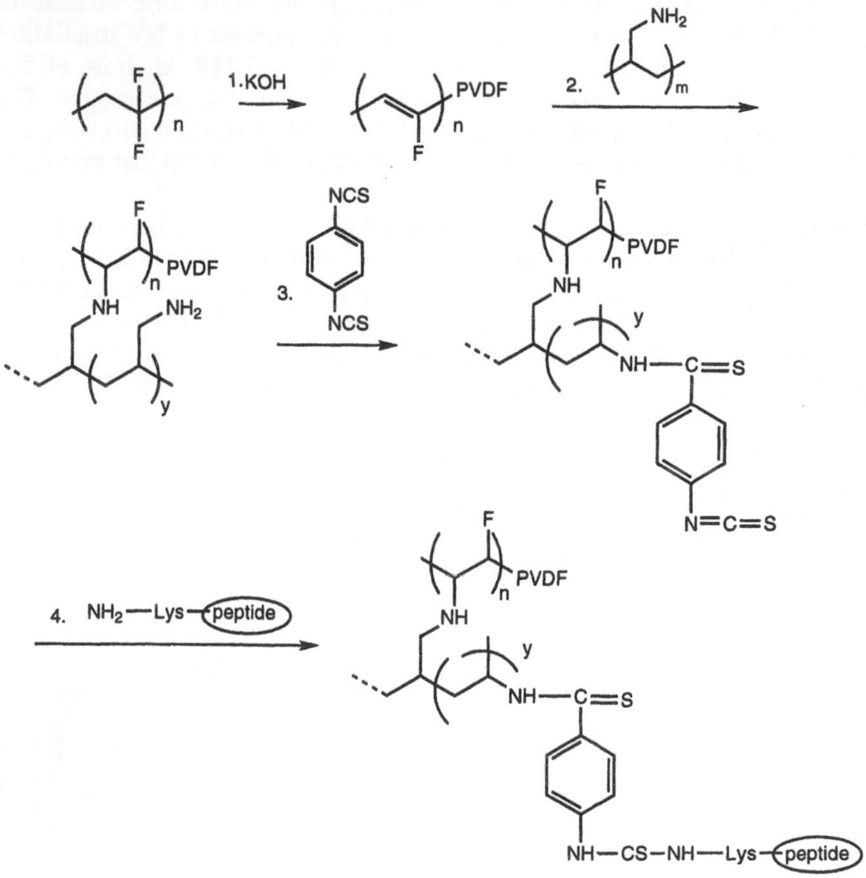

SCHEME 2   Covalent binding of peptides to PVDF membranes.

lysine-containing polypeptides gave derivatized membranes for solid phase sequence analysis [53]. Another method is available for activating hydrophilic PVDF membranes: the reaction with 1,1'-carbonyldiimidazole (Scheme 3). This was used for immobilizing human placental alkaline phosphatase on a cross-flow microfiltration membrane [54].

Recently, the sulfonation of ultrafiltration PVDF membrane has been carried out by immersion in SO_3-triethylphosphate solution. Further reaction with N-actyl ethanolamine gave N-(2-hydroxylethyl)sulfonamide derivative [55]. The same functionalization procedure was applied to polysulfone membranes (see Sec. II.B.3).

3. Polysulfone (PS) and Poly(ether sulfone) (PES)

The classical strategies for polysulfones functionalization are based on aromatic electrophilic substitution reactions. For instance, sulfonated alkyl segments could be introduced on PES ultrafiltration hollow fibers by heterogeneous reaction with propane sultone in the presence of a Friedel–Crafts catalyst (Scheme 4) [56]. Direct sulfonation, chloromethylation and aminomethylation reactions were also developed for rendering PS membranes

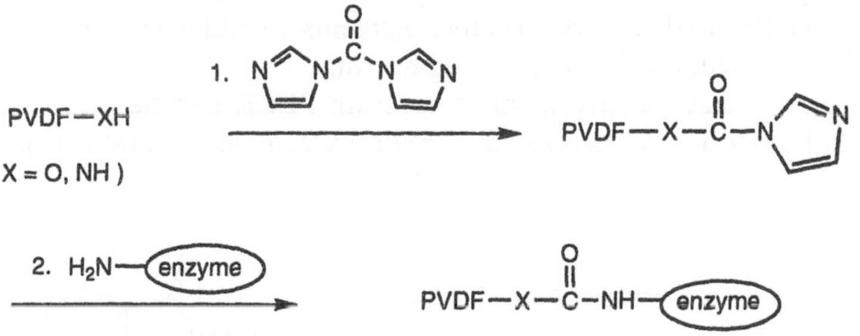

SCHEME 3   Enzyme immobilization on hydrophilic PVDF membranes.

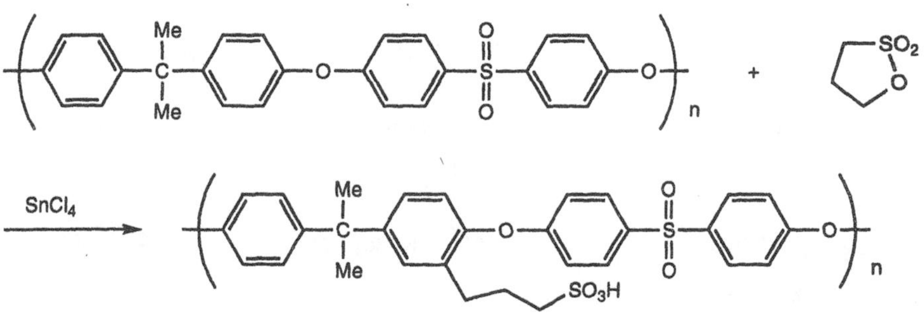

SCHEME 4   Friedel–Crafts alkylation of polyether sulfone membrane with propane sultone.

more "intelligent" (Scheme 5) [57]. All these modifications, and the subsequent derivatizations, transformed the neutral polymer into charged polymers ($-SO_3^-$, $-NH_3^+$, $-NMe_3^+$).

Recently, a novel approach for PS (and PES) membranes functionalization has been disclosed, involving the photochemical graft polymerization of acrylic acid [58]. The initiation consisted in H-abstraction by photoexcited benzophenone from the methyl side group, thus avoiding polymer chain scission (Scheme 6). The resulting PS surface displayed carboxylic acids, the activation of which (carbodiimide) allowed the covalent immobilization of various biomolecules. Poly(ether sulfone) (PES) is intrinsically photosensitive; thus no photoinitiator is required to initiate the graft-polymerization of hydrophilic vinyl monomers [59]. When PES membranes were irradiated while immersed in methanol (or water) containing monomers, polymerization of the monomers took place only at the membrane surface, no homopolymerization in solution being observed. A mechanism involving free radical cleavage of PES chains has been proposed (Scheme 7).

4. Poly(ether ether ketone) (PEEK)

Poly(ether ether ketone) is a high-performance thermoplastic exhibiting excellent mechanical properties, thermal stability and environmental resistance. This polymer, mainly used for constructive elements in industry, has found recently new developments in biomedical engineering.

The preparation of track-etched membranes from PEEK film has been considered [60]. Although not yet described, the surface functionalization of such

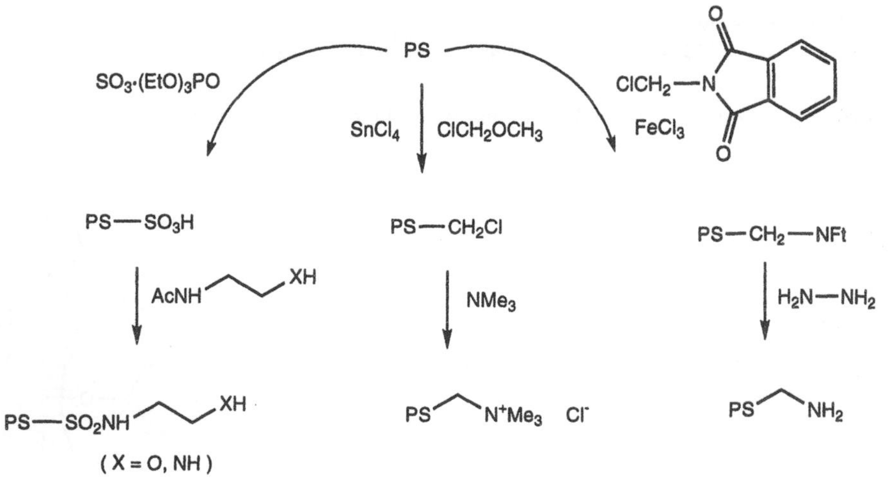

SCHEME 5 PS membrane functionalization by sulfonation, chloromethylation and aminomethylation.

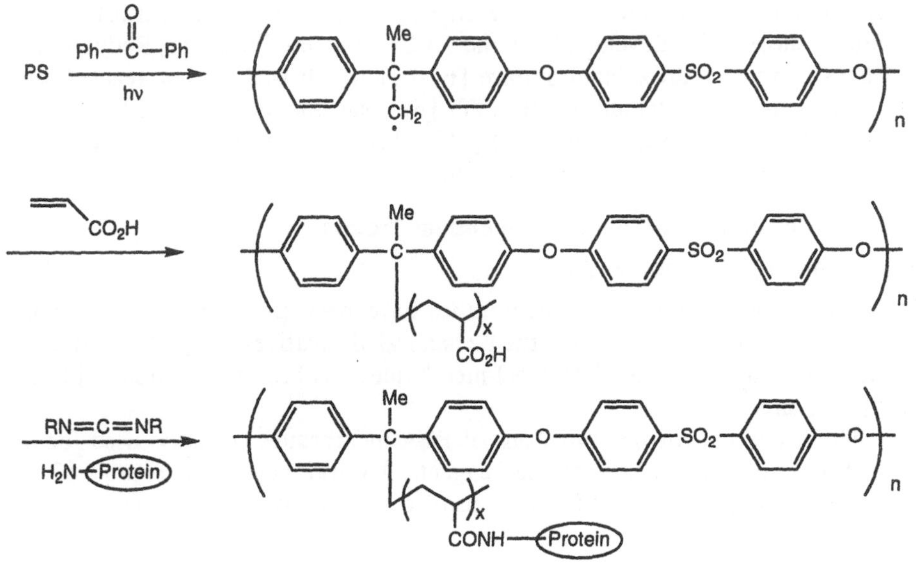

SCHEME 6 Photochemical functionalization of PES ultrafiltration membrane for covalent immobilization of biomolecules.

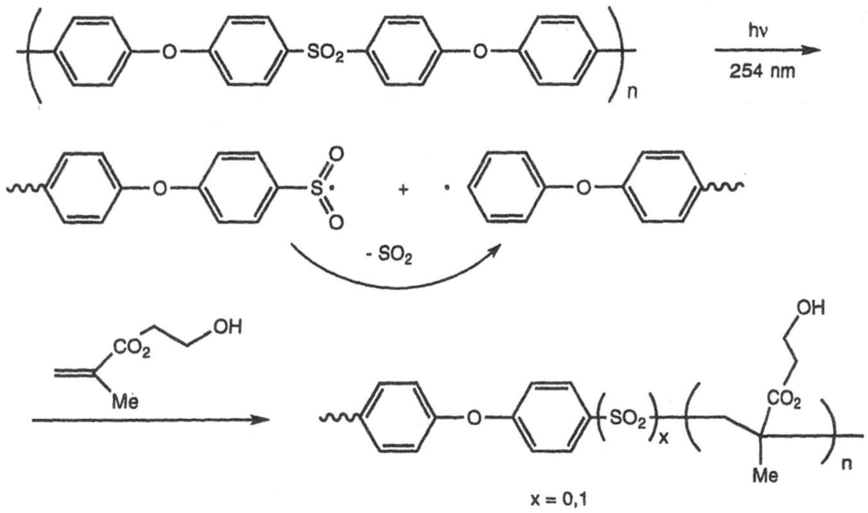

SCHEME 7 Photochemical functionalization of PES ultrafiltration membrane without photoinitiator.

hydrophobic membranes could be envisaged using the wet chemistry techniques successfully developed for the PEEK film modification. Reduction of PEEK gave a hydroxylated surface [61–63] which was further reacted with diethylaminosulfur trifluoride (DAST) [64], succinamic acid [65], or hexamethylene diisocyanate (Scheme 8) [66]. This later surface allowed the covalent coupling of aminoacids and proteins [67].

C. Derivatization of Pendant Functional Groups

1. Polyvinyl Alcohol (PVA)

For many years, functional membranes have been prepared from polyvinyl alcohol and copolymers, and their chemical derivatives [68]. An important therapeutic application of PVA gel membranes has been in the area of plasma separation.

The pendant hydroxyl functions of PVA membranes could be used for the anchorage of various electrophilic reagents. A novel membrane capable of performing bioseparations, specifically protein fractionations, was prepared from

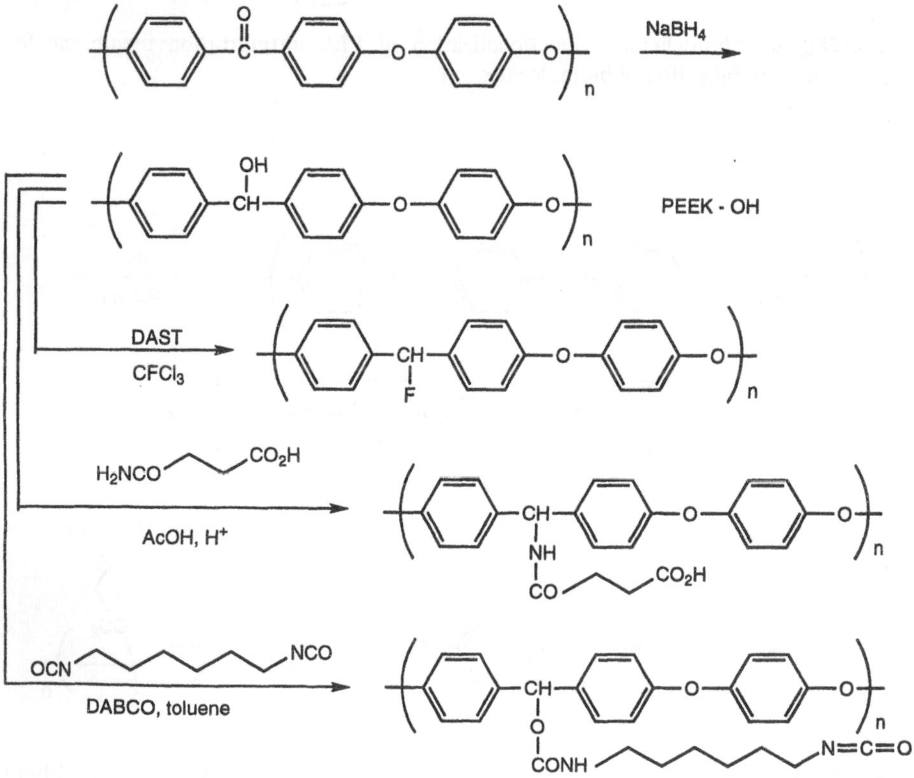

SCHEME 8   Surface wet chemistry on PEEK film.

PVA gel cross-linked with glutaraldehyde, and then surface modified by interfacial polymerization with toluene 2,4-diisocyanate (TDI) in hexane [69].

2. Polyacrylonitrile (PAN)

PAN-based membranes display pendant nitrile groups which can be transformed either into methylene amines, by reduction, or into carboxylic acids, by hydrolysis. Both types of chemical transformations have been successfully used for the grafting of poly(ethylene oxide) (PEO) on the surface of poly(acrylonitrile-co-vinyl chloride) (PAN/VC) anisotropic membranes [70].

After treatment with aqueous sodium borohydride, the resulting PAN/VC-NH$_2$ membranes were functionalized with PEO-succinimide (Scheme 9). Reaction of PAN/VC with concentrated hydrochloric acid gave PAN/VC-CO$_2$H membranes which were activated by a water soluble carbodiimide (WSC), then coupled to PEO-NH$_2$ (Scheme 9). These mild surface modifications carried out in aqueous solutions did not affect the pore structure and the transport properties of the material. PEO grafted PAN/VC membranes showed decreased protein adsorption and enhanced biocompatibility.

Ultrafiltration (UF) membranes prepared from PAN homopolymer, and copolymer with methyl acrylate, were similarly modified for immobilizing enzymes [71]. The membranes were treated with a hydroxylamine hydrochloride solution, and then further hydrolyzed with 2 M HCl (Scheme 10).

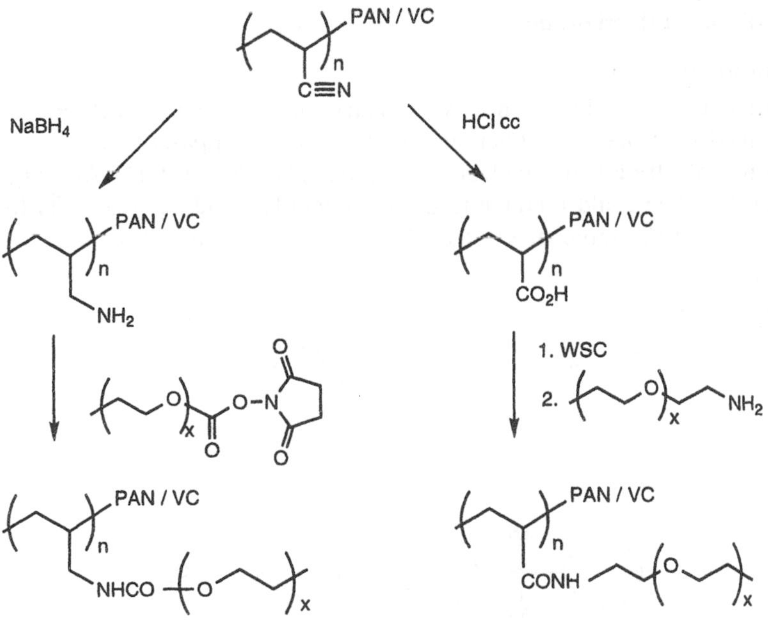

SCHEME 9   Grafting of poly (ethylene oxide) on PAN/VC membranes.

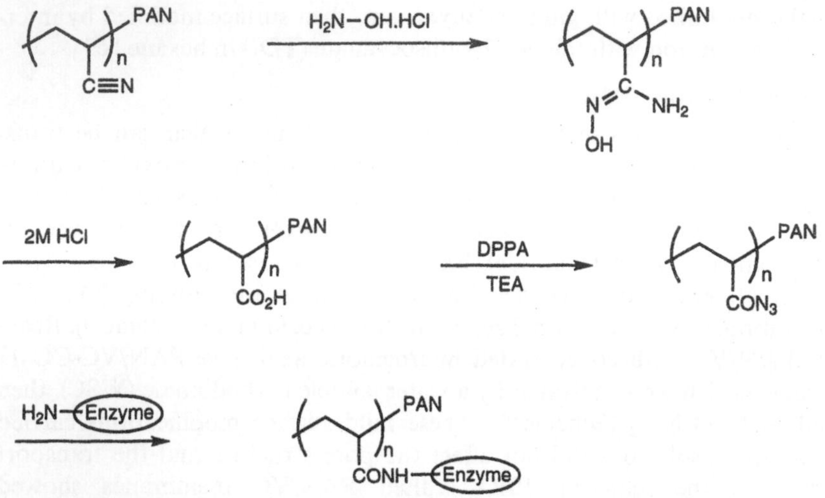

SCHEME 10   Enzyme immobilization on PAN ultrafiltration membranes.

Activation of the surface carboxyl functions resulted from the reaction with diphenyl phosphoryl azide (DPPA) and triethylamine (TEA) in acetonitrile; the acyl azide functions could rapidly fix enzymes.

D.   Chain-Ends Derivatization

1.   Polycarbonate (PC)

Membranes made from bis-phenol A polycarbonate films by track-etching treatment, should display new phenolic endings, on the apparent surface and the pore walls, resulting from the basic hydrolysis [12] (Scheme 11). Although not yet reported, one could imagine to use the phenolate endings reactivity for the coupling of various molecules (via acylation or etherification reactions).

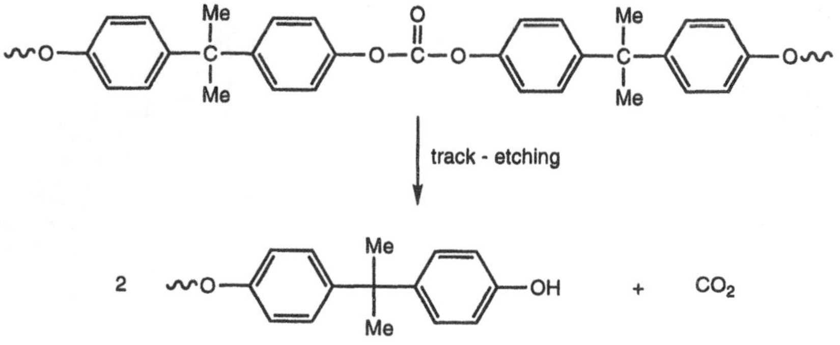

SCHEME 11   PC track-etched membrane.

PC membranes [72–74], activated by glow-discharge, were surface-grafted with poly (methacrylic acid) [75]; the anchorage site was not determined.

2. Poly(ethylene terephthalate) (PET)

Track-etched membranes made from poly(ethylene terephthalate) (PET) films expose new chain-ends created by the etching treatment [6]; they are carboxyl and hydroxyl functions (Scheme 12). The narrow pores of these membranes show many of the properties of biological ion channels, such as rapid switching, selectivity for cations over anions, and modulation by H^+ and divalent cations (Zn^{2+}, Ca^{2+}) [76,77]. Lowering of negative surface charge, by methylation of carboxyl residues with diazomethane, reduced the selectivity between cations and anions, and the sensitivity to protons. As expected, grafting with poly(2-methyl-5-vinyl-pyridine) (=polycation) reversed the selectivity and sensitivity to pH [76,77].

The amount of surface carboxyl chain-ends in PET track-etched membranes could be significantly increased by treatment with potassium permanganate in diluted sulfuric acid [78–80]; native hydroxyl chain-ends were oxidized into new carboxyl endings (Scheme 12). The inverse transformation of

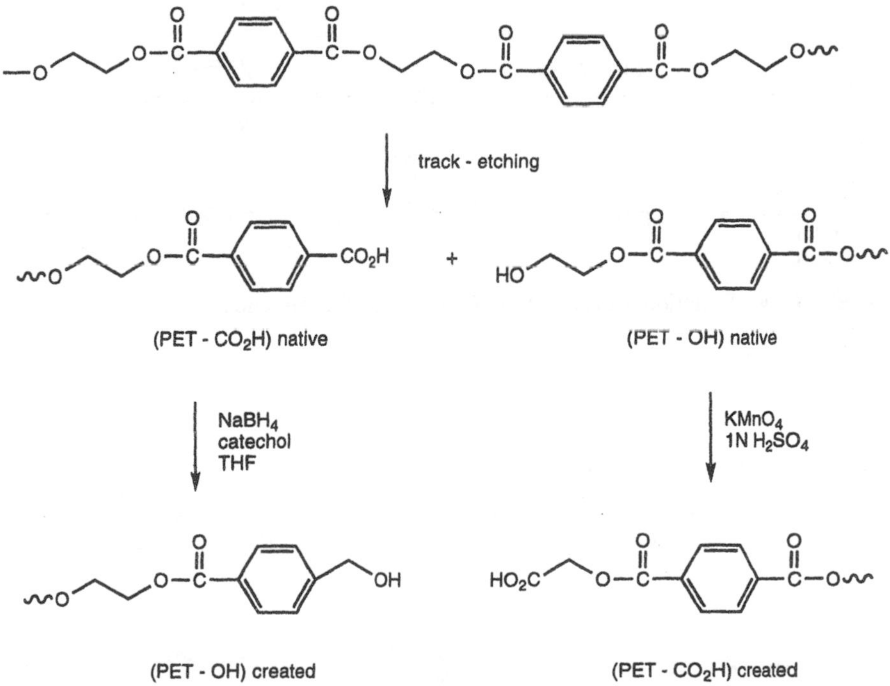

SCHEME 12 Naturally occurring and chemically created chain-ends of PET membranes.

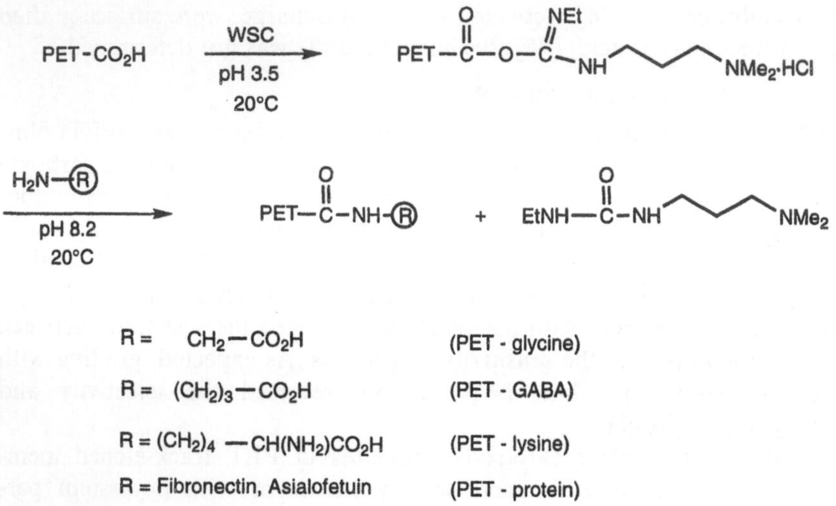

SCHEME 13 Functionalization of the PET carboxyl chain-ends.

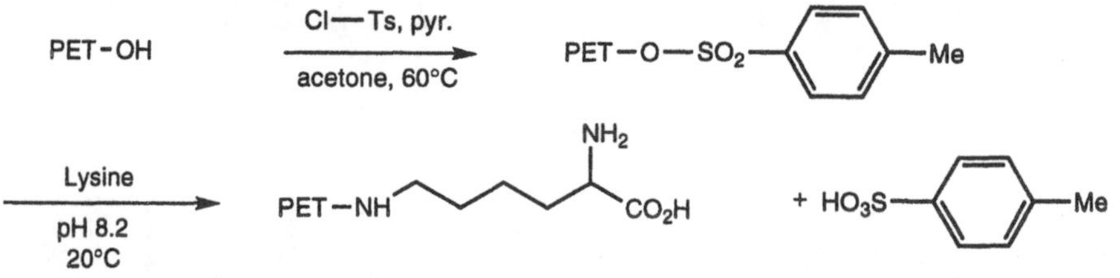

SCHEME 14 Functionalization of the PET hydroxyl chain-ends.

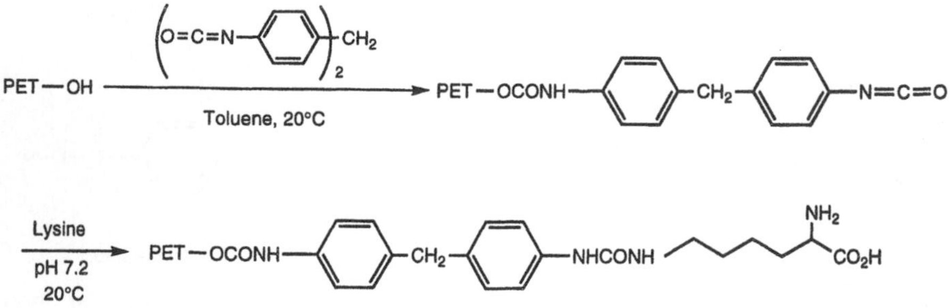

SCHEME 15 PET membrane functionalization via a diisocyanate spacer arm.

native carboxyl chain-ends into new hydroxyl endings, by reduction with the NaBH$_4$-catechol complex, readily applied to films only (Scheme 12) [80].

Activation of PET-CO$_2$H membranes with water soluble carbodiimide (WSC) allowed further functionalization with various aminoacid derivatives [78,79], and proteins [81] (Scheme 13). Similarly, activation of PET-OH membranes with p-toluenesulfonyl chloride followed by reaction with aminoacids gave new derivatized membranes [82,83] (Scheme 14). Finally, biomolecules could be immobilized on PET-OH via a diisocyanate spacer arm (Scheme 15) [82].

III. CHEMICAL ASSAYS OF FUNCTIONALIZED MEMBRANES

A. Surface Analysis Strategies

The characterization of a solid surface is intrinsically an arduous problem because the volume of matter concerned relative to the bulk is extremely low. Therefore, classical spectroscopic methods that probe the bulk as well as the surface, produce information (or signals) in which the surface contribution would appear like traces of impurities! Specific methods have been developed to analyze the outermost layers of a solid [16,84–86]; each of those investigates different extents in depth, from 1 to 3 atomic layers to about 10 μm (Table 1).

Physical microstructure information (morphologies, and topographic images) are provided by *scanning electron microscopy* (SEM) and *atomic force microscopy* (AFM) [87].

Contact angle measurements examine the angle made by a liquid drop (water or other solvent that does not penetrate the matter) on the solid

TABLE 1 Standard Surface Analysis Techniques

Method	Depth of analysis	Information	Surface sensitivity
SEM AFM	Outermost atomic layer	Morphology Topography Microstructure	High
Contact angle (Θ)	Outermost atomic layer	Wettability pH titration	High
SIMS	≤ 10 Å	Structure of characteristic fragments	High
XPS	10–100 Å	Elemental analysis Some structural analysis	Medium
FTIR (ATR)	1–10 μm	Functional groups analysis	Low

surface; the contact angle is a balance between the magnitudes of three inter-facial tensions (or surface free energies): air–drop, drop–membrane and membrane–air. This highly sensitive technique has been developed for the surface pH titration (i.e., observing the contact angle made on the solid surface by various aqueous buffers as a function of the pH) [88]. Surface free amine groups can be detected by a decrease in contact angle at lower pH. In contrast, surface free carboxylic acids can be detected by a decrease in contact angle at higher pH. These observations are consistent with the fact that charged sur-faces ($-NH_3^+$, $-CO_2^-$) are more hydrophilic, thus making a lower contact angle than the neutral forms.

The *spectroscopic techniques* widely used to analyse surfaces from a chemi-cal and structural point of view are the secondary ion mass spectrometry (SIMS), X-ray photoelectron spectroscopy (XPS), and Fourier transform infra-red spectroscopy (FTIR) in the attenuated total reflectance mode (ATR) [89]. SIMS provides informations about the composition and chemical structure of charged fragments ejected from the surface under bombardment with an ion beam. XPS spectra are obtained by irradiating the samples with an X-ray source; electrons (from the atom core levels) are emitted from the surface with different kinetic energies that can be correlated to the binding energy of the electrons to their respective nucleus. Thus, XPS gives a direct measure of the types of atoms and their relative amounts (i.e., surface elemental analysis) within an interface domain of about 5–20 atomic layers. The method can also distinguish different oxidation states for each type of atoms (small shifts in the binding energy). Accordingly, some functional groups may be identified. However, the most accurate method to analyse chemical functions remains the IR spectroscopy adapted for surface examination [59,71], even if this tech-nique samples an important interface domain of about 5 μm. Indeed, the surface-sensitivity of the spectroscopic techniques diminishes when the sam-pling depth increases (Table 1).

All the analytical tools mentioned above examine exclusively the apparent surface of the polymer samples. Now, as far as membranes are concerned, functional informations related to the hole walls may be of interest, particu-larly for the track-etched membranes in which new chain-ends are created. NMR [57,63,70,75] and UV [58,63] *spectra recorded after dissolution* of the samples can provide structural informations about the total open surface, despite the fact that the relevant signals are often partially masked by the bulk contribution. *Titration* methods, in solution, have been used for determining the amount of carboxylic and sulfonic acid functions grafted on PC [75], and PES [56,57] membranes, respectively; they involve the dyeing with rhodamin, brilliant blue or methylene blue, by the formation of salts (ion pairs).

Lastly, *covalent labeling* of functionalized membranes increasingly develops as a powerful method of analysis. Selective chemical derivatization procedures, performed on the solid samples by wet chemistry, are able to distinguish

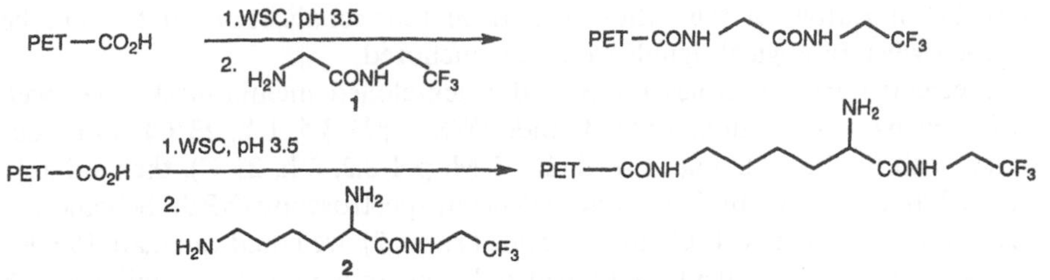

SCHEME 16 Covalent coupling of fluorine tags on activated PET-CO$_2$H membranes.

among different functionalities. Marking functional groups of interest with an elemental tag (i.e., a type of atom not already found in the surface; usually, fluorine) increases the XPS analysis performances [90] (see Sect. III.B). More interestingly, labeling functional groups with a radioactive tag (usually, tritium) allows the counting of the reactive functions displayed on the total open surface of membrane samples (i.e., apparent surface and internal surface of the pores) (see Section III.C).

The covalent labeling approach has been fully exemplified in our laboratory with the analysis of surface modified PEEK films [63–67], and track-etched PET membranes [67,79–83]. The labeling reactions have been conducted in water solution (near the physiological pH), at room temperature, a mild situation that mimics the conditions likely to be encountered in the covalent coupling of biologically active molecules (peptidomimetics, peptides, proteins ...). Thus, our chemical assays have established quantitative bases for the further development of biocompatibilization strategies (see Sect. IV).

The work devoted to the analysis of PET membranes is the subject of the following sections.

B. Surface Labeling for XPS Analysis

The microporous PET track-etched membranes display surface carboxyl functions, naturally occurring and/or created by an oxidative treatment [78] (Scheme 12).

The most often used fluorine labels for XPS characterization of carboxylated surfaces are 2,2,2-trifluoroethanol and trifluoroacetic anhydride, forming esters and mixed anhydrides, respectively [91–94]. Thus, the labels are fixed by means of water-sensitive linkages.

Labeling of surface carboxyl groups with fluorinated amines in aqueous solution to give water-stable derivatized surfaces, via the formation of amide bonds, has been reported by our group [79]. We selected aminoacid derivatives as starting materials for the construction of fluorine tags. N-(trifluoroethyl) glycinamide **1** and L-N-(trifluoroethyl) lysinamide **2** have been considered. Indeed, their reactivity towards various PET-CO$_2$H samples may be indicative of the ratios of surface functionalization that could be reached when biological signals would be anchored.

Pretreated PET samples (films and track-etched membranes) have been activated by water soluble carbodiimide (WSC, pH 3.5, 1 h, 23°C), and incubated with the fluorine tags 1 or 2 (10^{-3} M, pH 8.2, 2 h, 23°C), then suitably washed and analyzed by X-ray photoelectron spectroscopy (XPS) (Scheme 16). From the experimental F/C atomic ratios (Table 2), we could calculate [95,96] the percentages of covalently modified polymer units into the sampling depth (about 50 Å). Control experiments (entries 1, 3, 5, 7, 9, 11) showed that in the absence of WSC activation, the fluorine tag 1 could not be associated to the PET-CO_2H surface, but that the bulkier tag 2 was slighly adsorbed. Indeed the lysine derivative 2 is naturally able to create more effective polar and nonpolar interactions at the polymer interface. Accordingly, the F/C atomic ratios measured after WSC activation and labeling of the PET-CO_2H samples (entries 8, 10, 12) have been corrected by subtracting the contribution due to the noncovalent fixation of the fluorine tag 2. Pretreated (hydrolyzed and/or

TABLE 2 Derivatization of PET-CO_2H with Fluorine Tags and XPS Analysis

Entry	Sample (treatment)	Label	F/C × 100 (corrected)	%
1	Film (1 + 2 + 4)	1	0.00	
2	Film (1 + 2 + 3 + 4)	1	0.24	0.8
3	Membrane A (2 + 4)	1	0.00	
4	Membrane A (2 + 3 + 4)	1	0.39	1.3
5	Membrane B (2 + 4)	1	0.00	
6	Membrane A (2 + 3 + 4)	1	0.29	1.0
7	Film (1 + 2 + 4)	2	0.083	
8	Film (1 + 2 + 3 + 4)	2	0.363 (0.28)	0.9
9	Membrane A (2 + 4)	2	0.095	
10	Membrane A (2 + 3 + 4)	2	0.422 (0.33)	1.1
11	Membrane B (2 + 4)	2	0.114	
12	Membrane B (2 + 3 + 4)	2	0.428 (0.31)	1.0

Film: Mylar A (DuPont de Nemours); thickness of 12 μm.
Membrane A: obtained by track-etching treatment of the film; pore density: 1.45×10^6 pores/cm^2 (apparent surface); mean diameter of the pores: 0.49 μm.
Membrane B: obtained by track-etching treatment of the film; pore density: 9.8×10^7 pores/cm^2 (apparent surface); mean diameter of the pores: 0.41 μm.
Treatment: 1 = basic hydrolysis (NaOH, H_2O-CH_3CN, 60°C, 18 h); 2 = oxidation ($KMnO_4$, 1.2 N H_2SO_4, 60°C, 1 h); 3 = activation (WSC, 0.1 M MES buffer pH 3.5, 1 h, 23°C); 4 = coupling (tag 1 or 2, 10^{-3} M, phosphate buffer, pH 8.2, 2 h, 23°C).
%: percentage of covalently modified polymer units.

oxidized) films and membranes, with low or high density of pores, exhibited very similar reactivities, ranging within 0.8 to 1.3% of apparent surface functionalization [95,96].

The hydroxyl chain ends (PET-OH) displayed on the apparent surface of film precursors and native track-etched membranes of poly(ethylene terephthalate) have been similarly assayed [83] by derivatization with the fluorine tag **2** (Scheme 17A). After selective activation by tosylation (Ts-Cl, pyridine, acetone, reflux, 1 h), incubation with L-N-(trifluoroethyl) lysinamide **2** (10^{-3} M, phosphate buffer, pH 8.2, 23°C, 2 h), and appropriate washing, the samples were analyzed by XPS (Table 3). On the other hand, the direct coupling of PET-OH with heptafluorobutyl (p-isocyanatobenzoyl) glycinate **3** has been performed (Scheme 17B). This original fluorine tag **3** was prepared in a multistep convergent sequence using p-aminobenzoic acid, glycine and 2,2,3,3,4,4,4-heptafluorobutanol as building blocks [83]. Blank samples, for controlling the noncovalent fixation of the label, have been prepared by incubation of the PET samples into a solution of heptafluorobutyl [N-(tert-butyloxycabonyl)aminobenzoyl] glycinate **4**; **4** is a precursor of **3**, still containing the molecular skeleton and the perfluorinated substituent, but not the reactive isocyanate moiety. The XPS analysis data collected in Table 3 showed that the simple physical adsorption of the tags could not be detected (entries 1, 3, 5, 7, 9).

The ratios of apparent surface functionalization obtained with the lysine tag **2** range within 1.0 to 1.4% of the polymer units contained in a depth of about 50 Å [97]. Using the isocyanate tag **3**, the membranes appeared more functionalized (1.3 to 2%) [98]. This result is consistent with the fact that the coupling of **3** is conducted in dry organic medium, without preactivation of the PET samples. In contrast, the PET-OTs samples (i.e., the activated PET-OH samples) are treated with the tag **2** in aqueous medium; thus

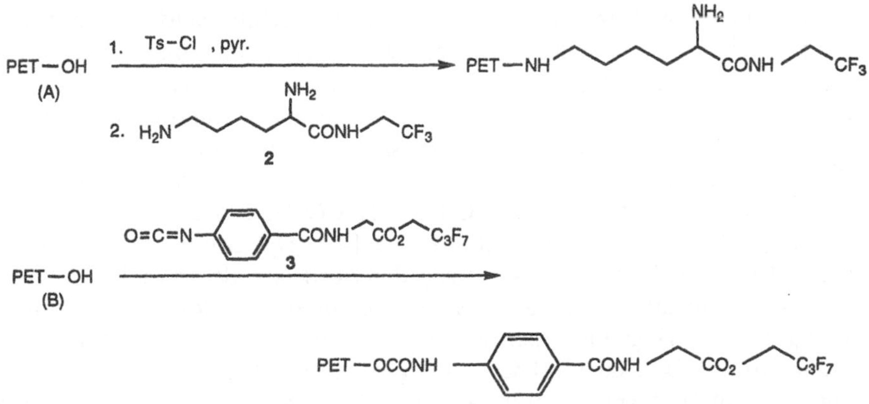

SCHEME 17 Covalent coupling of fluorine tags on (activated) PET-OH membranes.

TABLE 3 Derivatization of PET-OH with Fluorine Tags and XPS Analysis

Entry	Sample (treatment)	Label	F/C × 100	%
1	Membrane A (2)	2	0.00	
2	Membrane A (1 + 2)	2	0.28	1.0
3	Membrane B (2)	2	0.00	
4	Membrane B (1 + 2)	2	0.41	1.4
5	Film (3)	3	0.00	
6	Film (4)	3	0.41	0.6
7	Membrane A (3)	3	0.00	
8	Membrane A (4)	3	0.88	1.3
9	Membrane B (3)	3	0.00	
10	Membrane B (4)	3	1.38	2.0

Film, Membrane A, Membrane B, %: see Table 2.
Treatment: 1 = activation (Ts-Cl, pyridine, acetone, reflux, 1 h); 2 = coupling (tag **2**, 10^{-3} M, phosphate buffer, pH 8.2, 2 h, 23°C); 3 = noncovalent fixation (50 mM BOC—NH—C_6H_4—CONH—CH_2—$CO_2CH_2C_3F_7$ (**4**), acetone, 1 h, 22°C); 4 = coupling (tag **3**, 50 mM, acetone or THF, 1 h, 22°C).

basic hydrolysis of PET-OTs appreciably competes with the nucleophilic substitution.

The surface chemistry described in this section does not alter the pore calibration of the track-etched membranes, as confirmed by the scanning electron microscopy (SEM) controls.

C. Radiochemical Assays

The radiolabeling with tritium is a highly sensitive technique (detection in the range of 10^{-12} mol/cm^2) allowing the assay of reactive functions displayed on the membrane open surface, i.e., apparent surface and internal surface of the calibrated pores. The method appears to be the most suitable one for the chemical characterization of surfaces exposing tenuous amounts of functions; it is therefore particularly well adapted for the titration of polymer chain-ends.

After appropriate activation (WSC for PET-CO_2H, and Cl-Ts/pyridine for PET-OH), the membranes are reacted with L-[4,5-^{3}H]lysine (= lysine*) under the wet chemistry conditions previously described (see Schemes 13 and 14). The sample-associated radioactivity is measured by liquid scintillation counting (LSC) [78], giving experimental values that can be directly correlated with the ratio of fixed labels. The results given in the Tables are expressed in pmoles per sample (experimental values), and converted in pmoles per open surface unit (cm^2) [99]; taking into account the respective open surfaces of the membranes permits a rigorous comparison between the different samples. Each value is the average of, at least, four independent measurements performed with four samples similarly treated; the standard deviation is indicated in parenthesis.

Usually, appropriate washings allow to remove most of the unreacted lysine*; nevertheless, some irreversible adsorption or diffusion of the radioactive label into the polymer interface cannot be avoided. This contribution of nonspecific fixation of lysine* is estimated by the counting (LSC) of blank samples prepared by omitting the activation reagents (WSC or Cl-Ts) in the derivatization procedures. The corrected values (pmol/cm^2) given in the tables are obtained by subtracting the blank values.

The PET film precursor displays 6.3 pmol/cm^2 of reactive carboxyl functions (Table 4, entry 2); after an oxidative treatment, the amount of CO_2H is nearly doubled (entry 4, see Schemes 12 and 13). Surface hydrolysis, mimicking the etching treatment of the membranes, also increases the ratio of labeled CO_2H groups (entry 6). Complete pretreatment of the film (hydrolysis and

TABLE 4   Surface Radiolabeling of the PET Carboxyl Chain-Ends [78–80]

Entry	Sample (treatment)	Fixed ^{3}H-lysine (pmol)		
		Sample	cm^2	Corrected
1	Film (4)	4.8 (1.6)	1.8 (0.6)	
2	Film (3 + 4)	21.5 (4.2)	8.1 (1.6)	6.3
3	Film (2 + 4)	11.9 (3.2)	4.5 (1.2)	
4	Film (2 + 3 + 4)	42.0 (5.3)	15.8 (2.0)	11.3
5	Film (1 + 4)	2.7 (0.3)	1.0 (0.1)	
6	Film (1 + 3 + 4)	41.8 (0.5)	15.7 (0.2)	14.7
7	Film (1 + 2 + 4)	13.8 (7.2)	5.2 (2.7)	
8	Film (1 + 2 + 3 + 4)	98.1 (4.2)	36.9 (1.6)	31.7
9	Membrane A (4)	18.5 (3.8)	6.2 (1.2)	
10	Membrane A (3 + 4)	110.9 (13.8)	36.9 (4.6)	30.7
11	Membrane A (2 + 4)	37.4 (3.2)	12.4 (1.1)	
12	Membrane A (2 + 3 + 4)	192.5 (10.8)	63.9 (3.6)	51.5
13	Membrane B (4)	19.0 (9.2)	0.8 (0.4)	
14	Membrane B (3 + 4)	567.1 (3.7)	25.2 (0.2)	24.4
15	Membrane B (2 + 4)	67.1 (2.4)	3.0 (0.1)	
16	Membrane B (2 + 3 + 4)	685.5 (16.4)	30.5 (0.7)	27.5

Film, Membrane A, Membrane B; see Table 2.
Treatment: 1 = see Table 2; 2 = see Table 2; 3 = see Table 2; 4 = incubation with L-[4,5-^{3}H]lysine monohydrochloride, 10^{-3} M, phosphate buffer, pH 8.2, 2 h, 23°C.

oxidation) furnishes a carboxylated surface displaying 31.7 pmol/cm^2 of reactive functions (entry 8); this surface appears very similar to the one of membrane A (entry 10), and, therefore, can be considered as a model surface for the coupling of bioactive molecules. The membrane A with a low density of pores offers 30.7 pmol/cm^2 of reactive CO$_2$H functions; surface oxidation leads to a value of 51.5 pmol/cm^2 (entry 12). The membrane B with a high density of pores appears more fragile and susceptible to some erosion under the wet chemistry conditions. The native membrane B displays 24.4 pmol/cm^2 of CO$_2$H groups; this amount is practically unchanged after the oxidative treatment (entries 14 and 16), due to some surface degradation.

The assays of the PET surface hydroxyl groups (Scheme 14; Table 5) show similar results for the native samples: the film precursor, membrane A and membrane B offer 4.8, 26.3 and 32.5 pmol/cm^2 of reactive OH groups, respectively (entries 2, 10 and 14). Surface hydrolysis of the film significantly enhances the number of hydroxyl chain ends (20.5 pmol/cm^2, entry 6). On the

TABLE 5   Surface Labeling of the PET Hydroxyl Chain-Ends [80,82]

| Entry | Sample (treatment) | Fixed ^{3}H-lysine (pmol) | | |
		Sample	cm^2	Corrected
1	Film (4)	5.8 (1.6)	2.2 (0.6)	
2	Film (3 + 4)	18.9 (1.8)	7.0 (0.7)	4.8
3	Film (2 + 4)	11.7 (1.3)	4.4 (0.5)	
4	Film (2 + 3 + 4)	31.9 (4.5)	12.1 (1.7)	7.7
5	Film (1 + 4)	6.1 (1.6)	2.3 (0.6)	
6	Film (1 + 3 + 4)	60.6 (2.9)	22.8 (1.1)	20.5
7	Film (1 + 2 + 4)	26.3 (6.6)	9.9 (2.5)	
8	Film (1 + 2 + 3 + 4)	35.6 (6.4)	13.4 (2.4)	3.5
9	Membrane A (4)	9.5 (1.0)	3.1 (0.3)	
10	Membrane A (3 + 4)	88.6 (7.6)	29.4 (2.5)	26.3
11	Membrane A (2 + 4)	14.2 (3.1)	4.7 (1.0)	
12	Membrane A (2 + 3 + 4)	73.5 (10.5)	24.4 (3.5)	19.7
13	Membrane B (4)	29.5 (2.6)	1.3 (0.1)	
14	Membrane B (3 + 4)	759.5 (48.5)	33.8 (2.1)	32.5
15	Membrane B (2 + 4)	58.1 (24.5)	2.6 (1.1)	
16	Membrane B (2 + 3 + 4)	579.8 (157.6)	25.8 (7.0)	23.2

Film, Membrane A, Membrane B: see Table 2.
Treatment: 1 = basic hydrolysis (NaOH, H$_2$O—CH$_3$CN, 60°C, 18 h); 2 = reduction (NaBH$_4$-catechol, THF, 20°C, 17 h); 3 = activation (Ts-Cl, pyridine, acetone, reflux, 1 h); 4 = labeling (incubation with L-[4,5-^{3}H]lysine monohydrochloride, 10^{-3} M, phosphate buffer, pH 8.2, 2 h, 23°C).

other hand, the reductive treatment appears poorly efficient for all types of samples (entries 4, 12, and 16), giving some surface degradation (SEM analyses) [80].

Interestingly, the coupling of a diisocyanate spacer-arm (Scheme 15) on the hydroxyl chain-ends offers high levels of surface labeling (Table 6). Pretreated film (hydrolysis), and membranes A and B give values of fixed lysine* within 35–58 pmol/cm^2.

A simple model has been considered [78] for discussing the LSC measurements. Assuming that one PET repeated unit should occupy a three-dimensional box of $4.56 \times 5.94 \times 10.75$ Å^3, and that, at least, 10 atomic layers (the domain usually investigated by the XPS technique) should be affected by the surface wet chemistry, we calculate [100] the average of 1.72×10^{15} PET monomer units per cm^2 of film (membrane) sample, or about 2850 pmol/cm^2. Thus experimental values of 30–60 pmol/cm^2 of labeling mean that 1–2% of the surface monomer units consist of chain-ends that have fixed the lysine*.

D. Dual Labeling with ^{3}H/F Tags

In order to compare the LSC (open surface) and XPS (apparent surface) analytical techniques, we have derivatized the surface of various PET samples with the ^{3}H- and F-labeled reagents 2* and 3* (Schemes 16 and 17), prepared from ^{3}H-lysine (lys*) and ^{3}H-glycine (gly*), respectively [79,83].

TABLE 6 Surface Labeling of the PET Hydroxyl Chain-Ends via the Coupling of a Diisocyanate Spacer Arm

		Fixed ^{3}H-lysine (pmol)		
Entry	Sample (treatment)	Sample	cm^2	Corrected
1	Film (3)	6.7 (1.1)	2.5 (0.4)	
2	Film (2 + 4)	23.7 (2.4)	8.9 (0.9)	6.4
3	Film (1 + 3)	29.0 (4.3)	10.9 (1.6)	
4	Film (1 + 2 + 3)	119.7 (21.8)	45.0 (8.2)	34.1
5	Membrane A (3)	29.5 (3.6)	9.8 (1.2)	
6	Membrane A (2 + 3)	200.2 (18.1)	66.5 (6.0)	56.7
7	Membrane B (3)	58.4 (9.0)	2.6 (0.4)	
8	Membrane B (4 + 3)	1379.7 (530.3)	61.4 (23.6)	58.8

Film, Membrane A, Membrane B: see Table 2.
Treatment: 1 = see Table 5; 2 = coupling to MDPI (1.25% in toluene, 1 h, 18°C); 3 = labeling (10^{-3} M ^{3}H-lysine, pH 7.2, 4 h, 23°C); 4 = coupling to MDPI during 2 h.
Source: Ref. 82.

TABLE 7 Tandem Analysis of PET-CO$_2$H Derivatized Samples by XPS and LSC Using the Label 2*

Entry	Sample (treatment)	LSC (open surface) pmol/cm^2; corrected		XPS (%) (apparent surface) F/C × 100; corrected	
1	Film (1 + 2 + 4)	49.9 (7.4)		0.069	
2	Film (1 + 2 + 3 + 4)	151.9 (11.5)	102.0	0.373	0.30 (1.0%)
3	Membrane A (2 + 4)	31.2 (9.8)		0.014	
4	Membrane A (2 + 3 + 4)	153.8 (2.3)	122.6	0.389	0.37 (1.2%)
5	Membrane B (2 + 4)	35.2 (1.7)		0.027	
6	Membrane B (2 + 3 + 4)	127.7 (6.0)	92.5	0.264	0.24 (0.8%)

Film, Membrane A, Membrane B, Treatments 1 to 4 and %: see Table 2.
Label 2*: L-[4,5-^{3}H]trifluoroethyl-lysinamide (see Scheme 16).

The coupling of 2* to the surface carboxyl functions of fully pretreated films and oxidized membranes give nearly close XPS results, i.e., about 0.8–1.2% of derivatized monomer units (sampling depth of 50 Å) (Table 7, Scheme 16). From the LSC measurements, we obtain values within 90–120 pmol-cm^2, meaning that the open surfaces of the various samples are chemically very similar. Comparison between the LSC results of Table 4 (entries 8, 12 and 16) and Table 7 (entries 2, 4 and 6) clearly shows that the lipophilic character of the label strongly influences its reactivity; the lysinamide 2* appears three times more reactive than lysine* itself. Since the XPS results do not show such a difference in reactivity (compare Tables 2 and 7), we assume that the most lipophilic label 2* should penetrate more deeply into the polymer interface; according to our model (see section III.C), we can estimate a derivatized domain of about 150 Å in depth [79]. The coupling of 2* to the PET surface hydroxyl functions (Scheme 17A; Table 8, entries 1 to 6) has conducted to the same conclusions.

The direct fixation of the isocyanate label 3* (Scheme 17B; Table 8, entries 7–12), under anhydrous conditions, provides the highest levels of functionalization. From the comparison between the XPS values (1.3–2% of labeled monomer units in 50 Å depth) and the LSC values (90–140 pmol/cm^2), we can conclude that the membranes modification has occurred in a domain of about 125 Å in depth [83].

At last, we have examined the possibility to react the perfluorobutyl ester moiety, displayed on the PET-OH membranes derivatized with the label 3*, with lysine* (Scheme 18). After 4 H of reaction (10^{-3} M lysine*, pH 8.2, 22°C),

TABLE 8 Tandem Analysis of PET-OH Derivatized Samples by XPS and LSC Using the Labels 2* and 3*

Entry	Sample (treatment)	LSC (open surface) pmol/cm^2; corrected		XPS (%) (apparent surface) F/C × 100
1	Film (2)	25.7 (16.8)		—
2	Film (1 + 2)	33.4 (2.6)	7.7	—
3	Membrane A (2)	23.0 (2.2)		0.000
4	Membrane A (1 + 2)	51.6 (8.5)	28.6	0.284 (1.0%)
5	Membrane B (2)	12.3 (0.7)		0.000
6	Membrane B (1 + 2)	92.4 (3.8)	80.1	0.414 (1.4%)
7	Film (3)	0.6 (0.2)		0.000
8	Film (4)	15.7 (0.8)	15.1	0.406 (0.6%)
9	Membrane A (3)	4.2 (0.7)		0.000
10	Membrane A (4)	94.2 (15.1)	90.0	0.882 (1.3%)
11	Membrane B (3)	0.4 (0.1)		0.000
12	Membrane B (4)	143.7 (5.8)	143.3	1.379 (2.0%)
13	Membrane A (3 + 5)	13.9 (2.9)		
14	Membrane A (4 + 5)	118.3 (17.7)	104.4	0.363 (0.5%)
	Lys* contribution = entry14-entry10		14.4	

Film, Membrane A, Membrane B, Treatments 1–4 and %: see Table 3.
Treatment 5 = incubation with ^{3}H-lysine (10^{-3} M, pH 8.2, 4 h, 22°C).
Label 2*: see Table 8; Label 3*: heptafluorobutyl (p-isocyanatobenzoyl)-[2-^{3}H]glycinate (see Scheme 17).

most of the fluorine atoms have been removed from the surface (Table 8, entry 14, XPS analysis). This results from ester substitution and hydrolysis. The contribution of the nucleophilic displacement with lysine* has been counted by LSC (Table 8, entries 10 and 14); a value of 14.4 pmol/cm^2 has been found.

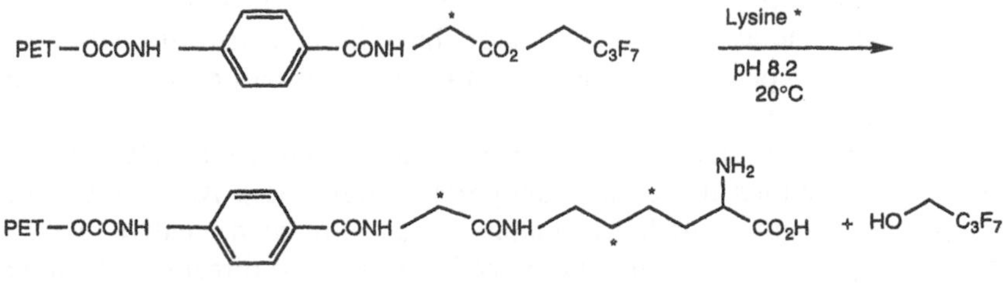

SCHEME 18 Dual labeling of PET-OH membranes.

This sequence of reactions (Schemes 17B and 18) constitutes an original strategy for anchoring bioactive molecules on PET membranes via a spacer-arm [83].

IV. NEW DEVELOPMENTS FOR FUNCTIONALIZED POLYMER MEMBRANES

Recently, new applications for membranes have appeared that do not make use of the membranes as simple separation barriers for filtrations [101].

Affinity membranes (grafted with affinity ligands) have been introduced in downstream processing of proteins as selective protein adsorbers [102].

Membranes are used as substrates for catalyst immobilization; for instance, lipase-immobilized capsule membranes work as efficient microreactors in ester syntheses and hydrolyses in organic solvents [103].

Supramolecular nano-engineering develops at functionalized surfaces to control protein organization [104].

Optical resolution membranes offer the possibility to treat large amounts of racemic compounds in one operation [105].

Controlled delivery systems utilize drugs loaded on polymer membranes; performant and stimuli-responsive systems has been developed (sensitivity to electricity, pH, glucose concentration, temperature) [106,107].

Polymer membranes have been integrated in in vitro culture systems of anchorage dependent animal cells [81,108–115]. This application opens the route towards tissue engineering, i.e., the development of functioning biological substitutes for damaged human tissues or organs [116,117].

Polymers are also widely used as biomaterials [118–122]; in particular, blood compatible devices and implants are made from surface modified polymer membranes [123,124]. The present development of polymer biomaterials are based on active biocompatibilization strategies which involve the surface immobilization of specific biological signals (heparin, RGD mimetics, growth factors ...) that are susceptible to selectively interact with proteins blood constituents, cells or tissues [125].

Lastly, calibrated microporous membranes have played a great part in the recent development of nanomaterials [126–128]; template syntheses of conductive polymers, metals, or semiconductors have been carried out within the membrane pores. Depending on the pore wall chemical nature, nanofibrils or nanotubules can be produced.

It is well established that surface chemistry and structure strongly influence the interfacial functions of polymer supports (membranes). Accordingly, the increasing requirement of intelligent materials has stimulated creative research in the field of polymer surface functionalization in view to direct specific interactions, and even, to generate selective recognition processes.

The aim of a better understanding of fundamental structure–property relationships needs the further development of sensitive analytical techniques for properly characterizing solid surfaces. For this purpose, the radiochemical assays we have setting up to analyze pore walls could be particularly helpful in the design of nanoreactors made of track-etched membranes.

REFERENCES

1. L. Cecille and J.-C. Toussaint (eds.), *Future Industrial Prospects of Membrane Processes*, Elsevier Applied Science, London 1989.
2. J. I. Kroschwitz (ed.), *Encyclopedia of Polymer Science and Engineering*, Wiley-Interscience Publication, New York, 1990 pp. 598–605.
3. M. C. Porter (ed.), *Handbook of Industrial Membrane Technology*, Noyes Publications, Park Ridge, New Jersey, 1990.
4. C. Dickenson, *Filters and Filtration Handbook*, Elsevier Advanced Technology, Oxford, 1992.
5. R. L. Fleischer, P. B. Price, and R. W. Walker, *Nuclear Tracks in Solids*, University of California Press, Berkeley, 1975.
6. E. Ferain and R. Legras, Nucl. Instrum. Methods Phys. Res. B, *84*: 331 (1994).
7. P. Y. Apel, Radiation Measurements 25: 667 (1995).
8. T. K. Rostovtseva, C. L. Bashford, G. M. Alder, G. N. Hill, C. McGiffert, P. Y. Apel, G. Lowe, and C. A. Pasternak, J. Membrane Biol., *151*: 29 (1996).
9. J. I. Calvo, A. Hernandez, P. Pradanos, and F. Tejerina, J. Colloid Interface Sci. *181*: 399 (1996).
10. J. I. Calvo, A. Hernandez, G. Caruana, and L. Martinez, J. Colloid Interface Sci. *175*: 138 (1995).
11. J. I. Calvo, A. Hernandez, P. Pradanos, L. Martinez, and W. R. Bowen, J. Colloid Interface Sci. *176*: 467 (1995).
12. E. Ferain and R. Legras, Nucl. Instrum. Methods Phys. Res. B *82*: 539 (1993).
13. W. J. Feast, H. S. Munro, and R. W. Richards (eds), *Polymer Surfaces and Interfaces II*, John Wiley and Sons, New York, 1993.
14. L. S. Penn and H. Wang, Polym. Adv. Technol. *5*: 809 (1994).
15. J. J. Pesek (ed), *Chemically Modified Surface*, The Royal Society of Chemistry, Special Publication 139, 1994.
16. F. Garbassi, M. Morra, and E. Occhiello, *Polymer Surfaces, from Physics to Technology*, John Wiley and Sons, New York, 1994.
17. J. J. Pesek, M. Matyska, and R. Abuelafiya (ed.), *Chemically Modified Surface, Recent Developments*, The Royal Society of Chemistry, Special Publication 173, 1996.
18. E. M. Tracey and R. H. Davis, J. Colloid Interface Sci. *167*: 104 (1994).
19. J. D. Le Roux, D. R. Paul, J. Kampa, and R. J. Lagow, J. Membr. Sci *94*: 121 (1994).
20. D. Mukherjee, A. Kulkarni, and W. N. Gill, J. Membr. Sci. *97*: 231 (1994).
21. G. Clarotti, A. A. Ben Aoumar, F. Schué, J. Sledz, K. E. Geckeler, D. Flösch, and A. Orsetti, Makromol. Chem. *192*: 2581 (1991).

22. A. Akelah and A. Moet, *Funtionalized Polymers and their Applications*, Chapman and Hall, London, 1990.
23. M. Lazár, T. Bleha, and J. Rychly, *Chemical Reactions of Natural and Synthetic Polymers*, Ellis Horwood Ltd, New York, 1989.
24. T. S. Godjevargova, A. R. Dimov, and N. Vasileva, J. Appl. Polym. Sci., *54*:355 (1994); J. Membr. Sci. *116*:273 (1996).
25. S. Pereira Nunes and K. V. Peinemann, J. Membrane Sci. 73:25 (1992).
26. K. Takata, H. Ihara, and T. Sata, Angew. Makromol. Chem. *236*:67 (1996).
27. L. E. S. Brink, S. J. G. Elbers, T. Robbertsen, and P. Both, J. Membr. Sci. *76*:281 (1993).
28. N. P. Desai and J. A. Hubbell, Macromolecules *25*:226 (1992); Biomaterials *13*:505 (1992).
29. H. V. Boenig, *Fundamentals of Plasma Chemistry and Technology*, Technomic Publishing Co. Inc., Lancaster, 1988.
30. J. Hopkins and J. P. S. Badyal, J. Phys. Chem. *99*:4261 (1995).
31. I. K. Meier, M. Langsam, and H. C. Klotz, J. Membr. Sci. *94*:195 (1994).
32. D. Jan, J. S. Jeon, and S. Raghavan, J. Adhesion Sci. Technol. *8*:1157 (1994).
33. S. Mok, D. J. Worsfold, A. Fouda, and T. Matsuura, J. Appl. Polym. Sci. *51*:193 (1994).
34. M. Ulbricht, A. Oechel, C. Lehmann, G. Tomaschewski, and H.-G. Hicke, J. Appl. Polym. Sci. *55*:1707 (1995).
35. M. Ulbricht, Reactive Functional Polym. *31*:165 (1996).
36. M. Ulbricht, H. Matuschewski, A. Oechel, and H.-G. Hicke, J. Membr. Sci. *115*:31 (1996).
37. T. Masuoka, O. Hirasa, Y. Suda, and M. Ohnishi, Radiat. Phys. Chem. (Int. J. Radiat. Appl. Instrum. Part C) *33*:421 (1989).
38. X. Libo, S. Tianyi, F. Yue'e, and L. Ming, Water Treatment *9*:41 (1994).
39. H. Thelen, R. Kaufmann, D. Klee, and H. Höcher, Fresenius J. Anal. Chem. *353*:290 (1995).
40. J.-Y. Lai, C.-W. Tseng, and K.-R. Lee, J. Appl. Polym. Sci. *61*:307 (1996).
41. M. Ulbricht and G. Belfort, J. Membr. Sci. *111*:193 (1996).
42. Y. Ito, L.-S. Liu, R. Matsuo, and Y. Imanishi, J. Biomed. Mater. Res. *26*:1065 (1992).
43. C. Nojiri, S. Kuroda, N. Saito, K. D. Park, K. Hagiwara, K. Senshu, T. Kido, T. Sugiyama, T. Kijima, Y. H. Kim, K. Sakai, and T. Akutsu, ASAIO J. *41*:M389 (1995).
44. T. J. McCarthy, Chimia *44*:316 (1990).
45. M. Pasternak, J. Appl. Polym. Sci. *57*:1211 (1995).
46. C. Nojiri, K. Hagiwara, K. Yokoyama, E. Kuribayashi, K. Hidaka, N. Ishida, K. Horiuchi, H. Oshiyama, A. Nogawa, T. Kido, T. Kijima, and T. Akutsu, ASAIO J. *41*:M561 (1995).
47. H. Kise and H. Ogata, J. Polym. Sci.: Polym. Chem. Edit. *21*:3343 (1983).
48. A. J. Dias and T. J. McCarthy, Polym. Mater. Sci. Eng. *49*:574 (1983); Macromolecules *17*:2529 (1984).
49. J. V. Brennan and T. J. McCarthy, Polym. Prepr. *29*:338 (1988); Polym Prepr. *30*:153 (1989).

50. R. Crowe and J. P. S. Badyal, J. Chem. Soc., Chem. Commun. 958 (1991).

51. J. Marchand-Brynaert, N. Jongen, and J.-L. Dewez, J. Polym. Sci., Part A: Polym. Chem. *35*: 1227 (1997).

52. C. Daubresse, T. Sergen-Engelen, E. Ferain, Y.-J. Schneider, and R. Legras, Nucl. Instr. Methods Phys. Res. *B105*: 126 (1995).

53. J. de Andrade Rodrigues, J. Combrink, and W. F. Brandt, Anal. Biochem. *216*: 365 (1994).

54. M. G. Roig, J. F. Bello, S. Rodriguez, J. M. Cachaza, and J. F. Kennedy, J. Mol. Catal. *93*: 85 (1994).

55. D. Düputell and E. Staude, J. Membr. Sci. *78*: 45 (1993).

56. A. Higuchi, N. Iwata, M. Tsubaki, and T. Nakagawa, J. Appl. Polym. Sci. *36*: 1753 (1988).

57. L. Breitbach, E. Hinke, and E. Staude, Angew. Makromol. Chem. *184*: 183 (1991).

58. M. Ulbricht, M. Riedel, and U. Marx, J. Membr. Sci. *120*: 239 (1996).

59. H. Yamagishi, J. V. Crivello, and G. Belfort, J. Membr. Sci. *105*: 237 and 249 (1995).

60. E. Ferain and R. Legras, Nucl. Instr. Methods Phs. Res. *B89*: 163 (1993).

61. N. L. Franchina and T. J. McCarthy, Macromolecules *24*: 3045 (1991).

62. N. L. Franchina and T. J. McCarthy, in *Chemically Modified Surfaces* (H. A. Mottola and J. R. Steinmetz, eds.), Elsevier Science Publishers, 1992, pp. 173–189.

63. O. Noiset, C. Henneuse, Y.-J. Schneider, and J. Marchand-Brynaert, Macromolecules *30*: 540 (1997).

64. J. Marchand-Brynaert, G. Pantano, and O. Noiset, Polymer *38*: 1387 (1997).

65. C. Henneuse, B. Goret, and J. Marchand-Brynaert, Polymer *39*: 835 (1998).

66. O. Noiset, Y.-J. Schneider, and J. Marchand-Brynaert, J. Polym. Sci., Part A: Polym. Chem. *35*: 3779 (1997).

67. J. Marchand-Brynaert, T. Boxus, M. Deldime-Rubbens, C. Henneuse, S. Jaumotte-Thelen, P. Mougenot, O. Noiset, and Y.-J. Schneider, ICPS-2 Proceedings, Namur, Belgium, 1997.

68. C. A. Finch (ed.), *Polyvinyl Alcohol—Developments*, John Wiley, New York, 1992.

69. R. H. Li and T. A. Barbari, J. Membr. Sci. *88*: 115 (1994).

70. M. S. Shoichet, S. R. Winn, S. Athavale, J. Milton Harris, and F. T. Gentile, Biotechnology Bioengineering *43*: 563 (1994).

71. H.-G. Hicke, P. Böhme, M. Becker, H. Schulze, and M. Ulbricht, J. Appl. Polym. Sci. *60*: 1147 (1996).

72. F. Martinez-Villa, L. Martinez, J. I. Arribas, and F. Tejerina, J. Membr. Sci. *36*: 31 (1988).

73. J. Mueller and R. H. Davis, J. Membr. Sci. *116*: 47 (1996).

74. I. M. Yamazaki, R. Paterson, and L. P. Geraldo, J. Membr. Sci. *118*: 239 (1996).

75. Y. Ito, M. Inaba, D.-J. Chung, and Y. Imanishi, Macromolecules *25*: 7313 (1992).

76. C. A. Pasternak, G. M. Alder, P. Y. Abel, C. L. Bashford, D. T. Edmonds, Y. E. Korchev, A. A. Lev, G. Lowe, M. Milovanivich, C. W. Pitt, T. K. Rostovtseva, and N. I. Zhitariuk, Radiation Measurements *25*: 675 (1995).

77. C. A. Pasternak, G. M. Alder, P. Y. Abel, C. L. Bashford, Y. E. Korchev, A. A.

Lev, T. K. Rostovtseva, and N. I. Zhitariuk, Nucl. Instr. Methods Phys. Res. *B105*:332 (1995).

78. J. Marchand-Brynaert, M. Deldime, I. Dupont, J.-L. Dewez, and Y.-J. Schneider, J. Celloid, Interface Sci. *173*:236 (1995).

79. M. Deldime, J.-L. Dewez, Y.-J. Schneider, and J. Marchand-Brynaert, Appl. Surface Sci. *90*:1 (1995).

80. T. Boxus, M. Deldime-Rubbens, P. Mougenot, Y.-J. Schneider, and J. Marchand-Brynaert, Polym. Adv. Technol. *7*:589 (1996).

81. S. Jaumotte-Thelen, I. Dozot-Dupont, J. Marchand-Brynaert, and Y.-J. Schneider, J. Biomed, Mater. Res. *32*:569 (1996).

82. P. Mougenot, M. Koch, I. Dupont, Y.-J. Schneider, and J. Marchand-Brynaert, J. Colloid Interface Sci. *177*:162 (1996).

83. P. Mougenot and J. Marchand-Brynaert, Macromolecules *29*:3552 (1996).

84. J. M. Walls (ed.) *Methods of Surface Analysis, Techniques and Applications*, Cambridge University Press, Cambridge, 1989.

85. D. R. Scheuing (ed.), *Fourier Transform Infrared Spectroscopy in Colloid and Interface Science*, ACS Symposium Series 447, Am. Chem. Soc., Washington, 1991.

86. J. Marchand-Brynaert, Chimie Nouvelle *14*:1613 (1996).

87. A. K. Fritzsche, A. R. Arevalo, M. D. Moore, V. B. Elings, K. Kjoller, and C. M. Wu, J. Membr. Sci. *68*:65 (1992).

88. C. C. Warmser and M. I. Gilbert, Langmuir *8*:1608 (1992).

89. D. Flösch, H.-D. Lehmann, R. Reichl, O. Inacke, and W. Göpel, J. Membr. Sci. *70*:53 (1992).

90. S. Zeggane and M. Delamar, Appl. Surf. Sci. *31*:151 (1988).

91. D. S. Everhart and C. N. Reilly, Anal. Chem. *53*:665 (1981).

92. Y. Nakayama, T. Takahagi, F. Soeda, K. Hatada, S. Nagaoka, J. Suzuki, and A. Ishitani, J. Polym. Sci. Part A: Polym. Chem. *26*:559 (1988).

93. A. Chiltoki, B. D. Ratner, and D. Briggs, Chem. Mater. *3*:51 (1991).

94. Y. Tamada and Y. Ikada, Polymer *34*:2209 (1993).

95. Considering the polymer repeated unit $-CO-C_6H_4-CO_2-CH_2CH_2-O-(C_{10}H_8O_4)$ and the derivatized chain end unit $-CO-C_6H_4-CO_2-CH_2-CONH-CH_2-CONH-CH_2-CF_3$ $(C_{14}H_{12}O_5N_2F_3)$, we calculate the percentage of labeled units as follows. For a mixture of 99.2% $(C_{10}H_8O_4)$ and 0.8% $(C_{14}H_{12}O_5N_2F_3)$, $F/C \times 100 = 2.4 \times 100/1003.2 = 0.239$ (experimental value = 0.24).

96. Considering the polymer repeated unit $(C_{10}H_8O_4)$ and the derivatized chain end unit $-CO-C_6H_4-CO_2-CH_2-CONH-(CH_2)_4-CH(NH_2)-CONH-CH_2-CF_3$ $(C_{18}H_{21}O_5N_3F_3)$, we calculate the percentage of labeled units as follows. For a mixture of 98.9% $(C_{10}H_8O_4)$ and 1.1% $(C_{18}H_{21}O_5N_3F_3)$, $F/C \times 100 = 3.3 \times 100/1008.8 = 0.327$ (experimental value = 0.33).

97. We considered the modified chain end unit $-CO-C_6H_4-CO_2-CH_2-CH_2-NH-(CH_2)_4-CH(NH_2)-CONH-CH_2-CF_3$ $(C_{18}H_{23}O_4N_3F_3)$. For a mixture of 98.6% $(C_{10}H_8O_4)$ and 1.4% $(C_{18}H_{23}O_4N_3F_3)$, $F/C \times 100 = 4.2 \times 100/1011.2 = 0.415$ (experimental value = 0.41).

98. We considered the modified chain end unit $-CO-C_6H_4-CO_2-CH_2$

$- CH_2 - OCONH - C_6H_4 - CONH - CH_2 - CO_2 - CH_2 - C_3F_7$ ($C_{24}H_{18}O_8N_2F_7$). For a mixture of 98% ($C_{10}H_8O_4$) and 2% ($C_{24}H_{18}O_8N_2F_7$), $F/C \times 100 = 14 \times 100/1028 = 1.36$ (experimental value = 1.38).

99. We used PET disks of 13 mm in diameter (12 μm thick). The open surface of film samples is 2.66 cm^2; of membrane A (low density of pores) is 3.01 cm^2; of membrane B (high density of pores) is 22.47 cm^2.

100. From the crystallographic data (H. F. Mark, N. M. Bikales, C. G. Overberger, G. Menges, and J. I. Kroschwitz, *Encyclopedia of Polymer Science and Engineering*, Wiley-Interscience, New York, 1985), we calculated that the PET monomer unit occupies a volume of 291 Å^3 or 2.91×10^{-22} cm^3. The volume covered by an apparent surface of 1 cm^2 and accessible to the chemical transformation was estimated to be 5×10^{-7} cm^3 (about 10 atomic layers). Therefore, this volume contains about 1.72×1015 monomer units, corresponding to 0.2856×10^{-8} moles of $C_8H_{10}O_4$ or 2856 pmoles. This calculation roughly applies to film and membrane samples. Indeed, the "empty volumes" of the calibrated membranes are negligible (0.3% for membrane A and 13% for membrane B) [79].

101. J. Haggin, Chem. Eng. October 1, 22 (1990).

102. T. C. Beeskow, W. Kusharyoto, F. B. Anspach, K. H. Kroner, and W.-D. Deckwer, J. Chromatogr. A. *715*:49 (1995).

103. K. Ijiro and Y. Okahata, J. Membr. Sci. *59*:101 (1991).

104. W. Knoll, L. Angermaier, G. Batz, T. Fritz, S. Fujisawa, T. Furuno, H.-J. Guder, M. Hara, M. Liley, K. Niki, and J. Spinke, Synthetic Metals *61*:5 (1993).

105. T. Aoki, A. Maruyama, K. Shinohara, and E. Oikawa, Polymer J. *27*:547 (1995).

106. Y. Moo Lee, S. Yoon Ihm, J. Kie Shim, J. Hong Kim, C. Soo Cho, and Y. Kiel Sung, Polymer *36*:81 (1995).

107. Y. Moo Lee and J. Kie Shim, J. Appl. Polymer Sci. *61*:1245 (1996).

108. T. Sergent-Engelen, C. Halleux, E. Ferain, H. Hanot, R. Legras, and Y.-J. Schneider, Biotechn. Techn. *4*:89 (1990).

109. J.-L. Dewez, A. Doren, Y.-J. Schneider, R. Legras, and P. G. Rouxhet, Surface Interface Anal. *17*:499 (1991).

110. J.-L. Dewez, A. Doren, Y.-J. Schneider, R. Legras, and P. G. Rouxhet, in *Interfaces in New Materials* (P. Grange and B. Delmon, eds.), Elsevier Applied Science, London, 1991, pp. 84–94.

111. C. Halleux and Y.-J. Schneider, In Vitro Cell. Dev. Biol. *27A*:293 (1991).

112. G. Schmid, C. R. Wilke, and H. W. Blanch, J. Biotechnol. *22*:31 (1992).

113. T. Sergent-Engelen, V. Delistrie, and Y.-J. Schneider, Biochem. Pharmacol. *46*:1393 (1993).

114. C. Halleux and Y.-J. Schneider, J. Cell. Physiol. *158*:17 (1994).

115. S. Thelen-Jaumotte, I. Dozot-Dupont, J. Marchand-Brynaert, and Y.-J. Schneider, J. Material Sci.: Materials in Medicine 7:162 (1996).

116. J. A. Hubbell and R. Langer, Chem. Eng. March 13, 42 (1995).

117. J. A. Hubbell, Biotechnol. *13*:565 (1995).

118. J. I. Kroschwitz (ed.), *Polymers: Biomaterials and Medical Applications*, Encyclopedia Reprint Series, John Wiley and Sons, New York, 1989, pp. 276–346.

119. D. Williams, *Concise Encyclopedia of Medical and Dental Materials*, Pergamon Press, Oxford, 1990, pp. 212–219.

120. S. W. Shalaby, Y. Ikada, R. Langer, and J. Williams (eds.), *Polymers of Biological and Medical Significance*, ACS Symposium Series 540, Am. Chem. Soc., Washington, 1994.
121. J. Marchand-Brynaert, Chimie Nouvelle *14*: 1580 (1996).
122. B. D. Ratner, Surface Interface Anal. *23*: 521 (1995).
123. C. Espadas-Torre and M. E. Meyerhoff, Anal. Chem. *67*: 3108 (1995).
124. J. R. Frautschi, R. Eberhart, J. A. Hubbell, B. D. Clark, and J. A. Gelfand, J. Biomater. Sci. Polymer Edn. *7*: 707 (1996).
125. J. A. Hubbell, Trends Polymer Sci. (TRIP) *2*: 20 (1994).
126. C. J. Brumlik and C. R. Martin, J. Am. Chem. Soc. *113*: 3174 (1991).
127. C. R. Martin, Adv. Mater *3*: 457 (1991).
128. C. R. Martin, Science, *266*: 1961 (1994).

4

Formation Process, Analysis and Structure of Silica Polymers, Fractal Aggregates and Membranes

BALAGOPAL N. NAIR Japan Chemical Innovation Institute, Tokyo, Japan

KLAAS KEIZER Department of Chemistry, Potchefstroom University for Christian Higher Education, Potchefstroom, Republic of South Africa

NORBERT MAENE VITO, Mol, Belgium

TATSUYA OKUBO and SHIN-ICHI NAKAO Department of Chemical System Engineering, University of Tokyo, Tokyo, Japan

Abstract

Microporous silica membranes are candidate materials for gas separation processes due to high selectivity, and high stability at enhanced temperatures and in chemically aggressive environments compared to their polymeric counterparts. Sol–gel synthesis of the polymeric silica sol and coating a substrate with that sol is the best known way to produce microporous silica membranes. The structure of silica polymers in the sol should be the most important parameter deciding the final properties of the membrane. Nevertheless no such structure–property correlation has so far been reported. This chapter aims to give the reader a systematic understanding of silica polymeric growth, synthesis chemistry and finally membrane characterization. Polymeric silica sols were prepared by hydrolysis and condensation of alkoxide. The fractal growth of the polymers during sol–gel transition is monitored with the help of Small Angle X-ray Scattering. Fractal dimensions and radii of gyration of sols and gels with different synthesis chemistry are compared. The type of aggregation mechanism prevailing in these systems is identified. The morphological formation of silica gels and membranes are evaluated by analyzing the porosity of the gel and gas permeation behavior of the membrane. The correlation between the sol synthesis parameters, fractal structure of the polymers, porosity of the gel and gas permeation/ separation behavior of the membrane are presented. It is shown that the optimization of sol synthesis parameters can lead to microporous silica membranes with molecular-sieving ability.

I. INTRODUCTION

Inorganic membranes are considered as candidate materials for gas separation. For high separation factors obviously the pore size of these membranes must lie in the microporous range at most. Amorphous silica, zeolite, porous glass and hollow carbon fibers are known to show such small pore sizes. The synthesis and processing of such membranes however is still a difficult task owing to the complications involved in packing these fine structures into a form which can withstand high temperature and pressure conditions during testing. This chapter is dedicated to an overview of the synthesis and processing conditions of one of these membranes, namely silica which has the maximum flexibility in synthesis and hence is projected to be the most interesting microporous membrane material.

A variety of silica membranes with amorphous structure are available for separation applications. Based on pore structure we can roughly characterize them into dense membranes made by chemical vapor deposition (CVD) processes, ultra microporous membranes made by polymeric sol–gel method and supermicroporous (and mesoporous) membranes made by colloidal silica method. More over, a number of silica glass membranes are widely studied for membrane applications.

The sol–gel process is the well known processing method as far as silica membranes are considered. Under moderate reaction conditions such processing leads to membranes with ultramicropores, as they are generally called, with high selectivity between small inorganic molecules such as He or H_2 and bigger inorganic or hydrocarbon counter parts. The present chapter is dedicated to detail the processing and structure of such membranes. However, before that, we would like to attract the attention of the readers to common amorphous silica composite membranes.

II. SILICA MEMBRANES

A variety of silica based membranes are available for gas separation purposes. These can broadly be classified into membranes with and without any composite structure. Microporous glass membranes have normally a symmetrical structure. Silica membranes with composite configuration are generally made by depositing an amorphous layer of silica over an inorganic support. Hence such structures can further be classified based on the structure of the depositing material and on the method of deposition.

A. Silica Membranes by Chemical Vapor Deposition (CVD)

Porous Vycor tubes with deposited silica in the pore are reported to be microporous (or dense). The deposition of silica was done by CVD. Gavalas and co-workers reported the formation of such a membrane capable of hydrogen separation in 1989 [1]. The composite inorganic membrane was developed by deposition of a 160 nm thick SiO_2 film in porous Vycor glass tube. The deposition was achieved by opposing reaction configuration, wherein the SiH_4 was allowed to flow through the porous tube and O_2 outside. The reactants diffused in opposite directions inside pores of the tube and the product was deposited in the pore wall. The developed film in turn plugged the flow of reactants thus stopping further deposition and hence unnecessary thickening of the deposition.

In a typical deposition process they used Vycor tube of 28% porosity and mean pore diameter 4 nm. The outer diameter of the tube was 7 mm and thickness 1.1 mm. 10% SiH_4/N_2 was flowing through the tube at a rate of 30 cm^3/min and 33% O_2/N_2 through the outside at a rate of 45 cm^3/min. The pressure was kept atmospheric. The tube was preheated at 450°C and cleaned by flushing with nitrogen. The oxidation of SiH_4 to SiO_2 happens inside the pores. The reaction was completed within 15 min. However, exposure to ambient atmosphere made the membrane densify and shrink introducing unwanted porosity into the deposited layer. A second CVD layer became necessary to plug these pores. The permeation of H_2 (at 100°C) decreased by a magnitude to 10^{-10} mol/m^2.s.Pa by this second deposition. The activation energy on the other hand has gone up from 22 kJ/mol to 34.7 kJ/mol. The final separation factor of H_2 at 450°C to nitrogen was reported as 115.

Asaeda has investigated [2] the possibility of repairing sol–gel made silica membranes by the CVD method. High separation factors could be obtained (He/N_2 573 at 300°C). The activation energy for diffusion went higher after the CVD to 8.1 kJ/mol for He and 12.2 for H_2 compared to the value of 4 and 8.3 before treatment. The CVD treatment was believed to plug pinholes. The CVD set-up used was nearly the same as that of Gavalas except the fact that O_2 mixture was flowing through the tube in this case and helium was used as the carrier gas.

Okubu and Inoue used CVD [3] of tetraethoxysilane (TEOS or tetra-ethyl-ortho-silicate) to modify porous glass membranes. H_2/N_2 selectivity equal to 11 was reported with a H_2 permeation of 5×10^{-9} mol/m$^2 \cdot$ s $\cdot$ Pa. The diffusion mechanism was identified to be in the transition region of Knudsen and microporous. Nakao et al. [4] also have employed porous Vycor tubes for the deposition of CVD silica layer by Opposing Reactant Geometry (ORG).

More recent reports from the group of Gavalas [5] show the synthesis of membranes by CVD of $SiCl_4$ or related compounds with H_2O at 600–800°C. The process can be arranged either in the ORG as described in the case of SiH_4 CVD or One Sided Geometry (OSG) wherein both the reactants stay in one side of the support. In ORG the formed layer has an asymmetric profile. The reaction is initiated at the surface silanols and is heterogeneous. In OSG the heterogeneous reaction occurring at the support surface as well as deposition of gas phase product clusters contribute to layer growth. This deposition from gas phase must be inside the pores for good membrane properties. The reactants in N_2 carrier gas were generated in bubblers and preheated to the temperature of the support before mixing approximately 5 cm before the support. Laminar flow conditions existed in the support conduit with a total flow rate of 200 cm^3/min. The Vycor support used was of 5 mm inside diameter, 1.1 mm thickness, 30% porosity and 5–7 cm length. The mean pore size was 4.4 nm.

The rate of deposition of the CVD layer was measured by H_2 and N_2 permeation. It is reported that H_2 permeation remained the same during a 20 min deposition at 600°C with a reactant concentration of 2.7% $SiCl_4$ and 13% H_2O in N_2. However, N_2 permeation dropped down by a factor of 50. It was stated that the growth of the deposited layer beyond the porous region, can create thermo-mechanical stress leading to crack formation. So adequate care has to be taken in the CVD process to use low enough concentration of reactants and to maintain control on deposition time. The hydrothermal stability of the membranes was also checked. The activation energy for H_2 permeation increased from about 10–15 kJ/mol to 25–30 kJ/mol by a treatment of the membrane at 550°C in the presence of 3 atm water vapor. The permeation dropped by a factor of 6 by this process to the range of 10^{-8} to 10^{-9} mol/$m^2 \cdot s \cdot Pa$ at 600°C.

The membrane structure was analyzed using defocus contrast electron microscopy and transmission electron microscopy (TEM). The analysis revealed an approximately 10 μm thick layer of deposit with a porosity distribution, giving maximum deposit density near the support surface. A dense layer of approximately 0.5 μm thickness and 10% trapped voids was detected close to the wall, which could be the barrier of permeation for gases other than H_2.

Recently CVD with TEOS precursor was used [6] to produce H_2 selective membranes. Alumina supports with 7 mm internal diameter and 3 mm thickness were used. γ-Alumina of 4 nm pore diameter and 3–5 μm thickness was coated on this before CVD. A 1.5–3 μm thick modified layer was formed by the deposition process. The resulting membrane showed activated diffusion for He and H_2 with an apparent activation energy of 17.3 kJ/mol for He and 20.4 for H_2. Hydrogen permeation of 3×10^{-9} mol/$m^2 \cdot s \cdot Pa$ was reported at 600°C with a perm-selectivity of 72.3 against N_2. However H_2 permeation as high as 2×10^{-6} could be realized on a membrane with permselectivity of 12.6 against N_2. Stability tests done on the membrane showed consistent permeation at continued exposure at 600°C for 150 h. However, permeation dropped by a factor of 3 for He and N_2 on exposing to moisture (20 mol% water/N_2) at 600°C for 2 h. Further drop in permeation, however, was very slow and negligible.

In short, CVD methods have shown to be successful in making membranes with a nearly dense separating layer. Even though the set-up for the processing of these membranes presents difficult engineering problems, the feasibility to automate the process makes CVD a successful method for commercial applications. Recent developments in the method have improved the membrane quality and consequently gas permeation values in the range of sol–gel membranes could be realized in these membranes with higher separation efficiency. However the application of these membranes is still restricted to separation of H_2 and He from larger molecules.

B. Colloidal Silica Membranes

The packing of colloidal particles into thin layer membranes is the most well known method of making inorganic membranes. Burggraaf et al. were the first to report the formation and characterization of colloidal membranes from boehmite particles [7,8]. On calcination boehmite converts into a stable γ-alumina structure. These membranes are mesoporous in structure and are widely used for ultrafiltration (UF) applications. Recently modified membranes of these kind are shown to be capable for nanofiltration (NF) applications [9,10]. Many other inorganic membranes with better chemical stability than alumina have been made since this first report. Zirconia [11], titania [12] and $BaTiO_3$ [13] membranes made from respective colloidal sols and heat treated to the crystalline counter parts are good examples.

Amorphous silica membranes have also been made by the colloidal sol method. Larbot et al. reported the formation of such mesoporous membranes from commercial silica sols [14]. A Spanish group, Muñoz-Aguado and Gregorkiewitz, has made colloidal silica based membranes using sol–gel procedures starting from sodium silicate solutions [15]. The pore size was measured as 1.6 nm and porosity as 35%. The membranes were thermally stable up to 873 K. Gas transport characteristics showed intermediate behavior between Knudsen and surface diffusion. The reproducibility of membrane synthesis was very high and this method seems suitable for making intermediate layers for possible surface modifications.

Asaeda et al. have reported the processing of silica membranes capable of separating propylene/propane mixtures [16]. However these membranes were made by a very distinct procedure. Colloidal silica sol was first hot-coated (160°C–180°C) in the support a number of times. Then a polymeric silica sol was used to finally coat the system. The resulting membrane system showed high selectivity between hydrocarbon molecules such as propylene/propane or n-butane/iso-butane. However the activation energy for helium transport was low in these membranes. The peculiar gas permeation and separation performance exhibited by such membranes are very typical and probably originates in the structure of the intermediate colloidal layer. As explained before these membranes were made by stacking layers with decreasing pore size. The last coating was made with polymeric sol. The layer before was colloidal in nature and had a pore size of 1 nm. It is possible that the polymeric coating in this case may not be a selective barrier, but rather serves to plug the defects in the underlying layer. This probability is mentioned to attract the attention of the readers to such interesting possibilities available with sol–gel processing.

The main disadvantage with the colloidal method of processing membranes is the limitation of available pore sizes. The nanometer size particles will undergo severe growth during the calcination stage. This will enhance pore growth and will limit porosity. Hence the main application of such membranes are in the UF and NF area. In gas separation applications, these membranes are generally used as intermediate layers on which microporous layers are deposited.

C. Synthesis of Membranes from Polymeric Silica Sols

Synthesis of polymeric silica sols for membranes are reported by a number of authors. The most prominent among these is the one step hydrolysis as reported by Uhlhorn et al. [17] and two-step synthesis reported by Brinker et al. [18]. One of the first efforts to make sol–gel silica microporous membrane was from Uhlhorn [19], synthesizing silica membranes showing activated diffusion for He and H_2. The thickness of the membrane was only 50 nm. A very high separation factor of 200 at 200°C was reported between H_2 and propylene. The sol in this case was made by acid catalyzed hydrolysis of TEOS in ethanol. de Lange [20] has made ultrathin (60 nm) microporous membranes with molecular dimensions of 0.5–0.7 nm. Gas transport was activated for hydrogen (E_{act} = 11 kJ/mol) and molecular sieve like separation factors were obtained for H_2/C_3H_6 mixtures (200 at 260°C).

Julbe et al. [21] has reported preparation of sol–gel unsupported membranes with very small pore sizes of the order of 0.5–0.6 nm on a variety of inorganic materials like ZrO_2, Al_2O_3, LaOCl, etc. They have also prepared catalytically active membranes like platinum [22] doped silica. The resulting porosity of the membrane was reasonably high. The second-phase dispersion was also shown to be of good quality. Maier et al. [23] have reported the sol–gel synthesis of a variety of microporous materials. They succeeded in obtaining average pore sizes of 0.6 nm for zirconia, 0.7 nm for titania and 1 nm for silica and alumina on unsupported membranes. Supported membranes of silica on alumina/silica supports of average pore radius of 1 nm showed activated diffusion. However the same on alumina (d_{av} = 20 nm) or Vycor glass (d_{av} = 4 nm) supports showed only Knudsen flow. The group of Brinker [18] have prepared sol–gel silica membranes with a pore radius less than 1 nm by a two-step hydrolysis of TEOS. The top layer was 20–120 nm thick in this case. However, permeability measurements on small molecule gases has not evidenced any activated transport. For readers interested in details such as formation of the thin layer, drying and shrinkage, stress development, etc. some of the publications from Brinker et al. will be worth reading [24–26].

Asaeda et al. [27] have reported the formation of microporous membranes capable of separating water/alcohol mixtures. They were among the first to report silica membranes showing activated transport for small molecules. He and H_2 showed increase in permeation with temperature while N_2 showed a decrease. The authors believed that this may because of the permeation of N_2 through some pinholes giving Knudsen diffusion. Activation energy for H_2 and He were estimated to be 8.3 kJ/mol and 4 kJ/mol. At 270°C a separation factor of 326 was obtained for He/N_2 mixture [16]. For those looking for excellent gas or liquid separation results the publications from Asaeda et al. [28–30] will be a useful guide. Several other publications on synthesis and characterization of microporous membranes are available [31–35].

D. Composite and Hybrid Membranes

Emerging applications of silica include synthesis of inorganic–silica and
organic–silica composite membranes. de Lange et al. [36] reported the formation of silica–alumina, silica–zirconia and silica–titania composite membranes
by sol–gel methods. Three synthesis routes were tested to make these binary
sols. In one case the binary mixture of the reactants were hydrolyzed in a
single step and in another case in two steps. In yet another case the sols were
made separately and mixed later on. Gas transport studies revealed that the
membranes made from the two-step hydrolysis method have high permeation
and high activation energy for H_2 diffusion. Mixing method gave membranes
with very high molecular sieving ability but permeation was low compared to
other composite membranes.

Silica incorporated polymer membranes are also investigated for enhanced
separation performance and stability. Koros et al. [37] reported selectivity
(O_2/N_2) enhancement of 6FDA-IPDA (hexafluorodianhydride-isopro-
pylidenedianiline) membranes in presence of silica particles. They have reported the significant increase in glass transition temperature of the polymer
suggesting restrictions in chain segmental mobility due to adsorption of the
polymer onto the silica particle. Effects such as these are observed on hybrid
or composite membrane by many other groups [38,39] and is an advocated
method for the high temperature stability of co-polymer membranes for petroleum component separation [40]. Recently, Raman et al. [41] suggested the
application of hybrid synthesis for the preparation of silica based microporous
membrane materials. They have made sols via the co-polymerization of
methyltriethoxysilane(MTES) and TEOS. On pyrolysis of the methyl ligands
membranes with microporous structure has been retained. A similar method
using 3-methacryloxypropyl trimethoxysilane (MPS) and TEOS was reported
by Cao et al. [42]. The synthesis of organic/inorganic hybrid networks [43]
with the capability to tailor-make pore sizes has been regarded as one of the
most promising membrane processing methods.

III. THEORY AND ANALYSIS OF SOL–GEL MEMBRANE
FORMATION

A. Sol–Gel Reaction Scheme

In general, polymeric sol structures for microporous membrane making are
prepared by acid catalyzed hydrolysis and condensation of tetra-ethyl-ortho-
silicate (TEOS) in presence of a mutual solvent. The sol–gel scheme can be
described by the following reactions in which OR represents an alkoxy group:

$$\text{hydrolysis} \rightarrow$$
$$\equiv\text{Si}-\text{OR} + \text{H}_2\text{O} \leftrightarrow \equiv\text{Si}-\text{OH} + \text{ROH}$$
$$\leftarrow \text{esterification}$$

$$\text{alcohol condensation} \rightarrow$$
$$\equiv\text{Si}-\text{OR} + \text{HO}-\text{Si}\equiv \leftrightarrow \equiv\text{Si}-\text{O}-\text{Si}\equiv + \text{ROH}$$
$$\leftarrow \text{alcoholysis}$$

$$\text{water condensation} \rightarrow$$
$$\equiv\text{Si}-\text{OH} + \text{HO}-\text{Si}\equiv \leftrightarrow \equiv\text{Si}-\text{O}-\text{Si}\equiv + \text{H}_2\text{O}$$
$$\leftarrow \text{hydrolysis}$$

The hydrolysis reaction proceeds through an electrophilic attack of the H^+-ion. This causes a decrease in reactivity as the number of OR groups on the Si decreases with the progress of hydrolysis [44]. Complete hydrolysis of silicon to Si(OH)_4 is thus small and the condensation reaction will start before the hydrolysis has been completed. As hydrolized molecules can directly polymerize with nonhydrolyzed alkoxyl groups, the acid catalyzed hydrolysis–condensation reactions can produce polymers in which the degree of cross-linking is low.

The degree of polymerization will depend on the ratio of the hydrolysis rate over the condensation rate [44]. Any change in the molar ratio of catalyst or water to alkoxide, synthesis time or temperature and the solvent concentration will influence the silica sol–gel structure, and hence the final membrane properties. The influence of each parameter, however, is different, just as in the case of selecting another set of reactants or catalysts. The structure of the resulting polymers can change from more or less linear to weakly branched polymers.

According to Aelion [45], the hydrolysis reaction rate increases linearly with increasing molar ratio of acidic catalyst to alkoxide (r_a). This has been confirmed by Boonstra and Bernards [46]. Higher hydrolysis reaction rates will lead to more hydrolyzed and therefore more branched polymers, while keeping the reaction time constant.

No literature presents a clear picture of the influence of the molar ratio of water to alkoxide (r_w) on the hydrolysis reaction rate. According to Uhlhorn et al. [19] the hydrolysis reaction rate will increase with increasing r_w, while the condensation rate is retarded. In contrast, Boonstra and Bernards [46] show results which suggest that the differences in hydrolysis reaction rate are minimal. Most authors [46,47] agree that the formation of more hydrolyzed species is favored with increasing r_w. Partlow and Yoldas [48] showed that the gelling volume of wet gels increases with increasing r_w. This reflects an increase in the degree of polymerization. Yoldas [49] states that a higher r_w promotes the formation of a higher ratio of bridging to nonbridging oxygen, thus yielding a stronger oxide network. Hence, with increasing r_w the formation of more hydrolyzed species is favored. After condensation, this will result in species with a more branched structure. This is confirmed by the viscosity measurements presented by Sakka and Kamiya [47]. They reported that, with a constant molar ratio of HCl to TEOS of 0.01, linear polymers are formed for $r_w < 4$ and branched polymers for $r_w > 4$.

B. Small Angle X-Ray Scattering (SAXS) Analysis of Silica Polymers

As we have observed in the previous section the hydrolysis and condensation of silica will lead to a variety of structures with shapes and sizes depending upon the synthesis parameters. Under acidic conditions ($< pH\ 2$) the structure is normally linear or weakly branched. For the formaton of microporous membranes, the ability of silica polymers to interpenetrate must be considerable. Short branched polymers are the best in this regard. However, the probability to form a dense structure is higher when the interpenetration becomes very high. On the other hand highly branched systems can lead to inefficient packing with resulting mesoporosity of the gel. The branching and interpenetration of silica polymers can very well be explained with the help of fractal concepts [50–59].

Fractal objects possess dilation symmetry compared to translation or rotation symmetry of ordinary Euclidean objects. Fractals can be characterized by a dimension (fractal dimension), which can take noninteger values to represent geometrical relationships. Silica polymeric systems grown by random processes are fractal objects and can be represented by a mass fractal dimension (D_f) related to mass M and size R. ($M \sim R^{D_f}$). D_f has a limiting value of three, where the object is Euclidean. As the fractal dimension decreases the structure will look sparser, giving essentially a linear configuration at $D_f = 1$ [60].

The mathematical concept of fractality is valid for an infinite range of similitude. However for physical systems cut-off values always exist. In a typical scattering curve (log I vs. log Q; $Q = 2\pi/\lambda \sin(2\theta)$), for cxample from a Small Angle X-ray Scattering (SAXS) experiment, three regions can be identified. The Guinier region, above the upper cut-off size (lower cut off Q value), the Porod region below the lower cut-off size and the intermediate fractal region. The Guinier region can provide information concerning polymer mass or radius, which is determined by the intercept and slope of log I vs. Q^2 plots. In the Porod region the scattered intensity decays showing power law behavior. The slope of the power law curve (P) can be correlated to the mass (D_f) and surface (D_s) fractal dimension according to the equation $P = -2D_f + D_s$. The cut-off Q values from fractal to Guinier region and from fractal to Porod region yield approximate values for respectively $1/\xi$ and $1/R_o$ [61]. The upper cut-off length ξ (shown as 'Ksi' in some figures in this chapter) can be correlated with the radius of gyration (R_g) according to the equation [52]:

$$R_g^2 = D_f(D_f + 1)\xi^2/2 \tag{1}$$

For D_f-values near one $R_g = \xi$ and for D_f-values larger than one $R_g > \xi$. For the D_f-values presented in this chapter the difference between R_g and ξ is not large. The lower cut-off length R_o can be correlated to the size of the primary building block. From the fractal range, where the intensity follows a power law, the dimension D_f can be calculated as the negative slope of the log I vs. log Q curve, where $I \propto Q^{-D_f}$ ($1/\xi \ll Q \ll 1/R_o$). The estimation of D_f and R_g can to a very good extent describe the structure of the gel.

The number of intersections between two mass fractals of radius R each placed independently of the other in the same region of space is given by the equation

$$M_{1,2} \propto R^{D_{f1} + D_{f2} - 3} \tag{2}$$

If the value of D_{f1} and D_{f2} is above 1.5, the probability of intersection will increase with the increase in size of the polymer. Such a condition will hinder the free interpenetration of the polymers (mutual opaqueness) and a heterogeneous microstructure can result [44]. Linear polymers with $D_f < 1.5$, on the other hand can pack efficiently (mutual transparency) leading to denser structures.

The mechanism of growth of silica aggregates depends on conditions such as pH and temperature. Under acid catalyzed conditions the hydrolysis rate is normally very high. Typical values reported for reaction rate constant for hydrolysis, is a factor 15–30 higher compared to the water-producing condensation reaction rate constant and at least 200 times higher than the reaction rate constant for the alcohol producing condensation reaction. As a consequence, a large amount of hydrolyzed species is present at the moment condensation becomes significant. The condensation at the beginning will happen between monomers, the concentration of which will drop eventually to very low values. Further condensation can only proceed through condensation between the bigger counterparts. Hence aggregation in the acid catalyzed system is termed as cluster–cluster aggregation.

Depending on the contraint there could be two types of cluster–cluster growth models. The colliding clusters stick together irreversibly in the first type of model. In other words, the rate limiting step for aggregation is the diffusion of the cluster. The model is called diffusion limited cluster–cluster aggregation (DLCCA) and will generate structures which are weakly branched. The mass fractal dimension of a typical DLCCA aggregate is only 1.8. In the case of silica polymerization, however, the functionality of the different species and the electron density distributions effectively limit the condensation rates. Hence the second type of model proposes that the reaction limitation is strong in silica systems and the model based on this (reaction limited cluster–cluster aggregation or RLCCA) leads to fractal structures with more compact structures ($D_f \sim 2.09$).

For the analysis of silica polymeric growth and aggregation by SAXS we have employed two types of instrumental systems. Preliminary measurements were performed using synchrotron radiation (X-ray wavelength $\lambda = 0.154$ nm) at the Non-Crystalline Diffraction beam line 8.2 of the SERC Synchrotron Radiation Source (SRS) in Daresbury, UK. The scattered X-ray intensities were recorded using a quadrant detector with camera length of 2 m and 0.6 m. The windows used were mostly Mylar but also Kapton was used for some of the measurements. The spectra obtained were corrected for background and parasitic scattering. In the scattering results shown the y-axis (log I) is scaled in arbitrary units and the x-axis (log Q) in nm^{-1}. In a later stage a SAXS set-up was designed especially for this purpose at VITO, Belgium. It consisted of an X-ray source with copper rotating anode equipped with double focusing. The power of the beam was 3 kW. A Siemens Xenon-filled wire camera recorded a two-dimensional image with a 0.01° angular resolution. For the in-situ measurement a 1 mm diameter boron glass capillary tube is filled with the sample liquid and mouned horizontally in the X-ray beam.

The interpretation of the result was achieved by a least squares program fitting data to a linear combination of two functions. The first function was proportional to the background correction and the second depended on two parameters related to R_g, D_f and a normalization factor. For the latter a Teixeira function [52] was selected on behalf of its simplicity and on the fact that it yields results which are not very sensitive to the angular interval over which the fitting was carried out. More details of the techniques adopted are reported by Maene et al. [62].

Finally it should be kept in mind that the structures which are formed under all synthesis conditions of silica detailed in this chapter might not be fractal in nature. For, e.g., a D_f value of 1 represents an object which is essentially a line. However we have mentioned values below 1 (slope of fractal region above -1) to show the continuity in growth of the sol constituents from beginning to gelation. Such a value of D_f has no physical meaning at all. Nevertheless for the easiness of classification we have grouped them all under fractal structures. Moreover a number of problems can in fact make the assessment of all the fractal parameters tricky. If the concentration of the polymer is high, underestimation of R_g will result because of entanglement. Near the percolation threshold the estimation of R_g is difficult too. Calculation of D_f must theoretically be done in a minimum fractality range of one decade ($\xi/R_o = 10$), which is difficult to find in some of the measured systems. Even with all these difficulties, estimation of the fractal dimension and cut-off radii may give a good indication of the structure of the gel as will be shown later in this chapter.

C. Methods of Characterization of the Gel and the Membrane

The transition of the polymeric sol into a gel is influenced by the drying rate and atmosphere to a great extent. Drying, shrinkage and associated structural changes in the gel are well detailed by Brinker and Scherer [44]. The effect of such changes can be efficiently monitored by evaluating the properties of the gel dried under different atmospheres as reported by de Lange et al. [20].

Thermogravimetric techniques are useful tools to compare the process of transformation of the dried gel into the membrane. As already stated the degree of condensation depends on the synthesis chemistry. Hence the shrinkage during calcination depends on the reaction parameters. In supported membranes this shrinkage is resisted by the support and hence create stresses in the membrane, leading to cracking. Hence an idea of weight loss during drying will be helpful in the design of membranes without significant cracking.

The structure and porosity of the calcined gel can be accurately estimated using gas adsorption techniques. N_2 adsorption at liquid N_2 temperature is the most well known method. The size of N_2 (kinetic diameter: 3.8 Å), however, limits its accessibility. Helium adsorption at liquid helium temperature is presently emerging as a better method. Analysis of pore size distribution can be made from these adsorption isotherms using methods like Horvath–Kawazoe (HK) or Dubinin–Radushkevich (DR) [63]. Details on the adsorption process and mechanisms can be found elsewhere [64–69]. However pore size calculations are rather empirical and difficult to justify completely by dynamic tests on supported membranes.

The dipping or coating process to make supported membranes has a very important influence on the characteristics of these membranes. Firstly, it involves the selection of the support substrate over which the membranes will be made. The substrate surface must be free from pinholes and such irregularities which will be difficult to heal by the thin active membrane layer. The surface finish of the support and the pore size and distribution are the two factors which can be used for deciding the selection criteria.

Secondly, the duration of polymeric silica sol coating is another parameter which has to be optimized with respect to factors such as the surface of the support, pore size, and the viscosity of the sol. Thin membranes are preferred since permeation decreases as the thickness increases. As the thickness increases the surface area of the membrane can also decrease (because of reduced roughness) altering permeation in its own way. This can have an influence on the selectivity as far as surface selective separation processes are concerned.

Atomic Force Microscopy (AFM) is a strong tool to characterize the surface of the support and the membrane. Evaluation of the surface with AFM can give details of the surface roughness as well as the distribution of second phase materials. Techniques like Field Emission Scanning Electron Microscopy (FESEM), Scanning AUGER (SAM) and X-ray Analytical Microscopy can also yield information on the details of silica membrane structure. Hence they also can give insight into the membrane formation process.

The best way to perform structural evaluation of silica membranes is to perform gas permeation studies. From the relationship of gas permeation to kinetic diameter of gas molecules an idea about the pore size of the membrane can be made. The activation energy for permeation of different gas molecules and the pressure dependency of permeation can highlight the effect of defects, if present. Selectivity between gas molecules is another useful factor. Hence, the factors which determine the final application of the membrane itself can to great extent elucidate the structure of the membranes.

This chapter is written to present the reader with a design concept. We will firstly explain the factors governing the formation of silica polymers with the help of fractal concepts. Then we will explain the relationship of such factors to the gel porosity and to the evolution of porosity from adsorption and thermogravimetric studies. The influence of parameters like drying atmosphere or rate are not explained here. It should be emphasized that some of these parameters are equally if not more significant than the factors controlled here to achieve the membrane design. The detailed mechanisms of drying and shrinkage or details of various evaluation techniques employed are also out of scope of this chapter. The synthesis of supported membranes was performed keeping many of the parameters like dipping time, temperature, concentration of the sol, etc. constant. The support used was of same kind throughout the course of investigation. As in the case of drying such parameters are influential and must be controlled before attempting to design molecular sieving membranes by the proposed route. The structure of the supported silica membrane has been detailed with the help of various scanning and analyzing tools. Finally we have introduced the method of confirmation of such a structure in the supported membrane with the help of gas permeation studies. Most of the research works mentioned in the rest of the chapter was performed in our groups [70–79]. But other related works are mentioned for the interested reader [80–84].

IV. SOL–GEL PROCESSING

A. Synthesis of Silica Sol and Measurement of Heat of Reaction

Polymeric sols were prepared by hydrolysis and condensation of tetra-ethyl-ortho-silicate (TEOS, Merck, p.a. grade) in ethanol with HNO_3 as catalyst. A mixture of HNO_3 (Merck, p.a. grade) and water was carefully added, using a dropping funnel, to a mixture of ethanol (ethanol absolute, Merck, p.a. grade) and TEOS under vigorous stirring. The reaction mixture was then refluxed for 3 h at $65°C \pm 5°C$ under stirring. The amount of ethanol added was kept constant during the present experiments.

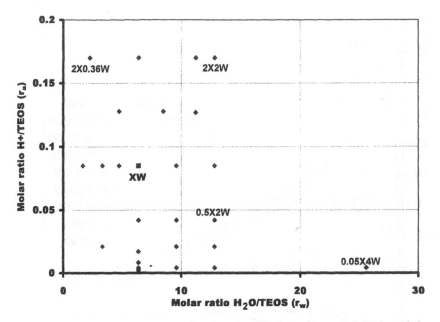

FIG. 1 Sample compositions and nomenclature of samples as a function of the water and acid content in the reaction mixture. Sample XW with 0.085 mol H^+ and 6.4 mol H_2O to each mole of TEOS is treated as the standard sample. The codes for other samples are derived from this.

In order to provide recipes for tailor-making silica membranes, the values of r_a (molar ratio of catalyst to TEOS) and r_w (molar ratio of water to TEOS) were varied. This variation is shown in Fig. 1. The standard sample is XW with a r_a-value of 0.085 and a r_w-value of 6.4. All other compositions are related to this standard composition. A sample $2X2W$ means the double amount of acid and water (compared to sample XW) in the reaction mixture so the r_a-value is 0.17 and the r_w-value is 12.8. For the sample $0.5X0.5W$ half the amounts of acid and water are in the reaction mixture and so on. About 30 reaction mixtures are shown in this Fig. 1. Some compositions of prepared reaction mixtures are outside the borders of this figure. The boundaries for the range of r_a and r_w are set by practical limitations. These practical limitations are defined as being those synthesis compositions which result in sols which are suitable for preparation of microporous supported membranes by dipping procedures.

The r_a-values have been changed over a wide range from 0.00085 to 0.34. For a molar ratio of catalyst to alkoxide of 0.021, or smaller ($<0.25X$ in Fig. 1), the sols yielded nitrogen dense gels. To the high r_a side no limiting composition was attained, even at $r_a = 0.34$ ($4X$) the obtained gel was microporous.

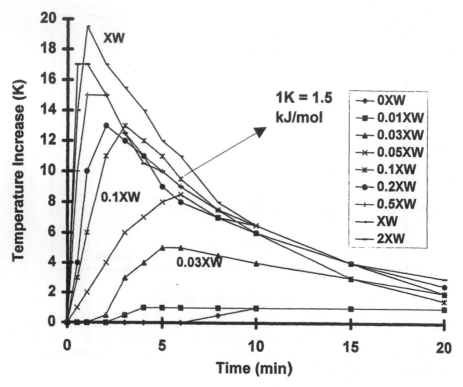

FIG. 2 Illustration of reaction heat after addition of different amounts of water and acid represented by temperature–time curves [62]. For sample compositions see Fig. 1.

The r_w-values have been varied over a range from 1.6 to 25.6 (0.25W to 4W). The 4W-sample is a two-phase liquid system which becomes homogeneous after 1 to 2 h reaction time. Only a single sample is prepared in this region because of this demixing. Although this sample can be suitable for the preparation of membranes a limitation for preparation was set at high values of r_w. At relatively low values of r_a (<0.25X) and high value of r_w the sol (0.25X2W) yielded a mesoporous structure for the unsupported membrane. This makes this sol unsuitable for the preparation of microporous membranes. Sols with compositions of relatively high values of r_a and high values of r_w were difficult to synthesize, as the sol 2X1.75W ($r_a = 0.17$, $r_w = 11.2$) did gelate during synthesis. Synthesis compositions with a high value for r_w and moderate values of r_a(0.06 < r_a < 0.15) produced sols which are suitable to prepare supported microporous membranes and hence the maximum of r_w was selected for practical considerations to 12.8 (2W) (Fig. 1).

All the prepared sols contained approximately 2 mol Si/L. Deviation from this molarity occurred in compositions with high values of r_w. Part of the sol

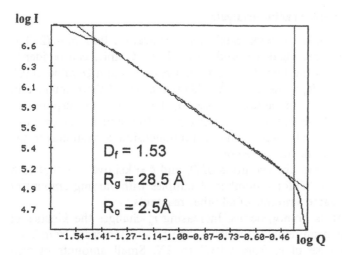

FIG. 3 A SAXS spectrum of sol $2XW$, in which Q is the scattering vector, I is the scattered intensity, D_f is the fractal dimension, R_o is the radius of the primary building unit and R_g is the radius of gyration [70]. (Room temperature aged.)

was diluted with ethanol to 0.2M, 0.1M and 0.05M. Sols were kept in closed glass bottles at room temperature (RT) for aging. In-situ SAXS measurements were carried out at 65°C on sols kept in capillary tubes.

Reaction heats of the samples were measured using noninsulated 10 ml test tubes. First, water was added to a mixture of TEOS and ethanol at room temperature to obtain the composition $0XW$. The instantaneous temperature increase of about 2°C involved in this addition, was considered to be caused by mixing enthalpy and was substracted from the heat effect obtained by addition of water containing a certain amount of acid. Figure 2 shows the curves for a number of samples containing a distinct amount of acid X. A rapid increase in temperature was observed for most of the samples and afterwards the temperature decreases by natural cooling. A similar type of heat effect was found in the experiments performed at 65°C. As is clear from the figure, for all samples containing more than $0.05X$, the rapid temperature increase approaches 10–20 K which is approximately 15–30 kJ/mol considering the heat capacity of the test tube plus liquids involved. Hence the hydrolysis of at least one ethoxy group occurs in a rapid first step when some protons are present. However, in the presence of small amounts ($X < 0.05$), of such protons the hydrolysis proceeds at a slower rate. When hydroxyl ions were involved instead of protons, no heat effect was detected. From this observation the conclusion is that hydrolysis of at least one ethoxy-group of the TEOS molecule is extremely fast compared with the time scale of polymer growth (condensation) experiments.

B. Polymer Growth and Fractal Analysis

The scattering curve of a sol with catalyst concentration 0.17 mol (2X) is shown in Fig. 3. The three regions Porod, Fractal and Guinier can be identified. The transition from the Porod to the fractal region is at a Q value of 0.4. This corresponds to an R_o value of 2.5 Å. This is the size of the primary unit from which the polymer is made up. The size of the polymer corresponds to the transition Q value from fractal to Guinier region. In the presented example this value was approximately 28.5 Å. The fractal dimension corresponds to the slope of the line, 1.53, in the fractal region.

Figures 4 and 5 illustrate the evolution of D_f and ξ = ksi over the first 15 h of reaction (in-situ at 65°C) for a number of samples with varying amount of protons but with the same amounts of all other reactants.

The fractal growth is homogeneous. Increasing r_a changes the kinetics of growth but the mechanism remains the same. The ξ value increased from 2 nm to 6 nm by an increase of r_a from 0.05X to 2X. Small amounts of acid ($X < 0.5$) lead only to a small increase in the size and fractal dimension of the silica polymers within 15 h at 65°C. Larger amounts of acid have substantially more effect on the growth kinetics in the first 15 h.

In measurements done with preprepared sol sample (XW), the slope of the log I vs. log Q curve in the intermediate region was measured as -0.41 after 1

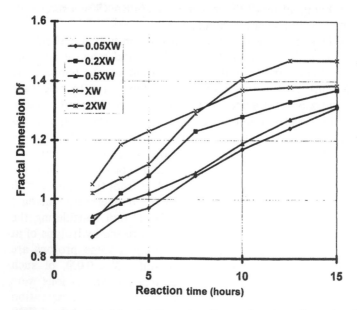

FIG. 4 Calculated fractal dimension D_f as a function of reaction time for samples with different amounts of acid [62]. For sample compositions see Fig. 1. (Temperature 65°C.)

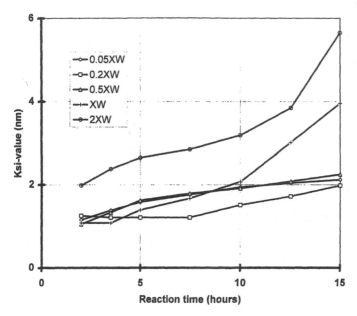

FIG. 5 Calculated value ξ (=Ksi) as a function of reaction time for samples with different amounts of acid. R_g is equal to ξ when $D_f = 1$, but is higher when $D_f > 1$. For sample compositions see Fig. 1. (Temperature 65°C.)

h and -0.63 after 2 h of synthesis. After 3 h a linear connected fractal has appeared with fractal dimension around 0.96 (this value is slightly less than in the in-situ reaction (Fig. 4), but the trends are the same). These sols were then aged in closed bottles at room temperature. After 6 days aging a fractal dimension of 1.4 was measured. The increase in fractal dimension and radius of gyration with time on room temperature aging is shown in Fig. 6. It can be seen that after a preliminary induction period of around 100 h the fractal dimension increases faster till it reaches a plateau. A final fractal dimension of 2.15 was measured after 8 months aging. R_g, however, could be measured only up to 3.6 nm.

Compared to the D_f value of 2.15 which was measured after room temperature aging, the fractal values of high-temperature aged systems are low. Figure 7 shows the increase in fractal dimension of two sols with extremely different degrees of reactivity ($2X2W$ and $0.05XW$). The kinetics in the initial hours are entirely different for the two samples. However after about 60 h of aging the fractal dimensions come closer to 1.8, although the value for the sample $0.05XW$ is somewhat smaller than that for the sample $2X2W$. This value (1.8) is similar to a diffusion limited aggregate. At high temperature obviously the reaction constraints are not so strict. The low-temperature value of $D_f = 2.15$ represents reaction limitations.

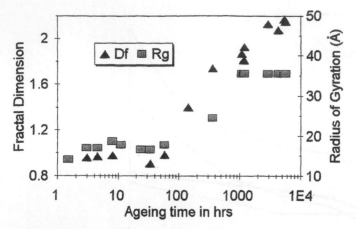

FIG. 6 Effect of aging on fractal growth is shown. The samples were aged at room temperature in closed bottles [70]. Sample composition was XW.

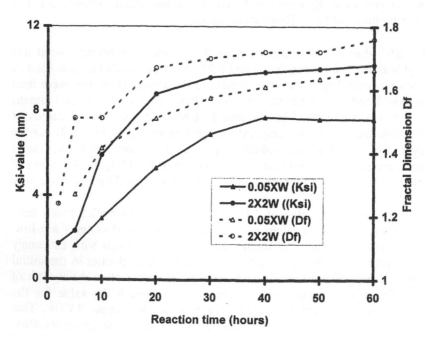

FIG. 7 ξ (=Ksi) and D_f as a function of reaction time for samples with different amounts of water and acid. (Temperature 65°C.)

Results of aging experiments (40 days) performed under different sample dilution are shown in Fig. 8. Sols with a wide range of reactivity was employed for the dilution study. The 0.2M, 0.1M and 0.05M sols showed smaller fractal dimensions than the 2M sol at all catalyst concentrations. Low and moderate concentrations of the sol apparently gave nearly the same structure under premature aging conditions. However it should be remembered that if sufficient time is provided these gels might grow to the same level as the concentrated sols.

The effect of water concentration on the morphological development at 65°C is shown in Fig. 9 (*0.5XW* and *0.5X2W*). As shown the effect can be rather large and higher amounts of water have accelerated the kinetics. When large amounts of water are added the concentrations of the sol will be smaller and hence the rate of growth should decrease. However at high temperature reactivity is rather high, reducing reaction limitations and favoring growth.

The effect of changing the mineral acid (HCl and HNO_3) is not very severe. As shown in Fig. 10 the change of acid from HNO_3 to HCl has caused some changes in the fractal dimension of the polymer but not in the size. These changes, even though they are weak, are in accordance with the earlier findings of Pope et al. [85]. They have observed that in TEOS systems the gelation time in HCl is 8% less than that in HNO_3 medium. Indeed growing kinetics seems somewhat faster using HCl instead of HNO_3.

The effect of the addition of hydroxyls instead of protons could not be interpreted in terms of fractal growth. No fast hydrolysis was observed and a

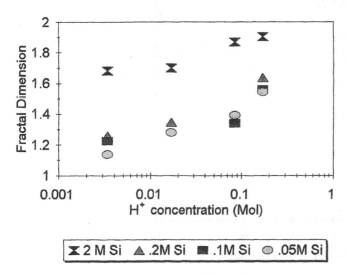

FIG. 8 Effect of concentration and H^+ amount (constant $r_w = 6.4$) on the gel structure [70]. The samples were diluted with ethanol after synthesis. (Room temperature aged.)

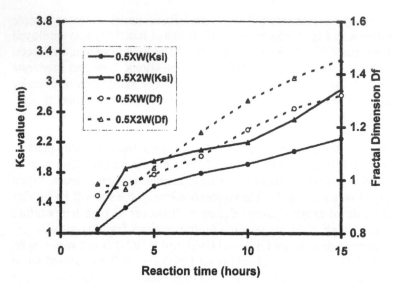

FIG. 9 ξ (=Ksi) and D_f as a function of reaction time for samples with different amounts of water. (Temperature 65°C.)

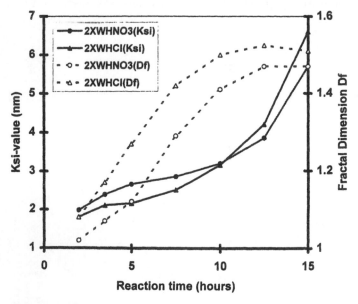

FIG. 10 ξ (=Ksi) and D_f as a function of reaction time for samples with different types of acid (HNO_3 vs. HCl). (Temperature 65°C.)

careful interpretation of the SAXS curves indicated the presence of plate-shaped particles in the nm-range after a short time. An extensive interpretation is not carried out since these sols were not suitable for preparation of membranes with molecular-sieving ability.

C. Thermogravimetric Analysis

Polymeric sols were dried in petri dish in ambient atmosphere. Gels obtained in this way (unsupported silica membranes) were characterized with thermogravimetric analysis. Figure 11 shows the TGA curves of a number of samples including the standard sample XW. For XW sample, the major part of the decomposition (15.5%) happens before 150°C mostly owing to the evaporation of water and ethanol remaining in the pores of the microporous gel. The total weight loss was about 20%. Between 150°C and 400°C, mostly removal of organic residues and further polymerization of the silica network takes place. At 400°C the total weight loss is about 19%. Above 400°C a further small weight loss ($\ll 1\%$) is related to removal of OH-groups from the surface [44]. Up to 600°C, the DTA-curves showed no sign of crystallization. A similar behavior was observed for most other gels [71].

Figure 11 shows also the dependence of decomposition profile on the synthesis chemistry of the sol. It is shown that the total relative weight loss of the dried gels (constant r_w of 6.4) increases with increasing r_a. One reason for the relatively large weight loss in the low temperature region (0–150°C) for the high r_a samples is the large pore volume of these gels as will be seen in the

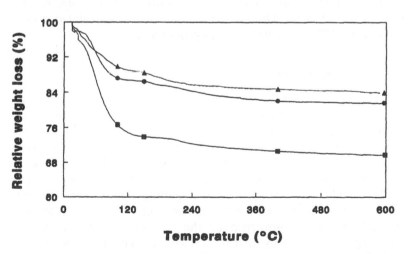

FIG. 11 Effect of molar ratio of HNO_3 to TEOS (r_a) on TGA-curves for sol $2XW$ (■), XW (●) and $0.01XW$ (▲), with constant molar ratio of H_2O to TEOS, $r_w = 6.4$ [71].

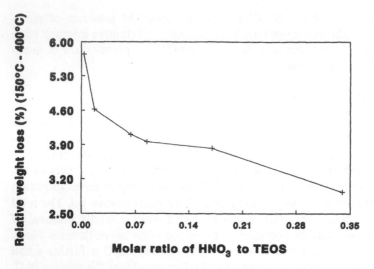

FIG. 12 Effect of molar ratio of HNO_3 to TEOS (r_a) on the relative weight loss of gels (%) between 150°C and 400°C (at constant $r_w = 6.4$) [71].

following section. As shown in Fig. 12 the weight loss between 150°C and 400°C was also sensitive to the chemistry of the sol. In this case with decreasing r_a the relative weight loss increased. Figure 13 presents the calculated weight loss between 150°C and 400°C for sols with varying r_a and r_w. The influence of r_a is very clear. The influence of r_w on the calculated relative weight loss between 150°C and 400°C is less pronounced.

D. Evaluation of Pore Morphology

Dried gels were calcined at 673 K under ordinary furnace conditions in air. The calcined unsupported membranes were characterized by nitrogen adsorption measurements at liquid nitrogen temperatures. Most of the samples showed type 1 isotherms [86]. Type 1 isotherm is a characteristic of microporous (pore width less than 2 nm) materials. Their shape is concave to the x-axis when the relative pressure of sorption is plotted against volume adsorbed. The volume adsorbed approaches a limiting value at very low pressures because of the enhanced adsorption in the micropores. The adsorption volume in such samples is governed by the accessible micropore volume (micropore filling) rather than by internal surface area. The nitrogen adsorbed volume in the low pressure region can be directly correlated to the micropore volume of the gel. Since this enhanced adsorption in the micropore is a func-

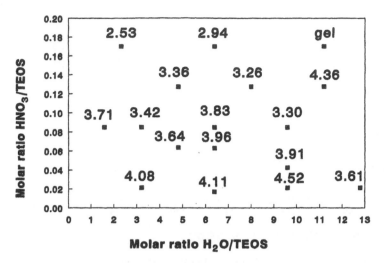

FIG. 13 Effect of the sol composition (with r_a and r_w changes) on the relative weight loss between 150°C and 400°C. % weight loss values are shown [71]. For corresponding sample codes see Fig. 1.

tion of pore size, probe molecule size and their interactions, care must be taken in deciding the type of adsorbate molecule for pore size measurement.

Most of the samples in our experiments showed type 1 isotherms and are thus microporous. Exceptions are samples with $r_a \sim 0.021$ and $r_w \sim 9.6$ (0.25X1.5W), which are nitrogen dense (no N_2 adsorption at 77 K), and sol W9 (0.25X2W), which only adsorbed nitrogen at relatively high pressures and is hence regarded to be mesoporous. It is shown in Fig. 14 that the microporosity has doubled for a gel while the r_a content increased from 0.75X to 4X. For $r_w > 4$, the porosity increases clearly with increasing r_a and tends to increase with increasing r_w, as can be seen in Fig. 15. For $r_w < 4$, the calculated porosities are surprisingly high, in contradiction with the low values of D_f obtained with SAXS-measurements for these sols. Low values of D_f indicate linear or very weakly branched polymers which would be expected to pack very well and form structures with very low porosity or even nitrogen dense structures. Samples with a low amount of protons ($r_a < 0.04$) showed nitrogen dense structures with low and moderate amounts of water in the mixture.

The method of Horváth and Kawazoe [87], based on describing adsorption with (10:4) Lennard-Jones potentials, has been applied to the data obtained from several samples to calculate the pore size. The model, derived for N_2 adsorption on microporous carbon with a slit shaped pore geometry, has been modified for cylindrical pore geometry by Saito and Foley [88]. This model was corrected for N_2 adsorption in oxide materials and applied here for calcu-

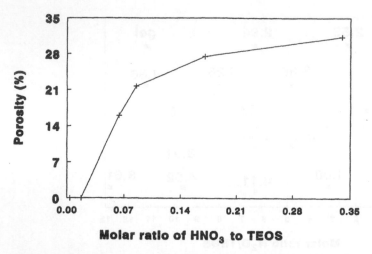

FIG. 14 Effect of the molar ratio of HNO_3 to TEOS on the microporosity of the gel, with constant molar ratio of H_2O to TEOS, $r_w = 6.4$ [71]. All the isotherms were Type 1.

lation of pore size. The details can be found elsewhere [63]. The peak positions and the widths of the peak of the obtained pore size distributions were more or less the same. An example of one of those pore size distributions is shown (for sol XW) in Fig. 16. The plot shows that the pore size distribution

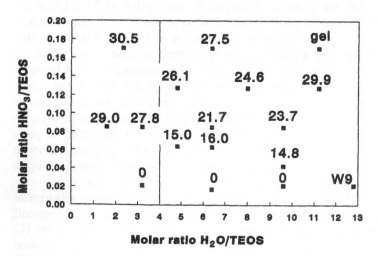

FIG. 15 Effect of the sol composition (with r_a and r_w changes) on the porosity. % porosity values are shown [71]. For corresponding sample codes see Fig. 1.

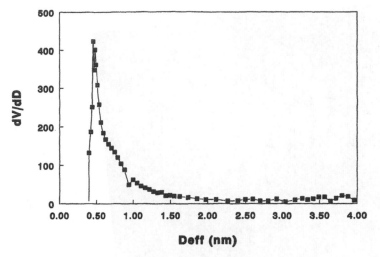

FIG. 16 Differential pore size distribution of sol XW according to the Horváth–Kawazoe model, in which D_{eff} is the effective pore diameter [71].

consists of a maximum at $D_{eff} = 0.5$ nm with a broad tail up to around $D_{eff} = 1.5$ nm, with a weak maximum at $D_{eff} = 0.75$ nm. D_{eff} is the effective pore diameter ($= 2r_p - d_E$) in which r_p is the calculated pore radius and d_E the diameter of an oxygen atom.

V. PROCESSING AND OBSERVATION OF SUPPORTED MEMBRANE STRUCTURE

The support for dipping polymeric silica sol was prepared as follows. α-Alumina powder of particle size 1 μm was pelleted by uniaxial pressing into cylindrical dimensions. This was then sintered at 1260°C to a density of 50%. The resulting support was cut into specific dimensions, one side was polished and then cleaned in an ultrasonic bath. The support thus formed has interconnected porosity with average pore size of 150 nm. The cleaned surface was free from pinholes and similar defects. This surface was then dip coated with γ-alumina sol.

γ-Alumina sol for this purpose was made by hydrolysis of aluminum-tri-sec-butoxide. This was added dropwise to water maintained at 90°C under vigorous stirring. The water alkoxide ratio was kept at 70 ~ 100:1. After hydrolysis the boehmite/water mixture was boiled for 1 h to clean up alcohol. This was then peptized with 1N HNO_3 by refluxing at 90°C for 12 h. The resulting sol had a pH of 4 and molarity 1.

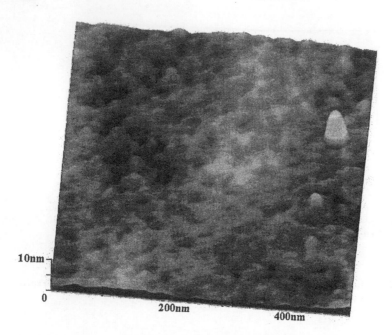

FIG. 17 AFM profile of silica membrane surface. (Courtesy; Seiko Instruments, Japan.)

Boehmite dip solution was prepared by mixing this sol with poly-vinyl acetate (PVA) solution (e.g., MW 66,000 ~ 79,200) to a concentration of 0.6 mol/L. The PVA solution can be prepared (for e.g.) by dissolving 3.5 g of PVA in 100 ml water in the presence of 0.005M HNO_3 at 90°C.

α-Alumina supports are then dip-coated with this sol. These were then dried in a climate chamber (40°C and 60% RH) followed by calcination at 600°C for 3 h. Then the membranes were tested for gas leakage. Crack free membranes showed Knudsen-type gas permeation behavior. The layer formed had a thickness of 2–3 μm, porosity 60% and mean pore size of 4 nm. To guarantee a crack free surface it is advisable to give a two-dip γ-alumina layer. The cracks in the first layer can be very well healed by the second dipping process carried out after the calcination of the first layer. The thickness of the membrane however, will increase by this process, reducing the gas permeation through the membrane. However, the resistance offered by these mesoporous layers is insignificant compared to the microporous silica layer to be prepared above it and hence a second layer may not appreciably change the final gas permeation properties of the membrane.

Dipping and drying of the microporous silica layer was carried out in the same way as that of the alumina intermediate layer. Calcination however was

FIG. 18 X-ray analytical microscopic image of a silica membrane surface. The membrane was previously used for permeation testing. Circular tracks in the picture represents deformations caused by O'ring while in the permeation cell.

carried out at a lower temperature of 400°C and at a lower heating rate of 25°C/min, just as in the case of gels for adsorption studies.

AFM measurements showed the roughness of the new surface as 20–40 nn, which is somewhat similar to the γ-alumina layer. The picture is shown (Fig. 17). The surface finish of the silica layer was dependent on that of the alumina layer. With γ-alumina the maximum surface finish that can be achieved is about 40 nm, which is limited by the size of the primary crystallite of alumina. This is an important design point. In order to make thinner silica membranes one needs to have intermediate layers with amorphous structure or crystallites with the least possible size, since the size of these crystallites (and hence the roughness of the layer) will be one of the limiting step in deciding the thickness of the top layer. But on the other hand it is clear from the AFM figure that the real area of the silica membrane is much higher than the area measured from the dimension of the surface since the membrane is a surface fractal by itself. This will have important implications when designing composite membranes with rate determining surfaces.

X-ray analytical microscopy (and X-ray fluorescent spectroscopy) is another useful tool in determining the structure and composition of these membranes.

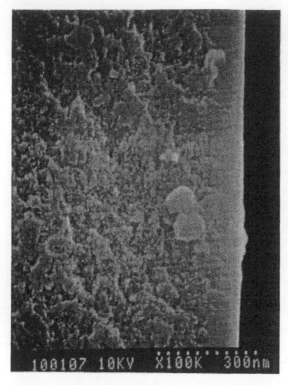

100107 10KV   X100K 300nm

FIG. 19   FESEM image of the cross-section of a silica membrane. Intermediate γ-layer is clearly visible. Silica layer is seen as a white line on top of gamma layer.

With a calibrated X-ray fluorescence analyzer (XrF), the area averaged thickness of the membrane can be measured, even though assumptions about the porosity have to be made. Since the gel porosity can be approximated by the membrane porosity, this is not a significant error. Another interesting use of the X-ray method is the microscopy which can determine the macro-distribution of ions in the membrane surface nondestructively. Figure 18 shows the image of a membrane scanned after gas permeation studies at high temperature. The circular tracks are the deformations produced by O'rings while testing. It has to be stated that such deformations do not have any significant impact on the permeation behavior of the membrane, as has been confirmed by further gas permeation tests after the microscopic measurements. This kind of observation method will be useful in finding the macro-distribution of second phases or the uniformity of coatings in the case of composite membranes.

Field Emission Scanning Electron Microscopy (FESEM) is one of the most powerful tools in determining the structure of amorphous membranes. Cross-sectional images of a silica membrane are shown in Figs. 19 and 20. Figure 19 shows the structure of a silica membrane over the intermediate alumina layer. The layer is interpenetrated but has a crack-free structure. Figure 20 shows a silica membrane sandwiched between two alumina layers. The topmost alumina layer in this case was not probably interpenetrated with silica during dipping. The fractal nature of the silica surface, however, can provide enough mechanical interpenetrating for the layer to hold on during drying. During further calcination it is highly possible that the interface should become inter-diffused. Such structures have shown to improve the selectivity to alkenes probably owing to surface selectivity at the interface and high adsorption capacity of alumina [89].

The supported membrane porosity and to some extent the pore size are functions of reactant concentrations and sol synthesis conditions as has been

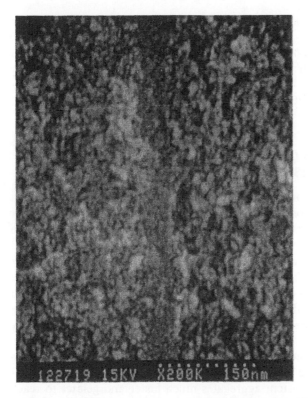

FIG. 20 FESEM image of a sandwiched silica layer between two gamma alumina layers is shown. The membrane was microporous [89].

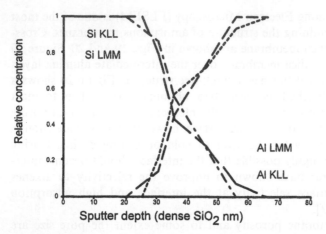

FIG. 21 SAM sputter profile of silica modified gamma alumina membrane [20].

discussed already. The thickness of the membrane however depends more on the dipping time and speed. Under the standard synthesis conditions (sol XW) a membrane thickness of 60 nm can be realized. However Scanning Auger Microscopy (SAM) sputter profiles showed the silica structure to be partly penetrated in the alumina mesoporous intermediate layer. Aluminum ions have been picked up from 30 nm onwards from the surface as shown in Fig. 21 [20].

VI. CORRELATION OF POLYMER AND MEMBRANE STRUCTURE: DISCUSSIONS

Hydrolysis and condensation reactions in silicon alkoxides depend on reactant concentrations as well as conditions such as the reaction temperature. Another variable which can change the pore structure of the gel is aging. Figs. 3–6 essentially indicates such developments in gel structure. The sol which showed a (fractal) slope of 0.4–0.6 during the growing stage, has developed more or less linear connected morphology by the end of synthesis with a fractal slope of 0.96. A fractal dimension of 1 theoretically represent linear connected fractal polymers [60]. Because of their mutual transparency, these polymers can give rise to well packed membranes. Consequently, smaller pore sizes or porosity are realized.

Aging of the sol as shown in Fig. 6 is rather slow at the beginning. The fractal dimension remained constant for the first few decades of hours. After this induction period, the system aggregates much faster and gelates to reach almost constant fractality. A final fractal dimension of 2.15 was observed after 8 months. This value is higher than expected for a classical tip–tip aggregate.

However Beelen et al. [90] has reported simulated fractal dimensions of 2.1 on DLCCA (diffusion limited cluster–cluster aggregation) aggregates with reaction constraints.

High temperature aging studies showed predominantly DLCCA effects. At high temperatures reaction limitations are low and hence the final fractal dimension is that of a DLCCA aggregate. Even with extremely low amounts of protons ($0.05XW$), the gel formed is more or less open structured. This is not completely unexpected since the heat of reaction of this sample was high enough for fast hydrolysis of at least one ethoxy group as we have already seen.

It is important to note that most of the samples reached gelation during the course of the high temperature measurement. From the growth curves it is difficult to distinguish this physical change. A thorough evaluation of growth curves in Figs. 4 and 5, however, reveals the following. Samples with higher amount of catalyst shows a transition point around 10 h. The rate of increase in D_f slows down where as ξ gains momentum around this point. This could correspond to percolation threshold. This increase in ξ corresponded well with the visual observation of gelation at some instants. However near the gel point, where the aggregates percolates to create the sol-gel transition, the synthesis chemistry of the sol is reportedly irrelevant [91]. It is also reported in the case of base catalyzed silica sol that the structure found by SAXS may not be representative of the macroscopic structure of the gel [44]. Nevertheless, in the discussion to follow we will show that the fractal structure of the polymer before gelation corresponds well with the final structure of the gel and the membrane made from them.

As can be seen in Fig. 8 the dilution can affect the kinetics of aggregation during aging. The effect of diffusion limitations on the aggregation during aging is clear. As already said the synthesis reported here all done at 65°C. This is the reason for the difference between the starting fractal dimensions of 0.96 (sample XW) to 1.3 between this work and that of de Lange et al. [20], even if the composition was nearly the same. In the case of de Lange's results the hydrolysis and condensation reactions are faster, because of the higher synthesis temperature. This large deviation of D_f by the end of 3-h synthesis clearly shows the reaction limitations on polymeric growth caused by temperature conditions.

Figure 3 presents the classical scattering spectra with Porod, fractal and Guinier regions. R_o values can be calculated to be in the region of 0.25 nm. This goes along with the findings of de Lange [20] and Kamiyama [92]. However contrary to Kamiyama's results the changes in R_o with synthesis chemistry were not that statistically significant under our experimental conditions. The primary building unit is most likely an oligometer built up from only a very limited amount of monomers since the Si-O bond length is 0.16–0.17 nm [20].

Figures 4, 5 and 9 present a systematic picture of fractality changes because of synthesis chemistry variations. D_f and R_g increases with catalyst concentration and water concentration in the reactant mixture. The increase in H^+ concentration increases the condensation rates, resulting in polymers with a higher degree of branching. In the area with $r_w > 4$, D_f is increasing with increasing r_a and r_w. This is in accordance with literature [45–49], where results indicated a linear relationship between r_a and the hydrolysis reaction rate. This leads to accelerated reaction rates, resulting in a higher degree of hydrolyzed groups on the species in the sol. After condensation, this will result in more polymerized and more branched structures of the species in the sol.

The relative weight loss during heating has increased with increasing r_a ($r_w = 6.4$). It is clear from Fig. 11 that the largest relative weight loss occurs in the temperature region of 0°C to 150°C. As the relative weight loss up to 150°C is attributed to the evaporation of water and ethanol [44], the samples with higher r_a contain higher amounts of fluid in their structure (per unit weight of the sample). Therefore this structure has to be more porous than the structures of samples with lower r_a. This conclusion is in accordance with results found from the nitrogen adsorption measurements, in which samples with increasing r_a show an increase in porosity.

In the range of 150–400°C, the relative weight loss is decreasing with increasing r_a at constant r_w ($r_w = 6.4$) as in Fig. 12. As higher r_a values leads to a higher degree of polymerization and branching of the polymer, the total number of ethoxy-groups in the polymer per unit weight of the sample will decrease. The TGA-curves were not notably affected by variation of r_w.

From Fig. 14 it becomes clear that the porosity increases with increasing r_a (constant $r_w = 6.4$). The same is found in Fig. 15, where the porosity increases for increasing r_a at several values of r_w. The structure of the polymer with higher r_a will be more polymerized and more branched, and thus more porous. From Fig. 14, it also becomes clear that with increasing r_a the increase in porosity becomes less, just as in the case of increase of D_f.

The samples with $r_a \sim 0.0021$ yielded nitrogen-dense gels. Because of the low r_a, these structures will most likely consist of linear polymers, which can pack very closely together. The pore number density obviously is insufficient to reach the percolation threshold of pore connectivity.

The present set of experiments indicates that, for $r_w > 4$, the porosity has a tendency to increase with increasing r_w. As already discussed earlier, the sols with $r_w < 4$ resulted in gels with a surprisingly high porosity. In this area the SAXS plots showed very low values for the fractal slope, $D_f < 0.8$. Comparable values for the fractal slope (<0.8) were generally found in the growing stages of other sols, indicating that at this low r_w-value the polymerization reactions are not completed within the synthesis time. Surprisingly these sols result in microporous structures with very high porosities. A logical assumption would be that the partially reacted species in the sol proceed with the condensation reactions during drying, resulting in a more open structure than was expected on basis of the SAXS results.

It also becomes clear from Fig. 15 that small changes in r_a results in relatively large changes in porosity, while large changes in r_w result in relatively small changes in porosity. Hence it can be concluded that most of the structures can be tailor-made by a mere variation of r_a alone without resorting to changes in r_w. Thus, for tailor-making membranes, changes in r_a have greater influence on the structure than changes in r_w.

A. Evaluation and Identification of Pore Morphology

From the study of SAXS spectra the method of aggregate formation in silica sols have been identified as a combination of Diffusion Limited Cluster–Cluster Aggregation (DLCCA) and Reaction Limited Cluster–Cluster Aggregation (RLCCA) [70,90]. The effect of RLCCA is predominant under low temperature or under nonstochiometric synthesis conditions. DLCCA, on the other hand, will be dominated under high temperatures. Under standard membrane processing conditions the high temperature synthesis of the sol and the low temperature drying will promote a structure influenced by both these mechanisms (DLCCA/RLCCA). The membrane properties hence depend on the synthesis conditions, concentration of the dipping solution and rate of drying. However the pattern of growth of silica polymers seems to be similar in the window of the present conditions. The kinetics are different but the mechanism remained the same, irrespective of moderate changes in r_a or r_w. Variables like changes in temperature of dilution changed the kinetics and sometimes the mechanism of aggregation. But none of these moderate changes initiated a morphological renovation.

Extreme conditions like highly-concentrated or nonstochiometric systems produced more aggressive changes. However, some of these conditions are unsuitable for synthesis of membranes without defects and cannot be accommodated in the present context of microporous membrane design.

From the trends we have seen so far, it seems as if tailor-making membranes with regard to permeation (porosity) is possible. With regard to selectivity (pore size) no quantitative understanding was available. Pore size calculations from adsorption isotherms (on gels) following the procedures of Horváth and Kawazoe (H–K) [87] generated bi-modal distribution with a strong maximum around 0.5 nm and a smaller and broader maximum around 0.7 nm. No significant changes were observed in pore size along with porosity changes.

B. Confirmation of Structure: Conclusions

Supported silica membranes were synthesized from sols with different synthesis history to make membranes with different porosity (gel). Figure 22 shows

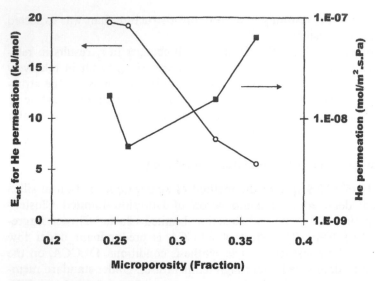

FIG. 22 Helium permeation (303 K and 1000 Torr) and activation energy of silica membranes with different synthesis history. Synthesis changes are reflected in the changes in gel porosity. (■), He permeation; (○), activation energy.

the helium permeation results of these membranes. It is shown that the permeation of helium increases proportional to the increase in porosity. However, the activation energy for helium permeation decreases as the porosity increases. From this point of view it looks as if the pore size really changes, since the activation energy in larger pores is indeed smaller than that in small pores. However, further results as shown in the kinetic diameter vs. permeation curves of Fig. 23, did not support this argument.

The shape of the curves, Fig. 23, is very important. It is clear that the porosity changes brings about changes in permeation only for very small values of the kinetic diameter. The drop in permeation as the molecular size increase from helium to N_2 became sharp as the porosity decreases. In case of molecules bigger than N_2 (w.r.t. kinetic diameter) the change in porosity did not make any appreciable differences in ratio of their permeation values (ideal selectivity). Furthermore N_2 permeation hasn't always been activated. The ratio of high (408 K) and low temperature (303 K) nitrogen permeation values decreased from 1.35 to 0.6 as the porosity went up from 24.6% to 36.2%. As a result of this nonactivated permeation the He/N_2 selectivity was extremely high at high temperatures for, e.g., the membrane with 24.6% porosity (Fig. 24).

The differences in mechanism of diffusion between the molelules (He vs. N_2 for example) and the high ideal selectivity (He/N_2) involved, suggests that the

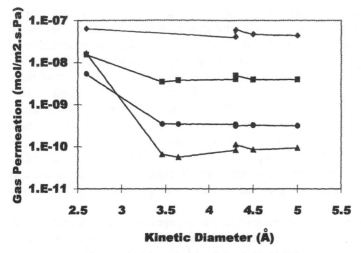

FIG. 23 Dependence of gas permeation to kinetic diameter of the permeating molecule and to the synthesis history of the membrane. Legend shows microporosity of the membrane material (gel) and activation energy for helium permeation (fitting range 303–373 K). Tested molecules were He(2.6 Å), O_2(3.46 Å), N_2(3.64 Å), C_3H_8(4.3 Å), n-C_4H_{10}(4.3 Å), C_3H_6(4.5 Å) and i-C_4H_{10}(5 Å). (◆), 36.23% 5.57 kJ/mol; (●), 26.03% 19.2 kJ/mol; (■), 33.04% 7.98 kJ/mol; (▲), 24.55% 19.55 kJ/mol [74].

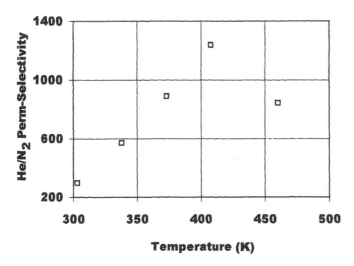

FIG. 24 The dependence of helium/nitrogen ideal selectivity on temperature is shown. The permeation behavior of this membrane for other gas molecules is shown in Fig. 23 (gel porosity; 24.6%) [75].

pore size distribution is bimodal in these membranes. Pores with sizes around 3 Å allow activated diffusion of He molecule and are capable of sieving all other molecules. Together with these small pores a sizable proportion of bigger pores are present. They are the leakage pores of the membrane and are responsible for the deterioration of molecular sieving ability. The size of these pores is not exactly known. The nonactivated transport of N_2 suggests that their size is in or above the Knudsen diffusion regime. Polymeric growth seems to amplify the presence of nonselective pores in the membrane. Hence these bigger pores might be the interaggregate voids produced by the opaqueness of the polymers. Controling the size and amount of this is crucial in tailor-making membranes with regard to pore size. Template based approaches, as detailed by Brinker et al. [41], is one way to control the size and distribution of such voids.

In the present level of understanding, the changes brought about by variations in the synthesis were in the cumulative pore volumes of pores with sizes smaller than those of N_2 molecular size and pores with much larger sizes, through which even larger molecules can easily diffuse. Permeation of molecules through these large pores is nonselective. The conclusion is that the majority of the pore sizes of these membranes lies between the molecular sizes of helium (0.26 nm) and nitrogen (0.364 nm). The very high helium activation energy of membranes with low porosities confirms the small pore sizes. This provides very high selectivity between these molecules as shown in Fig. 24, under the most suitable synthesis conditions. Controlling the synthesis chemistry can facilitate optimization of the molecular-sieving performance and tailor-make the membrane with respect to permeation.

ACKNOWLEDGMENTS

Our sincere gratitude to the colleagues and management of University of Tokyo, University of Twente, VITO and Japan High Polymer Center for the excellent atmosphere and help they have provided us during the course of this research work. A part of the work detailed in this chapter was performed by Dr. R. S. A. de Lange and Ms. J. W. Elferink during the course of their stay in Twente with K. Keizer. Our sincere thanks to them. B. N. Nair would like to acknowledge Prof. A. J. Burggraaf for the constant encouragement he has provided. A part of this work has been conducted by the support of the Petroleum Energy Center (PEC) subsidized from the Ministry of International Trade and Industry, Japan.

LIST OF SYMBOLS

d_{av} Average pore diameter of the membrane
D_{eff} Effective pore diameter calculated by H–K analysis

d_E Diameter of oxygen atom as used in H–K analysis
D_f Mass fractal dimension of the polymer
D_s Surface fractal dimension of the polymer
E_{act} Activation energy (apparent) for diffusion
I Intensity of scattered wave
$\xi(Ksi)$ Upper cut-off length of fractal region
λ Wave length of scattered radiation
M Mass of polymer
Q Scattering vector
R Size of the polymer
R_o Lower cut-off length of fractal region
R_g Radius of gyration
r_a Molar ratio of acid to TEOS
r_w Molar ratio of water to TEOS
r_p Calculated pore radius by H–K analysis
θ Scattering angle
W Represents 6.4 mol of H_2O for each mol of TEOS in the synthesis mixture
X Represents 0.085 mol of H^+ for each mol of TEOS in the synthesis mixture

REFERENCES

1. G. R. Gavalas, C. Megiris, and S. W. Nam, Chem. Eng. Sci. *44*: 1829 (1989).
2. S. Kitao and M. Asaeda, Gas separation of thin porous silica membrane prepared by sol–gel and CVD methods, ICIM 2, Montpellier, France 1991.
3. T. Okubo and H. Inoue, J. Membrane Sci. *42*: 109 (1989).
4. S-I. Nakao, Y. Satoh, and S. Kimura, Pore size control of porous glass membrane by TEOS/O_3 CVD in the opposite reactants geometry, Proceedings of ICIM 3 (Y. H. Ma, ed.), 1994, pp. 37–47.
5. M. Tsapatsis and G. Gavalas, J. Membrane Sci. *87*: 281 (1994).
6. J. C. S. Wu, H. Sabol, G. W. Smith, D. L. Flowers, and P. K. T. Liu, J. Membrane Sci. *96*: 227 (1994).
7. A. F. M. Leenaars, K. Keizer, and A. J. Burggraaf, J. Mater. Sci. *19*: 1077 (1984).
8. A. F. M. Leenaars and A. J. Burggraaf, J. Colloid Interface Sci. *105*: 27 (1985).
9. A. Larbot, S. Alami-Younssi, M. Persin, J. Sarrazin, and L. Cot, J. Membrane Sci. *97*: 167 (1994).
10. S. Alami-Younssi, A. Larbot, M. Persin, J. Sarrazin, and L. Cot, J. Membrane Sci. *91*: 87 (1994).
11. J. M. Zuter-Hofman, Chemical and thermal stability of modified mesoporous ceramic membranes, PhD thesis, University of Twente, Enschede, The Netherlands (1995).
12. K-N. P. Kumar, Nanostructured ceramic membranes, PhD thesis, University of Twente, The Netherlands (1993).
13. K. Kusakabe, K. Ichiki, and S. Morooka, J. Membrane Sci. *95*: 171 (1994).

14. A. Larbot, A. Julbe, C. Guizard, and L. Cot, Membrane Sci. *44*: 289 (1994).
15. M. J. Muñoz-Agudo and M. Gregorkiewitz, J. Membrane Sci. *11*: 7 (1996).
16. M. Asaeda, A. Yamamichi, M. Satoh, and M. Kamakura, Preparation of porous membranes for separation of propylene/propane gaseous mixtures, Proceedings of ICIM 3 (Y. H. Ma, ed.), 1994, pp. 315–324.
17. R. J. R. Uhlhorn, K. Keizer, and A. J. Burggraaf, J. Membrane Sci. *66*: 271 (1992).
18. C. J. Brinker, T. L. Ward, R. Sehgal, N. K. Raman, S. L. Hietala, D. M. Smith, D. W. Hua, and T. J. Headley, J. Membrane Sci. *77*: 165 (1993).
19. R. J. R. Uhlhorn, Ceramic membranes for gas separation, PhD thesis, University of Twente, The Netherlands (1990).
20. R. S. A. de Lange, Microporous sol–gel derived ceramic membranes for gas separation, Ph.D. Thesis, University of Twente, The Netherlands (1993).
21. A. Julbe, C. Guizard, A. Larbot, L. Cot, and A. Giroir-Frendler, The sol–gel approach to prepare candidate microporous inorganic membranes for membrane reactors, J. Membrane Sci. *77*: 137 (1993).
22. C. Balzer, A. Julbe, C. Guizard, A. Larbot, J. Peureux, A. Giroir-Frendler, J. A. Dalmon, and L. Cot, Silica based membranes designed for catalytic reators, Proceedings of ICIM 3, (Y. H. Ma, ed.), 1994, pp. 629–633.
23. W. F. Maier and H. O. Schramm, Mater Res. Soc. Proc. *271*: 493 (1992).
24. C. J. Brinker, A. J. Hurd, P. R. Schunk, G. C. Frye, and C. S. Ashley, J. Non-Crystalline Solids, *147/148*: 424 (1992).
25. C. J. Brinker, N. K. Raman, M. N. Logan, R. Sehgal, R. A. Assink, D. W. Hua, and T. L. Ward, J. Sol–Gel Sci. Technol., *4*: 117 (1995).
26. N. K. Raman, C. J. Brinker, L. Delattre, and S. S. Prakash, Sol–gel strategies for amorphous inorganic membranes exhibiting molecular sieving characteristics, Proceedings of ICIM 3, (Y. H. Ma, ed.), 1994, pp. 63–73.
27. M. Asaeda and L. D. Du, J. Chem. Eng. Japan *19*: 72 (1986).
28. S. Kitao, H. Kameda, and M. Asaeda, Membrane *15*: 222 (1990).
29. M. Azaeda, K. Okazaki, and A. Nakatani, Ceramic Transactions *31*: 411 (1992).
30. M. Asaeda, Y. Oki, and T. Manabe, Preparation of porous silica membranes for separation of inorganic mixtures at high temperature in *Energy Conversion and Utilization with High Efficiency*, 1993, pp. 253–258.
31. A. J. Burggraaf and L. Cot, *Fundamentals of Inorganic Membrane Science and Technology*, Elsevier, Amsterdam, 1996.
32. R. R. Bhave, *Inorganic Membranes*, Van Nostrand Reinhold, 1991.
33. A. J. Burggraaf, Key points in understanding and development of ceramic membranes, Proceedings of ICIM 3, (Y. H. Ma, ed.), 1994, pp. 1–16.
34. R. S. A. de Lange, K. Keizer, and A. J. Burggraaf, J. Membrane Sci. *99*: 139 (1995).
35. R. D. Noble and S. A. Stern, *Membrane Separations Technology, Principles and Applications*, Elsevier, Amsterdam, 1995.
36. R. S. A. de Lange, J. H. A. Hekkink, K. Keizer, and A. J. Burggraaf, J. Membrane Sci. *99*: 57 (1995).
37. M. Moaddeb and W. J. Koros, J. Membrane Sci. *125*: 143 (1997).
38. K. Kusakabe, K. Ichiki, and S. Morooka, Preparation of CO_2 permselective hybrid membranes by sol–gel process, Proceedings of Euromembrane 95, (W. R. Bowen, R. W. Field, and J. A. Howell, eds.), 1995, pp. 208–211.

39. T. Okui, Y. Saito, T. Okubo, and S. Sadakata, J. Sol-Gel Sci. Technol. *5*:127 (1995).
40. W. S. Ho, Hard/Soft segment copolymer membranes for pervaporation separation of aromatics from saturates, AIChE annual meeting, Chicago, 1996.
41. N. K. Raman, M. T. Anderson, and C. J. Brinker, Chem. Mater. *8*:1682 (1996).
42. G. Cao, Y. Lu, L. Delattre, C. J. Brinker, and G. P. Lopez, Adv. Mater. *8*:588 (1996).
43. J. Wen and G. L. Wilkes, Chem. Mater. *8*:1667 (1996).
44. C. J. Brinker and G. W. Scherer, *Sol–Gel Science: The Physics and Chemistry of Sol–Gel Processing*, Academic Press Ltd, London, 1990.
45. R. Aelion, A. Loebel, and F. Eirich, J. Am. Chem. Soc. *72*:5705 (1950).
46. A. H. Boonstra and T. N. M. Bernards, J. Non-Crystalline Solids *108*:249 (1989).
47. S. Sakka and K. Kamiya, J. Non-Crystalline Solids *48*:31 (1982).
48. D. P. Partlow and B. E. Yoldas, J. Non-Crystalline Solids *46*:153 (1981).
49. B. E. Yoldas, J. Mater. Sci. *14*:1843 (1979).
50. C. J. Brinker, R. Sehgal, S. L. Hietala, R. Deshpande, D. M. Smith, D. Loy, and C. S. Ashley, J. Membrane Sci. *94*: 85 (1994).
51. B. B. Mandelbrot, *The Fractal Geometry of Nature*, W. H. Freeman & Company, New York, 1983.
52. J. Teixeira, J. Appl. Cryst. *21*:781 (1988).
53. O. Glatter and O. Kratky, *Small Angle X-ray Scattering*, Academic Press, London, 1982.
54. C. Rottman, G. S. Grader, Y. Hazan, and D. Avnir, Langmuir *12*:5505 (1996).
55. P. Meakin, Phys. Rev. Lett. *51*:1119 (1983).
56. G. Dietler, C. Aubert, D. S. Cannell, and P. Wiltziux, Phys. Rev. Lett. *57*:3117 (1986).
57. H. E. Stanley and N. Ostrowsky, *On Growth and Form*, Martinus Nijhoff, Netherlands, 1986.
58. D. W. Schaefer and K. D. Keefer, Mater. Res. Soc. Symp. Proc. Vol. 73., Mater. Res. Soc. *73*:277 (1986).
59. P. Meakin, Ann. Rev. Phys. Chem. *39*:237 (1988).
60. J. E. Martin and A. J. Hurd, J. Appl. Cryst. *20*:61 (1987).
61. J. Zarzycki, J. Non-Crystalline Solids *121*:110 (1990).
62. N. Maene, B. B. Nair, P. d'Hooghe, S.-I. Nakao, and K. Keizer, J. Sol–Gel Sci. Technology *12,2*:in press (1998).
63. R. S. A. de Lange, K. Keizer, and A. J. Burggraaf, J. Porous Mater. *1*:139 (1995).
64. M. M. Dubinin, Carbon *27*:457 (1989).
65. S. J. Gregg and K. S. W. Sing, *Adsorption, Surface Area and Porosity*, Academic Press, London, 1982.
66. A. Lecloux and J. P. Pirard, J. Colloid Interface Sci. *70*:265 (1979).
67. S. W. Webb and W. C. Corner, Sorption of gases in microporous solids; Pore size characterization by gas adsorption, in *Characterization of Porous Solids II*, (F. Rodriguez-Reinoso, J. Rouquerol, K. S. W. Sing, and K. K. Unger, eds.) Elsevier, Amsterdam, 1991, pp. 31–40.
68. D. H. Everett and J. C. Powl, J. Chem. Soc. Faraday Trans. I, *72*:619 (1976).
69. J. H. de Boer, B. G. Linsen, and J. Osinga, J. Catalysis, *4*:643 (1965).

70. B. N. Nair, J. W. Elferink, K. Keizer, and H. Verwey, J. Colloid Interface Sci. *178*: 565 (1996).
71. J. W. Elferink, B. N. Nair, K. Keizer, and H. Verwey, J. Colloid Interface Sci. *180*: 127 (1996).
72. R. J. R. Uhlhorn, K. Keizer, and A. J. Burggraaf, J. Mater. Sci. *72*: 527/537 (1992).
73. B. N. Nair, J. W. Elferink, K. Keizer, and H. Verwey, J. Sol–Gel Sci. Technology *8*: 471 (1997).
74. B. N. Nair, K. Keizer, T. Okubo, and S-I. Nakao, Adv. Mater. *10*: 249 (1997).
75. B. N. Nair, K. Keizer, T. Okubo, and S-I. Nakao, J. Membrane Sci. *135*: 237 (1997).
76. R. S. A. de Lange, K. Keizer, and A. J. Burggraaf, J. Membrane Sci. *104*: 81 (1995).
77. K. Keizer, R. J. R. Uhlhorn, R. J. van Vuren, and A. J. Burggraaf, J. Membrane Sci. *39*: 285 (1988).
78. R. S. A. de Lange, K. Keizer, and A. J. Burggraaf, J. Non-Crystalline Solids *191*: 1 (1995).
79. B. N. Nair, K. Keizer, H. Verweij, and A. J. Burggraaf, Separation Sci. Technol. *31*: 1907 (1996).
80. T. W. Zerda, I. Artaki, and J. Jonas, J. Non-Crystalline Solids, *81*: 365 (1986).
81. L. C. Klein, Ann. Rev. Mater. Sci. *15*: 227 (1985).
82. C. Guizard, C. Mouchet, R. Vacassy, A. Julbe, and A. Larbort, J. Sol–Gel Sci. Technol. *2*: 483 (1995).
83. L. C. Klein and G. J. Garvey, J. Non-Crystalline Solids, *38/39*: 45 (1980).
84. R. K. Iler, *The Chemistry of Silica*, John Wiley & Sons Inc., New York, 1979.
85. E. J. A. Pope and J. D. Mackenzie, J. Non-Crystalline Solids *87*: 185 (1986).
86. K. S. W. Sing, Pure and Appl. Chem. *57*: 603 (1985).
87. G. Horváth and K. Kawazoe, J. Chem. Eng. Japan, *16*: 470 (1983).
88. A. Saito and H. C. Foley, AIChE Journal *37*: 429 (1991).
89. B. N. Nair, W. Elferink, M. J. Gilde, K. Keizer, H. Verweij, and A. J. Burggraaf, J. Membrane Sci. *116*: 161 (1996).
90. T. P. M. Beelen, W. H. Dokter, H. F. Van Garderen, and R. A. Van Santen, Adv. Colloid Interface Sci. *50*: 23 (1994).
91. J. E. Martin and J. Wilcoxon, Mater. Res. Soc. Symp. Proc. *180*: 199 (1990).
92. T. Kamiyama, M. Mikami, and K. Suzuki, J. Non-Crystalline Solids *150*: 157 (1992).

5

Fundamentals of Transport Phenomena in Polymer Solution–Diffusion Membranes

J. H. PETROPOULOS, M. SANOPOULOU, and K. G. PAPADOKOSTAKI
Physical Chemistry Institute, Democritos National Research Centre,
Athens, Greece

Abstract

The fundamental transport properties, namely permeability and permselectivity, of polymer solution–diffusion membranes in their most
important applications are discussed. The applications considered are
gas separation, vapor permeation/pervaporation and reverse osmosis. It
is emphasized that these physically diverse transport processes may be
formulated, and the relevant data analyzed, in a reasonably uniform

and, at the same time, rigorous manner. On the more practical side, attention is focused on the major common physicochemical parameters which govern transport behavior in these processes and the establishment of fundamental principles, which can serve as guidelines for the design of polymeric membrane materials with optimum permeability and permselectivity.

I. INTRODUCTION

Achievement of membrane separations of practical interest requires (a) suitable membrane configuration and module design, usually in the form of ultrathin "asymmetric" or "composite" membranes in hollow fibre or spirally wound sheet form [1,2], and (b) sufficiently high membrane permeability and permselectivity. Both asymmetric and composite polymeric membrane configurations to be considered here consist basically of an ultrathin polymer surface layer resting on a porous support. The latter is normally highly permeable and unselective; so that selective transport through the composite or asymmetric membrane is effectively controlled by dissolution of the penetrant molecules in, and subsequent diffusion through, the polymeric material composing the aforementioned surface layer; which, in effect, constitutes the real solution–diffusion membrane and will be referred to simply as "the membrane" in what follows.

Clearly, rational polymeric material selection for the achievement of optimum membrane permeability and permselectivity properties, presupposes fundamental understanding of the physical mechanisms of solution and diffusion and of the effect of the nature of the polymer and of the penetrant(s) on these processes. This, in turn, requires (i) properly defined permeability and permselectivity parameters, based on the formulation of penetrant transport through the membrane in terms of appropriate driving forces, and (ii) evaluation of the physical behavior of the said permeability and permselectivity parameters by means of suitable molecular models of the polymer–penetrant system.

Progress along these lines would obviously be facilitated by adoption of a unified approach to (i) and (ii) in studies of different separation processes. This is not commonly done at the present time. Here, we consider three such processes of topical interest, namely gas separation, vapor permeation/ pervaporation and reverse osmosis (hyperfiltration); which are usually formulated in terms of gas, vapor or hydrostatic pressure gradient driving forces, respectively (see Figs. 1a–c). It has frequently been pointed out [1–4] that penetrant transport may be formulated quite generally in terms of chemical potential gradient driving forces (see Fig. 1d); but few attempts have so far been made to carry this approach through to the establishment of actual working equations of a fundamental nature and wide applicability [2,5–7]. We

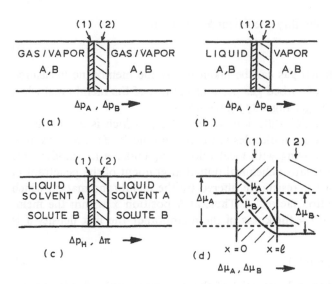

FIG. 1 Schematic illustration of the separation of a binary mixture AB by (a) gas or vapor permeation, (b) pervaporation, or (c) reverse osmosis (hyperfiltration), using a simple composite membrane configuration consisting of (1) an ultrathin polymer surface layer (the actual selective solution–diffusion membrane) and (2) a porous support layer (assumed to possess infinite permeability and no selectivity). Transport of A and B from the feed phase (on the left-hand side) to the permeate phase (on the right-hand side) is commonly regarded as the result of diverse driving forces (operating in the direction of the arrows), resulting from gas/vapor (Δp_A, Δp_B), or hydrostatic (Δp_H) and osmotic ($\Delta \pi$), pressure differences applied across the membrane. A unified picture is shown in (d), where all these processes are regarded as driven by forces resulting from the application of chemical potential differences $\Delta \mu_A$, $\Delta \mu_B$ across the membrane. Chemical potential profiles $\mu_A(x)$, $\mu_B(x)$ are set up within the solution–diffusion membrane and transport of A and B molecules, at any location $0 \leq x \leq l$ therein, is considered to be driven by the local chemical potential gradients ($\partial \mu_A / \partial x$, $\partial \mu_B / \partial x$).

present here another attempt at a (hopefully somewhat simpler, more general and/or rigorous) unified treatment of this kind. We further show that the dependence of permeability and permselectivity properties on salient polymer and penetrant molecular characteristics can be understood also on the basis of a uniform set of general principles.

II. GAS PERMEATION

A. Fundamental Transport Parameters

The permeability coefficient P, which controls the flux of gas through a homogeneous polymeric (or other) membrane, is the product of physically more fundamental thermodynamic and kinetic parameters, namely [3,4]:

(a) The sorption or solubility coefficient S defined by

$$S = C/f \approx C/p \tag{1}$$

which indicates how much gas can be taken up by the membrane (measured by the concentration C of sorbed gas per unit volume of the membrane) when equilibrated with a given gas fugacity f (pressure p).

(b) The "thermodynamic" diffusion coefficient D_T, which is a measure of the mobility of the penetrant molecules in the membrane. The sorbed gas molecules are regarded as moving with local velocity u_x under a thermodynamic driving force $-\partial\mu/\partial x$ (negative chemical potential gradient of the penetrant in the membrane) against the resistance offered by the membrane matrix, which is measured by a "friction factor" ζ. Thus, at a position x within the membrane ($0 \le x \le l$, where l = thickness of the membrane), the flux density J is given by [3,4]

$$J_x = u_x C = -(C/\zeta)(\partial\mu/\partial x) \tag{2}$$

Denoting by μ_g the chemical potential of the penetrant molecules in the gas phase which would be at equilibrium with C at x, we have

$$\mu = \mu_g = \mu_g^o + RT \ln f \approx \mu_g^o + RT \ln p \tag{3}$$

Then, inserting Eq. (3) in (2) and making use of the definition $D_T = RT/\zeta$ and of Eq. (1), we get

$$J_x = -(D_T C/f)(\partial f/\partial x) = -D_T S(\partial f/\partial x) = -P(\partial f/\partial x) \approx -P(\partial p/\partial x) \tag{4}$$

where $P = D_T S$ is the (differential) permeability coefficient.

In practice, we often use the Fick (or practical) diffusion coefficient defined by

$$J_x = -D(\partial C/\partial x) \tag{5}$$

which is known as Fick's law when D = const. Comparison of Eqs. (4) and (5) shows that

$$D = D_T S(df/dC) = P(df/dC) \approx P(dp/dC) \tag{6}$$

Equation (6) indicates that Fick's law is valid (D = const) only when both D_T = const and S = const and hence P = const. (Note that S = const implies $S(df/dC) = 1$, hence $D \equiv D_T$; otherwise $D \ne D_T$). We shall refer to such a system as ideal. Nonideal penetrant–membrane systems are characterized by P or D varying appreciably with C (or f) (due to either S or D_T or both being functions of C).

The permeability coefficient usually measured is the integral coefficient $\bar{P}$. obtained by integration of Eq. (2), under conditions of steady-state permeation ($J_x = J_S$ = const), i.e.

$$J_S l = \int_{f_1}^{f_0} P \, df = \bar{P}(f_0 - f_1) \approx \bar{P}(p_0 - p_1) \tag{7}$$

where f_0 (p_0), f_1 (p_1) denote the (constant) gas fugacity (pressure) maintained on the upstream or feed $(x = 0)$, and downstream or permeate $(x = l)$, sides of the membrane, respectively. Substitution from Eq. (6) into Eq. (7) yields the corresponding integral D, namely

$$J_S l = \int_{C_1}^{C_0} D \, dC = \bar{D}(C_0 - C_1) = \bar{P}(f_0 - f_1) \approx \bar{P}(p_0 - p_1) \tag{8}$$

where $C_0 = Sf_0$, $C_1 = Sf_1$ (i.e., the membrane surfaces are considered to be at equilibrium with the adjoining feed and permeate phases). Equation (8) shows that for $f_1 = C_1 = 0$, $\bar{P} = \bar{D}S(f_0)$.

Permeation of a binary gas mixture AB may be formulated as follows:

$$J_{AMS} = -P_{AM}(df_A/dx) = \bar{P}_{AM}(f_{AO} - f_{Al})/l \approx \bar{P}_{AM}(p_{AO} - p_{Al})/l \tag{9}$$

$$J_{BMS} = -P_{BM}(df_B/dx) = \bar{P}_{BM}(f_{BO} - f_{Bl})/l \approx \bar{P}_{BM}(p_{BO} - p_{Bl})/l \tag{10}$$

where the subscripts M have been introduced to allow for the fact that the permeability of one gas may be significantly affected by the other one (coupling effect). If this is so, the integral permeabilities $\bar{P}_{AM}$, $\bar{P}_{BM}$ must be derived from $P_{AM}(f_A, f_B)$, $P_{BM}(f_A, f_B)$ by simultaneous solution of Eqs. (9) and (10) [3,4] (see Sec. II.C.4 and 5 below for the relevant detailed treatments).

The intrinsic permselectivity of the membrane is conveniently defined as

$$\alpha_M^o = \bar{P}_{AM}/\bar{P}_{BM} \tag{11}$$

Under a given set of operating conditions, a separation factor α_M is used in practice to indicate the gas composition (n_{Al}/n_{Bl}) emerging on the permeate side relative to that (n_{AO}/n_{BO}) applied on the feed side (n = number of moles), namely

$$\alpha_M = n_{Al} n_{BO}/n_{AO} n_{Bl} \approx p_{Al} p_{BO}/p_{AO} p_{Bl} \tag{12}$$

Since $n_{Al}/n_{Bl} = J_{AMS}/J_{BMS}$, substitution from Eqs. (9)–(11) into (12) yields

$$\alpha_M \approx \alpha_M^o (1 - p_{Al}/p_{AO})/(1 - p_{Bl}/p_{BO}) \approx \alpha_M^o/[1 + (\alpha_M^o - 1)p_{Bl}/p_{BO}] \tag{13}$$

Equation (13) shows that (i) $\alpha_M \approx \alpha_M^o$, when $p_{Bl}/p_{BO} = 0$ $(p_{Al}/p_{AO} = 0)$ and (ii) $\alpha_M < \alpha_M^o (\alpha_M > \alpha_M^o)$, when $p_{Bl}/p_{BO} > 0$ $(p_{Al}/p_{AO} > 0)$, if $\alpha_M^o > 1$ $(\alpha_M^o < 1)$; i.e., α_M^o represents the upper limit of the degree of separation obtainable, which is approached as the operating downstream pressure is reduced. For ideal pure gas–membrane systems:

$$\alpha_M^o = \alpha^o = P_A/P_B = S_A D_A/S_B D_B = \alpha_S^o \alpha_D^o \tag{14}$$

Equation (14) indicates that $\alpha_M^o = \alpha^o$ is independent of feed composition and may be conveniently analyzed into solubility and diffusivity selectivity factors

α_S^o and α_D^o, respectively. In nonideal systems α_M^o cannot properly be analyzed in this way. However, it is often (e.g., in pervaporation) useful to compare α_M^o with the apparent solubility selectivity defined as $S_{AM}(f_{AO}, f_{BO})/S_{BM}(f_{BO}, f_{AO})$.

It is noteworthy that the fundamental (S, D_T) and derived (P, D, α_M^o) parameters may be defined perfectly generally and independently of the type of membrane (whether solution–diffusion or porous, for example); but the physical behavior of these parameters obviously depends critically on the nature of the membrane and the penetrant.

B. Sorption Properties

1. Simple Dissolution

Sorption of a micromolecular penetrant A by an amorphous flexible-chain polymer P (or the amorphous region of a partly crystalline polymer of this kind) is regarded as a process of dissolution closely analogous to that in liquid solvents [8–10]. For nonpolar or weakly polar systems, in which intermolecular interactions are principally of the nonspecific van der Waals type:

$$\ln(f_A/f_A^{sat}) = \ln v_A + (1 - \bar{V}_A/\bar{V}_P)(1 - v_A) + \chi_A(1 - v_A)^2 \tag{15}$$

where $f_A(\approx p_A)$, $f_A^{sat}(\approx p_A^{sat})$ denote the fugacity (pressure) of A vapor over the A–P solution and over pure liquid A, respectively; v_A is the volume fraction of A in the A–P solution; $\bar{V}_A$, $\bar{V}_P$ are the relevant molar volumes; and χ_A is the Flory–Huggins interaction parameter, which is given by

$$\chi_A = 1/Z + \overline{\Delta H}_{MA}/RT = 1/Z + K\bar{V}_A(\sqrt{E_{CA}} - \sqrt{E_{CP}})^2/RT \tag{16}$$

In Eq. (16), $\overline{\Delta H}_{MA}$ is the (partial molar) enthalpy of mixing liquid A with P; Z is approximately equal to the coordination number of the lattice used to model the A–P solution (but, in practice, serves as an empirical constant, usually put equal to 0.35) [11]; E_{CA}, E_{CP} are the relevant cohesive energy densities (E_C = molar energy of vaporization/molar volume) and K is a constant (≈ 1 for simple liquid solutions) [8]. Equation (16) is derived by considering that the mixing process involves breaking A–A and P–P intermolecular contacts to form an equal number of A–P contacts and then assuming that the intermolecular energy per A–P contact is the geometric mean of that per A–A and P–P contact. It predicts $\overline{\Delta H}_{MA} > 0$ (endothermic mixing), if $E_{CA} \neq E_{CB}$; and $\overline{\Delta H}_{MA} = 0$ (athermal mixing), if $E_{CA} = E_{CB}$. Equations (15) and (16) are only rough approximations; but more elaborate treatments would not be of immediate interest here, because they do not usually lead to explicit analytical results [12].

Using Eq. (1) and $v_A = C_A \bar{V}_A$, Eq. (15) becomes for $v_A \ll 1$ (neglecting terms in v_A^2)

$$\begin{aligned}
\ln S_A = \ln(C_A/f_A) &= -\ln \bar{V}_A - \ln f_A^{sat} - (1 + \chi_A) + (1 + 2\chi_A)\bar{V}_A C_A \\
&= \ln K_A + b_A C_A
\end{aligned} \tag{17}$$

where K_A, b_A are constants. The predicted variation of S_A with C_A or p_A is illustrated in Fig. 2a. At sufficiently low f_A/f_A^{sat} (simple gases at not too high pressures) $S_A = K_A$ (Henry's law). The (virtual for simple gases) parameter f_A^{sat} may be roughly evaluated through the (integrated) Clausius–Clapeyron equation [9]

$$\ln f_A^{sat} = \overline{\Delta H}_{VA}/RT_{bA} - \overline{\Delta H}_{VA}/RT = K_V - \overline{\Delta H}_{VA}/RT \tag{18}$$

where $\overline{\Delta H}_{VA}$ is the molar enthalpy of evaporation, T_{bA} is the boiling point and $K_V \approx$ const. On the basis of Eqs. (16)–(18), K_A can be expressed as

$$\begin{aligned}\ln K_A &= -(1 + 1/Z) - \ln \overline{V}_A - K_V + \overline{\Delta H}_{VA}/RT - \overline{\Delta H}_{MA}/RT \\ &= \ln K_0 + \overline{\Delta H}_{VA}/RT - \overline{\Delta H}_{MA}/RT = \ln K_0 - \overline{\Delta H}_A/RT \tag{19} \\ &= \ln K_0' + \overline{\Delta H}_{VA}/RT \tag{20}\end{aligned}$$

In Eq. (20), one may put ($K_C \approx$ const, $K_E \approx$ const)

$$\overline{\Delta H}_{VA}/R = K_V T_{bA} = K_C T_{CA} = K_E \varepsilon_A/k \tag{21}$$

to derive a correlation with either T_{bA} or T_{CA} (critical temperature) or ε_A/k (Lennard–Jones force constant). Note that $\overline{\Delta H}_A = -\overline{\Delta H}_{VA} + \overline{\Delta H}_{MA}$ is the enthalpy of sorption from the gas phase; and that terms which are insensitive to temperature or gas properties have been grouped into K_0 or K_0', respectively, to bring into evidence the approximate linear correlation between $\ln K_A$

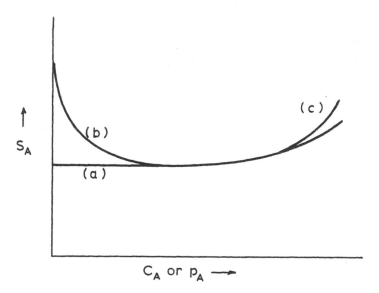

FIG. 2 Schematic illustration of the behavior of the sorption or solubility coefficient, as a function of gas/vapor pressure or concentration of sorbed species, under conditions of (a) simple dissolution (Eq. (17)), (b) dual mode sorption (Eq. (22)), and (c) clustering of dissolved molecules.

and $1/T$, or between $\ln K_A$ and the chosen gas property (T_{bA}, T_{CA} or ε_A/k) predicted by Eqs. (19) and (20), respectively.

Considering the drastic approximations involved, Eq. (20), in conjunction with (21), is remarkably well obeyed in practice [10]. As illustrated by the examples given in Table 1, the slope of these correlations is essentially independent of the solvent (whether micromolecular or polymeric) [13], as required by the theory; although wider variability is found in more extensive compilations of existing data [14]. This means that sorption selectivity (α_S^0) is primarily governed by gas properties and is in favor of the more condensable gas. The effect of the solvent medium is embodied in K_0'.

In the presence of polar or other specific solute–solvent interactions, S_A will be enhanced beyond what has been suggested above and the solvent medium will become correspondingly more selective for the more strongly interacting gas. This is illustrated in Table 2, where the selectivity for CO_2 (which has a quadrupole moment) over CH_4 clearly tends to increase with the polarity of the solvent. As was the case above, sorption selectivity (α_S^0) is much the same for polymeric media and their micromolecular liquid analogs [15].

2. Dual-Mode Sorption

Of particular interest for gas separation is the case of (reversible) chemical interaction of the penetrant gas with suitable moieties of the medium, referred

TABLE 1 Application of Eqs. (20) and (21) to Gases in Various Solvent Media (K_0' in cm³ STP/cm³ atm; K_E/T in K⁻¹)[a]

	$(K_E/T) \times 10^2$	$K_0' \times 10^{-2}$
Liquids (25°C)		
Benzene	0.95	2.98
n-heptane	0.94	1.69
Rubbers (25°C)		
Natural rubber	0.94	1.11
Silicone rubber	0.94	1.88
Butyl rubber	1.00	0.90
Amorphous polyethylene	0.94	0.72
Polychloroprene	0.97	1.10
Glasses (35°C)		
Polycarbonate	0.92	1.15
Polysulfone	0.96	0.93
Copolyester	0.96	1.03
Poly(phenylene oxide)	0.93	1.65

[a] *Source*: Ref. 13.

TABLE 2 Solution Selectivity (K_A/K_B or K_{A1}/K_{B1}) for CO_2/CH_4 in Various Solvent Media[a]

n-hexane	2.40	Amorphous Polyethylene	2.01
Benzene	4.68	Natural rubber	3.61
Methanol	7.63	Polysulfone	4.12
Methyl acetate	11.5	Cellulose acetate	11.4

[a] *Source*: Ref. 15.

to as "carriers"; because such interactions can be highly selective. This specific sorption mechanism (designated in what follows by the subscript 2) is governed by an affinity constant K_{A2} and occurs in parallel with the normal dissolution or nonspecific sorption mechanism (designated in what follows by the subscript 1). We thus have a dual mode sorption process, the overall sorption coefficient for which (S_A) is given by the sum of S_{A1} and S_{A2}, yielding for a simple gas ($S_{A1} = K_{A1}$)

$$S_A = C_A/f_A = (C_{A1} + C_{A2})/f_A = S_{A1} + S_{A2} = K_{A1} + s_{AO} K_{A2}/(1 + K_{A2} f_A)$$

$$(22)$$

In Eq. (22), s_{AO} denotes the concentration (in the same units as C_{A2}) of the moieties of the polymer (assumed univalent and equivalent, i.e., unaffected by any variability of their microenvironment) which participate in the specific sorption process; and the expression for S_{A2} follows from the usual definition of K_{A2}, namely

$$K_{A2} = C_{A2}/(s_{AO} - C_{A2})f_A \qquad (23)$$

Equation (22) has been applied, e.g., to sorption of SO_2 in a series of polymers containing groups of various basicities [16] and to O_2 sorption by membranes containing various concentrations of cobalt–porphyrin-complex carriers [17].

Equation (22) has also been widely applied to glassy polymers. It is well known that polymers below their glass transition temperature T_g are in a quasiequilibrium state, characterized by specific volume $\hat{V}_G$ in excess of the expected equilibrium value $\hat{V}_L$ (deduced by extrapolation from the $T > T_g$ region, cf. Fig. 3); the precise value of $\hat{V}_G$ at any $T < T_g$ depending on the previous history of the polymer. The excess free volume ($\hat{V}_G - \hat{V}_L$) is expected to be, at least partly, in the form of fixed microcavities dispersed in the polymer matrix. Such preformed (or partially preformed) microcavities can act as "sorption sites" for penetrant molecules; since less (or even no) energy must be expended in breaking interpolymer (P–P) contacts, when gas molecules are introduced therein. This sorption process (which should, according

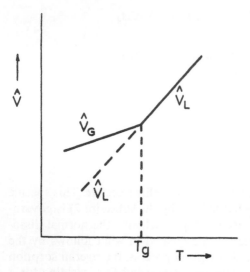

FIG. 3 Temperature dependence of polymer specific volume near the glass transition temperature (T_g).

to what has been said above, be considerably more exothermic than simple dissolution in the dense polymer matrix, i.e., $-\Delta H_{A2} > -\Delta H_{A1}$) is treated as simple Langmuir adsorption, which also fits the formalism of Eq. (22).

This model is obviously consistent with the tendency of S_A to decline with increasing gas pressure (as illustrated in Fig. 2b) commonly observed in glassy polymer–gas systems [3,13,18,19] and K_{A1}, K_{A2} and s_{AO} are routinely evaluated by curve-fitting Eq. (22) to the experimental data. However, the use of simple Langmuir adsorption theory entails a high degree of oversimplification; because the adsorption sites are thereby postulated to be independent, permanent and isoenergetic (i.e., $-\Delta H_{A2} = $ const). The latter condition is rarely realized in any kind of real adsorbent [3]; whereas the first two conditions together presuppose that the properties of the polymer are not appreciably modified by the penetrant. This premise becomes increasingly unrealistic with increasing gas pressure and adsorbability. Polymer properties may be modified in this manner both reversibly (plasticization) and semipermanently (conditioning) [3].

Although these limitations must constantly be kept in mind, there is nevertheless considerable evidence showing that this model is a useful and physically meaningful theory, as distinct from a mere curve-fitting exercise.

Thus, the correlation of K_{A1} (using the values obtained by curve-fitting Eq. (22) to a number of different glassy polymer-gas systems) with gas properties (ε_A/k), according to Eqs. (20) and (21), conforms well to the pattern discussed above for rubbery polymers (cf. lower lines of Table 1). An analogous correlation with ε_A/k is expected for K_{A2}. This has also been shown experimentally, though in less detail [3,19].

From the point of view of selectivity, it is clear that the adsorption mode in glassy polymers also favors the heavier gases (and it is noteworthy that s_{AO}, as well as K_{A2}, tends to be higher for heavier gases) [19]. Furthermore, in competition among the components of a gas mixture for the limited number of adsorption sites, the heavier gas will again be favored. So, no significant changes in the selectivity characteristics of simple dissolution are expected; although the solubility of both gases will, of course tend to be depressed, in accordance with the relevant mixed Langmuir isotherm, namely

$$S_{AM} = S_{A1} + S_{A2M} = K_{A1} + s_{AO} K_{A2}/(1 + K_{A2} f_A + K_{B2} f_B) \tag{24}$$

Equations (22) and (24) show that $S_{AM} < S_A$ (and similarly $S_{BM} < S_B$).

C. Diffusion Properties

In Sec. II.A, the diffusion process was described, from the macroscopic irreversible thermodynamic point of view, as motion under a (thermodynamic) driving force against the frictional resistance of the diffusion medium. From the microscopic viewpoint, micromolecular diffusion is regarded as a succession of random molecular jumps. More specifically (cf. Fig. 4), a sorbed gas molecule is normally trapped in a certain position by the surrounding polymer segments (initial state); until such time as the said segments happen, as a result of thermal fluctuations, to be displaced in such a way that a hole of suitable size opens up for the gas molecule to jump into ("activated" or "transition" state). The jump is completed by "closure" of the hole left behind by the displaced gas molecule; so that the latter is now trapped in its new position (final state). Random walk theory yields [4]

$$D_{TA} = \kappa v_A \lambda_A^2 \tag{25}$$

where κ is a geometrical constant ($= 1/6$ for a simple homogeneous random walk); λ_A is the mean jump length; and v_A is the frequency of jumping (constant in an ideal system), which corresponds to the frequency with which a hole of the minimum required size can open up at the appropriate location. The latter frequency can be expressed in terms of either energy or volume fluctuations, as described below.

1. Activation Energy Treatment

According to the Eyring activation—or transition—state treatment [10] of v_A, Eq. (25) becomes

$$D_{TA} = \kappa \lambda_A^2 (kT/h) \exp(\overline{\Delta S_A^*}/R) \exp(-\overline{\Delta H_A^*}/RT) \tag{26}$$

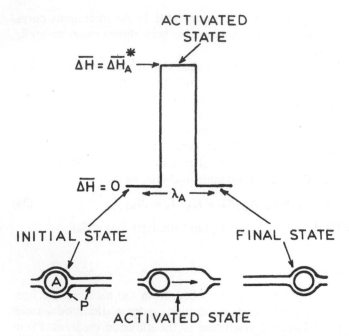

FIG. 4 Schematic pictorial representation of an elementary diffusion jump (assumed for convenience of representation to proceed along the polymer chains) and corresponding activation enthalpy profile. (From Ref. 4.)

where $\overline{\Delta H_A^*}$ and $\overline{\Delta S_A^*}$ represent the difference in partial molar enthalpy and entropy, respectively between activated and normal (ground) states (cf. Fig. 4). Comparison of Eq. (26) with the Arrhenius activation energy expression commonly employed in practice

$$D_{TA} = D_{TA}^o \exp(-E_{DA}/RT) \tag{27}$$

shows that $E_{DA} = \overline{\Delta H_A^*} + RT$ and that D_{TA}^o depends both on $\overline{\Delta S_A^*}$ and λ_A. $\overline{\Delta S_A^*}$ is positively correlated [10] with $\overline{\Delta H_A^*}$; but the exponential term is normally dominant, so that D_{TA} decreases with increasing E_{DA} ($\overline{\Delta H_A^*}$).

A very crude macroscopic evaluation of E_{DA}, on the basis of the energy E_{HA} required to open up one mole of cylindrical cavities of length λ_A and diameter equal to that of the gas molecule σ_A, in a medium of cohesive energy density E_{CP}, yields [20]

$$E_{DA} \approx E_{HA} = 0.25\pi\sigma_A^2 \lambda_A E_{CP} \tag{28}$$

Linear correlations between $\ln D_{TA}$ (where the value of D_{TA} for $C_{AO} \to 0$ is used in the case of nonideal systems) and σ_A^2 have proved very useful for the reduction of a large volume of experimental data [14]. Examination of the actual E_{DA} values, however, shows no consistent quantitative relation between E_{DA} and σ_A; although it is clear that E_{DA} increases (and hence D_{TA} decreases) with increasing molecular size of the penetrant less steeply in rubbers than in stiff-chain polymers, as illustrated in Fig. 5 [21]. It has also been pointed out [22] that E_{DA} is not correlated with E_{CP} as implied by Eq. (28), when dissimilar polymers are considered; and that the relevant plots often clearly extrapolate to $E_{DA} = 0$ at a finite value of $\sigma_A = \sigma_A^0 > 0$. The latter feature is particularly prominent in the case of stiff-chain polymers of low packing density (cf. Fig. 6) [23].

To understand the nature of the main factors which determine E_{DA} (and hence D_{TA}), one must refer to one of the more sophisticated, though still only semiquantitative, molecular models which have been proposed. According to Brandt [24], the process of hole formation requires (i) intramolecular energy $E_{\alpha A}$ (per mole) to bend two (initially straight at a distance d apart) polymer

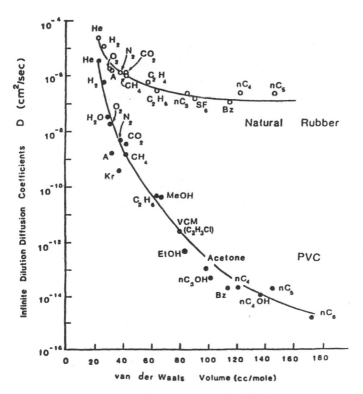

FIG. 5 Examples of the dependence of diffusivity on penetrant molecular size. (From Ref. 21.)

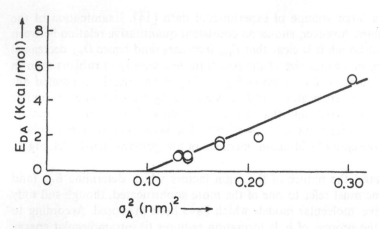

FIG. 6 Activation energies of gases diffusing in poly(1-trimethyl silyl-1-propyne) (PTMSP). (From Ref. 23.)

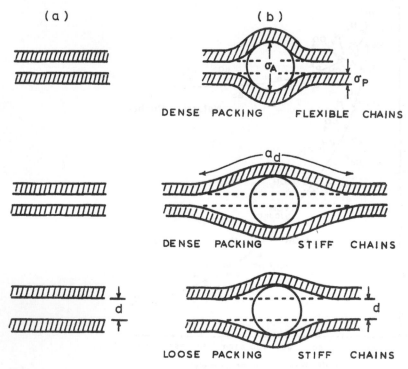

FIG. 7 Model representation of (a) normal and (b) activated, configuration of polymer chains for an elementary diffusion jump (proceeding in a direction normal to the chains), according to the approach of Ref. 24. (From Ref. 4.)

chain segments (of length a_d) away from each other (see Fig. 7) and (ii) intermolecular energy $E_{\beta A}$ (per mole) to overcome the repulsion of the bending segments by their neighbors. The former term is evaluated on the basis of partial rotation around each backbone chain bond (a $-C-C-$ backbone is assumed) against the potential energy barrier to internal rotation ψ_0 (per mole). The latter term corresponds to that assumed in Eq. (28) and is evaluated in terms of the internal pressure of the polymer p_I (which is closely related to E_{CP} but more accessible experimentally) and the molar activation volume $\overline{\Delta V_A^*}$ (which can be calculated by simple geometry in terms of a_d, σ_A, d and the diameter of the polymer chain σ_P): $E_{\beta A} = p_I \overline{\Delta V_A^*}$. For $a_d \gg \sigma_A - d$, it is found that

$$E_{HA} = E_{\beta A} + E_{\alpha A} = N_0 p_I \sigma_P a_d (\sigma_A - d)/2 + 18 \psi_0 b_0 (\sigma_A - d)^2 / a_d^3$$

$$= \phi_\beta (\sigma_A - d) + \phi_\alpha (\sigma_A - d)^2 \tag{29}$$

where σ_A is the diameter of the gas molecule (or the effective diameter of a nonspherical molecule, which should be close to the diameter of its smallest cross-section); b_0 is the length of a backbone chain bond projected on the chain axis; N_0 is the Avogadro number; and it is assumed that $E_{HA} = 0$ for $\sigma_A \leq d$. It will be noted that $E_{\beta A}$ increases directly, and $E_{\alpha A}$ inversely, with a_d; hence there is an optimum value of a_d (a_{d0}) which yields a minimum value of E_{HA} (E_{HA}^o). Assuming $E_{DA} \approx E_{HA}^o$, Eq. (29) is clearly consistent with the observation of a finite σ_A^o noted above and successfully predicts a weaker dependence of E_{DA} on σ_A for flexible-chain polymers ($\psi_0 \approx 0$). Also, the fact that E_{DA} does not correlate with E_{CP} for polymers which are dissimilar (and hence exhibit varying chain flexibility) now becomes understandable. (For a more detailed treatment the reader may consult Refs. 24 and 25).

2. Free Volume Treatment

By a (non-rigorous) extension of the free volume treatment of self-diffusion in a hard-sphere liquid [20], an expression for v_A in Eq. (25) has been derived [26] yielding

$$D_{TA} = A_{DA} \exp(-B_{dA}/v_f) = A_{DA} \exp(-B_D V_{hA}^*/v_f) \tag{30}$$

where A_{DA}, B_{dA} depend on penetrant molecular size (and shape), but the latter is the controlling parameter; B_D is treated as a constant, but, according to a more rigorous (and complex) treatment [27,28], depends on the size of the polymer jumping unit; V_{hA}^* represents the minimum size of hole required to permit a diffusion jump; and v_f is the fractional free volume of the polymer–penetrant system.

The free volume approach has proved particularly useful for a description of the effect of various factors on D_{TA} in polymers above T_g. Thus, V_{hA}^* in Eq. (30) is found to correlate well with penetrant molecular volume [28]. On the other hand, the effect of temperature, pressure and plasticization by the penetrant is embodied in the relation [29]

$$v_f(T, p, v_A) = v_{fs} + \alpha_f(T - T_s) - \beta_f(p - p_s) + \gamma_A v_A \qquad (31)$$

In Eq. (31), α_f, β_f, γ_A are positive constants characteristic of the particular system; and the subscript s denotes a suitable reference state, where $v_{fs} = v_f(T_s, p_s, 0)$ and $p_s = 1$ atm, $T_s = T_g$ are convenient choices [30]. The "plasticization coefficient" γ_A is physically interpreted in terms of the higher fractional free volume of the liquid penetrant v_{fA} relative to that of the pure polymer v_{fP} (on the basis of additivity of volumes upon mixing it is found that $\gamma_A = v_{fA} - v_{fP}$). It follows that for a binary penetrant mixture AB we have [31]

$$v_f = v_{f0} + \gamma_A v_A + \gamma_B v_B \qquad (32)$$

where v_{f0} refers to pure polymer.

Below T_g, the free volume approach described above assumes more of an empirical character; but retains at least some of its usefulness.

The correlative value of the free volume approach is enhanced by the fact that it enables us to draw close quantitative parallels between micromolecular transport and other (notably flow or mechanical) properties of the polymer [30]; but, as matters stand at present, it does not appear to offer prospects of relating transport properties to molecular structure comparable to those afforded by the energy-based treatment of the preceding subsection.

3. Diffusion Selectivity and Permselectivity

As indicated above and illustrated in Fig. 5, diffusion selectivity favors the penetrant molecule of smaller effective diameter σ_A and tends to be high in stiff-chain, and low in flexible-chain, polymers.

In contrast to this, sorption, in the absence of strong specific interactions, gives rise to moderate selectivity which works in favor of the larger (more condensable) gas molecule and is insensitive to the nature of the polymer (v.s.). Thus, the permselectivity of rubbers tends to be low and in favor of the larger gas molecule; whereas the permselectivity of stiff-chain polymers favors the smaller gas molecule and can be quite high. Accordingly, practical gas separation is typically based on stiff-chain polymer membranes. (Note, incidentally that in the practically important CO_2/CH_4 and O_2/N_2 separations, the first named component has lower σ_A but is also more condensable and is, consequently, favored by both sorption and diffusion selectivity). Figure 5 also illustrates the empirical "rule" that polymers which exhibit high (low) selectivity are characerized by low (high) diffusivity and vice versa. This "rule" is commonly expressed, in practice, in a less precise way, namely in terms of permselectivity and permeability [32,33], as illustrated for a typical gas separation in Fig. 8.

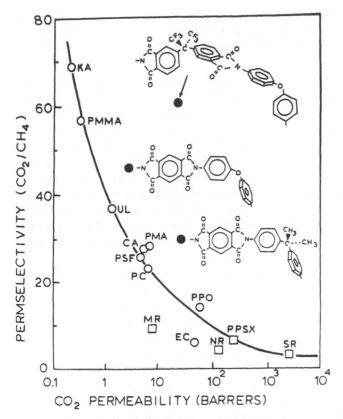

FIG. 8 Permselectivity (CO_2/CH_4)–permeability (CO_2) relation for conventional glassy (○) and some rubbery (□) polymeric membrane materials (KA = "Kapton" polyimide; UL = "Ultem" polyether imide; PMA = polymethyl acrylate; CA = cellulose acetate; EC = ethyl cellulose; NR = natural rubber; SR = silicone rubber; MR = methyl rubber; PPSX = polyphenyl siloxane; PMMA = polymethyl methacrylate; PSF = polysulfone; PC = polycarbonate; PPO = polyphenylene oxide). Filled points are examples of improved glassy polymer membrane materials, which combine reduced density of packing with higher overall chain stiffness. (Adapted from Ref. 32.)

Reference to Eqs. (27), (29), assuming $E_{DA} \approx E_{HA}^o$, shows that for given $\sigma_A \approx \sigma_B > d$

$$\ln(D_{TA}/D_{TB}) = \ln(D_{TA}^o/D_{TB}^o) - (E_{DA} - E_{DB})/RT \approx \ln(D_{TA}^o/D_{TB}^o) \\ + [\phi_\beta + \phi_\alpha(\sigma_B + \sigma_A - 2d)](\sigma_B - \sigma_A)/RT \tag{33}$$

where the second term is the dominant one. Equation (33) shows that a gain in selectivity can be achieved by increasing backbone chain stiffness (represented by ψ_0 which is incorporated in ϕ_α, cf. Eq. (29)) or the density of packing (i.e. lowering d and thereby also increasing p_I and hence ϕ_β, cf. Eq. (29)); but this inevitably leads (cf. Eqs. (27), (29)) to higher E_{DA}, E_{DB} and hence lower D_{TA}, D_{TB}.

Hence, Eqs. (29), (33) provide a sound theoretical interpretation of the aforementioned permselectivity–permeability (or, more precisely, diffusion selectivity–diffusivity) trade-off "rule". Furthermore, they also indicate the way to circumvent this "rule"! Note first that the equations in question lead naturally to the definition of a molecular sieve, by indicating that the optimum combination of high diffusivity with high selectivity requires (assuming $\sigma_A < \sigma_B$) adjustment of the interchain spacing to $\sigma_A < d < \sigma_B$ (hence $E_{DA} = 0$, $D_{TA} = D_{TA}^o$), in conjunction with maximum chain rigidity (to maximize E_{DB}). This ideal combination cannot, of course, be realized (or even closely approached) in amorphous polymer matrices, where a range of d values inevitably exists; but it has been shown [32] that marked gains in permeability without sacrifice of permselectivity can be achieved by "opening up" the tight structure of the common highly selective glassy polymers, which fall on the upper part of the permselectivity–permeability trade-off curve of Fig. 8, provided that chain rigidity is suitably increased at the same time. Hence, the above simple theory provides the proper fundamental guidelines for the design of polymer membranes with optimum gas separation properties.

The model of Eqs. (29) and (33) yields no quantitative information for the case of $\sigma_A < d$. However, the similarity of this case with diffusion in micropores, where selectivity in favor of the lighter gas is limited to $\sqrt{(M_B/M_A)}$ (M = gas molecular weight, $M_B > M_A$), suggests that gains in diffusivity realized by opening up the polymer structure to the point of $\sigma_A < \sigma_B < d$ are likely to be accompanied by heavy loss in selectivity (cf. the high gas permeability and low permselectivity of PTMSP [34], where $E_{DA} \approx 0$ for gases with $\sigma_A < 0.35$ nm, as illustrated in Fig. 6).

4.   Dual-Mode Transport

The permeability of glassy polymers, and other media where dual mode sorption occurs, may be expressed, in a simplified manner, as the sum of components due to dissolved and adsorbed (reversibly bound) gas molecules, designated by subscripts 1 and 2, respectively, i.e. [3,35,36]

$$P_A = P_{A1} + P_{A2} = S_{A1} D_{TA1} + S_{A2} D_{TA2} \tag{34}$$

where, in the absence of plasticization effects: D_{TA1}, D_{TA2} = const. The activation enthalpy profile for a gas molecule diffusing in such a medium is expected to be as illustrated in Fig. 9; where the shallow and deep wells represent "solution" and "adsorption" sites, respectively, the difference in well depth corresponding approximately to the difference in the respective enthalpies of sorption $-(\overline{\Delta H}_{A2} - \overline{\Delta H}_{A1})$. Since $(\overline{\Delta H}_{A2}^* - \overline{\Delta H}_{A1}^*) \approx -(\overline{\Delta H}_{A2} - \overline{\Delta H}_{A1})$ (cf. Fig.

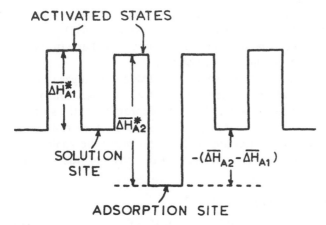

FIG. 9 Activation enthalpy profile according to the simple dual-mode transport model [35,36]. (From Ref. 4.)

9) and (cf. Eq. 26)

$$D_{TA2}/D_{TA1} = (\lambda_{A2}/\lambda_{A1})\exp[(\overline{\Delta S}^*_{A2} - \overline{\Delta S}^*_{A1})/R]\exp[-(\overline{\Delta H}^*_{A2} - \overline{\Delta H}^*_{A1})/RT]$$

(35)

where the last factor is dominant, it is expected that $D_{TA2}/D_{TA1} < 1$, with D_{TA2}/D_{TA1} becoming progressively lower for the more strongly sorbed gases. Good inverse correlations between D_{TA2}/D_{TA1} and ε_A/k have, in fact, been noted in glassy polymers [3,13]. In cases where the adsorption mode is due to the presence of a fixed carrier, it is similarly expected that D_{TA2} will vary inversely with the affinity of the carrier moiety for the relevant gas. However, the compound parameter $K_{A2} D_{TA2}$ tends, as a rule, to increase with rising K_{A2}.

Integration of Eq. (34) from zero (assuming $f_{AI} = 0$) to f_{AO}, after substitution from Eq. (22), yields in analogy to Eq. (7)

$$\bar{P}_A(f_{AO}, 0) = P_{A1} + P_{A2} = S_{A1} D_{TA1} + S_{A2}(f_{AO}, 0)D_{TA2}$$

$$= K_{A1} D_{TA1} + (s_{AO} D_{TA2}/f_{AO})\ln(1 + K_{A2} f_{AO})$$

(36)

Equation (36) shows that the experimentally measured integral permeability decreases from a value of $\bar{P}_A = K_{A1}D_{TA1} + s_{AO} K_{A2} D_{TA2}$ at $f_{AO} \to 0$ to a value of $\bar{P}_A = K_{A1}D_{TA1}$ as $f_{AO} \to \infty$. The corresponding integral diffusion coefficient $\bar{D}(C_{AO}, 0) = \bar{P}(f_{AO}, 0)/S_A(f_{AO})$ (see Eq. (8)) increases from a value of $\bar{D}_A = D_{TA1}(1 + s_{AO} K_{A2} D_{T2}/K_{A1} D_{TA1})/(1 + s_{AO} K_{A2}/K_{A1})$ at $f_{AO} \to 0$ to a value of $\bar{D}_A = D_{TA1}$ as $f_{AO} \to \infty$. The upper limiting values are approached rapidly when K_{A2} is high. Thus, in practice, $\bar{P}_A$ and $\bar{D}_A$ normally reflect very largely the properties of P_{A1} and D_{TA1}, respectively. On the other hand, D_{TA1}, D_{TA2} are similarly affected by various factors, such as the size and shape of the gas molecule or the fractional free volume of the polymer.

Hence, the presence of the second transport mode leads to changes in transport behavior, which are relatively minor for practical purposes and reflect primarily differences in sorption behavior. Thus, the depression of the sorption of one gas by the presence of another (v.s.) is reflected in a corresponding permeability effect (negative flow coupling) [3], as shown by the analogue of Eq. (36) for a binary gas mixture AB, obtained on the basis of Eqs. (24) and (34) (as described in Ref. 37), namely

$$\bar{P}_{AM} = K_{A1}D_{TA1} + D_{TA2}s_{AO}K_{A2}$$
$$\times \ln(1 + K_{A2}f_{AO} + K_{BO}f_{BO})/(K_{A2}f_{AO} + K_{B2}f_{BO}) \tag{37}$$

On this basis, the presence of the adsorption mode in glassy polymers is not expected to give rise to significant changes in permselectivity.

On the other hand, the possibility of enhancing selectivity through a chemically specific adsorption mode (v.s.) is of particular interest for a gas pair, like O_2/N_2, differing relatively little in condensability and molecular diameter but substantially in chemical properties. This is another way of circumventing the permeability–permselectivity trade-off rule; because ideally only P_A is increased by the introduction of S_{A2} (cf. Eq. (34)), the carrier moiety being essentially inert towards gas B ($S_{B2} = 0$), as in the practical example of Ref. 17 considered above. If the uptake of gas A by the carrier is fast, Eqs. (34), (36) apply. To those familiar with facilitated transport in liquid membranes, where the carrier–gas complex is itself mobile, it may appear strange that introduction of a *fixed* carrier can enhance gas transport. The answer is (cf. Fig. 9) that, according to the Eyring transition-state theory (v.s.), all gas molecules in the polymeric medium are normally confined in fixed positions (potential energy wells), out of which they jump when sufficiently activated. The frequency of jumping ν_A (cf. Eqs. (25), (26)) is higher (lower), i.e. the molecule is more (less) mobile, if the confining activation barrier ($\overline{\Delta H_A^*}$) is lower (higher). Thus, gas molecules reversibly bound by a fixed carrier, however strongly, possess small, but nonzero, effective mobility ($D_{TA2} > 0$). For example, the high-affinity oxygen carrier used in Ref. 17 gave $D_{TA2}/D_{TA1} = 0.02$. Even so, a more than threefold increase in $\bar{P}_A(p_{AO}, 0)$ was obtained (with $P_B \approx$ const), at $p_{AO} = 5$ torr, for the highest carrier concentration used. However, Eq. (36) shows that $\bar{P}_A(f_{AO}, 0)$ declines rapidly with increasing p_{AO}, when K_{A2} is high; and, in fact, little advantage remains at p_{AO} as low as 100 torr, as shown in Fig. 10. Thus, to extend the permeability gain to higher p_{AO} (as would be required for practical gas separation), the use of low affinity carriers is indicated and the gain which can be achieved is correspondingly limited.

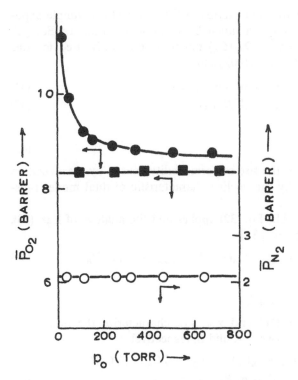

FIG. 10   Measured oxygen (●, ■) or nitrogen (○) permeability $\bar{P}(p_0, p_l = 0)$ of poly-butyl methacrylate membrane with attached cobalt–porphyrin-complex oxygen carrier in active (Co II; ○, ●) or inert (Co III; ■) form (25°C). (From Ref. 17.)

5.   Plasticization Effects

The permeability coefficient of light gases in rubbery polymers usually remains sensibly constant in the pressure range normally employed in practice. Heavy gases at higher pressures or vapors typically plasticize the polymer [29], causing primarily D_{TA} and secondarily S_A to increase with C_A, in accordance with Eqs. (30), (31) and with Eq. (17), respectively. For not too strong effects of this kind, expansion to first order in $\gamma_A v_A = \gamma'_A C_A$ and $b_A C_A$, followed by suitable combination of the aforesaid relations, yields [38]

$$S_A = K_A \exp(b_A C_A) \approx K_A(1 + b_A C_A) \approx K_A(1 + b_A K_A f_A) \tag{38}$$

$$D_{TA}/D_{TAO} = \exp[B_{dA} \gamma'_A C_A/(v_{fO}^2 + v_{fO} \gamma'_A C_A)] \tag{39}$$

$$\approx \exp[B_{fA} \gamma'_A K_A f_A(1 + b_A K_A f_A - \gamma'_A K_A f_A/v_{fO})]$$

$$\approx \exp(B_{fA} \gamma'_A K_A f_A) \tag{40}$$

where $D_{TAO} = D_{TA}(C_A = 0)$; v_{fO} is the fractional free volume of pure polymer under the specified experimental conditions; $B_{fA} = B_{dA}/v_{fO}^2$; $\gamma'_A = \gamma_A \bar{V}_A$; and the partial compensation of the small terms in Eq. (40) yields a simple exponential $D_{TA}(f_A)$ function, which is a much better approximation to Eq. (39) [38] than the simple exponential $D_{TA}(C_A)$ function commonly used for this purpose [39,40]. Equations (38) and (40) yield

$$P_A(f_A) = K_A D_{TAO} \exp(G_A f_A) = P_{AO} \exp(G_A f_A) \tag{41}$$

$$\bar{P}_A(f_{AO}, 0) = P_{AO}\{[\exp(G_A f_{AO}) - 1]/G_A f_{AO}\} \tag{42}$$

where

$$G_A = (B_{fA} \gamma'_A + b_A)K_A \tag{43}$$

Note that, in glassy polymers, the rise in permeability caused by plasticization may be initially superseded by the decline characteristic of dual mode transport [41].

For a binary gas mixture AB, Eq. (32) applies and the analogs of Eqs. (38), (39), (40) and (41) are respectively [38]

$$S_{AM} = K_A \exp(b_A C_A + b_{AB} C_B) \approx K_A(1 + b_A K_A f_A + b_{AB} K_B f_B) \tag{44}$$

where [39,42]

$$b_{AB} = (\chi_{AP} - \chi_{AB})\bar{V}_B + (1 + \chi_{BP})\bar{V}_A$$

$\chi_{AP} \equiv \chi_A$ was defined in Eq. (16) and χ_{BP}, χ_{AB} characterize the interaction between B and polymer and between A and B, respectively;

$$D_{TAM}/D_{TAO} = \exp[B_{dA}(\gamma'_A C_A + \gamma'_B C_B)/v_{fO}(v_{fO} + \gamma'_A C_A + \gamma'_B C_B)] \tag{45}$$

$$\approx \exp[B_{fA}(\gamma'_A K_A f_A + \gamma'_B K_B f_B)] \tag{46}$$

$$P_{AM} \approx K_A D_{TAO} \exp(G_A f_A + G_{AB} f_B) = P_{AO} \exp(G_A f_A + G_{AB} f_B) \tag{47}$$

where

$$G_{AB} = (B_{fA} \gamma'_B + b_{AB})K_B \tag{48}$$

According to Eq. (37), the effect of B on S_{AM} depends on the relative strength of the A–P, B–P and A–B interactions. On the other hand, Eqs. (45), (46) show that the diffusivity of the penetrants is always mutually enhanced. The latter effect normally dominates and determines the behavior of P_{AM}, P_{BM} (positive flow coupling).

The dependence of the integral permeabilities $\bar{P}_{AM}$, $\bar{P}_{BM}$ on f_{AO}, f_{BO} cannot, in general, be worked out analytically in analogy with Eq. (42). An analytical expression can be derived, however, for the intrinsic permselectivity (cf. Eq. (11)), namely [38,40]

$$\alpha^o_M = [P_{AO}(G_B - G_{AB})f_{BO}/P_{BO}(G_A - G_{BA})f_{AO}]$$
$$\times \{\exp[(G_A - G_{BA})f_{AO}] - 1\}/\{\exp[(G_B - G_{AB})f_{BO}] - 1\} \tag{49}$$

where the meaning of G_B, G_{BA} is obvious, on the basis of Eqs. (43) and (48), respectively, and the exponential terms may be expanded for small plasticizing effects.

To obtain a clearer picture of the predicted behavior of α_M^0, assume that A and B represent a light nonplasticizing gas and a heavier one which causes appreciable plasticization, respectively. This implies $B_{fB} > B_{fA}$, $G_A f_{AO} \approx 0$, $G_{BA} f_{AO} \approx 0$. Equation (49) then reduces to

$$\alpha_M^0 \approx (P_{AO}/P_{BO})[1 - (G_B - G_{AB})f_{BO}/2] \tag{50}$$

where the dominant first term in

$$G_B - G_{AB} = (B_{fB} - B_{fA})\gamma_B' K_B + (b_B - b_{AB})K_B$$

is positive. Hence α_M^0 tends to decrease with increasing f_{BO} and, according to whether $P_{AO} < P_{BO}$ (sorption selectivity dominant) or $P_{AO} > P_{BO}$ (diffusion selectivity dominant), the effect of plasticization will be enhancement or depression of permselectivity, respectively. Gas separation by means of stiff-chain polymer membranes obviously corresponds to the latter situation and should, therefore, be adversely affected by plasticization, a prediction in agreement with common experience.

III. VAPOR PERMEATION/PERVAPORATION

A. Permeability

The permeability behavior of vapors is governed by the basic principles presented in Sec. II, with some complications resulting from (i) the stronger polymer–penetrant (and penetrant–penetrant) interactions which are possible here and (ii) the range of penetrant concentration established in the polymer under the experimental conditions used (which is maximized in pervaporation, wherein the membrane is in contact with a liquid phase on the upstream side and near vacuum may be applied on the downstream side).

In particular, the treatments of sorption and diffusion based on Eq. (15) and Eqs. (30), (31) respectively are, in principle, applicable to nonpolar or weakly polar polymer–vapor systems; but, one should keep in mind that here sorption nonideality and plasticization effects will often be too pronounced (esp. in pervaporation) to justify the approximations used in Sec. II.C.5 to derive results in the simple form of Eqs. (38) and (40) (and their mixed-penetrant counterparts). Furthermore, considerations regarding the definition (frame of reference) of the diffusion coefficient [5,42] and the limitations of simple dissolution theory [43] acquire increasing significance.

Additional effects to be accounted for arise from the fact that strong polar polymer–penetrant and penetrant–penetrant interactions are frequently of importance. Water, in particular, is often one of the penetrants of interest (cf. removal of organics from aqueous streams, dehydration of organic solvents). Explicit inclusion of the effect of such complications on sorption behavior, is, at present, possible only at the empirical or (at best) semiempirical level [11,42,44–50]; and often involves the introduction of additional terms in Eq.

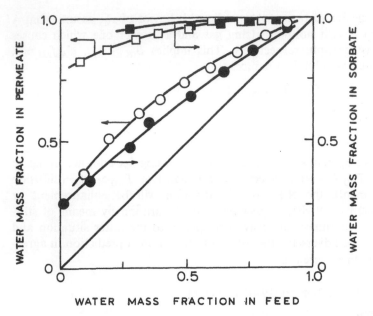

FIG. 11 Comparison of pervaporation (open points, $p_l = 0.1$ torr) and liquid sorption (filled points) data for water–ethanol mixtures in membranes ($l \approx 20$ μm) of poly-acrylonitrile ($\square$) or cellulose acetate containing 2.3 acetyl groups per glucose monomer unit ($\bigcirc$). (From Ref. 45.)

(15) [11,44,50] and/or (empirically determined) variation of the Flory–Huggins interaction parameter with composition [42,45,48,49].

As far as water sorption is concerned, the most prominent features which differentiate it from simple dissolution (Eq. (17)) include (i) specific interactions (incl. hydrogen bonding) with hydrophilic groups of the polymer (leading to deviations of the dual mode sorption type illustrated in Fig. 2b) and (ii) clustering, leading to deviations of the type illustrated in Fig. 2c. The latter deviations tend to be particularly in evidence in moderately hydrophobic polymers [51] (in strongly hydrophobic polymers the extent of sorption is normally too low to exceed the Henry's law limit significantly). The diffusion coefficient of water also does not appear to conform well to the behavior predicted by the plasticization theory embodied in Eq. (39). In particular, D_{H2O} increases markedly with concentration in hydrophilic polymers, in (at least qualitative) agreement with the said theory; but in moderately hydrophobic polymers, it may exhibit the opposite trend, which is attributed to the aforementioned tendency of water to form clusters in a nonpolar environment [51]. Here too no satisfactory fundamental theory exists and Eq. (40) must be applied in an empirical manner (see also below).

The above discussion indicates that a general (even approximate) fundamental physical treatment of permeability in pervaporation is as yet lacking; but a reasonably close approach to such a treatment can be achieved in the case of nonpolar or weakly polar systems, either in the form presented above or in the (generally more cumbersome and/or semiempirical) forms given in the literature [42,47,50,52,53].

B. Permselectivity

The special features of vapor permeability behavior noted here have an interesting impact on permselectivity. The main observation worth noting in this respect is that permselectivity in pervaporation is commonly dominated by sorption selectivity (as illustrated by the examples shown in Fig. 11), in contrast to what is normally the case in gas separation practice (cf. Sec. II.C.3). This is a consequence of the fact that sorption selectivity relies heavily on differences in polymer–penetrant interactions and is, therefore, particularly sensitive to differences in the chemical nature of the penetrants (as previously illustrated in Table 2). Such differences can obviously be much more pronounced among vapors (as in the case of water vs. apolar organic solvents) than among simple gases. Furthermore, the strong plasticization effects likely to occur in pervaporation tend to reduce diffusion selectivity, as indicated by the results of the treatment of such effects given in Sec. II.C.5.

IV. REVERSE OSMOSIS

Reverse osmosis (hyperfiltration) constitutes one of the most important transport phenomena involving solution–diffusion membranes. In this process a liquid solvent (A) and a solute (B) are transported, under hydraulic ($\Delta p_H = p_{HO} - p_{Hl}$) and osmotic ($\Delta \pi = \pi_0 - \pi_l$) pressure heads (with $\Delta p_H > \Delta \pi$), through a solvent-selective membrane from a feed, to a permeate, solution (the corresponding process which utilizes a solute-selective membrane is commonly referred to as piezodialysis). The best known application (which will be considered below) is the desalination of sea or brackish water by weakly polar (moderately hydrophobic) uncharged membranes.

A. Solvent Transport

Liquid transport under a hydraulic pressure head (hydraulic flow or filtration) is commonly described by a hydraulic permeability or filtration coefficient [54,55] (see below); but may be formulated, in a manner consistent with that used above, by suitable adaptation of Eqs. (2) and (3).

In particular, note that the chemical potential of a liquid phase (denoted by subscript s and assumed for simplicity to be incompressible) at 1 atm, consisting of pure solvent A, is given, according to Eq. (3), by

$$\mu_{sA}^{o} = \mu_{gA}^{o} + RT \ln f_{A}^{sat} \tag{51}$$

Application of a hydrostatic pressure head Δp_H causes an increase in chemical potential given by $\bar{V}_A \Delta p_H$, which is reflected in higher vapor pressure for the pressurized liquid ($f_{HA}^{sat} > f_A^{sat}$). Hence, following Eq. (51), we have

$$\mu_{sHA}^{o} - \mu_{sA}^{o} = RT \ln(f_{HA}^{sat}/f_A^{sat}) = \bar{V}_A \Delta p_H \tag{52a,b}$$

On the other hand, the addition of solute B to A depresses the chemical potential of A by $\bar{V}_A \pi$ (where π is the osmotic pressure) and this is reflected in a drop of the vapor pressure (under 1 atm pressure) from f_A^{sat} to f_A. Hence, following Eq. (51), we get

$$\mu_{sA} - \mu_{sA}^{o} = RT \ln(f_A/f_A^{sat}) = -\bar{V}_A \pi \tag{53a,b}$$

In reasonably dilute solutions, the osmotic pressure π is related to the concentration of solute c_B by

$$\pi = \zeta_B' RT c_B \approx RT c_B$$

where ζ_B' is the osmotic coefficient. The effects described by Eqs. (52), (53) are assumed to be effectively independent.

Under actual operating conditions, the downstream solution is at $p_{HI} = 1$ atm; while the upstream solution *and* the membrane (which is considered to rest on a rigid porous support) [5,6] are under the hydrostatic pressure head $\Delta p_H = p_{HO} - p_{HI}$. Thus, in order to express the chemical potential of A within the membrane μ_A in a convenient way, Eq. (3) is replaced by a combination of Eqs. (52) and (53), namely

$$\mu_A = \mu_{sA} = \mu_{sHA}^{o} + RT \ln(f_A/f_{HA}^{sat}) = \mu_{sHA}^{o} + RT \ln a_A' \tag{54a,b}$$

where a_A' is the activity of solvent defined with respect to pure pressurized liquid as standard state. At the upstream ($x = 0$) and downstream ($x = l$) surfaces of the membrane we have, respectively

$$\mu_{AO} = \mu_{sAO} = \mu_{sHA}^{o} + RT \ln(f_{AO}/f_{HA}^{sat}) = \mu_{sHA}^{o} - \bar{V}_A \pi_0 \tag{55a,b}$$

$$\mu_{Al} = \mu_{sAl} = \mu_{sHA}^{o} + RT \ln(f_{Al}/f_{HA}^{sat}) = \mu_{sHA}^{o} + RT \ln(f_{Al}/f_A^{sat})$$
$$- RT \ln(f_{HA}^{sat}/f_A^{sat}) = \mu_{sHA}^{o} - \bar{V}_A \pi_l - \bar{V}_A \Delta p_H \tag{56a,b}$$

where Eq. (56b) has been derived from Eq. (56a) by splitting the last term on the right-hand side of the latter into two terms reflecting the effects described by Eqs. (52) and (53). Subtraction of Eqs. (56) from Eqs. (55) then yields

$$\Delta \mu_A = \mu_{AO} - \mu_{Al} = RT \ln(f_{AO}/f_{Al}) = \bar{V}_A(\Delta p_H - \Delta \pi) \tag{57a,b}$$

Incorporation of f_{HA}^{sat} into μ_{sHA}^{o} in Eq. (54a) leaves the formalism of Eq. (4) intact; while Eq. (54b) leads to an alternative formulation in terms of a_A', which applies equally well to vapor permeation/pervaporation (and has also been extended to gases), namely

$$J_{xA} = u_{xA} C_A = -(D_{TA} C_A/RT)(\partial \mu_A/\partial x) = -(D_{TA} C_A/a_A')(\partial a_A'/\partial x)$$
$$= -(D_{TA} S_A')(\partial a_A'/\partial_x) = -P_A'(\partial a_A'/\partial x) \tag{58}$$

where $S_A' = C_A/a_A' = S_A f_{HA}^{sat}$ and $P_A' = D_{TA} S_A' = P_A f_{HA}^{sat}$. The advantage gained by the use of a_A' is that solvent uptake by the membrane (C_A) is primarily a function of a_A', not of hydrostatic pressure [5]. Thus, $S_A'(a_A')$ (and hence $P_A'(a_A')$, if the effect of hydrostatic pressure on D_{TA} indicated by Eqs. (30) and (31) is also a minor one) is insensitive to the value of Δp_H. Equations (7), (8) may also be rewritten in terms of a_A', i.e.

$$J_{AS} l = \int_{a_{Al}'}^{a_{AO}'} P_A' \, da_A' = \bar{P}_A'(a_{AO}' - a_{Al}') = \bar{D}_A(C_{AO} - C_{Al}) \tag{59}$$

where (cf. Eqs. (55) and (56))

$$a_{AO}' = \exp(-\bar{V}_A \pi_0/RT); \quad a_{Al}' = \exp[-\bar{V}_A(\Delta p_H + \pi_l)/RT]$$

showing that $a_{Al}' \to 0$ (hence $C_{Al} \to 0$, i.e., sorbed solvent is increasingly squeezed out of the membrane at the downstream side) [5] as $\Delta p_H \to \infty$. It follows that J_{AS} has an upper limit of $J_{AS}^{max} = \bar{P}_A' a_{AO}'/l = \bar{D}_A C_{AO}/l$, which is equivalent to the pervaporation flux obtained (see Eq. (8)) when vacuum is applied downstream (again provided that pressurization does not affect the magnitude of C_{AO} and D_{TA} significantly), as emphasized particularly by Paul [5].

On the other hand, the hydraulic permeability coefficient (P_{HA}) referred to above is given by [5,55,56]

$$J_{AS} l = P_{HA}(\Delta p_H - \Delta \pi)/\bar{V}_A \tag{60}$$

This definition is based on a different integrated form of Eq. (58), namely [55,56] Eq. (61a), into which one may introduce either Eq. (57b) or Eq. (57a) to obtain Eq. (61b) or Eq. (62), respectively

$$J_{AS} l = D_{THA} C_{AO} \Delta \mu_A/RT = D_{THA} \bar{V}_A C_{AO}(\Delta p_H - \Delta \pi)/RT \tag{61a,b}$$
$$= D_{THA} C_{AO} \ln(a_{AO}'/a_{Al}') \tag{62}$$

where the effective diffusion coefficient D_{THA} will, in general, differ from D_{TA}, unless $D_{TA} C_A$ does not vary appreciably across the membrane (i.e., $C_{Al} \to C_{AO}$) under the conditions of the experiment (see below). $D_{THA} C_{AO}$ or $D_{THA} C_{AO} \bar{V}_A = D_{THA} v_A$ are alternative hydraulic permeability parameters used to describe solvent transport [5,56].

The relation between the main alternative permeability parameters defined above follows from Eqs. (59), (60), (61b) and (62), which yield

$$RTP_{HA}/\bar{V}_A^2 = D_{THA}\,C_{AO} = \bar{P}'_A(a'_{AO} - a'_{Al})/\ln(a'_{AO}/a'_{Al}) \tag{63a,b}$$

In practice, the condition $C_{Al} \to C_{AO}$ (v.s.) is generally fulfilled, if $a'_{Al} \to a'_{AO}$ ($\Delta p_H \to \Delta \pi$); in which case $\bar{P}'_A \to P'_A(a'_{AO})$ and expansion of the right-hand side of Eq. (63b) yields

$$P'(a'_{AO}) = D_{TA}(a'_{AO})S'_A(a'_{AO}) = D_{THA}\,C_{AO}/a'_{AO} = D_{THA}\,S'_A(a'_{AO}) \tag{64}$$

Equation (64) confirms that, under the aforesaid condition, D_{THA} may be identified with $D_{TA}(a'_{AO})$ in all polymer–solvent systems; hence the hydraulic permeability parameter $D_{THA}\,C_{AO}$ or $D_{THA}\,v_{AO}$ is obviously to be preferred over P_{HA} for the purpose of the unified treatment pursued here.

Equation (64) is useful in practice, because it provides a good approximation to Eq. (63b) over wider activity intervals ($a'_{AO} - a'_{Al}$), provided that (i) ($a'_{AO} - a'_{Al})/a'_{AO}$ remains small and (ii) D_{TA} and S'_A do not vary significantly within this activity range. These conditions are usually satisfied tolerably well for the moderately hydrophobic polymeric membrane materials and hydrostatic pressure heads normally used in water desalination operations. Hence, in this case also, it is permissible to identify D_{THA} with D_{TA}. However, pertinent data are scarce, due to the fact that most reported filtration measurements relate to asymmetric or composite membrane configurations of unspecified surface layer thickness.

The most detailed fundamental work has been done using relatively thick dense cellulose acetate membranes [55–57]. As illustrated in Fig. 12b, the effective measured solvent (water) permeability $D_{THA}\,v_{AO}$ (which, in accordance to what has been said above, corresponds approximately to $\bar{V}_A P'_A$ at $a'_A = 1$) increases regularly with diminishing degree of acetylation (rising hydrophilicity) of the membrane and a large part of this is attributable to increase of D_{THA} with v_{AO} (cf. Figs. 12a and 12b). A concurrent study of D_{THA} and the tracer diffusion coefficient $D^*_{TA}(C_{AO})$ (measured at zero applied pressure head) in a series of polymers of widely varying hydrophilicity [54] showed that the dependence of both coefficients on v_{AO} is similar and is steeper in hydrophobic polymers than in hydrophilic ones. On the other hand, the value of D_{THA} is usually found to exceed that of $D^*_{TA}(C_{AO})$. The discrepancy tends to be relatively small in hydrophobic polymers but becomes large in hydrophilic ones [54,55] and is attributed to pressure-induced cooperative motion of water molecules, as seen in viscous flow through pores (but cf. also the considerations on the frame of reference used in the definition of D_{TA}, which have been advanced by Paul [5]).

Although simplified theoretical interpretations have been offered for the dependence of D^*_{TA} on the degree of hydration of the polymer v_{AO} (one of which is based on an analogy with the free-volume approach of Eq. (30) [54]),

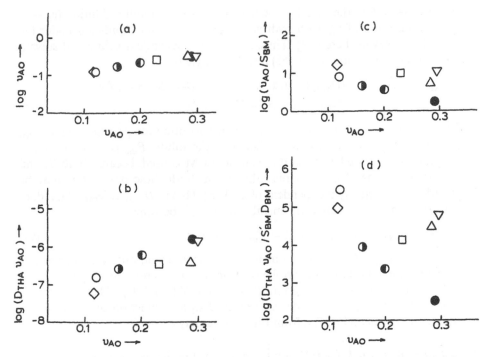

FIG. 12 (a) Water sorption, (b) water permeability, (c) water/NaCl sorption selectivity, and (d) water/NaCl intrinsic permselectivity, in dense membranes of: cellulose acetate containing 1.72 (●), 2.05 (◐), 2.24 (◑) or 2.57 (○) acetyl groups per glucose monomer unit (D_{BM} from immersion experiments) [56]; an aromatic polyimide (◇); an aromatic polyamide (□); a polybenzimidazopyrrolone (▽); and an aromatic polyamide–hydrazide (△). (See Ref. 58 for molecular structures; D_{BM} determined approximately [32] from the reverse osmosis data of Ref. 58.)

their success is bound to be limited, particularly in the case of moderately hydrophilic or hydrophobic polymers of interest here, in view of the fact that the microscopic distribution of the sorbed water in the polymeric material is also important. Comparison of the behavior of various polymer–water systems has shown [58] that, in fact, polymers wherein sorbed water molecules exhibit high (low) tendency to cluster are characterized by low (high) D_{THA}.

B. Solute Transport

To express the chemical potential of the (nonvolatile) solute in the membrane, Eq. (3) is replaced by

$$\mu_B = \mu_{sB} = \mu_{sB}^\circ + RT \ln a_B = \mu_{sB}^\circ + RT \ln \xi_B c_B \qquad (65)$$

where $a_B \to c_B$ (i.e. the activity coefficient $\xi_B \to 1$) at infinite dilution ($c_B \to 0$) and the variation of μ_{sB}° with hydrostatic pressure is not significant under the conditions relevant here [59]. Thus, assuming independent solute and solvent transport, introduction of Eq. (65) into Eq. (2) yields

$$J_{xB} = u_{xB} C_B = -(D_{TBM} C_B/a_B)(\partial a_B/\partial x) = -(D_{TBM} S'_{BM})(\partial a_B/\partial x)$$
$$= -P'_{BM}(\partial a_B/\partial x) \approx -P'_{BM}(\partial c_B/\partial x) \tag{66}$$

where $S'_{BM} = C_B/a_B = C_B/\xi_B c_B \approx C_B/c_B$ is the sorption (or partition), and D_{TBM} the (thermodynamic) diffusion, coefficient of the solute; P'_{BM} is the corresponding permeability coefficient; and the subscript M is used, because both S'_B and D_{TB} are functions of C_A. On the other hand, both these parameters may be regarded as effectively independent of C_B [56]. Hence, $D_{TBM} \equiv D_{BM}$. If C_A does not vary appreciably across the membrane, Eq. (7) becomes

$$J_{BS} l = J_{BS}^\circ l = P'_{BM}(a_{BO} - a_{Bl}) \approx P'_{BM}(c_{BO} - c_{Bl}) \tag{67}$$

If the variation of C_A across the membrane is significant, one can, in principle, determine the concentration profile of A across the membrane $C_A(x)$ from Eq. (58) by standard methods, given $P'_A(a'_A)$ and $S'_A(a'_A)$ [60]. Then, given the dependence of P'_{BM} on C_A, one can express P'_{BM} as a function of x and obtain an integral permeability $\bar{P}'_{BM}$ from Eq. (66), namely

$$J_{BS} l = J_{BS}^\circ l = l\left[\int_0^l P'_{BM}(x)^{-1} dx\right]^{-1}(a_{BO} - a_{Bl}) = \bar{P}'_{BM}(a_{BO} - a_{Bl})$$
$$\approx \bar{P}'_{BM}(c_{BO} - c_{Bl}) \tag{68}$$

C. Convection Effects

The assumption of independent solute and solvent transport made above tends to break down increasingly, as the degree of swelling of the polymer by the solvent rises. Accordingly, a convective velocity component (u_{xB2}) is added to the diffusive one (now designated by u_{xB1}) in Eq. (66) (the converse convective effect on the solvent flux being normally small). Thus, we get

$$J_{xB} = u_{xB} C_B = (u_{xB1} + u_{xB2})C_B = -P'_{BM}(\partial a_B/\partial x) + u_{xB2} C_B$$
$$\approx -P'_{BM}(\partial c_B/\partial x) + u_{xB2} C_B \tag{69}$$

In the case of transport through relatively wide pores (as in "Nuclepore" membranes), solute transport was successfully described [61] by means of Eq. (69) with $u_{xB2} = u_{xA}$. For a more general treatment, one may introduce a flow-coupling parameter β_B defined by

$$u_{xB2} = \beta_B u_{xA}$$

which can assume values between zero (independent solvent and solute fluxes) and unity ("complete" coupling of fluxes, as in the example quoted above).

Under experimental conditions where C_A does not vary appreciably across the membrane ($C_{AI} \approx C_{AO}$, $v_{AI} \approx v_{AO}$)

$$u_{xA} \approx u_{AO} = J_{AS}/C_{AO} = \text{const} \tag{70}$$

and Eq. (69) is easily integrated to

$$J_{BS} = \beta_B u_{AO} S_B'[\exp(\beta_B w_B)c_{BO} - c_{BI}]/[\exp(\beta_B w_B) - 1] \tag{71}$$

where u_{AO} follows from Eqs. (61b), (70); and

$$w_B = u_{AO} l/D_{BM} = D_{THA} \bar{V}_A(\Delta p_H - \Delta \pi)/D_{BM} RT \tag{72}$$

For $\beta_B w_B \ll 1$, Eq. (71) reduces to the simple sum of diffusive and convective components, in accord with the usual linear irreversible thermodynamic formulation of coupled flows (cf., e.g., Ref. 55), namely

$$J_{BS} = D_{BM} S_{BM}'(c_{BO} - c_{BI})/l + u_{AO} S_{BM}' \beta_B(c_{BO} + c_{BI})/2 \tag{73}$$

D. Permselectivity

The separation factor α_M for solvent over solute (cf. Eq. (12)), and its relation to the "solute rejection factor" (R_B) normally used in practice, is given by

$$\alpha_M = c_{BO}/c_{BI} = c_{BO} J_{AS} \bar{V}_A/J_{BS} = 1/(1 - R_B) \tag{74}$$

where c_{BO}, c_{BI} are expressed as molalities. Substitution from Eqs. (59) and (68) yields for the case of independent solvent and solute fluxes

$$\begin{aligned}
\alpha_M = \alpha_{MO} &\approx \bar{V}_A \bar{P}_A'(a_{AO}' - a_{AI}')/\bar{P}_B'(1 - c_{BI}/c_{BO}) \\
&= 1 + \bar{V}_A \bar{P}_A'(a_{AO}' - a_{AI}')/\bar{P}_B'
\end{aligned} \tag{75}$$

or, under conditions of $C_{AO} \approx C_{AI}$, use of Eq. (61b) yields the more familiar expression [56,57]

$$\alpha_M = \alpha_{MO} \approx 1 + (D_{THA} v_{AO}/D_{BM} S_{BM}')(\Delta p_H - \Delta \pi)\bar{V}_A/RT \tag{76}$$

In the presence of convection effects (with $C_{AO} \approx C_{AI}$), α_M becomes, in view of Eqs. (71), (72),

$$\alpha_M \approx [\exp(\beta_B w_B) - 1 + (\beta_B S_{BM}'/v_{AO})]/[\beta_B S_{BM}'/v_{AO})\exp(\beta_B w_B)] \tag{77}$$

which, for $\beta_B w_B \ll 1$, reduces to

$$\alpha_M = (w_B v_{AO}/S_{BM}')(1 - \beta_B w_B/2) + 1 - \beta_B w_B = \alpha_{MO} - \beta_B w_B(1 + \alpha_{MO})/2 \tag{78}$$

Note that v_{AO} in Eqs. (76) and (77) may be interpreted as a partition coefficient analogous to C_B/c_B, in view of the fact that the volume fraction of water in the liquid phase is approximately unity.

Equation (76) shows that the separation factor is governed by the intrinsic permselectivity of the membrane and the applied pressure head. Equation (78) further puts in evidence the reduction in the degree of separation caused by convective coupling and shows that this effect increases in line with the applied pressure head and with the diffusion selectivity of the membrane in favor of the solvent.

Note that, in the case of simple electrolyte solutes and weakly polar (moderately hydrophobic) uncharged membranes of interest here, both sorption and diffusion selectivity work against the solute, because of its markedly stronger polar character and larger (hydrated) molecular size, respectively.

The energy of interaction which determines the extent of sorption is primarily electrostatic and hence depends on the difference in dielectric constant between the polymeric medium and water. However, the observed values of S'_B (which appear to be close to those measured in chemically similar liquids; cf. the similarity of the partition coefficient of NaCl in cellulose acetate and in glycerol diacetate [62]) are usually markedly higher than might be expected on the basis of the macroscopic dielectric constant of the hydrated membrane [59,63]. This is attributed to clustering of the imbibed water around the sorbed ions, thus providing an energetically much more favorable microenvironment for the latter. (The converse effect, i.e., enhancement of water sorption due to the presence of sorbed ions, is generally not considered important). Consequently, sorption selectivity is, in practice, rather moderate and tends to deteriorate in polymers where the sorbed water exhibits a strong tendency to form clusters, as indicated by the "cluster functions" which can be deduced from the relevant water sorption isotherms [58].

Thus, for good permselectivity one must rely primarily on diffusion selectivity, which can be very high, as illustrated in Fig. 12. However, D_{BM} increases with the water content (v_{AO}) of the membrane, more steeply than D_{THA} [54,56,64]. There is thus a trade off between water permeability and the intrinsic permselectivity for water (as illustrated for the case of cellulose acetate in Figs. 12b and d); which will tend to be exacerbated, in practice, by the increasing importance of convection effects as v_{AO} increases. Attempts to correlate theoretically D_{BM} with v_{AO}, on the same basis as was discussed above for D_{TA}^{*}, have been made [64–68], but they are obviously subject to the limitations indicated in the aforesaid discussion and are of little help in understanding, e.g., the differences in diffusion selectivity illustrated in Fig. 12d.

On the other hand, the basic principles governing the effect of polymer molecular structure on gas diffusion selectivity previously discussed are useful, provided that due account is taken of the effect of imbibed solvent. Thus, here, the interchain spacing of the polymer d (cf. Eq. (29)) is not only a function of the inherent "packability" of the polymer chains but is also critically dependent on the degree of swelling v_{AO}. The latter may be adjusted by proper balancing of the nature and relative number of hydrophilic and hydrophobic groups in the polymer chain (note that some structural irregularity or steric hindrance is also necessary, in order to prevent crystallization of the unswollen polymer during membrane formation [69].

Another consideration, as explained previously, is that the best selectivity is achieved when d is uniform; hence a microscopically uniform distribution of the sorbed water in the polymer is desirable. In other words, diffusion selectivity (like sorption selectivity, v.s.) is enhanced by a low degree of water clustering. Stiff-chain polymers are not only inherently more diffusion–selective than rubbers (for the reasons indicated in Sec. II.C.3 on the basis of Eq. (29)), they are also more effective in keeping water clustering low, as demonstrated in Ref. 58. The reason for this is that in flexible-chain polymers extensive molecular rearragement can easily occur, thus permitting the (thermodynamically favored) formation of water clusters with participation of the polar groups of the surrounding polymer chains (especially noticeable in ionomers [70]). On the other hand, at not too high v_{AO}, the aforesaid clusters tend to be largely isolated, thus accounting for the fact that D_{THA} is also low.

Hence, moderately hydrophobic stiff-chain polymers are the obvious choice from the point of view of both permeability and permselectivity. The classical example is cellulose acetate (v.s. and Figs. 12b and d), wherein a composition of ~ 2.3 acetyl groups per glucose monomer unit appears to be optimum for single-pass seawater desalination to potable levels. (Note that the D_{BM} values used for Fig. 12d were determined by immersion experiments; the effective permselectivity obtained under reverse osmosis conditions is usually lower, presumably due to microscopic membrane structural nonhomogeneity effects) [57]. Examples of other materials of similar or better performance are given in Fig. 12.

V. CONCLUSION

Gas separation, vapor permeation/pervaporation and reverse osmosis have been considered as examples of physically diverse membrane separation processes, which may be formulated and studied in a unified manner. A treatment along these lines, aiming at formulations of reasonable simplicity and practical applicability combined with a minimum of simplifying assumptions and/or empiricism, has been presented. The behavior of the parameters which govern transport has been considered in relation to salient physicochemical characteristics of the polymer–penetrant system, with the aid of suitable idealized model representation of the latter. The primary aim of this study was to show that permeability and selectivity in the aforementioned separation processes may be understood also on the basis of a unified set of fundamental principles.

Solubility properties reflect primarily the strength of polymer–penetrant interactions; hence sorption selectivity is particularly sensitive to the chemical nature of polymer and penetrant. Diffusion selectivity, on the other hand, is the result of a molecular sieving process and is, thus, chiefly dependent on penetrant molecular size (and shape) in relation to appropriate polymer chain packing density and adequate chain stiffness, aptly described in semi-quantitative terms by the Brandt model discussed in Sec. II.C.3. Consequently, in nonpolar or weakly polar polymer–penetrant systems, sorption and diffusion selectivity tend to favor the larger or smaller penetrant molecule, respectively. The observation that sorption selectivity is usually dominant in vapor permeation/pervaporation, but not in gas separation, is primarily a consequence of the fact that vapors exhibit a much wider variety in chemical properties than gases (while the antagonistic effect of diffusion selectivity is minimized by positive flow coupling and by the choice of flexible-chain polymeric materials).

On the other hand, enhancement of sorption selectivity in specific gas separations (notably O_2/N_2) by the use of carriers was seen above to be of limited advantage under practical conditions, because of an accompanying drop in diffusivity of the specifically sorbed penetrant, resulting in only small gains in permselectivity. Thus, practical gas separation relies primarily on the diffusion selectivity obtainable from stiff-chain polymeric materials. The limitations imposed by the low permeabilities of the latter materials were reduced sufficiently to make the process commercially viable for a number of appplications, by developments in ultrathin-membrane-surface-layer and large-membrane-surface-area (hollow fiber) technology. More recently, attention has been focused on the development of materials of improved permselectivity vs. permeability properties, for which the principles discussed above provide useful guidelines.

The chief application of reverse osmosis, namely water desalination by uncharged hydrophobic membranes, which was chosen as the third example to be discussed here, also relies primarily on diffusion selectivity (thanks to the substantial difference in size between the hydrated ions of the solute and the solvent molecules); although sorption selectivity also favors the solvent. However, both these selectivities are inversely related to, and critically dependent on, the extent of solvent uptake; because the latter determines the density of polymer chain packing and the chemical environment for sorbed solute, which are effective in the desalination process. Thus, for the attainment of optimum permeability–permselectivity properties in this case, one is called upon to manipulate the hydrophilic–hydrophobic balance of the polymer chains (which determines the extent of solvent uptake), as well as their stiffness and packability.

One should not, of course, forget that from the point of view of practical application, material properties other than permeability and permselectivity are important; notably mechanical and rheological properties (formation of defect-free ultrathin membrane surface layers, durability under stress) and resistance to chemical degradation.

REFERENCES

1. P. Meares (ed.), *Membrane Separation Processes*, Elsevier, Amsterdam, 1976.
2. M. Mulder, *Basic Principles of Membrane Technology*, Kluwer, Dordrecht, 1991.
3. J. H. Petropoulos, Adv. Polym. Sci. *64*:93 (1985).
4. J. H. Petropoulos, J. Membrane Sci. *53*:229 (1990).
5. D. R. Paul, Separation Purification Meth. *5*:33 (1976).
6. C. H. Lee, J. Appl. Polym. Sci. *19*:83 (1975).
7. T. Kataoka, T. Tsuru, S. Nakao, and S. Kimura, J. Chem. Eng. Japan *24*:326 (1991).
8. H. Mark and A. V. Tobolsky, in *Physical Chemistry of High Polymeric Systems*, Wiley Interscience, New York, 1950; Chapter 8.
9. G. Gee, Quart. Rev. Chem. Soc. (Lond.) *1*:265 (1947).
10. V. T. Stannett, in *Diffusion in Polymers* (J. Crank and G. S. Park, eds.), Academic Press, New York, 1968, Chapter 2.
11. R. F. Blanks and J. M. Prausnitz, Ind. Eng. Chem. Fundam. *3*:1 (1964).
12. J. H. Petropoulos, Pure Appl. Chem. *65*:219 (1993).
13. K. Toi, G. Morel, and D. R. Paul, J. Appl. Polym. Sci. *27*:2997 (1982).
14. V. V. Teplyakov and S. G. Durgarian, Vysokomol. Soedin. A *26*:1498 (1984).
15. W. J. Koros, J. Polym. Sci., Polym. Phys. Ed. *23*:1611 (1985).
16. S. I. Smirnov, V. K. Belyakov, S. I. Semenova, and V. G. Karachevtsev, Vysokomol. Soedin. A *25*:2073 (1983).
17. H. Nishide, M. Ohyanagi, O. Okada, and E. Tsuchida, Macromolecules *20*:417 (1987).
18. W. R. Vieth, J. M. Howell, and J. H. Hsieh, J. Membrane Sci. *1*:177 (1976).
19. W. J. Koros, A. H. Chan, and D. R. Paul, J. Membrane Sci. *2*:165 (1977).
20. C. A. Kumins and T. K. Kwei, in *Diffusion in Polymers* (J. Crank and G. S. Park, eds.), Academic Press, New York, 1968, Chapter 4.
21. R. T. Chern, W. J. Koros, H. B. Hopfenberg, and V. T. Stannett, in *Material Science of Synthetic Membranes* (D. Lloyd, ed.), Am. Chem. Soc. Symp. Ser. 269, 1985, Chapter 3.
22. W. W. Brandt and G. A. Anysas, J. Appl. Polym. Sci. *7*:1919 (1963).
23. R. Srinivasan, S. R. Auvil, and P. M. Burban, J. Membrane Sci. *86*:67 (1994).
24. W. W. Brandt, J. Phys. Chem. *63*:1080 (1959).
25. R. J. Pace and A. Datyner, J. Polym. Sci., Polym. Phys. Ed. *17*:437, 453, 465 (1979).
26. H. Fujita, Fortschr. Hochpolym. Forsch. *3*:1 (1961).
27. J. S. Vrentas and J. L. Duda, J. Polym. Sci., Polym. Phys. Ed. *15*:403, 417 (1977).
28. J. S. Vrentas and J. L. Duda, J. Appl. Polym. Sci. *21*:1715 (1977).
29. H. L. Frisch and S. A. Stern, CRC Crit. Rev. Solid State Mater. Sci. *11*:123 (1983).
30. J. D. Ferry, *Viscoelastic Properties of Polymers*, 3rd Ed., Wiley, New York, 1980.
31. S. M. Fang, S. A. Stern, and H. L. Frisch, Chem. Eng. Sci. *30*:773 (1975).
32. W. J. Koros, G. K. Fleming, S. M. Jordan, T. H. Kim, and H. H. Hoehn, Progr. Polym. Sci. *13*:339 (1988).
33. L. M. Robeson, W. F. Burgoyne, M. Langsam, A. C. Savoca, and C. F. Tien, Polymer *35*:4970 (1994).
34. Y. Ichiraku, S. A. Stern, and T. Nakagawa, J. Membrane Sci. *34*:5 (1987).

35. J. H. Petropoulos, J. Polym. Sci., A2 *8*:1797 (1970).
36. J. H. Petropoulos, J. Polym. Sci., Part B *26*:1009 (1988).
37. J. H. Petropoulos, J. Membrane Sci. *48*:79 (1990).
38. J. H. Petropoulos, J. Membrane Sci. *75*:47 (1992).
39. M. H. V. Mulder and C. A. Smolders, J. Membrane Sci. *17*:289 (1984).
40. J. P. Brun, C. Larchet, G. Bulvestre, and B. Auclair, J. Membrane Sci. *25*:55 (1985).
41. J. S. Chiou and D. R. Paul, J. Membrane Sci. *32*:195 (1987).
42. J. W. Rhim and R. Y. M. Huang, J. Membrane Sci. *46*:335 (1989).
43. P. J. Flory, Disc. Faraday Soc. *49*:7 (1970).
44. C. M. Hansen and A. Beerbower, *Encyclopedia of Chemical Technology*, Suppl. Vol., Wiley Interscience, New York, 1971.
45. M. H. V. Mulder, T. Franken, and C. A. Smolders, J. Membrane Sci. *22*:155 (1985).
46. A. Heintz and W. Stephan, J. Membrane Sci. *89*:143 (1994)
47. A. Jonquieres, R. Clement, D. Roizard, and P. Lochon, J. Membrane Sci. *109*:65 (1996).
48. J. W. Rhim and Y. M. Huang, J. Membrane Sci. *70*:105 (1992).
49. K. Kargupta, D. Siddartha, and S. K. Sanyal, J. Membrane Sci. *124*:253 (1997).
50. S. J. Doong, W. S. Ho, and R. P. Mastondrea, J. Membrane Sci. *107*:129 (1995).
51. J. A. Barrie, in *Diffusion in Polymers* (J. Crank and G. S. Park, eds.), Academic Press, New York, 1968, Chapter 8.
52. C. K. Yeom and R. Y. M. Huang, J. Membrane Sci. *67*:39 (1992).
53. A. Heintz and W. Stephan, J. Membrane Sci. *89*:153 (1994).
54. H. Yasuda, C. E. Lamaze, and A. Peterlin, J. Polym. Sci., A2 *9*:1117 (1971).
55. G. Thau, R. Bloch, and O. Kedem, Desalination *1*:129 (1966).
56. H. K. Lonsdale, U. Merten, and R. L. Riley, J. Appl. Polym. Sci. *9*:1341 (1965).
57. H. K. Lonsdale, in *Desalination by Reverse Osmosis* (U. Merten, ed.), M.I.T. Press, Cambridge, MA, 1966, Chapter 4.
58. H. Strathmann, and A. S. Michaels, Desalination *21*:195 (1977).
59. U. Merten, in *Desalination by Reverse Osmosis* (U. Merten, ed.), M.I.T. Press, Cambridge, MA, 1966, Chapter 2.
60. J. Crank, *Mathematics of Diffusion*, 2nd Ed., Clarendon Press, Oxford, 1975.
61. C. P. Bean, in *Membranes 1, Macrosopic Systems and Models* (G. Eisenman, ed.), Marcel Dekker, New York, 1972, Chapter 1.
62. K. A. Kraus, R. J. Raridon, and W. H. Baldwin, J. Am. Chem. Soc. *86*:2571 (1964).
63. E. Glueckauf, Desalination *18*:155 (1976).
64. H. Yasuda, C. E. Lamaze, and L. D. Ikenberry, Makromol. Chem. *118*:19 (1968).
65. N. A. Peppas and C. T. Reinhart, J. Membrane Sci. *15*:275 (1983).
66. N. A. Peppas and H. J. Moynihan, J. Appl. Polym. Sci. *30*:2589 (1985).
67. K. C. Sung and E. M. Topp, J. Controlled Release *37*:95 (1995).
68. H. Matsuyama, M. Teramoto, and H. Urano, J. Membrane Sci. *126*:151 (1997).
69. H. Sumitomo and K. Hashimoto, Adv. Polym. Sci. *64*:63 (1985).
70. K. A. Mauritz, and A. J. Hopfinger, in *Modern Aspects of Electrochemistry* (J. O'M. Bockris, B. E. Conway, and R. E. White, eds.), Plenum, New York, 1982, Chapter 6.

6

Irreversible Thermodynamic Models for Pervaporation and Ultrafiltration

A. STEINCHEN Université d'Aix-Marseille, Marseille, France

Abstract

This paper gives a model of membrane transport based on the thermodynamics of irreversible processes (TIP). The membrane is considered as a single phase in which the fluxes of permeants are driven by their gradients of chemical (or electrochemical) potentials. The membrane material itself is considered as the "solvent" in the membrane phase. In the steady state, the gradients of chemical (or electrochemical) potentials of the permeant species are assumed to be constant through the membrane phase. This allows to define mean phenomenological coefficients in the membrane. These last coefficients account for the various interactions between all the components present in the membrane. They depend on the mean concentrations of permeants in the membrane and consequently, through a local equilibrium hypothesis at both membrane surfaces, they are related to the composition of the neighboring phases. Ultrafiltration and pervaporation data are analyzed in terms of this TIP approach. A major insight is then obtained in the understanding of the membrane resistance in terms of interactions between membrane–permeants and permeants–permeants.

I. INTRODUCTION

Transport through membranes has been widely studied since the earliest work of L. Vegard [1, 2] and W. S. Lazarus-Barlow [3]. Many attempts to find a coherent theory were developed during the last fifty years. The most popular ones are the irreversible thermodynamic theory of Kedem and Katchalsky [4, 5] and the frictional model developed by Spiegler [6] and by Kedem and Katchalsky [5, 7]. Hydrodynamic models based on the Brownian motion of particles in pores [8] or models of solution–diffusion [9] assume mechanisms on molecular scale to give an interpretation of the transport coefficients. Many other models were discussed and are reviewed by Soltanieh and Gill [10] and by Kesting [11].

The most interesting approach is the statistical–mechanical theory of membrane transport developed by Mason et al. [12–17]. It indeed gives the most general and most rigourous frame to the transport equations through membranes, moreover it has been shown [16] that the frictional model and the Katchalsky–Kedem model can in fact be derived from the statistical–mechanical equations by suitable algebra to reproduce the frictional coefficients. The notion of reflection coefficients introduced by Staverman [18] have also been generalized to solutions of arbitrary complexity with external forces and viscous flow [14].

Our present approach starts from the same premises: the dense membranes such as the reverse osmosis membranes, ultrafiltration membranes, pervaporation membranes may be considered as multicomponent mixtures in which the membrane material is one of the component of the mixture constrained to be stationary in space. In terms of the macroscopic description, it is a single volume phase in which the state variables are defined locally by a local averaging (coarse-graining) over membrane structure and smoothing over time intervals. The restrictions for using such local description are clearly detailed by Mason and Lonsdale [12].

The macroscopic local state variables obtained by such averaging are as for classical continuous systems the local temperature T, the local pressure p, and the local concentrations of all the species i present in the mixture. In each volume element δV in which the averaging has been performed, the density of Gibbs free enthalpy $g = \delta G/\delta V$ varies according to the local equilibrium law

$$dg = -s\,dT + dp + \sum \mu_i\,dC_i \tag{1}$$

where $s = \delta S/\delta V$ is the local density of entropy and $\mu_i = (\partial g/\partial C_i)_{T,\,p,\,C_{i\neq i}}$ the local chemical potential (or partial molal free enthalpy) of i in the mixture. According to the Euler theorem on functions of first order, we have

$$\sum C_i \mu_i = g \tag{2}$$

from Eqs. (1) and (2), the Gibbs–Duhem relation is easily derived

$$\sum C_i\,d\mu_i = -s\,dT + dp \tag{3}$$

For charged and polarized systems [19,20] the electric field $\bar{E}$ appears as additional variable. The Gibbs–Duhem relation reads then

$$\sum C_i\,d\mu_i = -s\,dT + dp - \bar{P}\,d\bar{E} \tag{4}$$

where $\bar{P}$ is the polarization by unit volume.

If the gradients are not too large, such continuous description already holds. It is not valid for very thin membranes such as bilayer membranes or biological membranes of molecular size.

II. TRANSPORT EQUATIONS FOR MEMBRANE PHASES

We will consider here the transport phenomena through the membrane itself, excluding all the transfer resistances due to boundary layers at the surfaces of the membrane. The two external solutions are assumed to be well stirred and uniform. Moreover, the components crossing the membrane are assumed to be in partition equilibrium at both solution–membrane interfaces.

In the frame of the continuum description depicted above, all the species present in the membrane are free to diffuse within the multicomponent mixture. One of the components, however is restricted to remain confined between the two boundaries of the membrane phase (impermeability boundary conditions for the membrane material). The other components may cross the membrane or may be partially "reflected". When the steady state is achieved, no further accumulation of any component occurs and the distribution of each component in the membrane remains constant. It means that all the fluxes become independent of the position and equal to the upstream and to the downstream fluxes. In this steady state, the membrane material flux has to be zero everywhere within the membrane. The volume flow (or barycentric flow) of the membrane itself is zero in the steady state. According to the general equation of the entropy production in charged and polarized media given by de Groot and Mazur [21] and by Sanfeld [20], the thermodynamic generalized forces are the negative of the gradients of electrochemical potentials of all the components of the mixture (diffusion forces), the gradient of the inverse temperature (heat transport) and the driving force for internal friction $-\partial v_k/\partial x_i$, responsible for the viscous stress π_{ik} (intrinsic viscosity of the medium).

When external constraints (of concentrations, of pressure or of electric potential) are applied to the boundaries of the membrane phase, gradients of chemical or electrochemical potentials resulting from the constraints exist in the membrane. The forces driving the transport through the membrane are all the gradients of chemical or electrochemical potentials of all the components present in the membrane, including the membrane material. In the absence of thermal gradient and for a barycentric velocity of the membrane phase equal zero, the general flux–force equation then reads, like for the diffusion process in multicomponent mixture

$$\phi_i = -\sum_{j=1}^{j=N+1} \frac{\mathscr{L}_{ij}}{T} \text{ grad } \tilde{\mu}_j \tag{5}$$

where ϕ_i is the flux of each component i (permeants and membrane material) and $\tilde{\mu}_j$ the local electrochemical potentials; the $\mathscr{L}_{ij}$ coefficients are the classical, locally defined, Onsager coefficients. If we call $i = 1$ the membrane material (considered as the solvent in the membrane phase) we may write for its flux

$$\phi_1 = 0 = -\frac{\mathscr{L}_{11}}{T} \text{ grad } \tilde{\mu}_1 - \sum_{i \neq 1} \frac{\mathscr{L}_{1i}}{T} \text{ grad } \tilde{\mu}_i \tag{6}$$

We eliminate the gradient of chemical potential of the membrane material and get then for all the other components

$$\phi_{i \neq 1} = \frac{-\mathscr{L}_{ii}}{T} \text{ grad } \tilde{\mu}_i - \frac{\mathscr{L}_{1i}}{T} \text{ grad } \tilde{\mu}_1 - \sum_{j \neq i} \frac{\mathscr{L}_{ji}}{T} \text{ grad } \tilde{\mu}_j$$

$$= \frac{-\left(\mathscr{L}_{ii} - \frac{\mathscr{L}_{1i}^2}{\mathscr{L}_{11}}\right)}{T} \text{ grad } \tilde{\mu}_i - \sum_{j \neq i} \frac{\left(\mathscr{L}_{ji} - \frac{\mathscr{L}_{1i}\mathscr{L}_{1j}}{\mathscr{L}_{11}}\right)}{T} \text{ grad } \tilde{\mu}_j \tag{7}$$

Another way to eliminate grad $\tilde{\mu}_1$ is to use the Gibbs–Duhem relation Eqs. (3) or (4); the present elimination, leading to Eq. (7) allows, however, easier simplifications for the applications that follow.

This equation allows to predict the flux of each permeant through the membrane if the local gradients of electrochemical or chemical potentials and the local phenomenological coefficients are known. As a first approximation, we take the gradients of chemical or electrochemical potentials of all the permeants as constant through the membrane. With the additional hypothesis of partition equilibrium at both membrane interfaces, we get

$$\phi_{i\neq 1} = \left(\frac{L_{ii} - \dfrac{L_{1i}^2}{L_{11}}}{eT}\right)\Delta\tilde{\mu}_i + \sum_{j\neq i}\left(\frac{L_{ij} - \dfrac{L_{1i}L_{1j}}{L_{11}}}{eT}\right)\Delta\tilde{\mu}_j \tag{8}$$

where the coefficients, L_{ii}, L_{11}, L_{ji}, L_{1i}, L_{1j}, are the mean values of the local phenomenological coefficients, e is the membrane thickness, and $\Delta\tilde{\mu}_i = \tilde{\mu}_i^{up} - \tilde{\mu}_i^{down}$, is the difference of electrochemical potential of the component i in the upstream and the downstream phase.

A. Ultrafiltration and Reverse Osmosis or Electroosmosis

The upstream and downstream phases are two solutions at the same temperature. The difference of electrochemical potentials then read

$$\Delta\tilde{\mu}_i = \bar{V}_i^{\circ}\Delta p + RT\Delta \ln a_i + z_i F\Delta\varphi \tag{9}$$

where $\bar{V}_i^{\circ}$ are the molal volumes, a_i the activities ($a_i = \gamma_i x_i$), $\Delta\varphi$ the electric potential difference between the two solutions, z_i the charge of the component i.

Combining Eqs. (8) and (9), yields for the flux of each permeant species

$$\phi_{i\neq 1} = \left[\sum_{j\neq 1}\frac{\left(L_{ji} - \dfrac{L_{1i}L_{1j}}{L_{11}}\right)}{eT}\bar{V}_j^{\circ}\right]\Delta p$$

$$+ RT\left[\sum_{j\neq 1}\frac{\left(L_{ji} - \dfrac{L_{1i}L_{1j}}{L_{11}}\right)}{eT}\Delta \ln \gamma_j x_j\right]$$

$$+ \left[\sum_{j\neq 1}z_j\frac{\left(L_{ji} - \dfrac{L_{1i}L_{1j}}{L_{11}}\right)}{eT}\right]F\Delta\varphi \tag{10}$$

The total volume flow across the membrane is given by

$$J_v = \sum_{i\neq 1}\phi_i\bar{V}_i^{\circ} \tag{11}$$

Most often, in the membrane separation processes the volume flow may be regarded as the velocity of the crossing species considered as "solvent" in the upstream solution (for instance water if the solution is an aqueous solution). Calling v_w the velocity of the solvent in the upstream solution we may write

$$J_v \simeq v_w = \phi_w\bar{V}_w^{\circ} \tag{12}$$

Combining now Eq. (12) with Eq. (10) written for the permeant solvent w, we get, for ideally dilute solutions with

$$\Delta \ln x_w \gamma_w = -\Delta \sum_{j \neq w} x_j \tag{13a}$$

$$\Delta \ln x_j \gamma_j = \Delta \ln x_j \qquad j \neq w \tag{13b}$$

where x_j are the mole fractions of the solutes in upstream and downstream dilute solutions

$$
J_v = \left[\sum_{j \neq 1} \frac{\left(L_{jw} - \dfrac{L_{1w} L_{1j}}{L_{11}} \right)}{eT} \bar{V}_j^o \right] \bar{V}_w^o \Delta p
$$

$$
+ \bar{V}_w^o RT \left[-\frac{\left(L_{jw} - \dfrac{L_{1w}^2}{L_{11}} \right)}{eT} \sum_{j=w} \Delta x_j + \sum_{j \neq w} \frac{\left(L_{jw} - \dfrac{L_{1w} L_{1j}}{L_{11}} \right)}{eT} \Delta \ln x_j \right]
$$

$$
+ \left[\sum_{j=1} z_j \frac{\left(L_{jw} - \dfrac{L_{1w} L_{1j}}{L_{11}} \right)}{eT} \right] \bar{V}_w^o F \Delta \varphi \tag{14}
$$

This last expression will be used later to rationalize the results of ultrafiltration of micellized solutions of ionic detergents [22]. It is also useful to understand the significance of the commonly used filtration and osmotic flow coefficients in terms of interactions inside the membrane.

B. Pervaporation

When the membrane is surrounded by two solutions, the flows of the crossing species are given by Eq. (10). In the pervaporation processes, the downstream phase is a gas, Eq. (8) still holds, but the chemical potentials in the gas have a different form. The flows through pervaporation membranes therefore, do not obey Eq. (10). The difference between the downstream and upstream chemical potentials of the permeants are now

$$
\Delta \mu_i = [\mu_i^{ol}(T) - \mu_i^{og}(T)] - RT \ln \frac{p_i}{p_{ref}} + \bar{V}_i^{ol} p^l + RT \ln a_i^l
$$

$$
= - RT \ln \frac{p_i}{p_i^o} + \bar{V}_i^{ol}(p^l - p_i^o) + RT \ln a_i^l \tag{15}
$$

where the superscript l refers to the upstream liquid and g to the downstream gas, p^l is the total pressure above the liquid, p_i^o the saturation pressure of the pure component i at temperature T while p_i is the partial pressure of i in the downstream gas. The solutions submitted to pervaporation are most often nonionic solutions and the different components in the upstream solution may have concentrations of the same order of magnitude. Therefore, we adopt here a symmetrical model of solution, i.e., that the standard molal volume $\bar{V}_i^{ol}$ appearing in Eq. (15) is the molal volume of the pure component i. (The gas may be assumed to be perfect, if not, we could introduce the fugacities.)

Combining Eqs. (8) and (15) we then get (see [24])

$$
\phi_{i \neq 1} = \frac{\left(L_{ii} - \dfrac{L_{1i}^2}{L_{11}}\right)}{eT}\left(-RT \ln \frac{p_i}{p_i^o} + \bar{V}_i^{ol}(p^l - p_i^o) + RT \ln a_i^l\right)
$$

$$
\times \sum_{j \neq i} \frac{\left(L_{ji} - \dfrac{L_{1i}L_{1j}}{L_{11}}\right)}{eT}\left(-RT \ln \frac{p_j}{p_j^o} + \bar{V}_j^{ol}(p^l - p_j^o) + RT \ln a_j^l\right) \quad (16)
$$

or introducing the mole fractions x_i^g in the gas phase

$$
\phi_{i \neq 1} = \frac{\left(L_{ii} - \dfrac{L_{1i}^2}{L_{11}}\right)}{eT}\left(-RT \ln \frac{p^g}{p_i^o} + \bar{V}_i^{ol}(p^l - p_i^o) - RT \ln \frac{x_i^g}{a_i^l}\right)
$$

$$
\times \sum_{j \neq i} \frac{\left(L_{ji} - \dfrac{L_{1i}L_{1j}}{L_{11}}\right)}{eT}\left(-RT \ln \frac{p^g}{p_j^o} + \bar{V}_j^{ol}(p^l - p_j^o) - RT \ln \frac{x_j^g}{a_j^l}\right) \quad (17)
$$

where p^g is the downstream total pressure in the gas phase. This last expression will be used later on in order to analyse the results of pervaporation experiments on binary solutions.

III. RELATION WITH THE CLASSICAL EQUATIONS OF MEMBRANE FLOW

The classical model of membrane flow [4,5] introduces two phenomenological coefficients: the mechanical filtration coefficient L_P and the coefficient of osmotic flow L_{PD}. In this model, the volume flow through the membrane reads, for two nonionic permeants

$$
J_v = L_P \Delta P + L_{PD} \Delta\pi \quad (18)
$$

where $\Delta\pi$ is the osmotic pressure difference. For a dilute binary solution, it reads

$$
\Delta\pi = \frac{RT\Delta\gamma_s x_s}{\bar{V}_w^o} \quad (19)
$$

where w is the permeant solvent and s the solute.

If we write Eq. (14) for a binary mixture of uncharged permeants, we obtain by identification of the coefficients of $\Delta\pi$ and Δ_p,

$$
L_p = \left[\frac{\left(L_{ww} - \dfrac{L_{1w}^2}{L_{11}} \right)}{eT} \bar{V}_w^o + \frac{\left(L_{sw} - \dfrac{L_{1w}L_{1s}}{L_{11}} \right)}{eT} \bar{V}_s^o \right] \bar{V}_w^o
\tag{20}
$$

and

$$
L_{PD} = \left(-\frac{\left(L_{ww} - \dfrac{L_{1w}^2}{L_{11}} \right)}{eT} + \frac{\left(L_{sw} - \dfrac{L_{1w}L_{1s}}{L_{11}} \right)}{eT\langle x_s \rangle} \right) \bar{V}_w^{o2}
\tag{21}
$$

where $\langle x_s \rangle$ is the mean molar fraction of the permeant solute in the membrane. For an ideal semi-permeable membrane,

$$
L_p = -L_{PD}
\tag{22}
$$

and we have consequently

$$
L_p = \left(\frac{(L_{ww}L_{11} - L_{1w}^2)}{eTL_{11}} - \frac{(L_{sw}L_{11} - L_{1w}L_{1s})}{eTL_{11}\langle x_s \rangle} \right) \bar{V}_w^{o2} > 0
\tag{23}
$$

or

$$
(L_{ww}L_{11} - L_{1w}^2) + \frac{1}{\langle x_s \rangle}(L_{1w}L_{1s} - L_{sw}L_{11}) > 0
\tag{24}
$$

From this relation, we may derive some considerations on the interactions responsible for the reflection of the solute by the membrane.

IV. APPLICATIONS TO SOME EXPERIMENTAL RESULTS

A. Ultrafiltration of Micellar Solutions

Let us start from Eq. (10) giving the volume flow. For a permeant dilute solution containing a dissociate univalent electrolyte in water, the electroneutrality condition in both downstream and upstream solutions requires that the fluxes of anions and cations are equal so that

$$
\Delta\varphi = \frac{\begin{array}{c} D_a(\bar{V}_a^o\Delta p + RT\Delta \ln x_a) + D_c(\bar{V}_c^o\Delta p + RT\Delta \ln x_c) \\ + D_w(\bar{V}_w^o\Delta p - RT\Delta x_a - RT\Delta x_c) \end{array}}{(D_a - D_c)F}
\tag{25}
$$

If micelles are present in the upstream solution and not in the downstream solution, the transmembrane potential reads

$$
\Delta\varphi = \frac{\begin{array}{c} D_a(\bar{V}_a^o\Delta p + RT\Delta \ln x_a) + D_c(\bar{V}_c^o\Delta p + RT\Delta \ln x_c) \\ + D_w(\bar{V}_w^o\Delta p - RT\Delta x_a - RT\Delta x_c - RTx_{mic}^{up}) \end{array}}{(D_a - D_c)F}
\tag{26}
$$

in which $\Delta x_a = \Delta x_c$ where x_{mic}^{up} is the mole fraction of micelles in the upstream solution, and where we have called

$$D_i = \frac{L_{ai}}{eT} - \frac{L_{ci}}{eT} - \frac{L_{a1}L_{1i}}{eTL_{11}} + \frac{L_{c1}L_{1i}}{eTL_{11}} \quad (i = \text{a anion}; i = \text{c cation}; i = \text{w water})$$

Introducing Eqs. (25) or (26) in Eq. (14), the volume flow now reads

$$J_v = \mathscr{A}\Delta p + RT\mathscr{B}\Delta x_c + RT\mathscr{C}\Delta x_a + RT\mathscr{D}x_{mic}^{up} \tag{27}$$

where the coefficients $\mathscr{A}$, $\mathscr{B}$, $\mathscr{C}$ and $\mathscr{D}$ are given in the appendix.

The data obtained for ultrafiltration of aqueous solutions of surfactants through zircon membranes [22] show a linear dependence of the volume flow with the pressure difference. Moreover, at zero pressure difference no osmotic flow is observed. The empirical law observed is thus a straight line corresponding to

$$J_v = \mathscr{A}\Delta p \tag{28}$$

From these experimental data, we may deduce that the terms $RT\mathscr{B}\Delta x_c + RT\mathscr{C}\Delta x_a + RT\mathscr{D}x_{mic}^{up}$ are negligible with regard to $\mathscr{A}\Delta p$. An evaluation of the coefficients $\mathscr{B}$, $\mathscr{C}$ and $\mathscr{D}$ (see Appendix) allows us to obtain a simplified expression of the volume flow in terms of phenomenological coefficients leading to

$$J_v \approx \left[L_{ww} - \frac{L_{w1}^2}{L_{11}} + \frac{\left(L_{wc} - L_{wa} + \frac{L_{w1}}{L_{11}}[L_{1a} - L_{1c}]\right)^2}{2L_{ac} - L_{cc} - L_{aa} + \frac{[L_{1a} - L_{1c}]^2}{L_{11}}} \right] \frac{\bar{V}_w^{o2}}{eT} \Delta p \tag{29}$$

for surfactant solutions below the cmc, and

$$a = L_{ww} - \frac{L_{w1}^2}{L_{11}}$$

$$b = \left(L_{wa} - L_{wc} + z_m L_{wm} + \frac{L_{w1}}{L_{11}}[L_{1c} - L_{1a} - z_m L_{1m}] \right)$$

$$c = -2L_{ac} + L_{cc} + L_{aa} + 2z_m L_{am} - 2z_m L_{cm} + z_m^2 L_{mm}$$

$$d = \frac{[L_{1a} - L_{1c}]^2 + z_m L_{1m}(2L_{1a} - 2L_{1c} + z_m L_{1m})}{L_{11}} \tag{30}$$

for micellized surfactant solutions, where the subscript m represents the micelles.

Many authors [25–29] have observed a lower permeability of the membrane for saline solutions than for pure water. This fact was explained either by adsorption effects or by specific interactions between ions and the membrane with opposite charges [28–31]. Our approach formally accounts for all these types of interactions, moreover, as the coupling coefficients L_{ik} may be positive or negative, the global influence of a dissociated electrolyte on the permeability may be as well a decrease or an increase, as also observed for some systems.

Permeation data for ultrafiltration through zircon membranes of two types of surfactant solutions were reported recently: a first series of experiments were carried on with a cationic surfactant, the cetyltrimethylammonium bromide (CTABr) [22] and a second set of measurements with the same membranes was performed on an anionic surfactant, the sodium dodecylsulfate (NaDS) [23].

For both types of surfactants, the measurements show a linear decrease of the permeability with the concentration of surfactant in the feed. Moreover, the lowering of permeability is much smaller above the cmc than below. The slope of permeability vs. surfactant concentration shows a break up at the cmc (see Figs. 1 and 2).

The experimental procedure used for the anionic and for the cationic surfactant was the same. The pressure difference was varied in a range of 1×10^5 Pa to 3.5×10^5 Pa, for surfactant concentrations ranging from 0 to 200 mol/m^3 for NaDS and from 0 to 100 mol/m^3 for CTABr. The circulation of the feed on the membrane was 4 m/s in both set of experiments.

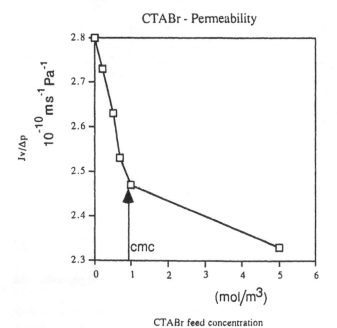

FIG. 1 Permeability vs. analytical concentration in the feed for CTABr solutions below and beyond cmc.

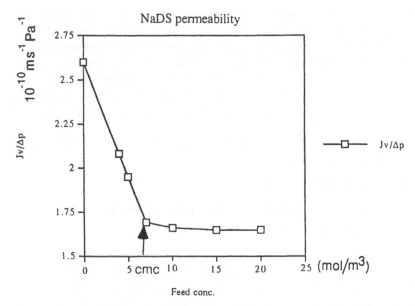

FIG. 2 Permeability vs. analytical concentration in the feed for NaDS solutions below and beyond cms.

The permeability $\prod = J_v/\Delta p$ was measured at 30°C for the CTABr solutions and at 25°C for NaDS. The permeability for pure water was 2.8×10^{-10} m/s Pa at 30°C and 2.6×10^{-10} m/s Pa at 25°C with an experimental accuracy of 10%. The results of permeability for pure water allow to relate $\prod$ to the phenomenological coefficients. When there is only one permeant (water) Eq. (29) reads

$$J_v = \left[L_{ww} - \frac{L_{w1}^2}{L_{11}} \right] \frac{\bar{V}_w^{o2}}{eT} \Delta p \tag{31}$$

and we have then

$$\prod = \left[L_{ww} - \frac{L_{w1}^2}{L_{11}} \right] \frac{\bar{V}_w^{o2}}{eT} \tag{32}$$

The molar volume of pure water, the temperature as well as the membrane thickness may be determined for each set of experiments. From the data of pure water permeability, a numerical value may be obtained for the combination of phenomenological coefficients under brackets $[L_{ww} - L_{w1}^2/L_{11}]$. These mean coefficients in the membrane depend on the mean concentration of water in the membrane. When small amounts of solutes are added to water, one may expect that the mean concentration of water in the membrane remains fairly the same as for pure water. The numerical value of $[L_{ww} - L_{w1}^2/L_{11}]$ then should remain the same. The permeability data obtained for dilute solutions of dissociated surfactants below the cmc seem indeed to confirm this assumption. The data of volume flow vs. pressure difference (See Tables 1 and 2) for various analytical concentrations of surfactant in the feed for the cationic surfactants as well as for the anionic surfactants, have been recently published [22, 23].

The two best fit laws obtained below the cmc for CTABr at 30°C and for NaDS at 25°C are respectively:

$$\prod = (2.8 - 0.45C_0)10^{-10} \text{ m/s Pa}$$

best fit permeation/concentration law for NaDS below cmc

$$\prod = (2.6 - 0.13C_0)10^{-10} \text{ m/s Pa}$$

with C_0 in mol/m^3.

We may now analyze these results in terms of the phenomenological coefficients through Eq. (29). The ordinate at the origin of these best fit laws may be identified with the volume flow for pure water given by Eq. (32). The C_0 linear

TABLE 1 CTABr at 30°C: Permeability vs. Analytical Concentration in the Feed

C_0 (mol/m^3)	$\Delta p = 1 \times 10^5$ Pa J_v (10^{-5} m/s)	$\Delta p = 2 \times 10^5$ Pa J_v (10^{-5} m/s)	$\Delta p = 3 \times 10^5$ Pa J_v (10^{-5} m/s)
0.2	2.6	5.4	8.2
0.5	2.5	5.2	7.9
0.7	2.4	5.1	7.6
1 (cmc)	2.3	5.0	7.4
5	2.3	4.8	7.0
10	2.2	4.7	6.8
20	2.1	4.4	6.3
30	2.0	4.1	5.8
40	1.8	3.9	5.5
50	1.7	3.6	5.1
60	1.6	3.4	4.9
70	1.4	3.2	4.6
80	1.3	3.0	4.4
90	1.3	2.9	4.1
100	1.2	2.7	3.9

Source: adapted from Ref. 22.

TABLE 2 NaDS at 25°C: Permeability vs. Analytical Concentration in the Feed

C_0 (mol/m³)	$\Delta p = 1 \times 10^5$ Pa J_v (10^{-5} m/s)	$\Delta p = 2 \times 10^5$ Pa J_v (10^{-5} m/s)	$\Delta p = 3 \times 10^5$ Pa J_v (10^{-5} m/s)
4	1.86	4.08	5.31
5	1.64	3.94	5.08
7	1.47	3.81	5.03
cmc			
10	1.42	3.64	4.97
15	1.39	3.47	4.94
20	1.39	3.36	4.94
30	1.39	3.33	4.94
40	1.39	3.31	4.94
50	1.39	3.31	4.81
60	1.39	3.19	4.67
70	1.39	3.03	4.53
cmc'			
100	1.19	2.67	4.03
130	0.97	2.31	3.6
160	0.78	2.03	3.11
200	0.56	1.64	2.67

Source: adapted from Ref. 23.

term may be identified with the term

$$\frac{\left(L_{wc} - L_{wa} + \dfrac{L_{w1}}{L_{11}}[L_{1a} - L_{1c}]\right)^2}{2L_{ac} - L_{cc} - L_{aa} + \dfrac{[L_{1a} - L_{1c}]^2}{L_{11}}} \frac{\bar{V}_w^{o2}}{eT}$$

in Eq. (29). So that we may write for CTABr at 30°C

$$\frac{\left(L_{wc} - L_{wa} + \dfrac{L_{w1}}{L_{11}}[L_{1a} - L_{1c}]\right)^2}{2L_{ac} - L_{cc} - L_{aa} + \dfrac{[L_{1a} - L_{1c}]^2}{L_{11}}} \frac{\bar{V}_w^{o2}}{eT} = -0.45 \times 10^{-10} C_o \tag{33}$$

and for NaDS at 25°C

$$\frac{\left(L_{wc} - L_{wa} + \dfrac{L_{w1}}{L_{11}}[L_{1a} - L_{1c}]\right)^2}{2L_{ac} - L_{cc} - L_{aa} + \dfrac{[L_{1a} - L_{1c}]^2}{L_{11}}} \frac{\bar{V}_w^{o2}}{eT} = -0.13 \times 10^{-10} C_o \tag{34}$$

Because of the electroneutrality condition of both upstream and downstream bulk solutions, the ion concentrations are identical to the analytical concentration of the surfactant in both bulk phases. In the membrane, for the same reason of electroneutrality, the mean ion concentration in the membrane must be equal to the mean analytical concentration of surfactant. For small concentrations, the mean phenomenological coefficients of ions in the membrane are linear functions of the mean ion concentrations and thus linear function of the mean analytical concentration of the surfactant. This last is proportional to the upstream analytical concentration C_0. The linear dependence of the volume flow with the upstream analytical concentration of surfactant is thus explained, through the phenomenological coefficients. Moreover, the various contributions of the membrane–solute interactions as well as the solute–solvent and solvent–membrane interactions appear explicitly. These interactions induce an overall effect on the permeability, linearly related to the amount of surfactant in the feed.

Above the cmc, the slope of the $\prod$ vs. C_0 curves shows a break up as seen on Figs. 1 and 2. The volume flow is still given by Eq. (29) if no micelle crosses the membrane. The permeability of the membrane is less influenced by the surfactant concentration than below in both systems studied here CTABr and NaDS through zircon membranes. The same behavior has been observed by Akay and Wakeman [25] on polymeric membranes. The analysis of the various terms in Eq. (29) allows to understand such behavior. Indeed, above the cmc, the monomeric ions concentration in the feed is almost constant and equals the cmc while the counterion concentration increases linearly with the surfactant concentration, but to a lesser extent than below the cmc. Above the cmc, the concentrations in the feed of the free monomer ion and of the counterion are different because of electroneutrality condition (the counterion concentration has to balance the total number of opposite charges carried by the monomers and by the micelles). In the membrane, however, the overall mean concentration of both cations and anions have to balance each one another. Their might exist local distributions of charges on both membrane interfaces but the integral charge density through the membrane phase and through the neighbouring double layers has to be zero. As the overall activity of the counter ion of the micellized detergent increases in the feed with the analytical concentration, the chemical diffusion driving force on the counter ion in the membrane increases. Consequently, the counter ion activity in the downstream solution increases as observed experimentally. By the electroneutrality condition in the downstream solution, the monomer detergent ion concentration has to equal the counterion concentration and, as observed experimentally, the monomer ion concentration in the downstream solution also increases with the upstream analytical concentration. Both ions concentration increasing in the downstream phase, it is worth assuming that the mean ion concentrations in the membrane follow the same evolution. The mean phenomenological coefficients in the membrane, for small concentrations in the membrane phase, are linear functions of the mean concentrations and thus also linear functions of the upstream analytical concentration. This allows to understand the linear behavior obtained for both systems NaDS and CTABr [see Eqs. (33) and (34)].

Beyond the cmc, in the two examples shown here above, the concentrations of monomeric ions in the upstream solution may be obtained in terms of the analytical concentration of detergent according to a mass balance assuming a mean aggregation number (the dispersion being quasi monodisperse) and a mean charge carried by the polymer ion. For CTABr, in the operating conditions of the above experimental results, the micelles are made of 90 monomers and the positive charge of the micelle is 14. The micelle upstream concentration, the bromide concentration and the CTA^+ concentration are then respectively

$$C_{mic} = \frac{C_o - cmc}{90}; \quad C_{Br^-} = cmc + 14\left(\frac{C_o - cmc}{90}\right); \quad C_{CTA^+} = cmc$$

For NaDS, the aggregation number is 60 and the charge 23, the concentrations of the micelle, of the sodium ion and of the dodecyl sulfate ion are then

$$C_{mic} = \frac{C_o - cmc}{60}; \quad C_{Na^+} = cmc + 23\left(\frac{C_o - cmc}{60}\right); \quad C_{DS^-} = cmc$$

An increase of analytical concentration beyond the cmc is thus responsible for an increase of the upstream concentration of the counter ion while the monomer ion concentration remains equal to the cmc. The overall concentrations of both negative and positive ions in the membrane increase when the upstream analytical concentration increases but to a smaller extent then below the cmc. For both systems reported in Refs. [22] and [23], the volume flows measured beyond the cmc show a linear dependence on the upstream analytical concentration of detergent (see Figs. 1 and 2) and a best fit equation for the permeability may be derived from the experimental results given in Tables 1 and 2.

best fit permeation/concentration law for CTABr beyond cmc

$\prod = (2.8 - 0.45 \text{ cmc} - 0.012C_o)10^{-10}$ m/s Pa

best fit permeation/concentration law for NaDS beyond cmc

$\prod = (2.6 - 0.13 \text{ cmc} - 0.00213C_o)10^{-10}$ m/s Pa

When micelles are crossing the membrane, Eq. (29) is no longer valid but it has to be replaced by Eq. (30) in which interaction terms involving the micelles in the membrane are taken into account. In NaDS solutions, for example, two forms of micelles may be present according to the value of the analytical concentration. A first cmc = 8 mol/m³ is observed corresponding to the formation of spherical negatively charged micelles. The second critical micellar concentration cmc' = 75 mol/m³ corresponds to the formation of rod-like micelles. As soon as the second critical micellar concentration is reached in the feed, rod-like micelles are crossing the membrane and the slope of the membrane permeability vs. analytical upstream concentration shows a new break up.

It is usual in engineering to introduce resistance coefficients to relate the volume flow to the pressure difference across the ultrafiltration membrane. The phenomenological law is then written for the crossflow of pure water (or pure upstream solvent) through the membrane

$$J_v = \frac{1}{\mu_o R_M} \Delta p \qquad (35)$$

where μ_o is the viscosity of pure water (or of the pure upstream solvent) and R_M, the membrane resistance.

When solutes are added to the solvent (for example electrolytes) the volume flow is reduced and it is classical to include an additional resistance R in Eq. (35) so that the phenomenological law reads

$$J_v = \frac{1}{\mu(R_M + R)} \Delta p \qquad (36)$$

where μ is the viscosity of the upstream solution. Comparing Eq. (35) to Eq.

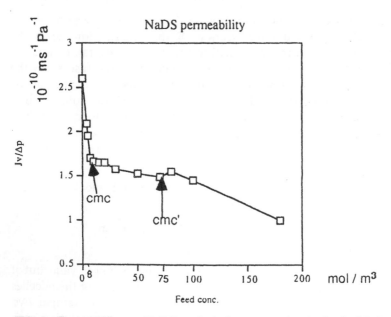

FIG. 3 Permeability vs. NaDS analytical concentration in the feed below and beyond cmc and beyond cmc'.

(31) and Eq. (36) to Eqs. (29) or (30), it is possible to obtain the resistance coefficients in terms of the mean Onsager coefficients in the membrane phase. These last coefficients allow us to relate the resistance coefficients to the interactions of all the components present in the membrane.

B. Pervaporation of Ethanolic Solutions of Linalool

An example of application of the TIP method for the analysis of the experimental results of pervaporation experiments of ethanolic solutions of linalool has been recently published [24]. The permeant species are linalool (3) and a pseudo solvent water–ethanol azeotropic mixture (2). The membrane (1) is a polydimethylsiloxane (PDMS).

The fluxes of both permeants read according to Eq. 17

$$\phi_2 = \frac{L_{22} - \dfrac{L_{12}^2}{L_{11}}}{eT}\left(-RT\ln\frac{p^g}{p_2^o} + \overline{V_2^{ol}}(p^l - p_2^o) - RT\ln\frac{x_2^g}{a_2^l}\right)$$

$$+ \frac{L_{23} - \dfrac{L_{12}L_{13}}{L_{11}}}{eT}\left(-RT\ln\frac{p^g}{p_3^o} + \overline{V_3^{ol}}(p^l - p_3^o) - RT\ln\frac{x_3^g}{a_3^l}\right) \qquad (37)$$

$$\phi_3 = \frac{L_{33} - \dfrac{L_{13}^2}{L_{11}}}{eT}\left(-RT\ln\frac{p^g}{p_3^o} + \overline{V_3^{ol}}(p^l - p_3^o) - RT\ln\frac{x_3^g}{a_3^l}\right)$$

$$+ \frac{L_{23} - \dfrac{L_{12}L_{13}}{L_{11}}}{eT}\left(-RT\ln\frac{p^g}{p_2^o} + \overline{V_2^{ol}}(p^l - p_2^o) - RT\ln\frac{x_2^g}{a_2^l}\right) \qquad (38)$$

and the total flux

$$\phi_T = \phi_2 + \phi_3 = \left(\frac{L_{33} - \dfrac{L_{13}^2}{L_{11}}}{eT} + \frac{L_{23} - \dfrac{L_{12}L_{13}}{L_{11}}}{eT}\right)$$

$$\times\left(-RT\ln\frac{p^g}{p_3^o} + \overline{V_3^{ol}}(p^l - p_3^o) - RT\ln\frac{x_3^g}{a_3^l}\right)$$

$$+ \left(\frac{L_{22} - \dfrac{L_{12}^2}{L_{11}}}{eT} + \frac{L_{23} - \dfrac{L_{12}L_{13}}{L_{11}}}{eT}\right)$$

$$\times\left(-RT\ln\frac{p^g}{p_2^o} + \overline{V_2^{ol}}(p^l - p_2^o) - RT\ln\frac{x_2^g}{a_2^l}\right) \qquad (39)$$

Using the relations $x_2^g = 1 - x_3^g$ and $x_3^g = \alpha(p^g/p_{ref})^\beta$ it is easy to transform Eq. (39) in order to obtain an explicit relation between the total flux and the downstream pressure. This last relation reads

$$\phi_T = A + B \ln \frac{p^g}{p_{ref}} + C \ln\left(1 - \alpha\left(\frac{p^g}{p_{ref}}\right)^\beta\right) \tag{40}$$

for small mole fractions of solute 3 in the downstream phase one gets

$$\phi_T \simeq A + B \ln \frac{p^g}{p_{ref}} - C\alpha\left(\frac{p^g}{p_{ref}}\right)^\beta \tag{41}$$

The reference pressure p_{ref} is 1 atm., the constants α and β are identified experimentally by linear regression, the constants A, B and C are combinations of the phenomenological coefficients multiplied by quantities independent on the downstream pressure

$$A = -\left(L_{23} + L_{33} - L_{13}\left(\frac{L_{12} - L_{13}}{L_{11}}\right)\right)$$

$$\times \left[\frac{R \ln \alpha \frac{p_{ref}\, a_3^l}{p_3^o}}{e} - \frac{\bar{V}_3^{ol}(p_3^o - p^l)}{eT}\right]$$

$$+ \left(L_{23} + L_{22} - L_{12}\left(\frac{L_{12} - L_{13}}{L_{11}}\right)\right)$$

$$\times \left[\frac{R \ln \frac{p_2^o\, a_2^l}{p_{ref}}}{e} - \frac{\bar{V}_3^{ol}(p_3^o - p^l)}{eT}\right] \tag{42}$$

$$B = -\left\{L_{22} + L_{33} + 2L_{23} - L_{12}\left(\frac{L_{12} + L_{13}}{L_{11}}\right) - L_{13}\left(\frac{L_{12} + L_{13}}{L_{11}}\right)\right.$$

$$\left. + \left[L_{23} + L_{33} - L_{13}\left(\frac{L_{12} + L_{13}}{L_{11}}\right)\right]\beta\right\}\frac{R}{e} \tag{43}$$

$$C = -\left\{L_{23} + L_{22} - L_{12}\left(\frac{L_{12} + L_{13}}{L_{11}}\right)\right\}\frac{R}{e} \tag{44}$$

The values of the coefficients A, B and C are determined by a fitting of the experimental values of the total flux vs. downstream pressure with Eq. (41). From these values, groups of phenomenological coefficients can be calculated. These latter are linearly dependent on the upstream amount of linalool within the experimental range investigated.

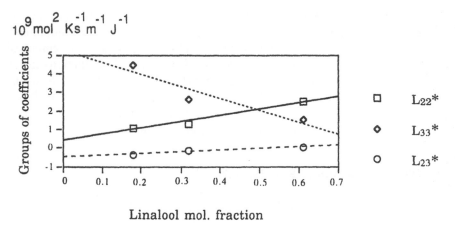

Linalool mol. fraction

FIG. 4 Groups of phenomenological coefficients in membrane vs. linalool mol fraction in the feed.

The interactions between linalool–solvent, linalool–membrane and solvent–membrane appear through the term $L_{23}^* = L_{23} - (L_{12}L_{13}/L_{11})$. This last term increases strongly with the linalool concentration in the feed but it is always smaller than the groups characterizing the solvent–solvent and solvent–membrane interactions $L_{22}^* = L_{22} - (L_{12}^2/L_{11})$ or the linalool–linalool and linalool–membrane interactions $L_{33}^* = L_{33} - (L_{13}^2/L_{11})$ as seen in Fig. 4.

The TIP method allows here to understand how the interactions in the membrane are modified when the mole fraction of the binary solution of permeants is changed. The method may also be applied to permeant mixtures with more than two components.

V. CONCLUSION

The present approach of studying the mass transfer through membranes considers the membrane as a phase with a fixed "solvent" the membrane material. The permeants are considered as solutes in this continuum. The membrane material is insoluble in both neighbouring phases. The classical TIP flux–force laws in the continuous membrane phase introduces the gradients of the chemical (or electrochemical) potentials of all the species present in the membrane as generalized forces. These local gradients are not measurable locally neither are the local phenomenological coefficients, however, assuming that in the steady state the gradients of chemical (or electrochemical) potentials are constant through the membrane, with the local equilibrium hypothesis of permeants at both membrane surfaces the gradients of permeants through the membrane are available and mean phenomenological coefficients in the membrane are defined. These last coefficients depend on the mean concentrations in the membrane phase and account for the interactions between all the components present in the membrane including the membrane material. The empirical resistance models may then now be explained in terms of interactions inside the membrane. While not entering in the detailed membrane structure, the model allows to give good predictions of the variations of fluxes with the composition of the feed solutions, in terms of interactions inside the membrane, as well for ultrafiltration as for pervaporation processes.

APPENDIX: COEFFICIENTS IN Eq. (27)

$$\mathscr{A} = W_w \bar{V}^\circ_w + W_a \bar{V}^\circ_a + W_c \bar{V}^\circ_c$$
$$- \frac{W_c - W_c}{D_c - D_a} (D_a \bar{V}^\circ_a + D_c \bar{V}^\circ_c + D_w \bar{V}^\circ_w)$$

$$\mathscr{B} = -W_w + \frac{W_a}{\langle x^m_a \rangle} + \frac{W_c - W_a}{D_c - D_a} \left(D_w - \frac{D_a}{\langle x^m_a \rangle} \right)$$

$$\mathscr{C} = -W_w + \frac{W_c}{\langle x^m_c \rangle} + \frac{W_c - W_a}{D_c - D_a} \left(D_w - \frac{D_c}{\langle x^m_c \rangle} \right)$$

$$\mathscr{D} = -W_w + \frac{W_c - W_a}{D_c - D_a} D_w$$

where

$$W_w = \frac{1}{eT} \left(L_{ww} - \frac{L^2_{w1}}{L_{11}} \right); \quad W_a = \frac{1}{eT} \left(L_{wa} - \frac{L_{w1} L_{1a}}{L_{11}} \right);$$

$$W_c = \frac{1}{eT} \left(L_{wc} - \frac{L_{w1} L_{1c}}{L_{11}} \right)$$

and

$$D_i = \frac{1}{eT} \left(L_{ai} - L_{ci} - \frac{L_{a1} L_{1i}}{L_{11}} + \frac{L_{c1} L_{1i}}{L_{11}} \right)$$

$$(i = \text{w water}; = \text{a anion}; = \text{c cation})$$

$\langle x^m_c \rangle$ and $\langle x^m_a \rangle$ are the mean mol fractions of cation and anion in the membrane.

REFERENCES

1. L. Vegard, Proc. Cambridge Phil. Soc. *15*: 13 (1908–1910).
2. L. Vegard, Proc. Cambridge Phil. Soc. *15*: 275 (1908–1910).
3. W. S. Lazarus-Barlow, J. Physiol. *19*: 140 (1895–1896).

4. O. Kedem and A. Katchalsky, J. Gen. Physiol. *45*: 143 (1961).
5. O. Kedem and A. Katchalsky, Biochim. Biophys. Acta *27*: 229 (1958).
6. K. Spiegler, Trans. Faraday Soc. *54*: 1409 (1958).
7. O. Kedem and A. Katchalsky, Trans. Faraday Soc. *59*: 1918 (1963).
8. H. Brenner and L. J. Gaydos, J. Colloid Interface Sci. *58*: 312 (1977).
9. H. K. Lonsdale, U. Merten, and R. L. Riley, J. Appl. Polym. Sci. *9*: 1341 (1965).
10. M. Soltanieh and W. N. Gill, Chem. Eng. Commun. *12*: 279 (1981).
11. R. E. Kesting, in *Synthetic Polymeric Membranes*, Wiley Interscience, New York, NY, 2nd Ed., 1985, Chapter 2.
12. E. A. Mason and L. A. Viehland, J. Chem. Phys. *68*: 3562 (1978).
13. L. F. del Castillo and E. A. Mason, Biophys. Chem. *12*: 223 (1980).
14. E. A. Mason and L. F. del Castillo, J. Membrane Sci. *23*: 199 (1985).
15. L. F. del Castillo, E. A. Mason, and H. E. Revercomb, Biophys. Chem. *10*: 191 (1979).
16. L. F. del Castillo and E. A. Mason, J. Membrane Sci. *28*: 229 (1986).
17. E. A. Mason and H. K. Lonsdale, J. Membrane Sci. *51*: 1 (1990).
18. A. J. Staverman, Rec. Trav. Chim. P. B. *70*: 344 (1951).
19. I. Prigogine, P. Mazur, and R. Defay, J. Chim. Phys. *50*: 146 (1953).
20. A. Sanfeld, in *Introduction to the Thermodynamics of Charged and Polarized Layers*, Monographs in Statistical Physics and Thermodynamics, Wiley Interscience, New York, 1968.
21. S. R. de Groot and P. Mazur, in *Non-Equilibrium Thermodynamics*, North-Holland, Amsterdam, 1962.
22. F. Charbit, A. Steinchen, Z. Sadaoui, and G. Charbit, J. Membrane Sci. *133*: 1 (1997).
23. C. Azoug, A. Steinchen, F. Charbit, and G. Charbit, J. Membrane Sci. in press (1998).
24. C. Molina, A. Steinchen, G. Charbit, and F. Charbit, J. Membrane Sci. *132*: 119 (1997).
25. G. Akay and R. J. Wakeman, Chem. Eng. Sci. *49*: 271 (1994).
26. E. Yildiz, T. Pekdemir, B. Keskindler, A. Cakici, and G. Akay, Trans. I Chem. E., Part A *74*: 517 (1996).
27. R. J. Wakeman and G. Akay, J. Membrane Sci. *91*: 145 (1994).
28. E. S. Tarleton and R. Wakeman, Trans. I. Chem. E *72*: 521 (1994).
29. J. A. Palmer, H. B. Hopfenberg and R. M. Felder, J. Colloid Interface Sci. *45*: 223 (1973).
30. P. M. Van der Velden and C. A. Smolders, J. Collid Interface Sci. *61*: 446 (1977).
31. A. S. Jonsson and B. Jonsson, J. Membrane Sci. *56*: 49 (1991).

7

Protein Adsorption on Ultrafiltration Membrane Surfaces and Effects on Transport

V. G. J. RODGERS Department of Chemical and Biochemical Engineering, The University of Iowa, Iowa City, Iowa

Abstract

Clearly, synthetic membrane separation can have a much more extensive impact on practical separation problems, from wastewater treatment to artificial organ designs, if fouling can be eliminated. Membrane fouling contributes significantly to a reduction in process separation efficiency. This is particularly true for protein fouling which occurs in nearly all bioprocessing separations. A significant amount of research has gone into understanding membrane fouling, particularly with respect to its effect on separation performance. This chapter will overview much of this work. It will begin with a discussion on the nature of proteins and synthetic membranes that are used in ultrafiltration and the basic models associated with membrane transport. Next a discussion follows on how membrane fouling can effect performance. Methods to determine whether fouling exists will also be discussed. Finally, methods to reducing and eliminating fouling are summarized.

I. INTRODUCTION

Separation of proteinaceous materials with membranes (ultrafiltration) has been an effective process for some time. However, the problem of membrane fouling, which effects both transport of solutes and solvents plagues ultrafiltration and substantially reduces both the process performance and predictability. The physical mechanisms of membrane fouling involve a buildup of protein on the external as well as the internal pore surface of the asymmetric membrane. As a result, the effective pore size and porosity of the membrane decrease, resulting in an alternation in membrane performance. This can be observed in both the permeate flux and the sieving capabilities of the membrane [1–8]. The flux decline for both solute and solvent is initially very rapid and then gradually reduces in rate over time. Figure 1 illustrates a typical solute flux reduction that is often observed in membrane separation of protein.

Generally speaking, the coupled effects of these many factors all can contribute to solute flux reduction, as illustrated in Fig. 1. Thus, in understanding the contributions of fouling on flux decline, it is first necessary to separate the effects of these other parameters. Often, however, this is not easy. Fortunately, mathematical modeling of transport and the associated time constants or

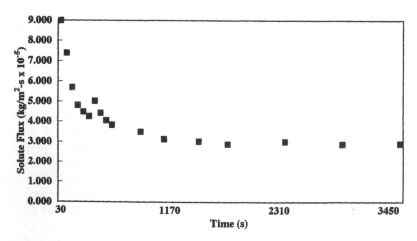

FIG. 1 Typical flux reduction that is observed in protein ultrafiltration. Adapted from Ref. 7.

characteristic times for many of these factors, including fouling, can be used to glean some insight to the impact of these factors to flux reduction. This chapter discusses the use of these tools in analyzing fouling effects on membrane performance. One should note that the subject of membrane fouling with respect to proteins is broad and a detailed presentation of the subject is not provided here. Rather, this chapter serves as a tutorial on the subject that can provide the reader with an overview of this important topic. The reader is urged to review the references cited for further detailed discussion of each subsection.

A. Protein Properties

Much of the problems with protein fouling in ultrafiltration is directly associated with the basic properties of proteins and the synthetic membrane's chemistry. This section provides a discussion of the two main properties of proteins that may contribute to protein–membrane interaction, size and charge. A more detailed discussion on protein structure can be found elsewhere [9].

Proteins are essentially large linear polymers made up of a combination of 20 amino acids. In the native state, the protein structure can be divided into four categories; primary, secondary, tertiary and quaternary. The primary structure describes the amino-acid residue sequence, the secondary structure refers to the hydrogen bonding of part of the molecule, the tertiary structure is the folding pattern and the quaternary structure represent the complex association of subunits. It is the association of the subgroups and the proteins three-dimensional structure that gives them their unique properties [9].

Since ultrafiltration is a size separation process, the most important property of proteins is physical dimension. This is because the minimum requirement for passing a protein through a pore is that the cross-sectional area occupied by the protein be less than the opening of the membrane pore. Often molecular weight, M_w, is used to characterize size of a protein. For proteins found in separation processes, the molecular weight can usually range from less than 10,000 to over 1,000,000 Da. Although molecular weight is often used to describe a protein's physical size, comparison of molecular weights to determine the potential selectivity of a process can be deceiving. This is because a protein's Einstein–Stokes radius is proportional to $M_w^{0.5}$ [10]. As shall be discussed below, most synthetic membranes usually have a distribution of pore sizes. Thus large differences in molecular weight are often necessary to provide a significant enough difference in protein separation. As an example, consider the separation of IgG (immuno gamma globulin) (156,000 Da) from albumin (66,500 Da). Although the molecular weight ratio of these two species is 2.4, the ratio of the Einstein–Stokes radii is only 1.5.

Perhaps the next most important aspect of aqueous soluble proteins is that they are electrostatic in nature. This is predominately because of the resonance of the peptide bonds between amino acids that establishes a permanent dipole moment and that reactive groups, such as terminal α-amino and carboxyl groups are present [9]. In aqueous media, these weakly acidic and basic side chains can react such as [11]

$$-COOH \rightleftharpoons -COO^- + H^+ \quad -NH_3^+ \rightleftharpoons -NH_2 + H^+ \tag{1}$$

These bonds are short range in aqueous solutions but once two or more surfaces come into contact, these forces can be quite strong. Combining the ionization capacity of groups on a single amino acid with the fact that a protein molecule is made up of hundreds to thousands of amino acids, results in a highly complex charged macromolecule. The charge distribution is not uniform, and because subgroups of amino acids can be effected by other local amino acids, the pK_a values for the residues can change with solution properties [9]. Thus their interaction with the solvent, surfaces and each other is expected to be a result of multiple interactions largely affected by charge. Since electrostatic interactions provide stability for the protein, breaking these bonds to link with other stronger ionic sites can result in protein denaturation which can result in further availability of interactive groups from the protein interior.

The net charge of the protein, Z, is the result of averaging the local surface charges along the macromolecule. This value is a function of the solution pH. The pH at which the net charge of the protein is zero is defined the isoelectric point. Thus, at pH values below the isoelectric point, the protein generally has a positive net charge, and at a pH above the isoelectric point, they generally have a negative net charge. However, the isoelectric point has been shown to depend somewhat on solution properties, such as buffers. This is due to contributions of the buffer ions in complex formations that ultimately affect the protein net charge [11].

Because soluble proteins are electrostatically charged, the osmotic pressure for these macromolecules tends to deviate significantly from ideality. This is primarily due to the electrostatic interaction of the macroions with one another, water and small ions in solution [12]. At low ionic strength, the interaction of the protein with H^+ and OH^- ions can alter the osmotic pressure due to the Donnan effect. However, at high ionic strength, an excluded volume effect is dominant and this interaction is minimized [11]. Ingham et al. [13] showed that the rejection of lysozyme in solution with albumin could be decreased by the addition of neutral salts.

Proteins also have the propensity to hydrogen bond with other surfaces such as membranes. Hydrogen bonding is also ionic interaction but the size of the hydrogen atom allows it easy access to negatively charged sites. This binding is short distanced but very strong. However, is aqueous solutions, hydrogen bonding readily occurs with water ions, therefore, this would not seem to add significantly to protein adsorption.

The apolar region of the protein can also result in hydrophobic interactions. Hydrophobic interaction is associated with entropic driving forces that minimize free energy. In aqueous solutions, the apolar regions of the molecule are generally turned toward the interior of the molecules since they cannot react with the polar solution. Polar groups also reside in the molecule interior and as a result tend to become ordered about a hydrophobic site. When hydrophobic groups bind, the entropic forces disorganize these polar groups. The alkyl groups are primarily responsible for hydrophobic interaction and the amino acids tryptophan, phenylalanine and tyrosine are the most hydrophobic. These apolar groups, located in the interior of the molecule, create a water cavity in order to react with another apolar group. The energy required to facilitate hydrophobic bonding is called the interfacial free energy. This bonding is very strong in aqueous solutions and is the strongest for protein adsorption on many surfaces.

Finally, proteins may interact with their environment via charge transfer. This is associated with excess electron density which may serve as an acceptor to a positive charge group. This interaction is associated with $\pi-\pi$ bonding in aqueous solutions [14].

B. Membrane Structure

As mentioned above, one of the most important factors in membrane separation of proteins is the size of the proteins relative to the membrane pores. In addition, the membrane chemistry is critical, since proteins can adsorb more easily on some surfaces as compared to others, resulting in blocked membrane pores. This section briefly describes these important properties of membranes. Details on membrane fabrication and other properties can be found elsewhere [15,16].

The first ultrafiltration membrane was developed in 1896 by gelatin impregnation of porous candle wax [17]. Since then, ultrafiltration membrane technology has moved from a period where only homogeneous membranes were used to development of anisotropic membranes which are used most often today. A history of membrane development has been provided by van Oss [17].

An anisotropic membrane consists of three regions; the ultrathin skin, which provides the dominant resistance to solute and permeate flux, the porous substructure, which has a chemistry similar to that of the skin, and a support backing, usually an inert material such as nonwoven polymer. The ultrathin skin layer contains the porous structure necessary for protein separation and usually has the highest surface area of all regions. An ideal membrane for protein ultrafiltration might be hydrophilic with neutral charge, have a high solvent permeability and possess a pore distribution which will pass proteins up to a particular cutoff and fully reject larger proteins. Often however, when manufacturing membranes, there are compromises. Consequently, some

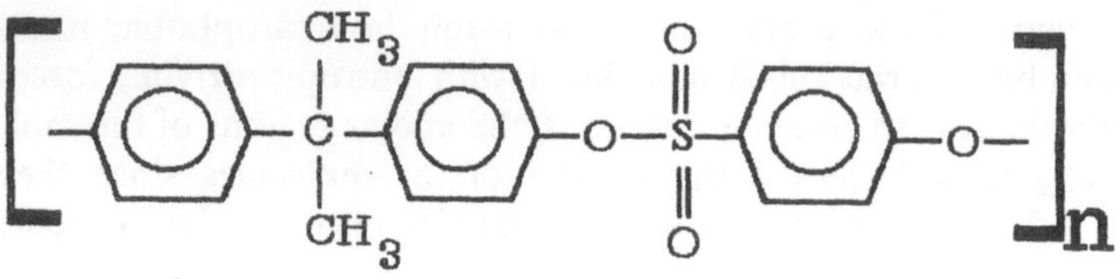

FIG. 2   Repeat unit structure for polyethersulfone.

membranes, which may be hydrophobic (and subsequently have a high adsorptivity for proteins) but of robust integrity are commonly found in protein separation processes. In addition, in practice, most anisotropic membranes have a wide distribution of pore sizes.

The separation characteristics of membranes are usually described by molecular weight cutoff (MWCO). The molecular weight cutoff value given to a membrane is usually the molecular weight of the solute where 90% is rejected by the membrane. Fane et al. [18] have determined from studies of some anisotropic membranes that 50% of the flow passes through only 20–25% of the pores. Thus, permeability is sensitive to large pore loss.

C.   Membrane Chemistry and Membrane–Protein Interaction

Membranes are made from a number of polymers. Typical polymers include; cellulose, cellulose diacetate and triacetate, polyacrylonitrile (PAN), polysulfone, polyethersulfone, and others. These polymers have been shown to provide the basic properties such as mechanical strength and ability to be cleaned that are necessary in preparing a membrane for practical use [16].

The chemical composition of the polymer can have a profound effect on the adsorbtivity of proteins. The property of the material that generally describes its interaction with proteins is classified as the relative hydrophobicity. As mentioned above, hydrophobicity is a generalized entropic effect that is best explained thermodynamically. Molecules that show poor solubility in water do so because they do not form hydration shells (a hydration shell occurs when a solute is surrounded by water molecules such that its charge or dipole interacts with the water dipole). Instead of hydration shells, the water forms cage-like structures known as clathrate. This gives the water more structure decreasing the randomness of the mixture [19]. The introduction of a protein near hydrophobic surfaces makes it thermodynamically favorable to interact and this allows the water to become more disordered. Usually hydrophilic surface groups such as hydroxyls, sulfonates and amines result in low protein fouling and hydrophobic groups (i.e., aromatic or aliphatic hydrocarbons) result in significant hydrophobic adsorption. However, this is not always the case. Many hydrophilic groups can contribute to extensive protein interaction due, possibly, to dipole–dipole or coulombic interaction [16]. This is exemplified by considering polyethersulfone and cellulose acetate. Figures 2 and 3 show the repeating unit structure for the polyethersulfone and the cellulosic membrane, respectively. As can be seen in Fig. 2, polyethersulfone is made up of diphenylen sulfone repeating units [20]. The oxygen molecules on the $-SO_2$ groups have two unshared electrons which can allow for significant hydrogen bonding. The acetylated D-glucose units of cellulose acetate (Fig. 3) also have the ability to hydrogen bond at the $-CO$ site. Despite these similarities, polyethersulfone induces order on the water and is, thus, considerably more interactive than cellulose and, thus, has a greater affinity for protein adsorption. Figure 4 shows the transient uptake of bovine serum albumin for cellulosic and polysulfone membranes with different pore sizes [21]. Clearly, the polysulfone has a much higher affinity for the protein than cellulose.

The interaction of proteins with ultrafiltration membranes is further complicated by the fact that most membranes are the results of polymer blends. While the chemistry of the single polymer can result in a number of reaction sites for interaction with the protein environment, polymer blends only further increase the membranes interaction diversity [16]. This can lead to lot-to-lot variations as well as local property differences on the same membrane.

To further complicate matters, all of the property variations of polymeric membranes can be considered to have a characteristic distance separation on the molecular scale. Coupling this with the different reactivity of residues that make up proteins, results in multiple heterogeneous interactions for proteins fouling of membranes. These phenomena make it difficult to directly determine dominant interactive forces in membrane fouling. However, it is possible to separate the general observation of fouling from deposition in many cases. This will be discussed later in this chapter.

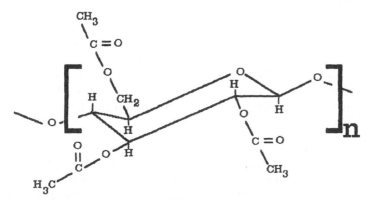

FIG. 3 Repeat unit substructure for cellulose acetate.

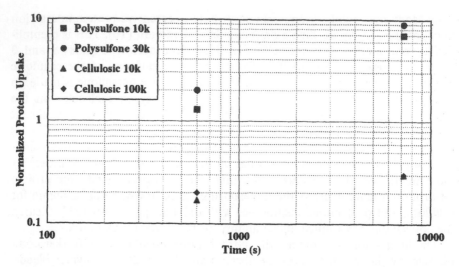

FIG. 4 Normalized transient uptake of bovine serum albumin on cellulosic and polysulfone membranes with different nominal pore sizes. Adapted from Ref. 21.

D. Elements of Transport Resistance

Knowing how membrane fouling contributes to flux loss is important in both, analyzing the process and in designing membranes and devices. Before we begin the discussion on fouling effects, it is important to discuss other factors that results in modified membrane performance. Figure 5 is a schematic of the various elements of transport resistance found in protein ultrafiltration. The following is a brief discussion of the transport resistance.

1. Compaction

Compaction is basically membrane compression that results from the continuous pressure drop across the membrane during operation. This compression can result in flux loss and possibly sieving reduction. Usually membranes are preconditioned to minimize compaction effects by operating with solvent (i.e., water) under pressure for several hours or days and monitoring permeate flux until it is essentially constant.

2. Concentration Polarization

Concentration polarization is an inevitable consequence of a flux balance of retained diffusible solutes at the membrane surface. This accumulation is an additional resistance in series with the membrane that reduces the permeate flux by as much as an order-of-magnitude or more [22–24]. However, it has

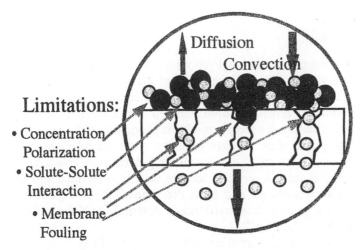

FIG. 5 Schematic diagram of various elements of transport resistance in protein ultra-filtration.

been shown that the increase in cross-flow shear rate can reduce the polariza-tion effect. This effect has been quantitatively modeled by several researchers [22,23,25–28]. Perhaps the most common expression for relating shear rate, γ, to permeate flux, J, in the ultrafiltration cross-flow module is that proposed by Michaels [22]. For the laminar cross-flow, for channel lengths, L_c, less than $0.1\gamma\, h^3/D_s$, where h is the channel height and D_s is the protein diffusivity in the bulk, he assumed steady-state film theory and obtained

$$J = k \ln\!\left(\frac{C_w}{C_b}\right) \tag{2}$$

where k is the mass transfer coefficient of the solvent defined as

$$k = C\!\left(\gamma\, \frac{D_s^2}{L_c}\right)^{1/3} \tag{3}$$

and C is a constant dependent on the geometry of the system. The values C_w and C_b denote wall and bulk concentrations, respectively. Thus it is expected that permeate flux will be proportional to $\gamma^{1/3}$ in the laminar flow regime. For turbulent flow cases, the mass transfer coefficient is approximated using empirical correlations of the Sherwood number, $\mathrm{Sh} = kd_h/D_s$ where d_h is the hydraulic diameter. Two common correlations are the Chilton–Colburn equa-tion

$$\mathrm{Sh} = 0.023\ \mathrm{Re}^{0.8}\ \mathrm{Sc}^{0.33} \tag{4}$$

and the Deissler equation

$$Sh = 0.023 \ Re^{0.875} \ Sc^{0.25} \tag{5}$$

where Re is the Reynolds number ($d_h V/v$) where V is the average cross-sectional velocity and v is the kinematic viscosity of the solution and Sc is the Schmidt number (v/D_s). The relationship to shear rate is coupled through the Reynolds number which is directly proportional to the cross-flow flowrate. These models provide qualitative agreement with experimental observations of limiting flux with respect to shear rate. In industry, often the relationship of flux to Re is tested to determine if concentration polarization resistance is dominant in fouling resistance. A series of test are usually performed and the power-law relationship between Re and Sh is determined. If the exponent is 0.8, one can assume that polarization resistance is dominating. If the value is less, this implies membrane fouling [29].

The characteristic time for concentration polarization, θ, is [30]

$$\theta \equiv \frac{D_s}{L_p^2(\Delta P - \sigma\Delta\pi)^2} \tag{6}$$

where L_p is the hydraulic permeability, ΔP is the hydrostatic pressure difference, σ is the reflection coefficient and $\Delta\pi$ is the osmotic pressure difference across the membrane. Typical values for θ are less than one second for ultrafiltration processes. Thus for cross-flow ultrafiltration, the initial flux decline is predominantly polarization development but it is unlikely that additional flux loss can be attributed to the development of the concentration polarization boundary layer alone.

3. Solute–Solute Interaction

Solute–solute interaction also affects the transport of solute through membranes. This is usually the result of electrostatic interactions that may form between proteins of varying charge. Solute–solute interaction can have a significant effect on solute rejection and solute flux. In a study involving the separation of human serum albumin and γ-globulin [23] it was shown that when small amounts of IgG were added to solutions containing albumin, the albumin retention coefficient increased markedly. This increase in albumin rejection significantly reduces the separation efficiency of this system. However modification of solution properties have been found to alter these effects. Ingham et al. [13] showed that modification of the interaction of lysozyme and albumin by adjusting ionic strength altered the rejection of lysozyme by polysulfone membranes. This interaction force can be modified by a change in solution properties.

4. Fouling

While concentration polarization can be controlled through modification of operating conditions, the other resistances, particularly adsorption, are not reversible with such changes and are often lumped under the general term of membrane fouling. Fouling from pore plugging, deposition and adsorption has been found to contribute significantly to solute flux reduction [3,8,31,32]. Fouling via deposition or adsorption, has been found to be the most significant resistance to solute flux [33] and adsorption appeared to have had a more pronounced effect on solute rejection than concentration polarization [34].

(a) *Adsorption.* Adsorption is actually a collection of distinctly different phenomena that cannot be treated as a single event. There are basically four general forces associated with adsorption of proteins on surfaces [11,35,36]. They are electrostatic force, hydrogen bonding, hydrophobic interaction and charge transfer. All of these phenomena have been mentioned above with respect to protein–membrane interaction.

(b) *Effects of Solution Properties on Adsorption.* While it was mentioned that protein–membrane interaction is generally heterogeneous, dominant aspects of adsorption can be altered via solution properties. For instance, depending on the surface charge, binding of proteins can be influenced by pH. Since protein charge is pH dependent, adsorption for electrostatic sites will be directly related to macromolecular charge. Examples have been shown where albumin and γ-globulin at their isoelectric points, adsorb at higher concentrations than at other pH values [36,37]. This is explained by the fact that when a protein is at its isoelectric point, its excluded volume is at its lowest and molecules can move closer to one another. In addition, since ionic interaction is minimized, hydrophobic forces can be more dominant.

(c) *Site Competition and Rate of Adsorption.* Adsorption of proteins on surfaces can be regarded as either completely reversible, partially reversible or irreversible. The reversible rate is generally found to vary for hydrophilic surfaces but it is usually slow for hydrophobic surfaces. Dillman and Miller [37] studied the adsorption of serum plasma on cation exchange cellophane, silicone–rubber and silicone–rubber–Lexan polymer membranes. Their results showed that two separate noninteracting adsorption processes were present. The first was hydrophilic and exothermic while the second was hydrophobic and endothermic. Furthermore, both processes seemed to demonstrate Langmuir-like adsorption behavior. However, adsorption can occur with either a monolayer or multilayers [38].

Site competition occurs in solutions containing two or more proteins. Lok et al. [39] reported that in solutions containing fibrinogen and albumin, on poly(dimethylsiloxane), albumin was found to adsorb first, but in time, fibrinogen was preferentially adsorbed. Beissinger et al. [40] found similar results when adsorbing albumin and γ-globulin on quartz. These observations of competition, along with other studies on adsorption rates, have determined that at least two adsorption states occur. The first state is considered loosely held. Molecules in this state can either desorb back into the bulk solution or remain attached to the site. In time however, molecules at the sites undergo conformational changes resulting in the second state, irreversible adsorption.

The rate of adsorption is key in understanding transient behavior of solute transport. The rate of protein adsorption has been extensively studied [36,38, 40,41]. Using visible wavelength total internal reflection fluorescence, changes due to adsorption in these cases were found usually to occur on the order of hours [36]. However, adsorption rate is strongly dependent on the surface materials used and thus, the above results, which were based on interaction with glass or mica, may have no direct application in ultrafiltration. In addition, the model considered transport across a flat surface which is quite different from the very narrow transport areas in the membrane pores.

(d) *Deposition and Pore Plugging.* Even when a particle does not adsorb, it is capable of blocking tortuous pores, and thus, can reduce observed transport through membranes. The rate of pore blockage is expected to be relatively fast [3]. It is associated with a probability, that, during the transport of the solute through the pore, the molecule can become trapped.

E. Transport Models

1. Permeate Flux

The remaining portion of this chapter discusses the effect fouling via adsorption or deposition has on membrane transport characteristics. The main factors used in describing membrane performance are permeate flux, and sieving coefficient. The following discusses how these factors are effected by fouling.

The first performance criterion of consideration is permeate flux. Permeate flux is basically the volumetric flowrate through a membrane of a specific nominal area. Since the mechanism for transport through ultrafiltration membranes is convection through pores, clearly, lodged and adsorbed proteins in these pores can effect the overall permeate flux.

Usually models for permeate flux begin with d'Arcy's Law [42] or the equivalent Kozeny–Carman equation [43]. The hydraulic, or d'Arcy, permeability can be written as

$$L_p = \frac{\varepsilon}{\tau} \frac{R_h^2}{2L} \tag{7}$$

where ε is the void fraction, or porosity of the membrane, R_h is the average hydraulic radius for the membrane pores, L is the effective membrane thickness, and τ is the tortuosity factor. The hydraulic permeability, L_p is the volumetric flux per driving force (pressure drop) across the membrane pore. To account for the reduction in overall pressure drop due to osmotic pressure and include the effect of fouling, the Kedem–Katchalsky model is often used [44],

$$J = \frac{\Delta P - \sigma \Delta \pi}{\mu(R_m + R_p)} \tag{8}$$

Here, μ is the solution viscosity. The osmotic pressure is a function of solute concentration at the membrane surface. The hydraulic permeability has now been written in terms of flux resistances where R_m is the membrane resistance during ultrafiltration, and R_p is the membrane resistance due to fouling. When the solute concentration in the permeate is low compared to the concentration of rejected solute at the membrane surface, or the sieving coefficient, $S_i \ll 1$, the reflection coefficient can be approximated as

$$\sigma \approx 1 - S_i, \tag{9}$$

where

$$S_i \equiv \frac{C_p}{C_w} \tag{10}$$

and C_p and C_w are the permeate and apparent wall concentration, respectively. The permeate concentration is easily determined from experiment. On the other hand, the concentration of rejected solute at the membrane surface, C_w, is often difficult to determine but, for cross-flow ultrafiltration, it can be estimated provided a relationship between osmotic pressure and solute concentration is known.

Although the porous structure of most asymmetric membranes is generally random, there have been a number of attempts to model the pores as straight cylinders in order to determine how adsorbed solutes effect permeate flux [e.g., 3,20,30,31,32,45]. Usually the ratio of the reduced permeability to the initial permeability is attributed to a change in the cylindrical pore radius due to adsorption or deposition and is written as

$$\frac{\Delta R_h}{R_{h,o}} = 1 - \left(\frac{L_p}{L_{p,o}}\right)^{1/4} \tag{11}$$

where the subscript o represents the clean membrane values.

However, this model frequently provides changes in pore radii that are substantially smaller than the solute molecular or particle size and lacks physical justification. As an alternative, Rodgers et al. [46], proposed models for adsorbed solute effects for arbitrary pore geometry. Based on a porous medium comprised of arbitrary shaped and tortuous pores of varying cross-section, the permeability ratio is written as

$$\frac{L_p}{L_{p,o}} = \left(\frac{\tau_o}{\tau}\right) \frac{(1 - q_s)^3}{(1 + \alpha q_s)^2} \tag{12}$$

and

$$\frac{L_p}{L_{p,\,o}} \approx \frac{(1 - q_s)^4}{(1 + \alpha q_s)^2} \tag{13}$$

Here q_s is the fraction of the membrane void volume occupied by the adsorbed solute particles and the shape dependent parameter α is defined as

$$\alpha \equiv \frac{a_s}{a_m}(1 - 2\gamma) \tag{14}$$

The parameter a_m is the pore surface area per unit void volume of clean membrane, and a_s is the specific surface of a solute particle, which is the surface area of the solute per solute volume. The parameter, γ, is defined as the fraction of the solute molecule surface area that is not wetted by the flowing fluid due to the fact that a part of the solute surface is adsorbed or adjacent to the pore wall. The value of γ is dependent upon the shape and rigidity of the solute particle, the pore geometry and rigidity, as well as the amount of solute adsorbed. These values range between 0 and 0.5 for monolayer coverage or less. For hard spherical solutes particles adsorbed on a hard pore surface, γ will have a value approaching zero, while pliable and strongly adsorbed species could have γ values near 0.5. For closely-packed, or multilayer adsorption, γ could be higher. Interestingly, when γ is equal to 0.5, the familiar cylindrical pore model (Eq. (11)) is equivalent to Eq. (13) with the same assumption. With $\gamma = 0.5$, the calculations for mass uptake were in good agreement with the mass uptake data measurements for the adsorption of BSA on polyethersulfone membranes [31].

Later it will be discussed how measured values for q_s are compared with permeate flux data to determine the significance of adsorption as compared to deposition.

2. Sieving

Sieving, defined by the sieving coefficient, S_i, is the parameter that relates the concentration of solute in the permeate with the concentration of the same species that is rejected by the membrane. Equation (10) defines the intrinsic sieving coefficient. Clearly as the membrane pore becomes more constricted or plugged due to fouling, the value of the sieving coefficient is reduced. One, approach to estimating how the adsorbed protein effects sieving is performed by using hindered transport theory. The theory of hindered transport is discussed in detail by Deen [47]. One concern with the use of hindered transport theory is that it has been developed for spherical particles in cylindrical pores and may not be representative of asymmetric membrane pores. However, Opong and Zydney [48] and Mochizuki and Zydney [49] demonstrated that hindered transport theory provides reasonable approximations for transport coefficients when analyzing the transport of macromolecules through asymmetric membranes.

Basically, hindered transport theory begins with the solute flux balance through the membrane where the cross-sectionally averaged one-dimensional solute flux through the membrane pore, $\bar{N}$, at steady state, can be expressed as [47]

$$\bar{N} = K_c \bar{V} \bar{C} - K_d D_\infty \frac{d\bar{C}}{dz} \tag{15}$$

where K_c and K_d are the cross-sectionally averaged convective and diffusive hindrance coefficients, respectively, $\bar{C}$ is the radially averaged concentration, $\bar{V}$ is the average solvent flux and D_∞ is the bulk solution protein diffusivity. The hindrance parameters express the perturbed effects in convective and diffusive flux that the protein experiences in the tight membrane pore. The sieving coefficient can be related to the hindrance parameters through a model developed by Spiegler and Kedem [50] where

$$S_i \equiv \frac{C_p}{C_w} = \frac{\phi K_c e^{Pe}}{\phi K_c + e^{Pe} - 1} \tag{16}$$

Here, the partitioning coefficient, ϕ, is approximated as

$$\phi = (1 - \lambda)^2 \tag{17}$$

where λ is the solute average radius to cylindrical pore radius ratio. The pore Peclet number is expressed as

$$Pe = \frac{K_c v L}{K_d D_\infty} \tag{18}$$

where v is the radially averaged velocity through the pore, L is the pore length. The relationship between the hindrance parameters and λ have been determined experimentally [i.e., 51].

The correct selection of λ results in the solute to pore ratio that is representative of the system in question. As an example, using the partitioning for a rigid spherical particle in a random arrangement of parallel planes, the hydraulic radius can be approximated as [52]

$$R_h = -\frac{\bar{L}}{2 \ln(\phi)} \tag{19}$$

where $\bar{L}$ is the mean external length of the solute. For fouled membranes, it is expected that the value of λ increases.

3. Selectivity

Because membrane fouling affects solute flux, it is also a significant factor in determining the overall selectivity of the separation process. The selectivity of a membrane system is a ratio of the permeabilities of the solutes [53]. The permeability for solutes is equal to the solute flux divided by the apparent concentration driving force. For species A the permeability can be written as

$$L_A = \frac{N_A}{(C_b - C_p)} \tag{20}$$

where N_A is the solute flux and C_b is the concentration of species A in the bulk solution.

Thus for species A and B the selectivity, may be defined as either

$$\alpha = \frac{L_A}{L_B} \quad \text{or} \quad \alpha = \frac{L_B}{L_A} \tag{21}$$

depending upon the reference solute. Other, more practical, models for selectivity also exist [16].

II. FOULING EFFECTS ON TRANSPORT

A. Amount of Protein Adsorbed

It has been generally accepted that during flux reduction, the initial rapid flux loss can be attributed to concentration polarization development (~ 1 s) followed by pore plugging and adsorbing macromolecules in its initial stages. Long-term fouling can be attributed to further development of fouling and possible compaction. The long-term uptake has been found to vary with solution properties and membrane material for both partially and totally retained membranes for ultrafiltration [3]. Generally it has been found that protein deposition, on the order of 0.5–200 μg/cm^2, can adsorb on the membrane over a long time (approximately 24 h) [31]. This large difference may be the result of many factors including different assumptions for the membrane nominal surface area and solution properties effects, such as pH that can alter adsorption. Robertson and Zydney [31] performed an extensive study for albumin adsorption on all layers of polyethersulfone membranes. They found that near monolayer adsorption (0.5 μg/cm^2) for long-term static adsorption.

B. Deposition vs. Adsorption

As mentioned, while deposition is considered the main contribution to flux decline in the initial stages of filtration, adsorption begins almost immediately as well. Determining the difference in the beginning of the filtration process can provide important insight on fouling. A recent study by Oppenheim et al. [54] investigated the short-term uptake of protein using electron paramagnetic resonance spectroscopy (EPR). In this study transient mass uptake, sieving and flux were correlated. Through a series of experiments these researchers compared the uptake of solute as measured by EPR with the calculated fouling resistance R_p. Generally, fouling resistance increased with increase in solute uptake. However, at the pH near the protein isoelectric point, the fouling resistance was higher for the same amount of mass uptake found at lower pH case. This implies that either the mass taken up during operations at pH values near the isoelectric point was adsorbed or deposited on the membrane in areas in which they effected the flux the most or that the protein structure was altered in such a manner as to increase its impact on flow. In either case, these observations relay the importance of analyzing the fouling phenomena. Figure 6 shows the results of this work.

One can also use this type of study to determine whether the solute uptake can be associated with deposition or adsorption. The logic is that, since the membrane is asymmetric, a number of regions are likely to exist where a protein can adsorb but will have no significance impact on overall permeate flux. This is particularly true in the porous substructure which has the same chemistry as the ultrathin skin directly above it. Using this as the basis for comparison, we can plot q_s (measured) (from direct measurement of mass on the membrane) vs. q_s (modeled) (determined from flux data). For systems in which the dominant form of solute uptake is deposition, one would expect a proportional relationship between the measured and modeled values for q_s. This is because all of the mass in the system would contribute to flux decline. For cases with adsorption dominance, the slope would be lower. Figure 7 shows a representation of this concept for bovine serum albumin on polysulfone membranes. The results imply that at pH 7 the uptake is primarily

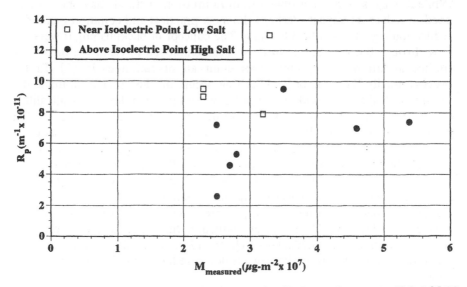

FIG. 6 Mass uptake of spin-labeled BSA on polysulfone membranes at pH 5, 0.05 M NaCl and pH 7, 0.15 M NaCl. Adapted from Ref. 54.

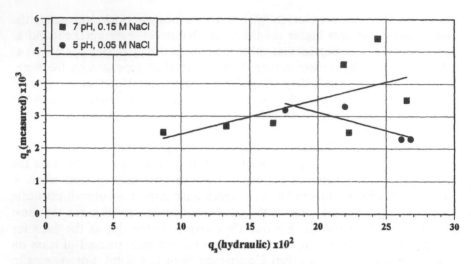

FIG. 7 Comparison of volume fraction occupied by solute as measured directly and as calculated by hydraulic theory. Adapted from Ref. 54.

deposition while at pH 5 (near the isoelectric point of 4.7), adsorption is a major contributor to solute mass uptake.

III. METHODS TO REDUCE FOULING

While fouling is a major problem in ultrafiltration, methods have been developed to reduce its impact. Perhaps the most practical and common method to reduce fouling effects is backflushing. The concept of backflushing (reversal of flow through the membrane) has also been employed to clean the membrane surface at intermittent points throughout an operation cycle [1]. In this process usually the cycle of backflushing occurs on the order of hours and is usually flushed for a period on the order of minutes. In hollow fiber ultrafiltration systems, reverse flow from the filtrate side back to fiber lumen is often performed quickly with little additional operating equipment. Von Baeyer et al. [55,56] demonstrated the use of on-line membrane regeneration in protein removal by monitoring hydraulic pressure in a flow controlled cascade plasmaphoresis apparatus. Other mechanisms for reduction of fouling include boundary-layer removal devices, pulsatile retentate flow and positive transmembrane pressure pulsing [57–61]. More recently negative transmembrane pressure pulsing and Dean vortex induction have also shown promise in reducing fouling [i.e., 7,30,33,62–64]. In addition, surface modification of membranes continues to make new strides in reducing fouling see [65,66, and Chap. 3].

In summary, as research continues, membrane separations will continue to reduce fouling resistance. With fouling reduced, the potential of new membranes with narrower pore size distributions will begin to arrive that will result in highly practical applications.

IV. NOTATION

a_m	pore surface area per unit void volume of clean membrane
a_s	specific surface of a solute particle
C	constant in Eq. (3)
C_b	bulk concentration
C_p	permeate concentration
C_w	apparent wall concentration
$\bar{C}$	radially averaged solute concentration
D_s	protein diffusivity
D_∞	bulk solution protein diffusivity
d_h	hydraulic diameter
h	channel height
J	solvent volumetric flux
K_c	cross-sectionally averaged convective hindrance coefficients
K_d	cross-sectionally averaged diffusive hindrance coefficients
k	mass transfer coefficient
$\bar{L}$	mean external length of the solute
L	membrane thickness
L_A	permeability of species A
L_B	permeability of species B
L_c	channel length in membrane module
L_p	hydraulic permeability
$L_{p,o}$	hydraulic permeability of clean membrane
M_w	molecular weight
N_A	solute flux of species A
$\bar{N}$	radially averaged solute flux though the membrane
Pe	Peclet number ($K_c vL/K_d D_\infty$)
q_s	fraction of the clean membrane void volume occupied by adsorbed solute particles
Re	Reynolds number ($d_h V/v$)
R_h	hydraulic radius
$R_{h,o}$	hydraulic radius of clean membrane
R_m	membrane resistance during ultrafiltration
R_p	membrane resistance due to fouling
Sc	Schmidt number (v/D_s)
Sh	Sherwood number
S_i	intrinsic sieving coefficient
$\bar{V}$	radially averaged solvent flux through the membrane
V	average cross-sectional velocity

v radially averaged velocity through the pore
Z net protein charge
z direction of flow through the membrane

α shape dependent parameter [Eqs. (12)–(14)]
α selectivity [Eq. (21)]
ΔP hydrostatic pressure difference
$\Delta \pi$ osmotic pressure difference across membrane
ΔR_h change in hydraulic radius due to fouling
ε void fraction
ε_0 void fraction or porosity of clean membrane
ϕ partitioning coefficient
γ shear rate [Eq. (3)]
γ fraction of the solute molecule that is not exposed to the fluid [Eq. (14)]
λ ratio of solute average radius to cylindrical pore radius
μ solution viscosity
v kinematic viscosity
θ characteristic time for polarization development
σ reflection coefficient
τ tortuosity factor for solute adsorbed membrane
τ_0 initial tortuosity factor for a clean membrane

REFERENCES

1. A. S. Michaels, in *Polymer Science and Technology, Ultrafiltration and Applications*, (A. R. Cooper, ed.), Plenum Press, New York, 1980, Volume 13.
2. T. Swaminathan, M. Chaudhury, and K. K. Sirkar, in *Polymer Science and Technology, Ultrafiltration and Applications*, (A. R. Cooper, ed.), Plenum Press, New York 1980, Volume 13, p. 247.
3. A. G. Fane, C. J. D. Fell, and A. G. Water, J. Membrane Sci. *16*:211 (1983).
4. C. Kleinstreuer and G. Belfort, in *Synthetic Membrane Processes*, Academic Press, Inc., 1984, p. 131.
5. A. Suki, A. G. Fane, and C. J. D. Fell, J. Membrane Sci. *21*:269 (1984).
6. H. Reihanian, C. R. Robertson, and A. S. Michaels, J. Membrane Sci. *16*:237 (1983).
7. V. G. J. Rodgers, Transmembrane pressure pulsing in protein ultrafiltration, D.Sc. Thesis, Washington University (1989).
8. W. S. Opong, Protein transport and deposition during size-selective membrane filtration, Ph.D. Thesis, University of Delaware (1991).
9. T. E. Creighton, *Proteins, Structure and Molecular Properties*, 2nd Ed., W. H. Freeman and Company, New York, 1993.
10. K. A. Granath and B. A. Kvist, J. Chromatogr. *28*:69 (1967).
11. C. Tanford, *Physical Chemistry of Macromolecules*, J. Wiley & Sons, New York, 1961.

12. V. L. Vilker, The ultrafiltration of biological macromolecules, Ph.D. Thesis, MIT (1976).
13. K. C. Ingham, T. F. Busby, Y. Sahlestrom, and F. Castino, in *Polymer Science and Technology, Ultrafiltration and Applications* (A. R. Cooper, ed.) Plenum Press, New York, 1980, Volume 13, p. 141.
14. S. Lapanje, *Physicochemical Aspects of Protein Denaturation*, Wiley Interscience, New York, 1978.
15. M. Cheryan, *Ultrafiltration Handbook*, Technomic, Lancaster, PA 1986.
16. L. J. Zeman and A. L. Zydney, *Microfiltration and Ultrafiltration, Principles and Applications*, Marcel Dekker, Inc., New York (1996).
17. C. J. van Oss, in *Progress in Separation and Purification*, (E. S. Perry and C. J. van Oss, eds.) Wiley Interscience, New York, 1970, Chapter 3, p. 97.
18. A. G. Fane and C. J. D. Fell, Desalination *62*: 117 (1987).
19. C. K. Mathew and K. E. van Holde, *Biochemistry*, Benjamin/Cummings, Redwod City, 1980.
20. E. Mathiasson and B. Sivik, Desalination *35*: 59 (1980).
21. S. F. Oppenheim, Protein ultrafiltration membrane fouling as examined by electron paramagnetic resonance spectroscopy, Ph.D. Thesis, The University of Iowa (1996).
22. A. S. Michaels, Chemical Engineering Progress *64*(12): 31 (1968).
23. W. F. Blatt, Arun Dravid, Alan S. Michaels, and Lita Nelsen, *Membrane Science and Technology*, (J. Flinn, ed.) Plenum Press, New York 1970, p. 47.
24. A. Jönsson and G. Trägårdh, Chemical Engineering Process *27*: 67 (1990).
25. J. Shen and R. F. Probstein, Ind. Eng. Chem. Fundam. *16*: 459 (1977).
26. D. R. Trettin and M. R. Doshi, Chem. Eng. Commun. *4*: 507 (1980).
27. K. Isaacson, P. Duenas, C. Ford, and M. Lysaght, in *Polymer Science and Technology, Ultrafiltration Membranes and Applications*, (A. R. Cooper, ed.) Plenum Press, New York 1980, Volume 13, p. 507.
28. V. Gekas and B. Hallstrom, J. Membrane Sci. *30*: 153 (1987).
29. W. Ekamp e-mail correspondence, membrane.ct.utwente.nl, supported by Membrane Technology Group at the University of Twente (1997).
30. V. G. J. Rodgers and R. E. Sparks, J. Membrane Sci. *68*: 149 (1992).
31. B. C. Robertson and A. L. Zydney, J. Colloid Interface Sci. *134*: 563 (1990).
32. K. J. Kim, A. G. Fane, C. J. D. Fell, and D. C. Joy, J. Membrane Sci. *68*: 79 (1992).
33. V. G. J. Rodgers and R. E. Sparks, AIChE Journal 37(10): 1517 (1991).
34. B. C. Robertson and A. L. Zydney, J. Membrane Sci. *29*: 287 (1990).
35. J. J. Andrade, in *Surface and Interfacial Aspects of Biomedical Polymers Protein Adsorption*, Plenum Press, New York, 1985, Volume 2, p. 1.
36. Y. Cheng, B. K. Lok, and C. R. Robertson, in *Surface and Interfacial Aspects of Biomedical Polymers Protein Adsorption*, Plenum Press, New York, 1985, Volume 2, p. 121.
37. W. Dillman and I. F. Miller, J. Colloid Interface Sci. *44*(2): 221 (1973).
38. A. Silberberg, *Surface and Interfacial Aspects of Biomedical Polymers Protein Adsorption*, Plenum Press, New York, 1985, Volume 2, p. 321.
39. B. K. Lok, Y.-L. Cheng, and C. R. Robertson, J. Colloid Interface Sci. *91*: 104 (1983).

40. R. L. Bessinger and E. F. Leonard, Trans. Am. Soc. Artif. Intern. Organs *XXVII*:225 (1981).
41. C-S. Lee and G. Belfort, Proc. Natl. Acad. Sci. USA *86*:8392 (1989).
42. R. Jackson, *Transport in Porous Catalysts*, Elsevier, New York, 1977.
43. J. Kozeny, *Hydralik*, Springer, Vienna, 1927.
44. O. Kedem and A. Katchalsky, Biochim. Biophys. Acta *27*:229 (1958).
45. A. M. Brites and M. N. de Pinho, J. Membrane Sci. *61*:49 (1991).
46. V. G. J. Rodgers, S. F. Oppenheim, and R. Datta, AIChE Journal *41*:1829 (1995).
47. W. M. Deen, AIChE Journal *33*:1409 (1987).
48. W. S. Opong and A. L. Zydney, AIChE Journal *37*:1497 (1991).
49. S. Mochizuki and A. L. Zydney, J. Membrane Sci. *68*:21 (1992).
50. K. S. Spiegler and O. Kedem, Desalination *1*:311 (1966).
51. P. M. Bungay and H. Brenner, Int. J. Multiphase Flow *1*:25 (1973).
52. J. C. Giddings, E. Kucera, C. P. Russel, and M. N. Myers, J. Phys. Chem. *72*:4397 (1968).
53. Vassilis Gekas, Division of Food Engineering, Lund University (1986).
54. S. F. Oppenheim, C. Phillips and V. G. J. Rodgers, J. Colloid Interface Sci. *184*:639 (1996).
55. H. von Baeyer et al., Trans ASAIO *XXIX*:739 (1983).
56. H. von Baeyer et al., J. Membrane Sci. *22*:297 (1985).
57. A. R. Ozdural and E. Piskin, J. Dialysis *3*:89 (1979).
58. M. R. Doshi, in *Polymer Science and Technology* (A. Cooper, ed.) Plenum Press, New York, 1980, Volume 13, p. 231.
59. M. Y. Jaffrin et al. Life Support Systems *2*:Suppl:207 (1984).
60. H. Bauer et al., J. Membrane Sci. *27*:195 (1986).
61. K. Abel, J. Membrane Sci. *133*:39 (1997).
62. K. Miller, S. Weitzel, and V. G. J. Rodgers, J. Membrane Sci. *76*:77 (1993).
63. K. Y. Chung, R. Bates, and G. Belfort, J. Membrane Sci. *81*:139 (1993).
64. H. Mallubhotla and G. Belfort, J. Membrane Sci. *125*:75 (1997).
65. A. Nabe, E. Staude, and G. Belfort, J. Membrane Sci. *133*:57 (1997).
66. H. Yamagishi, J. V. Crivello, and G. Belfort, J. Membrane Sci. *105*:237 (1995).

8

Diffusion of Dyes in Porous Membranes with Parallel Pore and Surface Diffusion

MASAKO MAEKAWA Division of Life Science and Human Technology, Nara Women's University, Nara, Japan

Abstract

The diffusion behavior of substances such as sulfonated azo dyes in porous cellulose membranes is interpreted on the basis of the parallel diffusion model. This consists of the dual mechanism of surface diffusion and pore diffusion. Diffusant adsorbed on the inner surface of the pore wall diffuses in the adsorbed state for surface diffusion while diffusant dissolved in the liquid phase in membranes diffuses in the dissolved state for pore diffusion. The procedure for obtaining the surface diffusivity and the pore diffusivity for the model is explained. In addition, the concentration–distance profile, effects of type of adsorption isotherm, the factors affecting or correlating the diffusivities and the effects of type of diffusion are discussed. The following conclusions are drawn. (1) The diffusion of substances which have an affinity on the substrate can be described on the basis of the parallel diffusion model. (2) Either Freundlich or Langmuir equations can be applied to the mass balance equation, provided the relationship between the concentrations of diffusant adsorbed on the inner surface of pore wall and diffusant dissolved in the liquid phase in the pores is suitably described. (3) The surface diffusivity for the parallel diffusion model is correlated with an affinity of the diffusant on the substrate. (4) The pore diffusivity for the parallel diffusion model is correlated with the molecular weight of diffusants except ones with anomalous properties such as high aggregation constant or high solubility.

I. INTRODUCTION

Recently much attention has been paid to the diffusion of various substances in membranes in view of their increasing importance in uses such as selective permeation, artificial dialysis and separation in medicine, chemical engineering and the food industry for example.

In particular diffusion in porous membranes has been of much interest for a long time and many studies have been carried out. For instance, the diffusion of dyes in polymers has been interpreted theoretically in studies of the kinetics of dyeing [1–12]. Many studies have been made using water-swollen cellulose membrane because it is available in sheet form. Dye molecules diffuse through the water-filled pores in the cellulose membrane and simultaneously adsorb on the pore wall. Although the diffusion of adsorbed dye on the pore wall along its surface has been considered, it has been regarded as negligible compared with the diffusion of dissolved dye (pore model). However, the apparent pore diffusivity based on the pore model was observed to depend on both the dye and salt concentrations in the bulk solution, which, as has been pointed out, contradicts the model [2,4,7,12].

On the other hand, surface diffusion in the adsorbed state in gaseous system has been known in the field of chemical engineering [13–16]. Then the adsorption rate from a solution by a solid adsorbent has attracted considerable attention in connection with advanced treatment of waste water, and the existence of surface diffusion in which volatile organics and poly(oxyethylene) diffuse in the adsorbed state on the inner surface of the activated carbon was demonstrated [17,18].

The parallel diffusion model consisting of surface diffusion and pore diffusion was proposed by combining the mathematical treatment of diffusion developed in the field of chemical engineering with the experimental procedure established in the field of dyeing chemistry [19]. Consequently, the procedure to determine the diffusivity for the model was established [20,21].

This chapter is intended to introduce the procedure for analysis of the diffusion in porous membranes based on the parallel diffusion model and to discuss the factors which influence diffusion behavior [19–28].

II. THEORETICAL ANALYSIS

When substances with an affinity to a substrate diffuse into porous membranes, two kinds of diffusion occur in parallel, i.e., diffusion of material dissolved in the liquid phase in the pores of membrane (pore diffusion) and diffusion of material adsorbed on the inner surface of pore wall (surface diffusion). Figure 1 shows a schematic diagram of concentration distribution of diffusant in the membrane–solution system. The concentration of diffusant dissolved in the bulk solution, $C_0(mol/m^3)$ is supposed constant at any distance. The concentration of diffusant adsorbed on the outer surface of membrane, $q_0(mol/m^3)$ is in equilibrium with C_0. The equilibrium between C_0 and q_0 is instantaneously established. The magnitude of q_0 is higher than that of C_0 because of an affinity of the diffusant to the substrate. The symbol C refers to the concentration of the diffusant dissolved in the pores per unit pore volume (mol/m^3); q refers to the concentration of the diffusant adsorbed on the inner surface of the pore wall based on total membrane volume (mol/m^3); $z(m)$ represents distance through membrane; $l(m)$ represents the thickness of the water-swollen membrane; the dashed line at $z = l$ represents an impermiable wall. Their units are as shown in the brackets.

In the theoretical development of the diffusion equations, it is assumed that: (1) surface and pore diffusion occur in parallel within membranes; (2) pore and surface diffusivities are constant during the adsorption process; (3) the pore diameter and the void fraction of the membrane are constant during the adsorption process; and (4) the concentration of the diffusant dissolved in the pores is in local equilibrium with the concentration of the diffusant adsorbed on the inner surface of the pore wall. These assumptions lead to the following mass balance equation:

$$\varepsilon_P \frac{\partial C}{\partial t} + \frac{\partial q}{\partial t} = \varepsilon_P D_P \frac{\partial^2 C}{\partial z^2} + D_S \frac{\partial^2 q}{\partial z^2} \tag{1}$$

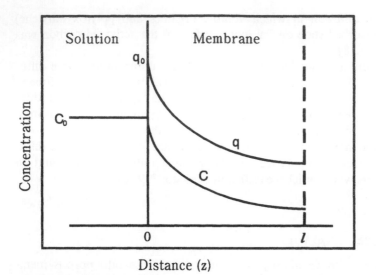

Distance (z)

FIG. 1 The concentration distribution of diffusant in the membrane–solution system. C_0 is the concentration of diffusant dissolved in the bulk solution; q_0 is the concentration of diffusant adsorbed on the outer surface of membrane in equilibrium with C_0; C is the concentration of diffusant dissolved in the pores; q is the concentration of diffusant adsorbed on the inner surface of pore wall; l is the thickness of membrane; the dashed line at $z = l$ represents an impermeable wall.

where t(s) represents diffusion time; ε_P is the void fraction of the membrane; $D_p(\mathrm{m}^2/\mathrm{s})$ and $D_S(\mathrm{m}^2/\mathrm{s})$ represent the pore and surface diffusivities, respectively. Using dimensionless variables, Eq. (1) is transformed to give Eq. (2)

$$\frac{\partial x}{\partial \tau_P} + \alpha \frac{\partial y}{\partial \tau_P} = \frac{\partial^2 x}{\partial \rho^2} + \beta \frac{\partial^2 y}{\partial \rho^2} \tag{2}$$

where $x = C/C_0$, $y = q/q_0$, $\tau_p = D_p t/l^2$, $\rho = z/l$, $\alpha = q_0/\varepsilon_P C_0$ and $\beta = \alpha D_s/D_p$; α indicates the degree of condensation of diffusant from liquid phase to solid phase (membrane surface); and β is an indicator of the type of controlling diffusion. There are two limiting cases, i.e., $\beta = 0$ (pore diffusion control) and $\beta = \infty$ (surface diffusion control). As Eq. (2) cannot be solved for $\beta = \infty$, Eq. (1) is transformed to Eq. (3):

$$\frac{\partial x}{\partial \tau_s} + \alpha \frac{\partial y}{\partial \tau_s} = \alpha \frac{\partial^2 y}{\partial \rho^2} \tag{3}$$

where $\tau_s = D_s t/l^2$.

When the relationship between x and y is calculated according to the equilibrium isotherm shown by Eq. (4), Eqs. (2) and (3) transform into Eqs. (5) and (6), respectively.

$$y = x^\gamma \tag{4}$$

$$\left[\alpha + \frac{1}{\gamma} y^{(1-\gamma)/\gamma}\right] \frac{\partial y}{\partial \tau_p} = \frac{1}{\gamma} \frac{\partial}{\partial \rho}\left[y^{(1-\gamma)/\gamma} \frac{\partial y}{\partial \rho}\right] + \beta \frac{\partial^2 y}{\partial \rho^2} \tag{5}$$

$$\left[\alpha + \frac{1}{\gamma} y^{(1-\gamma)/\gamma}\right] \frac{\partial y}{\partial \tau_s} = \alpha \frac{\partial^2 y}{\partial \rho^2} \tag{6}$$

The initial and boundary conditions (I.C. and B.Cs.) are given by Eq. (7):

(I.C.) $y = 0$ at $\tau_p = 0$ or $\tau_s = 0$
(B.Cs.) $y = 1$ at $\rho = 0$ $\partial y/\partial \rho = 0$ at $\rho = 1$ $\tag{7}$

The local concentration of the diffusant in the membrane (A_L) is shown as

$$A_L = q + \varepsilon_p C \tag{8}$$

However, the local concentration of the diffusant in the membrane differs according to the distance from the outer surface of the membrane. It decreases with increasing distance from the outer surface of the membrane. Then, the mean concentration of the diffusant in a membrane (A) is defined as

$$A = \int_0^l (q + \varepsilon_p C) \, dz/l \tag{9}$$

The fractional attainment of equilibrium (F) is expressed by

$$F = \frac{A}{q_0 + \varepsilon_p C_0} = \frac{\alpha \int_0^1 y \, d\rho + \int_0^1 x \, d\rho}{\alpha + 1} \tag{10}$$

When $\alpha = \infty$, Eq. (3) is reduced to Eq. (11) and the solutions are given by Eqs. (12) and (13).

$$\frac{\partial y}{\partial \tau_s} = \frac{\partial^2 y}{\partial \rho^2} \tag{11}$$

$$y = 1 - 2 \sum_{n=0}^{\infty} \frac{(-1)^n}{(n+0.5)\pi} \times \exp\{-(n+0.5)^2\pi^2\tau_s\}$$
$$\times \cos\{(n+0.5)\pi(1-\rho)\} \tag{12}$$

$$F = 1 - 2 \sum_{n=0}^{\infty} \frac{1}{(n+0.5)^2\pi^2} \times \exp\{-(n+0.5)^2\pi^2\tau_s\} \tag{13}$$

These equations are not affected by the concentration of the diffusant in the pores, because when $\alpha = \infty$, the concentration of the diffusant adsorbed on the inner surface of the pore wall is much higher than that in the pores. Therefore,

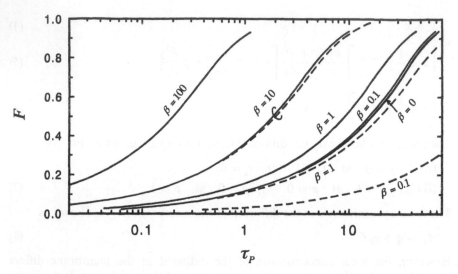

FIG. 2 Effects of β on uptake curves (both resistances exist). $\alpha = 100$; $\gamma = 0.5$; (———) Eq. (5); (– – –) Eq. (13) [19].

when α is large enough, the F–τ_s curve is unaffected not only by α but also by γ.

Equations (5) and (6) are transformed into finite difference equations and solved numerically. Figure 2 represents the effects of β on the uptake curves

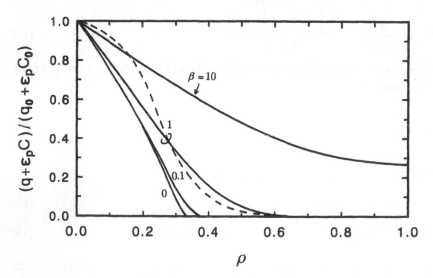

FIG. 3 Effects of β and γ on concentration–distance profiles (both resistances exist). [Eq. (5)]; $\alpha = 100$; $\tau_P = 2$; γ; (———) 0.5; (– – –) 0.1 [19].

for parallel diffusion when $\alpha = 100$ and $\gamma = 0.5$. As β increases, the adsorption rate increases. The broken lines indicate the analytical solution Eq. (13) for large α. The uptake curve in $\beta \geq 10$ can be estimated by the solution. When $\beta \leq 0.1$, the adsorption rate can be approximated by that for pore diffusion control ($\beta = 0$). Figure 3 shows the effect of β on the concentration–distance profile at $\tau_p = 2.0$. It is clear that the larger β is, the faster becomes the adsorption rate. The effect of γ on the concentration–distance profile is also presented for the case of $\beta = 1$. The concentration near the membrane surface for $\gamma = 0.1$ is higher than that for $\gamma = 0.5$. This means that the diffusant adsorbs well on the pore surface in the case of small γ and the concentration gradient of the diffusant in a membrane becomes steeper with a decrease of γ.

III. MEASUREMENT OF UPTAKE CURVES AND CONCENTRATION–DISTANCE PROFILES

Uptake curves (the relationship between concentration of diffusant in the membrane and diffusion time) and concentration–distance profiles (the relationship between concentration of diffusants in the membrane and diffused distance) are measured using an ultrafiltration-type cell with water jacket (Sartorius SM 165 26). The membrane is placed on a plastic plate at the bottom of the cylindrical cell. Then, the cell is filled by aqueous solution of diffusants such as dyes shown in Fig. 4. The solution is stirred by the magnetic stirrer which is designed to stir at 1 mm above the membrane surface at a rate high enough to prevent hydrodynamic boundary layer effects. The diffusant diffuses from the outer surface of membrane into the pores and nonstead-state diffusion is established. Uptake curves are generated by the integral step method using one sheet of the membrane. The concentration–distance profiles were measured by placing a stack of ten membranes together over a given period and separating them for concentration analysis. The units of concentration of diffusants in the membrane are converted into mol per volume from mol per weight using volume unit of water-swollen membrane per unit weight of dry membrane.

IV. DETERMINATION OF DIFFUSIVITIES FOR THE PARALLEL DIFFUSION MODEL

A. Concentration of Diffusant in the Membrane

The relationship between C_0 and q_0 can be obtained by measuring equilibrium adsorption isotherms. In many cases the relationship between q_0 and C_0 can be described by the Freundlich equation [Eq. (14)].

$$q_0 = kC_0^\gamma \tag{14}$$

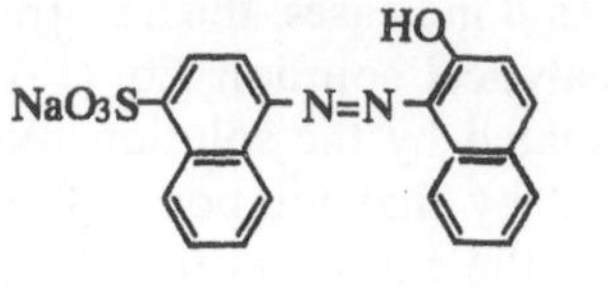

1. C.I. Acid Red 88 (MW=400.4)

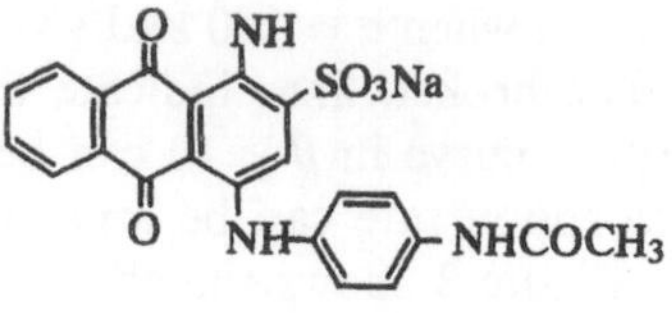

2. C.I. Acid Blue 40 (MW=473.4)

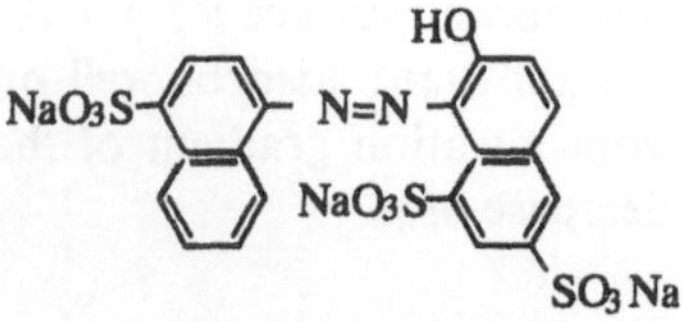

3. C.I. Acid Red 18 (MW=604.5)

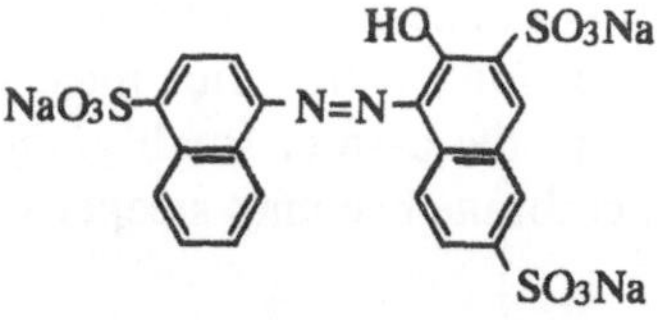

4. C.I. Acid Red 27 (MW=604.5)

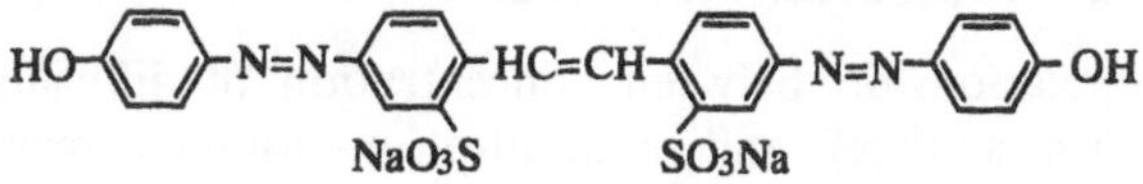

5. C.I. Direct Yellow 4 (MW=624.2)

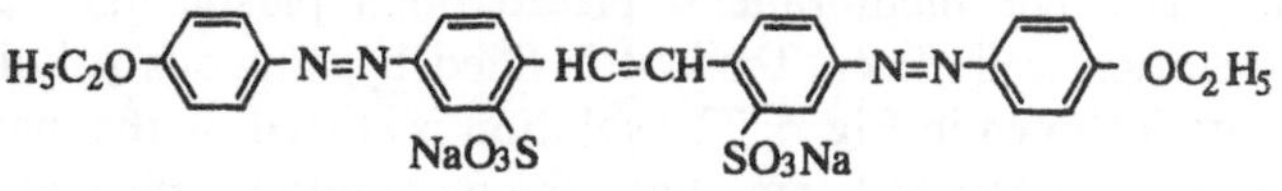

6. C.I. Direct Yellow 12 (MW=680.7)

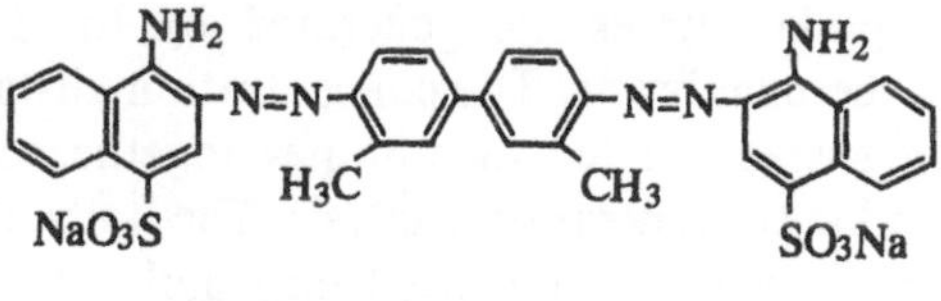

7. C.I. Direct Red 2 (MW=724.7)

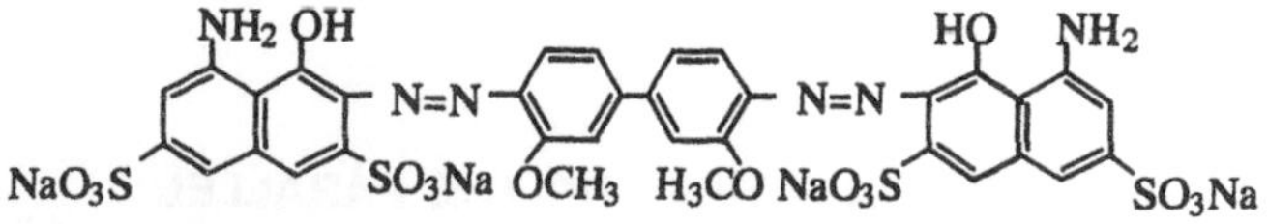

8. C.I. Direct Blue 15 (MW=992.8)

FIG. 4 Structural formulae of dyes used as diffusants.

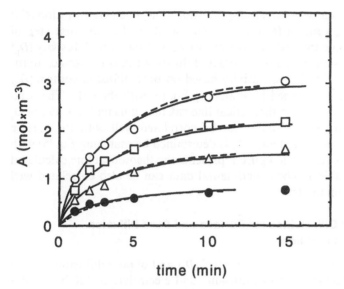

FIG. 5 Uptake curves of C.I. Acid Red 88 in the presence of different concentrations of $NaCl(C_E)$ at 55°C ($C_0 = 0.3$ mol/m^3). C_E; ($\bullet$) 10 mol/m^3, ($\triangle$) 30 mol/m^3, ($\square$) 50 mol/m^3, and ($\bigcirc$) 100 mol/m^3. (———) theoretical lines for surface diffusion control [Eq. (6)]; (–––) theoretical lines for pore diffusion control [Eq. (5)] [24].

where k is the coefficient which can be assumed as an index for an affinity of the diffusant to the substrate; γ is also a coefficient affected by the strength of adsorption. The values of k and γ are determined from the intercept and the slope of the line of the logarithmic plots of Eq. (14), respectively. When the affinity of a diffusant is high, k becomes large and γ becomes small. The adsorption is stimulated by the addition of electrolyte such as sodium chloride. The concentration of diffusant in a membrane consists of both diffusant adsorbed on the inner surface of pore wall (q) and diffusant dissolved in the liquid phase in the membrane (C). The values of q and C are low for large distances (z). As diffusion proceeds, q and C increase. The values of C and q at equilibrium are equal to C_0 and q_0. C is assumed to be in local equilibrium with q by assumption (4) in the theory. Therefore, the relation between q and C is represented by the following equation.

$$q = kC^\gamma \tag{15}$$

The values of k and γ are obtained from the equilibrium isotherm.

B. Diffusivities Based on Surface and Pore Diffusion Control

Figure 5 shows the experimental uptake curves of dye 1 in Fig. 4 measured using one sheet of cellulose membrane. The mean concentration of dye in the membrane (A) increases with increasing diffusion time, dye concentration (C_0) and electrolyte concentration (C_E) in the bulk solution. For the first step of procedure to determine the surface diffusivity (D_s) and the pore diffusivity (D_p) for the parallel diffusion model, the surface diffusivity based on surface diffusion control (D'_s) and the pore diffusivity based on pore diffusion control (D'_p) are introduced. D'_s is determined by matching Eq. (6) with the data. The solid line in the figure represents the theoretical line calculated using the value of D'_s in Table 1. The experimental data can be correlated well with the surface diffusion model. On the other hand, D'_p is determined by matching Eq. (5) with the data. The broken line in the figure represents the theoretical line calculated using D'_p given in Table 1. The experimental data can be also correlated well with the pore diffusion model.

C. Dependence of Diffusivities for Surface and Pore Diffusion Control on Concentration

Both diffusivities of surface diffusion control (D'_s) and of pore diffusion control (D'_p) depend on concentrations of diffusants and electrolyte in the bulk solution. Then the values of D'_s and D'_p are plotted against the concentration of NaCl in Figure 6 [21]. The value of D'_s depends on both dye concentration (C_0) and NaCl concentration (C_E) in the bulk solution. It increases with increasing C_0 and with decreasing C_E. The value of D'_p also depends on both dye concentration (C_0) and NaCl concentration (C_E) in the bulk solution. It increases with increasing C_E and with decreasing C_0. An increase of both C_0 and C_E is associated with increase of adsorption, and influences D'_s and D'_p in

TABLE 1 Physical Properties in the Cellulose Membrane—C.I. Acid Red 88 System at 55°C

C_0 mol/m^3	C_E mol/m^3	α	γ	$D'_s \times 10^{12}$ m^2/s	$D'_p \times 10^{11}$ m^2/s	$D_{eff} \times 10^{12}$ m^2/s
0.1	100	20.1	0.597	2.17	3.67	2.00
0.2	100	16.6	0.597	2.20	3.06	2.03
0.3	10	3.40	0.557	4.38	1.00	2.98
0.3	30	7.13	0.509	2.84	1.57	2.33
0.3	50	10.1	0.551	2.59	2.10	2.21
0.3	100	14.1	0.597	2.32	2.75	2.04
0.5	30	5.57	0.509	3.29	1.35	2.59
0.5	50	7.96	0.551	2.63	1.69	2.25
0.5	100	11.8	0.597	2.38	2.43	2.13
1.0	30	4.03	0.509	3.77	1.14	2.86

Source: Ref. 24.

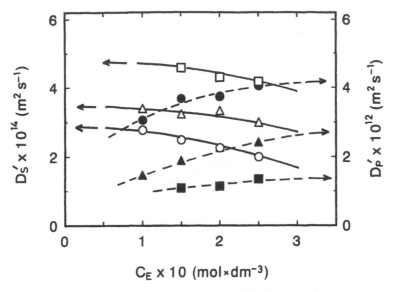

FIG. 6 Effects of concentrations of C.I. Direct Blue 15 (C_0) and NaCl(C_E) on the surface diffusivity determined assuming surface diffusion control (D_s'), and the pore diffusivity determined assuming pore diffusion control (D_p'). C_0; ($\bigcirc, \bullet$) 1×10^{-4} mol/dm^3), ($\triangle, \blacktriangle$) 3×10^{-4} mol/dm^3 and ($\square, \blacksquare$) 1×10^{-3} mol/dm^3 [21].

an contrasting manner. This is because an increase of C_0 is accompanied by decrease of α, on the contrary, an increase of C_E is accompanied by increase of α. Then, the plots of D_s' against α are shown in Fig. 7. It is apparent that D_s' decreases exponentially with increasing α. This indicates that the contribution of surface diffusion is enhanced, by contrast, that of pore diffusion diminishes with increasing α.

D. Diffusivities for the Parallel Diffusion Model

When the concentration of diffusant in a membrane is determined, the change of the total concentration of $q + C$ is measured experimentally over time. Then to determine the surface diffusivity (D_s) and the pore diffusivity (D_p) based on the parallel diffusion model, the effective diffusivity for the homogeneous model is calculated. Assuming Fickian diffusion with a constant effective diffusivity (D_{eff}), the mass balance equation in the membrane is given by Eq. (16) as

$$\frac{\partial A_L}{\partial t} = D_{eff} \frac{\partial^2 A_L}{\partial z^2} \tag{16}$$

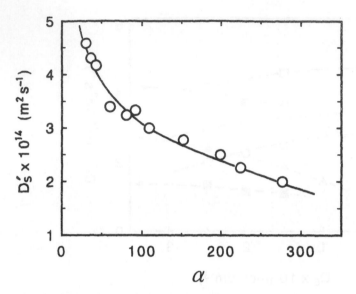

FIG. 7 Dependence of the surface diffusivity determined assuming surface diffusion control (D_s') on α.

A_L defined by Eq. (8) is used in Eq. (16). The initial condition (I.C.) and boundary conditions (B.Cs.) are given by

(I.C.) $A_L = 0$ at $t = 0$

(B.Cs.) $A_L = A_0$ at $z = 0$ (17)

$\qquad\qquad \dfrac{\partial A_L}{\partial z} = 0$ at $z = l$

where $A_0 = q_0 + \varepsilon_p C_0$. The solution is given by Eq. (18)

$$F = \frac{\displaystyle\int_0^l A_L \, dz}{A_0} = \frac{\displaystyle \alpha \int_0^1 y \, d\rho + \int_0^1 x \, d\rho}{\alpha + 1}$$

$$= 1 - 2 \sum_{n=0}^{\infty} \frac{1}{(n + 0.5)^2 \pi^2} \times \exp\left[-(n + 0.5)^2 \pi^2 \frac{D_{eff}\, t}{l^2} \right] \qquad (18)$$

When surface diffusion is the rate-controlling steps and $\alpha = \infty$, the mass balance equation, Eq. (1), is reduced to Eq. (19):

$$\frac{\partial q}{\partial t} = D_s \frac{\partial^2 q}{\partial z^2} \qquad\qquad\qquad\qquad\qquad\qquad\qquad (19)$$

When $\alpha = \infty$, Eq. (16) is also reduced to Eq. (20):

$$\frac{\partial q}{\partial t} = D_{\text{eff}} \frac{\partial^2 q}{\partial z^2} \tag{20}$$

From Eqs. (19) and (20), it appears that the effective diffusivity for $\alpha = \infty$ (or $1/\alpha = 0$) gives the surface diffusivity for the parallel diffusion model. On the other hand, Eq. (21) is derived from the relationship between the fluxes based on the parallel diffusion model and the Fickian model:

$$D_{\text{eff}}\left(1 + \varepsilon_p \frac{dC}{dq}\right) = D_S + \varepsilon_p D_p \frac{dC}{dq} \tag{21}$$

When $dC/dq \ll 1$, Eq. (21) is reduced to Eq. (22):

$$D_{\text{eff}} = D_S + \varepsilon_p D_p \frac{dC}{dq} \tag{22}$$

On activated carbon, it has been shown that there exist surface and pore diffusion resistances for adsorption of tetrahydrofuran vapor [29]. The measurements were made under steady-state conditions in a diaphragm cell. Their experimental effective diffusivities were correlated according to Eq. (23), which was derived by substituting $dC/dq = \Delta C/\Delta q$ into Eq. (22), and surface and pore diffusivities were obtained from the intercept and slope, respectively:

$$D_{\text{eff}} = D_S + D_p \varepsilon_p \frac{\Delta C}{\Delta q} \tag{23}$$

The intraparticle diffusivities were measured from uptake data for adsorption of several hydrocarbon gases on activated carbon particles by changing the bulk pressure differentially [30]. The successive amounts of adsorbate added were always small enough that the adsorption isotherm could be considered linear in the concentration range examined. The intraparticle diffusivity was plotted against a dimensionless mean slope of the equilibrium isotherm (K_D). The pore and surface diffusivities are given by the intercept and the slope according to Eq. (24):

$$D_{\text{eff}} = D_p + K_D D_S \tag{24}$$

For liquid phase adsorption, Takeuchi et al.'s [29] method may require a long experimental time for steady-state diffusion to be reached, and Costa et al.'s [30] method may produce more experimental error than a vapor phase adsorption system. It would be more useful to determine intraparticle diffusivities by an integral step method. Since, in the case of the integral step method, dC/dq may be a function of both the position within a particle and time, it can not be determined from the equilibrium isotherm only. By taking C_0/q_0 for the linear isotherm system as an approximation for dC/dq, Eq. (21) is transformed

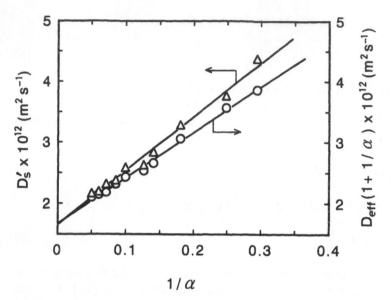

FIG. 8 Determination of the surface diffusivity for the parallel diffusion model (D_s) from the intercept of the line plotting D'_s or D_{eff} $(1 + 1/\alpha)$ vs. $1/\alpha$ for C.I. Acid Red 88 at 55°C [24,25].

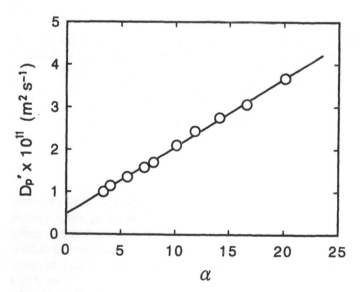

FIG. 9 Determination of the pore diffusivity for the parallel diffusion model (D_p) from the intercept of the line plotting D'_p vs. α for C.I. Acid Red 88 at 55°C [24].

TABLE 2 Physical Properties of Various Dyes in the Cellulose Membrane at 25°C

No. (Fig. 4)	Dye (C.I. number)	M.W.	Valency	C_E (mol/m^3)	k	$D_s \times 10^{14}$ (m^2/s)	$D_p \times 10^{13}$ (m^2/s)
1	Acid Red 88	400.4	1	10–30	1.93–5.17	36.4	1.97
2	Acid Blue 40	473.4	1	30–50	4.35–5.67	37.9	9.41
3	Acid Red 18	604.5	3	2000	3.46	54.3	94.1
4	Acid Red 27	604.5	3	500	3.54	49.1	64.5
				1000	4.82	48.4	35.3
5	Direct Yellow 4	624.2	2	20–50	13.3–22.1	2.37	6.12
6	Direct Yellow 12	680.7	2	20–30	15.9–25.4	1.52	3.00

Source: Ref. 26.

TABLE 3 Physical Properties of Various Dyes in the Cellulose Membrane at 55°C

No. (Fig. 4)	Dye (C.I. number)	α	$D_s \times 10^{15}$ (m^2/s)	$D_p \times 10^{13}$ (m^2/s)	D_s/D_p	β
1	Acid Red 88	3.4–20.1	1660	47.7	0.348	1.18–6.99
2	Aid Blue 40	7.86–20.2	1590	195	0.0815	0.641–1.65
5	Direct Yellow 4	27.5–84.8	133	86.9	0.0153	0.421–1.30
6	Direct Yellow 12	30–165	130	30.2	0.0430	1.29–7.10
7	Direct Red 2	128–406	3.04	1.73	0.0176	2.25–7.13
8	Direct Blue 15	30–277	20.5	5.13	0.0400	1.20–11.1

Source: Ref. 28.

into Eq. (25):

$$D_{eff}\left(1 + \frac{1}{\alpha}\right) = D_S + D_{pa}\frac{1}{\alpha} \tag{25}$$

where D_{pa} represents the approximate pore diffusivity. When $1/\alpha \to 0$ in Eq. (25), D_{eff} approaches D_S. However, the slope of the line when the left-hand side in Eq. (25) is plotted against $1/\alpha$ may not give an accurate pore diffusivity, because of the approximation of linear isotherm. D_{pa} is equal to D_p only when the isotherm is linear.

Figure 8 represents the plots of experimental effective diffusivity based on Eq. (25). D_{eff} is determined by matching Eq. (18) with the data. The line correlates well to a straight line. The intercept of the line provides D_S based on Eq. (25). In addition, the slope of the line provides an estimate of the pore diffusivity under the assumption of a linear isotherm. The relationship between D'_s and $1/\alpha$ is also plotted in Fig. 8. The line correlates to a straight line and its intercept coincides with that of line of Eq. (25), though their slopes are different. Accordingly, D_S can be obtained by plotting D'_s against $1/\alpha$ without using the homogeneous model.

Figure 9 shows the plots of D'_p against α for dye 1 [24]. It appears that D'_p also correlates with α. An increase of α is accompanied by an increase of D'_p, because the contribution of surface diffusion increases with increasing α. The pore diffusivity for the parallel diffusion model (D_p) is obtained from the intercept of the line $(\alpha = 0)$. Table 2 and 3 summarize D_S and D_p determined for dyes in Fig. 4.

V. DISCUSSION

A. Concentration–Distance Profiles in Membranes

Concentration–distance profiles of diffusant in membranes can be measured experimentally using a stack of membranes. On the other hand, theoretical values based on the parallel diffusion model can be calculated by Eq. (5), when the values of α, γ, D_s and D_p are known. Figure 10 represents the experimental concentration–distance profile measured using a stack of ten membranes and the theoretical curves calculated by Eq. (5) or Eq. (6) for 2-h diffusion for dye 1. Although the theoretical lines for surface diffusion control (broken line) and for pore diffusion control (dashed-and dotted line) disagree with the experimental data, the theoretical line for the parallel diffusion model (solid line) agrees well with the experimental data. Thus, it is possible to confirm in this matter whether the values of D_s and D_p determined in Sec. IV are proper or not. In addition, the profiles of diffusant in the membrane can be predicted by calculation using Eq. (5), when α, γ, D_s and D_p are known.

B. Effects of Type of Adsorption Isotherm

As described before, the relationship between q and C is assumed to be in local equilibrium and C is calculated according to an equilibrium isotherm such as

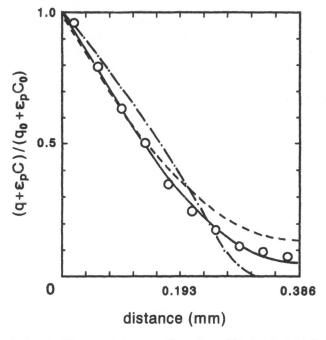

FIG. 10 The concentration–distance profile of C.I. Acid Red 88 in the stacked membrane at 55°C for 2-h diffusion time. Theoretical lines for; (– – –) surface diffusion control ($D'_s = 3.29 \times 10^{-12}$ m²/s); (— · —) pore diffusion control ($D'_p = 1.35 \times 10^{-11}$ m²/s); (———) the parallel diffusion model ($D_s = 1.66 \times 10^{-12}$ m²/s and $D_p = 4.77 \times 10^{-12}$ m²/s); $\alpha = 5.57$ and $\gamma = 0.509$ [24].

the Freundlich equation. In this section the effects of applying the Langmuir equation are discussed. Applying the Langmuir equation shown by Eq. (26), transforms Eqs. (2) and (3) and into Eqs. (27) and (28), respectively. The equilibrium constant K in Eq. (26) is evaluated from the constant K_L in the Langmuir isotherm from $K = 1/(C_0 K_L + 1)$:

$$y = \frac{x}{K + (1 - K)x} \tag{26}$$

$$\left[\alpha + \frac{K}{\{1 - (1 - K)y\}^2} \right] \frac{\partial y}{\partial \tau_P} = K \frac{\partial}{\partial \rho} \left[\frac{1}{\{1 - (1 - K)y\}^2} \frac{\partial y}{\partial \rho} \right] + \beta \frac{\partial^2 y}{\partial \rho^2} \tag{27}$$

$$\left[\alpha + \frac{K}{\{1 - (1 - K)y\}^2} \right] \frac{\partial y}{\partial \tau_S} = \alpha \frac{\partial^2 y}{\partial \rho^2} \tag{28}$$

The initial and boundary conditions are the same as for Eq. (7).

The value of K is small for diffusants with a high affinity and depends on C_0. The Langmuir equation is applicable at a lower concentration range, for example, at $C_0 \leqq 0.3$ mol/m^3 for dyes 6 and 8 [23]. There is no difference between theoretical lines of uptake curves for surface diffusion control when applying either the Langmuir or Freundlich equations. Accordingly, D_s' obtained by curve fitting with both theoretical values is the same. On the other hand, there is a little difference between the theoretical lines of uptake curves for pore diffusion control when applying either the Langmuir or Freundlich equations. However, the difference in D_p' is comparable to the experimental error, and consequently the plots of D_p' against α provide the same intercept which represents D_p. In addition there is little difference between the concentration–distance profiles when both equations are applied [25]. Thus, it is assumed that any isotherm can be applied provided the relationship between q and C is suitably described.

C. Contributed Factors for Diffusivity

The factors which influence diffusion, molecular-size, affinity and the aggregation of diffusants are known [10]. When diffusants have a high affinity to the substrate, their movement must be retarded. In the recent study on the parallel diffusion model, the good correlation between the diffusivities (D_S and D_p) and molecular weight was observed for some dyes (2, 5, 6, 8 in Fig. 4) as shown in Fig. 11 [28]. However, there are some exceptions, i.e., D_p of dyes 1 and 7, and D_S of dye 7 deviate below the line as shown in Fig. 11. Furthermore, D_S and D_p for dyes 3 and 4 are much higher than the values expected from their molecular weight [26]. Dyes 3 and 4 have high solubility because of three sulfonic acid groups, however, they adsorb in the presence of high concentrations of NaCl. Dyes 1 and 7 are known to have a strong tendency of aggregate [31–33], which is usually associated with a high affinity. And aggre-

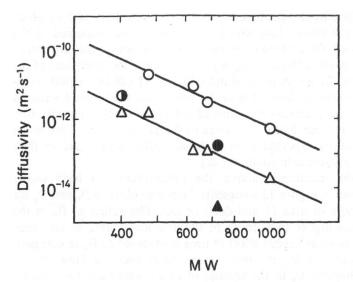

FIG. 11 Correlation of diffusivity with molecular weight; (○,◑,●) the pore diffusivity for parallel diffusion model (D_p) and (△,▲) the surface diffusivity for parallel diffusion model (D_s) at 55°C for dyes 1, 2 and 5–8 in Fig. 4; (◑) C.I. Acid Red 88 and (●,▲) C.I. Direct Red 2 [28].

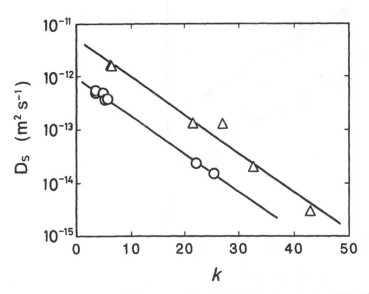

FIG. 12 Relationship between surface diffusivity for the parallel diffusion model (D_s) and the coefficient of the Freundlich isotherm (k) as an index of affinity at (○) 25°C and (△) 55°C [26,28].

gation is accompanied by the decrease of diffusivity. The affinity of dyes which have high solubility is usually low. And high solubility is accompanied by the increase of diffusivity. Thus, these facts lead to the conclusion that D_S correlates to the affinity of the diffusants. D_S is plotted against the coefficient of the Freundlich isotherm (k), an index of affinity, in Fig. 12 [26,28]. Good correlation is observed between them. It must be noted that the larger k value at higher C_E must be used, because the value of k depends on the concentration of electrolyte. On the other hand, the values of D_p for dyes 1 and 7 are much smaller than the values expected from their molecular weight due to their strong tendency to aggregate in solution [28].

In the discussion mentioned above, the temperature has been tacitly assumed to be constant. Figure 13 represents Arrhenius plots of D_S and D_p for dye 1 in the presence of urea (1 mol/dm³) or not. The values of D_S in the presence of urea are higher than those in the absence of urea at any temperature, in which more enhanced effect of urea is observed to D_p in comparison to D_S. The value of D_p at lower temperatures becomes large by the addition of urea although D_p in the absence of urea is extremely low because

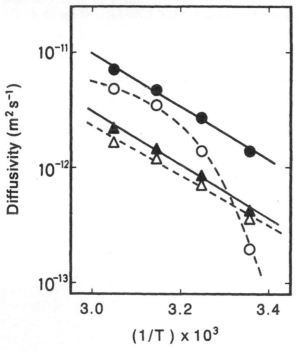

FIG. 13 Arrhenius plots of the surface diffusivity ($\triangle$ and $\blacktriangle$) and the pore diffusivity ($\bigcirc$ and $\bullet$) for the parallel diffusion model in the absence ($\bigcirc$ and $\triangle$) and presence ($\bullet$ and $\blacktriangle$) of urea (1 mol/dm³) for C.I. Acid Red 88 [27].

of high aggregation of the dye in the solution, and the resulting plots reveal a straight line. The reason for this may be attributed to the entropy change in the system brought about by the addition of urea. The addition of urea (1 mol/dm^3) accelerates pore diffusion of the dye to some extent, however, D_p for dye 1 in the presence of urea is still smaller than the value expected from the relationship in Fig. 11. The reason for this is assumed to be that the concentration of urea is not enough to prevent aggregation thoroughly and/or that the other factors exist in aggregation of dye 1. The activation energies of surface diffusion and pore diffusion in the presence of urea are 44.4 kJ/mol [27].

D. Effects of Type of Diffusion

The value of β which is an indicator for the type of controlling diffusion is defined as the product of α and D_S/D_p. Then, it increases proportionally with increasing α when D_S and D_p are constant. The lines in Fig. 14 represent β calculated using α, D_S and D_p of dye 1 at 25–55°C against $1/\alpha$. The symbols show ones in which D_S and D_p are confirmed by the measurements of concentration–distance profiles. As described in the theoretical analysis, diffusion is controlled by surface diffusion for $\beta > 10$. On the other hand, diffusion

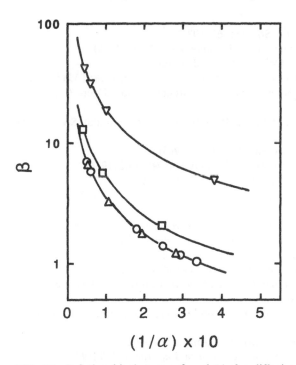

FIG. 14 Relationship between β and $1/\alpha$ for diffusion of C.I. Acid Red 88 at various temperatures; (∇) 25°C, ($\square$) 35°C, ($\triangle$) 45°C and ($\bigcirc$) 55°C [24].

is almost controlled by pore diffusion for $\beta < 0.1$. Parallel diffusion occurs for $0.1 \leq \beta \leq 10$. The plots of β at 45 and 55°C lie on the same line; this indicates that the contribution of both diffusion is similar at both temperatures. The plots of β at 35°C lie above them, and β for large α is more than 10. Furthermore, the value of β at 25°C is larger than 10 for a wide range of $\alpha(>5)$, which means surface diffusion is dominant at this temperature. Table 3 represents the range of β for some dyes at 55°C. The values of β for dyes 1, 6, 7 and 8 are nearly the same, where the contribution of surface diffusion is larger than that of pore diffusion. The value of α for dye 1 is approximately less than a tenth of those of dyes 6, 7 and 8, but its small D_p makes β large. Although the value of α for dye 7 is much larger than those of the others, small D_S/D_p makes β small. The contribution of both surface diffusion and pore diffusion is similar for dyes 2 and 5.

In conclusion, parallel diffusion occurs in the porous membrane for most dyes, but surface diffusion is dominant for some cases. Examples where pore diffusion is dominant are not shown here, because the procedure described in this chapter may be adapted when some extent of adsorption occurs.

REFERENCES

1. T. H. Morton, Trans. Faraday Soc. *31*:262 (1935).
2. W. N. Garvie and S. M. Neale, Trans. Faraday Soc. *34*:335 (1938).
3. T. H. Morton, J. Soc. Dyers Colourists *62*:272 (1946).
4. H. A. Standing, J. O. Warwicker, and H. F. Willis, J. Text. Inst. *38*:T335 (1947).
5. R. H. Peters, J. H. Petropolous, and R. McGregor, J. Soc. Dyers Col. *77*:704 (1961).
6. R. McGregor, R. H. Peters, and J. H. Petropolous, Trans. Faraday Soc. *58*:1045 (1962).
7. J. O. Warwicker, J. Polym. Sci. Part A, *1*:3105 (1963).
8. R. McGregor and R. H. Peters, Trans. Faraday Soc. *60*:2062 (1964).
9. P. B. Weize and H. Zollinger, Trans. Faraday Soc. *64*:1963 (1968).
10. J. Crank and G. S. Park, *Diffusion in Polymers*. Academic Press, London, 1968, 325.
11. T. Hori, M. Mizuno, and T. Shimizu, *Colloid Polym. Sci. 258*:1070 (1980).
12. Z. Morita, T. Tanaka, and H. Motomura, *J. Appl. Polym. Sci. 31*:777 (1986).
13. K. Kawazoe and Y. Fukuda, *Kagaku kogaku 29*:374 (1965).
14. P. Schneider and J. M. Smith, *AIChE Journal 14*:886 (1968).
15. C. N. Satterfield, *Mass Transfer in Heterogeneous Catalysis*. M.I.T. Press, Cambridge, Massachusetts, 1970.
16. D. M. Ruthven, *Principle of Adsorption and Adsorption Precesses*. John Wiley, New York, 1984.
17. M. Suzuki and K. Kawazoe, *J. Chem. Eng. Jap. 8*:379 (1975).
18. M. Suzuki, T. Kawai, and K. Kawazoe, *J. Chem. Eng. Jap. 9*:203 (1976).
19. H. Yoshida, T. Kataoka, M. Nango, S. Ohta, N. Kuroki, and M. Maekawa, *J. Appl. Polym. Sci. 32*:4185 (1986).

20. H. Yoshida, M. Maekawa, and M. Nango, *Chem. Eng. Sci. 46*:429 (1991).
21. M. Maekawa, K. Murakami, and H. Yoshida, *J. Colloid Interface Sci. 155*:79 (1993).
22. M. Maekawa, H. Yoshida, and M. Nango, *J. Chem. Soc. Jap. 1989*:1178 (1989).
23. H. Yoshida, T. Kataoka, M. Maekawa, and M. Nango, *Chem. Eng. J. 41*:B1 (1989).
24. M. Maekawa, M. Tanaka, and H. Yoshida, *J. Colloid Interface Sci. 170*:146 (1995).
25. M. Maekawa, K. Murakami, and H. Yoshida, *Colloid Polym. Sci. 273*:793 (1995).
26. M. Maekawa and M. Kondo, *Colloid Polym. Sci. 274*:1145 (1996).
27. M. Maekawa, M. Ohmori, A. Yamashita, and M. Nango, *Colloid Polym. Sci. 275*:784 (1997).
28. M. Maekawa, K. Kasai, and M. Nango, *Colloid Surf. A 132*:173 (1998).
29. Y. Takeuchi, E. Furuya, and H. Ikeda, *J. Chem. Eng. Jap. 17*:304 (1984).
30. E. Costa, G. Calleja and F. Domingo, *AIChE Journal 31*:982 (1985).
31. K. Hamada and M. Mitsuishi, *Dyes Pigm. 19*:161 (1992).
32. C. Robinson and H. Mills, *Proc. Roy. Soc. London A131*:576 (1931).
33. C. Robinson, *Proc. Roy. Soc. London A148*:681 (1935).

9

Osmotic Properties of Polyelectrolyte Gels

DIETRICH WOERMANN   Institute of Physical Chemistry, University of Köln, Köln, Germany

Abstract

The phenomena of positive and negative osmosis observed with polyelectrolyte gel membranes separating two aqueous electrolyte solutions are analyzed. The analysis is focused on two aspects: treatment of the osmotic phenomena in terms of the linear laws of the thermodynamics of irreversible processes of discontinuous systems and in terms of a model, the model of the membrane with narrow pores. This approach makes it possible to predict the experimental conditions under which positive and negative osmosis will be observed. The predictions of the model are compared with experimental data.

I. DESCRIPTION OF THE MEMBRANE SYSTEM

Let us consider an isothermal system in which a cross-linked polyelectrolyte gel membrane separates two dilute aqueous solutions of the same electrolyte. The concentrations of the solute in the bulk phases are different. The concentration in the left bulk phase [phase (')] is higher than that in the right bulk phase [phase (")]. Figure 1 shows such a system schematically. The symbol 0 refers to the solvent and the symbol 1 to the solute. The membrane is assumed to be permeable to both components. But the effective permeability of the two components is different. The system reaches its thermodynamic equilibrium state by an exchange of matter across the membrane. The molar flows of the components 0 and 1 are measured by determining the amount of substance of the two components in the bulk phases as function of time.

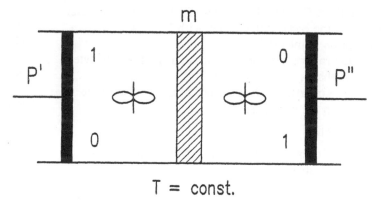

FIG. 1 Isothermal membrane system (schematically). The bulk phases (left bulk phase, phase ('); right bulk phase, phase (")) of the membrane m are two aqueous solutions of the same solute (electrolyte). Solvent, index 0; solute, index 1). The position of the symbols 0 and 1 indicate that the concentration of the solute in the left bulk phase is higher than that in the right. The membrane is formed by a cross linked polyelectrolyte gel. It is permeable to the solvent and to the solute. But the effective diffusion coefficients the two components are different. A hydrostatic pressure difference can be applied across the membrane using two pistons. P' and P'' is the hydrostatic pressure in the left and right bulk phase, respectively. The bulk phases are stirred mechanically to keep their composition homogeneous.

After the start of an experiment, the membrane system reaches a stationary state after a certain transition time. In the stationary state the amount of substance of the components 0 and 1 within the membrane does not change with time anymore. The same is true of the molar flows across the membrane. The bulk phases are vigorously stirred and their volumes are chosen so that the relation given by Eq. (1) holds. Under this condition each bulk phase remains in local thermodynamic equilibrium although flows of the component 0 and 1 across the membrane take place.

$$\frac{c_1^{(\alpha)}}{(dc_1^{(\alpha)}/dt)} \gg \frac{\delta^2}{\tilde{D}_1} \tag{1}$$

The symbol (α) refers to the left bulk phase $(')$ and the right bulk phase $('')$, respectively. c_1 is the molar volume concentration of component 1. t is the time and δ the thickness of the membrane. $\tilde{D}_1$ is the effective diffusion coefficient of component 1 within the membrane.

Which combinations of directions of the molar flows of the components 0 and 1 across the membrane can be observed in such a system? Which direction of the volume flow across the membrane results from these molar flows?

II. PHENOMENOLOGICAL TREATMENT

A. Entropy Production

From a phenomenological point of view this question can be answered by writing down the entropy production of the system in the stationary state in terms of the thermodynamic of irreversible processes of discontinuous systems [1–4]. It is given by Eq. (2)

$$T \frac{d_{int} S}{dt} = J_0'' \Delta \mu_0 + J_1'' \Delta \mu_1 \geq 0 \tag{2}$$

$d_{int} S/dt$ is the internal entropy production (S, entropy) of the system in the stationary state caused by the irreversible diffusion of the components 0 and 1. T is the thermodynamic temperature. J_j'' is the molar flow of component j ($j = 0, 1$) across the membrane into the right bulk phase relative to the membrane ($J_j^{(\alpha)} = dn_j^{(\alpha)}/dt$; $n_j^{(\alpha)}$, amount of substance of component j in bulk phase $(\alpha) = ('), ('')$. In the stationary state the $J_j^{(\alpha)}$ are related by $J_j' + J_j'' = 0$. μ_j is the chemical potential of component j. Δ is the difference between the left and the right bulk phase [$\Delta = (') - ('')$].

The second law of thermodynamics demands that for irreversible processes the entropy production is positive. The entropy production vanishes when the system has reached its thermodynamic equilibrium state (thermodynamic equilibrium at constant temperature and pressure: $\mu_j' = \mu_j''$, $j = 0, 1$).

The entropy production given by Eq. (2) is the sum of two terms. Each term is the product of a flow and a driving force conjugate to it. The flows are time derivative of extensive state parameters (amount of substance, $n_j^{(\alpha)}$) and the driving forces are differences of intensive state parameter (chemical potential, $\mu_j^{(\alpha)}$; thermodynamic field). The driving forces characterize the "distance" of the system from its thermodynamic equilibrium state. Flows and driving forces are independent from each other and disappear in the equilibrium state.

As already stated, the concentration of component 1 in the left bulk phase of the isothermal and isobaric system is assumed to higher than that in the right bulk phase. The opposite is true for component 0. The corresponding differences of the chemical potentials $\Delta\mu_j$ of the two components have opposite signs. Therefore, the driving force $\Delta\mu_0$ conjugate to J_0'' is smaller than zero ($\Delta\mu_0 < 0$ (assuming $(c_1 f_1)' > (c_1 f_1)''$; f_1, activity coefficient of the solute). The opposite is true for the driving force $\Delta\mu_1$ conjugate to J_1'' ($\Delta\mu_1 > 0$).

On the basis of Eq. (2) it is concluded that three combinations of directions of molar flows of the components 0 and 1 are thermodynamically possible in the membrane system shown in Fig. 1. They are shown schematically in Fig. 2 [5,6]. The arrows indicate the direction of the molar flows. A flow of a component in the direction of its conjugate driving force is called a "congruent"

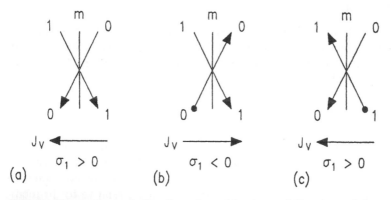

FIG. 2 Thermodynamically allowed combinations of directions of the molar flows of the components 0 and 1 across the membrane under isobaric conditions in the system shown in Fig. 1. The slanted arrows indicate the direction of the molar flows. Arrows carrying no black dots indicate flows which follow the direction of the conjugate concentration gradient ("congruent" transport). The arrows carrying a black dot indicate flows which are directed against their conjugate concentration gradient. ("incongruent" transport). The horizontally oriented arrows J_V give the direction of the osmotic volume flow across the membrane under isobaric conditions. Positive osmosis: $J_V\leftarrow$, $L_{V1} < 0$, $\sigma_1 > 0$; (a) and (c). Negative osmosis: $J_V\rightarrow$, $L_{V1} > 0$, $\sigma_1 < 0$; (b).

flow (see Fig. 2a) [7]. The arrows marked by a black dot (see Figs. 2b) and Fig. 2c) indicate that these flows take place against their conjugate driving force ("incongruent"flows) [7]. The incongruent flows are caused by a coupling of the flows within the membrane (momentum transfer). A combination of two incongruent flows is thermodynamically forbidden.

The flows J_0'' and J_1'' of the components 0 and 1 cause a volume flow across the membrane which is given by Eq. (3).

$$J_V'' = V_0 J_0'' + V_1 J_1'' \tag{3}$$

V_j is the partial molar volume of component j. It is assumed to be independent of concentration. The volume flow $J_V^{(\alpha)}$ across the membrane is given by $J_V^{(\alpha)} = dV^{(\alpha)}/dt((\alpha) = (\prime), (\prime\prime))$. In the stationary state J_V' and J_V'' are related by $J_V' + J_V'' = 0$.

The volume flows $J_V^{(\alpha)}$ can be measured by connecting calibrated horizontally oriented capillaries to the bulk phases and by observing the movement of the meniscus of the solution in the capillaries. In dilute solutions of the solute the term $(V_1 J_1'')$ in Eq. (3) is small compared with the term $(V_0 J_0'')$. It can be neglected for a qualitative discussion of the direction of the osmotic volume. The volume flow and the flow of the solvent have the same direction.

The directions of the volume flow across the membrane associated with the three thermodynamically possible combinations of the directions of the molar flows of the components 0 and 1 are also shown in Fig. 2. Systems (a) and (c) exhibit "positive" osmosis (volume flow into the bulk phase with the higher concentration of the solute). System (b) shows "negative" osmosis (volume flow into the bulk phase with the lower concentration of the solute). Often the word "anomalous" is added to the expressions positive and negative osmosis for two entirely different reasons: (a) in the case of positive osmosis, to indicate that the volume flows across a polyelectrolyte membrane in contact with dilute electrolyte solutions are large compared with that of a semipermeable membrane with a matrix carrying no charged groups under identical experimental conditions; (b) in the case of negative osmosis, to indicate that this phenomenon is an unexpected phenomenon at first sight. Anomalous osmosis does not lead to an osmotic equilibrium state of the system because the membrane is permeable to both components forming its bulk phases (osmotic equilibrium: $\mu_0'(P', T) = \mu_0''(P'', T); P' > P''$).

B. Linear Laws

The phenomenological considerations have to be taken one step further to see that the transition from a positive to a negative osmotic volume flow is associated with a change of sign of the phenomenological transport coefficient characterizing the coupling of the flow of the solute relative to the volume flow with the osmotic volume flow.

The entropy production [Eq. (2)] is transformed linearly by introducing two new flows, the volume flow J_V'' and the flow $(J_1^*)''$ of the solute relative to the volume flow. These new flows replace the old flows J_0'' and J_1''. The new flows are introduced because they can be measured experimentally more easily than the flows J_0'' and J_1''. As already mentioned, J_V'' can be measured using capillaries. $(J_1^*)''$ can be determined by measuring the change of the concentration of component 1 with time $((J_1^*)'' = V''(dc_1''/dt)$ (stationary state: $(J_1^*)'$ + $(J_1^*)'' = 0)$.

The volume flow J_V'' is given by Eq. (3) and the flow relative to the volume flow $(J_1^*)''$ by Eq. (4).

$$(J_1^*)'' = J_i'' - \bar{c}_1 J_V'' \tag{4}$$

with

$$\bar{c}_1 = (c_1' + c_1'')/2.$$

The new flows are linear combinations of the old flows. Corresponding new driving forces are constructed in such a way that the entropy production remains unchanged [1–4,8,9].

The entropy production in terms of the now flows J_V'' and $(J_1^*)''$ and the conjugate new driving forces ΔX_V and ΔX_1^* are given by Eqs. (5a–5c).

$$T\frac{d_{int}S}{dt} = J_V''\Delta X_V + (J_1^*)''\Delta X_1^* \geq 0 \tag{5a}$$

with

$$\Delta X_V = \bar{c}_0\,\Delta\mu_0 + \bar{c}_1\Delta\mu_1 = \Delta P + \bar{c}_1\left[\Delta_c\mu_1 - \frac{V_1}{V_0}\,\Delta\mu_0\right] + \frac{\Delta_c\mu_0}{V_0} \tag{5b}$$

$$\Delta X_1^* = -\frac{V_1}{V_0}\,\Delta\mu_0 + \Delta\mu_1 = -\frac{V_1}{V_0}\,\Delta_c\mu_0 + \Delta_c\mu_1 \tag{5c}$$

In writing down the second form of the right-hand side of Eqs. (5b) and (5c) the difference $\Delta\mu_i$ of the chemical potential of component i ($i = 0, 1$) is split into a pressure and a concentration dependent (subscript "c") part ($\Delta\mu_i = V_i\Delta P + \Delta_c\mu_i$).

It can be shown that for systems close to equilibrium in which the bulk phases are formed by dilute solutions the expression of the driving force ΔX_V takes on the form given by Eq. (6) and that of the driving force ΔX_1^* the form given by Eqs. (7a) and (7b) if the bulk phases are ideal dilute electrolyte solutions. Details are given in Appendix A. Deviations from the property of an ideal solution can be taken into account by introducing osmotic coefficients.

$$\Delta X_V = \Delta P \tag{6}$$

$$\Delta X_1^* = \Delta\Pi_1/\bar{c}_1 \tag{7a}$$

with

$$\Delta\Pi_1 = (v_+ + v_-)RT \, \Delta c_1 \qquad (7b)$$

Δc_1 is the concentration difference of the electrolyte between the bulk phases and $\Delta\Pi_1$ the corresponding osmotic difference. v_i is the number of ions of species i which are formed by the dissociation of one molecule of the electrolyte. R is the universal gas constant.

It is assumed that each of the flows J_V'' and $(J_1^*)''$ are a function of both driving forces ΔX_V and ΔX_1^* [i.e., $J_V''(\Delta P, \Delta X_1^*)$, $(J_1^*)''(\Delta P, \Delta X_1^*)$]. To derive an expression for the dependence of the flows on the driving forces for a membrane system close to its equilibrium state [i.e. $(.\Delta P/\bar{P}) \ll 1$; $(\Delta X_1^*/\bar{X}_1^*) \ll 1$; $\bar{P} = (P' + P'')/2$; $\bar{X}_1^* = (\bar{X}_1^{*'} + \bar{X}_1^{*''})/2$] the flows $J_V''(\Delta P, \Delta X_1^*)$ and $(J_1^*)''(\Delta P, \Delta X_1^*)$ are developed into a power series in terms of ΔP and ΔX_1^* around the equilibrium state. The series is broken off after terms linear in the driving forces. The resulting linear laws of J_V'' and $(J_1^*)''$ for ideal dilute solutions are given by Eqs. (8) and (9).

$$J_V'' = L_{VV} \Delta P + L_{V1} \Delta X_1^* \qquad (8)$$

$$(J_1^*) = L_{1V} \Delta P + L_{11} \Delta X_1^* \qquad (9)$$

The range of the driving forces in which the flows J_V'' and $(J_1^*)''$ are linear function of the driving forces ΔP and ΔX_1^* has to be established in separate experiments. The L_{jk} are phenomenological transport coefficients which can be arranged in form of a 2×2 matrix. They are a function of temperature, of pressure and of the mean concentration $\bar{c}_1$. They are independent of the driving forces. The set of L_{jk} describes completely the transport properties of a given membrane system close to its equilibrium state at the given values of T, P and $\bar{c}_1$.

The phenomenological transport coefficients of the linear laws derived from the entropy production form a symmetric matrix (Onsager symmetric relation $L_{jk} = L_{jk}$). This reduces the number of independent transport coefficients which have to be determined experimentally. On the other hand, the Onsager relations can be used to check the internal consistency of experimentally determined transport coefficients L_{jk}. The diagonal terms L_{VV} and L_{11} are called permeabilities (L_{VV}, mechanical permeability, L_{11} permeability of the solute) which have positive values for thermodynamic reasons $(dS_{int}/dt \geq 0)$. The off-diagonal terms L_{1V} and L_{V1} ($L_{IV} = L_{V1}$) can have positive or negative values or can be zero. They are different from zero when the flows J_V'' and $(J_1^*)''$ are coupled. For thermodynamic reasons the values of L_{VV}, L_{11} and L_{1V} ($= L_{V1}$) are related by the inequality $(L_{VV}L_{11} - L_{1V}^2) > 0$ (see, e.g., Refs. 1–4, 8, 9).

If $\Delta X_1^* (= \Delta\Pi_1/\bar{c}_1)$ is larger than zero and the coupling coefficient L_{V1} has a negative value, the volume flow will be directed from the more dilute bulk phase ('') into the more concentrated bulk phase (') under isobaric conditions [see Eq. (8) and Figs. 2a and 2c; positive osmosis]. If the coupling coefficient

L_{V1} is positive under the same experimental conditions the volume flow is directed from the more concentrated bulk phase (') into the more dilute bulk phase (") [see Eq. (8) and Fig. 2b; negative osmosis].

A theoretical analysis of osmotic volume flows across membranes in terms of the irreversible thermodynamics of continuous systems is given in Refs. 10 and 11.

An incongruent transport of the solute takes place under isobaric conditions (see Fig. 2c) when the ratio $(J_1''/\Delta\Pi_1)_{\Delta P=0}$ is smaller than zero. It follows from the Eqs. (4), (8) and (9) that this is the case if the transport coefficient L_{V1} has sufficiently large negative values $((L_{V1} + L_{11}/\bar{c}_1) < 0)$. The permeability L_{11} has always a positive value.

C. Reflection Coefficient

For a more quantitative discussion of the osmotic properties of the membrane system shown in Fig. 1, the hydrostatic pressure difference ΔP is determined experimentally which has to be applied across the membrane to suppress the osmotic volume flow $(J_V = 0)$ generated by the osmotic difference $\Delta\Pi_1$. The ratio $(\Delta P/\Delta\Pi_1)_{J_V=0}$ is called the reflection coefficient σ_1 of the membrane for the solute 1 [see Eq. (10a)] [12–14]. The reflection coefficient σ_1 is related to the phenomenological transport coefficient L_{VV} and L_{V1} by Eq. (10b). It follows from Eq. (8) taking into account the definition of the reflection coefficient [Eq. (10a)]. It has to be checked experimentally that the reflection coefficient σ_1 determined at a given mean concentration $\bar{c}_1$ of the solute is independent of the applied osmotic difference $\Delta\Pi_1$

$$\sigma_1 \equiv \left(\frac{\Delta P}{\Delta\Pi_1}\right)_{J_V=0} \tag{10a}$$

$$\sigma_1 = -\frac{1}{\bar{c}_1}\frac{L_{V1}}{L_{VV}} \tag{10b}$$

If the membrane is impermeable to the solute 1 the reflection coefficient σ_1 has the value $\sigma_1 = 1$. The pressure difference ΔP which has to be applied to suppress the volume flow across the membrane is equal to the osmotic difference $\Delta\Pi_1$ and the system is in its osmotic equilibrium state. If the membrane is permeable to the solute as well as to the solvent the system cannot reach its osmotic equilibrium state. σ_1 is different from 1 and changes with time because the composition of the bulk phases changes with time. Positive osmosis is associated with a positive value of the reflection coefficient $(\sigma_1 > 0; L_{V1} < 0; L_{VV} > 0)$ and negative osmosis with a negative value of the reflection coefficient $(\sigma_1 < 0; L_{V1} > 0; L_{VV} > 0)$ (see Fig. 2). An interpretation of σ_1 in terms of friction coefficients is given in Ref. 15.

The coupling coefficient L_{V1} can vary in a wide range limited by the thermodynamic condition $(L_{VV}L_{11} - L_{V1}^2) > 0$. A priori no upper and lower bound of σ_1 can be given on the basis of these considerations. That means the reflection coefficient σ_1 of a leaky membrane can have values $|\sigma_1| > 1$.

Introducing the reflection coefficient σ_1 into the linear law of J_V'' leads to Eq. (11).

$$J_V'' = L_{VV}[\Delta P - \sigma_1 \Delta \Pi_1] \tag{11}$$

If the dependence of the transport coefficients L_{VV} and σ_1 on $\bar{c}_1$ is known the dependence of J_V'' on $\bar{c}_1$ at constant pressure can be calculated ($J_V = -L_{VV}\sigma_1\Delta\Pi_1$) can be calculated.

D. Hyperfiltration

In a hyperfiltration experiment the sign of the reflection coefficient σ_1 of a solute for a given membrane determines the sign of the concentration difference (osmotic difference) of the solute between the solution of the high pressure phase [phase (')] and the filtrate [phase (")] in the stationary state. Such a state is established after a certain transition time if the volume of the high pressure phase is large enough so that the concentration of the solute in phase (') does not change with time during the hyperfiltration experiment (i.e., $dc_1'/dt = 0$). Then, the composition of the solution passing the membrane reaches a time independent value $((J_1^*)'' = 0)$ and the hyperfiltration ratio $[\Delta X_1^*/\Delta P]_{(J_1^*)''=0}$ is given by Eq. (12) which follows from Eq. (9).

$$\left[\frac{\Delta X_1^*}{\Delta P}\right]_{(J_1^*)''=0} = -\frac{L_{V1}}{L_{11}} = \sigma_1 \bar{c}_1 \frac{L_{VV}}{L_{11}} \tag{12}$$

The ratio of the permeabilities (L_{VV}/L_{11}) has always a positive value and the hyperfiltration ratio and the reflection coefficient must have the same sign. This prediction has been confirmed experimentally, e.g., [15-19]. It is found that for $\sigma_1 > 0$ the concentration of the solute in the filtrate is smaller than in the high pressure phase. For $\sigma_1 < 0$ the concentration of the solute in the filtrate is higher than that in the high pressure phase. Hyperfiltration of aqueous electrolyte solutions using membranes with a reflection coefficient of the solutes close to 1 are of practical importance to remove electrolytes from aqueous electrolyte solutions from solutes ("reverse osmosis").

III. PREDICTIONS OF THE OSMOTIC PROPERTIES OF A POLYELECTROLYTE GEL MEMBRANE ON THE BASIS OF THE MODEL WITH NARROW PORES

A. Description of the Model

The preceding section is devoted to a treatment of the osmotic phenomena of a membrane system in terms of the thermodynamic of irreversible processes in discontinuous systems. The membrane is considered a "black box". In order to gain more insight into the cause of the observed osmotic phenomena it is necessary to construct a suitable model of the membrane. The real membrane is replaced by a fictitious model which is amenable to a theoretical analysis. The model reflects only the typical properties of the membrane. Simplifying assumptions are made to keep the number of the parameter of the model small. For polyelectrolyte gel membranes such a model has been developed by Teorell [20–23], Meyer and Sievers [24–26]; and Schmid [27–32]. It has been worked out in great detail by Schlögl [6]. It is the "model of the membrane with narrow pores". This model has also been treated by Läuger and Kuhn [33].

The model is based on a number of simplifying assumptions:

1. The matrix of the cross-linked polyelectrolyte gel carries electric charges (covalently bound fixed ionic groups) and has a homogeneous structure (i.e. constant local concentration of crosslinks and fixed ionic groups). In contact with water the solution within the pores contains only mobile ions of a sign opposite to that of the fixed charges (counterions) to maintain electroneutrality. In equilibrium with an aqueous electrolyte solution the pore fluid contains also mobile ions of the same sign as the fixed charges (coions) and the additional counterions.

    The mobile ions (ionic species i) are distributed homogeneously over the cross-section of the pores by the thermal motion of the ions. This is the case when the characteristic length ξ of the pore structure has a value of the order of the radius of the ion cloud of the Debye–Hückel theory of strong electrolytes (i.e., 0.5 nm $\lesssim \xi \lesssim$ 10 nm; "narrow pores") [34–38].

3. The solution present in the pores of the matrix of the membrane is so dilute that it can be treated as an ideal dilute solution.

4. The concentration of all components of the medium within the pores are only a function of the coordinate x running perpendicular to the phase boundary membrane/solution.

5. A coupling between the transport of dissolved ionic particle species i is neglected. Coupling effects between the transport of the solvent molecules and dissolved particles species are taken into account to a first approximation by adding a convection term $(\tilde{C}_i \cdot j_V)$ to the transport equation of the dissolved particle species [see Eq. (13)]. This term assumes a tight coupling between the transport of the solvent molecules and that of the dissolved species. A coupling between the transport of the dissolved particles and the membrane matrix is also taken into account by introducing an effective diffusion coefficient $\tilde{D}_i$ [see Eq. (13)] of the dissolved species in the transport equations and by a mechanical permeability $(\tilde{d}_h)$ in the equation of transport of volume [see. Eq. (14)].

The equations of transport of the model of the membrane with narrow pores are given by Eq. (13) (extended Nernst–Planck equation) and Eq. (14) [6].

$$j_i = \tilde{C}_i j_V - \tilde{D}_i \left[\frac{d\tilde{C}_i}{dx} + z_i \tilde{C}_i \frac{F}{RT} \frac{d\tilde{\phi}}{dx} \right] \tag{13}$$

$$j_V = \tilde{d}_h \left[\frac{d\tilde{P}}{dx} + F\omega\tilde{X} \frac{d\tilde{\phi}}{dx} \right] \tag{14}$$

j_i is the molar flow density of the solute particle species i across the membrane. j_V is the volume flow density across the membrane. The quantities marked by a tilde ($\tilde{\ }$) refer to the membrane phase. $\tilde{D}_i$ is the effective diffusion coefficient of ionic species i in the membrane. $\tilde{d}_h$ is the specific mechanical permeability of the membrane. $\tilde{C}_i$ is the concentration of the ionic species i per unit volume of the solution within the pores. z_i is the valency of the species i including its sign (cation, $z_i > 0$; anion $z_i < 0$). F is the Faraday number. $\tilde{\phi}$ is the electrical potential in the membrane phase. $\tilde{P}$ is the hydrostatic pressure in the membrane phase which is higher than the ambient (atmospheric) pressure ("osmotic swelling" pressure). $\tilde{X}$ is the concentration of the fixed ionic groups per unit volume of the solution within the pores. The symbol ω represents the sign of the charge of the fixed ionic groups (cation exchange membrane, $\omega = -1$; anion exchange membrane, $\omega = +1$). The space coordinate is x. It runs perpendicular to the phase boundary [membrane phase/bulk phase].

Equations (13) and (14) show that the model contains the system specific parameters $\tilde{D}_i$, $\tilde{C}_i$, $\tilde{d}_h$, ω and $\tilde{X}$. The concentrations $\tilde{C}_i$ and the fixed ion concentration $\tilde{X}$ are related by the condition of electroneutrality in the membrane phase. They can be determined in independent experiments. The sign of the fixed charges ω and the fixed ion concentration $\tilde{X}$ can be determined by ion exchange experiments. The method of determination of the mechanical permeability $\tilde{d}_h$ can be read from Eq. (14) ($\tilde{d}_h = \delta \cdot j_V/\Delta P)_{\Delta\phi = 0; \, \Delta c_1 = 0}$; δ, thickness of the membrane). The effective diffusion coefficient $\tilde{D}_i$ can be determined from measurements of the molar flow density j_i^* of a radioactive tracer of the ionic species i^* across the membrane separating two bulk phases of the same concentration ($c_1' = c_1''$) [39–41]. Three methods are available to obtain values of the concentrations $\tilde{C}_i$ within the membrane phase: analytical determinations; radioactive tracer ion exchange experiments (i.e., $\tilde{C}_i/c_1 = \tilde{C}_i^*/c_1^*$); calculations using the Donnan relation if the fixed ion concentration is known.

The expressions for $\tilde{C}_+$ and $\tilde{C}_-$ for a single (1, -1) valent electrolyte (e.g., KCl or HCl) and a membrane with a fixed ion concentration $\omega\tilde{X}$ is given by Eqs. (15). They are derived by combining the condition of electroneutrality of the membrane phase ($\tilde{C}_+ - \tilde{C}_- + \omega\tilde{X} = 0$) with the Donnan relation [$\tilde{C}_+ \cdot \tilde{C}_- = (c_1)^2$]. It is assumed that the solution is ideally dilute.

$$\frac{\tilde{C}_+}{c_1} = \sqrt{\left(\frac{\tilde{X}}{2c_1} \right)^2 + 1} - \frac{\omega\tilde{X}}{2c_1} \tag{15a}$$

$$\frac{\tilde{C}_-}{c_1} = \sqrt{\left(\frac{\tilde{X}}{2c_1}\right)^2 + 1} + \frac{\omega \tilde{X}}{2c_1} \tag{15b}$$

The total concentration of the mobile ions $\tilde{C}(=\tilde{C}_+ + \tilde{C}_-)$ in the pore fluid is always larger than the corresponding concentration in the bulk phase because the charges of the fixed ionic groups are electrically compensated by counterions. Therefore, there exists an osmotic pressure jump $\delta P(=\tilde{P} - P)$ and a jump of the electrical potential $\delta \phi(=(\tilde{\phi} - \phi)$; Donnan potential) at each of the two phase boundaries [membrane phase/bulk phase]. The pressure jump δP is given by Eq. (16). The pore fluid is under higher hydrostatic pressure (swelling pressure). The pressure jump δP is not measurable quantities but it can be calculated if the concentrations $\tilde{C}_i$ of the mobile ions in the pore fluid at the phase boundary (membrane phase/bulk phase) are known.

$$\delta P = (\tilde{P} - P) = RT \sum_i (\tilde{C}_i - c_i) \tag{16}$$

If the electrolyte concentration of the bulk phases is different and the bulk phases are under equal pressure there exists an (osmotic) pressure drop cross the membrane given by Eq. (17). This pressure difference is independent of the sign of the fixed charges ω.

$$\Delta \tilde{P} = \delta \tilde{P}' - \delta \tilde{P}'' = RT \left[\sum_i (\tilde{C}_i' - c_i') - \sum_i (\tilde{C}_i'' - c_i'') \right] \tag{17}$$

The corresponding electrical potential jump $\delta \phi(=\tilde{\phi} - \phi)$ is given by Eq. (18) for ideal dilute solutions. This equation follows from the condition of the electrochemical equilibrium of ionic species i between the membrane phase and the bulk phase ($\eta_i = \tilde{\eta}_i$; η_i, electrochemical potential of ionic species i; $\eta_i = \mu_i + z_i F\phi$).

$$\delta \phi = \frac{RT}{z_i F} \ln \frac{\tilde{C}_i}{c_i} \tag{18}$$

If the electrolyte concentrations in the bulk phases is different there exists an electrical potential difference $\Delta \phi(=(\phi' - \phi''))$ between the bulk phases (membrane potential) given by Eq. (19).

$$\Delta \phi = -\delta \phi' + \Delta \tilde{\phi} + \delta \phi'' \tag{19}$$

$\Delta \tilde{\phi}(=(\tilde{\phi}' - \tilde{\phi}''))$ is the electrical potential drop within the membrane between the left and the right interface. It is caused by the difference of the effective diffusion coefficients of the mobile ions of the pore fluid (diffusion potential). If the pore fluid contains only counter ions of the same species ($c_1/X \ll 1$) the membrane phase is impermeable to the electrolyte the electrical potential difference between the bulk phases is given by ($\Delta \phi = -\delta \phi' + \delta \phi''$).

B. Osmotic Properties in the Presence of a Single Electrolyte in the Bulk Phases

1. Qualitative Discussion

The experimental conditions under which positive or negative osmosis will be observed under isobaric condition ($P' = P''$) are discussed using a polyelectrolyte gel membrane with negatively charged fixed ionic groups ($\omega = -1$) as an example.

The starting point of the discussion is the integrated form of Eq. (14) which is given by Eq. (20).

$$j_V = j_V(\Delta \tilde{P}) + j_V(\Delta \tilde{\phi}) \tag{20}$$

with

$$j_V(\Delta \tilde{P}) = \frac{\tilde{d}_h}{\delta} \Delta \tilde{P} \quad \text{and} \quad j_V(\Delta \tilde{\phi}) = \frac{\tilde{d}_h}{\delta} F \tilde{X} \Delta \tilde{\phi}$$

The term $j_V(\Delta \tilde{P})$ represent the contribution of the hydrostatic pressure difference $\Delta \tilde{P}(= \tilde{P}' - \tilde{P}'')$ between the left and right interphase of the membrane to the observed osmotic volume flow density j_V. The term $j_V(\Delta \tilde{\phi})$ represents the corresponding contribution of the electrical potential difference $\Delta \tilde{\phi}(= \tilde{\phi}' - \tilde{\phi}'')$. The magnitude and the direction of $j_V(\Delta \tilde{\phi})$ changes with the magnitude and the sign of the diffusion potential $\Delta \tilde{\phi}$. $\Delta \tilde{\phi}$ can act as a driving force of a volume flow because the pore fluid of the gel membrane carries a charge density $\tilde{\rho} = -F\omega \tilde{X}$ (here $\omega = -1$).

Under the chosen experimental conditions the electrolyte concentration in the left bulk phase is higher than that in the right bulk phase. Therefore the pressure difference $\Delta \tilde{P}$ within the membrane phase has a negative value (see Eq. (17); $\sum_i (\tilde{C}_i' - c_i') > \sum_i (\tilde{C}_i'' - c_i''))$. $j_V(\Delta \tilde{P})$ is directed from the more dilute to the more concentrated bulk phase. It would lead to a positive osmosis if it would act in the absence of the contribution $j_V(\Delta \tilde{\phi})$.

The prediction of the conditions under which positive and negative osmosis will be observed with a leaky polyelectrolyte gel membrane with negatively charged fixed groups ($\omega = -1$) under isobaric conditions in terms of Eq. (20) are summarized in Fig. 3 [42]:

1. Positive osmosis will be observed when the diffusion potential $\Delta \tilde{\phi}$ has a negative value ($\Delta \tilde{\phi} < 0$; $\tilde{D}_+ > \tilde{D}_-$). Then $j_V(\Delta \tilde{P})$ as well as $j_V(\Delta \tilde{\phi})$ are directed from the more dilute to the more concentrated bulk phase (see Fig. 3a).
2. Positive osmosis will be observed when $j_V(\Delta \tilde{P})$ and $j_V(\Delta \tilde{\phi})$ have opposite directions ($\Delta \tilde{\phi} > 0$; $\tilde{D}_+ < \tilde{D}_-$) as long as $|j_V(\Delta \tilde{P})| > |j_V(\Delta \tilde{\phi})|$ (see Fig. 3b). Both cases corresponds to the types of transport (a) and (c) in Fig. 2.

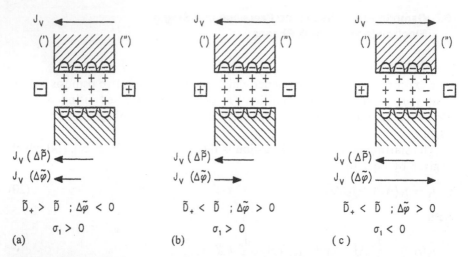

FIG. 3 Model of the membrane with narrow pores: The osmotic phenomena observed with a polyelectrolyte gel membrane with negatively charge fixed ionic groups ($\omega = -1$) are analyzed qualitatively in terms of Eq. (20). The membrane is presented by a single horizontally oriented pore. The concentration of the solute (electrolyte) in the left bulk phase is higher than that in the right ($c_1' > c_1''$). J_v is the volume flow across the membrane. The bulk phases are under equal pressure ($P' = P''$). For details see the text.

3. Negative osmosis is observed when $j_v(\Delta\tilde{P})$ is directed from the dilute to the concentrated bulk phase ($\Delta\tilde{P} < 0$) and $j_v(\Delta\tilde{\phi})$ is directed in the opposite direction ($\Delta\tilde{\phi} > 0$; $\tilde{D}_+ < \tilde{D}_-$) but $|j_v(\Delta\tilde{P})| < |j_v(\Delta\tilde{\phi})|$ (see Fig. 3c). This situation corresponds to the type of transport in Fig. 2b.

2. Quantitative Discussion of the Osmotic Properties

The quantitative treatment of the osmotic properties in term of the model of the membrane with narrow pores begins with the definition of the reflection coefficient [see Eq. (10a)].

$$\sigma_1 = \left(\frac{\Delta P}{\Delta\Pi_1}\right)_{J_v = 0} \tag{10a}$$

To keep the presentation simple it is assumed that the aqueous bulk phases contain a single $(1, -1)$ valent electrolyte (e.g., NaCl or HCl) under isobaric conditions. The volume flow density across the membrane is given by Eq. (21).

$$j_v = [\tilde{d}_h/\delta][\Delta\tilde{P} + F\tilde{X}\,\Delta\tilde{\phi}] \tag{21}$$

It describes a superposition of two contributions to the isobaric volume across the membrane. To suppress it a pressure difference $\Delta P(=P' - P'')$ is applied across the membrane which—according to Eq. (21)—is given by Eq. (22).

$$\Delta P = -[\Delta \tilde{P} + F\tilde{X} \, \Delta\tilde{\phi}]_{J_V=0} \tag{22}$$

A combination of Eqs. (10a) and (22) leads to Eq. (23) which can be used to calculate the dependence of the reflection coefficient σ_1 of the parameter $(c_1/\tilde{X})$ using the model of the membrane with narrow pores.

$$\sigma_1 = -\left[\frac{\Delta \tilde{P} + F\tilde{X} \, \Delta\tilde{\phi}}{\Delta\Pi_1}\right]_{J_V=0} \tag{23}$$

The pressure difference $\Delta \tilde{P}$ can be calculated from Eq. (17) and the potential difference $[\Delta\tilde{\phi}]_{J_V=0}$ from Eq. (24) (see Appendix B).

$$\left[\frac{F}{RT} \, \Delta\tilde{\phi}\right]_{J_V=0, \, I=0} = \tilde{U} \ln\left\{\frac{\tilde{D}_+ \, \tilde{C}_+'' + \tilde{D}_- \, \tilde{C}_-''}{\tilde{D}_+ \, \tilde{C}_+' + \tilde{D}_- \, \tilde{C}_-'}\right\} \tag{24}$$

with

$$\tilde{U} = \frac{\tilde{D}_+ - \tilde{D}_-}{\tilde{D}_+ + \tilde{D}_-}$$

I is the electric current flow.

The value of $[\Delta\tilde{\phi}]_{J_V=0, \, I=0}$ depends on the ratio $(\tilde{D}_-/\tilde{D}_+)(=(\tilde{D}_{co}/\tilde{D}_{counter}))$. The concentrations $\tilde{C}_+$ and $\tilde{C}_-$ at the phase boundaries [membrane phase/ bulk phase] can be calculated using the Eqs. (15).

The dependence of the reflection coefficient σ_1 on the concentration ratio $(c_1/\tilde{X})$ calculated in this way for of a $(1, -1)$ valent electrolyte for fixed values of the ratio $(\tilde{D}_-/\tilde{D}_+)$ is shown in Fig. 4. The curve refers to a gel membrane with $\omega = -1$. Also shown in Fig. 4 is a σ_1 vs. $(c_1/\tilde{X})$ curve for a $(2, -1)$ valent electrolyte for the same type of membrane. This curve is calculated using a more general equivalent expression of the reflection coefficient of a (z_+, z_-) valent electrolyte given by Schlögl [6]. It can be expressed in a form given by Eq. (25) (see Appendix C).

$$\sigma_1 = 1 - \frac{z_+^2(\tilde{D}_+ \, \tilde{C}_+/\tilde{D}_- \, \tilde{C}_-)(\tilde{C}_-/c_-) + z_-^2(\tilde{C}_+/c_+)}{z_+^2(\tilde{D}_+ \, \tilde{C}_+/\tilde{D}_- \, \tilde{C}_-) + z_-^2} \tag{25}$$

The concentrations $\tilde{C}_+$ and $\tilde{C}_-$ are calculated from the Donnan relation for a $(2, -1)$ valent electrolyte for a given fixed ion concentration $\tilde{X}$ [41,44]. The ratio $\tilde{D}_-/\tilde{D}_+$ is kept constant for each calculated σ_1 vs. $(\tilde{c}_1/\tilde{X})$ curve.

If the ratio $(\tilde{c}_1/\tilde{X})$ is small compared with 1 (i.e., $(\tilde{c}_1/\tilde{X}) \ll 1$) the membrane contains practically no coions but only counter ions. Under this condition the membrane has the properties of semipermeable membrane. But it is permeable to the solvent. The reflection coefficient approaches the value 1 (see Fig. 4;

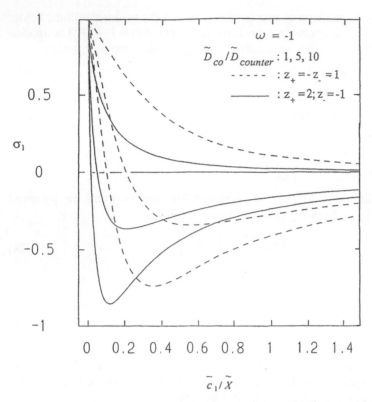

FIG. 4 Model of the membrane with narrow pores: The theoretically predicted dependence of the reflection coefficient σ_1 of a $(1, -1)$ valent electrolyte (e.g., NaCl) and a $(2, -1)$ valent electrolyte (e.g., $BaCl_2$) is shown as a function of the concentration ratio $(\tilde{c}_1/\tilde{X})$ for a polyelectrolyte gel membrane with negatively charged fixed ionic groups $(\omega = -1)$. $\tilde{c}_1$ is the mean molar volume concentration of the electrolyte $(\bar{c}_1 = (c'_1 + c''_1)/2)$. $\tilde{X}$ is the concentration of the fixed ionic groups (mol/dm^3 pore fluid). Parameter of the calculation is the ratio $(\tilde{D}_{co}/\tilde{D}_{counter})$ (upper curve: $(\tilde{D}_{co}/\tilde{D}_{counter}) = 1$; middle curve $(\tilde{D}_{co}/\tilde{D}_{counter}) = 5$; lowest curve $(\tilde{D}_{co}/\tilde{D}_{counter}) = 10$; coions Cl^- ions; counter ions, Na^+, Ba^{2+}). For details of the calculation see the text.

$\lim(\tilde{c}_1/\tilde{X}) \to 0$, $\sigma_1 \to 1$). With increasing values of $(\tilde{c}_1/\tilde{X})$ the concentration of the coions in the pore fluid increases [see Eqs. (15)] and the membrane becomes permeable to the solute. The reflection coefficient decreases. For $(\tilde{c}_1/\tilde{X}) \gg 1$ the membrane has lost its selectivity almost completely. $(\tilde{c}_1/\tilde{X}) \gg 1$, $\sigma_1 \to 0$). Whether there is a change of sign of the reflection coefficient depends on the ratio of the effective diffusion coefficients of the coions and the counter ions $(\tilde{D}_-/\tilde{D}_+)$ (see Fig. 4).

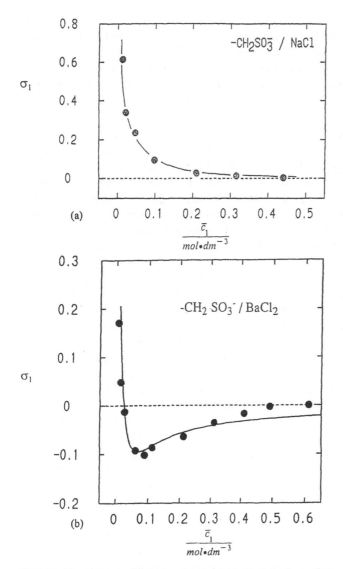

FIG. 5 Experimentally determined concentration dependence of the reflection coefficient $\sigma(NaCl)$ of NaCl (Fig. 5a, [20]) and the reflection coefficient $\sigma(BaCl_2)$ of $BaCl_2$ (Fig. 5b, [23]) for a membrane $[-CH_2 \cdot SO_3^-]$. Data characterizing the membrane are: water content $y(H_2O, Na^+) = 0.77$ (mass fraction of water, gel loaded with Na^+ ions); analytical fixed ion concentration $\tilde{X}_a(Na^+) = 0.51$ mol/dm^3 pore fluid; mechanical permeability $\tilde{d}_h = 1.3 \times 10^{-5}$ cm^5/J/s; thickness, $\delta = 0.1$ cm. The drawn out line in the Fig. 5b represents Eq. (25). The following parameter values are used for the calculation: $\tilde{D}_-/\tilde{D}_+ = 2.40$. The concentrations $\tilde{C}_+$ and $\tilde{C}_-$ are calculated using the Donnan relation for a 2, -1 valent electrolyte [23] with an effective fixed ion concentration $\tilde{X}_{eff} = 0.14$ mol/dm^3 pore fluid.

Two typical experimental σ_1 vs. $\tilde{c}_1$ curve is shown in Fig. 5. They demonstrate that the concentration dependence of the reflection coefficient is qualitatively in good agreement with the theoretical predictions. More experimental data are given in Refs. 41, 43 and 44 which support this statement.

Most of the experimental data available for a quantitative test of the theoretical predictions of osmotic properties of polyelectrolyte membranes using the model of the membrane with narrow pores are membranes formed by condensation products of substituted phenols and formaldehyde (p-phenolsulfonic acid/formaldehyde $-SO_3^-$ membranes [45] and (hydroxyphenyl) methansulfonic acid/formaldehyde $-CH_2 \cdot SO_3^-$ membranes [46]. For these gels it is found that the ratio of the effective diffusion coefficient $(\tilde{D}_-/\tilde{D}_+)$ of the coion and the counter ions of a given electrolyte has about the same value as the corresponding ratio $(D_-/D_+)_\infty$ of the ions in free solution at infinite dilution [47]. This finding is taken into account to compare quantitatively the experimental determined concentration dependence of σ_1 with the prediction of the model.

The experimental $\sigma_1(\tilde{c}_1)$ curves are represented quantitatively to a good approximation by the model of the membrane with narrow pores [Eq. (25)] if concentration independent values of the ratio $(\tilde{D}_-/\tilde{D}_+)(=(D_-/D_+)_\infty)$ are used and the fixed ion concentration is taken as a parameter of the fit (see Fig. 5b and Ref. 44). It turns out that the effective fixed ion concentration $\tilde{X}_{eff}$ obtained in this way is considerably smaller than the analytically determined value $\tilde{X}_a(\tilde{X}_{eff}/\tilde{X}_a \approx 0.3)$ [41,44,48]. The value of $\tilde{X}_{eff}$ is close to the value of the fixed ion concentration obtained from an evaluation of independent electroosmotic experiments with the same membranes in terms of the model of the membrane with narrow pores $((J_V/I)_{\Delta P=0,\,\Delta c_1=0} = F \cdot \tilde{X} \cdot \tilde{d}_h/\tilde{\kappa}$, $\tilde{\kappa}$ is the electrical conductivity of the membrane $[\Omega^{-1}/cm]$. I is the electric current which passes the membrane in the electroosmotic experiment. The difference between the analytically determined fixed ion concentration and the effective fixed ion concentration is assumed to be caused primarily by structural inhomogenieties of the $-SO_3^-$ and the $-CH_2 \cdot SO_3^-$ gel membrane used for the experiments [41,44]. The results of small-angle and ultrasmall-angle X-ray scattering experiments with $-SO_3^-$ and $-CH_2 \cdot SO_3^-$ gels have been interpreted by assuming that the matrix is composed of regions with higher and lower degree of cross links (i.e., locally changing values of the fixed ion concentration and the mechanical permeability) [49,50]. This means that one essential simplifying assumption on which the model of the membrane with narrow pores is based, is not fulfilled, namely the assumption of a homogeneous structure of the gel matrix. There are reports in the literature suggesting that structural inhomogenieties in polyelectrolyte gel membranes are a common feature [51].

The model of the membrane with narrow pores can also be used to find the experimental conditions under which an incongruent transport of the electrolyte (see Fig. 2c) will be observed under isothermal conditions [6,33,42].

Results of a calculation for a polyelectrolyte membrane with negatively charged ionic groups ($\omega = -1$) and a $(1, -1)$ electrolyte in the aqueous bulk phases are shown in Fig. 6. The effective diffusion coefficient of the counter ion have to be much larger than that of the coion (i.e., $(\tilde{D}_+/\tilde{D}_-) \gg 1$) and the ratio $(\tilde{D}_+/\tilde{D}^{\cdot})$ smaller than 1 ($\tilde{D}^{\cdot} = \tilde{d}_h RT\tilde{X}$). An incongruent transport of an electrolyte in a (polyelectrolyte gel membrane/single electrolyte, water)-system has

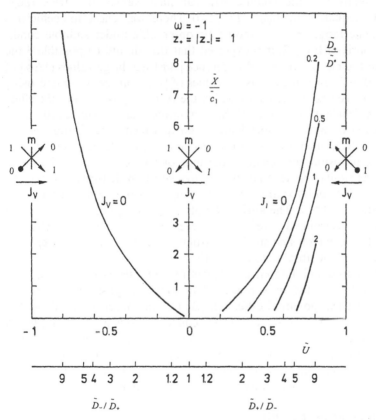

FIG. 6 Model of the membrane with narrow pores: Parameter fields for the observation of the thermodynamically allowed combinations of directions of the molar flow J''_0 of the solvent (index 0) and of the molar flow J''_1 of a single $(1, -1)$ valent electrolyte (index 1) across a polyelectrolyte membrane with negatively charged groups ($\omega = -1$) under isobaric conditions (see Fig. 1). $\tilde{D}_i$, effective diffusion coefficient of ionic species i. $\tilde{D}^{\cdot}$, measure of the hydrodynamic permeability of the membrane ($\tilde{D}^{\cdot} = \tilde{d}_h RT\tilde{X}$). $\tilde{d}_h$, mechanical permeability; $\tilde{X}$, fixed ion concentration; $\bar{c}_1$, mean concentration of the electrolyte in the bulk phases.

not been found up to now. The stated conditions $(\tilde{D}_+/\tilde{D}_-) \gg 1$; $\tilde{D}_+/\tilde{D}^{\cdot} < 1$; $(\tilde{D}^{\cdot} = \tilde{d}_h \tilde{X} RT)$ to observe an incongruent transport of an electrolyte could not be met with $-SO_3^-$ and $-CH_2 \cdot SO_3^-$ membranes (see below).

C. Osmotic Properties in the Presence of Mixed Electrolyte Solutions in the Bulk Phases

The phenomenological treatment of the osmotic properties of a membrane shows that the coupling coefficient L_{V1} between the volume flow and the flow of the solute relative to the volume flow can have values in a wide range limited by the inequality $(L_{11}L_{VV} - L_{V1}^2) > 0$. Therefore, reflection coefficients of a solute in the range $|\sigma_1| > 1$ should be observable under suitable conditions. On the basis of Eq. (22) it is expected that this should be possible if the absolute value the electric potential difference $|\Delta\tilde{\phi}|$ has large values ($|\Delta\tilde{\phi}|$ of the order of 10 mV). In principle, large values of $|\Delta\tilde{\phi}|$ can be generated using an electrolyte for the experiments for which the ratio $(\tilde{D}_{co}/\tilde{D}_{counter})$ of the effective diffusion coefficient of its ions in the membrane phase is sufficiently large and small compared with 1, respectively. The experimental realization of this concept using $-SO_3^-$ membranes appears to be not possible because the ratio of the effective diffusion coefficient of the ions of an electrolyte in the membrane phase has similar values than that in free solution. It turns out that the corresponding values of $|\Delta\tilde{\phi}|$ are not large enough to observe reflection coefficients with values $|\sigma_1| > 1$. The author is not aware of a publication in which experimentally determined reflection coefficients $|\sigma_1| > 1$ with a [polyelectrolyte gel membrane/single electrolyte, water] system are reported except for "mosaic" membranes (see Sec. IV).

The electrical potential difference $|\Delta\tilde{\phi}|$ can be increased strongly by adding a second electrolyte to the bulk phases. This makes it possible to generate values of the electrical potential difference $|\Delta\tilde{\phi}|$ of the order of 10 mV within the membrane phase even at low electrolyte concentrations in the bulk phases. They are generated by the diffusion of the counter ion species of the two electrolytes within the membrane in opposite directions (counter diffusion). For experiments with a cation exchange membrane ($\omega = -1$) it is convenient to choose pairs of electrolytes which have a common anion (e.g., HCl and NaCl).

1. Reflection Coefficient of HCl

Let us consider a system which has been studied experimentally [52]. A cation exchange membrane ($-SO_3^-$ membrane) with an effective fixed ion concentration $\tilde{X}_{eff}$ of about 0.4 mol/dm^3 pore fluid separates two aqueous solutions containing HCl and NaCl. For HCl there exists a concentration difference between the bulk phases ($c'(HCl) = 5 \times 10^{-3}$ mol/dm^3; $c''(HCl) = 2 \times 10^{-2}$ mol/dm^3). The concentration of NaCl in both bulk phases has the same value $c'(NaCl) = c''(NaCl) = c(NaCl)$. It is varied in the range $0 \leq c(NaCl) \leq 5$ mol/

dm^3. The concentration difference of HCl is maintained constant. This experimental situation is symbolized by [HCl Δc/NaCl)].

The reflection coefficient of HCl in such a system is defined by Eq. (26) which corresponds to that given by Eq. (10a).

$$\sigma(HCl) = \left[\frac{\Delta P}{\Delta\Pi(HCl)}\right]_{\Delta\Pi(NaCl)=0; \, J_V=0} \tag{26}$$

It describes also the experimental procedure of the determination of $\sigma(HCl)$.

Experimental results are shown in the upper part of Fig. 7 in which $\sigma(HCl)$ is plotted as function of the concentration ratio $c(NaCl)/\bar{c}(HCl)$. The curve starts at $\sigma(HCl) = 1$ for $c(NaCl)/\bar{c}(HCl) = 0$. With increasing values of ratio $c(NaCl)/\bar{c}(HCl)$ the reflection coefficient $\sigma(HCl)$ becomes larger than 1 reaches a maximum of $\sigma(HCl) \approx 2.5$ at $c(NaCl)/\bar{c}(HCl) \approx 5$ and decreases again.

This concentration dependence of $\sigma(HCl)$ can be understood in terms of the model of the membrane with narrow pores. The analysis is based on Eq. (27) which is analogous to Eq. (23).

$$\sigma(HCl) = -\left[\frac{\Delta\tilde{P} + F\tilde{X}\,\Delta\tilde{\phi}}{\Delta\Pi(HCl)}\right]_{\Delta\Pi(NaCl)=0; \, J_V=0} \tag{27}$$

The dependence of $[\Delta\tilde{P}]$ and $[F\tilde{X}\Delta\tilde{\phi}]_{J_V=0}$ on the concentration ratio $c(NaCl)/\bar{c}(HCl)$ is calculated using the model of the membrane with narrow pores.

The ratio of the concentrations of the Na^+ and the H^+ counter ions in the membrane phase has about the same value as the same ratio in the bulk phase [i.e., $c(H^+)/c(Na^+) = \tilde{C}(H^+)/\tilde{C}(Na^+)$]. This is found experimentally and is in agreement with the simplifying assumption on which the model of the membrane with narrow pores is based (Donnan relation for ideal dilute electrolyte solutions). Under the chosen condition of the experiment the ratio $[c(H^+)/c(Na^+)]$ is smaller in the left bulk phase than in the right bulk phase. Consequently at the two phase boundaries [membrane phase/bulk phase] the inequality $[\tilde{C}(H^+)/\tilde{C}(Na^+)]' < [\tilde{C}(H^+)/\tilde{C}(Na^+)]''$ holds. Therefore H^+ counter ions diffuse in the direction of their concentration gradient within the membrane phase from the right to left bulk phase. For Na^+ there exists a concentration gradient within the membrane in the opposite direction although the concentration of the Na^+ in both bulk phase has the same value. This counter diffusion of H^+ and Na^+ ions generates a comparatively large diffusion potential within the membrane. The ratio of the effective diffusion coefficients $\tilde{D}(H^+)/\tilde{D}(Na^+)$ has a value of about 7. Assuming that the membrane phase contains only ions belonging to one class of valency (single valent cations, H^+, Na^+) the electrical potential difference $[\Delta\tilde{\phi}]_{J_V=0}$ can be calculated using Eq. (28) [6].

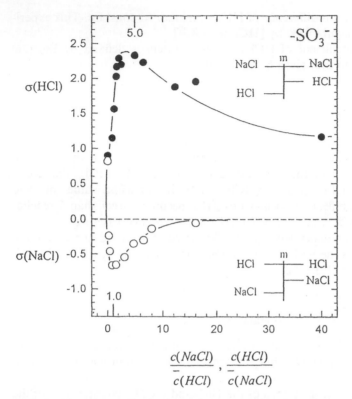

FIG. 7 Experimentally determined concentration dependence of the reflection coefficient of HCl (σ(HCl)) and NaCl (σ(NaCl)) with a phenolsulfonic acid/formaldehyde ($-SO_3^-$) membrane separating two aqueous electrolyte solutions containing HCl and NaCl. Upper part of Fig. 7: System HCl (Δc)/NaCl. The concentrations of HCl are kept constant. The concentration of NaCl which has the same value in both bulk phases is varied. Experimental conditions: c'(HCl) $= 5 \times 10^{-3}$ mol/dm^3; c''(HCl) $= 2 \times 10^{-2}$ mol/dm^3; c'(NaCl) $= c''$(NaCl) $= c$(NaCl); $0 \leq c$(NaCl) ≤ 5 mol/dm^3. $\bar{c}$(HCl) is the mean concentration of HCl between the bulk phases ($\bar{c}$(HCl) $= (c'$(HCl) $+ c''$(HCl))/2), $\bar{c}$(HCl) $= 1.25 \times 10^{-2}$ mol/dm^3. $T = 25°$C. Lower part of Fig. 7: System NaCl (Δc)/HCl. The concentrations of NaCl are kept constant. The concentration of HCl which has the same value in both bulk phases is varied. Experimental conditions: c'(NaCl) $= 5 \times 10^{-3}$ mol/dm^3; c''(NaCl) $= 2 \times 10^{-2}$ mol/dm^3; c'(HCl) $= c''$(HCl) $= c$(HCl); $0 \leq c$(HCl) ≤ 5 mol/dm^3. $\bar{c}$(NaCl) is the mean concentration of HCl between the bulk phases ($\bar{c}$(NaCl) $= (c'$(NaCl) $+ c''$(NaCl))/2), $\bar{c}$(NaCl) $= 1.25 \times 10^{-2}$ mol/dm^3. Data characterizing the membrane: water content y(H$_2$O, Na$^+$) $= 0.64$ (mass fraction of water); analytical fixed ion concentration $\tilde{X}_a$(Na$^+$) $= 1.37$ mol/dm^3 pore fluid; thickness, 0.1 cm.

$$[\Delta\tilde{\phi}]_{J_V=0} = \frac{RT}{F} \ln\left\{\frac{\sum_i \tilde{D}_i \tilde{C}_i''}{\sum_i \tilde{D}_i \tilde{C}_i'}\right\} \tag{28}$$

$$i = H^+, Na^+$$

Under that condition the flows of the H^+ and the Na^+ ions are coupled by the conditions of electroneutrality. But actually the membrane phase contains ions of two classes of valencies (single valent cations, H^+, Na^+ and single valent anions, Cl^-). A procedure has been worked out to calculate $[\Delta\tilde{\phi}]_{J_V=0}$ for this case [6].

A good estimate of $[\Delta\tilde{\phi}]_{J_V=0}$ can be obtained from the Nernst–Planck equation [see Eq. (13)] neglecting the convection term $(\tilde{c}_i j_V)$, using the constant electric field assumption (i.e., $[\Delta\tilde{\phi}]_{J_V=0}(x) = ([\Delta\tilde{\phi}]_{J_V=0} / \delta))$ [53]. This leads to Eq. (29) which is solved numerically for $[\Delta\tilde{\phi}]_{J_V=0}$.

$$\sum_i z_i \tilde{D}_i \frac{[\tilde{C}_i' - \tilde{C}_i'' \exp\{(z_i F/RT)\Delta\tilde{\phi}_{J_V=0}\}]}{1 - \exp\{(z_i F/RT)\Delta\tilde{\phi}_{J_V=0}\}} = 0 \tag{29}$$

Figure 8a shows the dependence of the term $[F\tilde{X}_{eff}\Delta\tilde{\phi}]_{J_V=0}$ on the concentration ratio $c(NaCl)/\bar{c}(HCl)$. The drawn out line represents $[\Delta\tilde{\phi}]_{J_V=0}$ data taking into account that the pore fluid contains H^+, Na^+ and Cl^- ions. The parameter values used for the calculation are $\tilde{X}_{eff} = 0.4$ mol/dm^3, $\tilde{D}(H^+) = 9.0 \times 10^{-5}$ cm^2/s, $\tilde{D}(Na^+) = 1.3 \times 10^{-5}$ cm^2/s, $\tilde{D}(Cl^-) = 2.0 \times 10^{-5}$ cm^2/s. The dashed line represents calculated $[\Delta\tilde{\phi}]_{J_V=0}$ data using Eq. (28) with $\tilde{X} = 0.4$ mol/dm^3, $\tilde{D}(H^+) = 9.0 \times 10^{-5}$ cm^2 s $\tilde{D}(Na^+) = 1.3 \times 10^{-5}$ cm^2/s. It is concluded that the presence of the coions (Cl^- ions) within the membrane phase has only a small influence on $[\Delta\tilde{\phi}]_{J_V=0}$.

Figure 8b shows the dependence of pressure $[\Delta\tilde{P}]$ on the concentration ratio $c(NaCl)/\bar{c}(HCl)$. $\Delta\tilde{P}$ is calculated using Eq. (15) in combination with the Donnan relations given by Eqs. (30) for $\omega = -1$.

$$\left(\frac{\tilde{C}_+}{c_+}\right) = \left\{1 + \left[\frac{\tilde{X}}{2c(HCl) + 2c(NaCl)}\right]^2\right\}^{1/2}$$
$$+ \frac{\tilde{X}}{2c(HCl) + 2c(NaCl)} \tag{30a}$$

$$\left(\frac{\tilde{C}_-}{c_-}\right) = \left\{1 + \left[\frac{\tilde{X}}{2c(HCl) + 2c(NaCl)}\right]^2\right\}^{1/2}$$
$$- \frac{\tilde{X}}{2c(HCl) + 2c(NaCl)} \tag{30b}$$

From the curves shown in Fig. 8 it is concluded that the term $[\Delta\tilde{P}]$ is small compared with term $[F\tilde{X}_{eff}\Delta\tilde{\phi}]_{J_V=0}$. This reflects the fact that for a gel with a fixed ion concentration of $\tilde{X} = 1$ mol/dm^3 pore fluid the driving force of an

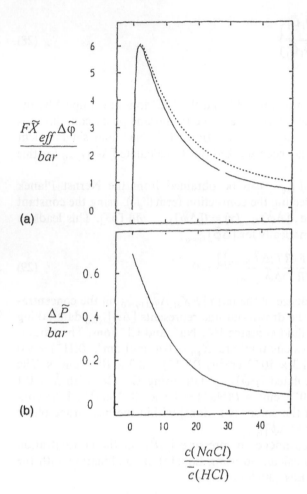

FIG. 8 Model of the membrane with narrow pores. System: HCl(Δc)/NaCl. Dependence of the quantities $[F\tilde{X}_{eff}\Delta\tilde{\phi}]_{Jv=0}$ and $[\Delta\tilde{P}]$ on the concentration ratio $[c(NaCl)/\bar{c}(HCl)]$ calculated on the basis this model for the membrane system described in the caption of the upper part of Fig. 7. ($\tilde{X}_{eff} = 0.4$ mol/dm^3 pore fluid.) For further details see text.

osmotic volume flow in form of an electrical potential difference $|\Delta\tilde{\phi}| = 1$ mV is equivalent to the driving force of a hydrostatic pressure difference of about 1 bar ($\Delta\tilde{P} = F\tilde{X}\Delta\tilde{\phi}$).

For values of the concentration ratio $[c(NaCl)/\bar{c}(HCl)] > 2.5$ the calculated $[F\tilde{X}_{eff}\Delta\tilde{\phi}]_{jv=0}$ vs. $[c(NaCl)/\bar{c}(HCl)]$ curve as well as the calculated $[\Delta\tilde{P}]$ vs. $[c(NaCl)/\bar{c}(HCl)]$ curve decrease monotonically with increasing values of

$[c(NaCl)/\bar{c}(HCl)]$. This indicates that the concentration difference of the mobile ions between the pore fluid and the bulk phase decreases with increasing values of $c(NaCl)/\tilde{X}$. This is expected on the basis of Eqs. (15).

The curve corresponding to the upper experimental $\sigma(HCl)$ vs. $[c(NaCl)/\bar{c}(HCl)]$ curve in Fig. 7 calculated from Eq. (27) is shown in the upper part of Fig. 9. At $[c(NaCl)/\bar{c}(HCl)] = 0$ there exists only a concentration difference of HCl between the bulk phases. The ratio $\bar{c}(HCl)/\tilde{X}$ is small compared to 1 and the membrane is impermeable to HCl. $\sigma(HCl)$ has the value $\sigma(HCl) \approx 1$. The term $[F\tilde{X}_{eff}\Delta\tilde{\phi}]_{J_V = 0}$ is close to zero and the ratio $[\Delta\tilde{P}/\Delta\Pi(HCl)]$ has the value 1. Adding NaCl makes a counter diffusion of H^+ and Na^+ possible. The

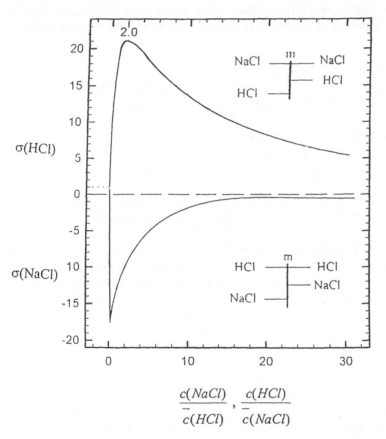

$$\frac{c(NaCl)}{\overline{c(HCl)}}, \frac{c(HCl)}{\overline{c(NaCl)}}$$

FIG. 9 Model of the membrane with narrow pores: Concentration dependence of the reflection coefficient of HCl ($\sigma(HCl)$) in the system HCl (Δc/NaCl) (upper curve) and that of NaCl $\sigma(NaCl)$ in the system NaCl (Δc)/HCl for the experimental condition given in the caption of Fig. 7. The calculation is based on Eqs. (27) and (31), respectively in combination with Eqs. (29) and (30).

term $[F\tilde{X}_{eff}\Delta\tilde{\phi}]_{Jv=0}$ becomes different from zero and positive. It has the same sign as the term $[\Delta\tilde{P}]$. The reflection coefficient $\sigma(HCl)$ becomes larger than 1. With increasing values of the concentration of NaCl the reflection coefficient $\sigma(HCl)$ increases because the term $[F\tilde{X}_{eff}\Delta\tilde{\phi}]_{Jv=0}$ increases, reaches a maximum and decreases again. It is evident that the concentration dependence of $\sigma(HCl)$ is mainly determined the concentration dependence of the term $[F\tilde{X}_{eff}\Delta\tilde{\phi}]_{Jv=0}$.

The dependence of the $\sigma(HCl)$ on $[c(NaCl)/\bar{c}(HCl)]$ is in qualitative agreement with the theoretical prediction. But the calculated values of $\sigma(HCl)$ are considerably larger than the experimentally determined values. The discrepancy is assumed to be caused mainly by the mentioned structural inhomogenieties of the membrane matrix of the $-SO_3^-$ membranes which could lead to local short circuiting of electrical potential differences within the membrane matrix.

2. Reflection Coefficient of NaCl

In the lower part of Fig. 7 the experimental data of the coefficient $\sigma(NaCl)$ of NaCl obtained with a $-SO_3^-$ membrane separating two bulk phases containing mixed electrolyte solutions (NaCl Δc/HCl) are shown. The reflection coefficient of NaCl in this system is defined by Eq. (31).

$$\sigma(NaCl) = -\left[\frac{\Delta\tilde{P} + F\tilde{X}\,\Delta\tilde{\phi}}{\Delta\Pi(NaCl)}\right]_{\Delta\Pi(HCl)=0;\,Jv=0} \tag{31}$$

For NaCl there exists a concentration difference between the bulk phases $(c'(NaCl) = 5 \times 10^{-3}$ mol/dm^{-3}, $c''(NaCl) = 2 \times 10^3$ mol/dm^3. The concentration of HCl in the bulk phases has the same value $(c'(HCl) = c''(HCl) = c(HCl); 0 \le c(HCl) \le 5$ mol/dm$^3)$. The concentration difference of NaCl is kept constant and the concentration of HCl is varied. On the basis of the model of the membrane with narrow pores a change of sign of $\sigma(NaCl)$ is expected to occur because $j_v(\Delta\tilde{P})$ and $j_v(\Delta\tilde{\phi})$ have different signs [54]. It is also predicted that the value of the absolute values of the reflection coefficient $\sigma(NaCl)$ in the system NaCl Δc/HCl at its minimum will be larger than the corresponding value in membrane systems with negative reflection coefficient and a single electrolyte in the solution forming the bulk phases (see Fig. 5b). Both predictions are in qualitative agreement with the experimental findings. The quantitative agreement between the theoretical predictions and the experimental data is again poor probably for the reasons given above. Reflection coefficients of NaCl smaller than $\sigma(NaCl) = -1$ were not observed in that system.

Results of hyperfiltration experiments with aqueous mixed HCl/NaCl solutions show that the sign of the hyperfiltration coefficient, see Eq. (12), is determined by the sign of the reflection coefficient of $\sigma(HCl)$ and $\sigma(HaCl)$, respectively [55].

There are many reports in the literature in which a transport of an electrolyte against its concentration difference in the bulk phases across polyelectrolyte gel membranes has been observed when the bulk phases contain a mixture of two electrolytes [56,57]. The experimental condition are especially simple if the two electrolytes have one ionic species in common (e.g., electrolytes HCl, KCl; membrane with $\omega = -1$). Teorell was the first to study such systems [58–61].

IV. MOSAIC MEMBRANES

Reflection coefficients of a solute smaller than $\sigma_1 = -1$ have been observed with composite gel membranes consisting of small patches with negatively charged fixed ionic groups ($\omega = -1$) and positively charged fixed ionic groups ($\omega = +1$) forming a mosaic like structure [62,63]. The mosaic membranes separate two aqueous solutions of a single electrolyte of different concentrations. A treatment of such a system in terms of the thermodynamic of irreversible processes is given in Ref. [64]. The hyperfiltration using mosaic membranes is discussed in Ref. 19.

The model of the membrane with narrow pores is used to analyse qualitatively the process causing a large negative osmotic volume flow (as well as a large electrolyte flow) under isobaric conditions which lead to reflection coefficient of the solute $\sigma_1 < -1$. It is assumed that the left bulk phase of a mosaic membrane [phase (')] is more concentrated than the right bulk phase [phase (")]. They are formed by dilute solutions of the same $(1, -1)$ valent electrolyte (e.g., NaCl). To make the arguments as simple as possible the following additional assumptions are made [65]:

1. The fixed ion concentration of the regions with negatively charged groups ($\omega = -1$) and that of the regions with positively charged groups ($\omega = +1$) has the same value ($\tilde{X}_{\omega=-1} = \tilde{X}_{\omega=+1} = \tilde{X}$). The fixed ion concentration $\tilde{X}$ of the two regions is large compared with the electrolyte solution in the bulk phases ($c_1/\tilde{X} \ll 1$). Then the patches are impermeable to the respective coions ($\tilde{C}_{+,\omega=-1} = \tilde{X}, \tilde{C}_{-,\omega=-1} = 0; \tilde{C}_{-,\omega=+1} = \tilde{X}, \tilde{C}_{+,\omega=+1} = 0$).
2. The effective diffusion coefficient of the counter ions in the region with $\omega = -1$ has the same value as that in the region with $\omega = +1$ ($\tilde{D}_{counter,\omega=-1} = \tilde{D}_{counter,\omega=+1} = \tilde{D}_{counter}$). The same is true for the mechanical permeability ($\tilde{d}_{h,\omega=-1} = \tilde{d}_{h,\omega=+1} = \tilde{d}_h$).
3. The area of the two kinds of regions in contact with the bulk phases has the same value ($a_{\omega=-1} = a_{\omega=+1} = a$; total membrane area, $a_{total} = 2a$).

The qualitative analysis of the osmotic properties of mosaic membranes proceeds in two steps. It is assumed that the regions forming the mosaic mem-

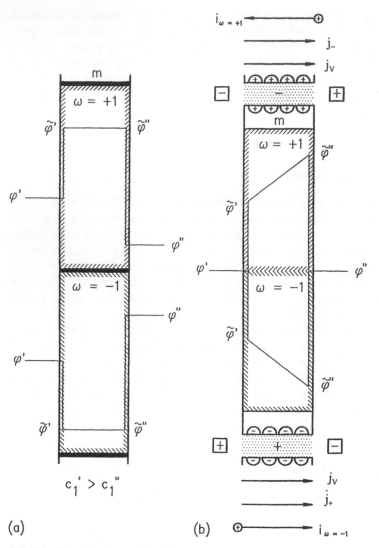

FIG. 10 Negative osmosis with a mosaic membrane consisting of patches with negatively charged fixed groups ($\omega = -1$) and positively charged fixed groups ($\omega = +1$). Two of these patches are shown schematically under two experimental conditions. In Fig. 10a the patches are assumed to be electrically isolated from each other. In Fig. 10b the patches are electrically short circuited by the electrically conducting bulk phases. For details see the text. $\rightarrow i_\omega$ indicates the direction of the local electric current density through membrane patches with fixed charges of sign ω carried by positively charged particles. The electric current densities $\rightarrow i_{\omega=-1}$ and $i_{\omega=+1}\leftarrow$ are caused by short circuiting of the membrane potentials of the different membrane patches by the electrically conducting bulk phases.

brane are electrically isolated from one another (see Fig. 10a):

At the phase boundaries (membrane patch with $\omega = -1$/bulk phase] the Donnan potentials $[\delta\phi = \tilde{\phi} - \phi]_{\omega=-1}$ have negative values. The absolute value of $|\delta\phi'|$ at the left phase boundary is smaller than the corresponding value $|\delta\phi''|$ at the right phase boundary because the concentration c_1' is larger than c_1''. The electrical potential difference $[\Delta\phi = \phi' - \phi'']_{\omega=-1}$ between the bulk phases has a negative value $(\Delta\phi_{\omega=-1} = (RT/F)\ln(c_1''/c_1'))$. The electrical potential difference $[\Delta\tilde{\phi} = \tilde{\phi}' - \tilde{\phi}'']_{\omega=-1}$ within each membrane patch is zero because the membrane is assumed to be impermeable to the coions (Cl^- ions).

For membrane patches with $\omega = +1$ the Donnan potentials $[\delta\phi = \tilde{\phi} - \phi]_{\omega=+1}$ are positive. The electrical potential jump $[\delta\phi']_{\omega=+1}$ at the left phase boundary [membrane phase/bulk phase) is smaller than the corresponding potential jump $[\delta\phi'']_{\omega=+1}$ at the right phase boundary. The electrical potential difference $[\Delta\phi = \phi' - \phi'']_{\omega=+1}$ between the bulk phases has a positive value $([\Delta\phi_{\omega=+1} = (RT/F)\ln(c_1'/c_1''))$. The potential difference $[\Delta\tilde{\phi} = \tilde{\phi}' - \tilde{\phi}'']_{\omega=+1}$ within the membrane is zero because the membrane is assumed to be impermeable to the coions (Na^+ ions).

The regions of a mosaic membrane are electrically short circuited (see Fig. 10b). The electrical isolation between the areas of the mosaic membrane with $\omega = -1$ and $\omega = +1$ is removed. The local electrical potential differences at the two interfaces [mosaic membrane/external bulk phase] are short circuited because the bulk phases are electrically conducting media. Under the assumed properties of the patches the electrical potential difference between the bulk phases vanishes $(\Delta\phi = (\phi' - \phi'') = 0)$. This generates a drop of the electrical potential within the regions with $\omega = -1$ and $\omega = +1$ $((\tilde{\phi}' - \tilde{\phi}'')_{\omega=-1} > 0$; $(\tilde{\phi}' - \tilde{\phi}'')_{\omega=+1} < 0$; $(\tilde{\phi}' - \tilde{\phi}'')_{\omega=-1} + (\tilde{\phi}' - \tilde{\phi}'')_{\omega=+1} = 0$; $(\tilde{\phi}' - \tilde{\phi}'')_{\omega=-1} = (RT/F)\ln(c_1'/c_1''))$. This situation is shown schematically in Fig. 10b. Local circulating electrical currents pass the mosaic membrane. In the membrane regions with $\omega = -1$ the electric current is carried selectively by cations (Na^+ ions) and in the membrane regions with $\omega = +1$ selectively by anions (Cl^-). Both ion flow are coupled by the condition of electroneutrality. The electric potential differences within the membrane phase $(\tilde{\phi}' - \tilde{\phi}'')_{\omega=-1}$ and $(\tilde{\phi}' - \tilde{\phi}'')_{\omega=+1}$ are driving forces of an volume flow density across the short circuited regions of the mosaic membrane $([J_v(\Delta\tilde{\phi})]_\omega = [a\tilde{d}_h/\delta][-F\omega\tilde{X}\Delta\tilde{\phi}]_\omega)$. The result is a comparatively large negative osmotic volume flow directed from the more concentrated into the more dilute bulk phase (total volume flow density under the stated conditions: $J_{v,\,total} = 2a(\tilde{d}/\delta)[F\tilde{X}|\Delta\tilde{\phi}|]$. Coupled with this comparatively large volume flow is an enhanced salt flow (see Fig. 10b).

The concept of local electric currents circulating through a membrane composed of regions with negative and positive charged fixed groups has been studied in detail [66–68].

V. EARLY STUDIES OF OSMOSIS WITH "LEAKY" MEMBRANES IN CONTACT WITH AQUEOUS ELECTROLYTE SOLUTIONS

Osmotic membrane phenomena were first described in the literature by Nollet in 1748 [69]. The first quantitative measurements of osmotic volume flows across membranes were carried out about 100 years later by Dutrochet [70–74], Vierrodt [75] and Graham [76]. In these experiments an animal membrane (pig's bladder) separated an aqueous electrolyte solution from water. Using an osmometric device phenomena were observed which are now called positive and negative osmosis. These terms were first used by Graham (1854). Dutrochet (1827) called them endosmosis (positive osmosis) and exosmosis (negative osmosis). The results of the experiments established that the volume flow density across the membranes depends on the nature of electrolyte and on its concentration. Further experiments demonstrated that the nature of the membrane does also influence on the observed osmotic phenomena and that both components of the bulk phases, the electrolyte and water, pass the membrane ("leaky" membranes).

The observation that the properties of the membrane influence the osmotic phenomena led Graham to use membranes for the separation of different substances by dialysis and to the characterization of substances as "crystalloids" and "colloids". The existence of membranes which were permeable to crystalloids and more or less impermeable to colloids triggered the search for membranes in which the osmotic volume flow is caused only by the transport of water. Traube (1867) found that certain types of precipitation membrane (e.g., copper ferrocyanide membranes) have the desired property [77]. This discovery and Pfeffer's procedure (1877) to form copper ferrocyanide membrane in a ceramic wall made studies of the osmotic equilibrium pressure possible [78–80]. The results of these measurements stimulated Van't Hoff to develop his theory of solutions [81]. He introduced the term semipermeable membrane ("halb durchläßige Wand") for a membrane which is permeable to only one component of a binary solution. The existence of semipermeable membranes helped to understand the water transport phenomena in biological cells [82].

Only few publications dealing with the osmotic properties of "leaky" membranes in contact with aqueous electrolyte solutions appeared in the literature at the turn of the 19th century. At that time, interest was focused on studies of the osmotic equilibrium in binary solutions using semipermeable membranes instigated by Van't Hoff's theory of solutions. The situation changed around 1910 with a series of publications by Loeb [83–95] and Bartell and coworkers [96–101]. The experimental set up used for the experiments was simple: A membrane (e.g., collodion, unglazed porcelain, gold beaters skin (cattle cecum), calves bladder, and parchment paper) in form of a sack or a flat membrane closed one side of a glass tube and separated an aqueous electrolyte solution of known concentration from water or a more dilute electrolyte solution. A vertically oriented capillary was attached to the sack or the glass tube and the height of the meniscus of the more concentrated solution in the capillary was measured after fixed times. The pressure difference which developed between the bulk phases was only transient because the membranes were permeable to the solvent and the solute. Such experiments were carried out as function of the electrolyte concentration. Usually, the composition of only one of the external phases was changed and that of the other was kept constant. The effective pore radius of the different membranes varied and covered a wide range from "narrow" to "wide" pores. In most experiments no efforts were made to keep the composition of the bulk phases homogeneous during the experiment. Investigations of Preuner and Roder (1923) demonstrated the strong influence of unstirred layers on the osmotic data [102]. Concentration polarizations at the membrane surface change the effective osmotic differences between the bulk phases. This makes a quantitative analysis of the older osmotic data in which the bulk phases were not stirred impossible.

The conjecture that electrokinetic processes play central role in the physics of positive and negative osmosis with "leaky" membranes was first started out by Graham [76]. This idea was taken up again by Bartell. He assumed that the pore wall of the membrane carries electric charges which are electrically compensated by mobile counter ions of opposite sign. This gives the pore fluid an electrical charge density with positive and negative sign, respectively, depending on the sign of the charges at the pore wall. In the osmotic experiments the concentration of the electrolyte in the bulk phases has different values and an electrical potential difference (diffusion potential) develops between the bulk phases. This potential difference acts as the driving force for a volume flow across the membrane. Depending on the sign of this potential difference and the sign of the charges on the pore wall positive or negative osmosis will be observed.

Freundlich (1916) had the opinion, at least for a certain time [103], that an electro-osmotic volume flow across the membrane assumed by Bartell is only possible if a closed electric current passes the membrane [104]. Bartell thought that the local electric currents in forward and backward direction passes through the same pore, in forward direction through the electrical double layer and in backward direction through the centre of the pore [101]. Sollner (1930) criticized this assumption of Bartell that positive or negative osmosis can take place in a single pore. He thought that an electroosmotic volume flow can only be generated by electric currents driven by an external source [104–106].

Söllner assumed that several neighbouring pores with different pore radii form an electroosmotic circuit. Following his arguments this concept leads for example to the following situations in two neighbouring pores of a membrane with a negatively charged matrix:

1. Two narrow pores with different radii are considered. The fixed ion concentration (per unit volume of the pore fluid) in the narrower pore is larger than that in wider pore. Therefore, the electrical potential difference between the ends of the narrower pore is larger than that of the wider pore. The presence of more coions in the wider pore lowers the electrical potential difference between the ends. The higher electrical potential difference at the narrower pore acts as an electric current source for an electroosmotic volume flow through the wider pore. Positively charged carrier of electric current pass the wider pore from the more dilute to the more concentrated bulk phase and cause a positive osmosis.

2. Two wide pores of different radii are considered. In pores diffusion potentials with different values are generated. It is assumed that the mobility of the coions in the pores is higher than that of the counterions. In this case the drop of the electric potential in the more narrow pore is smaller than that in the wider pore. The higher potential difference at the wider pore acts as an electric current source for an electroosmotic volume flow through the more narrow pore. Positively charged carrier of electric current pass the narrower pore from the more concentrated to the more dilute bulk phase and cause a negative osmosis.

Schlögl objected to this explanation of the osmotic phenomena with leaky membrane for reasons which are given in detail in Ref. 42. Using the model of the membrane with narrow pores he could show that positive and negative osmosis can occur in a single pore of a membrane without invoking the concept of local circulating local electric currents. His theoretical treatment and that of Kuhn and Läuger is in very good agreement with all experimental osmotic data obtained with polyelectrolyte gels.

VI. CONCLUSION

It is concluded that the physics of the anomalous positive and negative osmosis observed with aqueous electrolyte solutions and polyelectrolyte gel membranes is very well understood in terms of the model of the membrane with narrow pores. The essential requirement of the applicability of the model is that the characteristic length of the porous structure of the membrane be small compared to the Debye length so that the counter ions and the coions present in the pore fluid are distributed homogeneously over the cross-section of the voids by the thermal motion of the ions (i.e., for membrane with a fixed ion concentration $\bar{X}$ of about 1 mol/dm^3, characteristic length, order of magnitude, 1 nm).

ACKNOWLEDGMENT

This manuscript is based on a series of lectures the author has given as a Carl Schurz Professor in the Department of Chemistry of the University of Wisconsin in Madison, Wisconsin in the summer of 1997. He thanks Professor H. Yu for his generous hospitality and the Carl Schurz Professorship Committee of the University of Wisconsin for its support.

VII. LIST OF SYMBOLS

a	membrane area [cm^2]
c_i	molar volume concentration of species i[mol/dm^3], [mol cm/dm^3]
$\tilde{c}_i$	arithmetic mean value of the molar volume concentration of species i[mol/dm^3], [mol/cm^3]
$\bar{C}_i$	molar volume concentration of species i in the membrane phase [mol/dm^3 pore fluid], [mol/cm^3 pore fluid]
$\tilde{d}_h$	specific mechanical permeability of the membrane phase [cm^5/J/s]
$\tilde{D}_i$	effective diffusion coefficient of species i in the membrane phase [cm^2/s]
$\tilde{D}^{\cdot}$	measure of the mechanical permeability, $\tilde{D}^{\cdot} = \tilde{d}_h \tilde{X} RT$[cm^2/s]
F	Faraday number, $F = 96{,}487$ A/s/mol
I	electrical current [A]
j_i	molar flow density of species i[mol/cm^2/s]
j_V	volume flow density [cm/s]
J_i	molar flow of species i relative to the membrane [mol/s]
J_i^*	molar flow of species i relative to the volume flow [mol/s]
J_V	volume flow [cm^3/s]
L_{ii}, L_{ik}	phenomenological transport coefficients
n_i	amount of substance of species i[mol]
P	pressure [bar], [J/cm^3]
R	universal gas constant, $R = 8.314$ J/K/mol
S	entropy [J/K]
t	time [s]
T	thermodynamic temperature [K]
V	volume [cm^3]
V_i	partial molar volume [mol/cm^3]
x	space coordinate [cm]
$\tilde{X}$	fixed ion concentration [mol/dm^3 pore fluid] [mol/cm^3 pore fluid]
z_i	valency of the charged species i including the sign; $z_+ > 0$; $z_- < 0$.

α	phase index (') ('')
δ	thickness of the membrane [cm]
Δ	differences of thermodynamic parameters between the bulk phases $\Delta = (') - ('')$
$\tilde{\kappa}$	specific conductivity of the membrane phase $[\Omega^{-1}/\text{cm}]$
μ_i	chemical potential of species $i[\text{J/mol}]$
ν_i	stoichiometric number of an electrolyte $A_{\nu+}B_{\nu-}$
ξ	characteristic length of the porous structure of the gel forming the mem brane [nm]
Π_i	osmotic value of species $i[\text{J/cm}^3]$; 1 J/cm^3 = 10 bar
σ_i	reflection coefficient of species $i[1]$
ϕ	electrical potential [mV]
ω	sign of the fixed charges [1]
0 (index)	solvent
1 (index)	solute
~ (superscript)	membrane phase
⁻ (superscript)	mean value

APPENDIX

A. Simplification of Eqs. (A1) and (A2)

The expressions of the driving forces ΔX_V and ΔX_1^* given by Eqs. (A1) [see Eq. (5b)] and (A2) [see Eq. (5c)] have a complex form.

$$\Delta X_V = \bar{c}_0 \, \Delta\mu_0 + \bar{c}_1 \Delta\mu_1 = \Delta P + \left\{ \bar{c}_1 \left[\Delta_c \mu_1 - \frac{V_1}{V_0} \Delta_c \mu_0 \right] + \frac{\Delta_c \mu_0}{V_0} \right\} \tag{A1}$$

$$\Delta X_1^* = \Delta_c \mu_0 - \frac{V_1}{V_0} \Delta_c \mu_1 \tag{A2}$$

For membrane systems close to equilibrium separating two bulk phases formed by dilute solutions these equations take on a simple form.

1. Simplification of Eq. (A1)

It will be shown that for the membrane systems just mentioned the term in brackets { } in Eq. (A1) vanishes for the special choice of $\bar{c}_1$ given by Eq. (A3) and ΔX_V takes on the simple form $\Delta X_V = \Delta P$ (see Eq. (6)).

$$\bar{c}_1 = \frac{\Delta \cdot c_1}{\ln(c_1'/c_1'')} \approx 2 \frac{\Delta \cdot c_1}{c_1' + c_1''} \tag{A3}$$

Taylor series expansion of $\ln(c_1'/c_1'')$ which is broken off after the first term

$$\left(\ln z = 2 \frac{z-1}{z+1} \quad \text{with } z = c_1'/c_1'' \right).$$

The starting point is the Gibbs–Duhem equation (T, P = const.) in an averaged form given by Eq. (A4).

$$\bar{c}_0 \Delta_c \mu_0 + \bar{c}_1 \Delta_c \mu_1 = 0 \qquad (A4)$$

$\Delta_c \mu_0$ and $\Delta_c \mu_1$ are given by Eqs. (A5) and (A6).

$$\Delta_c \mu_0 = -RTV_0 \Delta c_1 \qquad (A5)$$
$$\Delta_c \mu_1 = RT \ln(c_1'/c_1'') \qquad (A6)$$

Substitution of Eqs. (A5) and (A6) into Eq. (A3) leads to Eq. (A7).

$$\bar{c}_0 = \frac{1}{V_0} \qquad (A7)$$

If it is assumed that $\bar{c}_1 V_1 \ll 1$ Eq. (A7) follows immediately from the thermodynamic relation $\bar{c}_0 V_0 + \bar{c}_1 V_1 = 1$.
Taking into account Eq. (A7) in Eq. (A1) the expression in brackets { } vanishes: $\Delta X_V = \Delta P$ [see Eq. (6)].

2. Simplification of Eq. (A2)

It will be shown that for the membrane systems close to equilibrium separating two bulk phases formed by dilute two component Eq. (2) takes on a simple form $\Delta X_1^* = \Delta\Pi_1/\bar{c}_1$ [see Eq. (7a)].
For dilute solutions ($\bar{c}_1 V_1 \ll 1$) and small concentration differences $\Delta_c \mu_1$ is given by Eqs. (A8).

$$\bar{c}_1 \Delta X_1^* = \bar{c}_1 \Delta_c \mu_1 - \frac{\bar{c}_1 \cdot V_1}{V_0} \Delta_c \mu_0 \approx \bar{c}_1 \Delta_c \mu_1 \qquad (A8a)$$

with

$$\Delta_c \mu_1 = RT \ln(c_1'/c_1'') \approx RT \, \Delta c_1/\bar{c}_1 \qquad (A8b)$$

and $c_1'' \approx \bar{c}_1$.
If component 1 is an strong electrolyte $C_{v_+} A_{v_-}$ Eqs. (A8) are transformed to Eqs. (A9).

$$\bar{c}_1 \Delta X_1^* = \Delta\Pi_1 \qquad (A9a)$$

with

$$\Delta\Pi_1 = RT(v_+ + v_-)\Delta c_1 \qquad (A9b)$$

B. Derivation of an Expression of the Electrical Potential Difference at Zero Electrical Current Flow $[\Delta\tilde\phi]_{J_V=0}$ Within a Gel Membrane with Fixed Charges of Sign $\omega(= +1, -1)$ Separating Two Aqueous Solutions of a Single (z_+, z_-) Valent Electrolyte on the Basis of the Model of the Membrane with Narrow Pores

The starting point is the Nernst–Planck equation for ionic species $i(= +, -)$:

$$j_i = -\tilde D_i\left[\frac{d\tilde C_i}{dx} + z_i\,\tilde C_i\,\frac{F}{RT}\frac{d\tilde\phi}{dx}\right] \tag{A10}$$

No electric current passes the membrane and the molar flow densities of the cations and the anions are related by Eq. (A11).

$$z_+\,Fj_+ + z_-\,Fj_- = 0 \tag{A11}$$

Combination of Eqs. (A10) and (A11) leads to Eq. (A12).

$$[z_+\,\tilde D_+\,d\tilde C_+ + z_-\,d\tilde C_-]$$
$$+ [z_+^2\,\tilde D_+\,\tilde C_+ + z_-^2\,\tilde D_-\,\tilde C_-]\frac{RT}{F}\,[d\tilde\phi]_{J_V=0} = 0 \tag{A12}$$

$\tilde C_+$ and $\tilde C_-$ are related by the condition of electroneutrality in the pore fluid. Differential changes of the concentrations of $\tilde C_+$ and of $\tilde C_-$ in the pore fluid cause differential changes of the total concentration $\tilde C(=\tilde C_+ + \tilde C_-)$ of the mobile ions in the pore fluid. They are given by Eqs. (A13).

$$d\tilde C_+ = -\frac{z_-}{z_+ - z_-}\,d\tilde C \quad\text{and}\quad d\tilde C_- = \frac{z_+}{z_+ - z_-}\,d\tilde C \tag{A13}$$

Combination of $\tilde C = \tilde C_+ + \tilde C_-$ with $z_+\tilde C_+ + z_-\tilde C_- + \omega\tilde X = 0$ leads to Eqs. (A14).

$$\tilde C_+ = -\frac{z_-\,\tilde C + \omega\tilde X}{z_+ - z_-} \tag{A14a}$$

$$\tilde C_- = \frac{z_+\,\tilde C + \omega\tilde X}{z_+ - z_-} \tag{A14b}$$

Combination of Eqs. (A12), (A13) and (A14) gives Eq. (A15) which can rearranged to given Eqs. (A16).

$$(\tilde D_+ - \tilde D_-)d\tilde C + \left[(z_+\,\tilde D_+ - z_-\,\tilde D_-)\tilde C\right.$$
$$\left. + \left(\frac{z_+}{z_-}\,\tilde D_+ - \frac{z_-}{z_+}\,\tilde D_-\right)\omega\tilde X\right]\frac{RT}{F}\,[d\tilde\phi]_{J_V=0} \tag{A15}$$

$$\frac{F}{RT}\,[d\tilde\phi]_{J_V=0} = -\tilde U\,\frac{d\tilde C}{\tilde C - \tilde V\omega\tilde X} \tag{A16a}$$

with

$$\tilde{U} = \frac{\tilde{D}_+ - \tilde{D}_-}{z_+ \tilde{D}_+ - z_- \tilde{D}_-} \quad \text{and} \quad \tilde{V} = \frac{-\dfrac{z_+}{z_-} \tilde{D}_+ + \dfrac{z_-}{z_+} \tilde{D}_-}{z_+ \tilde{D}_+ - z_- \tilde{D}_-} \tag{A16b}$$

Integration of Eq. (A16a) between the two phase boundaries [membrane phase/bulk phase] results in Eq. (A17).

$$\left[\frac{F}{RT} \Delta\tilde{\phi} \right]_{J_V=0, I=0} = (\tilde{\phi}' - \tilde{\phi}'')_{J_V=0} = \tilde{U} \ln \frac{\tilde{C}'' - \tilde{V}\omega\tilde{X}}{\tilde{C}' - \tilde{V}\omega\tilde{X}} \tag{A17}$$

C. Derivation of an Expression of Reflection Coefficient σ_1 of Single (z_+, z_-) Valent Electrolyte for a Gel Membrane with Fixed Charges of Sign $\omega(=+1, -1)$ on the Basis of the Model of the Membrane with Narrow Pores

The pressure difference $\Delta P(= P' - P'')$ which has to be applied between the bulk phases of a gel membrane to suppress the osmotic volume flow caused by an osmotic difference $\Delta\Pi_1(= RT(v_+ + v_-)\Delta c_1)$ of a single binary (z_+, z_-) valent electrolyte is given by Eq. (A18).

$$\Delta P = -[\Delta\tilde{P} - F\omega\tilde{X} \Delta\tilde{\phi}]_{J_V=0} \tag{A18}$$

The pressure difference $\Delta\tilde{P}$ is given by Eq. (A19) which follows from Eq. (17).

$$\Delta\tilde{P} = RT[(\tilde{C}' - \tilde{C}'') - (c' - c'')] = \left[\frac{\tilde{C}' - \tilde{C}''}{c' - c''} - 1 \right]\Delta\Pi_1 \tag{A19}$$

with $\tilde{C} = \tilde{C}_+ + \tilde{C}_-$ and $c = c_+ + c_-$. The electrical potential difference $[\Delta\tilde{\phi}]_{J_V=0, I=0}$ is given by Eq. (A17) (see Appendix B). Combining Eqs. (A17), (A18), and (A19) leads to Eq. (A20).

$$\sigma_1 = \left[\frac{\omega\tilde{X}\tilde{U}}{c' - c''} \ln\left\{ \frac{\tilde{C}'' - \tilde{V}\omega\tilde{X}}{\tilde{C}' - \tilde{V}\omega\tilde{X}} \right\} - \frac{\tilde{C}' - \tilde{C}''}{c' - c''} + 1 \right]_{J_V=0} \tag{A20}$$

with $\Delta\Pi_1 = RT(c' - c'')$.

It is assumed that the concentration difference of the electrolyte between the bulk phases is small. In this case the term $\tilde{C}' - \tilde{C}''/c' - c''$ in Eq. (A20) can be written in the form given by Eq. (A21c) and the logarithmic term in the same equation can be developed into a power series which can be broken off after the second term [see Eq. (A22)].

The derivation of Eq. (A21c) starts with Eq. (A21a)

$$\frac{\tilde{C}' - \tilde{C}''}{c' - c''} = \frac{d\tilde{C}}{dc} = \frac{d\tilde{C}_+}{dc_+} = \frac{d\tilde{C}_-}{dc_-} \tag{A21a}$$

The Donnan relation of a z_+, z_- valent electrolyte is given by Eq. (21b).

$$(\tilde{C}_+)^{z_-} \cdot (\tilde{C}_-)^{-z_+} = (c_+)^{z_-} \cdot (c_-)^{-z_+} \tag{A21b}$$

Taking the logarithm of Eq. (A21b) and differentiation of the resulting expression leads to Eq. (A21c) if the condition of the electroneutrality in its differential form in the membrane phase $(z_+ d\tilde{C}_+ + z_- d\tilde{C}_- = 0)$ and in the bulk phase $(z_+ dc_+ + z_- dc_- = 0)$ is taken into account.

$$\frac{d\tilde{C}_+}{dc_+} = \frac{d\tilde{C}}{dc} = \frac{\tilde{C}' - \tilde{C}''}{c' - c''} = \frac{(z_+^2 c_+ + z_-^2 c_-)\tilde{C}_+ \tilde{C}_-}{(z_+^2 \tilde{C}_+ + z_-^2 \tilde{C}_-)c_+ c_-} \tag{A21c}$$

$$\ln\left\{\frac{\tilde{C}'' - \tilde{V}\omega\tilde{X}}{\tilde{C}' - \tilde{V}\omega\tilde{X}}\right\} = \ln\left\{1 + \frac{\tilde{C}'' - \tilde{C}'}{\tilde{C}' - \tilde{V}\omega\tilde{X}}\right\} \approx \frac{\tilde{C}'' - \tilde{C}'}{\tilde{C}' - \tilde{V}\omega\tilde{X}} \tag{A22}$$

Combining Eqs. (A20), (A21c), and (A22) leads to Eq. (A23).

$$\sigma_1 = 1 - \left[\frac{(z_+^2 c_+ + z_-^2 c_-)\tilde{C}_+ \tilde{C}_-}{(z_+^2 \tilde{C}_+ + z_-^2 \tilde{C}_-)c_+ c_-} \cdot \frac{\tilde{C} + (\tilde{U} - \tilde{V})\omega\tilde{X}}{\tilde{C} - \tilde{V}\omega\tilde{X}}\right] \tag{A23}$$

with

$$\tilde{U} - \tilde{V} = \frac{z_+ + z_-}{z_+ z_-} \quad \text{and} \quad \tilde{C} = \tilde{C}_+ + \tilde{C}_-$$

Equation (A23) takes on the form given by Eq. (A24) when the condition of the electroneutrality in the membrane phase $(z_+ \tilde{C}_+ + z_- \tilde{C}_- + \omega\tilde{X} = 0)$ and in the bulk phases $(z_+ c_+ + z_- c_- = 0)$ are taken into account.

$$\sigma_1 = 1 - \frac{z_+^2(\tilde{D}_+ \tilde{C}_+/\tilde{D}_- \tilde{C}_-)(\tilde{C}_-/c_-) + (\tilde{C}_+/c_+)}{z_+^2(\tilde{D}_+ \tilde{C}_+/\tilde{D}_- \tilde{C}_-) + z_-^2} \tag{A24}$$

REFERENCES

1. A. Katchalsky and P. F. Curran, *Nonequilibrium Thermodynamics in Biophysics*, Harvard University Press, Cambridge, Massachusetts, 1965.
2. R. Haase, *Thermodynamics of Irreversible Processes*, Dover Publications, New York, 1969.
3. S. R. de Groot and P. Mazur, *Nonequilibrium Thermodynamics*, Dover Publications, New York, 1984.
4. K. S. Forland, T. Forland, and S. K. Ratje, *Irreversible Thermodynamics*, John Wiley Chichester, 1989.
5. R. Schlögl, Naturwissenschaften 50: 169 (1963).
6. R. Schlögl, *Stofftransport durch Membranen*. Steinkopff Verlag, Darmstadt, 1964.
7. F. A. H. Schreinemakers, *Lectures on Osmosis*. G. Naeffe, The Hague, 1938.
8. P. Meixner and H. G. Reik, *Handbuch der Physik*, Springer Verlag, Berlin, 1959, Vol. III, p. 413.
9. F. Sauer, in *Handbook of Physiology*, American Physiological Society, 1973, p. 399.

10. Y. Kobatake, J. Chem. Phys. *28*: 146 (1958).
11. Y. Kobatake, J. Chem. Phys. *28*: 442 (1958).
12. A. J. Stavermann, Rec. Trav. Chim. Pays. Bas. *70*: 344 (1951).
13. A. J. Stavermann, Rec. Trav. Chim. Pays. Bas. *71*: 623 (1952).
14. A. J. Stavermann, Trans. Faraday. Soc. *48*: 176 (1952).
15. L. O. Kedem and A. Katchalsky, J. Gen. Physiol. *45*: 143 (1961).
16. E. Hofer and O. Kedem, Desalination *5*: 167 (1968).
17. W. Pusch and D. Woermann, Naturwissenschaften *55*: 228 (1968).
18. W. Pusch and D. Woermann, Ber. Bunsenges. Phys. Chem. *74*: 444 (1970).
19. F. B. Leitz, in *Membrane Separation* (P. Meares, ed.), Elsevier Scientific, Amsterdam, 1976, p. 261.
20. T. Teorell, Proc. Soc. Exp. Biol. Med. *334*: 282 (1935).
21. T. Teorell, Trans. Faraday Soc. *33*: 1053, 1086 (1937).
22. T. Teorell, Ber. Bunsenges. Phys. Chem. Z. Elektrochem. *55*: 460, (1951).
23. T. Teorell, Prog. Biophys. *3*: 305 (1953).
24. K. H. Meyer and J. F. Sievers, Helv. Chim. Acta. *19*: 649 (1936).
25. K. H. Meyer and J. F. Sievers, Helv. Chim. Acta. *19*: 665 (1936).
26. K. H. Meyer and J. F. Sievers, Helv. Chim. Acta. *19*: 987 (1936).
27. G. Schmid, Ber. Bunsenges. Phys. Chem. Z. Elektrochem. *54*: 424 (1950).
28. G. Schmid, Ber. Bunsenges. Phys. Chem. Z. Elektrochem. *55*: 229 (1951).
29. G. Schmid and H. Schwarz, Ber. Bunsenges. Phys. Chem. Z. Elektrochem. *55*: 295 (1951).
30. G. Schmid and H. Schwarz, Ber. Bunsenges. Phys. Chem. Z. Elektrochem. *55*: 684 (1951).
31. G. Schmid and G. Schwarz, Ber. Bunsenges. Phys. Chem. Z. Elektrochem. *56*: 35 (1952).
32. G. Schmid, Ber. Bunsenges. Phys. Chem. Z. Elektrochem. *56*: 181 (1952).
33. P. Läuger and W. Kuhn, Ber. Bunsenges. Phys. Chem. *68*: 4 (1964).
34. Extensive work has been devoted to the development of a model to treat the transport processes across membranes with a charged matrix and wide pores.
35. W. Kuhn, P. Läuger, H. Voellmy, R. Bloch, and H. Mayer, Ber. Bunsenges. Phys. Chem. *67*: 364 (1963).
36. P. Läuger, Ber. Bunsenges. Phys. Chem. *68*: 352 (1964).
37. T. S. Sørensen and J. Koefoed, J. Chem. Soc. Farad. Trans. II *70*: 665 (1974).
38. V. Sasidhar and E. Ruckenstein, J. Colloid Sci. *85*: 332 (1982).
39. R. Schlögl and F. Helfferich, Ber. Bunsenges. Phys. Chem. Z. Elektrochem. *56*: 644 (1952).
40. F. Helfferich, Ber. Bunsenges. Phys. Chem. Z. Elektrochem. *56*: 947 (1952).
41. H. Röttger and D. Woermann, Langmuir *9*: 1370 (1993).
42. R. Schlögl, Z. Phys. Chem. N.F. *3*: 73 (1955).
43. M. Schönborn and D. Woermann, Ber. Bunsenges. Phys. Chem. *71*: 843 (1967).
44. J. Schink, H. Röttger, and D. Woermann, J. Colloid Interface Sci. *171*: 351 (1995).
45. G. Manecke, Z. Phys. Chem. *20*: 193 (1952).
46. E. Philipsen and D. Woermann, *17*: 139 (1984).
47. Ngoc-Ty and D. Woermann, J. Chem. Soc. Faraday Trans. *90*: 875 (1994).
48. G. Wiedner and D. Woermann, Ber. Bunsenges. Phys. Chem. *79*: 868 (1975).

49. J. Schink, L. Belkoura, D. Woermann, F. Yeh, Y. J. Li and B. Chu, Ber. Bunsenges. Phys. Chem. *100*:1103 (1996).
50. O. Hahn and D. Woermann, Ber. Bunsenges. Phys. Chem. *101*:703 (1997).
51. K. Chakravarti, B. Christensen, and B. Langer, J. Membrane Sci. *22*:111 (1985).
52. A. E. Yaroshuk, H. Röttger, and D. Woermann, Ber. Bunsenges. Phys. Chem. *97*:676 (1993).
53. R. Schlögl, Ber. Bunsenges. Phys. Chem. *70*:400 (1966).
54. O. Hahn and D. Woermann, J. Membrane Sci. *117*:197 (1996).
55. O. Hahn and D. Woermann, Ber. Bunsenges. Phys. Chem. *100*:1791 (1996).
56. T. Teorell, Proc. Natl. Acad. Sci. USA *21*:152 (1935).
57. T. Teorell, J. Gen. Physiol. *21*:107 (1937).
58. R. Neihoff and K. Sollner, J. Phys. Chem. *61*:159 (1957).
59. S. Salimen, Nature *200*:1069 (1963).
60. D. Woermann, J. Am. Chem. Soc. *90*:3020 (1968).
61. P. Schwahn and D. Woermann, Ber. Bunsenges. Phys. Chem. *90*:773 (1986).
62. J. N. Weinstein and S. R. Caplan, Science *161*:273 (1984).
63. M. Tasaka, T. Okono, and T. Fujimato, J. Membrane Sci. *19*:273 (1984).
64. O. Kedem and A. Katchalsky, Trans. Faraday Soc. *59*:1931 (1963).
65. D. Woermann, Ber. Bunsenges. Phys. Chem. *71*:87 (1967).
66. R. Neihof and K. Sollner, J. Phys. Chem. *94*:157 (1950).
67. R. Neihof and K. Sollner, J. Gen. Physiol. *39*:613 (1955).
68. K. Söllner, S. Dray, E. Grim, and R. Neihof, in *Transport across Membranes*, (H. T. Clark and D. Nachmanson, eds.), Academic Press, New York, 1954, p. 144.
69. J. A. Nollet, Histoire de la Académie Royale des Science, p. 57 (1748). Translation of some pages in J. Membrane Sci. *100*:1 (1995).
70. M. Dutrochet, Ann. Chim. Phys. *35*:393 (1827).
71. M. Dutrochet, Ann. Chim. Phys. *37*:191 (1828).
72. M. Dutrochet, Ann. Chim. Phys. *49*:411 (1832).
73. M. Dutrochet, Ann. Chim. Phys. *51*:159 (1832).
74. M. Dutrochet, Ann. Chim. Phys. *60*:337 (1835).
75. K. Vierrodt, Ann. Phys (Poggen. Ann.) *73*:519 (1848) abstract from Arch. Physiol Heilkunde *5*:479 (1846).
76. T. Graham, Phil. Trans. Roy. Soc. London *A144*:177 (1854).
77. M. Traube, Arch. Anat. Physiol. wiss. Med. 87 (1867).
78. W. Pfeffer, *Osmotische Untersuchungen*, Engelmann, Leipzig (1877).
79. A. Findlay, *Osmotic Pressure*. Longmans, Green and Co, London, (1913).
80. J. C. W. Frazer, in *A Treatise on Physical Chemistry Vol. 1*, (H. S. Taylor, ed.), New York, van Nostrand, 1931, 2nd ed. Chapter VII, pp. 353–414.
81. J. H. Van't Hoff, Z. Phys. Chem. *1*:481 (1887).
82. R. Höber, *Physikalische Chemie der Zelle und der Gewebe*, 6th Ed., Engelmann, Leipzig (1926).
83. J. Loeb, J. Gen. Physiol. *1*:717 (1919).
84. J. Loeb, J. Gen. Physiol. *2*:87 (1920).
85. J. Loeb, J. Gen. Physiol. *2*:173 (1920).
86. J. Loeb, J. Gen. Physiol. *2*:273 (1920).
87. J. Loeb, J. Gen. Physiol. *2*:387 (1920).
88. J. Loeb, J. Gen. Physiol. *2*:563 (1920).

89. J. Loeb, J. Gen. Physiol. *2*: 577 (1920).
90. J. Loeb, J. Gen. Physiol. *2*: 659 (1920).
91. J. Loeb, J. Gen. Physiol. *2*: 673 (1920).
92. J. Loeb, J. Gen. Physiol. *4*: 213 (1922).
93. J. Loeb, J. Gen. Physiol. *4*: 463 (1922).
94. J. Loeb, J. Gen. Physiol. *5*: 89 (1923).
95. J. Loeb, *Proteins and the Theory of Colloidal Behavior*, McGraw Hill, New York, 1923.
96. F. E. Bartell, J. Am. Chem. Soc. *36*: 646 (1914).
97. F. E. Bartell and C. D. Hocker, J. Am. Chem. Soc. *38*: 1032 (1916).
98. F. E. Bartell and C. D. Hocker, J. Am. Chem. Soc. *38*: 1036 (1916).
99. F. E. Bartell and L. B. Sims, J. Am. Chem. Soc. *44*: 289 (1922).
100. F. E. Bartell and D. C. Carpenter, J. Phys. Chem. *27*: 101 (1923).
101. F. E. Bartell, Colloid Symp. Monogr. *1*: 120 (1923).
102. G. Preuner and O. Roder, Z. Elektrochem. *29*: 54 (1923).
103. H. Freundlich, Kolloid Z. *18*: 11 (1916).
104. K. Söllner, Ber. Bunsenges. Phys. Chem. Z. Elektrochem. *36*: 36 (1930).
105. K. Söllner, Ber. Bunsenges. Phys. Chem. Z. Elektrochem. *36*: 234 (1930).
106. K. Söllner and A. Grollmann, Ber. Bunsenges. Phys. Chem. Z. Elektrochem. *38*: 274 (1932).

10

Electrochemical Characterization of Membranes and Membrane Surfaces by EMF Measurements

TORBEN SMITH SØRENSEN*   Physical Chemistry, Modelling & Thermodynamics/DTH, Vanløse (Copenhagen), Denmark

SERGIO ROBERTO RIVERA†   Departamento de Físico-Química, Universidad de Concepción, Concepción, Chile

---

* Also affiliated with The Danish National Museum, Department of Conservation, Brede, Denmark, as a senior scientist.
† *Current affiliation*: SQM-Salar, Atacama Desert, Antofagasta, Chile.

Abstract

A survey is given of the kind of information which can be drawn from electromotive force studies of electrolyte concentration cells with membranes as separators. The theoretical analysis spans from the most general formalism of irreversible thermodynamics (in practice only useful in the case of two kinds of ions only) to a generalized Nernst–Planck–Donnan treatment able to yield approximate information about ratios of ion diffusion coefficients and Nernst distribution coefficients. The methodologies are exemplified with studies of weak ion exchange or nonionic membranes. Dense and asymmetric cellulose acetate membranes are examples of the first kind of membranes, since these membranes contain a small "fixed charge" of dissociated glucuronic acid groups. It is important to realize that such membranes inserted between two aqueous solutions of, e.g., NaCl cannot, in general, be treated as a two ion + membrane system, since either H^+ or OH^- or both ions participate in the diffusion process and in the Donnan equilibrium process. Also, the glucuronic acid groups may be neutralized by protons or bind divalent ions, so that the "fixed charge" changes sign. The redissociation of such bound, divalent ions is often an extended kinetic process with relaxation times of the order of weeks, depending on temperature and ionic strength. In the case where the influence of the "third ion" can be neglected, general irreversible thermodynamics leads to a method for the characterization not only of the "mean transport numbers" of the membrane but also of the "surface transport numbers" which are generally different for the two sides of an asymmetric membrane. The difficulties of measuring correctly such surface transport numbers are discussed by a critical evaluation of recent experimental studies of this kind. Completely new measurements on a strongly asymmetric, supported polyether sulfone membrane are presented. In one series of experiments, three different kinds of measuring cells have been used with NaCl as the electrolyte in order to check any influence of "unstirred layers" on surface and mean transport numbers. In another set of experiments, the surface and mean transport numbers of Ba^{2+} in $BaCl_2$ have been measured. The different concentration dependence of the two surface transport numbers reflects the asymmetry of the membrane.

I. INTRODUCTION

Since the proposition of the theories of Teorell, Meyer and Sievers [1–3], electromotive force (emf) studies of concentration cells with membranes as separators have been used to elucidate the internal structure of the membrane material [4–8]. For example, ratios between the diffusion coefficient of ions, ion Nernst distribution coefficients, the concentration of fixed charge at varying pH, and even the kinetics of ion exchange and of the binding/dissociation of divalent cations have been estimated in cellulose acetate membranes in previous studies by one of the present authors with coworkers [9–15]. The characterization is even more powerful when combined with impedance spectroscopy, in which case the ion diffusion coefficients themselves may be estimated together with the average size of the water-rich "alveoles" and their average permittivity [16–19].

The experimental techniques and the physicochemical models have not yet been brought to complete perfection. A complete physicochemical model for the electrochemical and dielectric response of "wet" (two-phase) membraneous material necessarily calls for a careful analysis of the interaction between the conductivity and dynamical electric double layer effects on one side with the internal dielectric relaxation of the polymers making up the membrane on the other side. Such an analysis have recently been attempted for "dry" (one-phase) polymers with ionic impurities [19–22]. Nevertheless, emf and impedance methods already seem to provide a good supplement to other characterization methods of micro- and macroheterogeneities (asymmetry) such as radiotracer autoradiography and tracer sorption experiments [23–25] or electron microprobe/X-ray spectroscopy, small-angle X-ray and neutron scattering spectroscopy, electron spin resonance and Mössbauer spectroscopy [25].

In a related though somewhat distinct line of electrochemical membrane research are some recent studies by our group using transient emf methods to characterize asymmetric membranes. Experimental studies [26–28] backed up by general irreversible thermodynamics [29–30] as well as theoretical models based on a generalized Nernst–Planck–Donnan approach [31,32] have been published. It was suggested that "initial time" emf studies may be used to provide information concerning the transport numbers of the ions in the *surface layers* of asymmetric membranes.

The method is the following: The membrane is soaked with a single electrolyte solution until equilibrium. Then, either the left-hand side (l.h.s.) or the right-hand side (r.h.s) of the membrane is suddenly exposed to a solution of the same electrolyte but at a different concentration. Since the concentration profile is initially exclusively situated to the left or to the right in the membrane, respectively, the average transport number of the cation (or the anion) in the surface layer will be determining for the initial emf. In the following we shall for brevity speak about *surface transport numbers*, when transport numbers are evaluated from initial emf data.

The measurement of emf in concentration cells is very simple in principle. A sketch of the experimental arrangement and the "potential jumps" contributing to the emf is shown in Figs. 1a and 1b, respectively. In the present chapter we shall attempt to give a general survey of the theory and some practical examples of emf characterization of homogeneous or inhomogeneous (asymmetric) membranes in electrolyte concentration cells. The above-mentioned studies of impedance and dielectric properties of membranes are relegated to another chapter [19]. Because of the apparent simplicity of emf characterization there are innumerable quite uncritical studies in the literature measuring emf, calculating "transport numbers" and drawing conclusions comparing such transport numbers. The simplicity of emf experiments in membrane concentration cells is deceiving, however, and the detailed theory behind such emf studies seems to be fully understood by few researchers.

Therefore, we begin with quite extensive theoretical considerations in Sec. II. The section also serves as an elaborate (though far from exhaustive) literature guide through the history and development of the concepts involved. First, we treat the *diffusion potential* generated to compensate the differences in ion diffusivities and being a substantial component in the total emf. The basic phenomenology of the diffusion potential is described in Sec. II.A from the general point of view of irreversible thermodynamics and from the much more restricted point of view of the Nernst–Planck electrodiffusion equations. The latter have to be formulated such that they include differences in the standard chemical potentials into the "driving forces" for the ions. The *Donnan potentials* at the two membrane–solution interfaces (see Fig. 1b) are two other major components in the total emf and these are treated in Sec. II.B. Adding the diffusion potential, the Donnan potentials and the electrode potentials we find the total emf of the cell, and in Sec. II.C we shall see that the so-called "quasi-thermostatic method" yields the final result much more quickly than any other method. Finally, in Sec. II.D we shall have a look at the irreversible thermodynamic theory of *surface transport numbers* in general, inhomogeneous or asymmetric membranes where only *two diffusing ions* are of significance.

In Sec. III we exemplify the practical use of the simplified Nernst–Planck–Donnan theory by the results found earlier for *cellulose acetate membranes* with different kinds of electrolytes. Cellulose acetate membranes are weak ion exchange membranes due to a small, but significant, number of glucuronic acid groups stemming from the oxidation of some of the primary alcohol

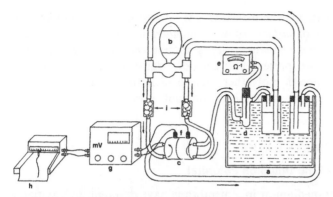

FIG. 1a Typical experimental setup for emf measurements over a membrane. The membrane is placed between the two half cells of the measuring cell (c). The circulation of the two solutions is done by either a doubly functioning peristaltic pump (b), or by two centrifugal pumps. The pressure dashpots (i) are only necessary with peristaltic pumps and thin, delicate membranes. The conductivity is followed in the most dilute solution (d,e).

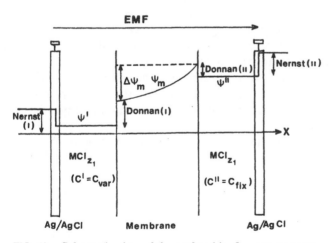

FIG. 1b Schematic view of the emf and its five components.

groups in the original cellulose. We shall have a critical look of what can really be deduced from such data about the structure of the membrane material. One of the very interesting features of these membranes is the strong binding of some divalent ions to the glucuronic acid groups (Sec. III.E).

In Sec. IV we treat examples of measurement on asymmetric membranes, in particular measurements of *surface transport numbers* in *initial value emf* measurements. In Sec. IV.A we evaluate critically some recent measurements, and in Sec. IV.B and IV.C we present entirely new transitory emf data for an uncharged, highly asymmetric polyether sulfone membrane using NaCl electrolyte and three different measuring cells for control in Sec. IV.B and $BaCl_2$ electrolyte in Sec. IV.C.

II. THEORETICAL CONSIDERATIONS

A. Phenomenology of the Diffusion Potential

When ions in a solvent medium or in a membrane have different diffusivities, a local electric field is generated during diffusion (without net electric current) to compensate for this difference, since the ions have to yield almost balancing contributions to the galvanic current in order for the external solutions and the membrane to stay very close to electroneutrality. The integration of the negative electric field through the membrane gives rise to the diffusion potential—an integral but unmeasurable part of the total emf.

From the end of last century many authors have discussed the diffusion potential—especially in the case of liquid–liquid junctions—theoretically in terms of the Nernst–Planck electrodiffusion equations (with or without the a priori assumption of electroneutrality) [33–40] as well as experimentally (measurements of emf in cells with transference) or both theoretically and experimentally [41–54]. One motivation for such studies is an attempt to understand better the KCl bridge, or more generally the salt bridge, which has a status as a kind of "Achilles' heel" in the definition of the functioning of ion selective electrodes and even in the definition of normal oxidation potentials of electrochemical redox systems.

The Nernst–Planck equations have also been used extensively for the study of electrodiffusion in membranes. Some few examples are given in Refs. 1–7, 14, 55–57. In a major part of the cellulose acetate studies of the group of Sørensen [9–13], the Nernst–Planck equations were also the basis but an explicit solution of these (for example for the steady state)—which is nontrivial in the case of three or more diffusing ions—was circumvented by the use of the Henderson assumption [34,35] of linear concentration profiles or, to be more precise, the Guggenheim assumption of a "continuous mixture zone" [43]. In such a zone, intermediary compositions in the zone are described as linear combinations of the terminal solutions (just inside the two membrane faces) by means of a single "mixing parameter" with arbitrary spatial variation. The differences between continuous mixture emf values and the more correct Pleijel–Schlögl [36,55] emf values, solving the Nernst–Planck equations for the stationary state, are usually small except for large concentration differences over the membrane or the diffusion zone [13,14,50,54].

Recently it has been demonstrated for inhomogeneous or asymmetric membranes [31,32,58] that it is extremely important to include the variation in the standard chemical potentials (or the Nernst distribution coefficients) of the ions from point to point in the membrane in the local "driving forces" for the ions. The "generalized" Nernst–Planck equation for electrodiffusion of an ion of species k in inhomogeneous (one-dimensional) diffusion zones should then be written:

$$J_k(x, t)/D_k(x) = -\partial c_{k, m}/\partial x + c_{k, m}(x, t)d \ln K_k(x)/dx$$
$$- (z_k F/RT)c_{k, m}(x, t)\partial \psi_m/\partial x \qquad (1)$$

In Eq. (1), $J_k(x, t)$ is the flux density of ion species no. k (mol k per unit area and unit time) at position x and time t, $D_k(x)$ is the diffusion coefficient of ion k in the membrane at position x, $c_{k, m}(x, t)$ is the concentration in the membrane (mol k per unit volume) of ion k, $K_k(x)$ is the Nernst distribution coefficient of ion k (membrane/external solution) at position x in the membrane, z_k is the valency with sign of ion k, F is the Faraday, R the gas constant, T the absolute temperature and $\psi_m(x, t)$ the electric potential in the membrane at position x and time t. The second term on the r.h.s. of Eq. (1) means that there is a "drive" for an ion to move towards regions in the membrane with high Nernst distribution coefficient for that ion even without any gradients in electric potential or concentration.

If one forgets the second term on the r.h.s. of eq. (1), one runs into problems with the second law of thermodynamics as pointed out in Refs. 31 and 32. For example, Takagi and Nakagaki [59] have argued for the possibility of "facilitated" as well as "reverse" transport in asymmetric ion exchange membranes. By "facilitated transport" is meant a nonzero steady state salt flux in a situation with two identical solutions on the two sides of the membrane. This evidently violate the second law of thermodynamics, since there cannot be an irreversible process without an overall driving force. The case is even worse with "reverse transport", where electroneutral salt is transported against its external concentration difference.

Manzanares, Mafé and Pellicer [60] have shown that neither "facilitated" nor "reverse" transport is possible in a simple model of an ion exchange membrane with asymmetric charge distribution. However, these authors, like Higuchi and Nakagawi [58], suggest that the reason for the erroneous results of Takagi and Nakagaki [59] is the fact that these authors use the Henderson hypothesis in their theory. In the paper of Manzanares, Mafé and Pellicer, however, there is no question of the lacking of the $d \ln K_k(x)/dx$ term in Eq. (1) since they put all Nernst distribution coefficients to unity everywhere in the membrane. In a generalization of their work to asymmetric membranes with gradients in fixed charge as well as in diffusion coefficients and in Nernst distribution coefficients, it was subsequently shown by Sørensen and Compañ [31,32] that neither "facilitated" nor "reverse" transport could ever occur in any such membranes solely because of the inclusion of the $d \ln K_k(x)/dx$ term.

The "generalized" Nernst–Planck equations represent of course, though compatible with thermodynamics, a very simplified description of reality: the ions behave ideally and do not interact with each other neither thermodynamically (through activity coefficients) nor irreversibly (through the phenomenological cross-coefficients of irreversible thermodynamics). The simplicity of the Nernst–Planck equations allows in optimal cases for approximate estimations of structural details of the membrane such as fixed charge density, ratios of diffusion coefficients and ratios of Nernst distribution coefficients, see Sec. III. In contrast, the general phenomenological equations of irreversible thermodynamics are exact but complicated to use, it is normally very difficult to find all the phenomenological coefficients from experiments and the coefficients found do not lend themselves easily to interpretation in terms of the structure of the membrane. Nevertheless, we shall make use of this approach in the present chapter in discussing the measuring of so-called "surface transport numbers" in asymmetric membranes with two diffusing ions only, see Sec. II.D and IV. Therefore, a short discussion of what can be said about the diffusion potential on the exact ground of irreversible thermodynamics will be appropriate here.

The basis of traditional, irreversible thermodynamics is a local description of "fluxes" (J) and "forces" (X) so that the product sum of fluxes and forces are either the local entropy production intensity or the local dissipation (of useful energy) [61–67]. Linear, symmetric matrix relations are found locally connecting fluxes and forces, the so-called phenomenological equations. A specialized treatment of certain pedagogical advantages has recently been put forward for vectorial transport processes in isotropic media with or without membranes in terms of "generalized friction forces" [29,30]. We may express the local dissipation density as

$$T\sigma = J_S \cdot (-\nabla T) + \sum_k J_k \cdot (-\nabla \mu_{\mathrm{grav, el,} k}) \tag{2}$$

where σ is the local rate of entropy production per unit of volume, J_S is the vector flux of entropy relative to a specified Galileian reference frame—for membranes most suitably the membrane matrix (for details, see for example the discussion in Ref. 30)—and the gravi-electrochemical potential of ion k is defined as:

$$\mu_{\mathrm{grav, el,} k} \equiv \mu_k + M_k \Phi + z_k F \psi \tag{3}$$

The chemical potential (per mol) is μ_k, the molar mass M_k and the gravitational potential Φ. In this chapter we neglect gravitational effects compared to electrical and chemical effects and we shall also only treat isothermal systems. The local dissipation is then given as

$$T\sigma = \sum_k J_k^{(m)} \cdot (-\nabla\mu_{el,\,k}) \tag{4}$$

and the phenomenological equations links the fluxes (relative to the membrane matrix) together with the forces by linear relations

$$J_k^{(m)} = \sum_p L_{kp}(-\nabla\mu_{el,\,p}) \quad (k = 1 \ldots N; \, p = 1 \ldots N) \tag{5}$$

and the symmetry conditions

$$L_{kp} = L_{pk} \quad (k = 1 \ldots N; \, p = 1 \ldots N) \tag{6}$$

We have assumed (local) isotropy and the presence of N ions or neutral species (apart from the membrane species). The matrix of phenomenological coefficients $\mathbf{L}$ is symmetric due to the reciprocity relations of Onsager [61,62] based on the microscopic reversibility of the fundamental equations of dynamics or in the present special case simply because of detailed momentum conservation during mutual "generalized friction", see Ref. 30.

The Onsager symmetry is preserved for so-called congruent transformations of forces and fluxes. For example, we may define "new" fluxes as a linear combination of the "old" ones

$$J_r^{(new)} \equiv \sum_k P_{kr} J_k^{(m)} \quad (r = 1 \ldots M; \, k = 1 \ldots N) \tag{7}$$

and, congruently, define the "old" forces in terms of the "new" ones (X_r) and the transpose of the $\mathbf{P}$ matrix $(\mathbf{P}^{T})$

$$-\nabla\mu_{el,\,k} \equiv \sum_r P_{kr}^T X_q = \sum_r P_{rk} X_r \quad (r = 1 \ldots M; \, k = 1 \ldots N) \tag{8}$$

(Evidently, it is not necessary that the transformation matrix $\mathbf{P}$ be quadratic). It is easily demonstrated that (1) the dissipation is invariant to the shift in fluxes and forces

$$T\sigma = \sum_k J_k^{(m)} \cdot (-\nabla\mu_{el,\,k}) = \sum_r J_r^{(new)} \cdot X_r \quad (r = 1 \ldots M; \, k = 1 \ldots N) \tag{9}$$

and that (2) the new phenomenological equations

$$J_r^{(new)} = \sum_s L_{rs}^{(new)} X_s \quad (r = 1 \ldots M; \, s = 1 \ldots M) \tag{10}$$

are also Onsager symmetric:

$$L_{rs}^{(new)} = L_{sr}^{(new)} \quad (r = 1 \ldots M; \, s = 1 \ldots M) \tag{11}$$

If $M > N$ the transformation is expanding, if $M < N$ the transformation is reducing.

In electrochemical applications, the galvanic current density J_q is an important variable and we want to include it as a new flux. So we perform an expanding, congruent transformation-choosing the $\mathbf{P}$ matrix as the following $(N + 1) \times N$ matrix:

$$\mathbf{P} \equiv \begin{pmatrix} 1 & 0 & 0 & 0 & \ldots & 0 \\ 0 & 1 & 0 & 0 & \ldots & 0 \\ 0 & 0 & 1 & 0 & \ldots & 0 \\ \cdots & \cdots & \cdots & \cdots & \cdots & \cdots \\ 0 & 0 & 0 & 0 & \ldots & 1 \\ z_1 F & z_2 F & z_3 F & z_4 F & \ldots & z_N F \end{pmatrix} \tag{12}$$

The "new" fluxes are then $\{J_1^{(m)}, J_2^{(m)}, \ldots, J_N^{(m)}, J_q^{(m)}\}$ and the corresponding "new" forces are $\{-\nabla\mu_1, -\nabla\mu_2, \ldots, -\nabla\mu_N, -\nabla\psi\}$, i.e. the negative gradients in the N chemical potentials expanded with the local electric field $-\nabla\psi$.

We now specialize to one-dimensional systems and write the phenomenological equations in terms of the expanded variables:

$$J_k^{(m)} = \sum_{p=1\ldots N} L_{kp}^{(new)}(-\partial\mu_p/\partial x) + L_{k,\,N+1}^{(new)}(-\partial\psi/\partial x) \quad (k = 1 \ldots N) \tag{13a}$$

$$J_q^{(m)} = \sum_{p=1\ldots N} L_{N+1,\,p}^{(new)}(-\partial\mu_p/\partial x) + L_{N+1,\,N+1}^{(new)}(-\partial\psi/\partial x) \tag{13b}$$

In emf studies, the galvanic current density relative to the membrane is zero

$$J_q^{(m)} = 0 \tag{14}$$

and it would be nice to have it as an independent variable (on the r.h.s. of the phenomenological equations). Also in many other electrochemical applications with nonzero current, the galvanic current density is often the variable under control. Since the matrix $\mathbf{L}^{(new)}$ is nonsingular it is possible to perform a partial inversion of $\mathbf{L}^{(new)}$ to a new matrix $\mathbf{Q}$ corresponding to an isolated change of side in the phenomenological equation of $J_q^{(m)}$ and $-\partial\psi/\partial x$:

$$J_k^{(m)} = \sum_{p=1\ldots N} Q_{kp}(-\partial\mu_p/\partial x) + Q_{k,\,N+1}J_q^{(m)} \quad (k = 1 \ldots N) \tag{15a}$$

$$-\partial\psi/\partial x = \sum_{p=1\ldots N} Q_{N+1,\,p}(-\partial\mu_p/\partial x) + Q_{N+1,\,N+1}J_q^{(m)} \tag{15b}$$

In such a partial inversion, matrix calculations show that an original symmetry in the $\mathbf{L}^{(new)}$ matrix is preserved as symmetry between variables not inverted or between inverted variables (in case more variables were partially inverted). However, there will be *antisymmetry* between inverted and non-inverted variables. We may write Eq. (15a) as

$$J_i^{(m)} = \sum_{p=1\ldots N} Q_{ip}(-\partial\mu_p/\partial x) + (t_i/z_i)(J_q^{(m)}/F) \quad (i = 1 \ldots I \le N) \tag{16a}$$

for a *charged* species i and

$$J_n^{(m)} = \sum_{p=1\ldots N} Q_{np}(-\partial\mu_p/\partial x) + t_n(J_q^{(m)}/F) \quad (n = I + 1 \ldots N) \tag{16b}$$

for an *uncharged* species n using the usual definition of the local *transport numbers* t_k. For an ion, the transport number is the fraction of the galvanic current carried by the ion when there are no gradients in chemical potentials (no diffusion). For a neutral species, it is the number of moles carried by the transfer of one Faraday under the same conditions. Equations (15b) can now be written (ρ = local specific resistance):

$$
\begin{aligned}
-\partial\psi/\partial x = - &\sum_{i=1\dots I} (t_i/z_i F)(-\partial\mu_i/\partial x) \\
- &\sum_{n=I+1\dots N} (t_n/F)(-\partial\mu_n/\partial x) + \rho J_q^{(m)}
\end{aligned} \tag{16c}
$$

In Eq. (16c) we have used the antisymmetry between the phenomenological equations linking the coefficients $Q_{N+1, p}(p = 1 \dots N)$ in Eq. (15b) to the coefficients $Q_{k, N+1}(k = 1 \dots N)$ in Eq. (15a), i.e., the coefficients linking inverted and noninverted variables.

For the diffusion potential, i.e., the difference in electrical potential between a point just inside the right face of the membrane (at $x = d_-$) and the electric potential just inside the left face of the membrane (at $x = 0_+$), under emf conditions (no galvanic current) we may therefore write:

$$
\begin{aligned}
\Delta\psi_m = - \int_{x=0_+}^{x=d_-} &\left[\sum_{i=1\dots I} (t_i/z_i F)(\partial\mu_i/\partial x) \right. \\
&\left. + \sum_{n=I+1\dots N} (t_n/F)(\partial\mu_n/\partial x) \right] dx
\end{aligned} \tag{17}
$$

The *ionic* transport numbers are not all independent, since all the ions together carry all the current (at constant chemical potentials). Thus, the ionic transport numbers are linked by the relation:

$$
\sum_{i=1\dots I} t_i = 1 \tag{18}
$$

Equation (17) is an exact equation but in general very difficult to use. The transport numbers are generally functions of the position in the membrane (x) as well as functions of the actual ionic concentrations at this position (at time t). The gradients in the chemical potentials are also functions of x and t. Normally, therefore, the diffusion potential is a complicated *functional* of the entire concentration profiles, and it will be time dependent. Although the diffusion potential is not measurable separately, it is a substantial part of the measurable emf, and emf will carry the same features. In Eq. (17) there will at least be one neutral species in membranes (the solvent, for example water) with associated transport number. Furthermore, one less independent ionic transport number than the number of ions present. In membrane-free solvents there is no solvent transport number, since the frame of reference is taken to be the solvent itself (Hittorf definition of the ionic transport number). There may be other neutral species than solvent, however.

In the subsequent sections we shall discuss simplifying conditions or assumptions which make easier the calculation of the diffusion potential. At this place we shall only mention the following restricted situation: If there are only *two diffusing ions* and one neutral species (the solvent o) there is only one independent ionic transport number, t_2 for the cation say, and (in a membrane) we have in addition one solvent transport number (t_o). If these transport numbers are *independent of position* (corresponding to a *homogeneous* membrane or a membrane-free solution) but dependent on a single composition variable (for example the external salt concentration c_s with which the corresponding spot in the membrane would be in equilibrium) we have from Eq. (17):

$$\Delta\psi_m = -(\Delta\mu_1/z_1 F) - \{1/[v_2 z_2 F]\} \int_{x=0}^{x=d} t_2(\partial\mu_s/\partial x)\, dx$$

$$- (1/F) \int_{x=0}^{x=d} t_o(\partial\mu_o/\partial x)\, dx \tag{19}$$

We have used Eq. (18), the formal eletroneutrality of the salt

$$v_1 z_1 + v_2 z_2 = 0 \tag{20}$$

(v_1 and v_2 are stoichiometric coefficients), and the definition of the chemical potential of the salt:

$$\mu_s \equiv v_1\mu_1 + v_2\mu_2 \tag{21}$$

Now, the chemical potential of the salt in the membrane at position x, and the chemical potential of the solvent at the same position are both equal to the corresponding chemical potentials in the external solution (with salt concentration c_s and solvent concentration c_o) with which the selected membrane spot would be in equilibrium. Furthermore, in this external solution the variations of these two chemical potentials are linked by the equation of Gibbs–Duhem (assuming that the temperature and pressure are both constant):

$$c_s\,\delta\mu_s + c_o\,\delta\mu_o = 0 \tag{22}$$

Correspondingly, we have in the membrane

$$\partial\mu_o/\partial x = -(c_s/c_o)\partial\mu_s/\partial x$$

(where in fact c_o is also determined thermodynamically by c_s). From Eq. (19):

$$\Delta\psi_m = -(\Delta\mu_1/z_1 F) - \{1/[v_2 z_2 F]\} \int_{x=0}^{x=d} [t_2 - (c_s/c_o)t_o]_{c_s}(\partial\mu_s/\partial x)\, dx \tag{23}$$

We introduce the so-called "apparent transport number" τ_2 (at external salt concentration c_s) by the definition:

$$\tau_2(c_s) \equiv [t_2 - (c_s/c_o)t_o]_{c_s} \tag{24}$$

We can then express Eq. (23) as follows:

$$\Delta\psi_m = -(\Delta\mu_1/z_1 F) - \{1/[\nu_2 z_2 F]\} \int_{x=0}^{x=d} \tau_2(c_s)(d\mu_s/dc_s)(\partial c_s/\partial x)\, dx \qquad (25)$$

The integrand in Eq. (25) is of the form $f(c_s)(\partial c_s/\partial x)$. At any given time, $c_s(x, t)$ is a given function of x and $(\partial c_s/\partial x)\, dx$ is the differential of this function dc_s. The integral is then independent of the course of the salt concentration profile and is loosing its character of a functional. The diffusion potential is not a function of time in this special case. We write finally:

$$\Delta\psi_m = -(\Delta\mu_{1,m}/z_1 F) - \{1/[\nu_2 z_2 F]\} \int_{\mu_s(L)}^{\mu_s(R)} \tau_2(\mu_s)d\mu_s \qquad (26)$$

For future reference we have added a subscript m in the first term on the right-hand side to remember that the chemical potentials of the ion 1 has to be taken in the membrane, *not* in the external solution.

B. Phenomenology of the Local Donnan Equilibrium

When an ion exchange membrane with a given fixed charge density c_q (in mol per unit volume) is put into contact with an external solution, a Donnan equilibrium is set up (after some time) where the ions are in electrochemical equilibrium across the membrane–solution interface (same electrochemical potentials) and where the chemical potential of the solvent is the same in the solution and in the membrane. The original theory we owe to Donnan [68,69], but here we shall neglect the so-called "Donnan pressure" caused by the relatively small pressure contributions to the chemical potentials.

Even in situations with irreversible electrodiffusion we consider the membrane layers immediately adjacent to the two external solutions to be in *local Donnan equilibrium* with the external solutions. The Donnan equilibrium has been treated repeatedly by many authors with various degrees of sophistication [1–6,9–11,15–18,68–79]. There is one "sin of omission" which is committed by most authors treating the Donnan equilibrium in *ideally dilute* systems, however, which we want to point out here: the lack of inclusion of individual Nernst distribution coefficients (membrane/solution) of the ions. This amounts to disregarding the fact that the differences in the standard state chemical potentials of the ions are not equal in the solution and in the membrane, and that these differences have individual values for each ion. For example, in the present monography, the chapters on "Ion Equilibrium and Transport in Weak Amphoteric Membranes" [80] and "Osmotic Properties of Polyelectrolyte Gels" [81] are restricted by the assumption of Nernst distribution coefficients equal to unity.

In the original membrane emf studies of Meyer and Sievers [1,2] and in the work of the group of Sørensen et al., individual Nernst distribution coefficients *have* been taken into account. In the latter case, this "extended Donnan theory" was used in emf studies [9–16,31,32] as well as in electric impedance studies [16–18], see Sec. III in this chapter and also the chapter "Interfacial Electrodynamics of Membranes and Polymer Films" [19]. One striking new feature in the more realistic systems with individual Nernst distribution coefficients for the ions is that Donnan potentials may exist at membrane–solution interfaces where the membrane carries no fixed charge! The differences in the affinities of the ions for the membrane are sufficient to generate an electric potential difference to preserve electroneutrality. The modified theory of ion exchange for general, ideal multi-electrolyte mixtures was put forward in Ref. 11 and repeated in Ref. 32. For quick reference we shall resume the theory below.

We consider a completely arbitrary (but electroneutral) mixture of ions with valencies arranged on a "charge axis" in the following way:

$$z_1 = z_{min}, z_2, z_3 \ldots z_{an}, 0, z_{an+1}, z_{an+2}, \ldots z_{an+cat} = z_{max} \tag{27}$$

The number of different anions are $= an$, and the number of different cations $= cat$. The mixture is in electrochemical equilibrium with a phase with fixed charge density $\omega \cdot c_q$, where $\omega = 1$ for a positive fixed charge (an anion exchange membrane) and $\omega = -1$ for a negative fixed charge (cation exchange membrane). If the mixture is considered to be ideally dilute, we may express the equilibrium between the two phases as follows (neglecting any influence of pressure differences):

$$\mu_i^o + RT \ln c_i + z_i F\psi = \mu_{i, m}^o + RT \ln c_{i, m} + z_i F\psi_m$$
$$(i = 1, 2 \ldots an + cat) \tag{28}$$

In Eq. (28), μ_i^o is the standard chemical potential per mol of ionic species no. 1. The subscript "m" means "in the membrane". Introducing the Donnan potential

$$\Delta\psi_D = \psi_m - \psi \tag{29}$$

and the definitions

$$\alpha \equiv \exp(-F\Delta\psi_D/RT) \tag{30}$$
$$K_i \equiv \exp([\mu_i^o - \mu_{i, m}^o]/RT) \tag{31}$$

the equilibrium conditions (28) can be written as:

$$c_{i, m}/c_i = K_i \alpha^{z_i} \quad (i = 1, 2 \ldots an + cat) \tag{32}$$

We have electroneutrality in the membrane:

$$\sum_{1 \ldots an} z_i c_i K_i \alpha^{z_i} + \omega \cdot c_q + \sum_{(an+1) \ldots cat} z_i c_i K_i \alpha^{z_i} = 0 \tag{33}$$

Multiplying Eq. (33) by $\alpha^{|z_1|}$ we obtain:

$$
\begin{aligned}
P_D(\alpha) &\equiv z_1 c_1 K_1 + z_2 c_2 K_2 \alpha^{|z_1|-|z_2|} + \cdots + z_{an} c_{an} K_{an} \alpha^{|z_1|-|z_{an}|} \\
&\quad + \omega \cdot c_q \alpha^{|z_1|} + z_{an+1} c_{an+1} K_{an+1} \alpha^{|z_1|+z_{an+1}} + \cdots \\
&\quad + z_{an+cat} c_{an+cat} K_{an+cat} \alpha^{|z_{min}|+z_{max}} = 0
\end{aligned}
\tag{34}
$$

The polynomial $P_D(\alpha)$ may be called the *Donnan polynomial*. It is of degree $|z_{min}| + z_{max}$, and the Donnan potential is given by one (or more) of the real positive roots of this polynomial through Eq. (30). Having found α, the calculation of the Donnan distribution of the various ions between the phases in straightforward through Eq. (32).

We now proceed to prove, that there is always one and only one real positive root of the Donnan polynomial. The proof uses the rule of Descartes: Let N be the number of changes of sign of the coefficients of the polynomial, when we proceed systematically from the left to the right. The number of real, positive roots is then either N or $N-2$ or $N-4$ ..., and so on down to 1 or 0. It is obvious from Eq. (34), that there is only one change of sign. For $\omega = 1$ this takes place before the term $\omega \cdot c_q \alpha^{|z_1|}$ for $\omega = -1$ after. Thus $N = 1$ and there is only one real, positive root to any thinkable Donnan polynomial. The Donnan potential and distribution is *uniquely* defined and bifurcation into several values is an impossibility in spite of the nonlinear character of the problem.

The formalism given here is simple and symmetric, but not operational in the sense that the fixed charge density and all these Nernst distribution coefficients cannot be found from emf measurements. For each type of electrolyte or electrolyte mixture it is necessary to transform the Donnan polynomial to a form with a minimum number of combinations of these parameters which *can* be found from measurements of emf, see Refs. 9–18, 31,32 and Sec. III.

C. Electromotive Force (EMF) of Concentration Cells

Only the emf of a concentration cell is a measurable quantity. This emf is composed of a diffusion potential, two Donnan potentials at the two membrane–solution interfaces and two electrode potentials, see Fig. 1b. In order to simplify the discussion a little, we restrict here ourselves to the case of one common anion (Cl^-, no. 1), a "primary" cation (Na^+, no. 2), a "secondary" cation (H^+, no. 3) and water (o). The treatment of other cases follows straightforwardly along the same lines. In this case, the general Eq. (17) for the instantaneous diffusion potential (at time θ) reduces to the following expression (we add subscript m to remember that the chemical potentials for the ions, the electrolytes and water are the ones prevailing at the given position in the membrane):

$$\Delta\psi_m(\theta) = -(\Delta\mu_{1,\,m}/z_1 F) - \{1/[v_2 z_2 F]\} \int_{x=0}^{x=d} t_2(\partial\mu_{21,\,m}/\partial x)\, dx$$

$$- \{1/[v_3 z_3 F]\} \int_{x=0}^{x=d} t_3(\partial\mu_{31,\,m}/\partial x)\, dx$$

$$- (1/F) \int_{x=0}^{x=d} t_o(\partial\mu_{o,\,m}/\partial x)\, dx \qquad (35)$$

We have used Eq. (18) to eliminate t_1, the formal electroneutrality of the electrolytes 21 and 31 (NaCl and HCl)

$$v_1 z_1 + v_2 z_2 = 0; \quad v_1 z_1 + v_3 z_3 = 0 \qquad (36)$$

and the definition of chemical potentials of the electrolytes in the membrane:

$$\mu_{21,\,m} \equiv v_1\mu_{1,\,m} + v_2\mu_{2,\,m}; \quad \mu_{31,\,m} \equiv v_1\mu_{1,\,m} + v_3\mu_{3,\,m} \qquad (37)$$

Notice, that the definitions (37) do *not* imply that the composition at position x in the membrane can be considered to be an electroneutral mixture of (for example) NaCl and HCl. In an ion exchange membrane with a fixed charge density this is not the case. Nevertheless, the relations (37) are a little more than definitions, since an *external* mixed solution with chemical potentials of the salts 12 and 13 fixed by

$$\mu_{21}(x, \theta) = \mu_{21,\,m}(x, \theta); \quad \mu_{21}(x, \theta) = \mu_{21,\,m}(x, \theta) \qquad (38)$$

is in Donnan equilibrium with the membrane at position x at time θ, if the Donnan potential is chosen so as to *produce* (quasi) electroneutrality in the membrane *including* the "fixed charge" c_q (eqv/unit volume) at this position:

$$z_1 c_{1,\,m}(x, \theta) + z_2 c_{2,\,m}(x, \theta) + z_3 c_{3,\,m}(x, \theta) + \omega \cdot c_q(x, \theta) = 0 \qquad (39)$$

The Eqs. (38) can be derived from the equality of the electrochemical potential for each of the ions. The stoichiometric electroneutrality conditions for the two electrolytes Eqs. (36) lead to a cancellation of the electric parts of the electrochemical potentials. Also, the chemical potential of water is the same in the membrane as in an external solution in Donnan and osmotic equilibrium with the membrane at (x, θ). As a consequence we may remove the subscripts m in the three integrands in Eq. (35):

$$\Delta\psi_m(\theta) = -(\Delta\mu_{1,\,m}/z_1 F) - \{1/[v_2 z_2 F]\} \int_{x=0}^{x=d} t_2(\partial\mu_{21}/\partial x)\, dx$$

$$- \{1/[v_3 z_3 F]\} \int_{x=0}^{x=d} t_3(\partial\mu_{31}/\partial x)\, dx - (1/F) \int_{x=0}^{x=d} t_o(\partial\mu_o/\partial x)\, dx \quad (40)$$

The chemical potentials are now chemical potentials of the (fictituous) external solutions without any membrane and therefore the usual Gibbs–Duhem equation applies, i.e.

$$\partial\mu_o/\partial x = -(c_{21}/c_o)\partial\mu_{21}/\partial x - (c_{31}/c_o)\partial\mu_{31}/\partial x \tag{41}$$

where c_{21}, c_{32} and c_o are the concentrations of electrolyte 21, electrolyte 31 and water in the *external* solution associated with (x, θ) in the membrane. Introducing (as in Sec. II. A) "apparent transport numbers"

$$\tau_k(c_{21}, c_{31}, x) \equiv [t_k - (c_{21}/c_o)t_o]_{c_{21}, c_{31}, x} \quad (k = 2, 3) \tag{42}$$

Eq. (40) may be written:

$$\Delta\psi_m(\theta) = -(\Delta\mu_{1,m}/z_1 F)$$
$$- \{1/[v_2 z_2 F]\} \int_{x=0}^{x=d} \tau_2(\partial\mu_{21}/\partial x)\, dx$$
$$- \{1/[v_3 z_3 F]\} \int_{x=0}^{x=d} \tau_3(\partial\mu_{31}/\partial x)\, dx \tag{43}$$

The Donnan potential at the left (L) solution/membrane interface can be expressed using, for example, the equality of the electrochemical potential of ion no. 1 (Cl^-):

$$\Delta\psi_L = \psi(x = 0_+) - \psi(L) = [\mu_1(L) - \mu_{1,m}(x = 0_+)]/\{z_1 F\} \tag{44a}$$

Similarly at the right (R) membrane/solution interface:

$$\Delta\psi_R = \psi(x = d_-) - \psi(R) = [\mu_1(R) - \mu_{1,m}(x = d_-)]/\{z_1 F\} \tag{44b}$$

The two Donnan potentials contribute to emf with the amount

$$\Delta\psi_{net} = \Delta\psi_L - \Delta\psi_R = [\mu_1(L) - \mu_1(R)]/\{z_1 F\} + [\mu_{1,m}(x = d_-)$$
$$- \mu_{1,m}(x = 0_+)]/\{z_1 F\} = [\mu_1(L) - \mu_1(R)]/\{z_1 F\} + (\Delta\mu_{1,m}/z_1 F) \tag{45}$$

If the electrodes are ion selective electrodes for ion no. 1 (for example Ag/Cl electrodes for Cl^-) the difference in electrode potentials (E.P.) are

$$\Delta(E.P.) = [\mu_1(R) - \mu_1(L)]/\{z_1 F\} \tag{46}$$

The emf (at time θ) is then given as:

$$emf (\theta) = \Delta\psi_m(\theta) + \Delta\psi_{net} + \Delta(E.P.)$$
$$= -\{1/[v_2 z_2 F]\} \int_{x=0}^{x=d} \tau_2(\partial\mu_{21}/\partial x)\, dx - \{1/[v_3 z_3 F]\} \int_{x=0}^{x=d} \tau_3(\partial\mu_{31}/\partial x)\, dx \tag{47}$$

It is seen that the emf is expressed solely through an integration involving the two "apparent transport numbers" for the cations in the membrane and the profiles of the "external" solutions in Donnan equilibrium with the integration point in the membrane. These are all observable quantities in principle, but in practice $c_{21} (x, \theta)$ and $c_{31} (x, \theta)$ will not be known in details.

However, since both transport numbers are functions of c_{21} and c_{31}, and since these external electrolyte concentrations vary according to how the internal ion profiles vary with space and time, the emf will normally be time dependent in a diffusion system (with or without membrane) with three ions (or more) until some stationary state of electrodiffusion is reached.

In inhomogeneous or asymmetric membranes, the apparent transport numbers depend also *explicitly* on the position x. In that case, emf will be time dependent before the steady state even in a two ion system. Only in the case of homogeneous membranes (as described in Sec. II. A) and in the case of "initial value emf measurements" on asymmetric membranes ([Sec. II. D and V), the measured emf will be independent of the profile of the single diffusing salt.

For diffusion in pure solvent, the only difference with Eq. (47) is that the apparent transport numbers are replaced by the Hittorf transport number. In two ion + solvent systems (or rather: one salt + solvent systems), the measured emf is completely independent on the profile of the salt as described in Sec. II. A for homogeneous membranes. With two (or more) diffusing salts, emf is time dependent. In diffusion zones with "free boundaries" [37,40,43,47–51] another type of "stationarity" is now possible. When all salt profiles after some time become dependent on a single "Boltzmann parameter"

$$y \equiv (x - x_0)/\sqrt{(\theta - \theta_0)} \qquad (48)$$

(where x_0 and θ_0 are constants to be found in each experiment or simulation), rather than on position and time explicitly, then the emf also becomes independent of time: the emf of "free diffusion", see ref. [40].

It is a bit ironic that expressions like Eq. (47) can be derived very simply and directly (compared to the long-winded method of irreversible thermodynamics presented here) by the so-called "quasi-thermostatic" method. This method originates in Lord Kelvin's treatment of the thermoelectric force [82] and Hermann von Helmholtz's treatment of emf of cells with transference [83]. A "virtual quantity" of electric charge is sent through a nonequilibrium system with zero galvanic current and all the energetic changes are supposed to cancel each other since the charge is "in partial equilibrium". Wagner [84] made a completely general demonstration for isothermal concentration cells (without membranes but with all combinations of electrolyte mixtures and electrodes) that the results of irreversible thermodynamics (using the Onsager relations locally) and the results of "sending one Faraday through" the elements are always completely equivalent. Sørensen and Jensen [9] showed the same for emf of concentration cells with ion exchange membranes and a single electrolyte, and very recently Sørensen, Compañ and Rivera [30] showed the same identity between the emf results of complicated irreversible thermodynamics and simple "quasi-thermostatic" considerations in non-isothermal electrochemical cells. Normally, the quasi-thermostatic method is depreciated in the literature of irreversible thermodynamics [61–64,85], but the methods are of great pedagogical value emphasizing electroneutrality from the beginning and also a formulation in terms of measurable quantities. Furthermore, it may perhaps be asked if such methods aren't more in the vein of traditional (macroscopic) thermodynamic reasoning than the statistical mechanical fluctuation arguments of Onsager.

The considerations in the present subsection have until now been completely general. Now, however, we specialize to ideally dilute membrane-electrolyte systems. In the traditional TMS treatment (Teorell, Meyer, Sievers, [1–3]) the emf is derived adding the diffusion potential derived from the Nernst–Planck equations to the two ideal Donnan potential contributions of the interface and the two ideal Nernst electrode contributions. The same procedure was used in the emf studies of cellulose acetate membranes of Sørensen et al. [9–16] and in the model emf studies of asymmetric membranes of Sørensen and Compañ [31,32], in both cases using the "extended Donnan theory" described in Sec. II. B.

Looking at the general, thermodynamic derivation above, it might seem that the Donnan potential theory described in Sec. II. B is not of much use. Indeed, one might for a NaCl + HCl system take as point of departure Eq. (47), where the contributions from the Donnan potentials and the electrode potentials have already been "built in". In the Nernst–Planck approximation we neglect the transport number of water, and the transport numbers of the cation 2 (Na^+) and the cation 3 (H^+) are given as:

$$\tau_k = t_k = c_{k,\,m} z_k^2 D_k / [c_{1,\,m} z_1^2 D_1 + c_{2,\,m} z_2^2 D_2 + c_{3,\,m} z_3^2 D_3] \quad (k = 2,\,3) \quad (49)$$

Inserting this into Eq. (47) we see that the Donnan problem sneaks in through the backdoor, since all the ion concentrations in the membrane have to be expressed in terms of the concentrations in a fictituous external solution in Donnan equilibrium with the membrane at position x. In the ideal approximation this can be done by means of the Eqs. (32) and (34) in Sec. II.B.

Whether or not the "building block method" of the TMS theory or the more direct "thermodynamic" method is used, the final result for emf in the ideal approximation is the same, of course. We shall later give examples of such expressions in special situations. The combination of Eqs. (47) and (49) shows us another important feature, however. There are three functions to be specified in Eq. (49) at any given time θ: $c_{k,\,m}(x)$, $k = 1 \ldots 3$. One can be calculated by the condition of electroneutrality in the (ion exchange) membrane, so two independent functions have to be specified corresponding to the two "external" profiles of electroneutral electrolytes. The relative course of these two functions determine the value of emf at time θ. Thus, even in homogeneous membranes and even under ideal conditions the emf is a complicated *functional* of electrolyte profiles when we have three (mobile) ions or more present in the membrane. In inhomogeneous (but still one-dimensional) membranes, the ion diffusion coefficients in Eq. (49) have also to be specified as functions of the position, and emf is a time dependent functional even in a two ion system.

Two procedures have been used to cut the Gordian Knot of the ion profiles which are very seldomly known experimentally:

1. The Nernst–Planck electrodiffusion equations may be solved in the stationary state, for example by solving the transcendental equations of Pleijel and Schlögl [13,14,36,55].

2. A Henderson–Guggenheim "continuous mixture zone" [34,35,43] may be assumed for simplicity. For a NaCl + HCl system, for example we write for the ion concentrations at position x in the membrane

$$c_{Na^+, m}(x) = c_{Na^+, m}(x = 0_+) + [c_{Na^+, m}(x = d_-) - c_{Na^+, m}(x = 0_+)]\delta(x) \quad (50a)$$

$$c_{H^+, m}(x) = c_{H^+, m}(x = 0_+) + [c_{H^+, m}(x = d_-) - c_{H^+, m}(x = 0_+)]\delta(x) \quad (50b)$$

where the "continuous mixture parameter" $\delta(x)$ is an *arbitrary*, smooth function of x satisfying the boundary conditions:

$$\delta(x) = 0 \quad \text{for} \quad x = 0_+; \quad \delta(x) = 1 \quad \text{for} \quad x = d_- \quad (51)$$

Since all the concentration profiles are now expressed through a single function $\delta(x)$, the emf can be integrated independently of the detailed course of $\delta(x)$, and simple *analytical* formulae for emf are found, see Sec. III.

D. Membranes with Inhomogeneities and Two Kinds of Ions

In inhomogeneous or asymmetric membranes, the apparent transport numbers depend not only on concentration but also explicitly on the position variable (x). Let us restrict ourselves to the case of a diffusing, binary strong electrolyte. In analogy with Eqs. (25) we may write

$$\Delta\psi_m = -(\Delta\mu_1/z_1 F) - \{1/[v_2 z_2 F]\} \int_{x=0}^{x=d} \tau_2(c_s, x)(d\mu_s/dc_s)(\partial c_s/\partial x)\, dx$$

and for the emf we have:

$$\text{emf}(\theta) = -\{1/[v_2 z_2 F]\} \int_{x=0}^{x=d} \tau_2(c_s, x)(d\mu_s/dc_s)(\partial c_s/\partial x)\, dx \quad (52)$$

As mentioned in the introduction, the idea in performing so-called "initial time" emf measurements [26–28] is to locate the entire jump in concentration near one or the other membrane/solution interface. Let us assume that the concentration jump is located almost entirely in the right (R) surface layer of the membrane. We definite the right "apparent surface transport number" of the cation as

$$\tau_{2, \text{surface R}}(c_s) \equiv \text{Mean}\{\tau_2(c_2, x \in [d - \varepsilon \,|\, d])\}; \quad \varepsilon \ll d \quad (53)$$

Since we may replace the transport number by a mean value in the right surface layer of the membrane, the emf in Eq. (52) loses its character of a functional and we have in analogy with Eq. (26):

$$\text{emf (init, R)} = - \{1/[\nu_2 z_2 F]\} \int_{\mu_s(L)}^{\mu_s(R)} \tau_{2,\,\text{surface R}}(\mu_s) d\mu_s \tag{54}$$

At constant pressure and temperature we have

$$d\mu_s \equiv RTd \ln a_s = \nu RTd \ln a_\pm; \quad \nu \equiv \nu_1 + \nu_2 \tag{55}$$

where a_s is the salt activity and $a_\pm$ the mean ionic activity. Inserting Eq. (55) into Eq. (54) and differentiating the integral with respect to its upper boundary we obtain:

$$[\partial\{F \cdot \text{emf (init, R)}/RT\}/\partial \ln a_{\pm,\,\text{R}}]_{a_{\pm,\text{L}}} = - \{\nu/[\nu_2 z_2]\}\tau_{2,\,\text{surface R}}(a_{\pm,\,\text{R}}) \tag{56}$$

This equation forms the mathematical basis for an *experimental method*: Measure the initial value emf's for the r.h.s. of the membrane varying the r.h. electrolyte concentration and fixing the l.h. electrolyte concentration. Plot the initial emf's vs. the logarithm of the mean ionic activity in the r.h.s. electrolyte. By numeric differentiation of the curve, one obtains the r.h. surface transport number of the asymmetric membrane as a function of the concentration of the electrolyte in the whole range of concentrations, in which the initial emf values have been measured. An expression completely analogous to Eq. (56) may be derived for the l.h. surface transport number, so that the asymmetry of the membrane can be analyzed by exact electrochemical methods. We shall look at experimental examples in Sec. IV.

Very recently [31,32], Nernst–Planck–Donnan models have been analyzed to investigate the properties of some model asymmetric ion exchange membranes with either 1:1 or 2:1 electrolytes. In Ref. 31 a situation was modelled resembling NaCl in a cellulose acetate membrane with a dense skin layer. The purpose was especially to support the initial value emf method with model calculations. The local value of the electroneutral *salt flux* through the membrane at zero galvanic current are found from the generalized Nernst–Planck equations (1) to be given as [see Ref. 31, Eq. (14)]

$$J_s(x) = - 2c_s(x)\{K_s(x)\}^2[\{c_{1,\,\text{m}}(x)/D_2(x)\} + \{c_{2,\,\text{m}}(x)/D_1(x)\}]^{-1}\partial c_s/\partial x \tag{57}$$

where $c_s(x)$ is the salt concentration in an "external" solution in Donnan equilibrium with the membrane point at position x, and $K_s(x)$ is the Nernst distribution coefficient of the salt:

$$K_s(x) \equiv [K_1(x)K_2(x)]^{1/2} \quad (1:1 \text{ electrolyte}) \tag{58}$$

The ion profiles $c_{1,\,\text{m}}(x)$ and $c_{2,\,\text{m}}(x)$ follows from $c_s(x)$ from Eq. (32). It is seen from Eq. (57) that the salt flux always "runs downhill" no matter how the salt profile is chosen, and neither "facilitated" nor "reverse" transport—such as postulated by Takagi and Nakagaki [59]—is possible in asymmetric membranes.

For the emf of ideal $1:1$ electrolytes in asymmetric membranes are also found from Eqs. (1) [see Ref. 31, Eq. (27)]:

$$(F/RT)\, emf = \ln[c_{s,\,L}/c_{s,\,R}] + (1/2) \int_{x=0}^{x=d} F(x)\{\partial \ln c_s/\partial x\}\, dx \tag{59a}$$

$$F(x) \equiv \frac{\{s(x)^2/D_{21}(x)\} - \{D_{21}(x)/s(x)^2\}}{1 + (1/2)(\{s(x)^2/D_{21}(x)\} + \{D_{21}(x)/s(x)^2\})} \tag{59b}$$

$$s(x) \equiv q(x)[\{1 + q^{-2}(x)\}^{1/2} - 1] \tag{59c}$$

$$q(x) \equiv c_q(x)/\{2K_s(x)c_s(x)\} \tag{59d}$$

We have in (59b) also introduced the relative diffusivity:

$$D_{21}(x) \equiv D_2(x)/D_1(x) \tag{60}$$

We just state the formulae here and postpone examples of calculations to Sec. IV.A.

For ideal $2:1$ electrolytes in asymmetric membranes we obtain similar equations for the salt flux and the emf, see Ref. 32, eqs. (23), (36), (37), (44)–(46):

$$J_s(x) = -D_s(x)K_s(x)\partial c_s/dx \tag{61}$$

In Ref. 32, the divalent cation was chosen as ion no. 1 and the univalent anion (reversible to the electrodes) as no. 2. We maintain this numeration in Eqs. (62–66) below. The *salt distribution coefficient* and the *salt diffusion coefficient* are defined as

$$K_s(x) \equiv [K_1(x) \cdot K_2^2(x)]^{1/3} \tag{62}$$

$$D_s(x) \equiv 3\{[\beta(x)^2 D_1(x)]^{-1} + 2\beta(x)/D_2(x)\}^{-1} \tag{63}$$

$$\beta(x) \equiv [K_1/K_2]^{1/3}\alpha(x) = [2c_{1,\,m}(x)/c_{2,\,m}(x)]^{1/3} \tag{64}$$

$$(F/RT)\, emf = \ln(c_{s,\,L}/c_{s,\,R})$$
$$+ \int_{x=0}^{x=d} G(c_{1,\,m}, c_{2,\,m}, x)[\partial \ln c_s/\partial x]\, dx \tag{65}$$

$$G(c_{1,\,m}, c_{2,\,m}, x) \equiv [\{1/[1 + 2D_{21}^{-1}(x)\beta^3(x)]\}$$
$$- \{1/[2 + D_{21}(x)\beta^{-3}(x)]\}] \tag{66}$$

In the paper on $2:1$ electrolytes in asymmetric membranes the focus was set on calculation of salt fluxes, emf's and ion profiles in the *stationary state* of electrodiffusion (at zero galvanic current). Sample calculations will be presented in Sec. IV.A.

III. SURVEY OF EARLIER STUDIES OF EMF OVER CELLULOSE ACETATE MEMBRANES

A. Experimental Setup and Cells with a Single Electrolyte

In the present section we attempt to survey some earlier studies of Sørensen et al. on emf of concentration cells with cellulose acetate membranes as separator [9–16]. This survey serves to exemplify which kind of structural information about weak ion exchange membranes one can obtain using the simplified Nernst–Planck–Donnan theory (rather than the general theory of irreversible thermodynamics). The basic idea is to extract the information using first the simplest two ion system (HCl), after which three ion systems as LiCl + HCl and even four ion systems as LiCl + HCl + CaCl$_2$ or NaCl + NaF + HCl may be treated. The reason why only aqueous solutions of HCl–but not solutions of e.g., NaCl or LiCl—is a real two ion system, is that it was discovered that H$^+$ from the self dissociation of water plays a considerable role in dilute binary electrolytes in competing with the other cation as a counterion to the negative fixed charge in cellulose acetate. For brevity, we shall from now on refer to the studies in Refs. 9–16 as "the Danish emf studies".

The experimental setup in these studies was equivalent to the one shown in Fig. 1a. However, in all other experiments than the ones referred to in Ref. 9, centrifugal circulation pumps were used instead of peristaltic pumps, since the latter sometimes created ruptures in the relatively thin CA membranes. The two stock solution flasks had a volume of ~1 L and they were thermostatted to 25.0 ± 0.1°C. The measuring cell used is a perspex cell shown in Fig. 2. It is designed to have a high flow velocity laterally along the two sides of the membrane because of the specially designed narrow, rhomboidic gaps between the cell walls and the membrane surfaces. The Ag/AgCl electrodes were high precision electrodes delivered to us by the department of fundamental standardization of pH at the Danish firm Radiometer A/S. They were placed in side chambers not to be affected by the streaming of the electrolyte solutions.

The high flow velocity and the highly turbulent flow in the narrow gaps in conjunction with the relatively low salt diffusivity in the dense CA membranes used is believed to eliminate practically completely the problems with "unstirred layers" which plague many other investigations in this field. With flows between 10 ml/min to 120 ml/min no changes in the measured stationary state emf were observed. Below 10 ml/min, some changes could be seen. In consequence, the flow rate was fixed to 70 ml/min corresponding to a mean, linear velocity in the gaps of about 30 cm/s. Generally, the stationary state of electrodiffusion in the membrane was reached within 3–5 h from the start of the experiment. Initial values of emf were not recorded in the Danish emf experiments. The first measurements of these experiments were made using a dense CA membrane which was not completely symmetric. When asymmetry was seen in the stationary emf measurements, the emf values treated in the

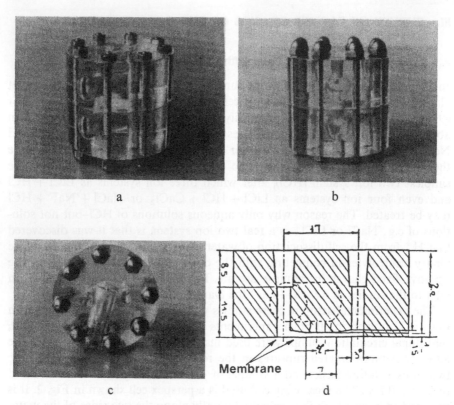

FIG. 2 The perspex cell used in the "Danish emf studies" on cellulose acetate membranes. The measures indicated are in mm. The "Danish cell" mentioned in Sec. IV.B is similar but with all linear dimensions multiplied by 2 [9].

models were the mean of two measurements with the membrane in one or in the other direction relative to the solutions.

The dense cellulose acetate membranes were cast from a solution of 25 wt% of 2.5-cellulose acetate (Eastman-Kodak E-398-3) in acetone on a glass plate in a layer originally 100 μm thick and the acetone were evaporated to complete dryness before quenching the membrane in deionized water at room temperature. Between the experimental series, the membranes is kept in formalin solution at 4°C. The thickness of the dense cellulose acetate membranes was ~ 30 μm.

The structure of the cellulose acetate chains is shown in Fig. 3, showing the acetylated primary and secondary alcohol groups, a nonacetylated alcohol group (only tri-cellulose acetate is fully acetylated) and a secondary alcohol group which has been oxidized to a carboxyl group (glucuronic acid group). There are very few of the latter in the cellulose acetetate E-398-3, much less

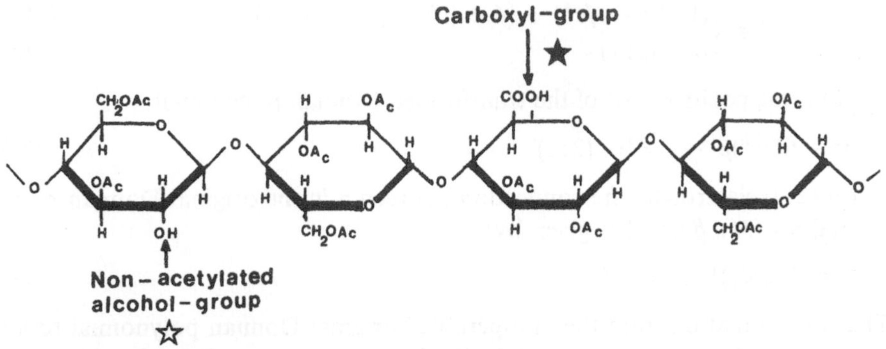

Carboxyl–group

Non–acetylated alcohol–group

FIG. 3 Part of a cellulose acetate (CA) polymer chain showing acetylated primary and secondary alcohol groups, a nonacetylated alcohol group and a glucuronic acid group (oxydized primary alcohol group) responsible for the cation exchange properties of CA.

than one carboxyl group per polymer molecule of degree of polymerization 100–300, see Ref. 86. Nevertheless, these glucuronic acid groups have a pronounced influence on emf, when one or both of the terminal solutions were dilute solutions of electrolytes different from HCl.

In Ref. 9 "apparent transport numbers" were defined for membrane experiments with one electrolyte only as derivatives of the curves of emf vs. $\ln a_{\pm}$ (variable), analogous to Eq. (56) for the "surface transport number" but with emf(init) replaced by emf(stationary) (or simply the time independent emf for completely homogeneous membranes). Since we have used here the word "apparent transport numbers" in a somewhat different context, we shall prefer the word "differential transport number":

$$\tau_{2,\,\text{diff}}(a_{\pm,\,\text{var}}) \equiv \pm(\nu_2 z_2/\nu)[\partial\{F \cdot \text{emf}/RT\}/\partial \ln a_{\pm,\,\text{var}}]_{a_{\pm,\,\text{fix}}} \tag{67}$$

The + sign is used when the l.h.s. solution is varied, the − sign when the r.h.s. solution is varied. The differential transport number is equal to the apparent transport number for the cation (ion no. 2) in the membrane soaked by the variable concentration at which the derivative is taken. In the Nernst–Planck approximation there is no difference between the apparent transport number (corrected for solvent flow) and transport number, and in Ref. 9 the Nernst–Planck–Donnan expressions were derived for the differential transport numbers in ion exchange membranes with $1:1$ and $2:1$ electrolytes:

$$t_{2,\,\text{diff}}(c^*) = [1 + D\{1 - (\xi c^*)^{-1}\}]^{-1} \tag{68}$$

$$D \equiv \begin{cases} D_{12} = D_1/D_2 & (1:1) \\ (D_{12}/2) & (2:1) \end{cases} \tag{69}$$

$$c^* \equiv \begin{cases} K_s c_s/c_q & (1:1) \\ 2K_s c_s/c_q & (2:1) \end{cases} \tag{70}$$

$$\xi \equiv \begin{cases} (1/2)[(-\omega/c^*) + \{4 + (c^*)^{-2}\}^{1/2}] & (1:1) \\ \beta^2 & (2:1) \end{cases} \quad \begin{matrix} (71a) \\ (71b) \end{matrix}$$

β is the real, positive root of the transformed Donnan polynomial:

$$\beta^3 + (\omega/c^*)\beta - 1 = 0 \quad (2:1) \tag{72}$$

For a $(2:1)$ electrolyte, the connection between α in the original Donnan polynomial Eq. (34), β and ξ is given by:

$$\beta \equiv (K_2/K_1)^{1/3}\alpha = \sqrt{\xi} \tag{73}$$

The transformation from the "inoperable" original Donnan polynomial to an "operable" Donnan polynomial (with the minimum number of measurable parameters) may be done in many ways, in fact the Donnan polynomial in Ref. 9 was different from Eq. (72): a third-order polynomial in ξ with a nonzero second-order term. The Donnan polynomial in Eq. (72) is the one used in Refs. 11 and 32. In Ref. 11 it was shown that the two Donnan polynomials have identical roots. An analytical solution for the real, positive root of Eq. (72) was discussed in Ref. 32.

Figures 4a and 4b show for $1:1$ and $2:1$ electrolytes the (differential) transport number of the cation in ideal Nernst–Planck–Donnan cation exchange membranes ($\omega = -1$) as a function of the dimensionless salt concentration c^* at different values of the ratio D_1/D_2. It is seen that very low salt concentration (relative to c_q) leads to a transport number equal to unity. In this case, the anion is completely *Donnan excluded* from the membrane and the cation transports all the galvanic current, i.e., the membrane is an *ideal cation exchanger*, Eq. (74a). In contrast, very high salt concentration (relative to c_q) makes insignificant the Donnan effects and the transport number becomes independent of salt concentration and given by Eq. (74b):

$$t_2 = 1 \qquad\qquad\qquad\qquad (c^* \ll 1) \tag{74a}$$

$$t_2^o = (z_2^2 D_2)/(2z_1^2 D_1 + z_2^2 D_2) = (1 + D)^{-1} \quad (c^* \gg 1) \tag{74b}$$

The last transformation in Eq. (74b) is valid for $1:1$ and $2:1$ electrolytes with the diffusion ratio D defined in Eqs. (69). In the intermediate region with $c^* \approx 1$ there is a strong dependence on the salt concentration. In the Nernst–Planck–Donnan approximation, the (differential) transport number of the cation in a cation exchange membrane always decreases with salt concentration.

In Ref. 9 emf values were reported for HCl experiments on a dense CA membrane where the l.h.s. concentration varies from 0.001 mol/L of 0.1 mol/L whereas the r.h.s. concentration is always fixed to 0.001 mol/L. (emf is always r.h. electrode minus l.h. electrode.) The values of $(F/2RT)\cdot$emf have been plotted vs. $\ln[c_s(\text{vac})/c_s(\text{fix})]$ and are very well fitted by a least-square polynomial of second degree passing through $(0, 0)$. By derivation of this poly-

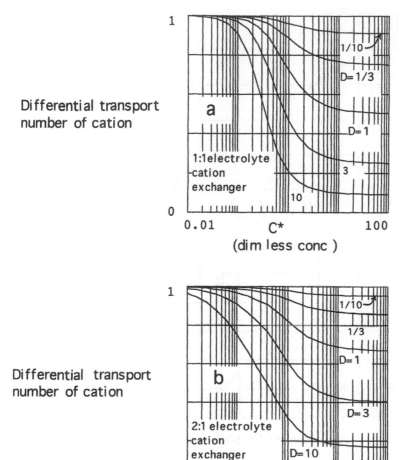

Differential transport number of cation

Differential transport number of cation

FIG. 4 Differential transport numbers of the cation for (a) 1:1 ideal electrolytes and (b) 2:1 ideal electrolytes. The ratio of membrane diffusion coefficients D is given in Eq. (69) and the dimensionless electrolyte concentration c^* by Eq. (70).

nomial, the (differential) transport number of H^+ (assuming electrolyte ideality) can be calculated as a linearly decreasing function of $\ln[c_s(\text{var})/c_s(\text{fix})]$. The transport number varies from ~ 0.975 at 0.001 mol/L to ~ 0.91 at 0.1 mol/L, see Fig. 5a.

In terms of the above Nernst–Planck–Donnan model, this variation can

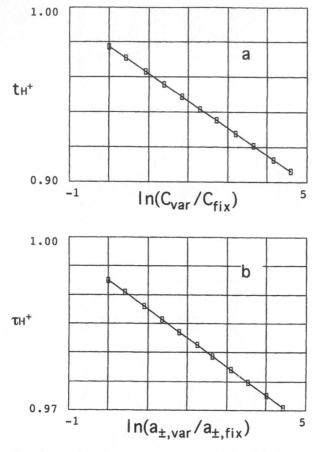

FIG. 5 (a) The transport number of H^+ in a dense CA membrane with aqueous HCl solutions at 25°C as a function of the concentration as calculated from experiments assuming ideality ($c_{fix} = 0.001$ mol/L). (b) The true, apparent transport number of H^+ determined by numeric differentiation of the experimental emf vs. $\ln a_{\pm, var}$ curve.

be due to a very small fixed charge density c_q. In fact the variation in t_{H+} may be fitted with $t_{H+}^0 = 0.909$ ($D = 0.1$) and a $c^* \approx 0.63$ at a HCl concentration $= 0.001$ mol/L. From Eq. (70) we then have that $c_q/K_s \approx 0.0016$ eqv./L. The value of c^* at 0.1 mol/L would then be ~ 6.3. According to Fig. 4a, the curve with $D_{12} = D = 0.1$ has almost, but not completely, reached the value t_2^0 at $c^* \approx 6$. However, the glucuronic acid groups in the CA membrane are probably almost all in the uncharged form at pH ≈ 1: Therefore, the real value of c^* at 0.1 mol/L is probably much greater than 6 and the value of t_{H+} should have reached constancy.

Since the value of t_{H+} still seems to vary at 0.1 mol/L, there have to be other explanations involved than just the fixed charge. The most natural objection is that emf should be plotted vs. $\ln[a_{\pm}(\text{var})/a_{\pm}(\text{fix})]$ instead of $\ln[c_s(\text{var})/c_s(\text{fix})]$. The exact apparent transport number τ_{H+} found by differentiation of the new least square, second order polynomial through (0, 0) is shown as a function of $\ln[a_{\pm}(\text{var})/a_{\pm}(\text{fix})]$ in Fig. 5b. This transport number varies very little with concentration. The variation is from 0.993 at 0.001 mol/L to 0.971 at 0.1 mol/L. This is very well in accordance with the more recent EMF measurements of Plesner, Malmgren-Hansen and Sørensen of HCl in another dense CA membrane where the mean apparent transport number were found to be $\tau_{H+} = 0.978 \pm 0.004$ by fitting a straight line to a plot of $(F/2RT) \cdot$ emf vs. $\ln[a_{\pm}(\text{var})/a_{\pm}(\text{fix})]$ in the region from 0.01 mol/L to 1.0 mol/L, see Fig. 5a in [18]. (By close inspection this plot is in reality slightly curved, however, and the apparent transport number decreases slightly with concentration just as stated here.)

It is a weakness in the analysis of emf data alone as it is performed in Refs. 9–16 that there is a considerable uncertainty of how much faster than Cl$^-$ the proton diffuses in the CA matrix. This is inevitably so, since the transport number of H$^+$ is quite close to unity. In Ref. 9 the point of view was taken that ideality should be assumed throughout, and the differential transport number of H$^+$ was taken from the emf vs. $\ln[c_s(\text{var})c_s(\text{fix})]$ plot at the high values of $c_s(\text{var})$ where the influence of any remaining fixed charge can be disregarded. Then the transport number for the proton was found to be 0.91 corresponding to a diffusion coefficient of the proton equal to ~ 10 times the diffusion coefficient of the chloride. This factor of 10 was maintained in the subsequent studies with mixed electrolytes, but this can easily be corrected for (see the discussion in Sec. III. B).

However, the apparent transport number τ_{H+} from the activity plots has a greater physical reality, since it is the real transport number of H$^+$ if (electroosmotic) water transport can be neglected. A value of $\tau_{H+} = 0.975$ corresponds (with a Nernst–Planck interpretation) to a diffusion of H$^+$ ca. ~ 40 times faster than that of Cl$^-$ in the CA matrix! In the emf experiments of the mixed electrolytes to be discussed in the next subsections the data can be fitted almost equally well with the ratio $D_{H+}/D_{Cl-} = 10$ as well as 40 since there is a considerable *covariance* between the parameters to be determined from the emf plots. Thus, in reality we need other experiments than emf experiments to settle the question. Such experiments could be electric impedance measurements on membranes bathed in uniform (but variable) electrolyte solutions, see the discussion in Refs. 15–19. Even these experiments could be roughly fitted with a ratio $D_{H+}/D_{Cl-} = 10$ at a fixed external pH = 5, see Refs. 15–17. First when more extensive studies were performed also at lower values of pH, evidence accumulated that the ratio D_{H+}/D_{Cl-} is probably quite close to 40 and certainly above 10.

In Ref. 9 the emf with the electrolytes NaCl, KCl and $CaCl_2$ and the same membrane specimen was also investigated with $c_s(\text{fix}) = 0.01$ mol/L. The emf vs. $\ln[c_s(\text{var})/c_s(\text{fix})]$ plots for NaCl and KCl both had a strong downward curvature except in the range 0.001 mol/L to 0.01 mol/L. This means strongly decreasing cation transport number in accordance with Fig. 4a. From the limiting high concentration transport number, the value of D_{12} can be found and the fit to the intermediate concentrations determines the other dimensionless parameter c_q/K_s. At the lower concentrations, an upward curvature is seen in the plots, see Figs. 10 and 11 in Ref. 9. This curvature cannot be understood in the framework of the two-ion Nernst–Planck model. We shall return to the question in the subsequent sections.

The emf curve with $CaCl_2$ showed almost no curvature, however, see Fig. 12 in Ref. 9. In the two-ion model, this could be interpreted in terms of a very small fixed charge caused by binding of Ca^{2+} to some of the glucuronic acid groups. The emf curve corresponded to a fixed concentration equal to 0.01 mol/L $CaCl_2$, and the variable molarity varied from 0.001 mol/L to 1 mol/L. In retrospect we can see that it was lucky that the $CaCl_2$ measurements were the last in the series, since the Ca^{2+} ions bind very strongly to the $-COO^-$ groups of the CA-matrix, so strongly indeed that it may take 14 days or more to dissociate at a concentration of $CaCl_2$ equal to zero, see Ref. 15 and Sec. III.E.

The parameters obtained for the four types of electrolytes using the Nernst–Planck–Donnan theory for a single electrolyte are listed in Table 1.

B. Concentration Cells with XCl + HCl (X = Li, Na, K)

Since the electrolytes are dissolved in water, it is necessary in dilute solutions to take the self dissociation of this medium into account. Furthermore if the circulating solutions are not protected from the atmosphere, absorption of

TABLE 1 Fitted Parameters in the Single Salt Approximation Dense Cellulose 2.5 Acetate Membrane, 25°C

Electrolyte	$D_{\text{cation}}/D_{Cl^-}$	c_q/K_s (negative eqv/L)
HCl	10–40	very low
NaCl	0.294	0.063
KCl	0.269	0.050
$CaCl_2$	0.069	very low

Source: data adapted from Ref. 9 and from the present analysis.

more or less carbon dioxide from the atmosphere will influence the pH of the solution which will generally be between 6 and 7. Therefore if one or both terminal solutions are dilute, it is necessary to take into account at least the presence of the H^+ ion so that the "two-ion systems" described in the previous sections (except the one with HCl) really are "three-ion systems" ($XCl + HCl$ or $XCl_2 + HCl$). For such systems, we obtain from Eq. (47) the following *analytical* expression for the emf—using the "continuous mixture" (CM) approximation (50a,b) and the ideal Nernst–Planck–Donnan model with individual distribution coefficients, see Refs. 10 and 11 and Sec. II.B

$$[F/RT] \cdot \text{emf (CM)} = \ln[c^*(L)x_{Cl,\,L}/\{c^*(R)x_{Cl,\,R}\}]$$
$$+ (1/z_X)\ln[\xi(R)/\xi(L)] + (F/RT)\Delta\psi_m \qquad (75)$$

with the diffusion potential

$$(F/RT)\Delta\psi_m = - (P_1/P_2)\ln[c^*(R)Q(R)/\{c^*(L)Q(L)\}] \qquad (76a)$$
$$P_1 \equiv z_{Cl}\Delta\{x_{Cl}c^*\xi^{(zCl/zX)}\} + z_X D_{X,\,Cl}\Delta\{c^*\xi\}$$
$$+ z_H D_{H,\,Cl}k_{H,\,x}\Delta\{x_H c^*\xi^{(zH/zX)}\} \qquad (76b)$$
$$P_2 \equiv z_{Cl}^2\Delta\{x_{Cl}c^*\xi^{(zCl/zX)}\} + z_X^2 D_{X,\,Cl}\Delta\{c^*\xi\}$$
$$+ z_H^2 D_{H,\,Cl}k_{H,\,x}\Delta\{x_H c^*\xi^{(zH/zX)}\} \qquad (76c)$$
$$\Delta\{\text{quantity}\} \equiv \text{quantity (R)} - \text{quantity (L)} \qquad (76d)$$
$$Q \equiv z_{Cl}^2 x_{Cl}\,\xi^{(zCl/zX)} + z_X^2 D_{X,\,Cl}\xi + z_H^2 D_{H,\,Cl}k_{H,\,x}x_H\,\xi^{(zH/zX)} \qquad (76e)$$

The dimensionless salt concentration c^* is defined by

$$c^* \equiv c_X/[c_q/K_s(XCl_n)] \qquad (77)$$

In the external solutions we define the concentration ratios as:

$$x_{Cl} \equiv c_{Cl}/c_X; \quad x_H \equiv c_H/c_X \qquad (78)$$

Furthermore we have introduced the Nernst distribution ratio

$$k_{H,\,x} \equiv K_H/K_X \qquad (79)$$

and the ratios of diffusion coefficients:

$$D_{X,\,Cl} \equiv D_X/D_{Cl}; \quad D_{H,\,Cl} \equiv D_H/D_{Cl} \qquad (80)$$

The variable ξ is the real, positive root in the transformed Donnan polynomial which—in the case of mixtures of two 1:1 electrolytes—is given by:

$$(1 + k_{H,\,x}x_H)\xi^2 - (1/c^*)\xi - (1 + x_H) = 0 \qquad (81)$$
$$\xi \equiv \sqrt{(K_X/K_{Cl})} \cdot \alpha \qquad (82)$$

In Refs. 10 and 11 this formalism was fitted to emf data for the same membrane specimen as investigated in Ref. 9 with NaCl, KCl and LiCl as the "variable salt". The value of pH was regulated by addition of HCl. At the higher concentrations of the variable salt, the determination of $D_{X, Cl}$ and c_q/K_s can be done by the two-ion model as before and pH has only indirect influence (titration of the fixed charge). If there is some asymmetry in the membrane, the stationary state emf values may depend on the direction of diffusion in the membrane, however, see Figs. 1 and 2 in Ref. 11. At the lower concentrations, the emf values are quite sensitive to pH but not to the direction of diffusion. The lower the pH the more significant is the upward curvature at low concentrations of XCl, see Fig. 6. Thus, a CA membrane may be used as a kind of "pH-meter" near neutrality.

The solid curves in Fig. 6 for pH = 5, 6 and 7 have been calculated by the above formulae using the parameters $c_q/K_s = 0.054$ (pH = 5), 0.077 (pH = 6) and 0.081 (pH = 7) [all values in eqv./L]. Furthermore, the value of $D_{Li, Cl}$ was

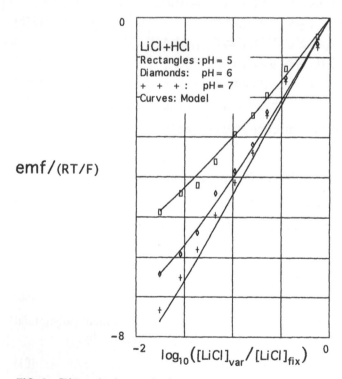

FIG. 6 Dimensionless emf values with variable concentrations less than 0.01 mol/L for LiCl experiments on a dense CA membrane at 25°C. Fixed background concentrations of HCl corresponding to pH(conc.) = 5, 6 and 7 are used. The curves correspond to model fits. See the text.

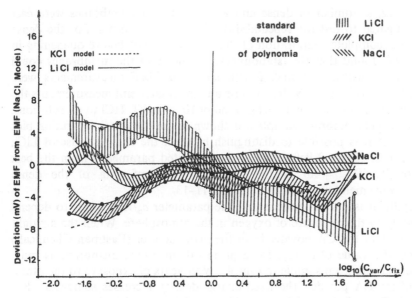

FIG. 7   The selectivity of a dense CA membrane for different cations at 25°C. The emf values have all been subtracted from the values calculated with the model fitted to the NaCl data, so the abscissa represents emf(NaCl, model). The three "uncertainty belts" shown are results of polynomial fittings to the experimental data. The most significant least square polynomials at the 95% significance level were fitted to the emf data. The belts are the polynomial smoothed values ± the calculated standard error of these smoothed values [12].

set to 0.12. The last two parameters were set to either

$$D_{H, Cl} = 10; \quad k_{H, Li} = 10 \tag{83a}$$

or

$$D_{H, Cl} = 40; \quad k_{H, Li} = 2.5 \tag{83b}$$

The solid curves are completely *identical* if we just keep the product $D_{H, Cl} \cdot k_{H, Li}$ constant. This is so for the following physical reason: even if the total galvanic current is zero, the contributions from each kind of ion to the current are different from zero. The upward curvatures of the emf curves at low variable concentrations are caused by the contribution to the current from the protons and this contribution is determined by the product of the diffusion coefficient and the concentration (the Nernst distribution coefficient) of the proton. Thus, we see that we cannot see from emf measurements alone if the proton diffuses 10 or 40 times as fast as the chloride ion in a dense CA membrane, cf. the discussion in the preceding section.

In Ref. 12, a number of dense and asymmetric CA membranes were cast and investigated to test the repeatability of the measurements. For the dense membranes (complete evaporation of the acetone solvent before quenching in water) it was found that the (stationary) asymmetry of the membranes could be maintained within ± 1 mV. Furthermore, all EMF measurements were repeatable to within ± 5 mV. In all these and in all later emf measurements the pH was fixed by addition of a background of 10^{-5} mol/L HCl to all solutions. For one specific membrane sample it is shown in the statistical separation plot in Fig. 7 that it is possible to distinguish between the emf response of LiCl, NaCl and KCl. Table 2 lists some of the evaluated parameters from the best fits (with $D_{H+}/D_{Cl-} = 40$) of the model to the emf data of the dense (homogeneous) membranes studied in Refs. 11–13.

Generally, it is our experience that the parameter c_q/K_{12} seems to depend very slightly to the exposure of oxygen in the atmosphere. When the air-tight plastic bag with the CA powder from the manufacturer (Eastman Chemicals) is broken, the value of c_q/K_{12} for a given salt in a cast membrane is quite small but varying from sample to sample. With years of exposure to the atmosphere of the CA powder, the fixed charge density increases somewhat. For example in Table 2 the membrane A (the membrane also used to produce the data in Table 1) was cast in 1980–1981 but the membrane B3II was cast in 1987 from a newly opened package of CA powder. This powder has "aged" a couple of years before the membranes B24II, B24III and B26II were cast. In the impedance measurements of Plesner, Malmgren-Hansen and Sørensen [18] on dense CA membranes, NaCl + HCl and KCl + HCl systems, the membranes were again cast from a new sample of powder, and the c_q/K_{12} found dropped to the low value 0.023 like for B3II in Ref. 12.

It is seen from Table 2 that the fixed charge is partially titrated at lower pH. However, this titration is only approximately accounted for with a "fixed charge density" which is constant in each experimental series. In reality, the concentration of the protons in the membrane is dependent on the external concentration of XCl even at a fixed external level of HCl. It was shown in Ref. 18 that when the titration is taken explicitly into account in the Donnan equilibrium, the Donnan polynomial becomes of third order even in 1:1 electrolyte systems. Instead of Eq. (81) we obtain

$$(1 + k_{H, x} x_H)(1 + k_{H, x} x_H)(c_H/K_a^*)\sqrt{(k_{H, x})}\xi^3 + (1 + k_{H, x} x_H)\xi^2$$
$$- [(1/c^*) + x_{Cl}(c_H/K_a^*)\sqrt{(k_{H, x})}]\xi - (1 + x_H) = 0 \quad (84)$$

where K_a^* is an effective dissociation constant of the glucuronic acid groups constituting the "fixed" charge. It is related to the "intrinsic" dissociation constant K_a, based upon the H^+ concentrations in the membrane, by:

$$K_a^* = K_a/K_{HCl} \quad (85)$$

TABLE 2 Fitted Parameters in XCl = HCl Systems. Dense Cellulose 2.5 Acetate Membrane, 25°C

Electrolyte mixture	Membrane	pH	c_q/K_{XCl} (neg. eqv./L)	D_{X+}/D_{Cl-}	D_{H+}/D_{Cl-}	$k_{H+,X+}$	Emf data from
LiCl + HCl	A	5	0.054	0.12	40	2.5	[11]
LiCl + HCl	A	6	0.077	0.12	40	2.5	[11]
LiCl + HCl	A	7	0.081	0.12	40	2.5	[11]
LiCl + HCl	B3II	5	0.030	0.19	40	2.5	[12]
NaCl + HCl	A	3	0.0010	0.30	40	≈12	[11]
NaCl + HCl	A	4	0.030	0.30	40	≈12	[11]
NaCl + HCl	B3II	4.5	0.022	0.25	40	2.5	[12]
NaCl + HCl	B3II	5	0.029	0.25	40	2.5	[12]
NaCl + HCl	B24II	5	0.043	0.25	40	2.5	[13]
NaCl + HCl	B24III	5	0.041	0.25	40	2.5	[13]
NaCl + HCl	B25IV	5	0.038	0.25	40	2.5	[13]
NaCl + HCl	B26II	5	0.042	0.25	40	2.5	[13]
KCl + HCl	B3II	5	0.023	0.28	40	≈2	[12]
KCl + HCl	B24II	5	0.035	0.28	40	2.5	[13]

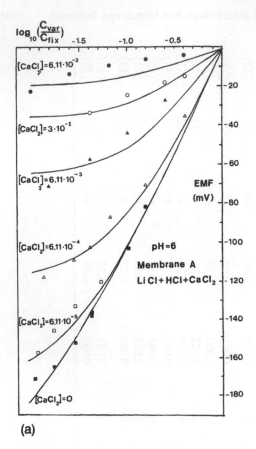

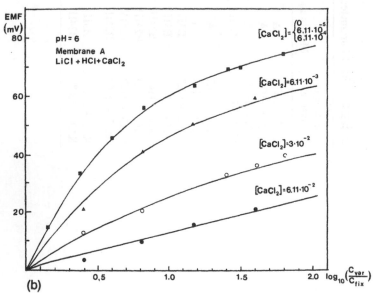

Although Eq. (84) was used in Ref. 18 for fitting membrane conductivities in experiments with the same XCl + HCl solutions on both sides of the membrane (but varying these solutions from experiment to experiment), no attempts have yet been made to apply Eq. (84) in connection with emf experiments. The situation in such experiments is much more complicated due to the variation of the electrolyte composition through the membrane. The best fit to the membrane conductivities was $pK_a^* = 2.8$ or $pK_a = 4.2$. This value may be compared to the value $pK_a = 4.65 \pm 0.30$ estimated in Ref. 11 using only the c_q/K_{HCl} values obtained from the second-order Donnan polynomial at varying background pH.

Finally, it should be noticed that all the parameter fits in Table 2 have been made assuming that the diffusion zone is a "continuous mixture" (CM) zone. In a number of cases this assumption was checked using the in principle more correct Pleijel–Schlögl integration of the Nernst–Planck equations and stationarity [13,14]. The "best fits" do not differ very much using the two methods, however. Taking, as an example, the CM parameters for membrane B24II with NaCl + HCl for comparison, one set of Pleijel–Schlögl values of the parameters were found to the values below:

B24II, Pleijel–Schlögl: $\{c_q/K_{NaCl}; D_{Na, Cl}; D_{H, Cl}; k_{H, Na}\} = \{0.042; 0.27; 10; 9.0\}$

As before, the two last numbers may just as well be 40 and 9/4.

C. Concentration Cells with YCl$_2$ + HCl + XCl (Y = Mg, Ca, Ba)

It was mentioned in Sec. III.A that Ca^{2+} ions seemed to lower the observed fixed charge perhaps by binding to the glucuronic acid groups. Indeed, Malm et al. [87] have reported on an increase in viscosity of CA-solutions in acetone, when the resin had been subjected to a prior washing with solutions of salts with divalent cations and when the pH was not too low. They interpreted this as formation of intermolecular bridges between the polymer chains with the divalent cations as the bridge formers.

In order to investigate this binding more closely, emf measurements were performed in concentration cells with YCl$_2$ + HCl + XCl with Y = Mg, Ca, Ba and X = Li, Na [11,13]. The concentration of HCl in all measurements was 10^{-6} or 10^{-5} mol/L. In Ref. 11, the "variable salt" was LiCl, pH was 6 and uniform "backgrounds" of CaCl$_2$ were added with concentrations ranging from $\sim 6 \times 10^{-5}$ mol/L to $\sim 6 \times 10^{-2}$ mol/L. Figures 8a and 8b show the

---

FIG. 8 (a) Values of emf for experiments with LiCl on a dense CA membrane at 25°C with variable concentrations less than 0.01 mol/L. The background pH(conc.) = 6 in all experiments and the background concentration of CaCl$_2$ is varied from one series to the next. (b) Similar curves for [LiCl] > 0.01 mol/L. [11].

results for low and high variable concentrations, respectively. A qualitative explanation of the appearance of the curves is the following:

With no added Ca^{2+} ions the emf curve is the usual one for LiCl, i.e., saturating at high LiCl concentrations at the differential transport number for Li^+ in a membrane with no fixed charge and approaching at intermediate LiCl concentrations the transport number unity in an ideal cation exchanger except for the H^+ induced upward bend at very low variable concentrations. When more Ca^{2+} ions are added, the chemical equilibrium

$$\text{Cellulose Acetate} -COO^- + Ca^{2+} = \text{Cellulose Acetate} -COO \cdots Ca^+ \quad (86)$$

is shifted more and more to the right. The overall fixed, negative charge is diminished in value. This means that the limiting transport number of Li^+ is reached at lower concentrations which explains the behavior in Fig. 8b. On the other hand, the added concentration of free Ca^{2+} ions contribute to the galvanic current (which is zero in total) just like HCl and gives rise to an increasing "plateau" in the emf at low concentrations of LiCl, see Fig. 8a.

The full curves in Figs. 8a and b were calculated from the Nernst–Planck–Donnan model (assuming CM-zone) with the parameters given in Table 3. The Donnan polynomial is of third order but we shall not write it down here, see the general description in Ref. 11. There are two additional dimensionless parameters, namely $D_{Ca^{2+}}/D_{Cl^-}$ and

$$k_{Ca^{2+},\,Li^+} \equiv (K_{CaCl_2}/K_{LiCl})^3 \quad (87)$$

If enough divalent cations are added, the membrane should convert itself to an *anion exchange membrane* (with a positive fixed charge and $\omega = +1$). This was studied in Ref. 13, where a dense CA membrane (B24III) was pretreated in a stirred solution of 1 mol/L $BaCl_2$ or $MgCl_2$ during one day. Assuming that the dissociation of the bound divalent ions is a very slow process (see Sec. III.E), the structural parameters of the membrane in anion exchange form may be evaluated from the emf curve using $BaCl_2$ or $MgCl_2$ as the "variable salt", see Fig. 9 and Table 3. Figure 9 also shows that it is impossible to fit the emf curves with $\omega = -1$. Indeed, the fact that an emf very close to zero is measured between 10^{-4} and 10^{-1} mol/L NaCl (with 10^{-2} mol/L NaCl as the fixed concentration) shows us that the membrane in that region is an *ideal anion exchanger* (with complete exclusion of cations). Using the quasi-thermostatic method and sending one (virtual) Faraday through the cell, it is seen that the chloride ion originates at one electrode, passes through the membrane and disappears at the other electrode. This amounts of a $\Delta G = 0$ for the net chemical transport (being nil) and the emf is zero.

D. Concentration Cells with KCl + KF + HCl

In Ref. 13, emf curves for the same dense CA membrane specimen (B24II) were compared using KCl and equimolar mixtures of KCl and KF as the "variable

TABLE 3 Fitted Parameters in YCl_2 + HCl + XCl and Pretreated YCl_2 + HCl Systems. Dense Cellulose 2.5 Acetate Membrane, 25°C

Mixture	Membrane	pH	pY	c_q/K_{XCl} (eqv./L)	D_{X^+}/D_{Cl^-}	D_{H^+}/D_{Cl^-}	$D_{Y^{2+}}/D_{Cl^-}$	k_{H^+,X^+}	k_{Ca^{2+},Li^+}	Ref.
Y = Ca²⁺										
X = Li⁺	A	6	4.21	−0.086	0.12	40[a]	0.1	2.5[b]	6 × 10⁻⁴	[11]
X = Li⁺	A	6	3.74	−0.086	0.12	40	0.1	2.5	6 × 10⁻⁴	[11]
X = Li⁺	A	6	3.21	−0.086	0.12	40	0.1	2.5	6 × 10⁻⁴	[11]
X = Li⁺	A	6	2.52	−0.086	0.12	40	0.1	2.5	6 × 10⁻⁴	[11]
X = Li⁺	A	6	2.21	−0.083	0.12	40	0.1	2.5	6 × 10⁻⁴	[11]
X = Li⁺	A	6	2.00	−0.080	0.12	40	0.1	2.5	6 × 10⁻⁴	[11]
X = Li⁺	A	6	1.52	−0.076	0.12	40	0.1	2.5	6 × 10⁻⁴	[11]
X = Li⁺	A	6	1.21	−0.042	0.12	40	0.1	2.5	6 × 10⁻⁴	[11]
Y = Ba²⁺	B24III	5	var	+0.085	—	40[a]	0.035	≈2.5[b]	—	[13]
Y = Mg²⁺	B24III	5	var	+0.20	—	40	0.050	≈2.5	—	[13]

[a] Original fit multiplied by 4.
[b] Original fit divided by 4.

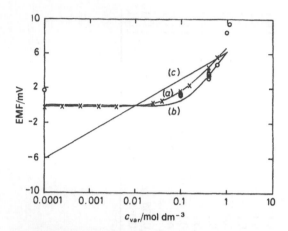

FIG. 9 Values of emf as a function of the variable concentration of 2:1 electrolytes for a dense CA membrane at 25°C. Crosses: $BaCl_2$. Circles: $MgCl_2$. The fixed concentration is 0.01 mol/L and pH(conc.) = 5. The curves (a) and (b) are calculated from the model assuming the membrane to be an anion exchanger ($\omega = +1$). Curve (a), $BaCl_2$: $D_{H+}/D_{Cl-} = 10$; $D_{Ba2+}/D_{Cl-} = 0.035$; $c_q/K_{BaCl_2} = 0.085$ eqv./L; $k_{H+, Ba2+} = 1$. Curve (b), $MgCl_2$: $D_{H+}/D_{Cl-} = 10$; $D_{Ba2+}/D_{Cl-} = 0.050$; $c_q/K_{BaCl_2} = 0.20$ eqv./L; $k_{H+, Ba2+} = 1$. Curve (c) is for the model for a cation exchanger ($\omega = -1$) and $D_{H+}/D_{Cl-} = 10$; $D_{Y2+}/D_{Cl-} = 0.018$; $c_q/K_{YCl_2} \leq 10^{-5}$ eqv./L; $k_{H+, Y2+} \leq 0.01$. It is not possible to fit the data in any way to the model for a cation exchange membrane even if it is assumed as in curve (c) that the fixed charge has been practically eliminated by the binding of divalent cations to the glucuronic acid groups [13].

salt" with pH kept at 5. Figure 10a—where the ideal Nernst potential difference has been subtracted from the measured emf values—shows that there can be up to 25 mV difference between the two systems. This considerable difference cannot be ascribed to differences in the electrode potentials of the Ag/AgCl electrodes between the KCl system and the KCl + KF system at the same total concentration, since a detailed experimental and theoretical study of activity coefficients in KCl–KF mixtures [88–92] has revealed that there is no significant difference between the mean ionic activity coefficient of KCl in solutions of pure KCl and in mixed equimolar KCl–KF solutions at the same total salt concentration. Furthermore, Monte Carlo studies [90–92] have shown that the difference between the natural logarithm of the single ion activity coefficient of Cl^- and the natural logarithm of the mean ionic activity coefficient for KCl (both values for a 1 mol/L equimolar mixture) is less than 0.02 corresponding to ~0.5 mV, see for example Fig. 9 in Ref. 90. This difference is without significance in the present context.

Figure 10b shows the model fit to the experimental emf data for the equimolar mixture. The Donnan polynomial is of second degree and in addition to

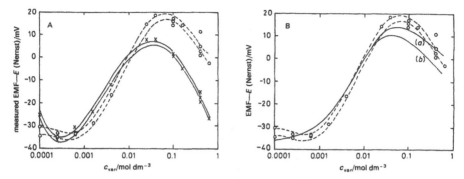

FIG. 10 Emf values after subtraction of the ideal contribution from the Ag/AgCl electrodes (to see more clearly the differences). Fixed concentration: 0.01 mol/L. Fig. 1a: Distinguishing between Cl^- and F^- ions for a dense CA membrane at 25°C with pH(conc.) = 5. Crosses: KCl solutions. Circles: Equimolar KCl–KF solutions. Dashed and full curves: Uncertainty belts of most significant least square polynomials at the 95% significance level. Fig. 1b: KCl–KF experiment, only, compared to model fits. The model values (assuming a CM diffusion zone) are $D_{K+}/D_{Cl-} = 0.28$; $D_{H+}/D_{Cl-} = 10$; $c_q/K_{KCl} = 0.035$ eqv./L; $k_{H+, K+} = 9.5$. Curve (a) is calculated with $D_{F-}/D_{Cl-} = 0.1$; $k_{F-, Cl-} = 0.83$. Curve (b) is with $D_{F-}/D_{Cl-} = 0.4$; $k_{F-, Cl-} = 1.18$ [13].

the parameters in the last line of Table 2, two more parameters were very approximately determined in Ref. 13:

$$k_{F-, Cl-} \equiv K_{F-}/K_{Cl-} = (K_{KF}/K_{KCl})^2 \approx 0.6; \quad D_{F-}/D_{Cl-} \approx 0.1 \qquad (88)$$

To demonstrate the sensitivity on these parameters, the solid curve (a) in Fig. 10b corresponds to $k_{F-, Cl-} = 0.83$ and $D_{F-}/D_{Cl-} = 0.1$ and the solid curve (b) corresponds to $k_{F-, Cl-} = 1.18$ and $D_{F-}/D_{Cl-} = 0.4$. It is probable that the much lower diffusion coefficient of F^- than that of Cl^- in the membrane is due to the strong hydration of the former ion. Thus, emf measurements over a dense CA membrane is very sensitive to the size difference between the two anions in marked contrast to direct measurements of emf in aqueous solutions with ion specific electrodes [88–90].

E. Binding/Dissociation of Divalent Ions to/from CA Membranes

We have already mentioned the strong binding of divalent cations to the glucuronic acid groups in Sec. III.A and III.C. The binding process is rapid, the dissociation slow. In Refs. 13, 15, the conversion of dense CA membranes to anionic exchangers by the binding of divalent ions and the subsequent slow dissociation of divalent ions in solutions free of such ions were studied. Especially, the rates of dissociation were studied as a function of the temperature and the ionic strength of the bathing solution.

We have already seen an example of anion exchange behavior of a dense CA membrane pretreated with Ba^{2+} or Mg^{2+} ions where $BaCl_2$ or $MgCl_2$

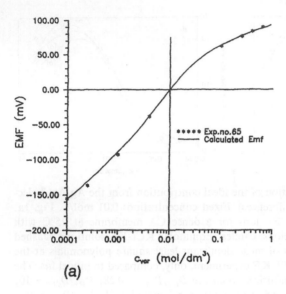

(a)

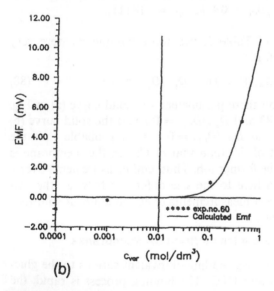

(b)

FIG. 11 Emf curves before and after binding of Ba^{2+} for a dense CA membrane at 25°C with NaCl as the variable salt and pH(conc.) = 5. (a) Before binding of Ba^{2+}, the curve is the usual one for a cation exchange membrane with $c_q/K_{NaCl} = 0.044$ eqv./L (with negative sign of fixed charge). $D_{Na+}/D_{Cl-} = 0.25$; $D_{H+}/D_{Cl-} = 10$; $k_{H+, Na-} = 9.5$. (b) After binding of Ba^{2+}, the curve corresponds to an anion exchange membrane with $c_q/K_{NaCl} = 0.29$ eqv./L (with positive sign of fixed charge). The other parameters as before [15].

TABLE 4 Characteristic Parameters for the Release of Bound Ba^{2+} Ions in Slow Release Experiments with Dense Cellulose 2.5 Acetate Membranes

Exp. no.	Membrane	[NaCl] (mol/L)	Temp. (°C)	Time until charge inversion (days)	Time for obtaining 60 mV (days)	$Q(0)$ (eqv./L)	$Q(\infty)$ (eqv./L)	Q_2 (eqv./L)	k_2 (days^{-1})	k_1/k_2
61	B24III	0.01 | 0.4	25	12	25	0.290	−0.0408	0.0820	0.0563	11.8
63	B24III	0.4 | 0.4	25	5	9.5	0.290	−0.0408	0.0594	0.1016	7.9
68	B26III	0.01 | 0.01	25	6	16	0.257	−0.0408	0.0668	0.0770	16.9
69	B24III	0.4 | 0.4	25	4	6	0.300	−0.0440	0.0675	0.1730	6.0

$Q(0) = Q_1 + Q_2 + Q(\infty)$ in Eq. (89).
Source: Ref. 15.

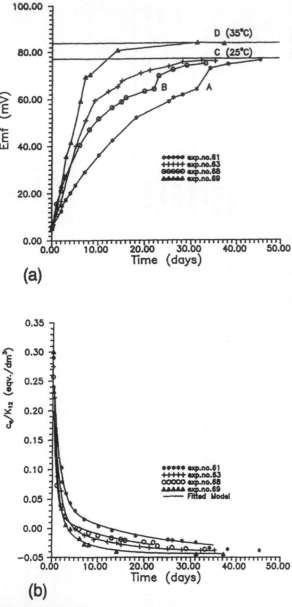

FIG. 12 (a) Emf as a function of time for dense CA membranes initially on Ba-form. During emf measurements (short times compared to the time scale shown in the curve) the concentrations of NaCl are $[NaCl]_{l.h.s.} = 0.4$ mol/L and $[NaCl]_{r.h.s.} = 0.01$ mol/L. Apart from these short times, the conditions of the dissociation of the bound Ba^{2+} ions

were used as "variable salt" (Fig. 9). In Ref. 15 the same membrane (B24III) was studied with NaCl as "variable salt" (and pH = 5) before and after "doping" with Ba^{2+} ions. Figure 11a shows the now well-known cation exchange behavior with a fixed charge corresponding to $c_q/K_{NaCl} = -0.044$ eqv./L in contrast to the anion exchange behavior (Fig. 11b) with a fixed charge corresponding to $+0.29$ eqv./L. Thus, the Ba^{2+} ions seem to bind not only to the $-COO^-$ groups but also to other "sites". Of course, it would not be possible to perform a series of emf experiments as that in Fig. 11b, if the dissociation of the Ba^{2+} ions from the sites in the bathing NaCl solutions were not quite slow. (Between every emf measurement in Fig. 11b the membrane is placed in 1 mol/L $BaCl_2$).

If membranes in "Ba^{2+}-form" are placed in bathing NaCl + HCl solutions (pH = 5) of various temperatures and ionic strengths, and if the membrane is from time to time taken out and measured in a standard concentration cell with NaCl concentrations 0.4 mol/L (left) and 0.01 mol/L (right) and pH = 5, we can follow the change in emf of the standard cell with time in a so-called *slow release experiment*, see Fig. 12a. Figure 12b shows the evaluated value of $c_q(\theta)/K_{NaCl}$ as a function of time θ. It is seen that it may take more than one month before the initial (cation exchange) membrane is reestablished. The process is speeded up with increasing temperature (35°C) and with increasing ionic strength in the bathing solution, see also Table 4. The decay of the fixed charge towards the original value are well fitted by a bi-exponential function:

$$c_q(\theta)/K_{NaCl} = Q_1 \exp(-k_1\theta) + Q_2 \exp(-k_2\theta) + Q(\infty) \tag{89}$$

This indicates two binding sites for Ba^{2+}, one site (1) with loosely bound Ba^{2+} ions (probably ion–dipole interactions with the O-atoms in the CA) and another site (2) with strongly bound Ba^{2+} ions (probably strong ion–ion inter-

---

are as follows: ***, membrane B24III, 25°C, $[NaCl]_{r.h.s.} = 0.01$ mol/L, $[NaCl]_{l.h.s.} = 0.4$ mol/L; $+++$, membrane B24 III, 25°C, $[NaCl]_{r.h.s.} = 0.4$ mol/L, $[NaCl]_{l.h.s.} = 0.4$ mol/L; $\bigcirc\bigcirc\bigcirc$, membrane B26III, 25°C, $[NaCl]_{r.h.s.} = 0.01$ mol/L, $[NaCl]_{l.h.s.} = 0.01$ mol/L; $\triangle\triangle\triangle$, membrane B26III, 35°C, $[NaCl]_{r.h.s.} = 0.4$ mol/L, $[NaCl]_{l.h.s.} = 0.4$ mol/L. The "jumps" denoted A and B in two of the curves are provoked by a sudden increase in concentration $[NaCl]_{r.h.s.}$ from 0.01 to 0.4 mol/L for the experiment *** (after 31 days) and a sudden increase in $[NaCl]_{r.h.s.}$ as well as in $[NaCl]_{l.h.s.}$ to 0.4 mol/L for the experiment $\bigcirc\bigcirc\bigcirc$ (after 22 days). Thus, it is seen that increased temperature as well as increased ionic strength promote the dissociation of divalent ions bound to the glucuronic acid groups. From Ref. 15, but the correlation of experiments with the symbols below Fig. 5 in this reference was not quite correct. (b) Calculated values of c_q/K_{NaCl} (with sign) as a function of time for the slow release of Ba^{2+} ions for the same four experiments as above. Parameters: $D_{Na+}/D_{Cl-} = 0.25$; $D_{H+}/D_{Cl-} = 10$; $k_{H+, Na+} = 9.5$. The curves are fittings of the bi-exponential relaxation, see Eq. (89) and Table 4 [15].

actions with the glucuronic acid groups). In the case of the second type of binding, it is quite difficult for a Ba^{2+} ion to escape from the "electrostatic capture" of a $—COO^-$ group with the relatively low permittivity prevailing in the CA membrane. It helps with thermal activation or formation of more narrow "ionic clouds" around each of the ions at higher ionic strengths. For more details, see Ref. 15.

IV. EMF OVER ASYMMETRIC MEMBRANES

A. Recent Studies of Asymmetric Membranes with Two Ions

In Sec. II.D an experimental method (based upon initial time emf measurements and general irreversible thermodynamics) was outlined. With this method, the transport number of the cation for each of the two *surface layers* of an inhomogeneous or asymmetric membrane can in principle be evaluated as a function of the salt concentration of the adjacent solution. In the present subsection we review recent experimental studies of this kind together with earlier measurements in the stationary state on asymmetric cellulose acetate membranes and recent model studies of asymmetric membranes. In the next two subsections, completely new results are presented for NaCl and $BaCl_2$ in polyether sulfone (PES) membranes.

In Ref. 12 several asymmetric CA membranes were cast by only partial evaporation of the acetone solvent before quenching in water, in some cases with addition of nonsolvents as formamide or water to the casting solution. The results were CA membranes with a skinlayer, similar in properties to the dense CA membranes and of thickness of ~ 1 μm or less and a thick porous layer dominated by phase-inversed water-rich "alveoles". For details about the phase-inversion procedure for producing asymmetric membranes for desalination and other purposes, the classical papers of Loeb and Sourirajan [93] and Strathman, Scheible and Baker [94] should be consulted. References 95–97 with many electron micrographs of asymmetric membranes prepared in different ways are also highly useful.

The asymmetric membranes cast in Ref. 12 were characterized by stationary emf measurements (using the cell shown in Fig. 2 and LiCl + HCl solutions) and the data were approximately fitted to the model described in Sec. III.B. This is clearly not a very satisfying procedure since the model is for homogeneous membranes only. However, the "average parameters" determined seemed more determined by the highly swollen, porous layer than by the skin layer. For example, the parameter c_q/K_{LiCl} is found to be only $\approx 1/50$ of the value found for dense membranes, and the ratios of diffusion coefficients were close to the ratios for the limiting conductivities of the ions in water. The average values were determined from mean emf values for the two orientation of the membrane to "eliminate" the asymmetry. Before this averaging, a differ-

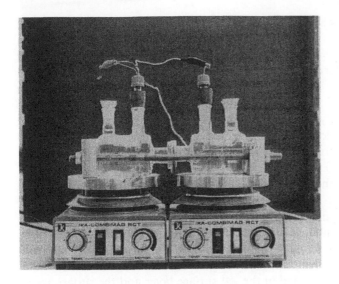

(a)

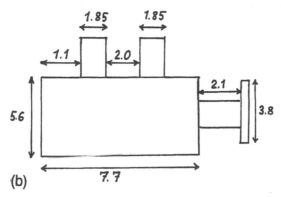

(b)

FIG. 13 (a) The "Spanish cell" used for the experiments in Refs. 26–28 and also, for comparison with other cells for the new NaCl experiments reported in Sec. IV.B. The cell is a noncirculation cell with double magnetic stirring (or propeller stirring through the second sets of side tubes. The temperature is ambient temperature. (b) The dimensions of one half cell of the "Spanish cell" in cm.

ence up to ±7 mV in the stationary state with the two orientations of the membrane was found, however.

Turning now to the initial time emf method, the first systematic study is the one of Compañ, López, Sørensen and Garrido [26]. In this study, asymmetric cellulose acetate (CA) and polysulfone (PS) membranes were studied using the initial emf values and a very simple measuring cell shown in Figs. 13a and b. The two membrane specimens were prepared at the Department of Nuclear and Chemical Engineering of the Universidad Politécnica de Valencia. The polysulfone membrane was cast from a solution of 15% of Polysulfone Ultralon-s from BASF in dimethylamide poured onto a polyester support (Freudemberg and Hollytex). The film formed was immersed in distilled water at 10°C for 10 min. Afterwards, the film was allowed to dry at ambient temperature. The asymmetric cellulose acetate membrane was made according to Ref. 12. It contains ~ 30 wt% water.

Figure 14 sketches the principle of an initial time emf measurement on an asymmetric membrane. The membrane is first immersed in one and the same aqueous solution of a single electrolyte (for example NaCl), and after some time the salt chemical potential is uniform everywhere, $\mu_{salt}(R)$ say. At the time $\theta = 0$, the l.h. solution is replaced by a solution of the same salt but with another concentration. Then, initially, the gradient in chemical potential and the diffusion potential is located in the left surface layer and the surface transport number in that layer may be found from emf measurements with Ag/AgCl electrodes. In Ref. 26, the emf measurements were made in concentration series with a *constant difference* (Δc) between the right and the left concentration of NaCl. Concentration series were made with $\Delta c = 0.04, 0.02,$

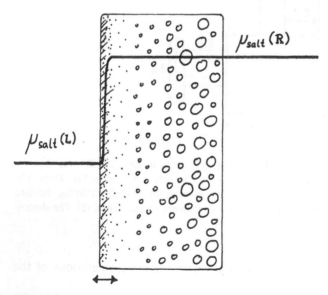

FIG. 14 Principle sketch of an "initial value emf" experiment characterizing one face of an asymmetric membrane.

0.004, and 0.002 mol/L. The concentrations varied over an interval from 0.001 to 0.12 mol/L. It was assumed that the "average surface transport number" found corresponded roughly to a concentration equal to $c_{mean} = c_L + (\Delta c/2)$. The average surface transport number of the right surface of the membrane was found in a similar way, changing the right solution at $\theta = 0$.

It was found for the PS membrane (Fig. 15) that for the series with $\Delta c = 0.04$ and 0.02 mol/L that the apparent surface transport number of Na^+ for the two membrane faces decreased linearly with increasing mean concentration, and that the transport numbers (for the same surface) were practically the same when calculated from each of the two series. However, the series with $\Delta c = 0.004$ and 0.002 mol/L lead to different transport numbers and concentration dependencies when the two series are compared, see Table 3 in Ref. 26. The reason is probably that these measurements are made at mean concentrations which are a factor of 10 lower than the series with $\Delta c = 0.04$ and 0.02 mol/L. At these low concentrations, the H^+ ions from the autoprotolysis of water may intefer considerably and a three-ion model is necessary. However, apparent surface transport numbers can only be rigorously determined in asymmetric membranes with only two ions as explained in Sec. II.D. In the measurements in Ref. 26 no attempt was made to stabilize pH.

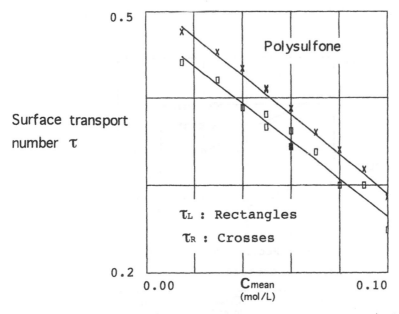

FIG. 15 Estimated variation of the surface transport numbers for Na^+ with the mean concentration $(c_L + c_R)/2$ for a polysulfone membrane using the "Spanish cell" and the "small Δc method", see the text. An asymmetry is shown between the left hand and the right hand face of the membrane. Ambient temperature.

For the asymmetric CA membrane (Fig. 16) a linear decrease of τ_{Na^+} with increasing mean concentration were also found but the decrease was much less than in the case of the PS membrane. The decrease in the apparent transport numbers may be interpreted in terms of the two-ion Nernst–Planck–Donnan model of ion exchange membranes (Sec. III.A). The fit was only a modest success since the model decrease in τ_{Na^+} is not straight but curved upwards, see Fig. 12 in Ref. 26. Making the best fit anyway the values below were obtained:

Left hand surface, CA: $c_q/K_{NaCl} = 0.005$ eqv./L;

$$D = D_{Cl^-}/D_{Na^+} = 1.7 \quad (90a)$$

Right hand surface, CA: $c_q/K_{NaCl} = 0.006$ eqv./L;

$$D = D_{Cl^-}/D_{Na^+} = 2 \quad (90b)$$

The value of c_q/K_{NaCl} is much less than the typical values found for dense CA membranes (see Sec. IV.A–D). In fact, the value is more consistent with the earlier "average values" obtained using the three-ion model on the stationary emf measurements on the more swollen, asymmetric CA membranes, see above and Ref. 12. The values of D are lower than in dense CA membranes where this value is typically ≈ 4. The ratio D for NaCl in infinite aqueous

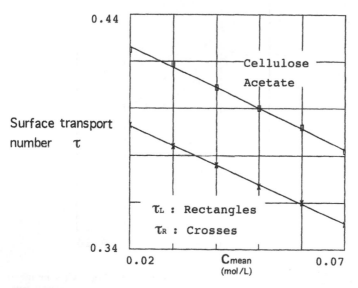

FIG. 16 Estimated variation of the surface transport numbers for Na^+ with the mean concentration $(c_L + c_R)/2$ for an asymmetric CA membrane using the "Spanish cell" and the "small Δc method". Ambient temperature.

dilution is 1.51 which is quite close to the value 1.7 found for the left hand surface. The r.h. surface seems to be more "dense" with a $D = 2$ and is probably the skin layer + possibly some adjacent more porous layer.

The transport numbers of the PS membrane in Fig. 15 may also be fitted to the two-ion model but the fit is not impressive (too much upwards curvature in the model, see Fig. 13 in Ref. 26). We only fit to the mean values:

Mean transport numbers, PS: $c_q/K_{NaCl} = 0.015$ eqv./L;

$$D = D_{Cl^-}/D_{Na^+} = 1.3 \quad (91)$$

This membrane appears to be quite swollen and with more fixed charge than the CA membrane, although it is still a weak cation exchanger.

Compañ, Sørensen and Rivera [27] measured initial emf values as well as stationary emf values using a phenol sulfonic acid (PSA) membrane in NaCl solutions. Once more, the above mentioned Δc method was applied with $\Delta c = 0.02$ mol/L. In contrast to the study in Ref. 26, the membrane was first soaked with the lower of the two solutions and then contacted with the higher solution at the interface to be investigated. The membrane was prepared at the Institut für Physikalische Chemie in Köln (Germany) by a condensation and cross-linking reaction between PSA and formaldehyde [98–100]. Such membranes possess microregions of highly cross-linked PSA interspaced by more open channels, see Fig. 7 in Ref. 98. Apart from this isotropic microheterogeneity with a length scale of the order of 10 nm, these membranes should be quite homogeneous at greater length scales, since they are formed by a uniform chemical reaction rather than by a casting procedure or by irradiation grafting as some of the membranes investigated by Pinéri [25]. The fixed charge density is 1.1 mol/kg and the membrane is highly swollen with 60 wt% water.

The surface transport numbers found are plotted vs. the natural logarithm of the mean ionic activity of the contact solution in Fig. 17. These transport numbers have been calculated directly from the experimental data using (for the right surface transport number)

$$\text{emf (init, R)} \approx \{2RT/F\}\tau_{Na^+,\text{ surface R}}(a_{\pm,R})\ln(a_{\pm,L}/a_{\pm,R}) \quad (92)$$

which is approximately correct due to the small concentration difference applied. In Figs. 16 and 17 the transport numbers were calculated from linear regressions of emf vs. $\ln(a_{\pm,L}/a_{\pm,L})$, see Fig. 5 in Ref. 26. From Fig. 17 it is evident that the membrane is quite close to ideal permselectivity of Na$^+$. This is because the fixed charge of this membrane is quite high and the dimensionless salt concentration $c^* \ll 1$ for all concentrations used in Ref. 27, see Fig. 4a of Sec. III.A. The surface transport number of the cation decreases with increasing concentration as expected for a cation exchanger. It is seen that there is a small, but significant, asymmetry in the membrane—in spite of the way of manufacturing of this membrane.

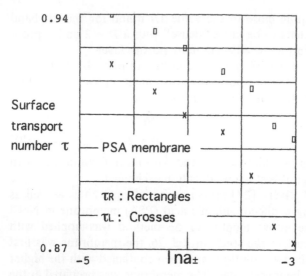

FIG. 17 Estimated surface transport numbers for Na^+ for the two faces of an asymmetric polyphenol sulfone acid (PSA) membrane as a function of the logarithm of the mean ionic activity of the contact solution to the face characterized. The "small Δc method" was used.

If the apparent transport number were given by the function $\tau_L(a_\pm)$ *throughout the entire membrane*, the emf would be time independent and given by the area under a smoothed curve fitted to the crosses in Fig. 17. Alternatively, if the apparent transport number were given by $\tau_R(a_\pm)$, the emf would be determined from the area under a curve fitted to the rectangles in Fig. 17. Performing the integration from $c_L = 0.01$ mol/L to $c_R = 0.08$ mol/L the values found are 77.3 and 79.3 mV, respectively. The mean value is 78.3 mV.

In reality, the transport number is a function of concentration as well as position and the emf is a functional. In the *stationary state* of diffusion one should expect to have some kind of mean value if the membrane properties are not deviating too much in the middle from the surface properties. Furthermore, the stationary mean value should depend on the direction of diffusion in an asymmetric membrane. For the two directions of diffusion, the stationary emf was measured in Ref. 27 to 78.5 ± 0.5 mV and 80.5 ± 0.3 mV. The first value is statistically identical to the mean value obtained from the integration of the two surface transport number functions. The second value is outside the interval between these two values, however.

There is reason to be somewhat sceptical about these results, however. The cell used (Figs. 13a and b) is not ideally suited for long-run emf measurements. It is not thermostatted, the volume of solution in the two chambers is small and the stirring quite inefficient due to the two "bottlenecks" close to the membrane. The two figures of emf vs. time shown in Ref. 27 correspond to "vigorous stirring" and "no stirring at all". In the latter case, a slow and continued decrease of emf was followed up to 200 min after contact. In the former case, there seemed to be a plateau from 15 min to 80 min, but emf was not followed after that time. We shall take up these questions in an improved study of an asymmetric membrane, comparing the results of three different measuring cells in Sec. IV.B

Very recently, Compañ, Sørensen, Andrio, López and de Abajo [28] studied two nonionic membranes, namely a dense and a porous, asymmetric membrane made of a polyether sulfone (PES). The electrolyte was NaCl and the measuring cell the same as before (Figs. 13a and b). The structure of the PES is shown in Fig. 18. The *dense* (pore free) membrane was prepared by casting polymer solutions (8% wt/vol in *N,N*-dimethylformamide) on glass plates. The solvent was evaporated in an air-circulating oven at 110°C under vacuum for 8 h. Residual solvent was removed by rinsing the polymer film in methanol for 24 h and by subsequent drying in vacuum at 80°C until constant weight. The *asymmetric, porous* membrane with a *skin layer* was prepared by casting polymer solutions (16% wt/vol in *N,N*-dimethylacetamide) on a flat glass plate and subsequently quenching the cast film in water at 10°C. The membrane was kept in the coagulation bath for 20 min and then transferred to a running water bath, where it was washed for 2 h. In the study of Compañ et al., the differentiation method (mentioned in Sec. II.D) was used to obtain surface transport numbers from initial value emf measurements. One external concentration was always $c_{fix} = 0.01$ mol/L with which the membrane was first brought to equilibrium. The emf(init) vs. $\ln(a_{\pm, \text{var}}/a_{\pm, \text{fix}})$ data were fitted with a least square polynomial through (0, 0) and the surface transport numbers as a function of $a_{\pm, \text{var}}$ or c_{var} were found by differentiation.

In Ref. 28 least square *third-order* polynomials for emf(init) were used. The idea was to have some more flexibility than just linear variation of $\tau_{\text{Na}+}$ with $\ln(a_{\pm, \text{var}})$. However, the quality and the number of data points did not really justify such a high degree of polynomial and the variations with concentration of $\tau_{\text{Na}+}$ reported in this work is probably spurious. *Second-order* polynomials fit just as well with the variance given. Therefore, we have refitted the data for emf(init) from Tables 1 and 2 in Ref. 28 with second-order polynomials

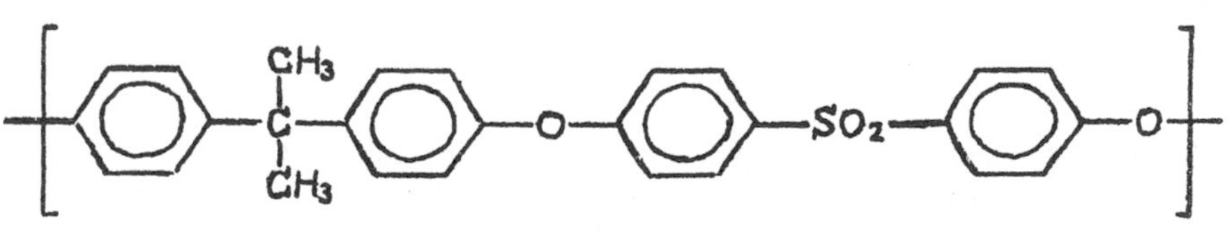

FIG. 18 Repetition unit of polyether sulfone (PES) used for the membranes in Ref. 28 and in Sec. IV.B and C.

through (0, 0) and plotted τ_{Na^+} in Figs. 19 and 20. The dense PES membrane (Fig. 19) exhibits little variation with concentration and small asymmetry. The asymmetry of the porous membrane is substantial, however, as seen in Fig. 20. One face has approximately the same decrease in τ_{Na^+} with increasing concentration as one of the faces of the dense membrane. The other face has *increasing* τ_{Na^+} with increasing concentration. In aqueous solutions of NaCl, the value of t_{Na^+} at 25°C varies from 0.393 at 0.005 mol/L to 0.385 at 0.1 mol/L, see Ref. 101, Tables 6–6-2. The values shown in Fig. 19 are not far from the water values. Therefore, for some reason the restrictions imposed by a dense PES membrane on the diffusion of Na^+ and Cl^- (compared to the diffusion in water) must be roughly the same.

In retrospect, we have difficulties in believing in at least some of the experimental data for the *stationary* emf values listed in Tables 1 and 2 in Ref. 28. They are mostly far outside the interval between the two initial emf values. For example, for the asymmetric membrane and $c_{var} = 0.5$ mol/L the two initial values of emf were 66.0 and 67.0 mV, but the two stationary emf values (for the two directions of diffusion) were reported to be 81.1 and 88.3 mV. Even worse, at $c_{var} = 0.001$ mol/L, the initial values of emf were −44.0 and −45.0 mV, but the two stationary emf values were stated as −85.0 and −91.0 mV. The similar values for the dense membrane lied also far outside the interval between the two initial values. We do not know precisely what went wrong in the stationary experiments. The nature of the measuring cell (which we call

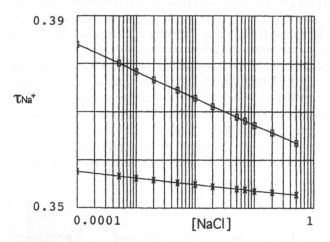

FIG. 19 Estimated surface transport numbers for Na^+ for the two faces of a dense PES membrane as a function of the concentration of NaCl in contact with the surface characterized. There is little asymmetry and little variation with concentration. The emf differentiation method is used, fitting a least square, second order polynomial through (0, 0) to the emf vs. $\ln(a_{\pm, var}/a_{\pm, fix})$ data.

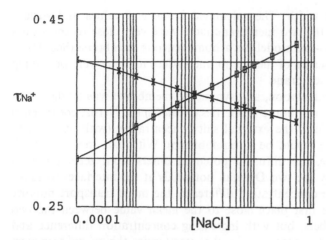

FIG. 20 Estimated surface transport numbers for Na^+ for the two faces of a porous, asymmetric PES membrane as a function of the concentration of NaCl in contact with the surface characterized. There is substantial asymmetry between the two faces and substantial (and inverse) variation with concentration. The emf differentiation method is used with a second-order polynomial through (0, 0).

the "Spanish cell") is not ideal as mentioned, but we shall see in the next subsection—by comparison with other types of emf cells—that it *is* possible to make more consistent measurements of stationary emf using that cell.

We finish this subsection by a summary of some results obtained with model Nernst–Planck–Donnan calculations for emf and salt diffusion flux in asymmetric membranes [31,32]. In Sec. II.D, the formalism for calculating the emf and the local salt flux at any time for a 1:1 and a 2:1 electrolyte was described [vide Eqs. (57)–(66)]. In Ref. 31, the somewhat unclear literature on the possible existence of "asymmetry potentials"—measured with asymmetrical membranes in contact with identical solutions at both sides [59,102–105]—was reviewed and demystified, generalizing earlier results of Higuchi and Nakagawa [58] and of Manzanares, Mafé and Pellicer [60]. Apart from this, Ref. 31 focused on 1:1 electrolytes in model asymmetric membranes mimicking NaCl in asymmetric cellulose acetate membranes. The asymmetry was modelled by means of exponential profiles in the membrane properties: diffusion coefficients, Nernst coefficients and fixed charge density.

The initial emf method was investigated for membranes with exponential profiles of $D_{21}(x)$ and $c_q(x)$, respectively, but constant Nernst coefficients. The initial sharp concentration profiles were simulated by very sharply decaying exponentials for the salt concentration $c_s(x)$ near one or the other interface. Whereas the "decay length" of the exponentials for $D_{21}(x)$ and $c_q(x)$ were chosen to be the width of the membrane, the decay length for $c_s(x)$ was rather

1/50 of the membrane width. The calculated initial emf values and surface transport numbers for the two membrane faces were very close to the values calculated from the two-ion model for a homogeneous membrane (Sec. III.A) assuming that the properties of the membrane surface in focus were prevailing throughout the whole membrane.

In another sample calculation, an asymmetric membrane was studied with a linear variation of all membrane properties (*including* the Nernst coefficients) and also a linear profile in the external salt concentration (with which each point in the membrane would be in equilibrium). With 0.01 mol/L at both sides of the membrane, the diffusion potential differs from zero, but it is exactly balanced out by the two Donnan potentials at the interfaces to make emf = 0. Increasing the concentration difference, the mean transport number for the cation is in the first place close to the mean value between the two surface transport numbers, but with increasing concentration difference and increasing mean salt concentration in the membrane, the mean transport number did not decrease towards the limit of negligible fixed charge [Eq. (74b)]. On the contrary, the mean transport number of the cation *increased*. The calculations in Ref. 31 showed that the reason for this relied upon the fact that the most important electric potential gradients in the model membrane studied were found near the part of the membrane wherein the concentration was very low.

Asaka [106] has commented that in membrane emf studies "it is difficult to establish which layer determines the electrochemical properties", since Horigome and Taniguchi [107] concluded that the membrane emf should be attributed to the dense layer, whereas Malmgren-Hansen, Sørensen and Jensen [12] stated that the porous layer was determining. In light of the above model calculations it is probably more sound to state that it simply in general is wrong to calculate emf values for an asymmetric membrane by means of a homogeneous model—except under the special conditions of the initial time emf method.

In Ref. 32, model calculations for 2:1 electrolytes in asymmetric membranes were performed. In this work, focus was on the *stationary* state of electrodiffusion. Thus, the salt concentration profile is not assumed as above but calculated for each stationary value of the salt flux by integration of Eqs. (61–64). Three model membranes were investigated: A very weak cation exchange membrane (VWC), a weak anion exchange membrane (WA) and a strong anion exchange membrane (SA). The words "weak" and "strong" refer to the magnitude of the absolute value of the fixed charge density (in equivalents) relative to the external salt concentrations. All the three model membranes had linear profiles of $D_{2+}(x)$, $D_-(x)$, $K_s(x)$ and $\omega c_q(x)$.

Examples of salt concentration profiles as well as profiles for the two ions individually are shown in the figures in Ref. 32. The electric field profile may also be calculated but only when special assumptions concerning $K_{2+}(x)$ and

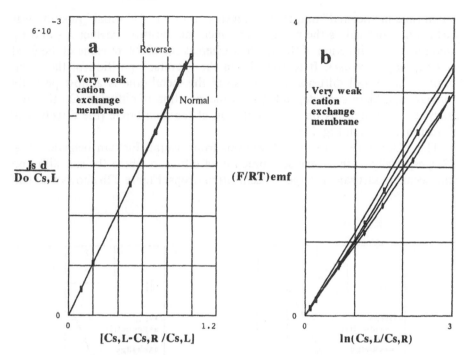

FIG. 21 Model study (Nernst–Planck–Donnan) of an asymmetric membrane with stationary diffusion of 2:1 electrolytes. Very weak, asymmetric cation exchange membrane. (a) Dimensionless salt flux as a function of dimensionless concentration drop. The behaviour is almost Fickian and there is practically no difference between "normal" and "reverse" direction of diffusion. (b) Dimensionless emf as a function of the logarithm of the concentration ratio (=the overall "driving force"). There is some asymmetry at high values of the driving force (up to ~10 mV). The lines with slopes 1.00 and 1.13 are shown, too. The first value seems approximately to be the asymptotic slope for the emf in both directions for small "driving forces" (global linearization à la Onsager [61,62]). The corresponding "Onsager transport number" for the divalent cation (call it Y^{2+}) is ~0.67 corresponding to some "Onsager average" of the ratio $D_{Cl^-}/D_{Y^{2+}}$ equal to ~1 for an uncharged membrane. (In the model asymmetric membrane this ratio varies linearly from 0.53 to 3 through the membrane). The line with slope 1.13 corresponds to an uncharged membrane with the ratio $D_{Cl^-}/D_{Y^{2+}}$ replaced by the mean value of this quantity through the membrane. Data adapted from Ref. 32.

$K_-(x)$ are made. For the calculation of emf and the concentration profiles such assumptions are not necessary, however, only $K_S(x)$ has to be known. This is also the case with 1:1 electrolytes although it was not explicitly stated in Ref. 31.

Figures 21a shows the (dimensionless) salt diffusion flux (from left towards right) as a function of the (dimensionless) concentration drop over the VWC-membrane in "normal" and in the "reverse" position. "Normal" position was (arbitrarily) defined as the position in which the diffusion coefficients and K_s *increases* in the direction of the salt flux whereas the absolute value of the fixed charge, ωc_q, *decreases*. It is opposite in the "reverse" position of the membrane. The overall diffusional response of the membrane is almost perfectly Fickian, and there is no dependence on the direction of diffusion. On the contrary, the emf depends on the orientation of the membrane (the direction of diffusion) as seen in Fig. 21b.

The WA-membrane shows deviations from overall Fickian behavior (Fig. 22a), especially in the "reverse" direction of diffusion where the salt diffusion flux seems to saturate at large concentration drops. Figure 22b shows that emf

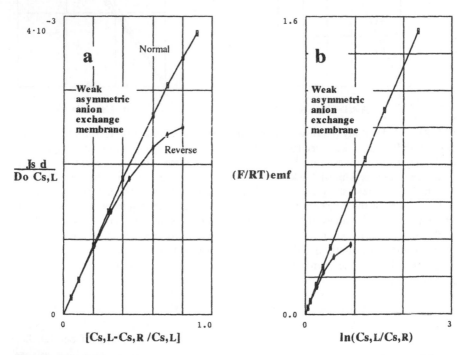

FIG. 22 Model study (Nernst–Planck–Donnan) of an asymmetric membrane with stationary diffusion of 2:1 electrolytes. Weak, asymmetric anion exchange membrane. (a) Dimensionless salt flux as a function of dimensionless concentration drop. The behaviour is nonFickian and with considerable asymmetry between "normal" and "reverse" direction of diffusion. (b) Dimensionless emf as a function of the overall "driving force". There is large asymmetry at high values of the driving force. The two curves have an "Onsager line" as common asymptote for small driving forces. Data adapted from Ref. 32.

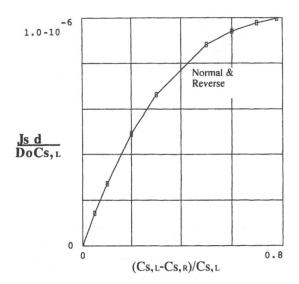

FIG. 23 Model study (Nernst–Planck–Donnan) of an asymmetric membrane with stationary diffusion of 2:1 electrolytes. Strong, asymmetric anion exchange membrane. Dimensionless salt flux as a function of dimensionless concentration drop. The behaviour is strongly nonFickian but with no asymmetry between "normal" and "reverse" direction of diffusion. The salt fluxes are very small (and emf is very close to zero) since the membrane is an almost ideal anion exchange membrane for all the concentrations shown. Data adapted from Ref. 32.

also behaves very asymmetrically. For the SA-membrane, the salt flux is strongly nonFickian (Fig. 23) and, remarkably, there is again no difference between the two directions of diffusion. The emf values are not shown since they are mostly equal to zero inside the computational error. This is so, since the membrane is very close to be an ideal anion exchanger.

Sending a "virtual" Faraday through the system makes the anion (Cl^-) participate in a ring process with no change in Gibbs' free energy. The interesting thing is, however, that the salt flux is not zero as in a completely ideal anion exchanger but has very small, well defined values depending on the overall concentration drop, see Fig. 23.

B. Asymmetric Polyether Sulfone Membrane with NaCl Using Three Cells

In view of the uncertainty with regard to the measurements with the "Spanish cell" (Figs 13a and b) mentioned in the previous section, the two authors of the present chapter decided to perform control measurements using different kinds of emf cells to test the reproducibility of surface and mean transport numbers. These measurements were made at the Universidad de Concepción during 1996–1997. The results reported in this subsection (NaCl) and in the subsequent subsection (BaCl$_2$) have not been published before.

1. Experimental

(a) *Chemicals.* NaCl was 99.5%, analytical grade, Merck. It was heated in an oven at 90°C until constant weight (1 h) and dissolved in distilled water to 0.2 mol/L. The other concentrations were made by dilution. The BaCl$_2 \cdot 2H_2O$ used in the study in Sec. IV.C was also Merck, analytical grade. It is quite strongly hygroscopic and has to be predried at 50°C for a week to be sure that there are two moles crystal water per mol BaCl$_2$.

(b) *Membrane Preparation, Asymmetry, Structure and Orientation.* The membrane used was based on a technical polysulfone polymer (UDEL P3500) which is the same nonionic polyether sulfone polymer used in Ref. 28, see the chemical structure of the repeating unit in Fig. 18. The preparation of the highly asymmetric membrane was performed in the following way: a solution of 16% w/v of polymer in *N,N*-dimethylacetamide was cast as a film on a nonwoven fabric of polyester fibres and immediately after quenched in water at 15°C. This produces a dense skin layer at the surface directly exposed to water. The membrane was kept in the coagulation bath for 20 min and then transferred to a running water bath and washed for 2 h.

The skin layer (smooth face of the membrane) was in all cells always oriented towards the "right" electrode whereas the support layer (rugged face of the membrane) was oriented towards the "left electrode". Three different circular cuttings from the same membrane preparation were used in the three measuring cells, so that the experiments could be performed simultaneously. Figure 24a shows a SEM microphotograph of the "smooth" side of the membrane at 400 × magnification. The "rugged" side (support side) is shown in Fig. 24b at the same magnification clearly exhibits the irregular fiber structure of the support layer.

(c) *Measuring Cells and Measuring Procedures.* The "Spanish cell" is the one shown in Figs. 13a and b. This is a nonflow, nonthermostatted cell with two bottleshaped glass chambers clamped together with the membrane sandwiched in between. In each chamber there are two side tubes, one for the Ag/AgCl electrode and one (with stopper) for the replacement of solution. Two magnetic stirrers provide the circulation of the solution on each side of the membrane. The membrane was first soaked in 0.01 mol/L NaCl solution (in both chambers) during at least 12 h. The asymmetry potential between the two electrodes (if any) was then measured. The emf measurements were started emptying either the left or the right chamber and refilling it with a NaCl solution with another molarity and recording the measured potentials vs. time.

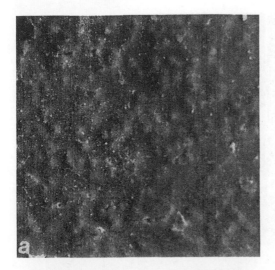

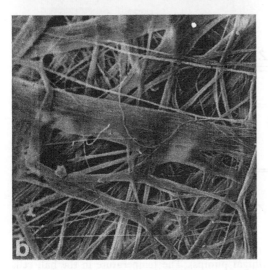

FIG. 24 SEM micrographs, of the two faces of the supported, asymmetric PES membrane used in Sec. IV.B and C. (a) The "smooth" side of the membrane (skin layer). (b) The rugged side of the membrane (support layer). Magnification 400 ×.

All previous initial emf's on asymmetric membranes were measured with this "Spanish cell". Dr. V. Compañ, Universitat Jaume I, Castellón, Spain, kindly provided us with one of the copies of this cell for comparison with the other types of cells.

A photograph of the "Chilenian cell" and its accessories is shown in Fig.

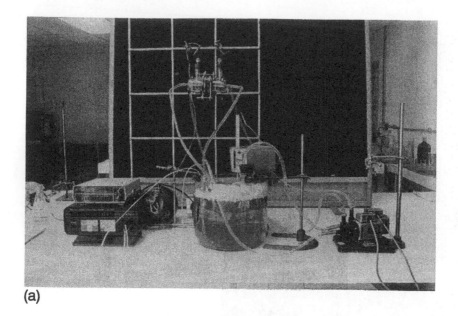

(a)

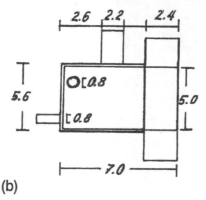

(b)

FIG. 25 (a) The "Chilenian" cell with accessories (voltmeter, conductometer, thermostat, solution reservoirs, two centrifugal pumps). The temperature in the half cells can be kept inside $25.0 \pm 0.1°C$. The flow in each half cell chamber is highly turbulent. (b) The dimensions of one half cell in cm.

25a. The dimensions of the half cell are shown in Fig. 25b. This cell is a flow cell made of two glass half cells. The two half cells are clamped on both sides of the membrane. They have not the "bottlenecks" of the "Spanish cell" and highly turbulent liquid flow is maintained in both chambers by means of two centrifugal pumps (Charles Austen Pumps, Ltd., model 016/301) connected to a variotransformer. The two solution reservoir flasks (1 L) were thermostatted in a thermostat bath to $25.0 \pm 0.1°C$ (using a Gallenkamp Thermostirrer). The most dilute of the two solutions were monitored by a conductimeter (Microprocessor Meter LF200, WTW, TÜV BAYERN) to detect any change in the concentration of NaCl during experiments of many hours of duration. The soaking of the membrane in 0.01 mol/L, NaCl was performed like in the Spanish cell. The emf measurements were begun immediately after the transference of the electrode (used to measure at the variable concentration) from a thermostatted solution at the variable concentration to the right or left half cell and the starting of the circulating flow of solution with variable concentration. These operations could be performed in less than one minute.

The "Danish cell" is the same as that described earlier in connection with the stationary state emf measurements on CA membranes, see Fig. 2. However, all dimensions were multiplied by a factor 2. The cell is a thermostatted flow cell consisting of two half cells of perspex clamped around the membrane. Each flow chamber is a very narrow channel of rhomboid shape (seen perpendicularly to the membrane). The channel first expands in the flow direction and then contracts. The NaCl solutions—kept thermostatted $(25.00 \pm 0.05°C$, Techne Tempunit TU-16D) in two 1 L flasks—are driven along the membrane surfaces with a relatively high speed by means of a double, peristaltic pump (Cole-Parmer instrument Co., model no. 7521-10). The Ag/AgCl electrodes are kept aside from the streaming solution in the channels in two side pockets bored out in the perspex cell halves. Apart from these details, the experiments with the "Danish cell" were carried out in the same way as the experiments with the "Chilenean cell".

The flow channel in each of the half cells of the new Danish cell has a volume of ~ 0.6 cm^3 and with a length of solution–membrane contact along the flow direction equal to ~ 4 cm, the average cross sectional area of the flow channel is 0.15 cm^2. In most experiments, a flow rate of 130 cm^3/min was used which then corresponds to an average linear velocity of ~ 870 cm/min or 14.4 cm/s along the membrane surface.

The voltages of all three cells were measured with a Keithley 177, microvolt DMM voltmeter calibrated against a Weston normal element, and the voltage–time data were collected automatically by computerized datalogging.

(d) *Ag/AgCl Electrodes and Asymmetry Potentials.* The preparation of the Ag/AgCl electrodes followed the receipt given in Ref. 49 with slight modifications: a Pt-thread was cleansed in concentrated nitric acid evolving in turns hydrogen and oxygen from the surface by electrolysis with changing polarity. The Pt-thread was rinsed in distilled water and surrounded by a silver spiral at a distance of 2–3 mm. The two electrodes were placed in a well stirred aqueous solution of $KAg(CN)_2$, 10 g/L, mixed with an equimolar amount of KOH. Purified nitrogen had been bubbled through the solution for at least 1 h in advance. The Pt-electrode was cathodically coated by silver with the Ag-spiral serving as an anode. The current density was kept at 5 mA/cm^2 in 60 min.

The silver coated Pt thread was rinsed in distilled water, and a part of the silver layer was converted to AgCl by electrolysis in an aqueous 0.1 mol/L HCl solution with a current density of 5 mA/cm^2 in 5 min. The Ag/AgCl electrode was now ready for use. A pair of electrodes just prepared, normally deviated less than 0.1 mV in the same NaCl solution after an equilibration time which should not exceed 15 min. The AgCl layer is slowly removed by use of the electrodes because of complexation of AgCl with chloride ions.

In the emf measurements, the asymmetry potential of the two electrodes in 0.01 mol/L NaCl was always measured before and after the experiment, and the emf values were corrected with the mean asymmetry potential. The electrode to be immersed in the new solution (different from 0.01 mol/L) was placed at least 15 min in a thermostatted sample of the new solution. Then it was rapidly transferred in wet state to the cell chamber, and the membrane was immediately after put in contact at this side with the new solution at the same temperature (flowing or not).

If the asymmetry potentials grew greater than 0.5 mV or if the time of electrode equilibration became excessively long, the electrodes were electrolyzed again in 0.1 mol/L HCl to renew the AgCl layer. If this did not help, residual AgCl was dissolved by prolonged exposure to 2 mol/L NaCl solution, and the silver layer was removed in ammonium hydroxide solution, whereafter the complete procedure described above was repeated.

(e) *Influence of the Flow Velocity on emf (Danish cell).* With the Danish cell we have performed measurements of emf (right electrode minus left electrode) of the same concentration cell at different flow rates. In Table 5 we have listed the initial and stationary emf values of the concentration cell

Ag | AgCl | 0.01 mol/L NaCl | support ... skin layer

$$| \text{0.2 mol/L NaCl} | \text{AgCl} | \text{Ag} \quad (93)$$

TABLE 5 Influence of Flow Rate on the EMF of Cell (93) Danish Cell

Flow rate (cm^3/min)	$-\text{emf}_{\text{initial}}$(mV)	$-\text{emf}_{\text{stationary}}$(mV)
47	47.9 ± 0.5	52.7 ± 0.2
60	53.7 ± 0.2	56.2 ± 0.2
87	56.2 ± 0.3	56.9 ± 0.1
110	55.6 ± 0.5	56.5 ± 0.5
165	56.5 ± 0.1	56.5 ± 0.2

EMF values corrected for asymmetry potentials.

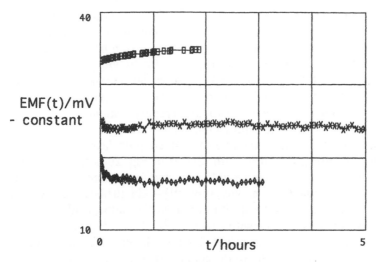

FIG. 26 Transients of the "Spanish cell". Skin layer experiments. NaCl. Ambient temperatures. EMF = right(skin) electrode-left (support) electrode. (a) skin(0.02 mol/L) → sup (0.01 mol/L); EMF(t)/mV + 20 (rectangles). (b) sup(0.01 mol/L) → skin(0.001 mol/L); EMF(t)/mV − 40 (diamonds). (c) sup(0.01 mol/L) → skin (0.0005 mol/L); EMF(t)/mV − 50 (crosses).

varying the flow rate simultaneously on both sides (double peristaltic pump).

These data show definitively that 47 cm^3/min (corresponding to 5.2 cm/s average linear velocity) is too small a flow rate. The low absolute values of both emf values must be ascribed to unstirred layers near the two membrane–solution interfaces. The average value of the stationary emf value for the higher four flow rates is −56.5 ± 0.3 mV. The stationary value seems to be flow independent above 60 cm^3/min. The average value of the initial emf for the higher three flow rates is −56.1 ± 0.4 mV and there is probably no flow dependence above 87 cm^3/min (corresponding to 9.6 cm/s). It is quite likely that in this special case there is very little difference between the initial and the stationary emf, since most of the resistance for diffusion is in the dense skin layer. Thus, the stationary state resembles the initial state since most of the concentration profile is situated over the skin layer. All other experiments in this paper have been performed at a flow rate in the neighborhood of 130 cm^3/min where the influence of unstirred layers should be minimized.

2. Examples of Transient EMF Curves

Since, in all cells, the smooth skin layer of the membrane turns to the right and the rugged support layer turns to the left, initial emf values should produce information about the skin layer in experiments where the variable concentrations were found in the right chamber. On the contrary, information about the layer with support is obtained in experiments with the variable concentration in the left chamber (and the fixed concentration 0.01 mol/L in the right chamber). The first kind of experiments will for brevity be called "skin layer experiments" and the second kind "support layer experiments". For each cell, a concentration series of variable concentrations was performed first for "skin layer experiments", then for "support layer experiments".

Figures 26 and 27 show some representative emf transients for the Spanish cell in the case of skin layer experiments and support layer experiments, respectively. For example, the curve with crosses in Fig. 26 is the emf values (= "skin electrode" − "support electrode", corrected for asymmetry potential) for the experiment denoted for brevity sup(0.01) → skin(0.0005). By this we mean an experiment with overall salt diffusion from the support side with 0.01 mol/L NaCl towards the skin side with 0.0005 mol/L NaCl. Figures 28 and 29 show similar representative emf transients for the Chilenian cell and Figs 30 and 31 for the Danish cell. We refer to the comments below the curves.

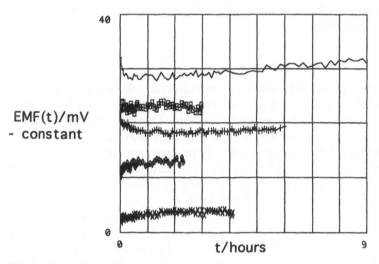

FIG. 27 Transients of the "Spanish cell". Support layer experiments. NaCl. Ambient temperatures. EMF = right(skin) electrode-left (support) electrode. (a) sup(0.2 mol/L) → skin(0.01 mol/L); EMF(t)/mV − 40 (rectangles). (b) sup(0.1 mol/L) → skin(0.01 mol/L); EMF(t)/mV − 35 (diamonds). (c) sup(0.05 mol/L) → skin(0.01 mol/L); EMF(t)/mV − 30 (× × ×). (d) skin(0.01 mol/L) → sup(0.001 mol/L); EMF(t)/mV + 75 (+ + +). (e) skin(0.01 mol/L) → sup(0.0005 mol/L); EMF(t)mV + 100 (line). Especially the curve (e) shows an almost linear long time asymptote due to diffusion equalization. The stationary values of such experiments are found extrapolating back the asymptote to time 0.

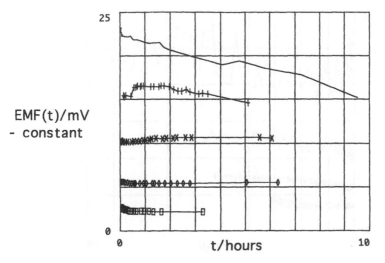

FIG. 28 Transients of the "Chilenian cell". Skin layer experiments, NaCl, $25.0 \pm 0.1°C$. EMF = right(skin) electrode-left (support) electrode. (a) skin (0.05 mol/L) → sup(0.01 mol/L; EMF(t)/mV + 35 (rectangles). (b) skin(0.02 mol/L) → sup(0.01 mol/L); EMF(t)/mV + 20 (diamonds). (c) sup(0.01 mol/L) → skin(0.005 mol/L); EMF(t)/mV − 5 (× × ×). (d) sup(0.01 mol/L) → skin(0.001 mol/L); EMF(t)/mV − 55 (+ + +). (e) sup(0.01 mol/L) → skin(0.0005 mol/L); EMF(t)/mV − 55(line).

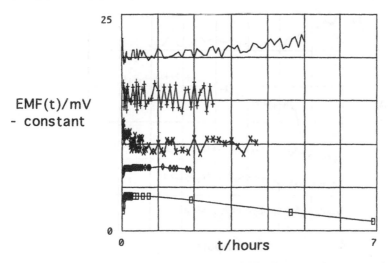

FIG. 29 Transients of the "Chilenian cell". Support layer experiments. NaCl. $25.0 \pm 0.1°C$. EMF = right(skin) electrode-left(support) electrode. (a) sup(0.2 mol/L) → skin(0.01 mol/L); EMF(t)/mV − 57 (rectangles). (b) sup(0.1 mol/L) → skin(0.01 mol/L); EMF(t)/mV − 40 (diamonds). (c) sup(0.02 mol/L) → skin(0.01 mol/L); EMF(t)/mV − 5 (× × ×). (d) skin(0.01 mol/L) → sup(0.001 mol/L); EMF(t)/mV + 58 (+ + +). (e) skin(0.01 mol/L) → sup(0.0005 mol/L); EMF(t)/mV + 90 (line).

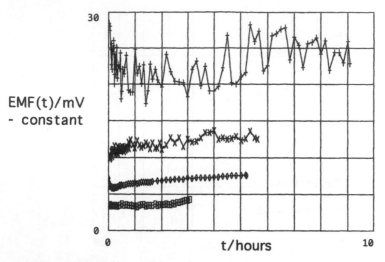

EMF(t)/mV
- constant

t/hours

FIG. 30 Transients of the "Danish cell". Skin layer experiments. NaCl. 25.00 ± 0.05°C. EMF = right(skin) electrode-left(support) electrode. (a) skin(0.2 mol/L) → sup(0.01 mol/L); EMF(*t*)/mV + 60 (rectangles). (b) skin (0.05 mol/L) → sup (0.01 mol/L); EMF(*t*)/mV + 37 (diamonds). (c) sup (0.01 mol/L) → skin(0.005 mol/L); EMF(*t*)/mV − 5 (× × ×). (d) sup(0.01 mol/L) → skin(0.0005 mol/L); EMF(*t*)/mV − 50 (+ + +).

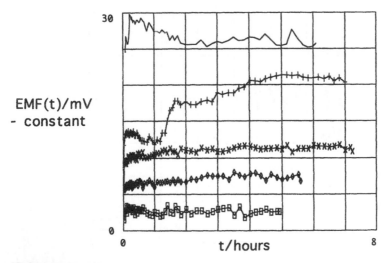

EMF(t)/mV
- constant

t/hours

FIG. 31 Transients of the "Danish cell". Support layer experiments. NaCl. 25.00 ± 0.05°C. EMF = right(skin) electrode-left(support) electrode. (a) sup(0.2 mol/L) → skin(0.01 mol/L); EMF(*t*)/mV − 58 (rectangles). (b) sup(0.05 mol/L) → /skin(0.01 mol/L); EMF(*t*)/mV − 25 (diamonds). (c) skin (0.01 mol/L) → sup(0.005 mol/L); EMF(*t*)/mV + 25 (× × ×). (d) skin(0.01 mol/L) → sup(0.001 mol/L); EMF(*t*)/mV + 70 (+ + +). (e) skin(0.01 mol/L) → sup(0.0005 mol/L); EMF(*t*)/mV + 100 (line).

3. Finding Surface Transport Numbers and Mean Transport Numbers

In the present experiments, when we characterize the right surface (the skin layer), we fix the salt concentration (and the salt chemical potential) in the left chamber to 0.01 mol/L and vary the concentration in the right. Using Eq. (56) and the corresponding equation for the characterization of the left surface (the support layer) we have for the *apparent surface transport numbers*:

$$\tau_{\text{cat, surface}}(c_{\text{s, surface}}) = \pm \{F/[2RT]\}[\partial \text{ EMF}_{\text{initial}}/\partial \ln a_{\pm, \text{surface}}]$$
$$\times (+ \sim \text{left, sup}; - \sim \text{right, skin}) \tag{94}$$

We also define *mean transport numbers* (for each direction of diffusion) using the equation:

$$\tau_{\text{cat, mean}}(c_{\text{s, L}}, c_{\text{s, R}}) \equiv (F/[2RT])\{\text{EMF}_{\text{stationary}}/[\ln(a_{\pm, \text{L}}/a_{\pm, \text{R}})]\} \tag{95}$$

In contrast to the surface transport numbers, these mean transport numbers have no clear physical meaning, except that they are the transport numbers one would obtain disregarding the fact that the transport number in the membrane is a function of position and concentration. Therefore, the mean transport number will in general be a function of the salt concentrations at *both* membrane phases.

The procedure followed is for each type of measuring cell to fit the initial or stationary emf values (corrected for any asymmetry potential) to a second degree, least square polynomial in the parameter:

$$p \equiv \ln(a_{\pm, \text{right}}/a_{\pm, \text{left}}) \tag{96}$$

We use least square polynomials with the restriction that the polynomial *has* to be zero when $p = 0$. By differentiation of the polynomials with respect to p the values of the surface transport number as a function of surface concentration can be found using Eq. (94). Thus, if we have

$$(F/RT) \text{ EMF}_{\text{initial, skin}} = A_1 p + A_2 p^2 \tag{97a}$$
$$(F/RT) \text{ EMF}_{\text{initial, sup}} = B_1 p + B_2 p^2 \tag{97b}$$
$$(F/RT) \text{ EMF}_{\text{stationary, skin}} = C_1 p + C_2 p^2 \tag{97c}$$
$$(F/RT) \text{ EMF}_{\text{stationary, sup}} = D_1 p + D_2 p^2 \tag{97d}$$

we obtain immediately:

$$\tau_{\text{cat, skin}} = - [(A_1/2) + A_2 p] \tag{98a}$$
$$\tau_{\text{cat, sup}} = - [(B_1/2) + B_2 p] \tag{98b}$$
$$\tau_{\text{cat, mean, skin}} = - (1/2)[C_1 + C_2 p] \tag{98c}$$
$$\tau_{\text{cat, mean, sup}} = - (1/2)[D_1 + D_2 p] \tag{98d}$$

By $\text{EMF}_{\text{stationary, sup}}$ we mean the stationary emf measured in an experiment beginning as an initial value emf experiment characterizing the support surface layer of the membrane. The corresponding mean transport number is $\tau_{cat, mean, sup}$.

The present method can only detect a linear dependence of the apparent transport numbers on $\ln a_{\pm}$ (variable). The number of data in each experimental series and the statistical errors in the measurements do not permit a polynomial of the third degree to be fitted significantly. In particular, such a polynomial would not yield reliable derivatives.

The transformation from molar concentrations of NaCl (and of $BaCl_2$ in the next subsection) in aqueous solutions at 25°C to activities may be made by any interpolation of compiled literature values. We have used the empirical ASPEV formulae which have been critically fitted to literature values of 1:1 and 2:1 electrolytes at various temperatures, see Eqs. (86)–(94) and Table 5 in Ref. 108.

In Tables 6–8, the four emf values found for each value of the variable concentration are listed, one table for each measuring cell. The uncertainties indicated are estimated uncertainties, looking at the statistical fluctuations in each experimental run. The calculated apparent transport numbers are shown as a function of the variable concentration in Figs. 32–35. In all cases, the transport number decreases with increasing concentration and (except in some cases in the high concentration end) they are always higher than the transport number of Na^+ in water at 25°C. The latter values have been indicated in all the four figures for easy comparison (curve with crosses). A highly swollen membrane without ion exchange properties would be expected to have approximately the same transport number as the free aqueous solution, since the mobility of the cation and anion is reduced by the same (tortuosity) factor.

In Fig. 32, the surface transport numbers for the skin layer are shown. The Spanish, Chilenian and Danish cell yield practically the same values, and these values should then be considered very reliable—given all the different circumstances of measuring. The transport number decreases steeply from ~0.60 to

TABLE 6 Measured EMF as a Function of NaCl Concentration. Spanish Cell

c_s(mol/L)	emf$_{int, skin}$(mV)	emf$_{stat, skin}$(mV)	emf$_{int, sup}$(mV)	emf$_{stat, sup}$(mV)
0.2	-55.1 ± 0.5	-56.4 ± 0.5	$+62.0 \pm 0.8$	$+62.0 \pm 0.8$
0.1	-43.7 ± 0.2	-45.4 ± 0.5	$+45.4 \pm 0.5$	$+48.0 \pm 0.7$
0.05	-31.5 ± 0.1	-32.8 ± 0.2	$+32.3 \pm 0.5$	$+33.7 \pm 0.5$
0.02	-14.0 ± 0.1	-15.6 ± 0.2	$+12.5 \pm 0.3$	$+13.5 \pm 0.3$
0.005	—	—	-15.1 ± 0.7	-15.1 ± 0.7
0.001	$+58.4 \pm 0.5$	$+56.7 \pm 0.5$	-54.6 ± 0.5	-56.8 ± 0.5
0.0005	$+77.3 \pm 2.0$	$+74.3 \pm 0.5$	-69.5 ± 0.5	-71.5 ± 0.7

EMF values corrected for asymmetry potentials. The fixed salt concentration was always 0.01 mol/L.

TABLE 7   Measured EMF as a Function of NaCl Concentration. Chilenian Cell

c_s(mol/L)	$emf_{init,\ skin}$(mV)	$emf_{stat,\ skin}$(mV)	$emf_{init,\ sup}$(mV)	$emf_{stat,\ sup}$(mV)
0.2	-57.5 ± 0.5	-60.0 ± 2.0	$+59.3 \pm 0.1$	$+61.0 \pm 0.2$
0.1	-44.9 ± 0.1	-44.7 ± 0.1	$+46.2 \pm 0.1$	$+47.3 \pm 0.1$
0.05	-32.3 ± 0.1	-32.8 ± 0.4	$+33.2 \pm 0.1$	$+33.6 \pm 0.1$
0.02	-14.43 ± 0.02	-14.56 ± 0.02	$+17.6 \pm 0.5$	$+14.7 \pm 0.8$
0.005	$+15.2 \pm 0.1$	$+15.69 \pm 0.03$	—	—
0.001	$+69.9 \pm 0.5$	$+71.5 \pm 0.1$	-41.0 ± 1.5	-42.7 ± 1.5
0.0005	$+77.8 \pm 0.5$	$+73.8 \pm 1.0$	-63.2 ± 5.0	-69.7 ± 0.5

EMF values corrected for asymmetry potentials. The fixed salt concentration was always 0.01 mol/L.

~ 0.32 with increasing NaCl concentration. This should be compared to the transport numbers in aqueous solution which are in the range 0.38–0.39.

The surface transport numbers for the support layer are not very consistent, see Fig. 33. The Chilenian cell yield transport numbers parallel to the transport numbers in water, but with values about 0.4 above the latter. The Spanish cell shows a higher slope with a variation from 0.50 to 0.40. The Danish cell show transport numbers with a steep variation almost like the values for the skin layer. The most we can say is that the initial emf values at the support side are very sensitive to the flow conditions in the cell.

Figure 34 shows the mean transport numbers calculated from the stationary emf values for the skin layer experiments. The Chilenian cell and the Danish cell yield parallel variations of the transport numbers with concentration. The "Chilenian values" are higher than the "Danish values" with about 0.15–0.20, however. The "Spanish values" lie a little below the Danish at low concentrations but merge with the "Danish values" at the higher concentrations. The Danish as well as the Chilenian cell seem both to yield quite reliable

TABLE 8   Measured EMF as a Function of NaCl Concentration. Danish Cell

c_s(mol/L)	$emf_{init,\ skin}$(mV)	$emf_{stat,\ skin}$(mV)	$emf_{init,\ sup}$(mV)	$emf_{stat,\ sup}$(mV)
0.2	-56.5 ± 0.1	-56.5 ± 0.2	$+60.8 \pm 0.5$	$+60.6 \pm 0.5$
0.1	-46.0 ± 0.3	-45.3 ± 0.1	$+49.0 \pm 0.5$	$+52.2 \pm 0.2$
0.05	-31.5 ± 0.5	-30.6 ± 0.2	$+29.6 \pm 0.3$	$+32.6 \pm 0.6$
0.005	$+14.7 \pm 0.2$	$+18.0 \pm 0.7$	-15.8 ± 0.3	-13.8 ± 0.3
0.001	$+65.4 \pm 3.0$	$+64.4 \pm 3.0$	-56.7 ± 1.0	-49.2 ± 0.5
0.0005	$+78.5 \pm 2.0$	$+74.5 \pm 3.0$	-69.8 ± 0.5	-73.8 ± 1.0

EMF values corrected for asymmetry potentials. The fixed salt concentration was always 0.01 mol/L.

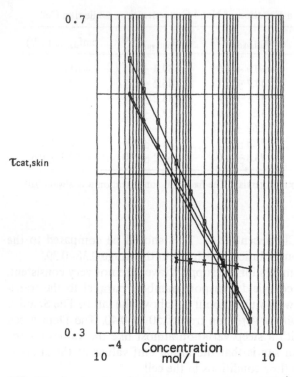

FIG. 32 Apparent surface transport numbers of Na$^+$ in the skin layer measured by three different cells. Line without symbols: Spanish cell, Rectangles: Chilenian cell. Diamonds: Danish cell, Crosses: NaCl in water, 25°C.

mean transport numbers decreasing from about 0.54 to about 0.40. Thus, the variation is less than for the surface transport numbers for the skin layer.

Figure 35 show similar mean transport numbers for stationary state experiments starting as support layer experiments. The variations are within a more narrow range than the surface and mean transport numbers for the skin layer experiments. All values in Fig. 38 are in the range 0.49–0.42. The steepest and highest are the "Spanish values", then comes the "Danish" and finally the "Chilenian" having a slope approximately as the water transport number. However, it is not sure that the three cells really differ significantly from each other.

4.   Discussion of Experiments Using Different Cells

The three cells yield reasonably consistent values of the surface and mean transport numbers in all cases except for the initial value emf measurements attempting to characterize the support face of the membrane. In the latter case, the flow conditions near the membrane seems to influence the measured

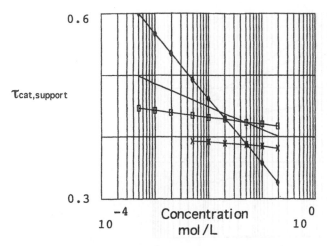

FIG. 33 Apparent surface transport numbers of Na$^+$ in the support layer measured by three different cells. Line without symbols: Spanish cell. Rectangles: Chilenian cell. Diamonds: Danish cell. Crosses: NaCl in water, 25°C.

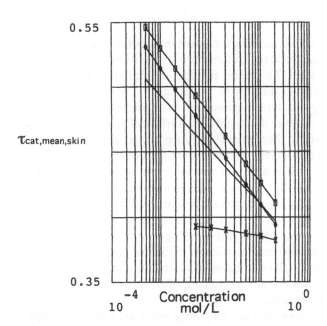

FIG. 34 Apparent, stationary mean transport numbers of Na$^+$ for the skin layer experiments measured by three different cells. Line without symbols: Spanish cell. Rectangles: Chilenian cell. Diamonds: Danish cell. Crosses: NaCl in water, 25°C.

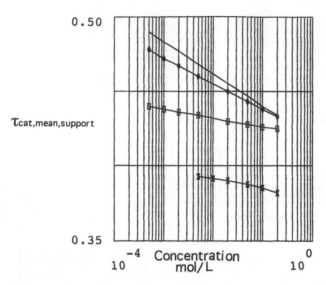

FIG. 35 Apparent, stationary mean transport numbers of Na$^+$ for the support layer experiments measured by three different cells. Line without symbols: Spanish cell. Rectangles: Chilenian cell. Diamonds: Danish cell. Crosses: NaCl in water, 25°C.

emf values (and the calculated surface transport numbers) in a critical way. Much more experiments under many different flow conditions would be necessary to clarify this question. The reason for the anomalous behavior of the support face is perhaps not so difficult to understand: The irregular support creates a semi-macroscopic complex geometry with pockets of liquids with stagnant flow distributed all over the membrane surface. Thus, it might require very high flow rates to remove these pockets of stagnant solution.

Even the basic assumption of one-dimensional diffusional geometry is challenged in the support layer. Of course, one can interpret one-dimensionality to be "in the mean"—taking the average over many random fibres of the support. One problem arising here, however, is that even if the mean galvanic current density is zero, the local current densities are not necessarily zero, since *ring galvanic currents* may form. This challenges the other basic assumption behind the irreversible thermodynamics of diffusion potentials: The condition of zero current density. (To our knowledge, the only theory dealing with the possibility of having ring current is the simplified one briefly discussed in Chapter 12 Sec. IV by Woermann.)

Comparing Figs. 32–35, however, the following conclusion for the comparison of skin layer and support layer transport numbers seems plausible: The skin layer shows a very high variation of the surface transport number with concentration (Fig. 32). The corresponding mean transport numbers also vary

TABLE 9 Initial EMF Values as a Function of NaCl Concentration. Spanish Cell. Castellón Data

c_s(mol/L)	$emf_{init,\ skin}$(mV)	$emf_{init,\ support}$(mV)
0.5	−61.0	+68.0
0.1	−37.0	+45.0
0.05	−28.0	+25.1
0.01	−0.3	+1.2
0.005	+19.0	−18.0
0.001	+61.0	−45.0
0.0005	+70.0	−63.0

No correction for asymmetry. The fixed salt concentration was always 0.01 mol/L.

but to a lesser extent. The mean transport numbers for the support face experiments show very little variation with concentration, and it would therefore not be surprising if the "true" surface transport numbers for the support face also vary little with concentration (as the "Chilenian" and "Spanish" values in Fig. 33). If the support surface is dominated by stagnant pockets of external solution the transport numbers and/or their variation should be close to the transport numbers in aqueous solution (as the "Chilenian" values in Fig. 33).

It should also be remembered that the flow experiments with the Danish cell (Table 5) were all "skin experiments" and not "support experiments". It might well be so that linear, average lateral velocities much above the applied 14 cm/s is required to remove the stagnant solution in the "mesh pockets". On the other hand, the liquid flow in the Spanish and, especially, in the Chilenian cell has a high, pulsating component perpendicular to the membrane at a short distance from the surface and this might be more efficient to remove stagnant pockets of solution.

It should be remarked that in Refs. 9, 13 and 15 where the "Danish cell" was used (with half the linear dimensions of the cell used here), the linear flow rate was estimated to be about 30 cm/s, and this was found much more than sufficient for stationary state emf measurements in concentration cells with smooth faced cellulose acetate membranes as separators. Indeed, no differences in the measured emf's were observed between 10 ml/min to 120 ml/min flow rate (corresponding to 4 cm/s to 53 cm/s for the original Danish cell), see Refs. 9 and 10. The initial value emf values were not studied in these papers, however. Neither were membranes with a support layer. The Danish cell is less suited for *initial* value emf experiments than the Spanish or the Chilenian cell since the electrodes are placed in side pockets to the streaming solution in the channel near the membrane. There is a considerable risk of initial "dead volumes" around the electrodes, and we did indeed observe strange jumps in the measured EMF values in the beginning of the experiment in some cases. The "dead volume problem" is increased when the linear dimensions of the cell are multiplied by a factor two.

We may compare the above mentioned surface transport numbers obtained in Concepción (Chile) using the Spanish cell with independent earlier measurements with the same cell in Castellón (Spain). The latter measurements were performed simultaneously with the measurements reported in Ref. 28 using two membranes of the same polymer (but without support layer). The data for the PES membrane with support layer were not reported in Ref. 28 but are useful here for comparison. The data are given in Table 9.

The variation of the surface transport numbers with concentration calculated by these data are shown in Fig. 36. The skin surface transport numbers (rectangles) are practically identical to the skin surface numbers from the Spanish and Danish cell in Fig. 32. (And the Chilenian cell yields skin surface numbers very close). The support surface transport numbers calculated from the Castellón data (diamonds) show much less variation with concentration than the Concepción data with the Spanish cell (Fig. 27).

Compared to Fig. 33, the Castellón surface transport numbers for the support layer are close to the values given by the Chilenian cell at 0.0005 mol/L and close to the values given by the Danish cell at 0.2 mol/L. Thus, the two independent measurements with the Spanish cell do not lead to identical results for the support surface transport number. This points once more to the

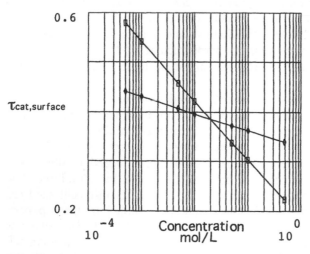

FIG. 36 Apparent surface transport numbers of Na^+ measured by the Spanish cell at ambient temperature (Castellón data). Rectangle: Skin layer. Diamonds: Support layer.

sensitivity of the initial emf measurements for the support layer to the precise flow conditions in the cell.

We observe, at low electrolyte concentrations, always *higher* transport numbers in the present nonionic polysulphone membrane than the transport numbers in aqueous solution. The highest transport numbers at low concentrations are found for the dense skin layer where the Na^+ ion seems to have a higher mobility than the Cl^- ion in contrast to the situation in aqueous NaCl. The skin layer also shows the greatest decrease in transport number with increasing salt concentration. In the cases where the more porous parts of the membrane are involved, the transport numbers come closer to the transport number in aqueous solution as would be expected.

It should be mentioned that the concentration behaviour seen for the cation transport number of the present membrane, namely a decrease from values above 0.5 to values below 0.5 is not possible in the framework of the ordinary interionic attraction theory of conductivity (Onsager, Fuoss). According to this theory it can be demonstrated that if the cationic transport number at infinite dilution is above 0.5, it will increase with increasing concentration. If it is below 0.5, it will decrease with increasing concentration. Finally, it will remain practically constant if the transport number is close to 0.5, see Robinson and Stokes, Ref. 109, pp. 156–159. The variation with concentration of experimental transport numbers of many 1:1 electrolytes in water at 25°C follow quantitatively from this theory, see Ref. 109, Table 7.7. Thus, the transport number can never cross 0.5 in such systems. Therefore, the skin layer in the present membrane cannot simply be represented just as a "solvent" with low permittivity in which we have usual Debye–Hückel–Onsager interactions. The specific physicochemical interactions of the ions with the membrane polymer have to be taken into account.

We should also remember that, according to Eq. (24), the apparent transport numbers contain a contribution from electroosmotic water transfer. Such a contribution should be more strongly felt in not too dense membranes with fixed charge, but oriented dipole layers near to the polymer chains may have a similar effect as a fixed charge. Therefore, it cannot be completely excluded that some contribution from electroosmosis is incorporated into the apparent transport numbers reported here.

C. Asymmetric Polyether Sulfone Membrane with BaCl₂

A series of experiments with $BaCl_2$ as electrolyte were run at the University of Concepción subsequently to the NaCl experiments described in the previous subsection. However, only the Chilenian cell was used for these experiments at 25.0 ± 0.1°C. The membrane was the same as before, and the transient emf experiments over long duration were carefully analyzed like in the NaCl experiments. The results are summarized in Table 10. It is seen from the table

TABLE 10   Measured EMF as a Function of $BaCl_2$ Concentration. Chilenian Cell

c_s(mol/L)	$emf_{init, skin}$(mV)	$emf_{stat, skin}$(mV)	$emf_{init, sup}$(mV)	$emf_{stat, sup}$(mV)
0.2	-42.2 ± 0.2	-41.2 ± 0.2	$+43.0 \pm 0.5$	$+43.3 \pm 0.2$
0.2	-40.5 ± 0.2	-39.2 ± 0.8	—	—
0.1	-33.1 ± 0.2	-32.8 ± 0.2	$+33.2 \pm 0.4$	$+33.4 \pm 0.4$
0.1	-32.3 ± 0.2	-30.1 ± 0.1	$+32.7 \pm 0.3$	$+33.0 \pm 0.2$
0.05	-24.7 ± 0.3	-24.1 ± 0.2	$+23.4 \pm 0.2$	$+23.7 \pm 0.2$
0.05	-22.3 ± 0.5	-19.5 ± 1.0	—	—
0.02	-11.5 ± 0.2	-10.8 ± 0.3	$+8.4 \pm 0.3$	$+8.2 \pm 0.5$
0.02	-10.5 ± 1.0	-11.5 ± 0.3	$+10.0 \pm 0.5$	$+11.3 \pm 0.5$
0.005	$+9.2 \pm 0.5$	$+10.0 \pm 0.5$	-10.8 ± 0.5	-7.2 ± 0.3
0.005	$+14.0 \pm 1.0$	$+11.8 \pm 0.3$	—	—
0.001	$+41.5 \pm 1.5$	$+39.5 \pm 1.0$	-38.0 ± 0.5	-36.5 ± 0.5
0.0005	—	—	-43.0 ± 0.5	-40.5 ± 0.5

EMF values corrected for asymmetry potentials. The fixed salt concentration was always 0.01 mol/L.

that the deviations between two repeated experiments are often greater than the uncertainty estimated from analysis of the single emf vs. time curve.

The surface transport numbers were calculated from the initial emf values by the differentiation method, fitting second order least square polynomials in $\ln(a_{\pm, \text{right}}/a_{\pm, \text{left}})$ through (0,0) to the emf data. The conversion from molar concentration to activities was done using the empirical formulae in Ref. 108. Mean transport numbers for "skin layer and support layer stationary state experiments" (defined as in Sec. IV.B) were also calculated. Equations (97a–d) are the same but instead of Eqs. (98a–d) we now have:

$$\tau_{\text{cat, skin}} = -(2/3)[A_1 + 2A_2 p] \tag{99a}$$

$$\tau_{\text{cat, sup}} = -(2/3)[B_1 + 2B_2 p] \tag{99b}$$

$$\tau_{\text{cat, mean, skin}} = -(2/3)[C_1 + C_2 p] \tag{99c}$$

$$\tau_{\text{cat, mean, sup}} = -(2/3)[D_1 + D_2 p] \tag{99d}$$

The results are shown in Figs. 37–40. For comparison, the transport numbers (at 18°C) for the Ba^{2+} ion in aqueous solutions of $BaCl_2$ are shown as a function of concentration [110]. The transport numbers at 25°C would probably not differ very much from those at 18°C (partially cancelling activation energies). It is seen that the apparent skin layer transport numbers for the membrane follow the transport numbers in free water quite closely at the higher concentrations (Fig. 37). At the lower concentrations, the membrane transport numbers are higher, however. This feature, and also the decrease in $\tau_{Ba^{2+}, \text{skin}}$ with inceasing concentration, resemble the situation for the NaCl experiments (Fig. 32) but for some reason the concentration dependence of

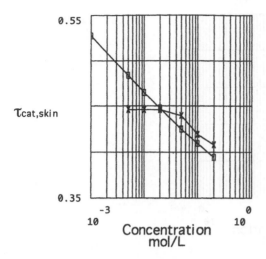

FIG. 37 Apparent surface transport numbers of Ba^{2+} for the skin layer measured by the Chilenian cell at $25.0 \pm 0.1°C$ (rectangles, estimated from Concepción data). Crosses: Transport number of Ba^{2+} in aqueous $BaCl_2$ at $18°C$.

$\tau_{Na^+, skin}$ is much more steep than for $\tau_{Ba^{2+}, skin}$. The variation of $\tau_{Ba^{2+}, sup}$ with concentration is less than for $\tau_{Ba^{2+}, skin}$ and the variation is the inverse (an increase with the concentration, see Fig. 38). The asymmetry between the two faces of the membrane seems to be more marked for $BaCl_2$ than for $NaCl$. But

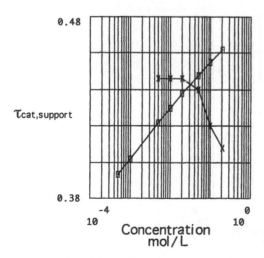

FIG. 38 Apparent surface transport numbers of Ba^{2+} for the support layer measured by the Chilenian cell at $25.0 \pm 0.1°C$ (rectangles, estimated from Concepción data). Crosses: Transport number of Ba^{2+} in aqueous $BaCl_2$ at $18°C$.

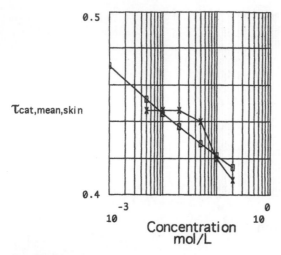

FIG. 39 Apparent, stationary mean transport numbers of Ba^{2+} for the skin layer experiments measured by the Chilenian cell at $25.0 \pm 0.1°C$ (rectangles, estimated from Concepción data). Crosses: Transport number of Ba^{2+} in aqueous $BaCl_2$ at $18°C$.

still, the values of $\tau_{Ba^{2+}, sup}$ are "in the neighbourhood of" the transport numbers in water. The stationary, mean transport numbers for skin layer experiments (Fig. 39), do hardly differ from the transport numbers in water. The similar mean transport numbers for the support layer, however, increases

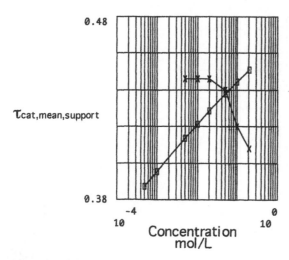

FIG. 40 Apparent, stationary mean transport numbers of Ba^{2+} for the support layer experiments measured by the Chilenian cell at $25.0 \pm 0.1°C$ (rectangles, estimated from Concepción data). Crosses: Transport number of Ba^{2+} in aqueous $BaCl_2$ at $18°C$.

with concentration (Fig. 40) quite similar to the surface transport numbers. When judging the uncertainty of the calculated transport numbers, one should remember that the "uncertainty belt" of the second-order least-square polynomials is wider near the extremes in the concentrations than in the middle.

V. DISCUSSIONS AND CONCLUSIONS

We have currently discussed the findings throughout this chapter. Therefore, we shall finish with a short, critical account of the main results which have been presented and also point out remaining research to be done.

Basically, there are two approaches to emf measurements over membranes (ion exchange or noncharged): One may derive exact expressions for the emf of concentration cells from irreversible thermodynamics, or one may introduce simplifications of ideality (Nernst–Planck–Ideal Donnan models). The first method is only really useful in cases where there is only one diffusing electrolyte and when the dimensionality of electrodiffusion is one. Then, however, the method may be extended to asymmetric membranes and "surface transport numbers" may be found. The recent investigations reported and discussed in this chapter are not quite definitive, however. The problem of finding the ideal measuring cell for initial value emf measurements has not yet been settled. Especially there are problems of separating electrode effects from membrane effects in the very initial stages and problems in connection with "unstirred layers". There may also be unsettled questions with respect to interference of other ions (notoriously H^+) and deviations from one-dimensionality at "rugged" membrane solution. Only few and simplified theories exist including the possibility of "ring galvanic currents", and such theories would indeed be difficult to compare with experiments.

Even with an experimental method working perfectly, the (apparent) surface transport numbers measured are just numbers, and so what? In order to interpret the results in terms of structural parameters of the membrane and the ions, it is necessary to simplify. Therefore we have, parallelly with the "exact" methods of irreversible thermodynamics, treated simple Nernst–Planck–Donnan models for homogeneous and inhomogeneous (e.g., asymmetric) membranes. We have stressed the necessity of including into the Donnan formalism the individual Nernst distribution coefficients for the ions which is very seldom done in the literature. We have also stressed the necessary transformations of variables in order to obtain the minimum number of determinable parameters from series of emf experiments with various electrolyte mixtures. Such parameters are the fixed charge density of the membrane divided by a Nernst distribution coefficient of a salt, ratios of ionic diffusion coefficients and ratios of ionic Nernst distribution coefficients.

The example with dense cellulose acetate membranes demonstrates, however, that even this minimum number of parameters cannot be determined without ambiguity from emf measurements alone. We need the help from other kinds of measurements such as electroosmosis, diffusion measurements, thermodynamic phase distribution experiments and, especially, from impedance measurements and the theories of such measurements [16–18,20–22,111]. See also the chapters by Sørensen [19], by Coster and Chilcott [112] and by Zholkovskij [113] in the present monograph. The chapter of Manzanares and Kontturi [114] deals with an interesting alternative of the interpretation of mean transport numbers from emf measurements in ternary electrolyte systems (also based on the Nernst–Planck equations).

We may conclude that although the collection of emf data from concentration cells with membranes as separators is easy (and indeed a widespread pastime for researchers worldwide) the interpretation of such data is often quite subtle, and emf data should not stand alone but should rather be used in connection with other experimental techniques before definite conclusions are drawn.

REFERENCES

1. K. H. Meyer and J.-F. Sievers, Helvetica Chim. Acta 19: 649 (1936).
2. K. H. Meyer and J.-F. Sievers, Helvetica Chim. Acta 19: 665 (1936).
3. T. Teorell, Zeitschr. Elektrochem. 55: 460 (1951).
4. F. Helfferich, Ion Exchange, McGraw-Hill, New York, 1962.
5. N. Laksminarayanaiah, Transport Phenomena in Membranes, Academic Press, New York, 1969.
6. N. Laksminarayanaiah, Equations of Membrane Biophysics, Academic Press, New York, 1984.
7. H.-U. Demisch and W. Pusch, J. Colloid Interface Sci. 69: 247 (1979).
8. W. Pusch, Desalination 59: 105 (1986).
9. T. S. Sørensen and J. B. Jensen, J. Non-Equilib. Thermodyn. 9: 1 (1984).
10. J. B. Jensen, T. S. Sørensen, B. Malmgren-Hansen, and P. Sloth, J. Colloid Interface Sci. 108: 18 (1985).
11. T. S. Sørensen, J. B. Jensen, and B. Malmgren-Hansen, J. Non-Equilib. Thermodyn. 13: 57 (1988).
12. B. Malmgren-Hansen, T. S. Sørensen, and J. B. Jensen, J. Non-Equilib. Thermodyn. 13: 193 (1988).
13. F. Skácel, B. Malmgren-Hansen, T. S. Sørensen, and J. B. Jensen, J. Chem. Soc. Faraday Trans. 86: 341 (1990).
14. S. Laursen, B. Malmgren-Hansen, and T. S. Sørensen, J. Non-Equilib. Thermodyn. 15: 223 (1990).
15. T. S. Sørensen, J. B. Jensen, and B. Malmgren-Hansen, Desalination 80: 293 (1991).
16. T. S. Sørensen, in Capillarity Today. Lecture Notes in Physics, vol. 386 (G. Pétré and A. Sanfeld, eds.). Springer, Berlin, 1991, pp. 164–221.
17. B. Malmgren-Hansen, T. S. Sørensen, J. B. Jensen, and M. Hennenberg, J. Colloid Interface Sci. 130: 359 (1989).

18. I. W. Plesner, B. Malmgren-Hansen, and T. S. Sørensen, J. Chem. Soc. Faraday Trans. *90*: 2381 (1994).
19. T. S. Sørensen, in *Surface Chemistry and Electrochemistry of Membranes* (T. S. Sørensen, ed.), Marcel Dekker, New York, 1998, Chapter 18.
20. T. S. Sørensen and V. Compañ, J. Chem. Soc. Faraday Trans. *91*: 4235 (1995).
21. T. S. Sørensen, V. Compañ, and R. Diaz-Calleja, J. Chem. Soc. Faraday Trans. *92*: 1947 (1996).
22. T. S. Sørensen, R. Diaz-Calleja, E. Riande, J. Guzman, and A. Andrio, J. Chem. Soc. Faraday Trans. *93*: 2399 (1997).
23. R. Wódski, A. Narebska, and J. Ceynova, J. Angew. Makromol. Chem. *78*: 145 (1979).
24. J. H. Petropoulos, J. Membrane Sci. *52*: 305 (1990).
25. M. Pinéri, in *Coulombic Interactions in Macromolecular Systems* (A. Eisenberg and F. E. Bailey, eds.), ACS Symposium Series 302, American Chemical Society, Washington DC, 1986, pp. 159–175.
26. V. Compañ, M. L. López, T. S. Sørensen, and J. Garrido, J. Phys. Chem. *98*: 9013 (1994).
27. V. Compañ, T. S. Sørensen, and S. R. Rivera, J. Phys. Chem. *99*: 12553 (1995).
28. V. Compañ, T. S. Sørensen, A. Andrio, M. L. López, and J. de Abajo, J. Membrane Sci. *123*: 293 (1997).
29. T. S. Sørensen and V. Compañ, Electrochim. Acta *42*: 639 (1997).
30. T. S. Sørensen, V. Compañ, and S. R. Rivera, Electrochim. Acta *43*: 951 (1998).
31. T. S. Sørensen and V. Compañ, J. Phys. Chem. *100*: 7623 (1996).
32. T. S. Sørensen and V. Compañ, J. Phys. Chem. *100*: 15261 (1996).
33. M. Planck, Ann. der Physik *40*: 561 (1890).
34. P. Henderson, Z. physik. Chem. *59*: 118 (1907).
35. P. Henderson, Z. physik. Chem. *63*: 325 (1908).
36. H. Pleijel, Z. physik. Chem. *72*: 1 (1910).
37. P. B. Taylor, J. Phys. Chem. *31*: 1478 (1927).
38. L. Bass, Trans. Faraday Soc. *60*: 1914 (1964).
39. D. Hafemann, J. Phys. Chem. *69*: 4226 (1965).
40. T. S. Sørensen and K. F. Jensen, J. Chem. Soc. Faraday Trans. 2 *71*: 1805 (1975).
41. G. N. Lewis and L. W. Sargent, J. Am. Chem. Soc. *31A*: 363 (1909).
42. A. C. Cumming and E. Gilchrist, Trans. Faraday Soc. *9*: 174 (1913).
43. E. A. Guggenheim, J. Am. Chem. Soc. *52*: 1315 (1930).
44. D. A. MacInnes and L. G. Longsworth, Cold Spring Harbor Symposia on Quantitative Biology *4*: 18 (1936).
45. K. V. Grove-Rasmussen, Acta Chem. Scand. *3*: 445 (1949).
46. M. Spiro, Electrochim. Acta *11*: 569 (1966).
47. W. H. Smyrl and J. Newman, J. Phys. Chem. *72*: 4660 (1968).
48. T. S. Sørensen, Studier over fysisk–kemiske systemers statik, dynamik, kinetik, Ph.D. dissertation, Danmarks Tekniske Højskole, Copenhagen, 1973, Chapter 3.
49. N. O. Østerberg, J. B. Jensen, and T. S. Sørensen, Acta Chem. Scand. *A32*: 721 (1978).
50. N. O. Østerberg, J. B. Jensen, T. S. Sørensen, and L. D. Caspersen, Acta Chem. Scand. *A34*: 523 (1980).

51. N. O. Østerberg, T. S. Sørensen, and J. B. Jensen, J. Electroanal. Chem. *119*:93 (1981).
52. A. K. Covington and M. J. F. Rebelo, Ion-Selective Electrode Rev. *5*:93 (1983).
53. E. Néher-Neumann, The liquid junction emf. Doctor Technices dissertation, Kungliga Tekniska Högskolan, Stockholm, 1987.
54. E. E. Johnsen, On liquid junction potentials and a solid state pH electrode, Ph.D dissertation, Norges Tekniske Höjskole, Trondheim, 1989, Chapters 1–5.
55. R. Schlögl, Z. physikal. Chem. (Neue Folge) *1*:305 (1954).
56. V. M. Aguilella, J. Garrido, S. Mafé, and J. Pellicer, J. Membrane Sci. *28*:139 (1986).
57. V. M. Aguilella, S. Mafé, and J. Pellicer. *Descripción de los procesos de transporte en disoluciones de electrolitos.* Universidad de Murcia, 1989, Chapter 3.
58. A. Higuchi and T. Nakagawa, J. Chem. Soc. Faraday Trans. 1 *85*:3609 (1989).
59. R. Takagi and M. Nakagaki, J. Membrane Sci. *27*:285 (1986).
60. J. A. Manzanares, S. Mafé, and J. Pellicer, J. Phys. Chem. *95*:5620 (1991).
61. L. Onsager, Phys. Rev. *37*:405 (1931).
62. L. Onsager, Phys. Rev. *38*:2265 (1931).
63. I. Prigogine, *Etude Thermodynamique des Phénomènes Irreversibles.* Dunod, Paris, 1947.
64. S. R. de Groot and P. Mazur, *Non-Equilibrium Thermodynamics,* Dover Publications, New York, 1984 (originally, North-Holland 1962).
65. R. Haase, *Thermodynamics of Irreversible Processes,* Dover Publications, New York, 1990. (Original in German *Thermodynamik der irreversiblen Prozesse.* Dr. Dietrich Steinkopff Verlag, Darmstadt, 1963).
66. A. Katchalsky and P. F. Curran, *Nonequilibrium Thermodynamics in Biophysics,* Harvard University Press, Cambridge, Massachusetts, 1969.
67. H. J. M. Hanley (ed.), *Transport Phenomena in Fluids,* Marcel Dekker, New York, 1969.
68. F. G. Donnan, Zeitschr. Elektrochemie *17*:572 (1911).
69. F. G. Donnan, Zeitschr. physikal. Chemie A *168*:369 (1934).
70. T. L. Hill, Discussions of the Faraday Soc. *21*:31 (1956).
71. G. Stell and C. G. Joslin, Biophys. J. *50*:855 (1986).
72. Y. Zhou and G. Stell, J. Chem. Phys. *89*:7010 (1988).
73. P. Chartier, B. Mattes, and H. Reiss, J. Phys. Chem. *96*:3556 (1992).
74. T. S. Sørensen and P. Sloth, J. Chem. Soc. Faraday Trans. *88*:571 (1992).
75. S. Mafé, J. A. Manzanares, and H. Reiss, J. Chem. Phys. *98*:2408 (1993).
76. S. R. Rivera and T. S. Sørensen, Molecular Simulation *13*:115 (1994).
77. T. S. Sørensen and S. R. Rivera, Molecular Simulation *15*:79 (1995).
78. S. Mafé, P. Ramfrez, A. Tanioka, and J. Pellicer, J. Phys. Chem. *101*:1851 (1997).
79. R. Schlögl, *Stofftransport durch Membranen,* Dietrich Steinkopff Verlag, Darmstadt, 1964.
80. P. Ramírez and S. Mafé, in *Surface Chemistry and Electrochemistry of Membranes* (T. S. Sørensen, ed.), Marcel Dekker, New York, 1998, Chapter 12.
81. D. Woermann, in *Surface Chemistry and Electrochemistry of Membranes* (T. S. Sørensen, ed.), Marcel Dekker, New York, 1998, Chapter 12.
82. W. Thomson, Proc. Roy. Soc. (Edinburgh) *3*:225 (1854).

83. H. von Helmholtz, Ann. Phys. *3*: 201 (1878).
84. C. Wagner, in *Advances in Electrochemistry and Electrochemical Engineering*, Vol. 4 (P. Delahay and C. W. Tobias, eds.), Interscience, New York, 1966, pp. 1–46.
85. D. G. Miller, Chem. Rev. *60*: 15 (1960).
86. H. K. Lonsdale, in *Desalination by Reverse Osmosis* (U. Merten, ed.), The M.I.T. Press, Cambridge, Massachusetts, 1966, pp. 93–160.
87. C. J. Malm, L. J. Tanghe, and G. D. Smith, J. Ind. Eng. Chem. *42*: 730 (1950).
88. J. B. Jensen, M. Jaskula, and T. S. Sørensen, Acta Chem. Scand. *41*: 461 (1987).
89. T. S. Sørensen and J. B. Jensen, Acta Chem. Scand. *43*: 421 (1989).
90. T. S. Sørensen, J. B. Jensen, and P. Sloth, J. Chem. Soc. Far. Trans. 1 *85*: 2649 (1989).
91. T. S. Sørensen, Molecular Simulation *14*: 83 (1995).
92. T. S. Sørensen and V. Compañ, Molecular Simulation *18*: 225 (1996).
93. S. Loeb and S. Sourirajan, Advan. Chem. Ser. *38*: 117 (1962).
94. H. Strathman, P. Scheible, and R. W. Baker, J. Appl. Polym. Sci. *15*: 811 (1971).
95. H. Strathman, K. Kock, and P. Amar, Desalination *16*: 179 (1975).
96. H. Strathman and K. Kock, Desalination *21*: 241 (1977).
97. W. Pusch, J. Membrane Sci. *10*: 325 (1982).
98. D. Pfenning and D. Woermann, J. Membrane Sci. *32*: 105 (1987).
99. G. Manecke, Z. Phys. Chem. *201*: 193 (1952).
100. R. Schlögl and U. Schödel, Z. Phys. Chem. N. F. *5*: 372 (1964).
101. H. S. Harned and B. B. Owen, *The Physical Chemistry of Electrolytic Solutions*, 3rd Ed., Reinhold, New York/Chapman and Hall, London, 1958.
102. A. M. Liquori and C. Botré, J. Phys. Chem. *71*: 3765 (1967).
103. S. Ohki, J. Colloid Interface Sci. *37*: 319 (1971).
104. N. Kamo and Y. Kobatake, J. Colloid Interface Sci. *46*: 85 (1974).
105. J. Garrido and V. Compañ, J. Phys. Chem. *96*: 2721 (1992).
106. K. Asaka, J. Membrane Sci. *52*: 57 (1990).
107. S. Horigome and Y. Taniguchi, J. Appl. Polym. Sci. *21*: 343 (1977).
108. T. S. Sørensen, P. Sloth, and M. Schröder, Acta Chem. Scand. *A38*: 735 (1984).
109. R. A. Robinson and R. H. Stokes, *Electrolyte Solutions*, Butterworths, London, Rev. Ed., 1968, Table 7-7, p. 158.
110. H. Falkenhagen, *Theorie der Elektrolyte*, S. Hirzel Verlag, Leipzig, 1971, p. 193, Tabelle 32.
111. T. S. Sørensen, J. Chem. Soc. Faraday Trans. *93*: 4327 (1997).
112. H. G. L. Coster and T. C. Chilcott, in *Surface Chemistry and Electrochemistry of Membranes* (T. S. Sørensen, ed.), Marcel Dekker, New York, 1998, Chapter 19.
113. E. K. Zholkovskij, in *Surface Chemistry and Electrochemistry of Membranes* (T. S. Sørensen, ed.), Marcel Dekker, New York, 1998, Chapter 20.
114. J. A. Manzanares and K. Kontturi, in *Surface Chemistry and Electrochemistry of Membranes* (T. S. Sørensen, ed.), Marcel Dekker, New York, 1998, Chapter 11.

11

Transport Numbers of Ions in Charged Membrane Systems

JOSÉ A. MANZANARES Department of Thermodynamics, University of Valencia, Burjasot, Spain

KYÖSTI KONTTURI Department of Chemical Engineering, Helsinki University of Technology, Espoo, Finland

Abstract

Transport numbers have been extensively used over the last decades to characterize ion transport in charged membranes. In spite of their conceptual simplicity, a number of difficulties arise in the interpretation of experimental results because of the influence of the operating conditions. The meaning of the transport numbers measured with different methods is here explained by relating them to the local migrational transport numbers and the concentration profiles. The important effects of the diffusion boundary layers and the electric current density used (in the case of Hittorf's method) are then analyzed. Although electromembrane processes often involve multicomponent systems, the characterization of the transport properties of the membrane is often made in terms of binary electrolyte systems. The definitions of potentiometric transport numbers in ternary systems are worked out and these numbers are computed from the solution of the transport equations. These transport numbers are compared to the apparent potentiometric transport numbers used in the literature (i.e., those obtained by assuming that the ternary system behaves as a binary system), and the benefits of their use are clearly shown. Finally, a brief account of the difference between transport numbers in the membrane-fixed and solvent-fixed reference systems is given, and a recent modification of Hittorf's method that makes use of countercurrent convective flow is reviewed.

I. INTRODUCTION

The efficiency of electromembrane processes requires quantitative information on transport of both ions and solvent in the membrane system. The counterion transport number (TN) and water transference number are then important characteristics provided by manufacturers of industrial membranes. The counterion TN is often found by Hittorf's method or by measuring concentration potentials. Hittorf's TN represent the fraction of current transported by a charged species in an ionic solution when no concentration gradients are present [1,2]. Thus, by Hittorf's method, the concentration change in the cathode and anode compartments is measured when a known amount of electrical current passes through the membrane system by the use of reversible electrodes. However, when electric conduction takes place across a membrane system, concentration gradients are inevitably present and this can lead to errors in TN determinations due to back diffusion. Modifications of Hittorf's method that avoid correction for back diffusion [3,4] and the use of radiotracers [5] have been suggested, though they are not easy to use in practice. Furthermore, the ordinary methods for TN determination in charged membranes are such that they actually measure properties of the membrane system, which incorporate the additional effect of the diffusion boundary layers, the influence of which is difficult to estimate [6].

The TN found by the emf method are known as potentiometric TN, and quite frequently do not coincide with Hittorf's TN because these two methods characterize the membrane system as a whole and the values they yield depend on the experimental conditions [7]. Since there is no satisfactory way at present to reliably determine TN, and Hittorf's method or its modifications are relatively laborious, the potentiometric method is often used.

One of the reasons why more extensive use of ion-exchange membranes has not been made is the lack of knowledge of their transport properties in the multicomponent case. Counterion TN measured when binary electrolyte solutions bath the membrane are then of limited value in the performance analysis of electromembrane process, where at least ternary systems are always involved. For instance, in the case of acid and alkali production with bipolar membranes, it is important to determine the TN through the monopolar membranes in systems such as NaCl–HCl or NaCl–NaOH [8].

The scope of this chapter is restricted to the theory of TN in dilute solutions of strong electrolytes. The details of experimental methods by means of which TN are determined will not be discussed. The literature on TN in charged membranes is very extensive and the early developments have been properly reviewed in authoritative monographs [5]. Thus, only a few pioneering works will be cited. The aim of the chapter is not to provide a complete account of the subject matter, but to explain the origin of important effects, such as that of the polarization layers, the electric current density or the changes in pH, and to show how they can be accounted for in terms of the Nernst–Planck formulation.

Section II is intended to serve as an introduction to the different TN definitions. The connection between TN and concentration profiles will be worked out in detail, which will enable for a relatively simple explanation of the effects of the diffusion boundary layers, and the driving forces (electric current density or concentration difference) used in the TN determination.

Section III endeavors to define potentiometric TN in ternary systems and presents simple theoretical expressions for their evaluation. The current use of apparent TN and the consequences of the fixed charge estimation are also discussed.

Finally, Sec. IV gives a brief account of the difference between TN in the membrane-fixed and solvent-fixed reference systems. A recent modification of Hittorf's method that makes use of a countercurrent convective flow is also reviewed.

II. BINARY ELECTROLYTES

A. Model System

Figure 1 presents a schematic view of the membrane system considered. The membrane is homogeneous and of thickness d. The concentration of fixed charge groups within the membrane is c_m and their charge number is z_m. The bathing solutions are of the same binary electrolyte at different concentrations, c_L and c_R. The electrolyte is considered to be completely dissociated and of $1:-1$ type. The two diffusion boundary layers (DBL) adjacent to the membrane have the same thickness δ.

The transport of ions is described by the Nernst–Planck equation [9]

$$J_i = -D_i\left(\frac{dc_i}{dx} + z_i c_i \frac{F}{RT}\frac{d\phi}{dx}\right) \tag{1}$$

where J_i, D_i and c_i are the flux density, diffusion coefficient and molar concentration of species i, respectively, ϕ is the local electric potential, F the Faraday constant, R the gas constant and T the absolute temperature. Alternatively, J_i can be presented as the sum of the salt flux density, J_{12}, and the ionic contribution to the electric current density [10]

$$J_i = -\frac{D_1 D_2}{D_1 c_1 + D_2 c_2}\frac{d(c_1 c_2)}{dx} + \frac{z_i D_i c_i}{D_1 c_1 + D_2 c_2}\frac{I}{F} = J_{12} + \frac{t_i}{z_i}\frac{I}{F} \tag{2}$$

where

$$t_i(x) \equiv \frac{z_i^2 D_i c_i(x)}{\sum_j z_j^2 D_j c_j(x)} \tag{3}$$

is the (differential) TN of species i [11], also called the *local migrational TN* because of its dependence on position within the membrane system.

In the absence of concentrations gradients, ion transport can be described

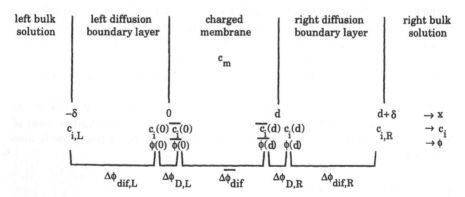

FIG. 1 Sketch of the membrane system and notations used for the ion concentrations and electric potential. Overbars denote membrane phase. The different potential drops in the system are also shown.

as a conduction process following Ohm's law, where every mobile charged species carries a fraction t_i of the electric current density. This statement, however, does not hold in the presence of concentration gradients. First, the electric current density

$$I = F \sum_i z_i J_i \tag{4}$$

does not obey Ohm's law but [2]

$$I = -\kappa \left(\frac{d\phi}{dx} - \frac{d\phi_{dif}}{dx} \right) \tag{5}$$

where

$$\kappa = \frac{F^2}{RT} \sum_j z_j^2 D_j c_j \tag{6}$$

is the electric conductivity and

$$\frac{d\phi_{dif}}{dx} = -\frac{RT}{F \sum_j z_j^2 D_j c_j} \sum_i z_i D_i \frac{dc_i}{dx} = -\frac{RT}{F} \sum_i \frac{t_i}{z_i} \frac{d \ln c_i}{dx} \tag{7}$$

is the gradient of the diffusion potential. That is, even in the absence of electric current, there may be ion migration due to the gradient of the diffusion potential. And second, the migrational TN $t_i(x)$ does not represent the fraction of current carried by species i [12], but the relative contribution of species i to the local electrical conductivity.

B. Permselectivity and Integral Transport Numbers

The permselectivity is the property of ion-exchange membranes most often used to describe its quality. Permselective membranes are those that exhibit selectivity with respect to the passage of charged species. In particular, an ideal permselective membrane only allows the passage of counterions (i.e., those having the opposite sign from the fixed groups). Due to Donnan exclusion, counterions have a concentration in the membrane which is higher than in the bathing solution, while coions (i.e., those having the same sign as the fixed groups) have a lower concentration than in the bathing solution. The permselectivity of a nonideal membrane is defined as the difference between the counterion TN in the membrane T_i and that in solution t_i divided by the same difference in the case of an ideal permselective membrane [13–15]

$$S = \frac{T_i - t_i}{1 - t_i} \tag{8}$$

But this simple statement requires a careful definition of the TN T_i.

Some authors consider that the TN T_i should only be defined in pure conduction processes (i.e., in absence of concentration gradients and convective flow) [1,16]. Then, the TN would represent the fraction of current transported by the species i [13]

$$T_i \equiv \left(\frac{z_i F J_i}{I}\right)_{dc_i/dx=0} \tag{9}$$

Unfortunately, concentration gradients develop in the membrane and in the adjacent DBL under nonequilibrium conditions, and Eq. (9) cannot be used in connection with Eq. (8). Therefore, another definition which provides an *integral* characterization of the fraction of current that is transported *in the membrane system as a whole* must be introduced; the migrational TN are position dependent and they cannot provide this integral characterization. It is then proposed to use

$$T_i \equiv \frac{z_i F J_i}{I} \tag{10}$$

where no restrictions apply [7], except for the requirement that current is transported under steady-state conditions, since only then the ion fluxes are constant throughout the membrane system.

Hittorf's method is intended to use directly the definition of integral TN. The membrane separates two electrolyte solutions of the same molarity, $c_L = c_R$ initially, and some electric current is passed across the system. Even though the passage of current causes slight changes in these concentrations, it is considered that Hittorf's method provides the result

$$T_i \equiv \left(\frac{z_i F J_i}{I}\right)_{c_L = c_R} \tag{11}$$

Thus, Eq. (11) is taken in the next section as the definition of the integral TN of species i.

The reliability of TN as permselectivity and fixed charge estimates depends on our ability to eliminate the influence of the experimental method used in their determination. In particular, the TN in the limit of small fluxes, T_i^{eq} (i.e., where the two bathing solutions are the same and no electric current crosses the membrane system) have to be extracted from the measurements. Since the ion concentrations are constant throughout the membrane in this limit, the migrational TN are also constant. However, the difference between the local migrational TN in the membrane and in the bathing solutions means that they are different from the integral TN T_i^{eq}. Note that T_i^{eq} characterizes the membrane system as a whole and taking the limit of small fluxes does not imply the disappearance of the DBL effects.

It is also very important to consider how well the permselectivity given by

Eqs. (8) and (11) describe the behavior of the membrane system under given operating conditions. The membrane permselectivity is routinely measured in laboratories without taking into account the particular electromembrane technique for which the membranes are to be used. The Hittorf's and potentiometric methods provide the permselectivity at the static or "zero gradient" condition. This means that the counterion TN for a membrane separating electrolyte solutions of the same molarity ($c_L = c_R$ at $t = 0$ in Hittorf's experiments) or at zero current ($I = 0$ in potentiometric experiments) are obtained. Unlike these laboratory experiments, the molarities of bathing solutions differ and an external electric field introduces an electric current to the operating electromembrane systems. As a result, the membrane permselectivity under operating conditions differs from that obtained in laboratory experiments [17]. Simple methods for the determination of the membrane performance for any concentration difference and current density have been presented by A. Narebska and S. Koter [14,17,18].

Note, however, that when the bathing solutions are of different concentrations, $c_L \neq c_R$, the ion fluxes are no longer proportional to the electric current and the TN T_i include a contribution from the salt flux. Furthermore, if this diffusional component is predominant, the TN T_i can be smaller than zero or larger than unity [7,19]. Obviously, they cease to represent the fraction of current transported by the species i.

To summarize, the permselectivity and the integral TN are in fact parameters which characterize the membrane system as a whole, i.e., they incorporate a contribution from the DBL. Furthermore, their values are not the same under equilibrium and nonequilibrium conditions, which means that the effect of electric current (in the case of Hittorf's method) or differences in electrolyte concentration in the bathing solutions (in the case of potentiometric method) must be studied.

Finally, it is interesting to comment that the homogeneity of the membrane also affects its permselectivity. In order to increase the membrane permselectivity either the diffusion coefficients or the concentration of fixed charged groups must be modified. The former requires changes in the membrane structure and the results are very limited. The latter (i.e., the increase in the fixed charge concentration) requires increasing cross-linking, with a prohibitive increase in the electrical resistance of the membrane. However, the total concentration of fixed charges is not the only factor influencing the ion permselectivity. The particular distribution of these groups inside the membrane can play a significant role [20]. The possibility of having permselectivities exceeding that of a homogeneous distribution was first considered by H. Reiss [21,22]. This pioneering work was followed by other studies which were able to predict the distributions that would lead to higher permselectivities [23,24]. More recently, the significant influence of the DBL has been demonstrated [20,25].

C. Integral Transport Number in Hittorf's Experiment

The condition $c_L = c_R \equiv c_b$ enables an important conclusion on membrane permselectivity to be made from Eq. (2). Since the product $c_1 c_2$ is constant across the membrane boundaries, Eq. (2) can be integrated from $x = -\delta$ to $x = d + \delta$ to yield

$$T_i = \frac{z_i^2 D_i \langle c_i \rangle}{\sum_j z_j^2 D_j \langle c_j \rangle} \tag{12}$$

where

$$\langle c_i \rangle = \frac{1}{d + 2\delta} \int_{-\delta}^{d+\delta} c_i(x)\, dx \tag{13}$$

is the average concentration of species i over the membrane system. Hence, T_i *is a constant which depends on the actual concentration profiles across the membrane system.* Moreover, its value lies between the migrational TN in solution (where $c_1 = c_2$)

$$t_i = \frac{D_i}{D_1 + D_2} \tag{14}$$

and the migrational TN in the membrane (where $\bar{c}_1 \neq \bar{c}_2$)

$$\bar{t}_i(x) = \frac{D_i \bar{c}_i(x)}{D_1 \bar{c}_1(x) + D_2 \bar{c}_2(x)} \tag{15}$$

which is position dependent.

When the diffusion coefficients in the membrane phase differ from those in the bathing solutions, Eq. (12) takes the form

$$T_i = \frac{\langle c_i / D_{3-i} \rangle}{\langle c_1 / D_2 \rangle + \langle c_2 / D_1 \rangle} \tag{16}$$

where the diffusion coefficients are considered to be position dependent in the form

$$D_i(x) = \begin{cases} D_i, & -\delta < x < 0,\ d < x < d + \delta \\ \bar{D}_i, & 0 < x < d \end{cases} \tag{17}$$

Equation (16) can be further simplified because the local electroneutrality condition $c_1 = c_2 = c$ implies that the concentration gradient is constant in the DBL and

$$\int_{-\delta}^{0} c_i(x)\, dx + \int_{d}^{d+\delta} c_i(x)\, dx = 2c_b \delta \tag{18}$$

Therefore

$$T_i = \frac{t_i r + \dfrac{\bar{\tau}_i \langle \bar{c}_i \rangle}{c_m}}{r + \dfrac{\bar{\tau}_1 \langle \bar{c}_1 \rangle + \bar{\tau}_2 \langle \bar{c}_2 \rangle}{c_m}} \quad \text{(counterion)} \tag{19}$$

where

$$\bar{\tau}_i \equiv \frac{\bar{D}_i}{\bar{D}_1 + \bar{D}_2} \tag{20}$$

is a constant (not to be confused with $\bar{t}_i$), and

$$\langle \bar{c}_i \rangle = \frac{1}{d} \int_0^d \bar{c}_i(x) \, dx \tag{21}$$

is the average concentration of species i within the membrane. The parameter r is defined as

$$r = \frac{2 \bar{D}_{12} c_b \delta}{D_{12} c_m d}, \tag{22}$$

with $D_{12} = 2 D_1 D_2 / (D_1 + D_2)$ and $\bar{D}_{12} = 2 \bar{D}_1 \bar{D}_2 / (\bar{D}_1 + \bar{D}_2)$ being the salt diffusion coefficients in solution and in the membrane, respectively.

The concentration $\langle \bar{c}_i \rangle$ can be easily evaluated in the limit of small fluxes. In particular, Eqs. (A1) and (A14) (see Appendix) yield

$$\langle \bar{c}_i^{eq} \rangle = \bar{c}_i^{eq} = -\frac{z_m c_m}{2 z_i} + \left[\left(\frac{c_m}{2} \right)^2 + c_b^2 \right]^{1/2} \tag{23}$$

where $c_b = c_L = c_R$. The counterion TN given by Eq. (19) in this limit has been represented in Fig. 2, against $\bar{D}_{12} \delta / D_{12} d$ which represents the ratio between the diffusional permeability of the DBL, D_{12}/δ, and that of the membrane, $\bar{D}_{12}/d$. The effect of both the membrane fixed charge concentration and the DBL thickness have been analyzed in Fig. 2. It is shown that $T_{\text{counterion}}$ varies from the migrational TN in the membrane to the migrational TN in the DBL when $\bar{D}_{12} \delta / D_{12} d$ decreases.

The concentration $\langle \bar{c}_i \rangle$ is also easily evaluated for the case of ideal permselective membranes, where total coion exclusion takes place. The local counterion TN within the membrane $\bar{t}_i$ equals unity, and

$$T_i = \frac{t_i r + \bar{\tau}_i}{r + \bar{\tau}_i} \quad \text{(counterion)} \tag{24}$$

Thus, the integral counterion TN varies between 1 when $r \ll 1$, i.e., when the DBL effects are negligible, and t_i when $r \gg 1$, i.e., when the transport across the membrane system is controlled by the DBL. In terms of the membrane permselectivity, which in this case takes the form $S = 1/(1 + r/\bar{t}_i)$, these two limits correspond to $S = 1$ and $S = 0$, respectively.

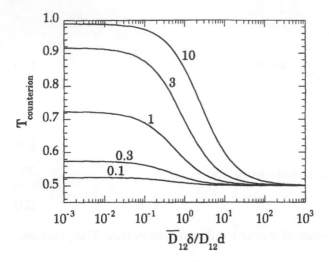

FIG. 2 Counterion transport number in the limit of small fluxes against the diffusional permeability of the DBL (relative to that of the membrane). The values of c_m/c_b are shown on the curves, and equal diffusion coefficients have been considered for coions and counterions, i.e., $D_1/D_2 = 1$ and $\bar{D}_1/\bar{D}_2 = 1$.

The application of Eq. (19) to nonideal membranes requires calculating $\langle \bar{c}_i \rangle$ from the solution of the Nernst–Planck equations. The description of this problem is conveniently made in terms of the TN ratio

$$\eta = \frac{T_1}{T_2} \tag{25}$$

Equations (A4) and (A5) in the Appendix can be easily transformed into

$$\eta = \frac{\bar{D}_1}{\bar{D}_2} \frac{\bar{c}_1(d) - e\bar{c}_1(0)}{\bar{c}_2(d) - e\bar{c}_2(0)} \tag{26}$$

where

$$e \equiv \exp\left\{ \frac{2[\bar{c}_1(d) - \bar{c}_1(0)] + d \sum_i \dfrac{J_i}{\bar{D}_i}}{\dfrac{z_m c_m}{z_1} \dfrac{\eta + \bar{D}_1/\bar{D}_2}{\eta - \bar{D}_1/\bar{D}_2}} \right\} \tag{27}$$

and the concentrations $\bar{c}_1(0)$ and $\bar{c}_1(d)$ are given by Eqs. (A14) and (A11). In particular, Eqs. (A11) take in this case the form

$$c_1(0) = c_b(1 - I/I_{lim}) \tag{28a}$$
$$c_1(d) = c_b(1 + I/I_{lim}) \tag{28b}$$

where

$$I_{\text{lim}} = \frac{\eta + 1}{\eta - D_1/D_2} \frac{2FD_1 c_b}{\delta} \tag{29}$$

is the limiting current density [26]. Equations (26) and (27) can be solved iteratively to obtain η, and thus also the TN T_i. This implies that the average concentrations $\langle \bar{c}_i \rangle$ are known [see Eq. (19)].

In Fig. 3, the local migrational TN is compared to the integral TN for different values of the DBL thickness. In the limit of high diffusional permeability of the DBL (relative to that of the membrane), $T_{\text{counterion}}$ equals the local migrational TN at $x = d$, i.e., the minimum value of $\bar{t}_i(x)$ inside the membrane. The explanation for this behavior can be found in Eqs. (2) (applied to membrane phase) and (10)

$$J_i = -\frac{\bar{D}_1 \bar{D}_2}{\bar{D}_1 \bar{c}_1 + \bar{D}_2 \bar{c}_2} \frac{d(\bar{c}_1 \bar{c}_2)}{dx} + \frac{\bar{t}_i}{z_i} \frac{I}{F} = \frac{T_i}{z_i} \frac{I}{F} \tag{30}$$

Since T_i is constant and the terms representing the diffusional salt flux inside the membrane and the ion migration have different signs, the local migrational TN has to be larger than T_i. Equality is possible only when there is no diffusional contribution to the ion flux, i.e., when the concentration profiles inside the membrane are flat. Indeed, Fig. 4 shows that the concentration profiles

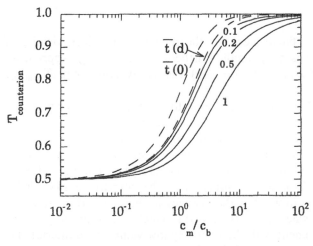

FIG. 3 The effect of the diffusional permeability of the DBL (values of $\bar{D}_{12} \delta / D_{12} d$ shown on the curves) on the counterion transport number in Hittorf's experiment. The electric current density amounts to 20% of the limiting value, $I/I_{\text{lim}} = 0.2$. Other parameters are $D_1/D_2 = 1$ and $\bar{D}_1/\bar{D}_2 = 1$. The dashed lines show the migrational counterion transport number at the membrane ends.

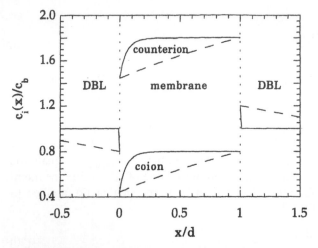

FIG. 4 The effect of the DBL thickness, at constant polarization ratio $I/I_{lim} = 0.2$, on the concentration profiles for $c_m/c_b = 1$, $\bar{D}_{12}/D_{12} = 1$, $D_1/D_2 = 1$, and $\bar{D}_1/\bar{D}_2 = 1$. The dashed lines correspond to $\delta/d = 1$ and show practically linear profiles. In this case, $\langle \bar{c}_{counterion} \rangle = 1.636$ and $T_{counterion} = 0.580$. The continuous lines correspond to $\delta/d = 0.01$, and show nonlinear concentration profiles inside the membrane, leading to an average concentration larger than in the case $\delta/d = 1$. In particular, $\langle \bar{c}_{counterion} \rangle = 1.780$ and $T_{counterion} = 0.692$. These values are to be compared to $\bar{c}_{counterion}(0) = 1.443$, $\bar{c}_{counterion}(d) = 1.800$, $\bar{t}_{counterion}(0) = 0.765$, $\bar{t}_{counterion}(d) = 0.692$.

inside the membrane are flat (except for the region in the close vicinity of $x = 0$) when $\bar{D}_{12}\delta/D_{12}d$ is very small. Furthermore, since $\langle \bar{c}_i \rangle$ approaches $\bar{c}_i(d)$ in the limit $\bar{D}_{12}\delta/D_{12}d \to 0$, Eq. (19) clearly explains that $T_{counterion}$ approaches $\bar{t}_i(d)$.

It was mentioned in Sec. II.B that TN have to be measured under nonequilibrium conditions (e.g., in the presence of electric current in Hittorf's method) and that the observed TN might depend on how far away is the system from the equilibrium state. In particular, since T_i depends on the actual concentration profiles across the membrane system [see Eq. (12)] and these are affected by the current density, T_i is also a function of the current density [20,24, 27]. For instance, Fig. 5 shows that the changes in the counterion transport are of the order of 10% when $\bar{D}_{12}\delta/D_{12}d = 0.1$, which is a common practical situation. This is in agreement with the relatively low values of counterion TN measured under limiting current conditions [28].

Experimentally, the TN may be observed to increase with increasing current density at low current densities [5,29]. This effect is due to back diffusion and cannot be accounted for by the above equations because of the condition $c_R = c_L$ imposed here.

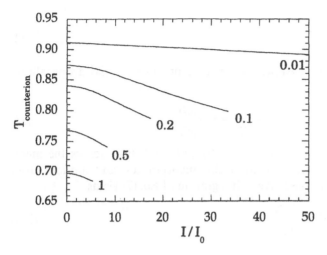

FIG. 5 The effect of the electric current on the counterion transport number in Hittorf's experiment for different values of the diffusional permeability of the DBL (values of $\bar{D}_{12}\delta/D_{12}d$ shown on the curves). The fixed charge concentration is $c_m/c_b = 3$, and the diffusion coefficients satisfy $D_1/D_2 = 1$ and $\bar{D}_1/\bar{D}_2 = 1$. The current has been normalized to $I_0 = FD_{12}c_b/d$, and ranges from zero to I_{lim}/I_0 (except for the case $\bar{D}_{12}\delta/D_{12}d = 0.01$, where $I_{lim}/I_0 = 333$).

D. Potentiometric Transport Numbers

In Sec. II.C, the integral TN under Hittorf's conditions, i.e., with $c_L = c_R = c_b$ and an electric current passing through the system, were introduced. In this section, a membrane system under zero electric current and where $c_L \neq c_R$ is considered and the integral TN under potentiometric conditions are introduced.

The diffusion potential drop in the membrane can be formally obtained by integrating Eq. (7)

$$\Delta\bar{\phi}_{dif} = -\frac{RT}{F}\int_0^d \sum_i \frac{\bar{t}_i}{z_i} \, d\ln \bar{c}_i \tag{31}$$

The actual integration requires the solution of the transport equations to find the concentration profiles, and therefore, the variation of t_i throughout the membrane. Alternatively, the variables t_i can be replaced by some average (constant) values, $\bar{T}_i$, which give the same diffusion potential. Thus, Eq. (31) is used to introduce the potentiometric TN $\bar{T}_i$ by means of the equation

$$\Delta\bar{\phi}_{dif} = -\frac{RT}{F}\sum_i \frac{\bar{T}_i}{z_i} \ln \frac{\bar{c}_i(d)}{\bar{c}_i(0)} \tag{32}$$

The property

$$\sum_i \bar{T}_i = 1 \tag{33}$$

together with Eqs. (A14) in Appendix for the Donnan potential drops, allows us to write

$$\Delta\phi_{D,L} + \Delta\bar{\phi}_{dif} + \Delta\phi_{D,R} = -\frac{RT}{F}\sum_i \frac{\bar{T}_i}{z_i} \ln \frac{c_i(d)}{c_i(0)} \tag{34}$$

In the presence of DBL effects, the total potential drop across the membrane system (or membrane potential) also incorporates contributions from the diffusion potential in these layers. Integration of Eq. (7) yields

$$\Delta\phi_{dif,L} = -\frac{RT}{F}\sum_i \frac{t_i}{z_i} \ln \frac{c_i(0)}{c_L} \tag{35a}$$

and

$$\Delta\phi_{dif,R} = -\frac{RT}{F}\sum_i \frac{t_i}{z_i} \ln \frac{c_R}{c_i(d)} \tag{35b}$$

so that the membrane potential is given by

$$\Delta\phi_M = -\frac{RT}{F}\sum_i \frac{\bar{T}_i}{z_i} \ln \frac{c_i(d)}{c_i(0)} - \frac{RT}{F}\sum_i \frac{t_i}{z_i} \ln \frac{c_i(0)c_R}{c_i(d)c_L} \tag{36}$$

where the concentrations $c_i(0)$ and $c_i(d)$ are

$$c_1(0) = c_2(0) = c_L - J_{12}\delta/D_{12} \tag{37a}$$
$$c_1(d) = c_2(d) = c_R + J_{12}\delta/D_{12} \tag{37b}$$

Equation (36) can be written, similarly to Eq. (34), in the form

$$\Delta\phi_M = -\frac{RT}{F}\sum_i \frac{T_i}{z_i} \ln \frac{c_R}{c_L} \tag{38}$$

which serves as a definition for the potentiometric TN T_i of the membrane system. Evidently, these TN are also required to satisfy the condition $\sum_i T_i = 1$. From a practical point of view, the TN T_i are evaluated by arranging Eq. (38) in the form

$$T_i = \frac{1}{2}\left[1 - \frac{z_i F \Delta\phi_M/RT}{\ln(c_R/c_L)}\right] \tag{39}$$

Note that the membrane potential $\Delta\phi_M$ must be calculated by subtracting the electrode potentials from the cell potential [15,30]. Comparison with Eq. (36) clearly shows that Eq. (39) must yield values between $\bar{T}_i$, when $J_{12}\delta/D_{12}c_L \ll 1$, i.e., when the DBL effects are negligible, and t_i, when the membrane effects are negligible and $c_i(0) \approx c_i(d)$.

From a theoretical point of view, the evaluation of T_i requires the solution of the transport equations in a binary system to calculate $\Delta\phi_M$. This solution can be easily derived from that worked out in the Appendix for a ternary system. In particular, the application of Eqs. (A4) and (A5) to a binary case gives

$$\Delta\bar{\phi}_{dif} = \frac{1}{z_1} \frac{RT}{F} \frac{\bar{D}_2 - \bar{D}_1}{\bar{D}_1 + \bar{D}_2} \ln \frac{\bar{c}_1(d) + \bar{\tau}_2 \dfrac{z_m c_m}{z_1}}{\bar{c}_1(0) + \bar{\tau}_2 \dfrac{z_m c_m}{z_1}} \tag{40}$$

and

$$J_{12} = -\frac{\bar{D}_{12}}{d}\left[\bar{c}_1(d) - \bar{c}_1(0) - \frac{z_m c_m}{2}\frac{F}{RT}\Delta\bar{\phi}_{dif}\right] \tag{41}$$

These equations, when combined to Eqs. (35), (37) and (A14), lead to the desired $\Delta\phi_M$ evaluation by following a simple iterative procedure.

The counterion TN given by Eq. (39) has been represented in Fig. 6, where both the effects of the membrane fixed charge concentration (values of c_m/c_L shown on the curves) and the DBL thickness have been analysed. When the diffusional permeability of the DBL (relative to that of the membrane) is small,

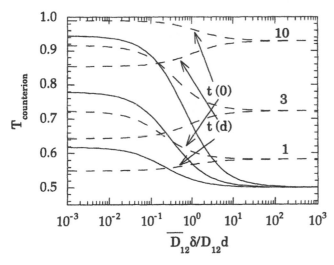

FIG. 6 Counterion potentiometric transport number in the limit of small fluxes against the diffusional permeability of the DBL (relative to that of the membrane) for membranes of different charge concentration (the values of c_m/c_L are shown on the curves). The concentration ratio has been set to $c_R/c_L = 5$, and the diffusion coefficients satisfy $D_1/D_2 = 1$ and $\bar{D}_1/\bar{D}_2 = 1$. The dashed lines show the migrational transport number of the counterion at the two ends of the membrane.

the concentration gradient is in the DBL, and $c_i(0) \approx c_i(d)$. The local migrational TN is constant within the membrane and the potentiometric TN equals the bulk value t_i. On the contrary, when the diffusional permeability of the DBL (relative to that of the membrane) becomes larger, the membrane phase is also polarized and $\bar{t}_i(x)$ can vary significantly over the membrane. In particular, it can be read from the curves with $c_m/c_b = 3$ that $\bar{t}_{counterion}(0) = 0.916$ and $\bar{t}_{counterion}(d) = 0.644$ when $\bar{D}_{12}\delta/D_{12}d \rightarrow 0$. The potentiometric TN $T_{counterion}$ takes approximately the average value of $\bar{t}_{counterion}(0)$ and $\bar{t}_{counterion}(d)$ at this limit. Note that this situation is different to that observed in the case of Hittorf's method, where $T_{counterion}$ approaches $\bar{t}_{counterion}(d)$ in the limit $\bar{D}_{12}\delta/D_{12}d \rightarrow 0$. The difference can be more easily appreciated by comparing Figs. 3 and 7.

Similarly to the Hittorf's integral TN, which is a function of the current density (see Fig. 5), the potentiometric TN varies with the concentration ratio c_R/c_L. This effect is more pronounced (see Fig. 8) in the case of high diffusional permeability of the DBL (relative to the membrane), i.e., low $\bar{D}_{12}\delta/D_{12}d$ values.

Figure 8 shows that the potentiometric TN depend on the two external concentrations and should be denoted as $T_i(c_R, c_L)$. It can be easily shown that,

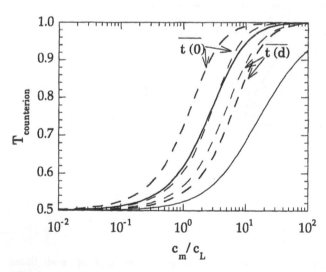

FIG. 7 The effect of the diffusional permeability of the DBL on the potentiometric transport number (continuous lines). The concentration ratio has been set to $c_R/c_L = 5$, and the diffusion coefficients satisfy $D_1/D_2 = 1$ and $\bar{D}_1/\bar{D}_2 = 1$. The dashed lines show the migrational transport number of the counterion at the two membrane ends. The bold lines correspond to $\bar{D}_{12}\delta/D_{12}d = 0.01$ and the thin lines to $\bar{D}_{12}\delta/D_{12}d = 1$.

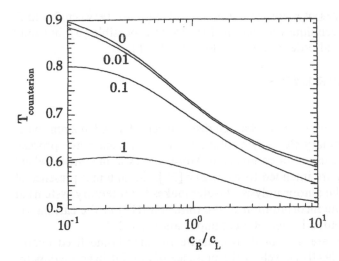

FIG. 8 The effect of the bulk concentration ratio on the potentiometric transport number for different values of the diffusional permeability of the DBL ($\bar{D}_{12}\delta/D_{12}d$ values are shown on the curves). The fixed charge concentration is $c_m/c_L = 1$, and the diffusion coefficients satisfy $D_1/D_2 = 1$ and $\bar{D}_1/\bar{D}_2 = 1$.

when $c_R > c_L$,

$$t_i^{eq}(c_R) < T_i(c_R, c_L) < t_i^{eq}(c_L) \quad \text{(counterion)} \tag{42}$$

where $t_i^{eq}(c)$ is the migrational TN inside the membrane corresponding to an equilibrium situation where the two external solution have the same concentration c. Equation (42) suggests that, in principle, the potentiometric TN could be referred to just one external solution concentration c_{av} such that

$$T_i(c_R, c_L) = T_i^{eq}(c_{av}, c_{av}) = t_i^{eq}(c_{av}) \quad \text{with} \quad c_L < c_{av} < c_R \tag{43}$$

In practice, this is not so straightforward due to the complicated dependence of $\Delta\phi_M$ on the ionic concentration differences [see Eq. (36)]. Several estimates have been proposed for c_{av} (e.g., c_R, c_L, $(c_R + c_L)/2$, $(c_R c_L)^{1/2}$, etc.) but they all lead to important systematic errors [31]. This problem can be easily overcome by using two potentiometric TN. In particular, it has been suggested [6,7] that $t_i^{eq}(c)$ could be estimated as

$$t_i^{eq}(c) = \tfrac{1}{2}[T_i(r_c c, c) + T_i(c/r_c, c)] + \varepsilon(t_i^{eq}) \tag{44}$$

where r_c is the ratio of external concentrations and $\varepsilon(t_i^{eq})$ is the error of this estimation. Since $T_i(r_c c, c)$ can be considered a linear function of $\ln r_c$ for small values of r_c, Eq. (44) leads then to an accurate determination of $t_i^{eq}(c)$. From the experimental point of view, however, it is required that r_c is not close to one, as $\Delta\phi_M$ would be small and could not be determined with sufficient accuracy. Satisfactory values of r_c for the estimation of $t_i^{eq}(c)$ are between 2 and 5. Other interpolation techniques to obtain $t_i^{eq}(c)$ are also possible [5], but only those accurate to second order in $\ln r_c$ should be used [31].

III. TERNARY ELECTROLYTES

A. Introduction

The counterion TN measured to characterize a given charged membrane is often obtained with binary electrolyte solutions. In electromembrane process, however, ternary systems are often involved. Moreover, even in systems where the bathing solutions are intended to be binary [32], the minimal presence of hydrogen ions from the autoprotolysis of water makes them ternary systems at high dilution [33]. The incorporation of the third ion (H^+) in the calculation of the membrane potential is then of great importance [34–38].

The measured TN are also used to estimate the membrane fixed charge concentration [28,33,39,40] as well as the presence of any intrinsic asymmetry present in the membrane [41–43]. Particularly interesting is the case of biological membranes such as cornea or skin. The recent interest in electro-assisted transdermal drug delivery processes has recalled the need for accurate determination methods of the TN of drugs [44]. Since biological membranes are often amphoteric, a change in bathing solution pH can alter the ratio of negatively charged to positively charged groups in the membrane [45] (see also Chap. 12). The TN determination is then carried out in the presence of an acid or a base that is added to adjust the pH of the bathing electrolyte solutions. The bathing solutions become then (at least) ternary systems, e.g., KCl–HCl or KCl–KOH.

The aim of this section is to study the effect of the acid or base addition on the potentiometric determination of TN. For the sake of clarity, the DBL effects will not be considered here. Firstly, the definition of potentiometric TN in ternary systems are worked out. Then, the local concentration and electrical potential profiles obtained from the solution of the transport equations are used to evaluate the potentiometric TN. These are compared to the apparent potentiometric TN, i.e., those obtained by assuming that the ternary system behaves as a binary system. Finally, some comments on the estimation of the membrane fixed charge concentration are given.

B. Apparent Potentiometric Transport Numbers

The analysis of TN in ternary electrolyte systems will be restricted to potentiometric TN. By extending Eq. (38) to the ternary case, the membrane potential can be written as

$$\Delta\phi_M = -\frac{RT}{F} \sum_i \frac{T_i}{z_i} \ln \frac{c_{i,R}}{c_{i,L}} \tag{45}$$

where $c_{i,R}$ and $c_{i,L}$ denote the ion concentrations in the bathing solutions, which are formed by mixing two completely dissociated binary electrolytes with a common ion. The common ion is denoted by subscript $i = 1$ and subscript $i = 3$ is used for the minority ion.

The potentiometric TN evaluation in ternary systems is complex both from a theoretical point of view as well as from an experimental point of view; note that the two independent TN cannot be obtained from a single membrane potential measurement. Then, some authors [45] have resolved to interpret the membrane potential measurements of ternary systems by using Eq. (45) in the binary system form, thus neglecting the effect of the acid or base added to adjust the pH. The potentiometric TN are then obtained as

$$T_{i,\,app} \equiv \frac{1}{2}\left[1 - \frac{z_i F \, \Delta\phi_M/RT}{\ln(c_{i,\,R}/c_{i,\,L})}\right] \tag{46}$$

and are named *apparent potentiometric TN*. This procedure constitutes an oversimplification in the study of ternary systems. The apparent TN so determined are not properties of the ions constituting the binary salt in the membrane but they also incorporate the effect of the acid or base added. Indeed, the introduction of Eq. (45) into Eq. (46) leads to

$$T_{1,\,app} = \frac{T_1}{2}\left[1 + \frac{\ln(c_{1,\,R}/c_{1,\,L})}{\ln(c_{2,\,R}/c_{2,\,L})}\right] + \frac{T_3}{2}\left[1 - \frac{\ln(c_{3,\,R}/c_{3,\,L})}{\ln(c_{2,\,R}/c_{2,\,L})}\right] \tag{47}$$

which coincides with T_1 only when $c_{1,R}/c_{1,L} = c_{2,R}/c_{2,L} = c_{3,R}/c_{3,L}$. Note, however, that $T_{2,\,app}$ does not coincide with T_2 unless $c_3 = 0$.

The apparent counterion TN in the ternary systems KCl–HCl and KCl–KOH is presented in Figs. 9 and 10. The two bathing solutions have the same pH, so that $c_{3,R} = c_{3,L} \equiv c_T = 10^{-pH}$ M. The membrane potential is calculated as described in the Appendix [see Eq. (A15)] for the particular case $\delta = 0$, i.e., in absence of DBL effects. Equation (46) is then used to obtain $T_{2,\,app}$. The infinite dilution values [46] have been employed for the diffusion coefficients: $D_{Cl^-} = 2.03 \times 10^{-5}$ cm^2/s, $D_{K^+} = 1.95 \times 10^{-5}$ cm^2/s, $D_{H^+} = 9.30 \times 10^{-5}$ cm^2/s, and $D_{OH^-} = 4.50 \times 10^{-5}$ cm^2/s.

Figure 9 corresponds to a negatively charged membrane ($z_m = -1$) and KCl–HCl bathing solutions. The fixed charge concentration is $c_m = c_{2,L}$, where subscript $i = 2$ is used for the potassium ion. It is observed that $T_{2,\,app}$ changes considerably with $c_T/c_{2,L}$ when $c_{2,R}/c_{2,L} = 0.1$ but not so much when $c_{2,R}/c_{2,L} = 10$ because these TN tend to ~ 0.5 at high bathing solution concentrations. Still, Fig. 10 shows that the influence of the third ion (H$^+$ or OH$^-$) on $T_{2,\,app}$ becomes more pronounced when higher values of the fixed charge concentration are considered. In this figure the situation of K$^+$ as coion ($z_m = 1$) has also been considered.

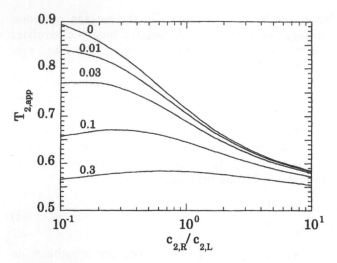

FIG. 9 Apparent transport numbers of potassium ion against its bulk solution concentration ratio $c_{2,R}/c_{2,L}$. The numbers on the curves give the value of $c_T/c_{2,L}$, where c_T is the H^+ concentration in the bathing solutions.

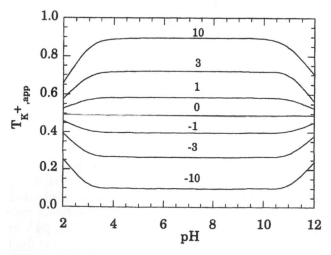

FIG. 10 The influence of the third ion (H^+ or OH^-) on the apparent transport number of potassium ion corresponding to $c_{2,R}/c_{2,L} = 10$. The values of $-z_m c_m/c_{2,L}$ are shown on the curves.

C. Potentiometric Transport Numbers

Even though Eq. (45) is sound due to its similarity to Eq. (38), the definition of the TN T_i is not straightforward. In contrast to the case for binary electrolytes, where there is only one independent TN and Eq. (38) constitutes the definition of the potentiometric TN, additional expressions are required when ternary systems are considered.

It has been shown [47] that Eq. (31) can be written in the form

$$\Delta\bar{\phi}_{\text{dif}} = -\frac{RT}{F}\left(\int_0^d \frac{d\ln\bar{c}_1}{z_1} + \int_0^d \frac{\bar{t}_2\,d\ln\bar{p}_{12}}{z_2} + \int_0^d \frac{\bar{t}_3\,d\ln\bar{p}_{13}}{z_3}\right) \tag{48}$$

where $\bar{p}_{12} \equiv \bar{c}_1\bar{c}_2$ and $\bar{p}_{13} \equiv \bar{c}_1\bar{c}_3$ are the ideal salt activities [48]. Equation (49) allows us to introduce the potentiometric TN in membrane phase as

$$\bar{T}_2 \equiv \frac{\displaystyle\int_0^d \bar{t}_2\,d\ln\bar{p}_{12}}{\ln[\bar{p}_{12}(d)/\bar{p}_{12}(0)]} \tag{49a}$$

$$\bar{T}_3 \equiv \frac{\displaystyle\int_0^d \bar{t}_3\,d\ln\bar{p}_{13}}{\ln[\bar{p}_{13}(d)/\bar{p}_{13}(0)]} \tag{49b}$$

while $\bar{T}_1$ is determined from Eq. (33).

In the DBL, equations similar to (48) and (49) can be obtained for the potentiometric TN and the diffusion potential drop. The membrane potential is then given by

$$\Delta\phi_M = -\frac{RT}{F}\left(\frac{1}{z_1}\ln\frac{c_{1,\text{R}}}{c_{1,\text{L}}} + \frac{T_2}{z_2}\ln\frac{p_{12,\text{R}}}{p_{12,\text{L}}} + \frac{T_3}{z_3}\ln\frac{p_{13,\text{R}}}{p_{13,\text{L}}}\right) \tag{50}$$

where

$$T_2 \equiv \frac{\displaystyle\int_{-\delta}^{d+\delta} t_2\,d\ln p_{12}}{\ln(p_{12,\text{R}}/p_{12,\text{L}})} \tag{51a}$$

$$T_3 \equiv \frac{\displaystyle\int_{-\delta}^{d+\delta} t_3\,d\ln p_{13}}{\ln(p_{13,\text{R}}/p_{13,\text{L}})} \tag{51b}$$

are the potentiometric TN in the membrane system. Note that Eq. (50) coincides with Eq. (45).

The T_i values where $c_{i,\text{R}} \neq c_{i,\text{L}}$ cannot be obtained from membrane potential measurements and require the solution of the transport equations for their evaluation (see Appendix). Figure 11 shows the apparent and exact TN of potassium ion for $c_{2,\text{R}}/c_{2,\text{L}} = 0.1$, 1 and 10. Once again, for the sake of clarity, DBL effects are not considered (i.e., $\delta = 0$). It is observed that the exact TN

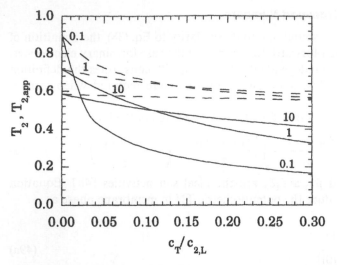

FIG. 11 Apparent (dashed lines) and exact (continuous lines) potentiometric transport number of potassium ion in the system KCl–HCl vs. $c_T/c_{2,L}$ for different values of $c_{2,R}/c_{2,L}$ (shown on the curves), $z_m = -1$ and $c_m/c_{2,L} = 1$.

take low values when $c_T/c_{2,L}$ increases, while the apparent TN remain close to 0.5 in this limit. It is also seen that the difference between exact and apparent values is significant, and increases with decreasing $c_{2,R}/c_{2,L}$.

D. Fixed Charge Estimation

The differences noted in the previous sections between the exact and the apparent TN suggest that the use of apparent TN to estimate the membrane fixed charge concentration could also lead to significant errors even when the third ion present has a relatively low concentration [47]. It is therefore necessary to identify the effect of the third ion by determining the relation between apparent and exact TN. However, this relation is very complicated (see Eq. (47) and note that T_1 and T_3 depend also on the ionic concentrations in the bathing solutions as well as on the unknown fixed charge concentration), and requires the solution of the transport equations (see Fig. 11). Fortunately, this situation changes when the limit of small fluxes (i.e., the equilibrium limit) is considered.

The equilibrium concentrations can be easily obtained from Eqs. (A1) and (A14) as

$$\bar{c}_1^{eq} = -\frac{z_m}{z_1}\frac{c_m}{2} + \left[\left(\frac{c_m}{2}\right)^2 + (c + c_T)^2\right]^{1/2} \tag{52a}$$

$$\frac{\bar{c}_2^{eq}}{\bar{c}_3^{eq}} = \frac{c}{c_T} \tag{52b}$$

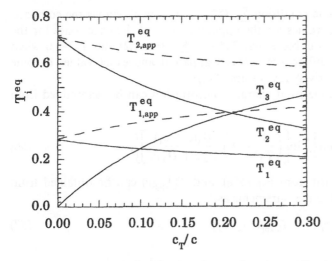

FIG. 12 Apparent (dashed lines) and exact (continuous lines) potentiometric transport numbers in the limit of small fluxes for the system KCl–HCl ($i = 1$ Cl$^-$, $i = 2$ K$^+$, $i = 3$ H$^+$).

where $c = c_{2,R} = c_{2,L}$ and $c_T = c_{3,R} = c_{3,L}$. Since no DBL effects are taken into account, the integral TN coincide with the migrational TN in the membrane, $T_i^{eq} = \bar{t}_i^{eq}$. Then, Eq. (52b) implies

$$\frac{T_2^{eq}}{\bar{D}_2 c} = \frac{T_3^{eq}}{\bar{D}_3 c_T} \tag{53}$$

Moreover, in the limit $c_{2,R}/c_{2,L} \to 1$, Eq. (47) reduces to

$$T_{1,app}^{eq} = T_1^{eq}\left(1 - \frac{1}{2}\frac{c_T}{c + c_T}\right) + \frac{T_3^{eq}}{2} \tag{54}$$

It is now possible to solve for T_1^{eq} and obtain

$$T_1^{eq} = \frac{2\left(1 + \dfrac{\bar{D}_2 c}{\bar{D}_3 c_T}\right)T_{1,app}^{eq} - 1}{2\left(1 + \dfrac{\bar{D}_2 c}{\bar{D}_3 c_T}\right)\left(1 - \dfrac{1}{2}\dfrac{c_T}{c + c_T}\right) - 1} \tag{55a}$$

and

$$T_2^{eq} = \frac{1 - T_1^{eq}}{1 + \dfrac{\bar{D}_3 c_T}{\bar{D}_2 c}} \tag{55b}$$

while T_3^{eq} is given by the condition $\sum_i T_i^{eq} = 1$. Figure 12 shows the comparison of the equilibrium values for the apparent TN and the exact ones for the case $z_m = -1$ and $c_m = c$. Note that $T_i^{eq} \to T_{i,\,app}^{eq}$ ($i = 1,2$) and $T_3^{eq} \to 0$ when $c_T \to 0$. However, the differences between apparent and exact values become significant even for relatively low values of c_T/c.

Finally, the membrane fixed charge concentration can be determined from Eqs. (52) and $T_i^{eq} = \bar{t}_i^{eq}$ as

$$c_m = \frac{2z_1}{z_m}(c + c_T)\sinh\left\{\frac{1}{2}\ln\left[\left(\frac{1}{T_1^{eq}} - 1\right)\frac{D_1(c + c_T)}{D_2 c + D_3 c_T}\right]\right\}, \tag{56}$$

where T_1^{eq} is determined from Eq. (55a), and $T_{i,\,app}^{eq}(c)$ can be obtained from two membrane potential measurements as

$$T_{i,\,app}^{eq} \approx \tfrac{1}{2}[T_{i,\,app}(r_c c, c) + T_{i,\,app}(c/r_c, c)] \tag{57}$$

where $r_c \equiv c_{2,\,R}/c_{2,\,L}$.

IV. CONVECTIVE FLOW

A. Reference System

Thus far the absence of bulk convective flow has been implicitly assumed. It is considered here the case of dilute solutions with nonzero solvent velocity. The reference system used to describe the relative average velocities of the different species now becomes of primary importance for the interpretation of experimental results [49]. The aim of this section is to briefly describe the effects of convective flow on ion transport in charged membranes. More thorough studies on the flux equations in these systems and the choice of reference frame can be found in Refs. 50–52.

Whenever the reference system is not made explicit, it must be assumed that the membrane-fixed or laboratory reference system is being used. In this reference system, the flux densities are given by

$$J_i = c_i v_i = -D_i\left(\frac{dc_i}{dx} + z_i c_i \frac{F}{RT}\frac{d\phi}{dx}\right) + c_i v_0 \tag{58}$$

where v_i is the velocity of species i and v_0 the solvent velocity (both defined with respect to the membrane).

The presence of bulk solvent flow inside a charged membrane gives rise to electrokinetic phenomena [16,53] (see also Chap. 15). Since the solution inside the membrane is not electrically neutral and has an electric charge per unit volume $-Fz_m c_m$, the mass transport also implies the presence of an electric current density, $I_{str} = -Fz_m c_m v_0$, which is called the *streaming current*.

When electric potential and concentration gradients are also present, the total current density is given by

$$I = -\kappa\left(\frac{d\phi}{dx} - \frac{d\phi_{\text{dif}}}{dx}\right) - Fz_{\text{m}} c_{\text{m}} v_0 = -\kappa\left(\frac{d\phi}{dx} - \frac{d\phi_{\text{dif}}}{dx} - \frac{d\phi_{\text{str}}}{dx}\right) \tag{59}$$

where κ was defined in Eq. (6) (some authors, however, use different definitions [53,54]). If the total current density is zero, the bulk flow inside the membrane implies that an electric potential gradient $d\phi_{\text{str}}/dx$ must appear, in addition to the diffusion potential gradient, to slow down the counterions and accelerate the coions and thus maintain electroneutrality. The electric potential drop in the membrane due to the bulk flow is called *streaming potential*, $\Delta\phi_{\text{str}}$.

In the next sections, the bulk flow is also described in terms of the velocity v_0 and the question of its origin is avoided. For the present discussion, it is sufficient to state that the velocity v_0 is proportional to the net force (other than viscous forces) acting on an elementary volume of the solution [55]

$$v_0 = d_{\text{h}}\left(-\frac{dp}{dx} + Fz_{\text{m}} c_{\text{m}} \frac{d\phi}{dx}\right) \tag{60}$$

where d_{h} is the hydrodynamic permeability. The electric potential gradient may be externally imposed but can also arise because of the solvent flow (i.e., the streaming potential gradient) or because of the concentration gradients (i.e., the diffusion potential gradient). Similarly, the pressure gradient maybe externally imposed or result from osmotic and electrosmotic phenomena. Further discussions on these topics maybe be found elsewhere [49,53].

In a reference system moving at velocity v with respect to the laboratory (i.e., with respect to the membrane), the flux density is [16]

$$J_i^{(v)} = c_i(v_i - v) = J_i - c_i v \tag{61}$$

In contrast to Eq. (58), Eq. (61) must also be applied to the charged groups fixed to the membrane matrix. Indeed, the electric current density is given by

$$I = F \sum_i z_i J_i^{(v)} \tag{62}$$

where the sum index runs over all charged species including the fixed groups, whose flux density inside the membrane is $J_{\text{m}}^{(v)} = -c_{\text{m}} v$. The local electroneutrality condition [Eq. (A1)] then leads to the important result that the electric current density is independent of the reference system used. Equation (59) is thus valid in any reference system.

Most of the classical experimental methods yield TN in the solvent-fixed reference system. The solvent velocity should then be determined by additional experimental arrangements for each particular case to provide a full description of the TN measured. Since the ion flux density in this reference system takes the form

$$J_i^{(0)} = -D_i \left(\frac{dc_i}{dx} + z_i c_i \frac{F}{RT} \frac{d\phi}{dx} \right) \qquad (63)$$

it could be thought that the expressions obtained in the previous sections were derived for the solvent-fixed reference system. However, this conclusion is valid only in the solution outside the membrane, where there is no contribution from the fixed charge (and no electrokinetic phenomena). Inside the membrane, $J_m^{(0)} = -c_m v_0$ and this means that their TN is not zero [56,57]. In fact, one of the difficulties associated with reference systems other than the membrane-fixed reference system is that TN change discontinuously at the membrane boundaries. But these reference systems must be used because TN measurements in the membrane-fixed system are extremely difficult.

B. Hittorf's Transport Numbers

The integral TN in any reference system is defined as [1,16]

$$T_i^{(v)} \equiv \frac{z_i F J_i^{(v)}}{I} \qquad (64)$$

The TN in the membrane-fixed and solvent-fixed reference systems thus follow the relationship

$$T_i^{(0)} = T_i - \frac{z_i F c_i v_0}{I} = T_i - \frac{z_i c_i \tau_0}{c_0} \approx T_i - \left(0.018 \frac{L}{mol} \right) z_i c_i \tau_0 \qquad (65)$$

where $\tau_0 \equiv F c_0 v_0 / I$ and c_0 are the transference number and molar concentration of water, respectively.

The continuity equation (i.e., the mass conservation equation) requires that J_i be independent of position under steady-state conditions. Hence, the TN in membrane-fixed reference system, T_i, are constant. On the contrary, Eqs. (61) and (64) show that $T_i^{(v)}$ is only independent of position if the concentration is homogeneous. When using TN such as $T_i^{(0)}$ it must therefore be understood that reference is made to the value at the bulk solution concentration. Accordingly, the concentration c_i in Eq. (65) is replaced by the bulk value.

From the experimental point of view, the flux $J_i^{(0)}$ is easily obtained from the observed change in concentration Δc_i in a time interval Δt as

$$J_i^{(0)} \approx \frac{V \Delta c_i}{A \Delta t} \qquad (66)$$

where A is the effective membrane area and V the volume of the compartment where Δc_i is measured. Transport numbers in solvent-fixed reference system are then reported from Hittorf's experiments [58].

The relevant question, however, is whether T_i or $T_i^{(0)}$ provides a value which characterizes the membrane. To answer this question, the transport equations [obtained from Eqs. (58) and (59)]

$$J_i = \bar{J}_{12} + \frac{\bar{t}_i}{z_i} \frac{I - I_{\text{str}}}{F} + \bar{c}_i v_0 \quad \text{(membrane)} \tag{67a}$$

$$J_i = J_{12} + \frac{t_i}{z_i} \frac{I}{F} + c_i v_0 \quad \text{(DBL)} \tag{67b}$$

are integrated from $x = -\delta$ to $x = d + \delta$, where the ion concentrations are $c_L = c_R \equiv c_b$. For the sake of simplicity, the diffusion coefficients are assumed to take the same value inside and outside the membrane. It is then obtained

$$T_i = \frac{z_i^2 D_i \langle c_i \rangle}{\sum_j z_j^2 D_j \langle c_j \rangle} + \frac{F v_0 \langle \bar{\kappa} \rangle}{I \langle \kappa \rangle} \left(z_i \langle c_i \rangle + \frac{d}{d + 2\delta} z_m c_m \bar{T}_i \right) \tag{68}$$

where

$$\bar{T}_i \equiv \frac{z_i^2 D_i \langle \bar{c}_i \rangle}{\sum_j z_j^2 D_j \langle \bar{c}_j \rangle} \tag{69}$$

The average values $\langle c_i \rangle$ and $\langle \bar{c}_i \rangle$ were defined in Eqs. (13) and (21), respectively. Similarly, $\langle \kappa \rangle$ and $\langle \bar{\kappa} \rangle$ are the average values of the electrical conductivity in the membrane system and inside the membrane.

Neglecting DBL effects, Eq. (68) simplifies to

$$T_i = \bar{T}_i + \frac{F v_0}{I} (z_i \langle \bar{c}_i \rangle + z_m c_m \bar{T}_i) \tag{70}$$

For the case of highly charged membranes, the sum inside brackets in Eq. (70) is of the order of c_b^2/c_m and can be neglected, thus giving $T_i \approx \bar{T}_i$ (see Fig. 13). However, for the case of weakly charged membranes, the sum inside brackets contributes to T_i and this number ceases to characterize accurately the migrational transport inside the membrane. On the contrary, the TN in the solvent-fixed reference system

$$T_i^{(0)} = T_i - \frac{z_i F c_b v_0}{I} \tag{71}$$

can be shown to be approximately equal to $\bar{T}_i$ for both highly and weakly charged membranes, thus providing a good characterization of the membrane.

C. Modified Hittorf's Method

The polarization of the DBL is responsible for the observed dependence of the TN determined by Hittorf's method on the current density (see Fig. 5) [5,59].

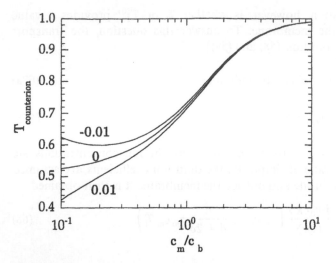

FIG. 13 Counterion Hittorf transport number in membrane-fixed reference system vs. c_m/c_b for different values of the ratio I_{str}/I (shown on the curves) and $\bar{D}_1/\bar{D}_2 = 1$. The central line corresponds to $\bar{T}_i$. DBL effects have not been incorporated.

Either the use of extrapolation methods or an estimation of the diffusional contribution are then required to obtain a value representative of the membrane system (which still would incorporate the effect of DBL) [60]. The problem of concentration polarization can be avoided by using a stack of membranes, but this method is tedious to use in practice [56,61] (see also Chap. 13, Sec. IV.B). More recently, the use of a convective flow opposed to the electric current has been proposed [4]. This modified Hittorf's method significantly reduces the concentration polarization and prevents the development of a concentration difference between the two bulk solutions.

When the conventional Hittorf's method is applied to a membrane system, the concentration changes in the two compartments are due to both the transport through the membrane system and the electrode reactions. Consider, e.g., a membrane bathed by KCl solutions where Ag/AgCl electrodes are immersed. Since the electrode reactions only involve chloride ions, there is a net salt flux $T_{K^+}I/F$ from the anode to the cathode compartment, where T_{K^+} is the integral TN of potassium ions. Then, the bulk concentrations change with time (i.e., the system is not under true steady-state conditions) and there is a contribution from back diffusion to the ion transport. In the modified Hittorf's method [4] the integral TN of the cation is zero due to the countercurrent convective flow, $T_{K^+} = 0$, i.e. for any given current density I, the convective velocity v_0 is adjusted so that $T_{K^+} = 0$ is satisfied. Obviously, the TN characterizing the membrane, $\bar{T}_{K^+}$ in Eq. (70), must be extracted from the current and convective flow measurements. When the fixed charge concentration is of the order or smaller than the bathing solution concentration, Eq. (71) gives $\bar{T}_{K+} = -Fc_b v_0/I$ where v_0 and I have opposite signs because the flow is opposed to the current. The determination of $\bar{T}_{K+}$ by this method consists then in adjusting the convective velocity v_0, for a given current density I, so that $T_{K+} = 0$ is satisfied and calculating $\bar{T}_{K+} \approx -Fc_b v_0/I$. Moreover, since the diffusional contribution to the ion transport through the membrane system is small, this TN $\bar{T}_{K+}$ does not depend on the electric current used in its determination.

D. Potentiometric Transport Numbers

The relationship between potentiometric TN and the reference system is difficult to make in practice because they are defined from the membrane potential expression and not from Eq. (64). In electrolyte solutions, it has long been discussed that potentiometric TN are essentially identical to Hittorf's TN, and therefore they are also relative to the solvent [62]. In the case of membrane systems, a good correlation between the TN determined by these two methods has also been observed [63], and thus it is widely accepted that both potentiometric and Hittorf's methods provide TN in the solvent-fixed reference system [17].

Equation (59) shows that in the presence of convective flow (and $I = 0$), the membrane potential is given by

$$\Delta\phi_M = \Delta\phi_{dif} + \Delta\phi_{str} = -\frac{RT}{F} \sum_i \frac{\bar{T}_i}{z_i} \ln \frac{c_R}{c_L} - Fz_m c_m v_0 \, d\langle\bar{\rho}\rangle \tag{72}$$

where $\bar{\rho} = 1/\bar{\kappa}$ is the local electrical resistivity in membrane phase, and $\langle\bar{\rho}\rangle$ its average value. In Eq. (72), DBL effects have been neglected for the sake of simplicity. This equation, however, if often written in the form

$$\Delta\phi_M = -\frac{RT}{F} \sum_i \frac{\bar{T}_{i,\,app}}{z_i} \ln \frac{c_R}{c_L} \tag{73}$$

where $\bar{T}_{i,\,app}$ is the so-called apparent potentiometric TN [5] note that the term apparent is used here for a different reason than in Sec. III.B).

The membrane potential $\Delta\phi_M$ can also be evaluated from nonequilibrium thermodynamics and written in the Scatchard–Staverman form [64–66]

$$\Delta\phi_M = -\frac{1}{F} \int \sum_{i=0}^{2} \tau_i \, d\mu_i = -\frac{RT}{F} \int \sum_{i=0}^{2} \tau_i \, d \ln c_i \tag{74}$$

where τ_0 is the transference number of water and $\tau_i \equiv \bar{T}_i/z_i$ is the transference number of ion species i (see also Chap. 10, Sec. II.A). Activities have also been replaced by concentrations for the sake of consistency with the above expressions. By using the Gibbs–Duhem equation, Eq. (74) can be transformed into Eq. (73), where $\bar{T}_{i,\,\text{app}}$ takes the form of a TN in the solvent-fixed reference system

$$\bar{T}_{i,\,\text{app}}^{(0)} = \bar{T}_{i,\,\text{app}} - z_i c_{\text{av}} \tau_0/c_0 \tag{75}$$

and c_{av} represents here the average $(c_R + c_L)/2$.

The equivalence of these two formulations [Eqs. (72) and (74)] can be shown by equating the convective terms in the Nernst–Planck and nonequilibrium thermodynamics formulations

$$c_i v_0 = -l_{i0} \frac{d\mu_0}{dx} \tag{76}$$

where l_{i0} is a phenomenological coefficient. It then follows that

$$\frac{d\phi_{\text{str}}}{dx} = -\frac{Fz_m c_m v_0}{\kappa} = \frac{F}{\kappa} \sum_i z_i c_i v_0$$
$$= -\frac{F}{\kappa} \left(\sum_i z_i l_{i0} \right) \frac{d\mu_0}{dx} = -\frac{\tau_0}{F} \frac{d\mu_0}{dx} \tag{77}$$

V. CONCLUDING REMARKS

Transport numbers have been extensively used over the last decades to characterize ion transport in charged membranes. In spite of their conceptual simplicity, a number of difficulties arise in the interpretation of experimental results because of the influence of the operating conditions. More effort should therefore be put to identify the effect of polarization layers and the driving force (i.e., the electric current density and/or the concentration difference) on the experimental results. Also, the use of simplified expressions for the TN (e.g., the application to ternary systems of equations valid only for binary systems) should be avoided.

Finally, attention must be called to the restrictions applying to the theoretical approach presented in this chapter. First, activities have been replaced by concentrations throughout, which limits the applicability of the equations to dilute solutions. Second, chemical partition coefficients have not been included, which amounts to consider only membranes with high water content. More important are the limitations associated with the homogeneous membrane assumption. Homogeneity is a spatial scale-dependent concept and all membranes deviate to some extent from homogeneity. If the membrane is inhomogeneous on a plane normal to the axis along which transport occurs, the introduction of a distribution of pore radii and charge densities will prove necessary when attempting to interpret experimental data [28]. Recent accounts of the effect of structural membrane inhomogeneity on transport properties can be found in Refs. 67–70.

APPENDIX: THE INTEGRATION OF THE NERNST–PLANCK EQUATIONS OVER THE MEMBRANE SYSTEM FOR THE CASE OF TERNARY ELECTROLYTE SOLUTIONS AND $|z_i| = 1$

In this appendix a procedure for the integration of the Nernst–Planck equations in ternary systems, under the assumption of local electroneutrality

$$\sum_i z_i \bar{c}_i(x) + z_m c_m = 0 \tag{A1}$$

is presented. The equations corresponding to binary systems can be easily obtained by taking $c_3 = 0$. Alternatively, the Schlögl integration procedure could also be used [36,71,72].

Since the electric potential gradient inside the membrane can be written as [73]

$$\frac{d\bar{\phi}}{dx} = \frac{RT}{F} \frac{\Gamma}{\sum_j z_j^2 \bar{c}_j + \Gamma z_m c_m} \sum_i \frac{d\bar{c}_i}{dx} \tag{A2}$$

where

$$\Gamma \equiv \frac{\sum_j z_j J_j/\bar{D}_j}{\sum_j J_i/\bar{D}_i} \tag{A3}$$

the diffusion potential drop in the membrane $\Delta\bar{\phi}_{dif}$ is given by

$$\Delta\bar{\phi}_{dif} \equiv \bar{\phi}(d) - \bar{\phi}(0) = \frac{RT}{F} \Gamma \ln \frac{\sum_i \bar{c}_i(d) + \Gamma z_m c_m}{\sum_j \bar{c}_j(0) + \Gamma z_m c_m} \tag{A4}$$

Alternatively, $\Delta\bar{\phi}_{dif}$ can also be obtained by integration of $\sum_i J_i/\bar{D}_i$ as

$$\Delta\bar{\phi}_{dif} = \frac{RT}{F} \frac{1}{z_m c_m} \sum_i \left[\bar{c}_i(d) - \bar{c}_i(0) + d \frac{J_i}{\bar{D}_i} \right] \tag{A5}$$

Equations (A4) and (A5) contain the sum $\sum_i \bar{c}_i$, which can be transformed into

$$\sum_i \bar{c}_i(x) = 2\bar{c}_1(x) + \frac{z_m c_m}{z_1} \tag{A6}$$

with the help of Eq. (A1) and observing that $z_2 = z_3 = -z_1$ because $i = 1$ is the common ion. The ion fluxes in Eqs. (A4) and (A5) are obtained by integration of the Nernst–Planck equations in Kramers' form [20,73–75] as

$$J_i = -\bar{D}_i \frac{\bar{c}_i(x)\exp\{z_i F[\bar{\phi}(x) - \bar{\phi}(0)]/RT\} - \bar{c}_i(0)}{\int_0^x \exp\{z_i F[\bar{\phi}(\xi) - \bar{\phi}(0)]/RT\} \, d\xi} \tag{A7}$$

and

$$\frac{J_2}{J_3} = \frac{\bar{D}_2}{\bar{D}_3} \frac{\bar{c}_2(d)\exp(z_2 F \Delta\bar{\phi}_{dif}/RT) - \bar{c}_2(0)}{\bar{c}_3(d)\exp(z_3 F \Delta\bar{\phi}_{dif}/RT) - \bar{c}_3(0)} \tag{A8}$$

where the equality $z_2 = z_3$ has been used.

In the DBL, the diffusion potential drops are given by

$$\Delta\phi_{dif, L} = \frac{RT}{F} \Gamma \ln \frac{c_1(0)}{c_{1, L}} \tag{A9a}$$

and

$$\Delta\phi_{dif, R} = \frac{RT}{F} \Gamma \ln \frac{c_{1, R}}{c_1(d)} \tag{A9b}$$

where

$$\Gamma \equiv \frac{\sum_j z_j J_j/D_j}{\sum_i J_i/D_i} \tag{A10}$$

$$c_1(0) = c_{1, L} - \frac{\delta}{2} \sum_i \frac{J_i}{D_i} \tag{A11a}$$

and

$$c_1(d) = c_{1, R} + \frac{\delta}{2} \sum_i \frac{J_i}{D_i} \tag{A11b}$$

The other two ion concentrations at the external side of the membrane/DBL interfaces are given by the local electroneutrality condition

$$c_1(x) = c_2(x) + c_3(x) \tag{A12}$$

and the analogous to Eq. (A8), i.e.

$$\frac{J_2}{J_3} = \frac{D_2}{D_3} \frac{c_2(0)\exp(z_2 F \Delta\phi_{dif, L}/RT) - c_{2, L}}{c_3(0)\exp(z_3 F \Delta\phi_{dif, L}/RT) - c_{3, L}} \tag{A13a}$$

and

$$\frac{J_2}{J_3} = \frac{D_2}{D_3} \frac{c_{2, R} \exp(z_2 F \Delta\phi_{dif, R}/RT) - c_2(d)}{c_{3, R} \exp(z_3 F \Delta\phi_{dif, R}/RT) - c_3(d)} \tag{A13b}$$

At the membrane/DBL interfaces, the Donnan potential drops are given by

$$\Delta\phi_{D, L} = -\frac{RT}{F} \frac{1}{z_i} \ln \frac{\bar{c}_i(0)}{c_i(0)} = \frac{1}{z_1} \text{arcsinh}\left(\frac{z_m c_m}{2z_1 c_1(0)}\right) \tag{A14a}$$

$$\Delta\phi_{D, R} = -\frac{RT}{F} \frac{1}{z_i} \ln \frac{c_i(d)}{\bar{c}_i(d)} = -\frac{1}{z_1} \text{arcsinh}\left(\frac{z_m c_m}{2z_1 c_1(d)}\right) \tag{A14b}$$

where Eqs. (A1) and (A9) have been used to obtain the last equalities.

The above equations form a closed system which enables the determination of values for ion fluxes and the different potential drops. The membrane potential is then obtained as

$$\Delta\phi_M = \Delta\phi_{\text{dif, L}} + \Delta\phi_{\text{D, L}} + \Delta\bar{\phi}_{\text{dif}} + \Delta\phi_{\text{D, R}} + \Delta\phi_{\text{dif, R}} \tag{A15}$$

The distributions of electric potential and the common ion concentration inside the membrane can be calculated from the system

$$\bar{\phi}(x) - \bar{\phi}(0) = \frac{RT}{F}\,\bar{\Gamma}\,\ln\frac{c_1(x) + (\bar{\Gamma} + 1/z_1)z_m\,c_m/2}{c_1(0) + (\bar{\Gamma} + 1/z_1)z_m\,c_m/2} \tag{A16}$$

and

$$\bar{\phi}(x) - \bar{\phi}(0) = \frac{RT}{F}\,\frac{1}{z_m\,c_m}\left\{2[c_1(x) - c_1(0)] + x\sum_i \frac{J_i}{\bar{D}_i}\right\} \tag{A17}$$

which are obtained by integration of Eq. (A2), and integration of $\sum_i J_i/\bar{D}_i$, respectively. The other two ion concentration profiles can be calculated from Eq. (A7).

The corresponding distributions in the DBL are finally given by

$$c_1(x) = c_{1,\,L} - \frac{x}{2}\sum_i \frac{J_i}{D_i}, \quad -\delta < x < 0 \tag{A18a}$$

$$c_1(x) = c_{1,\,R} + \frac{x}{2}\sum_i \frac{J_i}{D_i}, \quad d < x < d + \delta \tag{A18b}$$

$$\phi(x) - \phi(-\delta) = \frac{RT}{F}\,\Gamma\,\ln\frac{c_1(x)}{c_{1,\,L}}, \quad -\delta < x < 0 \tag{A19a}$$

$$\phi(x) - \phi(d + \delta) = \frac{RT}{F}\,\Gamma\,\ln\frac{c_1(x)}{c_{1,\,R}}, \quad d < x < d + \delta \tag{A19b}$$

$$\frac{J_2}{J_3} = \frac{D_2}{D_3}\frac{c_2(x)\exp\{z_2\,F[\phi(x) - \phi(-\delta)]/RT\} - c_{2,\,L}}{c_3(x)\exp\{z_2\,F[\phi(x) - \phi(-\delta)]/RT\} - c_{3,\,L}}, \quad -\delta < x < 0 \tag{A20a}$$

$$\frac{J_2}{J_3} = \frac{D_2}{D_3}\frac{c_2(x)\exp\{z_2\,F[\phi(x) - \phi(d + \delta)]/RT\} - c_{2,\,R}}{c_3(x)\exp\{z_2\,F[\phi(x) - \phi(d + \delta)]/RT\} - c_{3,\,R}}, \quad d < x < d + \delta \tag{A20b}$$

LIST OF SYMBOLS

c molar concentration [mol/cm^3]
D diffusion coefficient [cm^2/s]

d membrane thickness [cm]
e auxiliary constant defined in Eq. (27)
F   Faraday constant [C/mol]
I electric current density [A/cm^2]
J flux density [mol/cm^2/s]
p ideal salt activity [mol^2/cm^6 in the case of $1 : -1$ electrolytes]
R gas constant [J/(mol K)]
r auxiliary constant defined in Eq. (22)
r_c ratio of bulk solution concentrations
S membrane permselectivity
T absolute temperature [K]
t local migrational TN
T_i integral TN of species i
v velocity [cm/s]
x position [cm]
z charge number

δ DBL thickness [cm]
ϕ local electric potential [V]
Γ auxiliary constant defined in Eqs. (A3) and (A10)
η TN ratio
κ electrical conductivity [Ω^{-1}/cm]
ρ electrical resistivity [Ω cm]
τ transference number
$\bar{\tau}_i$ auxiliary constant defined in Eq. (20)
ξ dummy integration variable
$\tilde{\mu}$ electrochemical potential [J/mol]
μ chemical potential [J/mol]

$\langle\ \rangle$ average value
Δ difference over the bulk or interfacial region (right minus left)
DBL   diffusion boundary layer
TN   transport number
$^-$ membrane phase

Subscripts/Superscripts

0   solvent
12   binary electrolyte formed by ion species 1 and 2
13   binary electrolyte formed by ion species 1 and 3
app   apparent
b   bulk solution in L and R compartments
c   concentration ratio

D   Donnan
dif   diffusion potential
eq   small fluxes limit (i.e., equilibrium limit)
i ion species i ($i = 1,2,3$)
L   left compartment
lim   limiting current density
M   membrane potential
m   fixed charge groups within the membrane
R   right compartment
str   streaming
°   standard

REFERENCES

1. N. Ibl, Pure & Appl. Chem. *53*: 1827 (1979).
2. J. Newman, *Electrochemical Systems*, Prentice Hall, Englewood Cliffs, New Jersey, 1973, Sec. 70.
3. K. Kontturi, P. Forsell, and A. Ekman, Acta Chem Scand. *A39*: 271 (1985).
4. K. Kontturi, S. Mafé, J. A. Manzanares, J. Pellicer, and M. Vuoristo, J. Electroanal. Chem. *378*: 111 (1994).
5. N. Lakshminarayanaiah, *Transport Phenomena in Membranes*, Academic Press, New York, 1969, p. 232.
6. K. A. Lebedev, V. I. Zabolotsky, and V. V. Nikonenko, Sov. Electrochem. *23*: 555 (1987).
7. K. A. Lebedev, V. V. Nikonenko, and V. I. Zabolotsky, Sov. Electrochem. *23*: 459 (1987).
8. N. V. Shel'deshov, V. I. Zabolotsky, M. V. Shadrina, and M. V. Solov'eva, J. Appl. Chem. USSR *63*: 831 (1990).
9. R. P. Buck, J. Membrane Sci. *17*: 1 (1984).
10. V. M. Aguilella, J. A. Manzanares, and J. Pellicer, Langmuir *9*: 550 (1993).
11. F. Helfferich, *Ion Exchange*, Dover, New York, 1995, p. 326 and footnote.
12. Ref. 2, Sec. 4 and 70.
13. R. Hattenbach, *Terminology for Electrodialysis*, European Society of Membrane Science and Technology, 1988.
14. A. Narebska and S. Koter, in *Advances in Membrane Phenomena and Processes* (A. M. Mika and T. Z. Winnicki, eds.), Wroclaw Technical University Press, Wroclaw, 1989, pp. 111–127.
15. N. Rossignol, D. E. A. Thesis, Univ. Pierre et Marie Curie (Paris VI), 1995.
16. R. Haase, *Thermodynamics of Irreversible Processes*, Dover, New York, 1990, Sec. 4–16.
17. A. Narebska and S. Koter, Electrochim. Acta *38*: 815 (1993).
18. S. Koter and A. Narebska, Sep. Sci. Technol. *24*: 1337 (1989/90).
19. J. Goodisman, *Electrochemistry: Theoretical Foundations*, Wiley, New York, 1987, p. 35.
20. A. V. Sokirko, J. A. Manzanares, and J. Pellicer, J. Colloid Interface Sci. *168*: 32 (1994).

21. H. Reiss and I. C. Bassignana, J. Membrane Sci. *11*: 219 (1982).
22. C. Selvey and H. Reiss, J. Membrane Sci. *23*: 11 (1985).
23. S. Mafé, J. A. Manzanares, M. J. Hernández, and J. Pellicer, J. Colloid Interface Sci. *145*: 433 (1991).
24. J. A. Manzanares, S. Mafé, and J. Pellicer, J. Chem. Soc. Faraday Trans. *88*: 2355 (1992).
25. S. Koter, J. Membrane Sci. *108*: 177 (1995).
26. J. A. Manzanares, W. D. Murphy, S. Mafé, and H. Reiss, J. Phys. Chem. *97*: 8524 (1993).
27. Ref. 11, p. 408.
28. K. Kontturi, S. Mafé, J. A. Manzanares, L. Murtomäki, and P. Viinikka, Electrochim. Acta *39*: 883 (1994).
29. T. R. E. Kressman, P. A. Stanbridge, and F. L. Tye, Trans. Faraday Soc. *59*: 2129 (1963).
30. S. Koter, Polish J. Chem. *69*: 1213 (1995).
31. N. I. Zharkikh, Sov. Electrochem. *27*: 123 (1991).
32. T. S. Sørensen and J. B. Jensen, J. Non-Equilib. Thermodyn. *9*: 1 (1984).
33. J. B. Jensen, T. S. Sørensen, B. Malmgren-Hansen, and P. Sloth, J. Colloid Interface Sci. *108*: 18 (1985).
34. T. S. Sørensen, J. B. Jensen, and B. Malmgren-Hansen, J. Non-Equilib. Thermodyn. *13*: 57 (1988).
35. B. Malmgren-Hansen, T. S. Sørensen, and J. B. Jensen, J. Non-Equilib. Thermodyn. *13*: 193 (1988).
36. S. Laursen, B. Malmgren-Hansen, and T. S. Sørensen, J. Non-Equilib. Thermodyn. *15*: 223 (1990).
37. F. Skácel, B. Malmgren-Hansen, T. S. Sørensen, and J. B. Jensen, J. Chem. Soc. Faraday Trans. *86*: 341 (1990).
38. T. S. Sørensen, J. B. Jensen, and B. Malmgren-Hansen, Desalination *80*: 293 (1990).
39. N. Lakshminarayanaiah, *Equations of Membrane Biophysics*, Academic Press, New York, 1984, p. 124.
40. Y. Toyoshima and H. Nozaki, J. Phys. Chem. *74*: 2704 (1970).
41. T. S. Sørensen and V. Compañ, J. Phys. Chem. *100*: 7623 (1996).
42. T. S. Sørensen and V. Compañ, J. Phys. Chem. *100*: 15261 (1996).
43. V. Compañ, T. S. Sørensen, A. Andrio, M. L. López, and J. de Abajo, J. Membrane Sci. *123*: 293 (1997).
44. S. Numajiri, K. Sugibayashi, and Y. Morimoto, Chem. Pharm. Bull. *44*: 1351 (1996).
45. Y. Rojanasakul and J. R. Robinson, Int. J. Pharm. *55*: 237 (1989).
46. R. A. Robinson and R. H. Stokes, *Electrolyte Solutions*, Butterworths, London, 1959.
47. J. A. Manzanares, G. Vergara, S. Mafé, K. Kontturi, and P. Viinikka, J. Phys. Chem. B *102*: 1301 (1998).
48. J. Garrido, V. Compañ, and M. L. López, J. Phys. Chem. *98*: 6003 (1994).
49. A. I. Gorshkov and O. V. Oshurkova, Sov. Electrochem. *26*: 135 (1990) [Élektrokhimiya *26*: 144 (1990)].
50. D. C. Mikulechy and S. R. Caplan, J. Phys. Chem. *70*: 3049 (1966).

51. J. W. Lorimer, J. Membrane Sci. *14*: 275 (1983).
52. B. Baranowski, J. Membrane Sci. *57*: 119 (1991).
53. Ref. 5, Chapter 6.
54. P. Schaetzel, E. Favre, B. Auclair, and Q. T. Nguyen, Electrochim. Acta *42*: 2475 (1997).
55. R. Schlögl, Discuss. Faraday Soc. *21*: 46 (1956) and references therein.
56. P. Forssell, K. Kontturi, and A. Ekman, Acta Chem. Scand. *A39*: 279 (1985).
57. G. Scatchard, J. Am. Chem. Soc. *75*: 2883 (1953).
58. A. I. Gorshkov and O. V. Oshurkova, Sov. Electrochem. *24*: 1292 (1988) [Élektrokhimiya *24*: 1292 (1988)].
59. H. P. Gregor and M. A. Peterson, J. Phys. Chem. *68*: 2201 (1964).
60. T. R. E. Kressman and F. L. Tye, Discuss. Faraday Soc. *21*: 185 (1956).
61. K. Kontturi, P. Forssell, and A. Ekman, Acta Chem. Scand. *A39*: 271 (1985).
62. M. J. Pikal and D. G. Miller, J. Phys. Chem. *74*: 1337 (1970).
63. Y. Hirata, M. Date, Y. Yamamoto, A. Yamauchi, and H. Kimizuka, Bull. Chem. Soc. Jpn *60*: 2215 (1987).
64. G. Scatchard, J. Am. Chem. Soc. *75*: 2883 (1953).
65. F. Danes, S. Sternberg, and S. Danes, Rev. Roumaine Chim. *26*: 11 (1981).
66. T. S. Sørensen and J. B. Jensen, J. Non-Equilib. Thermodyn. *9*: 1 (1984).
67. J. H. Petropoulos, J. Membrane Sci. *52*: 305 (1990).
68. V. I. Zabolotsky and V. V. Nikonenko, J. Membrane Sci. *79*: 181 (1993).
69. I. Tugas, G. Pourcelly, and C. Gavach, J. Membrane Sci. *85*: 183 (1993) and *85*: 195 (1993).
70. N. P. Berezina, N. P. Gnusin, O. Dyomina, and S. Timofeyev, J. Membrane Sci. *86*: 207 (1994).
71. R. Schlögl, Z. phys. Chem. N. F. *1*: 305 (1954).
72. H. U. Demisch and W. Pusch, J. Colloid Interface Sci. *69*: 247 (1979).
73. A. Guirao, S. Mafé, J. A. Manzanares, and J. A. Ibáñez, J. Phys. Chem. *99*: 3387 (1995).
74. H. A. Kramers, Physica *7*: 284 (1940).
75. K. Kontturi, J. A. Manzanares, and L. Murtomäki, Electrochim. Acta *40*: 2979 (1995).

12

Ion Equilibrium and Transport in Weak Amphoteric Membranes

PATRICIO RAMÍREZ Departament de Ciències Experimentals, Universitat "Jaume I" de Castelló, Castelló, Spain

SALVADOR MAFÉ Department of Thermodynamics, University of Valencia, Burjasot, Spain

Abstract

We present model calculations concerning the effect of pH on the ion equilibrium and transport in amphoteric membranes composed of weak polyelectrolytes where the charged groups are randomly distributed along the axial direction of the membrane. The theoretical approach employed is based on the Nernst–Planck equations. The complete system of electrical charges formed by: (i) the pH dependent, amphoteric membrane fixed charge, and (ii) the four mobile charges (the two salt ions and the hydrogen and hydroxide ions) have been taken into account without any additional assumption. The theoretical predictions show that the ionic fluxes and the membrane potential are very sensitive to the external pH. The potential use of these predictions for the analysis of experiments involving pH dependent passive transport through synthetic and biological membranes is emphasized. In particular, the model predictions are compared with recent experimental data obtained with a polymer membrane which contains succinyl chitosan as ampholyte and poly(vinyl alcohol) as supporting matrix. The results obtained explain satisfactorily the observed experimental trends (including the position of the membrane isoelectric point) in broad ranges of pH and electrolyte concentration.

I. INTRODUCTION

Amphoteric cross-linked polymer networks contain both positively and negatively fixed charge groups chemically bound to the polymer chains. Most physico-chemical applications of these polymer networks concern their swelling behavior when immersed in an electrolyte bath, especially in the case of polymer hydrogels [1,2]. It is also possible to prepare amphoteric membranes which show ion-exchange properties [3–12]. Early studies on amphoteric membranes were carried out by Söllner [13–15] and Weinstein and Caplan [16–18], who considered charge-mosaic membranes on the basis of the Non-equilibrium Thermodynamics formalism developed by Kedem and Katchalsky [19]. Amphoteric polymer membranes composed of weak polyelectrolytes where the charged groups are randomly distributed along the axial direction rather than on the normal plane of the membrane have been considered more recently by Yamauchi and co-workers [20,21] and by Tanioka and co-workers [22–24]. The membrane potential and piezodialysis properties of these membranes [22–24] were found to be very sensitive to the external pH and then the membranes could be of potential use for biochemical sensors and pH-controlled drug delivery systems.

Polymer membranes composed of silk fibroin have also been reported to have amphoteric properties [25,26] due to the existence of weakly acidic carboxyl groups and weakly basic amino groups. Since ionizable protein amino acid residues (i.e., carboxylic acid groups) and protonated amine groups are very common in biological systems, the study of ion transport in weak amphoteric membranes can also be of relevance for biological membranes. This is the case of the cornea, for instance, where the ion permselectivity appears to be controlled by the degree of protonation of ionizable sites within the tissue. In a recent study [27], the permselectivity of the rabbit cornea was analyzed in terms of diffusion and streaming potential measurements, and the effect of the external pH on these potentials suggested that the cornea contains acidic and basic charge groups that could be responsible for the observed differences in the permeabilities between cationic and anionic species.

Although the permselectivity of biological membranes is certainly a complicated phenomenon that involves not only passive electrostatic barriers (probably due to membrane fixed charges) but also active elements like carriers and pumps [28,29], we propose here to study theoretically an ideal case which considers only one major effect: the pH dependence of passive transport through a weak amphoteric membrane carrying both positive and negative fixed charge groups. This case serves as a simplified physical model for many real systems, and can be of relevance not only for the dialysis and piezodialysis properties of polymer weak amphoteric membranes but also for the pH controlled ion transport and drug delivery through membranes of biological interest.

The theoretical model employed for studying the pH dependence of ion transport in weak amphoteric membranes is based on the Nernst–Planck equations. The physical basis and limitations of these equations as applied to membrane systems can be found elsewhere [30,31]. All the electrical charges composed by: (i) the pH dependent, amphoteric membrane fixed charges, and (ii) the four mobile charges (the two salt ions and the hydrogen and hydroxide ions) have been fully taken into account in the model. The membrane characteristics studied are the ionic fluxes and the membrane potential, with particular emphasis on the membrane isoelectric point.

We believe that the model predictions presented here can be useful for the analysis of future experiments because of the following reasons: (i) experiments involving electrolyte transport through biomembranes, biochemical sensors and pH-controlled drug delivery systems are often conducted using buffer solutions and the measured ternary ion system properties are analyzed in many cases in terms of binary system equations [27,32]; (ii) most of the above experiments are conducted with the same pH value in the two external solutions bathing the membrane [22,23,27,32–34], and thus the effects of imposing a pH gradient through the membrane are not well-known; and (iii) simplifying assumptions such as equal pH values inside and outside the membrane and constant electrical field within the membrane [28,29] are sometimes used without a clear statement of the validity of these assumptions.

II. THEORETICAL MODEL

The system considered is shown schematically in Fig. 1. The amphoteric membrane extends from $x = 0$ to $x = d$, and separates two solutions of the same univalent electrolyte. The solutions are assumed to be perfectly stirred, and the whole system is isothermal and free of convective movements. $c_i(x)$ stands for the concentration of the ith-species at a point of coordinate x within the membrane ($i = 1$ for salt cations, $i = 2$ for salt anions, $i = 3$ for hydrogen ions, and $i = 4$ for hydroxide ions). c_{ij} denotes the concentration of the ith-species in the bulk of the jth-solution ($j = L$ for the left solution and $j = R$ for the right solution). pH_j ($j = L, R$) refers to the pH value in solution j.

The amphoteric membrane contains acidic (N) and basic (P) groups homogeneously distributed throughout its axial coordinate. These groups are assumed to be monovalent, and can be charged or not depending on the local value of the pH within the membrane. We denote by N_C and N_N the concentrations of the charged and neutral acidic groups, and by P_C and P_N the concentrations of the charged and neutral basic groups, respectively. The total

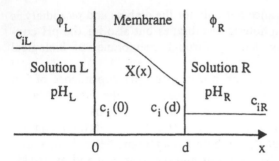

FIG. 1 Schematic representation of the amphoteric membrane and the membrane system.

concentrations of acidic and basic groups in the membrane are N_T and P_T, respectively. The following equilibria between *neutral* groups N_N or P_N and *charged* groups N_C or P_C are assumed:

$$N_N \xrightleftharpoons{K_N} N_C^- + H^+ \qquad\qquad\qquad (1a)$$

$$P_C^+ \xrightleftharpoons{K_P} P_N + H^+ \qquad\qquad\qquad (1b)$$

where K_N and K_P are the respective equilibrium constants, $N_T = N_N + N_C$ and $P_T = P_N + P_C$. From Eqs. (1), the local concentrations of charged groups within the membrane are

$$N_C = \frac{1}{1 + c_3/K_N}\, N_T \qquad\qquad\qquad (2a)$$

$$P_C = \frac{c_3/K_P}{1 + c_3/K_P}\, P_T \qquad\qquad\qquad (2b)$$

and the local concentration X of the net fixed charge in the membrane is defined as

$$X = P_C - N_C \qquad\qquad\qquad (3)$$

where we have included the sign (positive or negative) of this charge in the value of X. The concentrations of H^+ and OH^- ions verify the water dissociation equilibrium condition

$$c_3 c_4 = K_W \qquad\qquad\qquad (4)$$

with $K_W = 10^{-14}$ M^2 through the whole system.

The ion concentrations obey the electroneutrality conditions

$$c_{1j} + c_{3j} = c_{2j} + c_{4j}, \quad j = L, R \qquad\qquad\qquad (5a)$$

$$c_1 + c_3 + X = c_2 + c_4 \qquad\qquad\qquad (5b)$$

in the bulk of the two bathing solutions and in the membrane phase, respectively.

Assuming that all the ions are in thermodynamic equilibrium at the membrane/solution interfaces located at $x = 0$ and $x = d$, the ideal Donnan equilibria give the following relationships between the bulk solution and inner (membrane phase) concentrations [28,29]

$$\frac{c_1(0)}{c_{1L}} = \frac{c_{2L}}{c_2(0)} = \frac{c_3(0)}{c_{3L}} = \frac{c_{4L}}{c_4(0)} \tag{6a}$$

$$\frac{c_1(d)}{c_{1R}} = \frac{c_{2R}}{c_2(d)} = \frac{c_3(d)}{c_{3R}} = \frac{c_{4R}}{c_4(d)} \tag{6b}$$

From Eqs. (2)–(6), it follows that

$$\frac{c_{3j}}{K_P}\frac{c_{3j}}{K_N}u_j^4 + \left[\frac{c_{3j}}{K_P} + \frac{c_{3j}}{K_N} + \frac{c_{3j}}{K_P}\frac{c_{3j}}{K_N}\frac{P_T/c_{1j}}{1 + c_{3j}/c_{1j}}\right]u_j^3$$
$$+ \left[1 - \frac{c_{3j}}{K_P}\frac{c_{3j}}{K_N} + \frac{(P_T - N_T)/c_{1j}}{1 + c_{3j}/c_{1j}}\frac{c_{3j}}{K_P}\right]u_j^2$$
$$- \left[\frac{c_{3j}}{K_P} + \frac{c_{3j}}{K_N} + \frac{N_T/c_{1j}}{1 + c_{3j}/c_{1j}}\right]u_j - 1 = 0, \quad j = L, R \tag{7}$$

where $u_L \equiv c_1(0)/c_{1L}$ and $u_R \equiv c_1(d)/c_{1R}$. Equations (7) can be solved numerically for u_L and u_R using a standard procedure. Then, the inner membrane phase concentrations $c_i(0)$ and $c_i(d)$, $i = 2, 3, 4$, can be obtained from Eq. (6) in terms of the electrolyte concentrations and the pH values in the external bathing solutions. Once all the concentrations $c_i(0)$ and $c_i(d)$ have been determined, the Donnan potential differences at the left $(x = 0)$ and right $(x = d)$ interfaces, $\Delta\phi_L$ and $\Delta\phi_R$, can be computed as

$$\Delta\phi_L = \frac{RT}{F}\log\frac{c_{1L}}{c_1(0)} \tag{8a}$$

$$\Delta\phi_R = \frac{RT}{F}\log\frac{c_1(d)}{c_{1R}} \tag{8b}$$

The electric potential and the ion fluxes in the bulk of the amphoteric membrane can be calculated solving the Nernst–Planck equations [30,31,35]

$$J_i = -D_i\left[\frac{dc_i}{dx} + (-1)^{i+1}c_i\frac{F}{RT}\frac{d\phi}{dx}\right], \quad i = 1, \ldots, 4 \tag{9}$$

with the condition of zero total current

$$J_1 - J_2 + J_3 - J_4 = 0 \tag{10}$$

In Eq. (9), D_i and J_i stand for the diffusion coefficient in the membrane and the flux of the ith-species, respectively, ϕ is the local electric potential, and the constants F, R and T have their usual meaning.

Substituting Eq. (4) into Eq. (9) for $i = 3$ and 4, and taking into account Eq. (10), we obtain

$$J_3 = \frac{J_2 - J_1}{1 + K_W D_4/(D_3 c_3^2)} \tag{11a}$$

$$J_4 = -\frac{D_4 K_W}{D_3 c_3^2} J_3 \tag{11b}$$

Equations (11) show that the fluxes of H^+ and OH^- ions are not constant through the membrane if c_3 changes with x. However, in the case of very low pH values, Eqs. (2) and (11) give approximately

$$N_C \approx 0 \tag{12a}$$

$$P_C \approx P_T \tag{12b}$$

$$J_3 \approx J_2 - J_1 \tag{13a}$$

$$J_4 \approx 0 \tag{13b}$$

Integrating Eqs. (9) for ϕ through the membrane and summing up the two Donnan potentials of Eqs. (8), the membrane potential $\Delta\phi_M = \phi_L - \phi_R$ is obtained as

$$\Delta\phi_M = -\frac{RT}{F} \log \frac{\dfrac{D_1}{D_3} \dfrac{J_3}{J_1} - \dfrac{c_{3L}}{c_{1L}}}{\dfrac{D_1}{D_3} \dfrac{J_3}{J_1} - \dfrac{c_{3R}}{c_{1R}}} \frac{c_{1L}}{c_{1R}} \tag{14}$$

where the quotient J_3/J_1 is the solution of the transcendental equation

$$\Gamma \log \frac{c_2(d) - P_T \dfrac{1-\Gamma}{2}}{c_2(0) - P_T \dfrac{1-\Gamma}{2}} = \log \frac{\dfrac{D_1}{D_3} \dfrac{J_3}{J_1} - \dfrac{c_{3L}}{c_{1L}}}{\dfrac{D_1}{D_3} \dfrac{J_3}{J_1} - \dfrac{c_{3R}}{c_{1R}}} \frac{c_1(0)}{c_1(d)} \tag{15}$$

with

$$\Gamma \equiv \frac{\dfrac{D_2}{D_1} - 1 + \dfrac{J_3}{J_1}\left(\dfrac{D_2}{D_3} - 1\right)}{\dfrac{D_2}{D_1} + 1 + \dfrac{J_3}{J_1}\left(\dfrac{D_2}{D_3} + 1\right)} \tag{16}$$

Formally identical equations can also be derived for the opposite case of high pH values. In the case of intermediate pH values, however, the above equations are not valid, and a numerical procedure must be used to solve the exact Eqs. (9).

We have employed the following iterative procedure to integrate the system of differential equations given by Eqs. (9): first we assume some initial values for the ion fluxes and integrate Eqs. (9) using a fourth-order Runge–Kutta method with the boundary conditions at the interface $x = 0$. Then, we check if the solutions satisfy the boundary conditions at $x = d$ or not. If not, the initial estimation is changed until the boundary conditions at $x = d$ are satisfied. This allows to obtain the ion concentration and electric potential profiles, $c_i(x)$ and $\phi(x)$, as well as the ion fluxes J_i. Then, the profile of the fixed charge concentration $X(x)$ through the membrane can be determined from Eqs. (2) and (3). Finally, the membrane potential is computed as

$$\Delta\phi_M \equiv \Delta\phi_L + \Delta\phi_D + \Delta\phi_R \tag{17}$$

where $\Delta\phi_D \equiv \phi(d) - \phi(0)$ is the diffusion potential in the membrane.

III. RESULTS AND DISCUSSION

In this section we present a set of model calculations concerning the membrane fixed charge concentration profile, the membrane potential and the ionic fluxes in the amphoteric membrane [36]. We have considered first the symmetrical case $N_T = P_T = 5 \times 10^{-2}$ M, and assumed the values $d = 10^{-5}$ cm for the membrane thickness and $pK_N = 4$ for the pK value of the acidic groups in all the calculations in Figs. 2–8. Also, we have introduced the following values for the diffusion coefficients of the ionic species within the membrane: $D_1 = 10^{-7}$ cm^2/s, $D_2 = 2D_1$, $D_3 = 9D$, and $D_4 = 5D_1$.

The steady-state values for the membrane potential and the ion fluxes are zero when the pH values and the electrolyte concentrations in the left and right bathing solutions are equal ($pH_L = pH_R$ and $c_L = c_R$). In this case, the concentrations of charged acidic and basic groups are constant through the membrane, and the net fixed charge concentration X within the membrane is homogeneous. Figure 2 shows this membrane fixed charge concentration vs. $pH_L = pH_R \equiv pH$ in the case $c_L = c_R = 5 \times 10^{-2}$ M. The numbers in the curves corresponds to the pK_P values considered. The concentrations P_C and N_C have been calculated solving Eq. (7) for $u_L = u_R$ and substituting the result in Eqs. (6) and (2). As expected, $X \approx P_T(X \approx -N_T)$ for $pH < pK_N(pH > pK_P)$ and $X \approx P_T/2$ $(X \approx -N_T/2)$ for $pH \approx pK_N(pH \approx pK_P)$. It is also observed that the membrane becomes uncharged in the vicinity of the isoelectric point $pI = (pK_N + pK_P)/2$, and that the range of pH values where the net fixed charge concentration is practically zero becomes enlarged as the difference between pK_P and pK_N is increased.

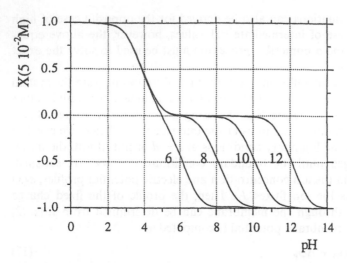

FIG. 2 Net fixed charge concentration X of the amphoteric membrane vs. $pH_L = pH_R \equiv pH$. We have considered the case $N_T = P_T = 5 \times 10^{-2}$ M, $c_L = c_R = 5 \times 10^{-2}$ M and $pK_N = 4$. The curves are parametric in pK_P [36].

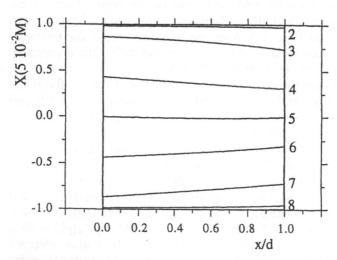

FIG. 3 Net fixed charge concentration profiles within the amphoteric membrane. We have considered $N_T = P_T = 5 \times 10^{-2}$ M, $c_L = 5 \times 10^{-2}$ M $= 5c_R$, $pK_N = 4$ and $pK_P = 6$ in the model calculations. The curves are parametric in $pH_L = pH_R \equiv pH$ [36].

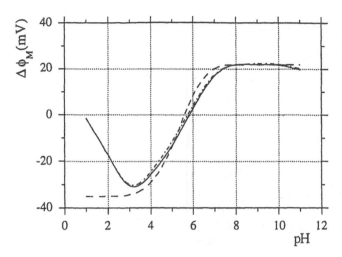

FIG. 4 Calculated membrane potential of the amphoteric membrane vs. pH for the same conditions as in Fig. 3. The continuous line corresponds to the exact numerical results. The dashed and dotted–dashed lines correspond to the approximations given by Eq. (18a), and Eqs. (12) and (19a), respectively [36].

Figures 3–5 illustrate the case $pH_L = pH_R \equiv pH$ and $c_L \equiv 5c_R$. The model calculations have been performed using $c_L = 5 \times 10^{-2}$ M and $pK_P = 6$. Figure 3 shows the net fixed charge concentration profiles within the membrane. The curves are parametric in the pH value, which is indicated in each

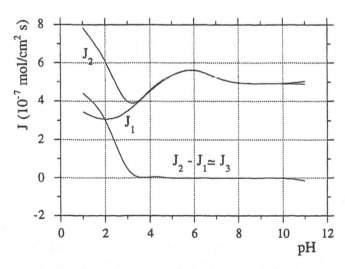

FIG. 5 Ion fluxes (exact numerical values) vs. pH for the same conditions as in Figs. 3 and 4 [36].

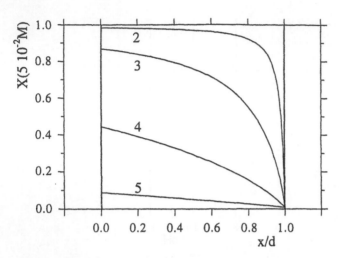

FIG. 6 Net fixed charge concentration profiles within the amphoteric membrane in the case $pH_L \neq pH_R$. We have used $N_T = P_T = 5 \times 10^{-2}$ M, $c_L = 5 \times 10^{-2}$ M $= 5c_R$, $pK_N = 4$ and $pK_P = 9$ in the model calculations. The curves are parametric in pH_L, with $pH_R = 6$. The case $pH_L = pH_R = 6$ gives $X \approx 0$ [36].

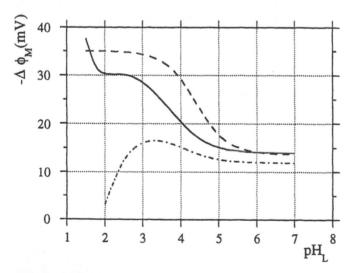

FIG. 7 Calculated membrane potential of the amphoteric membrane vs. pH for the same conditions as in Fig. 6. The curves correspond to numerical calculations (continuous line), results of Eq. (18a) (dashed line), and results of Eqs. (12) and (19a) (dotted–dashed line) [36].

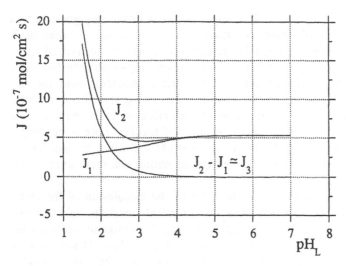

FIG. 8 Ion fluxes (exact numerical values) vs. pH for the same conditions as in Figs. 6 and 7 [36].

curve. Again, we see that $X \approx P_T(X \approx -N_T)$ for pH < pK_N(pH > pK_P) and that $X \approx 0$ near the isoelectric point pI = ($pK_N + pK_P)/2 = 5$. However, in the regions pH $\lesssim pK_N$ and pH $\gtrsim pK_P$ the net fixed charge concentration profiles become inhomogeneous due to the local variation of the pH within the membrane.

Figure 4 shows the calculated membrane potential vs. pH for the same conditions than in Fig. 3. The continuous line corresponds to the results obtained using the numerical procedure described in the previous section. The dashed line has been calculated assuming that the pH value within the membrane is equal to that of the bathing solutions and that the fluxes of the H^+ and OH^- ions can be neglected. Under these assumptions, the net fixed charge concentration X within the membrane is homogeneous, and can be calculated from Eqs. (2) and (3) for each pH value. The membrane potential and the fluxes of salt ions can be obtained using the equations [28]:

$$\Delta\phi_M \approx \frac{RT}{F} \left\{ \log \frac{c_L}{c_R} \frac{\sqrt{X^2 + 4c_R^2} - X}{\sqrt{X^2 + 4c_L^2} - X} + U \log \frac{\sqrt{X^2 + 4c_R^2} + UX}{\sqrt{X^2 + 4c_L^2} + UX} \right\} \quad (18a)$$

$$J_1 \approx J_2 \approx \frac{D_2 D_1}{D_2 + D_1} \frac{1}{d} \left\{ \sqrt{X^2 + 4c_L^2} - \sqrt{X^2 + 4c_R^2} \right.$$

$$\left. + UX \log \frac{\sqrt{X^2 + 4c_R^2} + UX}{\sqrt{X^2 + 4c_L^2} + UX} \right\} \quad (18b)$$

where $U \equiv (D_2 - D_1)/(D_2 + D_1)$. This approximation gives very good results in the range $8 < \text{pH} < 10$, where the membrane has a negative value of X ($X \approx -N_T$, see Fig. 3) and the membrane potential is nearly constant ($\Delta\phi_M \approx 22$ mV). Also, introducing $X \approx 0$ in Eq. (18) gives approximately the same value $\Delta\phi_M \approx -14$ mV obtained with the numerical procedure near the iso-electric point. However, the results obtained by using the above approximation deviate significantly from the exact numerical ones in the region of low pH values because in this region the flux of the H^+ ions is no longer negligible. The deviations in the pH range $4 < \text{pH} < 8$ must be ascribed to the fact that the net fixed charge concentration within the membrane is not homogeneous.

A more accurate analytical approximation of the calculation of the membrane potential can be achieved using the so-called constant field approximation [28,29] which assumes that $d\phi/dx \approx \Delta\phi_D/d = $ constant. In this case, Eqs. (9) can be readily integrated for $i = 1, 2$ and 3 in the low pH region [note that in this limit $J_4 \approx 0$ and $J_3 \approx J_1 - J_2 = $ constant, see Eqs. (10) and (11)]. Under these assumptions we obtain [28,29]:

$$\Delta\phi_D \approx \frac{RT}{F} \log \frac{D_3 c_3(0) + D_2 c_2(d) + D_1 c_1(0)}{D_3 c_3(d) + D_2 c_2(0) + D_1 c_1(d)} \tag{19a}$$

$$J_1 \approx \frac{F}{RT} \frac{D_1}{d} \Delta\phi_D \frac{c_1(0)\exp[-F\,\Delta\phi_D/RT] - c_1(d)}{1 - \exp[-F\,\Delta\phi_D/RT]} \tag{19b}$$

$$J_2 \approx -\frac{F}{RT} \frac{D_2}{d} \Delta\phi_D \frac{c_2(d)\exp[-F\,\Delta\phi_D/RT] - c_2(0)}{1 - \exp[-F\,\Delta\phi_D/RT]} \tag{19c}$$

$$J_3 \approx \frac{F}{RT} \frac{D_3}{d} \Delta\phi_D \frac{c_3(0)\exp[-F\,\Delta\phi_D/RT] - c_3(d)}{1 - \exp[-F\,\Delta\phi_D/RT]} \tag{19d}$$

Substituting Eq. (19a) in Eq. (12), the membrane potential can be calculated. A similar procedure can be followed in order to obtain the constant field approximation for the membrane potential in the limit $\text{pH} \gg 7$. The dotted–dashed line in Fig. 4 corresponds to the results given by this approximation.

Figure 5 shows the dependence of the ion fluxes on the pH for the same conditions than in Fig. 4. The results have been obtained using the numerical procedure described in the previous section. As expected, we see that $J_1 \approx J_2$ and $J_3 \approx J_4 \approx 0$ in the intermediate pH range $4 < \text{pH} < 10$. It can also be observed that the ion fluxes J_1 and J_2 attain a local maximum at the pH value where $\Delta\phi_M = 0$ in Fig. 4 (this pH value does not coincide exactly with $\text{pI} = 5$ because the pH within the membrane is not equal to the external pH). Again, the constant value $J_1 \approx J_2 \approx 4.9 \times 10^{-7}$ mol/cm^{2}s in the region $8 < \text{pH} < 10$ and the value $J_1 \approx J_2 \approx 5.3 \times 10^{-7}$ mol/cm^{2}s for $\text{pH} = \text{pI} = 5$ can be anticipated from Eq. (13b) taking $X \approx -N_T$ and $X \approx 0$, respectively. As we have mentioned above, we see that the fluxes J_3 and J_4 cannot be neglected for the case of low and high pH values, respectively (compare Figs. 4 and 5). In these limits, the constant field approximation given by Eqs. (19) can provide good analytical expressions for the ion fluxes.

The case $c_L = 5c_R$ and $pH_L \neq pH_R$ is considered in Figs. 6–8. We have fixed $c_L = 5 \times 10^{-2}$ M, $pH_R = 6$ and $pK_P = 9$ in the calculations. Figure 6 shows the profiles of the net fixed charge concentration within the membrane. The numbers close to each curve correspond to the pH_L value considered. We see that the profiles are highly inhomogeneous except for the case $pH_L \approx pH_R = 6$, where the membrane is practically uncharged ($X \approx 0$). As could be anticipated, the inhomogeneity of the membrane increases as pH_L decreases respect to the value in the right solution, $pH_R = 6$.

Figure 7 shows the membrane potential of the amphoteric membrane for the same case than in Fig. 6. The exact numerical results have been plotted in continuous line. The dashed and the dotted–dashed lines correspond to the approximations given by Eq. (18a), and by Eqs. (12) and (19a), respectively. The exact numerical results for the ion fluxes vs. pH_L are shown in Fig. 8. As in the previous case (see Figs. 4 and 5), the behavior of the membrane potential is closely related to the behavior of the ionic fluxes through the membrane. We can distinguish three different regions in Fig. 7: first, the membrane potential decreases with pH_L, then attains a plateau region characterized by a constant value $\Delta\phi_M \approx -30$ mV, and, finally, decreases again with pH_L. These regions correspond to $J_3 > J_1$, $J_3 \approx J_1$ and $J_3 \ll J_1 \approx J_2$ in Fig. 8, respectively. The approximated solution for $\Delta\phi_M$ given by Eq. (18a) deviates significantly from the exact solution except for the pH region $5 < pH_L < 7$, where $X \approx 0$, $J_1 \approx J_2 \approx 5.3 \times 10^{-7}$ mol/cm^{2}s and $J_3 \approx 0$ (see Figs. 6–8). The results for $\Delta\phi_M$ obtained using Eqs. (12) and (19a) do not agree with the exact numerical results over the entire range of pH_L values considered, and thus the constant field assumption constitutes a poor approximation when a pH gradient exists through the membrane.

In order to apply the above theoretical model to a particular experimental situation we have considered the results by Tanioka et al.[22–24], where the membrane potential and the solute (salt) permeability of a weak amphoteric polymer membrane composed by the succinyl chitosan chains supported by a poly(vinyl alcohol) matrix were reported. Since the water content of the membranes was very high, we can estimate the ion diffusion coefficients in the membrane as [37,38] $D_i = [H^2/(2 - H)^2]D_{i, \text{solution}}$, where $D_{i, \text{solution}}$ is the diffusion coefficient in a free aqueous solution and H is the degree of hydration. For these membranes, the pK_a values are $pK_N = 4.65$ and $pK_P = 6.3$ [24,39], so that the unknown parameters are only P_T and N_T in our case. In principle, the ratio N_T/P_T could be approximately estimated from the degree of substitution of carboxylic groups from amino groups [22–24], though the experimental uncertainties in the determination of the cationic/anionic capacity ratio of amphoteric membranes are usually relatively high [4,5].

The results of the membrane potential obtained by our numerical procedure are shown in Figs. 9 and 10. The points are the experimental results for the A-50 membrane [23,24], which has $H = 0.79$, and the lines represent the theoretical calculations. In the experiments, the KCl concentration of the left solution in Fig. 1 (c_0) was initially five times lower than that of the right solution ($5c_0$). Then, the pH of the solutions, which takes the same value in the two bulk solutions, was adjusted to the desired value by adding KOH or HCl.

The A-50 membrane had a degree of substitution from amino to carboxylic groups of 50% [23,24]. However, we see from Figs. 9 and 10 that we have to assume that $N_T \neq P_T$ in order to reproduce the experimental results. Indeed, Fig. 9 corresponds to the effective [22–24,40] charge densities $N_T = P_T = 4 \times 10^{-2}$ M and Fig. 10 to $N_T = 6 \times 10^{-2}$ M and $P_T = 4 \times 10^{-2}$ M. These latter values give the best fitting between theory and experiment. Since the experimental uncertainties in the cationic/anionic capacity ratio of amphoteric membranes can be relatively high [4,5], we conclude that a slight deviation from the equality $N_T = P_T$ could occur in our case, and could produce significant effects on the membrane potential (cf. Fig. 9 with Fig. 10).

Figure 11 shows the calculated pH dependence of the ion flux J_1. Again, we take the salt concentration of the right solution to be five times higher than that of the left solution. We see that there is a maximum in the salt flux at a

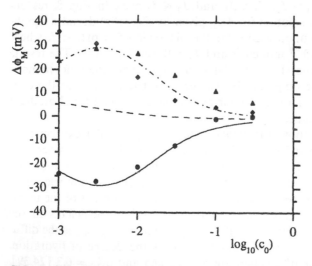

FIG. 9 Membrane potential $\Delta\phi_M$ vs. salt concentration c_0 for the A-50 membrane with $H = 0.79$ (see Ref. 13). The KCl concentration of the left solution in Fig. 1 (c_0) was initially five times lower than that of the right solution ($5c_0$). The symbols correspond to the experimental results of Ref. 13 and the lines correspond to the theoretical calculations with $N_T = P_T = 4 \times 10^{-2}$ M for pH = 2.8 (continuous line), pH = 5.6 (dashed line) and pH = 11.2 (dotted–dashed line) [24].

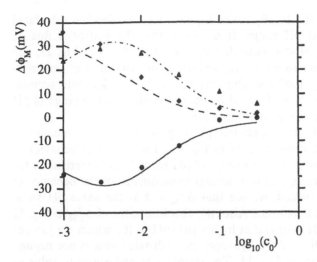

FIG. 10 Membrane potential vs. salt concentration c_0 for the same system of Fig. 9 when $N_T = 6 \times 10^{-2}$ M and $P_T = 4 \times 10^{-2}$ M in the theoretical calculations [24].

certain pH, which is in agreement with previous experimental results which showed that the solute permeability coefficient should reach a maximum (and then the reflection coefficient [23] should reach a minimum) near the iso-electric point [3,23]. It is also shown in this figure that the position of this

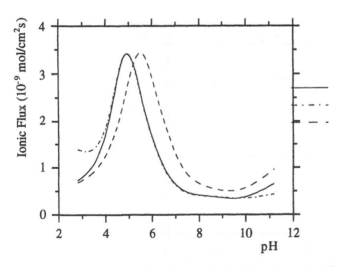

FIG. 11 Calculated ion flux J_1 vs. pH for $N_T = P_T = 4 \times 10^{-2}$ M (dashed line) and $N_T = 6 \times 10^{-2}$ M and $P_T = 4 \times 10^{-2}$ M (continuous line) in the case of $c_0 = 10^{-3}$ M. The calculated ion flux J_2 (dotted–dashed line) is also shown [24].

maximum changes with the N_T/P_T ratio. Figure 11 gives also the calculated ion flux J_2 over a broad pH range. It is shown that the hydrogen flux J_3 cannot be neglected for pH < 4 (note that $J_1 < J_2$ for pH < 4 in Fig. 11, and thus $J_1 + J_3 = J_2$ in order to ensure the experimental condition of zero electric current). Analogously, the hydroxide flux J_4 should be taken into account when pH > 10. Therefore, Fig. 11 could be useful to establish the range of pH values where the salt ions are the dominant ions.

Finally, Fig. 12 shows the predicted pH dependence of the membrane potential under the same conditions as in Fig. 11. The S-shaped behavior of the membrane potential over a broad range of pH value is characteristic of the weak amphoteric membrane, and is a natural consequence of the behavior of the ion flux in Fig. 11. Indeed, we see that $\Delta\phi_M = 0$ at the same pH value which makes the ion flux maximum. Also, the absolute value of $\Delta\phi_M$ in Fig. 12 decreases at lower pH (pH < 4) and at higher pH (pH > 10), which are just the pH values at which the flux of the hydrogen or hydroxide ions is not negligible, respectively, as shown in Fig. 11. The decrease in the absolute value of $\Delta\phi_M$ at pH < 4 and pH > 10 is due to a decrease in the Donnan potential. The latter is caused by an increase in the total ion concentration in the left or right bulk solution which occurs at very low or very high pH.

In summary, we have presented a set of model calculations concerning the membrane potential and the ionic fluxes in weak amphoteric membranes [24,36]. The whole system of equations including the four Nernst–Planck equations and the equations for the local dissociation equilibria within the

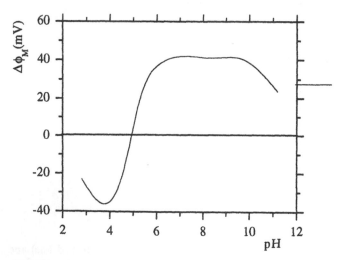

FIG. 12 Calculated membrane potential vs. pH for $N_T = 6 \times 10^{-2}$ M and $P_T = 4 \times 10^{-2}$ M in the case of $c_0 = 10^{-3}$ M [24].

membrane have been solved numerically without any additional simplifying assumption. The comparison of the exact theoretical results with those obtained by using several approximations as well as with previous experimental studies has shown the potential utility of the numerical solution, especially when a pH gradient is imposed through the membrane. Since the pH dependence of passive transport through weak amphoteric membranes constitutes a problem of great importance in dialysis and piezodialysis processes using polymer membranes [22–24], in ion transport through biological membranes [28,29], and in pH-controlled drug delivery systems [32–34], the model calculations presented here could be of interest for the analysis of future experiments.

ACKNOWLEDGMENTS

Financial support from the DGICYT, Ministry of Education and Science of Spain under Project No PB95-0018 is gratefully acknowledged. This chapter summarizes general results published by the authors in Refs. 24 and 36. The figures have been reprinted with permission from Elsevier Science. Part of this work was carried out during a summer stay by the authors to the laboratory of Prof. A. Tanioka, Department of Organic and Polymeric Materials, Tokyo Institute of Technology.

REFERENCES

1. A. E. English, S. Mafé, J. A. Manzanares, X. Yu, A. Yu. Grosberg, and T. Tanaka, J. Chem. Phys. *104*: 8713 (1996).
2. J. P. Baker, H. W. Blanch, and J. M. Prausnitz, Polymer *36*: 1061 (1995).
3. A. Yamauchi, S. Tsuruyama, H. Masumori, Y. Nagata, K. Kaibara, and H. Kimizuka, Bull. Chem. Soc. Jpn *55*: 3297 (1982).
4. K. Kaibara, H. Sonoda, Y. Nagata, and H. Kimizuka, Bull. Chem. Soc. Jpn *56*: 1346 (1983).
5. K. Kaibara, Y. Nagata, T. Kimotsuki, and H. Kimizuka, J. Membrane Sci. *29*: 37 (1986).
6. A. Yamauchi, H. Shinohara, M. Shinoda, M. Date, Y. Hirata, and H. Kimizuka, Bull. Chem. Soc. Jpn *60*: 1645 (1987).
7. Y. Hirata, M. Date, Y. Yamamoto, A. Yamauchi, and H. Kimizuka, Bull. Chem. Soc. Jpn *60*: 2215 (1987).
8. K. Kaibara, H. Inoue, S. Tsuruyama, and H. Kimizuka, Bull. Chem. Soc. Jpn *61*: 1517 (1988).
9. A. Yamauchi, M. Date, Y. Yamamoto, Y. Hirata, and H. Kimizuka, Bull. Chem. Soc. Jpn *61*: 793 (1988).
10. Y. Hirata, Y. Yamamoto, M. Date, A. Yamauchi, and H. Kimizuka, J. Membrane Sci. *41*: 177 (1989).
11. Y. Hirata and A. Yamauchi, J. Membrane Sci. *48*: 25 (1990).
12. K. Kaibara, K. Kumagai-Ueda, and H. Inoue, Bull. Chem. Soc. Jpn *66*: 77 (1993).
13. K. Söllner, Biochem. Z. *244*: 390 (1932).

14. R. Neihof and K. Söllner, J. Phys. Colloid Chem. *54*:157 (1950).
15. K. Söllner, Arch. Biochem. Biophys. *54*:129 (1955).
16. J. N. Weinstein and S. R. Caplan, Science *161*:70 (1968).
17. J. N. Weinstein, B. J. Bunow and S. R. Caplan, Desalination *11*:341 (1972).
18. J. N. Weinstein, B. W. Misra, D. Kalif, and S. R. Caplan, Desalination *12*:1 (1973).
19. O. Kedem and A. Katchalsky, Trans. Faraday Soc. *59*:1918, 1931 and 1941 (1963).
20. A. Yamauchi, Y. Okazaki, R. Kurosaki, Y. Hirata, and H. Kimizuka, J. Membrane Sci. *32*:281 (1987).
21. Y. Hirata, G. Sugihara, and A. Yamauchi, J. Membrane Sci. *66*:235 (1992).
22. K. Saito and A. Tanioka, Polymer *37*:2299 (1996).
23. K. Saito, S. Ishizuka, M. Higa, and A. Tanioka, Polymer *37*:2493 (1996).
24. P. Ramírez, S. Mafé, A. Tanioka, and K. Saito, Polymer *38*:4931 (1997).
25. C. Jianyong, A. Tanioka, and N. Minoura, Sen'i Gakkaishi *49*:486 (1993).
26. C. Jianyong, A. Tanioka, and N. Minoura, Sen'i Gakkaishi *50*:32 (1994).
27. Y. Rojanasakul and J. R. Robinson, Int. J. Pharm. *55*:237 (1989).
28. N. Laksminarayanaiah, *Equations of Membrane Biophysics*, Academic Press, New York, 1984.
29. S. G. Schultz, *Basic Principles of Membrane Biophysics*, Cambridge University Press, Cambridge, 1980.
30. R. P. Buck, J. Membrane Sci. *17*:1 (1984).
31. R. S. Eisenberg, J. Membrane Biol. *150*:1 (1996).
32. K. Kontturi, S. Mafé, J. A. Manzanares, B. L. Svarfvar, and P. Viinikka, Macromolecules *29*:5740 (1996).
33. Y. Osada, Adv. Polym. Sci. *82*:1 (1987).
34. M. Casolaro and R. Barbucci, Colloids Surf. A *77*:81 (1993).
35. T. S. Sørensen and J. B. Jensen, J. Non-Equilib. Thermodyn. *9*:1 (1984).
36. P. Ramírez, A. Alcaraz, and Mafé, J. Electroanal. Chem. *436*:119 (1997).
37. J. S. Mackie, and P. Meares, P. Proc. Royal Soc. London A*232*:498 (1955).
38. A. Tanioka, M. Natsuizaka, K. Saito, and K. Miyasaka, in *New Developments in Ion Exchange, Proceedings of the International Conference on Ion Exchange* ICIE'91, Tokyo, October 2–4, 1991.
39. Dr. K. Horiuchi, Katakura Chikkarin Co. Ltd., private communication.
40. T. Ueda, N. Kamo, N. Ishida, and Y. Kobatake, J. Phys. Chem. *76*:2447 (1972).

13

Water, Ion and Entropy Transport in Ion-Exchange Membranes

SIGNE KJELSTRUP   Department of Physical Chemistry, Norwegian University of Science and Technology, Trondheim, Norway

TATSUHIRO OKADA   Department of Polymer Physics, National Institute of Materials and Chemical Research, Ibaraki, Japan

MAGNAR OTTØY   The Membrane Research Group, Telemark Technical Research and Development Center, Porsgrunn, Norway

Abstract

Water, ion and entropy transport are described in two ion-exchange membranes, the homogeneous cation exchange membrane CR61 AZL 389 from Ionics and the inhomogeneous Nafion 117 membrane from DuPont. Irreversible thermodynamics is used to describe transports and design experiments. Transport properties are interpreted on the background of equilibrium data. While the water content of the Ionics membrane is almost constant, the water content of the Nafion membrane varies largely with membrane cation(s). There are two types of water in the Nafion membrane: one type that does not freeze, and one type that freezes. Ions distribute according to regular solution theory in both membranes. The equilibria for water and ion exchange are slow reactions; they are determined by small self-diffusion coefficients. The electric mobility of an ion in the membrane is smaller than in dilute water solutions; by one order of magnitude in the Ionics membrane. The electric mobility of a cation in a mixture with protons is constant, confirming small interactions between the proton, the other ion and the charged polymer chain. Interactions between two different alkali cations were quantified. A characteristic amount of water follows the bulk transport of a monovalent cation, also when it is in a mixture with another monovalent cation. This model has no microscopic analogue. The number of water molecules associated with reversible transport of an ion depends on the field strength of the ion, but seems uncorrelated with the water content in the membrane. The water permeability is larger than expected from self diffusion, and increases with increasing water content. The membrane surface is the source or sink for entropy changes during transport. Data relevant for fuel cell modeling are given. One may expect jumps in intensive variables at the membrane surface for the combination of large membrane fluxes and small thermal and electrical conductivities.

I.   INTRODUCTION

Ion-exchange membranes play an important role in an increasing number of processes in chemical and biochemical industry. Ion-exchange membranes are used, e.g., in electrodialysis and as separators in electrolytic cells and fuel cells. Electrodialysis is widely applied in the food, dairy, pulp and paper industries, in desalination of water and in recycling of plating bath rinse water. Other major applications are as separator in the chloro-alkali process and in the low-temperature polymer electrolyte membrane fuel cell (see Chapter 14). A process for salt splitting is based on the use of bipolar membranes. A bipolar membrane is composed of two ion-exchange membranes, one cationic and one anionic. The biopolar membrane will split water into protons and hydroxyl ions in an electrochemical cell. This membrane opens up a broad range of applications, e.g., the regeneration of acid and base constituents from aqueous salt solutions. Industrial processes using ion-exchange membranes are discussed in a recent book by Scott and Hughes [1].

The classic book on ion-exchange membranes is from 1962 by Helfferich [2]. An ion-exchange membrane has three major constituents, the polymer network, its cationic sites, and membrane water [2]. A membrane, that is a good electrical conductor, has a concentration of ionic sites similar to a highly concentrated salt solution, 1–2 M. The water content is high, typically between 30 and 50 wt% of wet resin. The membrane can in many aspects be regarded as a concentrated polyelectrolyte solution [3].

We distinguish between cation- and anion-exchange membranes. The cation-exchange membrane has covalently bound anionic sites, such as sulfonic acid or carboxylic acid groups. Cation transport is preferred in this membrane. The anion-exchange membrane has cationic sites such as alkyl ammonium groups. This membrane transports anions mainly. A high ion-exchange capacity exclude ions of the same charge (as the ion-exchange groups) and promote transport of ions with the opposite charge.

Knowledge on how and why water and ions are transported is important for application of ion-exchange membranes, e.g., in the fuel cell or in separation technology. The conduction mechanism in ion-exchange membranes is different from that in aqueous solutions. In the ion-exchange membrane ions must move via ion-exchange sites, and electrostatic as well as steric interactions (polymer cross-links) influence the transport [3]. Water transport is closely linked to transport of ions. During dehydration, the membrane resistance will increase dramatically [4]. Most membranes have a high water content in order to keep the ionic conductivity high.

The aim of this chapter is to give insight into water and ion transport in ion-exchange membranes that are selective to cations. Together with this mass transport, there will also be transport of entropy, and we shall describe this, in theory mainly. We have studied a Nafion membrane, that has both hydrophilic and hydrophobic parts, and a membrane from Ionics which is mainly hydrophilic [5–18]. We shall review data that explain how ions and water move together and separate (Sec. V–VII). How does water move; alone and in combination with ions? How does ion transport compare to water transport?

Answers to these questions benefit from information on the equilibrium state of the membrane, which is therefore discussed first, see Sec. II.

Water and ions can be transported by chemical, mechanical, electrical and thermal forces. Irreversible thermodynamics [18,19] deals with all forces systematically, see Sec. III. Another advantage offered by this theory is that alternative experimental routes are provided to the same variable. The theory is also useful for experimental design. We review recent experimental methods in Sec. IV that can be used to obtain high accuracy results for electric conductivity, transport numbers and transported entropies [9,10,12–17]. Our models for ion and water transport in Sec. V–VII are developed within the framework of irreversible thermodynamics [18].

Irreversible thermodynamics has now been developed to deal with surfaces as separate thermodynamic systems [20]. In Chapter 14 we show how the surface transport theory works for the electrode–membrane surfaces of a fuel cell, which has jumps in intensive variables across the surface. The present chapter is devoted to bulk membrane transport, mainly. To some extent we report also on effects that are special for the membrane surface, what they are, and when they are important. We shall deal with aspects of heat transport in Sec. VII.

The basic assumption of irreversible thermodynamics, is the assumption of local equilibrium. This assumption was tested and confirmed by nonequilibrium molecular dynamic simulations [21] in a bulk system with transport of heat and mass. The assumption of local equilibrium *in* a surface between two bulk phases has not yet been tested. Local equilibrium *across* the membrane surface, means that the intensive variables of the system are continuous at the surface.

II. THE EQUILIBRIUM STATE

The equilibrium state of the membrane should be known before we discuss membrane transport. We limit ourselves to systems without coions in the membrane. This means membranes with high ion-exchange capacity and low to moderate concentrations in the adjacent aqueous solutions. For water we have:

$$H_2O(aq) = H_2O(m) \tag{1}$$

An example of an ion-exchange reactions is:

$$KCl(aq) + HM = HCl(aq) + KM \tag{2}$$

Here (m) and M denote the membrane phase for water or ion, respectively. The equilibrium state of the membrane can be studied when the membrane is in equilibrium with a solution with known thermodynamic potentials.

A. The Membrane Polymer and the Membrane Water

The cation-exchange membrane CR61 AZL 389 from Ionics is a cross-linked sulfonated copolymer of vinyl compounds cast in homogeneous films on synthetic reinforced fabrics. This membrane has 1.6 kmol/m^3 sulfonated groups. The water contents is 43 wt% corresponding to $\lambda = 17$ moles of water per mole of sulfonic group. The number does not vary much with the cation in the membrane.

The Nafion 117 membrane consists of a polytetrafluoroethylene backbone and regularly spaced, long fluorovinyl ether pendent side chains, terminated by a sulfonate ionic group. The sulfonate concentration is 1.13 kmol/m^3. The membrane has thus hydrophobic and hydrophilic regions [22] and there are no cross-links between the polymers. Pores of diameter 4 nm are connected with channels of diameter 1 nm. The water content in the membrane was investigated by Xie and Okada [5], with alkali as well as alkali earth metal salts in the aqueous solution. The water concentration in the membrane, λ, varied between 10 and 20 molecules of water per sulfonic group, see Table 1. The value of λ in the table may be underestimated, as it is very difficult to remove the last water molecules from the polymer. Xie and Okada found signs of different states of water [5]. The infrared (IR) spectra of the membranes gave a broad band at 3450 cm^{-1}, typical for the hydrogen-bonded OH$^-$-stretch in bulk water. Differential scanning calorimetry showed that some water was freezing around $-20°C$, but some was not possible to freeze even at $-120°C$. The amount that freezes, n_w, was estimated using the enthalpy of freezing of bulk water, see Table 1. For the metal ions, there is a reduction in n_w and λ with the cation field strength. The ratio n_w/λ is also reduced, meaning that the varying amount of bulk-like, freezing water can be associated with the hydrophilic parts of the membrane.

Roorda et al. [23] studied nuclear magnetic relaxation of $H_2{}^{17}O$ in a charged hydrogel with $\lambda = 5$, and found a higher relaxation of water in the gel than in pure water. The rotational motion of water is therefore slower in the gel than in water. Van Keulen [24] reported self-diffusion constants of water

TABLE 1 Total Number of Water Molecules per Ionic Site, λ, and Number n_w, that Freezes at $-20°C$ in Nafion 117 [5]. The Transference Number for Water is taken from Ref. 16

Membrane form	HM	LiM	NaM	KM	RbM	CsM	MgM$_2$	CaM$_2$	SrM$_2$	BaM$_2$
λ	22.6	19.5	16.5	10.8	10.1	8.6	17.3	17.2	16.2	14.1
n_w	10.6	9.3	7.8	4.5	3.1	3.5	8.9	8.0	7.6	4.6
t_w	2.6	15.6	9.7	5.3	5.2	6.3				

between 1.3 and 1.5×10^{-9} m^2/s for a cross-linked phenol sulfonic acid membrane, while Springer et al. [25] measured values varying from 1 to 7×10^{-10} m^2/s for increasing water contents in Nafion 117. The self-diffusion constant in bulk water is 2.3×10^{-9} m^2/s [26]. Different states of water were not detected in the gel [23] on a ms time scale. (The gel does not have hydrophobic regions, in contrast to the Nafion membrane.)

Membrane water seems to distribute specifically around each ion and each charged group and counterion, and water moves slower in the membrane than in the aqueous solution. This is due to both the nature of the polymer, and the fact that it is dense and hinders translation.

B. Ionic Distributions Over a Quasi-Anion Lattice

We have studied thermodynamic mixing properties of the Ionics membrane mixtures of NaM–LiM, KM–NaM, KM–LiM, RbM–NaM [6,8], KM–SrM$_2$ [7], and HM–NaM, HM–CaM$_2$ in Nafion [17,27].

The mixtures KM–LiM, RbM–NaM, with different sized cations, have an enthalpy and entropy of mixing according to regular solution theory. The activity coefficient f for AM in the exchange reaction ACl + BM = BCl + AM is:

$$\ln f_{AM} = bx_{BM}^2/RT \tag{3}$$

where x_{BM} is the equivalent fraction of BM. When A$^+$ is smaller than B$^+$, the value of b is typically -1.6×10^3 [6]. This gives an activity coefficient smaller than unity for AM, meaning that the smaller cation is preferred. Høgfeldt [28] reported other experimental results that follow Eq. (3).

The equilibria NaM–LiM, KM–NaM, that have ions with similar sizes, have ideal distributions of cations over the anion-quasi lattice: The entropy of mixing is that of a statistical distribution, and there are no preferred bonds ($b = 0$). Self diffusion data for Li$^+$ and Na$^+$ in polystyrene sulfonate membranes support that these ions interact with the membrane in similar ways [3]. We therefore speculate that cations often distribute themselves almost randomly over the available cation sites in the membrane. If one of the cations is divalent, a cation vacancy plus the divalent ion may distribute together [7]. Useful activity coefficients models can thus be obtained from Eq. (3).

The dense packing of charged polymers, and a certain chain flexibility, make the cation sites appear like in a concentrated ionic solution. Since regular solution theory describes the thermodynamic properties of mixing, the fixed ionic charges must retain a structure.

The equilibria (1,2) across the membrane surface take hours to establish according to experimental experience [7–9]. The self-diffusion constants of Li$^+$ and Na$^+$ were an order of magnitude lower in the membrane than in a dilute water solution of the salt, decreasing further with increasing degree of cross-linking of the polymer [3]. The membrane hinders the movement of both water and ions. This can explain the time needed to establish equilibrium between a membrane and its adjacent solutions. Slow equilibration of ions in Eq. (2) slows down the establishment of the equilibrium (1) for water, and vice versa. When composition changes are fast, for instance by transport of ions (electric current) through the membrane, the assumption of equilibrium *across* the surface may therefore not hold.

III. IRREVERSIBLE THERMODYNAMIC DESCRIPTION

A. Coupled Transports in the Bulk Membrane Phase

The coupled transports of heat, two salts, water, and electric charge in the bulk of a cation-exchange membrane is fully determined by five fluxes and their conjugate forces. The dissipation function, $T\Theta$, is given by the product sum of the conjugate fluxes and forces in a system. For a volume element of the membrane, we choose the fluxes and forces which can be directly related to experiments; see de Groot and Mazur [19] and Førland et al. [18]:

$$T\Theta = -J_1\nabla\mu_{1,\,T} - J_2\nabla\mu_{2,\,T} - J_w\nabla\mu_{w,\,T} - J'_q\nabla \ln T - j\nabla\varphi \qquad (4)$$

The fluxes of two components 1 and 2, and water across the membrane are J_1, J_2 and J_w, respectively, while J'_q and j are the measurable heat flux and the electric current density. We choose as components the neutral electrolytes and water. The amount of electrolyte is everywhere given by the amount of one of the ions in the electrolyte or in the membrane. For instance, in a membrane composed of NaM and HM in equilibrium with NaCl(aq) and HCl(aq) it is practical to identify J_1 with J^+_{Na} and J_2 with J^+_H, in the presence of a nonzero electric current and Ag(s)|AgCl(s)-electrodes. (Another example of identification of components is given in Sec. IV.B) The conjugate forces for the neutral components are the chemical potential gradients at constant temperature:

$$\nabla\mu_{i,\,T} = \nabla\mu_i(c) + V_i\nabla P \qquad (5)$$

for $i = 1$, 2 and w. The first term to the right is the concentration dependent part of the chemical potential, V_i is the partial molar volume of i, and p is the pressure. The conjugate force for the heat flux is $-\nabla \ln T$. The electric force refer to the electrodes that are used in the experiments [9–16], meaning that it is an operational force (or operational electric potential). In order to define the operational electric potential everywhere in the membrane, we consider auxiliary electrodes at any location in the membrane, in a solution in equilibrium with the membrane [18]. The electric force is not conservative; it depends on the path of the process. Note, we follow Ref. [18] in their use of units and notation for $\nabla\varphi$.

The flux equations for the membrane follow from Eq. (4)

$$J_1 = -L_{11}\nabla\mu_{1,T} - L_{12}\nabla\mu_{2,T} - L_{13}\nabla\mu_{w,T} - L_{14}\nabla \ln T - L_{15}\nabla\varphi \qquad (6)$$

$$J_2 = -L_{21}\nabla\mu_{1,T} - L_{22}\nabla\mu_{2,T} - L_{23}\nabla\mu_{w,T} - L_{24}\nabla \ln T - L_{25}\nabla\varphi \qquad (7)$$

$$J_w = -L_{31}\nabla\mu_{1,T} - L_{32}\nabla\mu_{2,T} - L_{33}\nabla\mu_{w,T} - L_{34}\nabla \ln T - L_{35}\nabla\varphi \qquad (8)$$

$$J_q' = -L_{41}\nabla\mu_{1,T} - L_{42}\nabla\mu_{2,T} - L_{43}\nabla\mu_{w,T} - L_{44}\nabla \ln T - L_{45}\nabla\varphi \qquad (9)$$

$$j = -L_{51}\nabla\mu_{1,T} - L_{52}\nabla\mu_{2,T} - L_{53}\nabla\mu_{w,T} - L_{54}\nabla \ln T - L_{55}\nabla\varphi \qquad (10)$$

where L_{ij} are phenomenological coefficients and Onsager's reciprocal relations apply

$$L_{ij} = L_{ji} \qquad (11)$$

We describe the determination of the electrical conductivity, $L_{55} = \kappa$ in Sec. IV.A. The other coefficients are conveniently determined from the following set of equations:

$$J_1 = -l_{11}\nabla\mu_{1,T} - l_{12}\nabla\mu_{2,T} - l_{13}\nabla\mu_{w,T} - l_{14}\nabla \ln T + t_1 j \qquad (12)$$

$$J_2 = -l_{21}\nabla\mu_{1,T} - l_{22}\nabla\mu_{2,T} - l_{23}\nabla\mu_{w,T} - l_{24}\nabla \ln T + t_2 j \qquad (13)$$

$$J_w = -l_{31}\nabla\mu_{1,T} - l_{32}\nabla\mu_{2,T} - l_{33}\nabla\mu_{w,T} - l_{34}\nabla \ln T + t_w j \qquad (14)$$

$$J_q' = -l_{41}\nabla\mu_{1,T} - l_{42}\nabla\mu_{2,T} - l_{43}\nabla\mu_{w,T} - l_{44}\nabla \ln T + \pi j \qquad (15)$$

obtained by elimination of the electric force in Eqs. (6)–(10). The coefficients are related by:

$$I_{ij} = L_{ij} - \frac{L_{i5} L_{5i}}{L_{55}} \qquad (16)$$

The transference numbers of component i, t_i of Eqs. (12)–(14), is defined by the flux of the component divided by the electric current density in the uniform, isothermal system:

$$t_i = \left(\frac{J_i}{j}\right)_{\nabla\mu_l=0;\ \nabla \ln T=0} = \frac{L_{i5}}{L_{55}} \qquad i = 1, 2, w \qquad (17)$$

With anion reversible electrodes, the flux of electrolyte is most conveniently defined by the transport of the cation of the electrolyte. In an ideal cation exchange membrane mixture, for instance NaM–HM, the component transference numbers are then given by the ionic transference numbers; $t_1 = t_{Na^+}$ and $t_2 = t_{H^+}$. The sum of component transference numbers is not given, but the sum of ionic transference numbers is always unity [18]. In a perfectly selective cation exchange membrane, as in the present example, we have:

$$t_{Na^+} + t_{H^+} = 1 \qquad (18)$$

We describe the experimental determination of ionic transference numbers as a function of composition in Sec. IV.B and C.

The Peltier heat, π, of an interface is the heat that has to be removed (or added, if π is negative) to the interface to maintain constant temperature when positive electric current is transferred from left to right through the interface. The Peltier heat is, in this definition, a scalar property of the interface. In a system that has a uniform electrolyte and identical electrodes, we may speak of a (scalar) transport of heat from one side (of the membrane electrolyte) to the other side. The heat transferred per unit of charge in this manner can be related to the Peltier heat and a ratio of phenomenological coefficients:

$$\pi = \left(\frac{J'_q}{j}\right)_{\nabla \ln T = 0;\ \nabla \mu_i = 0} = \frac{L_{45}}{L_{55}} \tag{19}$$

The coefficient ratio thereby refer to the total process, removal of heat on one electrode and addition on the other. For an electrode, the contribution to the Peltier heat from the electronic conductor (the metal) is normally negligible [18]. The Peltier heat is then the temperature times the entropy changes that accompany the charge transfer. The value of the ratio L_{54}/L_{45} is more easily determined than L_{45}/L_{45}, see Eq. (23) below and Sec. IV.D.

The heat effect given by Eq. (19) is principally different from the irreversible Joule heat, because it changes sign with the direction of the electric current density. When the Peltier heat is a function of temperature, there is also a reversible heat effect in the bulk phase between the two interfaces (the Thomson heat). The Thomson heat is connected to the heat flux in the bulk membrane.

When $j = 0$, the membrane allows interdiffusion of (two) cations and water transport. The water permeability, according to Eqs. (12)–(14) is

$$L_p = -\left(\frac{J_v}{\Delta p}\right)_{j=0} = -\frac{1}{\Delta p}(J_1 V_1 + J_2 V_2 + J_w V_w) \approx L_{33} V_w / l_m \tag{20}$$

where l_m is the membrane thickness.

The water permeability and the transference number for water can be obtained together, when interdiffusion is kept negligibly small by choice of experimental conditions, see Sec. IV.C.

The heat of transfer, that is associated with water transport through the membrane, is defined by

$$q_w^* = \left(\frac{J'_q}{J_w}\right)_{\Delta \mu_{1,T} = \Delta \mu_{2,T} = 0;\ \Delta \ln T = 0,\ j = 0} = \frac{l_{43}}{l_{33}} \tag{21}$$

This definition is equivalent to the definition of the Peltier heat above, in the way that it also describes heat transferred across the system through scalar heat effects of opposite signs at two solution–membrane interfaces. Again, the coefficient ratio relate to a cell process. The difference between Eqs. (19) and (21) is that the heat transport in Eq. (21) is caused by mass (water) transport; while in Eq. (19), it is caused by the electric current density. Both heat effects are reversible, in the sense that they change sign with the change of direction in the mass flux or the electric current density. There may also be heat effects in the bulk membrane from transfer of water (a Dufour effect). This is mostly a small effect.

In order to relate Eqs. (5)–(15) to experiments, we need to integrate them over the membrane. We then assume that:

1. We can find a water phase in equilibrium with the membrane at any membrane location (Scatchard's assumption [2]) and integrate across these water solutions, which have known salt activities. Scatchard's assumption was already used to define the electric force in Eq. (4).
2. There is chemical, mechanical and thermal equilibrium *across* the surface of the membrane. The integration limits for intensive variables of the membrane are then given by the corresponding solution values adjacent to the membrane surfaces.

The phenomenological coefficients of the membrane are not continuous at the interface. Their values jump from the membrane value to the solution value. The total cell potential difference $\Delta\varphi_{obs}$ must be corrected for the potential difference of the electrodes, $\Delta V_{el}\Delta p$, to obtain the electric force over the membrane [18]:

$$\Delta\varphi = \Delta\varphi_{obs} + \Delta V_{el}\Delta p \qquad (22)$$

where $\Delta V_{el} = V_{Ag} - V_{AgCl}$.

Common boundary conditions for integration of Eqs. (4)–(15) over the membrane are given by assumptions (1) and (2) and zero gradients in intensive variables in the bulk solutions. In order to integrate, we also need to know how the coefficients depend on intensive variables. We show below (in Sec. IV.B) how we can obtain the concentration dependence of t_i from a measured (integral) emf, through the use of membrane stacks.

B. Further Comments on Surface Heat Effects vs. Bulk Heat Effects

We discussed above how the Peltier effect (or the heat of transfer) appear at membrane surfaces when charge (or mass) is transported across the membrane, and we mentioned the reversible heat Thomson and Dufour effects in the bulk membrane. Some further comments can be related to explicit formulas.

The Seebeck coefficient of a thermocell is equal to minus the Peltier heat of Eq. (19) divided by the temperature; by application of Eq. (11). Consider a cation exchange membrane in equilibrium with HCl(aq). The Ag(s)|AgCl(s)-electrodes in the two solutions have different temperatures. The dissipation function, Eq. (4), includes the temperature dependence of the chemical potential (the entropy) of HCl and water, in the term that contains the heat flux [15]. The Peltier heat, in terms of entropies, is therefore:

$$\left(\frac{\Delta\varphi}{\Delta T}\right)_{\Delta c = 0} = -\frac{\pi}{T} = S_{HCl} + t_w S_w + \Delta S_{el} - S_{HM}^* \tag{23}$$

Here S_{HCl} and S_w are the partial molar entropies of HCl and water, respectively, and S_{HM}^*, is the transported entropy of protons in the membrane. The electrode reactions contribute by

$$\Delta S_{el} = S_{Ag} - S_{AgCl} \tag{24}$$

[compare Eq. (22)]. The transported entropy of electrons is neglected. We distinguish between transported entropy and thermodynamic entropies in Eq. (23). The relevant thermodynamic entropies can be deduced from the molar fluxes in Eqs. (12)–(14), they are multiplied by the transference numbers of the components. The transported entropy, on the other hand, is connected with the process of charge transfer. The whole of Eq. (23) gives the Peltier effect for the electrode surface. The (bulk) Thomson effect is related to the temperature variation in S_{HM}^* and $t_w S_w$. The Thomson effect is a second-order effect to the Peltier effect.

The reversible heat associated with absorption of water into the membrane, is given from the energy balance across the membrane surface:

$$J'_q(l) + \sum_{i=1}^{3} J_i H_i(l) = J'_q(m) + \sum_{i=1}^{3} J_i H_i(m) \tag{25}$$

where (l) and (m) denote the solution and membrane sides of the surface, respectively. When the heat flux in the solution is small, $J'_q(l) = 0$, and the chemical potentials of the electrolytes, as well as their fluxes, are (approximately) zero, we can find an *estimate* for q_w^* of the surface from Eqs. (21) and (25):

$$\left(\frac{J'_q(m)}{J_w}\right)_{\Delta\mu_{1,T} = \Delta\mu_{2,T} = 0, \, \Delta T(s) = 0} = H_w(l) - H_w(m) = \Delta_{abs} H \tag{26}$$

In principle, the heat of transfer is a kinetic property. This expression shows that it can contain a thermodynamic part. The transport property, q^*, has been modeled by combinations of partial molar enthalpies [29] and by activation energies for viscous flow [30]. The heat flux $J'_q(m)$ can be used for J'_q in the integrated Eq. (9). The contribution to the heat of transfer from water transport in the bulk membrane is small [18].

Irreversible thermodynamics for surfaces distinguishes between bulk and surface effects, and gives flux equations also for the surface (see Chapter 14). When the surface is introduced as a separate thermodynamic system, we do not need assumption 2.

IV. EXPERIMENTAL DESIGNS

The definitions (17 and 19) describe experiments which are difficult to do;
Hittorf experiments and measurements of Peltier effects. Electroosmosis
experiments are also difficult. Through Eq. (11) we can replace these by emf-
experiments that yield accuracies better than 2%. We review such methods for
determination of transport properties, presented before in detail by Ottøy et
al. [9,12–14] and Okada et al. [10,11].

A. Membrane Conductivity from a Stack Method

The electric resistance is measured with uniform membrane composition. The
resistance of an ion-exchange membrane is comparable to that of the water
solution in a conductivity cell. It is therefore difficult to separate the resistance
of the membrane, R_m, from that of the solution. A membrane stack experiment can resolve the separation problem in a two-step procedure [13,14]. The
total resistance of a stack of n membranes with adjacent electrolyte solutions
is:

$$R(n) = R_o + nR_{ml} \qquad\qquad (27)$$

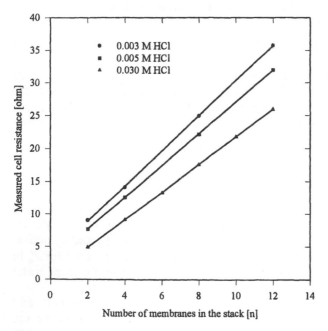

FIG. 1   Measured cell resistance $R(n)$ as a function of the number of membranes, n, in
the stack [14].

where R_{ml} is the resistance of one membrane plus its surface liquid layer, and R_o is the resistance of the liquid layers at the electrodes. From the plot of $R(n)$ vs. n (see Fig. 1), we first determine R_{ml} and R_o from the slope and intercept of the curve. The resistance R_{ml} is further equal to the membrane resistance, R_m, plus the resistance of the surface liquid layers of the membrane, R_1:

$$R_{ml} = R_m + R_1 \tag{28}$$

We can expect that R_m is constant within a range of solution concentrations. The variation in R_1 with composition can be found from tabulated values of the specific electrolyte conductivity. This gives the basis for the separation of terms in Eq. (28). Figure 2 shows the resistance R_{ml} for an Ionics membrane in contact with different solutions of HCl. At any concentration, a tangent to the curve can be found. From the intercept of this tangent with the y-axis, we find R_m.

At high external salt concentration, the membrane loses its selectivity, while at low concentration it starts to swell. These effects can obstruct the determination of R_m if a too broad concentration interval is chosen for the evaluation. They are, however, much more pronounced for HCl than for other salts, like KCl. The curve similar to Fig. 2, is linear over a relatively broad range of

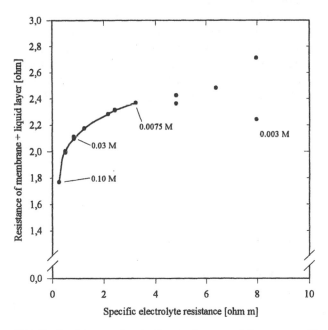

FIG. 2 Resistance of a single membrane and the surrounding electrolyte layer, R_1, as a function of the electrolyte resistance [14].

specific resistances for KCl-solutions. It was further shown that the interfacial liquid layer between the membranes in a stack varied with type of membrane. For the smooth and sticky Nafion membrane, the interfacial liquid layers became so thin that their contribution to the measured resistance could be neglected. The accuracy of the method is better than for other known methods, see Refs. 13 and 14 for further references, partly because the surface liquid layer contribution can run as high as 10% of the total resistance even at moderate concentrations.

B. Ion Transference Numbers from a Stack Method

The transference number of an ion depends on the membrane composition. The transference number is determined in a concentration cell experiment, where the membrane composition varies through the cell. We shall see how we can use a stack to keep a defined concentration gradient, and at the same time, find the concentration dependence of the transference number.

Consider an isothermal, isobaric, three-component system. The gradient in the operational electric potential for $j = 0$, is from Eqs. (10), (11) and (17):

$$\nabla\varphi = -t_1\nabla\mu_1 - t_2\nabla\mu_2 - t_w\nabla\mu_w \tag{29}$$

We can arrange the experimental conditions so that $\Delta\mu_w = 0$ by keeping the ionic strength constant on both sides. We assume that the chemical potential gradient of water inside the membrane is zero in this situation. Consider the system HM–KM and hydrogen reversible electrodes to measure $\Delta\varphi$. The amount of KM is everywhere given by the amount of K^+, n_K^+. The transference number of KM is therefore $t_2 = t_{K^+}$. The amount of HM that is transferred through the membrane per unit of charge transferred, the transference number of HM, is then $t_1 = -t_{K^+}$. By introducing this into Eq. (29) we obtain:

$$t_{K^+} = \frac{d\varphi}{d(\mu_{HCl} - d\mu_{KCl})} \tag{30}$$

When t_{K^+} is known, we can find t_{H^+} from Eq. (18). The first problem is to deal with diffusion that is superimposed on charge transfer. The next is to relate the measured emf, $\Delta\varphi$, to the local value of t_{K^+} in order to find $t_{K^+}(x_{KM})$. Both problems can be resolved by application of a membrane stack. The stack has so many membranes (usually 8–10), that the boundary solutions are not changed by diffusion during the experiment. The differential of Eq. (30) can be related to the difference values of the measured variables by

$$\frac{d\varphi}{d(\mu_{HCl} - d\mu_{KCl})} = \frac{d\Delta\varphi}{d\Delta(\mu_{HCl} - \mu_{KCl})} \tag{31}$$

when we choose a reference solution on one side of the stack, and vary the composition on the other side of the stack. We have taken advantage of assumption a) for the chemical potentials in Eq. (30). By plotting $\Delta\varphi$ as a function of $\Delta(\mu_{HCl} - \mu_{KCl})$, we find the transference number of Eq. (30) for a given composition. An example of such an experimental curve for determination of transference numbers is shown in Fig. 3. The transference number is obtained as a continuous function of concentration with 1% accuracy in this manner.

C. Water Transference Numbers from Streaming Potentials

Water transference numbers are determined for membranes of uniform composition. The emf method that can replace the Hittorf measurements is the streaming potential method. For $j = 0$, we have from Eqs. (5), (10), (11), (17) and (22):

$$\left(\frac{\Delta\varphi_{obs}}{\Delta P}\right)_{\Delta c = 0} = -\sum_i t_i V_i - \Delta V_{el} \tag{32}$$

The pressure difference, which is applied to the membrane in this experiment, leads to an electric potential difference, but also to a volume flow, that is

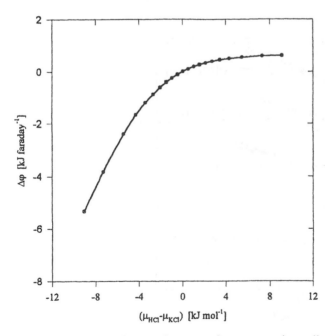

FIG. 3 The emf of the membrane stack concentration cell as a function of the difference in chemical potentials between the test solution and the reference solution. The curve is used for determination of t_{K^+}, according to Eqs. (28) and (29) [9].

mainly water flow. The solution on the low pressure side becomes more dilute, while the solution on the high pressure side becomes more concentrated. Contributions to the cell potential arise also from this. It was shown [10] that this variation in the chemical potential differences leads to a correction term in Eq. (32):

$$\Delta\varphi_{\text{obs}} \approx - (t_1 V_1 + t_2 V_2 + t_w V_w + \Delta V_{\text{el}})\Delta p + A\sqrt{t} \tag{33}$$

By plotting $\Delta\varphi_{\text{obs}} = EF$ vs. $\sqrt{t}$ we find the electric potential at zero time. An example of such a plot is shown in Fig. 4. This can next be used to find the streaming potential with high accuracy, by plotting EF vs. Δp. The water transference number can be calculated from Eq. (32) using known ionic transference numbers (the concentration variation must be known). The constant A can be related to the water permeability, L_p, when the water flux is constant, and the Nernst–Planck assumption is valid in the adjacent solution. For a solution with one chloride, we obtain:

$$A = -L_p \frac{8RTt_{\text{Cl}^-}}{\sqrt{\pi D_{\text{HCl}}}} \Delta p \tag{34}$$

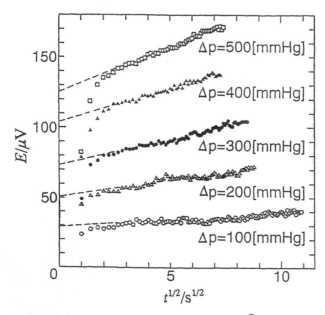

FIG. 4 The variation of the emf (E) with $\sqrt{t}$ in a Nafion membrane in contact with 0.03 M CaCl$_2$ [17]. The extrapolation to find the streaming potential for various pressure differences (in mm Hg) is also shown.

Streaming potential measurements can be used also to find the water permeability when the approximations leading to Eq. (33) are fulfilled.

Streaming potential measurements are accurate for membranes in contact with aqueous solutions, but cannot be used for membranes in contact with vapor. A method similar to the emf method for ionic transference number (Sec. IV.B) can then be used to find the water transference number [14]. This method is interesting for investigation of the fuel cell membranes, which operate in humidified hydrogen or oxygen atmospheres.

D. The Transported Entropy from Seebeck Coefficients

The experiment described by Eq. (23) is illustrated in Fig. 5. The figure shows that the electric potential, $\Delta\phi = EF$, follows the variation in $\Delta T(t)$. Heat leakage across the membrane is not important in this experiment, as long as the temperature can be kept constant on the two sides. From the constant ratio $\Delta\varphi/\Delta T$ we obtain the entropy combination of Eq. (23) for a given membrane and electrolyte composition. The result is valid for the average temperature of the cell.

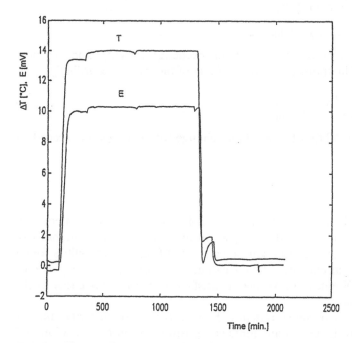

FIG. 5 The parallel variation in emf (E/mV) and the temperature difference (ΔT/°C) across the cell with time [12].

E. Thermal Osmosis Experiments

The easiest way to find an estimate for the heat of transfer of the membrane surface, $q*(s)$, is by the following procedure. We assume that the water permeability, l_{33}, is constant across the membrane and across the surface. The water permeability of the membrane is then determined, see Eqs. (20) and (34). A temperature difference is applied across the membrane and the resulting water flux is found, giving l_{34} for the membrane as a whole with uniform concentrations, see Eq. (14). We may then, to a first approximation, assume that the sole contribution to this black box value is due to the membrane surface, giving $\Delta_{ads} H$ in Eq. (26). Thermal osmosis results have been reported by several authors, see, e.g., Hanaoka et al. [31].

V. IONIC TRANSPORT

The experiments described in Sec. IV.A and IV.B concern ion transport in membranes. Such systems can be described in more detail by introducing the electric mobility of an ion in the membrane. When the membrane composition is known, u_i relates the conductivity, $\kappa = (l_m/A_m R_m)$ (see Sec. IV.A) and the transference numbers (see Sec. IV.B). With two cations A^+ and B^+, a membrane conductivity model is [18]:

$$L_{55} = \kappa/F^2 = cF(u_{A+} x_{A+} + u_{B+} x_{B+}) \tag{35}$$

where F is Faraday's constant, c is the ion exchange capacity, and the mole fraction of i, is x_i. The transport number of one of the ions is accordingly:

$$t_{A+} = \frac{L_{i5}}{L_{55}} = \frac{u_{A+} x_{A+}}{u_{A+} x_{A+} + u_{B+} x_{B+}} \tag{36}$$

We have proposed [18] that the mobilities change with composition according to:

$$\begin{aligned} u_{A+} &= u_{A+}^\circ(1 - kx_{BM}) \\ u_{B+} &= u_{B+}^\circ(1 - kx_{AM}) \end{aligned} \tag{37}$$

where u_{A+}° (u_{B+}°) is the mobility of the pure AM (BM), and k is an interaction constant, which describes how the presence of one ion reduces the mobility of the other. Transference numbers can be calculated from the mobilities found by conductivity measurements, but they can also be measured directly as outlined in Sec. IV.B. We have performed a satisfactory consistency check of the results in this manner.

We have seen that in some systems, the membrane conductivity changes almost linearly with the membrane ionic composition, in both the Nafion and the Ionics membrane, in spite of the high cationic site concentration (1.13 and 1.6 kmol/m^3, respectively). A linear relation means that the ionic mobilities can be taken as constant. This means that $k = 0$, and $u_i = u_i^{\circ}$ in Eq. (37). Okada et al. [17,27] found this for HM–NaM and HM–CaM$_2$ in a Nafion membrane, and Ottøy et al. [9] found the same for HM–KM and HM–NaM in the Ionics membrane. These systems are special in the way that they involve protons. The H^+ clusters seem to be too small to interact with other ionic clusters.

Ojala and Kontturi [32,33] investigated the Ionics membrane systems, NaM–KM, NaM–LiM and NaM–RbM. All these systems show that the ions do not move independent of each other; Eq. (35) does not give a straight line when plotted against composition. A value of k was typically 0.13 [14]. A nonlinear variation in the conductivity with composition was also found for KM–SrM$_2$, with $k = 0.28$ [18]. Ojala and Kontturi also found that the mobilities of two ions approached one another. One ion will have to change position with another ion when moving. The slower ion will then be accelerated whereas the faster ion will be retarded. Ionic mobilities are compared to electrolyte mobilities at infinite dilution in Table 2. We see from Table 2 that the membrane ionic mobilities are smaller than those in dilute aqueous solution by one order of magnitude for the Ionics membrane. The results for the Nafion membrane are somewhat larger.

In the Nernst–Einstein approximation, the mobility of an ion is proportional to its diffusion constant. In the present system, which allows interdiffusion only, it is not unreasonable that this assumption is true, as is also confirmed by experiments (see Ref. 18 and references therein). Validity of the approximation requires that the coupling between mass fluxes is small. In terms of Eqs. (6)–(10) this means that $L_{12} = 0$, and $L_{i5} = L_{ii}$, for $i = 1, 2$. When one can expect a relation between the interdiffusion coefficient, L_{ii}, and the electric mobility was given through L_{i5}, one can also expect a correlation between the electric mobility and the self diffusion constant for the ions. Indeed the self diffusion constant for ions varies [23] in a similar way as the mobility. A

TABLE 2 Selected Ionic Mobilities at 298 K

Cation A^+	Mobility $u_{A^+}^{\circ}/10^8$ m^2/V/s		
	Nafion	Ionics	Infinite dilution
H^+	14.8	2.30	36.3
Na^+	2.7	0.30	5.19
K^+		0.38	7.61
Ca^{2+}	2.5		6.16
Sr^{2+}		0.09	

Source: Refs. 9, 14, 17 and 27.

higher degree of cross-linkages lead to a reduction in u_i by orders of magnitude [23].

In Gierke's cluster network model for Nafion, the diameter of the conducting pore was estimated to 1 nm [22]. Xie and Okada [15] measured the membrane conductivity with ammonium derivative cations to examine this estimate. When the magnitude of the cation diameter approached 1 nm, the membrane resistance increased several orders of magnitude. Collisions between the polymer chain and counterions clearly obstruct the translational motion of the ion along the chain severely.

VI. WATER TRANSPORT

A. The Water Transference Number

In a membrane with one cation, the water transference number is constant as long as the membrane contains cations only. This fact, that is long known, is seen in Fig. 6 where t_w in KM (Ionics membrane) is plotted as a function of the concentration of KCl in the aqueous solution. The high constant value has been taken as the number of water molecules transported per K^+ across the membrane. The decrease in t_w around 0.1 kmol/m³ has accordingly been

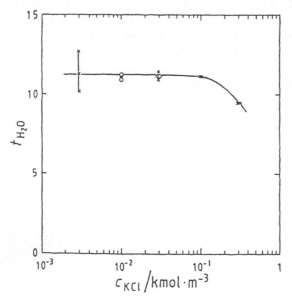

FIG. 6 The water transference number in the ionics membrane as a function of c_{KCl} in the aqueous solution [10].

associated with anion transport in the opposite direction. A similar decrease is found for t_w in Nafion at higher concentrations, 1 kmol/m^3 [16].

Water transference numbers for different ionic forms of Nafion are listed in Table 1. On the macroscopic level it looks like each ion carries a permanent number of water molecules. On a microscopic level, however, we cannot speak of a permanent number of water molecules transported with each ion. The water transport in electroosmosis or streaming potential measurements occur within seconds, common for all ions. The water molecules behaves very different, however, near the different cations in Table 1. For instance, the relaxation times for water rotation is in the picosecond (ps) range for water near all ions [26], but the *residence time* for water near an ion varies dramatically; from ps to weeks, increasing with the charge of the ion. It was shown that Na$^+$ in Nafion is surrounded in the nearest shell by less water molecules, than is transported by electroosmosis [33]. It is therefore not a permanent number of water molecules (for instance the waters of hydration) that follow an ion through the membrane. An average over all dynamic interactions along the transport path will, however, produce a reproducible number of water molecules per ion transported on the macroscopic level.

It is interesting to see from Table 1, that the ratio t_w/λ varies in the same manner as n_w/λ. It is likely that t_w for AM includes water, largely, but not exclusively (since $t_w > n_w$) from the hydrophilic domains of the membrane. Hydrophilic cations in the Nafion membrane, leads to an increase in t_w as well as in the water content. Surprisingly, the hydrophobic parts of the organic cations cause t_w to change largely, from 6 to 25, for an equilibrium water content, λ, that is almost constant [15]!

The trend for t_w in the Ionics membrane is similar to that in the Nafion membrane; t_w is higher in NaM (14.3) than in KM (10.7). The water transference numbers are higher in the Ionics than in the Nafion membrane. For KM we have 10.7 and 5.3, respectively. The water content in the Ionics membrane does not vary significantly [7].

In the HM membranes t_w is very small, even if the water content is large. Experiments with Nafion 117, show that the water transference number in the HM membrane, is also different when the membrane is in contact with a liquid system and when it is in contact with water vapor. The results are 2.6 [10,12,16] and 1.2 [14,25], respectively. Thermodynamically speaking, the water activity will be the same whether we have pure liquid water or saturated water vapor, and hence one should expect that the water content and water transference number in the membrane is the same in the two cases. One explanation is [14] that liquid water, starting from the surface, is able to rearrange the polymer chains in the membrane, thereby creating regions of higher polarity than water vapor can. Contact angle measurements by Zawodzinski et al. [34], support this explanation, showing that the surface of the Nafion 117 in contact with water vapor is very hydrophobic.

In two-component systems, a regularity appears for mixtures of monovalent cations. A linear relation is observed between t_w and the transference number of one of the ions [10]; meaning that transport of one of the ions does lead to transport of a certain amount of water, independent of the presence of the other ion. In asymmetric cation mixtures like for $KM-SrM_2$, the similar plot is non-linear; it even has a peak in $NaM-SrM_2$ at $t_{Na+} = 0.60$ [11]. This is shown in Fig. 7. No chloride was detected in the membrane. The water permeability is lower with SrM_2 than with NaM (see below). The enhancement in t_w must have its origin in a varying degree of cross-linkage and binding of Sr^{2+}. (See also Chap. 15, pp. 514–516.)

We have seen above that the transport of water in an electric field, as expressed by t_w, is largely determined by the nature of the ion, and not much by the water content in the membrane. Factors that increase the water transference number are hydrophobicity of the cation, valence, and/or membrane cross-linking. An explanation for the observed variation in t_w, must address the reversible nature of electroosmosis or its reciprocal phenomenon, the streaming potential experiment [as derived from Eq. (11)]. In the streaming potential experiment, water is forced through the membrane by a pressure gradient. We are concerned with the water transport that is reversibly linked

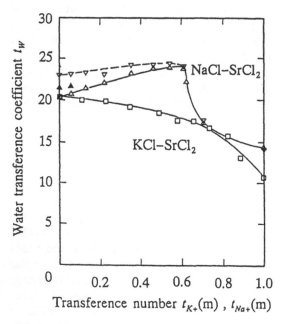

FIG. 7 The water transference number in $NaM-SrM_2$ and $KM-SrM_2$ ionics membranes [11].

to the ionic movement, that follows from the pressure gradient. Water that diffuses freely superimposed on charge transfer, is not relevant. We can explain the variation in the reversible water transfer, by a variation in the force (pressure difference) that is required to give current carrying ions a certain velocity. It is likely that strongly bound, divalent ions, or ions which are large and hydrophobic, require a larger force per ion moved, than ions that are loosely bound. The more cross-linked the membrane is, the higher the necessary force per cation. By changing the direction of the pressure difference, we can change the direction of the current (and the electric potential): The process is hence reversible. On the average, it follows that more water molecules should be transported per charge-carrying cation, with hydrophobic and divalent cations, than with monovalent cations. Similarly, t_w should increase with membrane tightness (the results for SrM_2–NaM). Also, one would expect that a relatively small force is required to move water with H^+. The source for water that accompanies the ions is clearly not only the membrane, since in some rare occasions one may also have $t_w > \lambda$.

B. Water Permeability

The water permeability, L_p, was determined for HM, KM, and SrM_2 as described in Sec. IV.C for the Ionics membrane. The value of L_p was larger in NaM than SrM_2, 2.4 and 0.9×10^{-14} m^2/s kg, respectively.

The water permeability in Nafion was higher than that in the Ionics membrane, by almost one order of magnitude [5]. When recalculated as a pressure diffusion constant, it gave values about 50 times higher than the self-diffusion constant of water. A smaller discrepancy was found for the Ionics membrane [16]. While the self-diffusion constant is a property of one molecule, diffusion is a bulk property. The pressure dependent part of the chemical potential, and the concentration dependent part should be equally effective per unit of force, see Eq. (5). When this is not so, the mechanism for water transport are not the same with the two forces. A pressure gradient can give extra contributions also from viscous forces. One would expect such contributions to vary with membrane water content, as described above.

The water permeability obtained in these measurements can be used to model transports with pressure gradients. They cannot be used to describe diffusion.

VII. ENTROPY TRANSPORT BY TRANSPORT OF IONS AND WATER

From the experiments described by Eq. (23) and Sec. IV.D [12] we determine the difference $S^*_{HM} - t_w S_w$ to be 13 J/K mol. Known values for S_w (69.9 J/K mol) and t_w(2.6) give $S^*_{HM} = 195$ J/K mol.

The calculated transported entropy is substantial, compared to that in water solutions. For HCl(aq) is reported $S^*_{HCl} = 22$ J/K mol, with water as the frame of reference for transport. The physical meaning of the transported entropy is still unclear. The meaning of a nonzero t_w is that protons are not transported without a simultaneous water transport. A distinction between the ionic contribution and the water contribution may therefore be artificial. More experiments are needed to study the variation of the transported entropy in membranes. In the meantime, knowledge of the experimental value can be used for modeling of thermal effects at the membrane surface (Chapter 14).

VIII. CONCLUSIONS

We have presented a systematic analysis of transport of heat, mass and charge in ion-exchange membranes using irreversible thermodynamics of bulk systems. With two cation exchange membranes as examples, one of them central for the fuel cell, we have shown how accurate transport properties can be obtained for the bulk membrane phase. Electrical transport properties of monovalent cation mixtures can be understood on the basis of a (nearly) statistical distribution of ions over the charged polymer, with the polymer network as a major obstruction for translational motion. The water transference number of the membrane is a linear function of the transport number of one ion in a mixture of monovalent ions. In the presence of divalent ions, this regularity breaks down. The water transference number seems to be determined by the relative ease of the ion's charge conducting ability. A possible contribution from viscous forces to the reported water permeabilities should be clarified. More data is needed to explain why the transported entropy in HM is so large.

The equations and data that are presented can be used to model ion-exchange membranes in operation. We have also discussed thermal sources at the interface. We shall use the data to model the polymer fuel cell in Chapter 14.

ACKNOWLEDGMENTS

We thank our co-authors who shared the efforts of producing the data.

LIST OF SYMBOLS

A   constant
A_m membrane area
b   constant in regular solution theory
c   molar concentration
D_i diffusion coefficient of i

E emf (in V)

F   Faraday's constant

f activity coefficient

H_i partial molar enthalpy

J_i flux of component (electrolyte) i

J'_q flux of measurable heat

J_V volume flux

j electric current density $[A/m^2 \ F]$

k interaction constant

L_p water permeability

L_{ij} phenomenological coefficient

l_m thickness of membrane

l_{ij} phenomenological coefficient for diffusion

n number of membranes

n_w moles water per moles sulfonic groups that freezes

p pressure

q^* heat of transfer

R universal gas constant

R_o resistant of liquid layer

R_m resistance of one membrane

R_{ml} resistance of one membrane and surrounding liquid layer

S entropy

S^* transported entropy

t time

t_i transference number of component i, or transport number of ion i

T absolute temperature

u_i electric mobility of ion i

V_i partial molar volume

x length

x_i mole fraction of component i

Δ a difference

$\Delta\varphi$ operational cell potential $(\Delta\varphi = EF)$

κ specific conductivity

λ number of water molecules per sulfonic acid group

μ_i chemical potential of component i

π Peltier heat

Θ entropy production per unit volume

REFERENCES

1. K. Scott and R. Hughes (eds.), *Industrial Membrane Separation Technology*, Chapmann and Hall, London, 1997.

2. F. Helfferich, *Ion-Exchange Membranes*, McGraw-Hill, New York, 1962.
3. R. H. Tromp, J. R. C. van der Maarel, J. de Bleijser, and J. C. Leyte, Biophys. Chem. *41*:81 (1991).
4. T. Okada, G. Xie, and Y. Tanabe, J. Electroanal. Chem. *413*:49 (1996).
5. G. Xie and T. Okada, Denki Kagaku *64*:718 (1996).
6. K. S. Førland, T. Okada, and S. Kjelstrup Ratkje, J. Electrochem. Soc. *140*:634 (1993).
7. T. Holt, T. Førland, and S. Kjelstrup Ratkje, J. Membrane Sci. *25*:133 (1985).
8. M. Skrede and S. Kjelstrup Ratkje, Z. Phys. Chem. Neue Folge. *155*:211 (1987).
9. M. Ottøy, T. Førland, S. Kjelstrup Ratkje, and S. Møller-Holst, J. Membrane Sci. *74*:1 (1992).
10. T. Okada, S. Kjelstrup Ratkje, and H. Hanche-Olsen, J. Membrane Sci. *66*:179 (1992).
11. T. Okada, S. Kjelstrup Ratkje, S. Møller-Holst, L. O. Jerdal, K. Friestad, G. Xie, and R. Holmen, J. Membrane Sci. *111*:159 (1996).
12. S. Kjelstrup Ratkje, M. Ottøy, R. Halseid, and M. Strømgård, J. Membrane Sci. *107*:219 (1995).
13. M. Ottøy and S. Kjelstrup Ratkje, Proceedings of the International Symposium of Electrochemical Science and Technology, August 24–26, Hong Kong, 1995.
14. M. Ottøy, Mass and heat transfer in ion-exchange membranes; applicable to solid polymer fuel cells, Dr.Ing. Thesis No. 47, Norwegian University of Science and Technology, Trondheim, 1996.
15. G. Xie and T. Okada, J. Chem. Soc. Faraday Trans. *92*:663 (1996).
16. G. Xie and T. Okada, J. Electrochem. Soc. *142*:3057 (1995).
17. T. Okada, N. Nakamura, M. Yuasa, and I. Sekine, J. Electrochem. Soc. *144*:2744 (1997).
18. K. S. Førland, T. Førland, and S. Kjelstrup Ratkje, *Irreversible Thermodynamics. Theory and Applications*, 2nd reprint, Wiley, Chichester, 1992.
19. S. R. de Groot and P. Mazur, *Nonequilibrium Thermodynamics*, North-Holland, Amsterdam, 1962, and Dover, New York, 1985.
20. A. M. Albano and D. Bedeaux, Physica. *147A*:407 (1988).
21. B. Hafskjold and S. Kjelstrup Ratkje, J. Stat. Phys. *78*:463 (1995).
22. T. D. Gierke, G. E. Munn, and F. C. Wilson, J. Polymer Sci. Polym. Phys. Ed. *19*:1687 (1981).
23. W. E. Roorda, J. de Bleijser, H. E. Junginger, and J. C. Leyte, Biomaterials *11*:17 (1990).
24. H. van Keulen, Solutions and applications of the Poisson–Boltzmann equation for the description of ion sorption and diffusion in charged systems of various geometries, Ph.D. Thesis, Leiden University, Netherlands, 1987.
25. T. E. Springer, T. A. Zawodzinski and S. Gottesfeld, J. Electrochem. Soc. *138*:334 (1991).
26. J. R. C. van der Maarel, Magnetic relaxation study of the structure and dynamics of water, Ph.D. Thesis, Leiden University, Netherlands, 1987.
27. T. Okada, S. Møller-Holst, O. Gorseth, and S. Kjelstrup, J. Electroanal. Chem. *442*:137 (1998).
28. E. Høgfeldt, Reactive Polymers *2*:19 (1984).

29. R. Haase, *Thermodynamics of Irreversible Processes*, Addison-Wesley, Reading, Massachusetts, 1969.
30. E. L. Dougherty and H. G. Drickamer, J. Phys. Chem. *59*:443 (1950).
31. K. Hanaoka, R. Kiyono, and M. Tasaka, J. Membrane Sci. *107*:219 (1993).
32. T. Ojala and K. Kontturi, Acta Chem. Scand. *42*:698 (1988).
33. T. Ojala and K. Kontturi, Acta Chem. Scand. *43*:340 (1989).
34. R. A. Komorski and K. A. Mauritz, J. Am. Chem. Soc. *100*:7487 (1978).
35. T. A. Zawodzinski, T. E. Springer, F. Uribe, and S. Gottesfeld, Solid State Ionics. *60*:199 (1993).

14

Irreversible Thermodynamics of Membrane Surface Transport with Application to Polymer Fuel Cells

SIGNE KJELSTRUP and PREBEN J. S. VIE   Department of Physical Chemistry, Norwegian University of Science and Technology, Trondheim, Norway

DICK BEDEAUX   Leiden Institute of Chemistry, Gorlaeus Laboratory, Leiden University, Leiden, The Netherlands

Abstract

Irreversible thermodynamics for bulk systems and surfaces is applied to the solid polymer fuel cell. The cell is composed of three bulk phases (the membrane and the electrodes) and two membrane–electrode interfaces. The electric potential profile in the cell is calculated, using literature data for the membrane and the electrode, for the isothermal, isobaric single, polymer fuel cell. The overpotential is defined. The temperature profile compatible with the emf measurement, is given for electrode backing materials that are thermostated on the outside.

I.   INTRODUCTION

Irreversible thermodynamics is a well established theory that describes transport in bulk systems, see e.g., de Groot and Mazur [1]. When this theory is used to describe membrane transport, one has frequently assumed that there is equilibrium across the membrane–electrolyte interface (for a discussion, see Chapter 13). This assumption need not be fulfilled in practice, in particularly not in electrochemical systems, when there is an electrode attached to the membrane. When heat, mass and charge is transported across the membrane–electrode interface, the interface may have an energy which is different from the surroundings. Bedeaux and coworkers [2,3] have extended the theory of irreversible thermodynamics so that it is capable of dealing with interfaces. Their theory introduces the surface or interface as a separate thermodynamic system following Gibbs [4]. By allowing the interface to have its own thermodynamic variables, it becomes possible to describe interfaces which are not in equilibrium with adjacent bulk phases. The versatility of irreversible thermodynamics has thus been increased. Bedeaux and coworkers have since 1990 used irreversible thermodynamics for bulk systems and for interfaces to model heat and mass transport across liquid–gas interfaces [5,6] and in electrochemical cells [7–9].

The solid polymer fuel cell is today the most promising fuel cell for the transport sector, alone or in combination with batteries (hybrid engines). The cell produces electric energy from hydrogen and oxygen, usually between 70 and 90°C. In the NECAR-model from Daimler–Benz, hydrogen is being supplied by water vapor reformation of methanol to a stack of fuel cells. Water is produced at the cathode, but must also be added to the anode at stationary state operation, to prevent the membrane from drying out. We shall study the energy conversion, and solve the coupled set of equations for heat, mass and charge transport in a one-dimensional single cell, using irreversible thermodynamics for the bulk parts of the cell [1] and for the electrode–membrane interfaces [2,3,7–9]. We have chosen to illustrate the method by applying it to the solid polymer fuel cell, because of its future potential. The cell has been modeled extensively in the literature, and the description using irreversible thermodynamics can therefore be compared to well documented descriptions, for instance Refs. 10 and 11.

There are three bulk parts in the single cell; the membrane and the backing materials for the electrode catalyst surface. There are two interfaces; the membrane–electrode interfaces between the backing materials and the membrane. The aim is to demonstrate irreversible thermodynamics for this heterogeneous system. This shall be done by a detailed calculation of the electric potential profile through the cell. The electric potential profile is also integrated to give the cell potential. From thermodynamic data for the electrode catalyst surface [12,13], we estimate the emf of the isothermal, isobaric cell. The definitions of the anode and cathode overpotentials that follow from the theory are presented. We shall see that we can address also the pressure and temperature gradients in the cell.

II. SYSTEM DESCRIPTION

A. The Membrane–Electrolyte Interface as a Thermodynamic System

The membrane–electrode interfaces in the polymer fuel cell are illustrated in Fig. 1, see parts labeled 2. Both membrane–electrode interfaces are regions of about 10 μm thick between the carbon backing material and the polymer membrane. In this region one has three-phase contacts; because the electrode reaction requires contact between the electronic conductor (platinum on carbon), the ionic conductor (membrane), and the gas. We assume that the interface regions are electroneutral. Interface polarization, from excess protons and compensating negative charges in the metal, is possible, however. This membrane–electrode interface can be regarded as a thermodynamic system, separate from the adjacent membrane or electrode backing material (parts 1 and 3 in Fig. 1, respectively) according to Gibbs [4]. The interface that we study is thicker than that Gibbs discussed, but this does not change the arguments for the method of treatment.

Gibbs introduced extensive variables of the surface as excess variables [4]. The excess internal energy of an interface is then obtained by integrating the

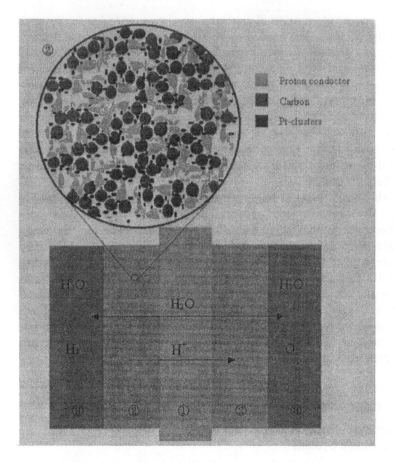

FIG. 1 The symmetric cell arrangement. (1) denotes the membrane, (2) the electrode catalyst region (see insert) and (3) is the electrode backing material. Transport of protons is from left to right. Courtesy of S. Møller-Holst [16].

internal energy across the interface and subtracting the extrapolated values of the internal energies of the adjacent bulk phases. Through such an integration procedure, we can obtain all excess densities per unit of interface area. These variables are denoted (s, a) and (s, c) in the present work; for the anode and cathode interface, respectively. The interface thickness of about 10 μm disappears as a variable by integration across the thickness. Gibbs [4] places the excess densities of an interface on an equal footing with the bulk phase densities, in his discussion of thermodynamics of heterogeneous media. As a frame of reference for the fluxes into and out of the interface, we take the nonmoving, equimolar surface of the Nafion membrane. This choice has the advantage that its location does not depend on the time in the experiment.

Existence of excess energy-, entropy- and mass densities, (u^s, s^s, n_i^s), implies that the surface also possesses its own temperature, $T^s = (\partial u^s/\partial s^s)_{n_i^s}$, and chemical potentials, $\mu_i^s = (\partial u^s/\partial n_i^s)_{s^s, n_j^s}$. The fundamental assumption in irreversible thermodynamics is that of local equilibrium [1]. By local equilibrium in an interface we mean that the normal thermodynamic relations are valid for the interface excess variables [2,3]. An assessment of this assumption should be done on the basis of the results that can be derived from it. In the present context we shall use surface thermodynamic variables to derive expressions for the overpotential of the electrodes. The variables of the expression are accessible by experiments which render the results open to independent experimental tests.

B. Fuel Cell Processes

A schematic picture of the solid polymer single cell was shown in Fig. 1. We described the electrode–membrane interfaces above. These interfaces are the anode and the cathode of the cell, respectively. The electrolyte is a water-containing, proton-conducting membrane (part 1). The electrode backing on each side consist of porous carbon impregnated with Teflon (parts 3).

Hydrogen gas diffuses to the interface through pores in the anode backing, and produces protons by oxidation of atomic hydrogen adsorbed in the interface [12,13]:

$$\tfrac{1}{2}H_2(g, a) \rightarrow H(s, a) \tag{1}$$

$$H(s, a) \rightarrow H^+(s, a) + e^-(s, a) \tag{2}$$

Here (g, a) denotes the gas phase in the pores close to the anode.

The membrane electrolyte contains between 10 and 15 molecules of water per ionic site [10]. Water must be supplied to the anode interface in order to prevent the membrane from drying out. In the stationary state there is a constant amount of water transported to the anode interface, calculated as t_w^a moles per Coulomb

$$t_w^a H_2O(g, a) \rightarrow t_w^a H_2O(s, a) \tag{3}$$

Proton conduction in the membrane electrolyte does not take place without water transport. The moles of water transported per Coulomb (the electro-osmotic effect) is t_w^m:

$$H^+(m, a) \rightarrow H^+(m, c) \tag{4}$$

$$t_w^m H_2O(m, a) \rightarrow t_w^m H_2O(m, c) \tag{5}$$

The side of the membrane facing the anode is denoted (m, a), while the side of the membrane facing the cathode is denoted (m, c).

At the cathode interface, protons react with adsorbed oxygen and produce water:

$$H^+(s, c) + \tfrac{1}{4}O_2(s, c) + e^-(s, c) \rightarrow \tfrac{1}{2}H_2O(s, c) \tag{6}$$

Oxygen gas migrates through the porous carbon backing on the cathode side:

$$\tfrac{1}{4}O_2(g, c) \rightarrow \tfrac{1}{4}O_2(s, c) \tag{7}$$

Water disappears from the cathode interface as vapor through the porous carbon:

$$t_w^c\, H_2O(s, c) \rightarrow t_w^c\, H_2O(g, c) \tag{8}$$

In the stationary state the amount of water vapor transported in carbon backing is t_w^c moles per Coulomb.

Diffusion in the carbon backing material is here taken to be fast. The Gibbs energy change of the cell reaction is normally written as:

$$\Delta_r G = \tfrac{1}{2}\mu_{H_2O}^{g,c} - \tfrac{1}{4}\mu_{O_2}^{g,c} - \tfrac{1}{2}\mu_{H_2}^{g,a} \tag{9}$$

Experience shows that not all of this chemical energy can be converted into electric energy, not even when very small currents are drawn from the cell. The ohmic losses in the cell are substantial for current densities of the order of 10^4 A/m². The overpotential, of the cathode mainly, reduces the cell potential similarly. It is one of the purposes of this work to describe interface potential drops and the anode and cathode overpotentials within the framework of irreversible thermodynamics. We shall thus locate, describe and explain the origin of the electric potential profile, as well as the sources of the dissipated energy. The temperature profile will also be discussed.

III. CONSERVATION OF CHARGE, MASS AND ENERGY IN THE INTERFACES AND THE BULK PHASES

The analysis of the system is restricted to stationary state conditions and transport in one direction only. The conservation equations of charge, mass and energy then take a simple form. It follows from electroneutrality that the electric current density j is constant throughout the cell. This is also true in the nonstationary state if one uses the condition of charge neutrality. Polarization is usually small in bulk phases [1]. At an interface, one may not neglect the polarization. For a constant electric current, the interface polarization is constant, however.

Furthermore, the flux of hydrogen gas in the carbon backing on the anode side (a), and oxygen gas in the carbon backing on the cathode side (c) are constant and given in terms of the electric current density by:

$$2J_{H_2}^a = -4J_{O_2}^c = j/F \tag{10}$$

The water flux is constant in the carbon backing on the anode side and in the bulk membrane, continuous through the anode interface and given by

$$J_w^a = J_w^m \tag{11}$$

At the cathode interface, water is produced according to Eq. (6) so that the constant water flux in the carbon backing on the cathode side is given by

$$J_w^c = J_w^m + j/2F \tag{12}$$

The total energy flux J_e in the system (cf. de Groot and Mazur [1] for a definition) is everywhere constant and continuous through the electrode interfaces. It is given in terms of the physical heat flux $J_q'^i$, where $i = $ a (anode side), m (membrane) or c (cathode side), in the bulk sections, the comoving partial enthalpies of formation, and the electric current times the potential ϕ:

$$
\begin{aligned}
J_e &= J_q'^{g,\,a} + J_{H_2}^a h_{H_2}^{g,\,a} + J_w^a h_w^{g,\,a} + j\phi^{g,\,a} = J_q'^{m,\,a} + J_w^m h_w^{m,\,a} + j\phi^{m,\,a} \\
&= J_q'^{m,\,c} + J_w^m h_w^{m,\,c} + j\phi^{m,\,c} \\
&= J_q'^{g,\,c} + J_{O_2}^c h_{O_2}^{g,\,c} + J_w^c h_w^{g,\,c} + j\phi^{g,\,c}
\end{aligned}
\tag{13}
$$

The total energy flux, which must not be confused with the internal energy flux, is transformed partly into electric power through the reactions that take place in the membrane–electrode interfaces. The transformations in the interface are described in Sec. IV.B and Sec. IV.C below. In the carbon backing material on both sides, the gas fluxes, the water flux and the electric current density are constant. In the membrane, the water flux and the electric current density are constant. The enthalpies here depend on local densities and temperatures. Because the total energy flux is constant throughout, the often substantial changes of the enthalpies when we are crossing an interface, lead to corresponding changes in the measurable heat flux.

IV. THE ENTROPY PRODUCTION RATE AND THE FLUX EQUATIONS

We consider transport per unit area in the x-direction across the membrane of a single cell, and start by finding suitable expressions for the entropy production rates. The frame of reference for the fluxes is the nonmoving surfaces (the equimolar surface of Nafion).

A. The Bulk Phases

In the bulk membrane, there is transport of heat, water and charge (protons). In the carbon backing charge is transported as electrons. The transport of hydrogen on the anode side, and of oxygen on the cathode side are both given in terms of the electric current in the stationary state. These elements therefore need not be considered separately. Thus in all three bulk phases, the entropy production rate is according to de Groot and Mazur [1]:

$$\sigma = J_q' \frac{d}{dx}\left(\frac{1}{T}\right) - J_w \frac{1}{T}\frac{d\mu_{w,T}}{dx} - j\frac{1}{T}\frac{d\phi}{dx} \tag{14}$$

where J_q' is the measurable heat flux, J_w is the water flux, and j is the electric current density. The conjugate forces of these fluxes are $(d/dx)(1/T) = -(1/T^2)(dT/dx)$, $-(1/T)(d\mu_{w,T}/dx)$, and $-(1/T)(d\phi/dx)$, where T is the temperature, $\mu_{w,T}$ the chemical potential of water at constant temperature and ϕ the (operational) electric potential that refer to given electrodes. The flux equations for the membrane are accordingly:

$$J_q' = -\frac{L_{qq}}{T}\frac{dT}{dx} - L_{qw}\frac{d\mu_{w,T}}{dx} - L_{q\phi}\frac{d\phi}{dx} \tag{15}$$

$$J_w = -\frac{L_{wq}}{T}\frac{dT}{dx} - L_{ww}\frac{d\mu_{w,T}}{dx} - L_{w\phi}\frac{d\phi}{dx} \tag{16}$$

$$j = -\frac{L_{\phi q}}{T}\frac{dT}{dx} - L_{\phi w}\frac{d\mu_{w,T}}{dx} - L_{\phi\phi}\frac{d\phi}{dx} \tag{17}$$

where L_{ij} are Onsager coefficients, and $L_{ij} = L_{ji}$ holds, see Ref. 1. The coefficients contain a factor $1/T$ from the forces.

In the pores of the carbon backing, we have transport of heat and gas, and in the carbon itself, electric charge is transported. We have assumed, as a first approximation, that diffusion of hydrogen and oxygen is fast, or that their chemical potential gradients are zero. We could in principle make the same approximation for the chemical potential of the water in the carbon backing. This reduces the set to two equations for J_q' and j. As we have to take J_w along in the membrane, we give the more general form for all three bulk phase, rather than giving specialized expressions for each bulk phase separately.

By solving the last equation for $d\phi/dx$, we can write the constitutive equations in the following form

$$J_q' = -\lambda\frac{dT}{dx} - l_{qw}\frac{d\mu_{w,T}}{dx} + \pi j \tag{18}$$

$$J_w = -\frac{l_{wq}}{T}\frac{dT}{dx} - l_{ww}\frac{d\mu_{w,T}}{dx} + t_w j \tag{19}$$

$$\frac{d\phi}{dx} = -\frac{\pi}{T}\frac{dT}{dx} - t_w\frac{d\mu_{w,T}}{dx} - rj \tag{20}$$

Here $\lambda = (L_{qq} - L_{q\phi}L_{\phi q}/L_{\phi\phi})/T$ is the (Fourier) thermal conductivity in W/m K, $l_{qw} = l_{wq} = L_{qw} - L_{q\phi}L_{\phi w}/L_{\phi\phi}$, $\pi = L_{q\phi}/L_{\phi\phi}$ is the Peltier coefficient in J/C, $l_{ww} = L_{ww} - L_{w\phi}L_{\phi w}/L_{\phi\phi}$, $t_w = L_{wq}/L_{\phi\phi}$ is the transference coefficient introduced earlier, and $r = 1/L_{\phi\phi}$ is the electrical resistivity in ohm m. We have chosen a definition of the transference coefficient such that its dimension is mol/C. This coefficient will then be given by the more usual transport number (which is dimensionless) multiplied by Faraday's constant (96,500 C/mol). The last equation gives the electric potential gradient in the bulk phases (in the unit V/m). The expression can be integrated to obtain the potential differences across these parts. The current density is given in A/m^2. It is common to model the potential drop across the membrane by the last term only, the resistance drop [10]. This means that the cell is normally taken to be isothermal and isobaric.

For the different bulk phases we have:

$$\pi^a = T[(S_e^* + \tfrac{1}{2}S_{H_2})/F + t_w^a S_w^a] \tag{21}$$

$$\pi^m = T[S_{H^+}^*/F - t_w^m S_w^m] \tag{22}$$

$$\pi^c = T[(S_e^* - \tfrac{1}{4}S_{O_2})/F - t_w^c S_w^c] \tag{23}$$

Here S_i is the entropy and S_i^* is the transported entropy of i. The first equation says that heat (entropy) is transported with electrons, hydrogen and water across the carbon backing on the anode side [15]. The second says that heat is transported with protons and water across the membrane. The third expresses that electrons, oxygen and water carry heat through the carbon backing on the cathode side.

The transference coefficients satisfy

$$t_w^a = t_w^m = t_w^c - \frac{1}{2F} \tag{24}$$

The first identity says that the need for water transport in the membrane determines the water transport to the anode interface. After the reaction at the cathode interface, half an additional molecule of water is carried along per charge carrier. We shall find the variation in ϕ, μ_w and T across the cell, for given different current densities j, and given boundary conditions. The membrane–electrode interfaces play an important role in the energy conversion and dissipation. They give the boundary conditions for integrations across the three bulk phases as will be explained below.

B. The Anode Interface

A schematic illustration of the fluxes into and out of the anode interface is given in Fig. 2. The entropy production rate is [2,3]:

$$\sigma^{s,a} = -J_q^{'g,a} \frac{T^{s,a} - T^{g,a}}{T^{s,a}T^{g,a}} - J_q^{'m,a} \frac{T^{m,a} - T^{s,a}}{T^{s,a}T^{m,a}} - J_w^{g,a} \frac{1}{T^{s,a}} (\mu_{w,T}^{s,a} - \mu_{w,T}^{g,a})$$

$$- J_w^{m,a} \frac{1}{T^{s,a}} (\mu_{w,T}^{m,a} - \mu_{w,T}^{s,a}) - j \frac{1}{T^{s,a}} \Delta\phi^{s,a} - v^{s,a} \frac{A^{s,a}}{T^{s,a}} \tag{25}$$

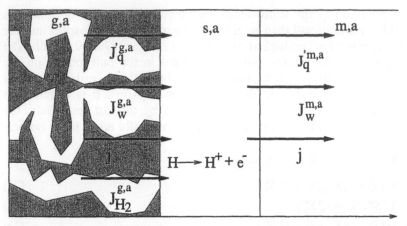

FIG. 2 Fluxes of heat (J'_q), water (J_w), current (j) and hydrogen (J_{H_2}) into and out of the anode interface. The carbon backing close to the interface is denoted (g, a), the anode interface (s, a) and the membrane close to the interface (m, a).

The thermodynamic variables for the interface were defined in Sec. II. There are two heat fluxes connected with an interface. One heat flux into (or out if the sign is negative) the interface from the carbon backing, $J'^{g,\,a}_q$, has the conjugate force $-(T^{s,\,a} - T^{g,\,a})/T^{s,\,a}T^{g,\,a}$. The other heat flux out of (or into, if the sign is negative) the interface into the membrane, $J'^{m,\,a}_q$, has the conjugate force $-(T^{m,\,a} - T^{s,\,a})T^{m,\,a}T^{s,\,a}$. Similarly, there are two water fluxes, $J^{g,\,a}_w$ and $J^{m,\,a}_w$ with conjugate forces $-(\mu^{s,\,a}_{w,\,T} - \mu^{g,\,a}_{w,\,T})/T^{s,\,a}$ and $-(\mu^{m,\,a}_{w,\,T} - \mu^{s,\,a}_{w,\,T})/T^{s,\,a}$, respectively. The electric current density, j, through the interface, has the conjugate force $-\Delta\phi^{s,a}/T^{s,\,a} = -(\phi^{m,\,a} - \phi^{g,\,a})/T^{s,\,a}$. We have assumed that the interface has a constant polarization for a given constant j. Thus, there is no contribution to σ^s from the displacement current.

According to Eqs. (1) and (2), the reaction $\frac{1}{2}H_2(g) \rightarrow H^+ + e^-$ goes in two steps via atomic hydrogen. The total reaction is also illustrated in Fig. 1. The contribution to the entropy production rate from the flux of $H_2(g)$ into the interface is contained in the last term. This term is the product of the electrode reaction rate, $v^{s,\,a}$, and the affinity, $A^{s,\,a}$, of the total reaction at the anode. The affinity is equivalent to Gibbs energy change for the anode reaction. The reaction rate is given in terms of the current density by:

$$v^{s,\,a} = j/F \tag{26}$$

This reaction rate refers to one mole electrons produced. The overall affinity is:

$$A^{s,\,a} = \mu^{s,\,a}_{H^+} + \mu^{s,\,a}_{e^-} - \frac{1}{2}\mu^{g,\,a}_{H_2} \tag{27}$$

Experimental data [12,13] support the view that hydrogen is adsorbed in atomic form at Pt, and that the chemical potential of the adsorbed atom is the same, whether it is chemisorbed or electrochemically adsorbed.

$$\mu_{H}^{s,\,a} = \mu_{H^+}^{s,\,a} + \mu_{e^-}^{s,\,a} \tag{28}$$

With Eq. (28), the rate limiting step is the first one, with the affinity:

$$A^{s,\,a} = \mu_{H}^{s,\,a} - \tfrac{1}{2}\mu_{H_2}^{g,\,a} \tag{29}$$

We estimate the affinity in Sec. V.

By introducing the assumptions and the flux dependencies of Eq. (26) into Eq. (25), we find:

$$\sigma^{s,\,a} = -J_{q}^{\prime g,\,a}\,\frac{\Delta T^{g,\,a}}{T^{s,\,a}T^{g,\,a}} - J_{q}^{\prime m,\,a}\,\frac{\Delta T^{m,\,a}}{T^{s,\,a}T^{m,\,a}} - J_{w}^{g,\,a}\,\frac{1}{T^{s,\,a}}\,\Delta\mu_{w,\,T}^{g,\,a}$$
$$- J_{w}^{m,\,a}\,\frac{1}{T^{s,\,a}}\,\Delta\mu_{w,\,T}^{m,\,a} - j\,\frac{1}{T^{s,\,a}}\left[\Delta\phi^{s,\,a} + \frac{A^{s,\,a}}{F}\right] \tag{30}$$

with $\Delta T^{g,\,a} = T^{s,\,a} - T^{g,\,a}$ and $\Delta T^{m,\,a} = T^{m,\,a} - T^{s,\,a}$. There are similar definitions for the chemical potential differences. The flux equations follow from the entropy production:

$$J_{q}^{\prime g,\,a} = -l_{qq}^{a,\,g}\,\frac{\Delta T^{g,\,a}}{T^{g,\,a}} - l_{qq}^{a,\,gm}\,\frac{\Delta T^{m,\,a}}{T^{m,\,a}} - l_{qw}^{a,\,g}\,\Delta\mu_{w,\,T}^{g,\,a} - l_{qw}^{a,\,gm}\,\Delta\mu_{w,\,T}^{m,\,a} + \pi^{a}j \tag{31}$$

$$J_{q}^{\prime m,\,a} = -l_{qq}^{a,\,mg}\,\frac{\Delta T^{g,\,a}}{T^{g,\,a}} - l_{qq}^{a,\,m}\,\frac{\Delta T^{m,\,a}}{T^{m,\,a}} - l_{qw}^{a,\,mg}\,\Delta\mu_{w,\,T}^{g,\,a} - l_{qw}^{a,\,m}\,\Delta\mu_{w,\,T}^{m,\,a} + \pi^{m}j \tag{32}$$

$$J_{w}^{g,\,a} = -l_{wq}^{a,\,g}\,\frac{\Delta T^{g,\,a}}{T^{g,\,a}} - l_{wq}^{a,\,gm}\,\frac{\Delta T^{m,\,a}}{T^{m,\,a}} - l_{ww}^{a,\,g}\,\Delta\mu_{w,\,T}^{g,\,a} - l_{ww}^{a,\,gm}\,\Delta\mu_{w,\,T}^{m,\,a} + t_{w}^{a}j \tag{33}$$

$$J_{w}^{m,\,a} = -l_{wq}^{a,\,mg}\,\frac{\Delta T^{g,\,a}}{T^{g,\,a}} - l_{wq}^{a,\,m}\,\frac{\Delta T^{m,\,a}}{T^{m,\,a}} - l_{ww}^{a,\,mg}\,\Delta\mu_{w,\,T}^{g,\,a} - l_{ww}^{a,\,m}\,\Delta\mu_{w,\,T}^{m,\,a} + t_{w}^{m}j \tag{34}$$

$$\Delta\phi^{A} = -\pi^{a}\,\frac{\Delta T^{g,\,a}}{T^{g,\,a}} - \pi^{m}\,\frac{\Delta T^{m,\,a}}{T^{m,\,a}} - t_{w}^{a}\,\Delta\mu_{w,\,T}^{g,\,a} - t_{w}^{m}\,\Delta\mu_{w,\,T}^{m,\,a} - r^{s,\,a}j \tag{35}$$

The coefficients include the common factor $1/T^{s,\,a}$. Their subscript indicate first the flux and then force that is relevant. Their superscripts indicate first the region (here the anode), then the side(s) of the interface that are involved (g, m or both; gm). We calculate the electric potential jump across the anode in terms of the effective electric potential $\Delta\phi^{A}$ from:

$$\Delta\phi^{s,\,a} = \Delta\phi^{A} - \frac{1}{F}\,A^{s,\,a} = \Delta\phi^{A} - \frac{1}{F}\left(\mu_{H}^{s,\,a} - \frac{1}{2}\mu_{H_2}^{g,\,a}\right) \tag{36}$$

The Peltier heats and the transference coefficients for the anode interface are identical to the bulk values in the adjacent bulk phase. The interface has an excess electric resistance, $r^{s,a}$. Due to Onsager symmetry the l-matrix is symmetric.

Mass and heat fluxes into the anode interface from the carbon backing have cross-coefficients similar to the same fluxes in the carbon backing. This is also true for fluxes from the interface into the membrane. The coupling coefficients across the interface are probably less important. We shall therefore neglect the coupling coefficients across the interface, i.e., we take $l_{qq}^{a,gm} = l_{qq}^{a,mg} = l_{qw}^{a,gm} = l_{wq}^{a,gm} = l_{qw}^{a,mg} = l_{wq}^{a,mg} = l_{ww}^{a,mg} = l_{ww}^{a,gm} = 0$. The constitutive relations then reduce to

$$J_q^{'g,a} = -l_{qq}^{a,g} \frac{\Delta T^{g,a}}{T^{g,a}} - l_{qw}^{ag} \Delta \mu_{w,T}^{g,a} + \pi^a j \tag{37}$$

$$J_w^{g,a} = -l_{wq}^{a,g} \frac{\Delta T^{g,a}}{T^{g,a}} - l_{ww}^{a,g} \Delta \mu_{w,T}^{g,a} + t_w^a j \tag{38}$$

for the heat and water fluxes in terms of the temperature jump, the chemical potential jump and the electric current into the anode interface from the carbon backing. On the membrane side of the interface one similarly obtains

$$J_q^{'m,a} = -l_{qq}^{a,m} \frac{\Delta T^{m,a}}{T^{m,a}} - l_{qw}^{a,m} \Delta \mu_{w,T}^{m,a} + \pi^m j \tag{39}$$

$$J_w^{m,a} = -l_{wq}^{a,m} \frac{\Delta T^{m,a}}{T^{m,a}} - l_{ww}^{a,m} \Delta \mu_{w,T}^{m,a} + t_w^m j \tag{40}$$

The expression for the electrical potential jump, Eq. (35), remains the same.

C. The Cathode Interface

The excess entropy production rate of the cathode interface is:

$$\sigma^{s,c} = -J_q^{'m,c} \frac{T^{s,c} - T^{m,c}}{T^{s,c} T^{m,c}} - J_q^{'g,c} \frac{T^{g,c} - T^{s,c}}{T^{s,c} T^{s,c}} - J_w^{m,c} \frac{1}{T^{s,c}} (\mu_{w,T}^{s,c} - \mu_{w,T}^{m,c}) \tag{41}$$

$$- J_w^{g,c} \frac{1}{T^{s,c}} (\mu_{w,T}^{g,c} - \mu_{w,T}^{s,c}) - \frac{1}{T^{s,c}} j \Delta \phi^{s,c} - \frac{1}{T^{s,c}} v^{s,c} A^{s,a} \tag{42}$$

The symbols have the same meaning as described above for the anode interface, they refer now, however, to the cathode interface. The stationary state reaction rate is again:

$$v^{s,c} = j/F \tag{43}$$

and the chemical reaction Eq. (6) has affinity:

$$A^{s, c} = \tfrac{1}{2}\mu_w^{g, c} - \mu_H^{s, c} - \tfrac{1}{4}\mu_{O_2}^{g, c} \tag{44}$$

where we have used again the assumption $\mu_H^{s, c} = \mu_{H^+}^{m, c} + \mu_{e^-}^{g, c}$. The entropy production rate becomes:

$$\sigma^{s, c} = -J_q'^{m, c}\frac{\Delta T^{m, c}}{T^{s, c}T^{m, c}} - J_q'^{g, c}\frac{\Delta T^{g, c}}{T^{s, c}T^{g, c}} - J_w^{m, c}\frac{1}{T^{s, c}}\Delta\mu_{w, T}^{m, c} \tag{45}$$

$$- J_w^{m, c}\frac{1}{T^{s, c}}\Delta\mu_{w, T}^{g, c} - j\frac{\Delta\phi^C}{T^{s, c}} \tag{46}$$

with the effective electric force, $\Delta\phi^C$. The effective electrical potential, in terms of the electric potential jump across the cathode interface, is:

$$\Delta\phi^{s, c} = \Delta\phi^C - \frac{1}{F}A^{s, c} = \Delta\phi^C - \frac{1}{F}\left(\frac{1}{2}\mu_w^{g, c} - \mu_H^{s, c} - \frac{1}{4}\mu_{O_2}^{g, c}\right) \tag{47}$$

Neglecting again the coupling coefficients *across* the interface for heat and water flow the constitutive relations become

$$J_q'^{m, c} = -l_{qq}^{c, m}\frac{\Delta T^{m, c}}{T^{m, c}} - l_{qw}^{c, m}\Delta\mu_{w, T}^{c, m} + \pi^m j \tag{48}$$

$$J_w^m = -l_{wq}^{c, m}\frac{\Delta T^{m, c}}{T^{m, c}} - l_{ww}^{c, m}\Delta\mu_{w, T}^{m, c} + t_w^m j \tag{49}$$

for the membrane side of the interface, and

$$J_q'^{g, c} = -l_{qq}^{c, g}\frac{\Delta T^{g, c}}{T^{g, c}} - l_{qw}^{c, g}\Delta\mu_{w, T}^{g, c} + \pi^c j \tag{50}$$

$$J_w^c = -l_{wq}^{c, g}\frac{\Delta T^{g, c}}{T^{g, c}} - l_{ww}^{c, g}\Delta\mu_{w, T}^{g, c} + t_w^c j \tag{51}$$

for the cathode side of the interface. The effective electrical potential is given by

$$\Delta\phi^C = -\pi^m\frac{\Delta T^{m, c}}{T^{m, c}} - \pi^c\frac{\Delta T^{g, c}}{T^{g, c}} - t_w^m\Delta\mu_{w, T}^{m, c} - t_w^c\Delta\mu_{w, T}^{g, c} - r^{s, c}j \tag{52}$$

This expression can be used with Eq. (47) to find the electric potential jump across the cathode interface.

V. THE CELL POTENTIAL AND THE ELECTRODE OVERPOTENTIALS

A. The Cell Potential

The local cell potential variation, $\phi(x)$, can be calculated for each part of the cell. The integration of the electric potential is carried out over the carbon backing on the anode side, Eq. (20); the anode interface, Eqs. (35) and (36); the membrane electrolyte, Eq. (20); the cathode interface, Eqs. (52) and (47), and the carbon backing on the cathode side, Eq. (20). The integration starts in the carbon backing at a point with a distance d^a from the anode interface. The temperature and the chemical potential of water at this point are T_0^a and $\mu_{w,\,o}^a$, respectively. The integration ends at a point in the carbon backing on the cathode side with a distance d^c from the cathode interface. The temperature and the chemical potential of the water at this point are T_0^c and $\mu_{w,\,o}^c$. We calculate the complete electric potential profile across the cell, using these equations and conditions in Sec. VII. We investigate the interface potential jumps in the next subsection, and the variations in the same in Sec. V.C.

The total cell potential is the sum of all contributions:

$$\Delta\phi = \int_a^{g,\,a} d\phi + \Delta\phi^{s,\,a} + \int_{e,\,a}^{e,\,c} d\phi + \Delta\phi^{s,\,c} + \int_{g,\,c}^{c} d\phi \tag{53}$$

By introducing all appropriate expressions, using constant entropies in the Peltier coefficients, and constant transference coefficients and electrical resistances, we obtain:

$$\begin{aligned}
\Delta\phi = & \left\{ -\left[\frac{1}{2F}\mu_w^{g,\,c} - \frac{1}{4F}\mu_{O_2}^{g,\,c} - \frac{1}{2F}\mu_{H_2}^{g,\,a} \right] + \frac{1}{F}[\mu_H^{s,\,c} - \mu_H^{s,\,a}] \right. \\
& - \left[\frac{1}{F}\left(S_{e^-}^* + \frac{1}{2}S_{H_2} \right) + \frac{t_w^a}{2}S_w^a \right](T^{s,\,a} - T_0^a) \\
& - \left[\frac{1}{F}S_{H^+}^* - t_w^m S_w^m \right](T^{s,\,c} - T^{s,\,a}) \\
& \left. - \left[\frac{1}{F}\left(S_{e^-}^* - \frac{1}{4}S_{O_2} \right) + \frac{t_w^c}{2}S_w^c \right](T_0^c - T^{s,\,c}) \right\} \\
& - t_w^a(\mu_{w,\,T}^{s,\,a} - \mu_{w,\,o}^a) - t_w^e(\mu_{w,\,T}^{s,\,c} - \mu_{w,\,T}^{s,\,a}) - t_w^c(\mu_{w,\,o}^c - \mu_{w,\,T}^{s,\,a}) \\
& - j(r^a d^a + r^{s,\,a} + r^e d^e + r^{s,\,c} + r^c d^c)
\end{aligned} \tag{54}$$

The cell emf is defined by $E = \lim_{j\to 0}(\Delta\phi)$. The classical cell emf is $E = -\Delta_r G/F$, with $\Delta_r G$ from Eq. (9). For a zero electric current, constant temperature and constant chemical potential of water, we find an additional contribution to E, $(\mu_H^{s,\,c} - \mu_H^{s,\,a})/F$, compared with the classical result. The classical result is recovered for $dT = 0$, $d\mu_{w,\,T} = 0$, $j \to 0$ and

$$\mu_H^{s,\,a} = \mu_H^{s,\,c} \tag{55}$$

Experimental values for E are about 0.2 V less than the emf (1.18 V for 70°C and 1 bar) calculated from Eq. (9) [16]. The discrepancy has been explained by mixed cathode potentials, or Pt-corrosion potentials, or low exchange current densities [17]. We see below that it can be explained, in terms of a difference between the chemical potentials of hydrogen at the anode and cathode surface. This would also explain the reproducible nature of the effect. We estimate the size of the term below, on the basis of known values for the chemical potential of H at the surface of Pt.

B. Maximum Interface Potential Jumps (Constant $\mu_{w, T}$ and T)

The maximum potential jumps across the electrode interfaces for constant temperature and chemical potential of water, are according to Eqs. (36) or (47), $\Delta\phi^s = -(1/F)A^s(j = 0)$. This is the potential jump in the emf-measurement. For the anode interface we have:

$$(\Delta\phi^s)_{j=0} = -\frac{1}{F}\left(\mu_H^{s,\,a} - \frac{1}{2}\mu_{H_2}^{g,\,a}\right) \tag{56}$$

The difference in chemical potentials is the Gibbs energy change for adsorption of hydrogen gas on Pt. The chemical potential of H in the μm thick layer that we define as the interface, $\mu_H^{s,\,a}$, is equal to the chemical potential of H at the Pt-surface, since H occurs only adsorbed at Pt in the interface region.

We can estimate the potential jumps at the anode and cathode from the standard Gibbs energy change for adsorption of H from an acid solution, reported for different surface coverages of hydrogen on Pt and Rh by Jerkiewicz and Zolfaghari [12]. One of their major findings was that the state of H for electrochemical adsorption from the solution was identical to the state of chemisorbed gas. The membrane side of our interface is also acid; we have a membrane polymer with a high proton concentration. In lack of other data, we shall use their value for $\mu_H^{s,\,a}$ for high surface coverage on Pt, for $T = 343$ K (-11 kJ/mol), with Eq. (56). This gives $(\Delta\phi^{s,\,a})_{j=0} = 0.11$ V for $p_{H_2(g)} = 1$ bar. This is illustrated later in Fig. 4. The data [12] indicate that $\mu_H^{s,\,a}$ will be more negative when the acidity increases. This means that our estimate of $(\Delta\phi^{s,\,a})_{j=0}$ may be too high.

The affinity for the reaction at the cathode surface is:

$$\begin{aligned} A^{s,\,c} &= \tfrac{1}{2}\mu_w^{g,\,c} - \mu_H^{s,\,c} - \tfrac{1}{4}\mu_{O_2}^{g,\,c} \\ &= \tfrac{1}{2}h_w^{g,\,c} - h_H^{s,\,c} - \tfrac{1}{4}h_{O_2}^{g,\,c} - T(\tfrac{1}{2}s_w^{g,\,c} - s_H^{s,\,c} - \tfrac{1}{4}s_{O_2}^{g,\,c}) \end{aligned} \tag{57}$$

At the cathode, the excess surface density of polarized hydrogen atoms (the surface coverage of H) must be much smaller than at the anode. We expect that it is virtually zero at low current densities. The data cited above [12] were extrapolated to zero surface coverage to give $\mu_H^{s,c} = -20$ kJ/mol. The other thermodynamic data were taken from standard tables, see Sec. VI.B. The results were $A^{s,c} = -94.6$ kJ/mol, giving $(\Delta\phi^{s,o})_{j=0} = 0.98$ V. In other words, the electrochemical reaction at the cathode is responsible for a major part of the cell's emf, see Fig. 4.

The sum of the anode and cathode potential jumps is the total emf, 1.09 V from these estimates. This is 0.11 V less the classical value. The origin of the reduction is the difference $\mu_H^{s,a} - \mu_H^{s,c} = -10$ kJ/mol.

The jumps in the electric potential for emf- conditions, reflects a *reversible* energy change in the interface during the electrochemical reaction. In the anode, the positive jump is due to the spontaneous adsorption of gas. When there is local equilibrium between the bulk gas and the surface, the term is of course zero. A higher acidity in the membrane than in the solution we have taken data from, will also make the anode potential jump smaller. At the cathode, however, the term is never zero. Here the jump reflects that the chemical reaction is not in equilibrium. This is not in conflict with the interface being in local *thermodynamic* equilibrium. The potential jumps across the interfaces do *not* represent a loss of energy, for a kinetically hindered discharge reaction (with a high activation energy). In the limit of zero current density, the chemical reaction is reversible, and the energy change is likewise.

C. Electrode Overpotentials (Constant $\mu_{w,T}$ and T)

The overpotential of an electrode surface is the potential between a current carrying electrode (working electrode) and a reference electrode of the same kind, which carries negligible current. We distinguish between the concentration overpotential, and the surface overpotential (see, e.g., Newman [8]). The concentration overpotential is due to gradient(s) in chemical potential(s) of component(s) accumulating in front of the working electrode. According to Newman, the concentration overpotential contains also a term due to excess electric resistance. The concentration overpotential derived from irreversible thermodynamics gives the same result. The surface overpotential is due to the *rate-limiting* electrochemical reaction [18]. The Butler–Volmer equation is normally used to describe the surface overpotential, but Newman states that the Gibbs energy change of the electrochemical reaction is equivalent to the Butler–Volmer equation (Ref. 18, p. 187). In irreversible thermodynamics, the differential change in Gibbs energy of the electrode reaction plus a resistance drop, gives the electrode surface overpotential at constant temperature. We shall see below how this can be derived for our interfaces.

Consider again the overpotential experiment. We examine such an experiment for both fuel cell electrodes. The chemical potential of water and the temperatures are constant across the interfaces. We assume that we are able to neglect (or correct for) contributions to the measurement from the membrane,

so that we deal only with the contribution from the membrane–electrode interface. The working electrode in the experiment, has its interface potential drop
from Eqs. (36) or (47):

$$\Delta\phi^s = -\frac{1}{F} A^s(j) - r^s j$$

The reference electrode has the opposite interface potential drop, taken for
$j = 0$. The overpotential is the sum of these potential drops:

$$\eta^s = \Delta\phi^s(j) - \Delta\phi^s(j = 0) = -[A^s(j) - A^s(j = 0)]/F - r^s j \tag{58}$$

The expression gives $\eta^s = 0$ when $j = 0$, as it should. The affinity is equal to
the Gibbs energy change of the reaction at constant temperature. When the
reaction for $j = 0$ is fast, there is local chemical equilibrium in the interface
and $A^s(j = 0) = 0$. The expression (58) contains a reversible contribution (from
the affinities) and a dissipative contribution (from the resistance term). Equation (58) will describe *the change* in the interface potential drop at the working
electrode, (here change in the Gibbs energy), from its value in the emf-
experiment.

For our anode reaction, Eq. (58) gives:

$$\eta^{s,\,a} = [\mu_H^{s_1\,a}(j = 0) - \mu_H^{s_1\,a}(j)]/F - r^{s,\,a} j \tag{59}$$

Experiments on fuel cells give the anode overpotential as a linear function of
current density [16]. This must then mean that $\eta^{s,\,a} = -r^{s,\,a} j$, with constant
$r^{s,\,a}$ and that $\mu_H^{s_1\,a}(j = 0) = \mu_H^{s_1\,a}(j)$ (the surface coverage of H varies little with j).
The resistance, $r^{s,\,a}$, is the resistance of the electrochemical reaction (2).

The similar expression of the cathode gives:

$$\eta^{s,\,c} = \frac{1}{F}\left(\frac{1}{2}\mu_w^{g,\,c} - \mu_H^{s_1\,c} - \frac{1}{4}\mu_{O_2}^{g,\,c}\right)_{j=0} - \frac{1}{F}\left(\frac{1}{2}\mu_w^{g,\,c} - \mu_H^{s_1\,c} - \frac{1}{4}\mu_{O_2}^{g,\,c}\right)_j - r^{s,\,c} j$$
$$\tag{60}$$

where $r^{s,\,c}$ is the resistance of reaction (6). The chemical potential of bulk water
and oxygen gas disappear from the expression, giving the same final form as
Eq. (59):

$$\eta^{s,\,c} = \frac{RT}{F}\ln\frac{a_H^{s_1\,c}(j)}{(a_H^{s_1\,c})_{j=0}} - r^{s,\,c} j \tag{61}$$

It is likely that the chemical potential of H in the polarized interface depends
on j.

Measurements indicate, however, that $\eta^{s,\,c}$ depends on the oxygen pressure
in the bulk phase [13]. This means that the assumptions we have used to

derive Eq. (60) are not valid. When the assumption $\mu_{O_2}^{s,c} = \mu_{O_2}^{g,c}$ is removed, we obtain

$$\eta^{s,c} = \frac{RT}{F} \ln \frac{a_H^{s,c}(j)[p_{O_2}^{s,c}(j)]^{1/4}}{[a_H^{s,c}(p_{O_2}^{s,c})^{1/4}]} - r^{s,c}j \tag{62}$$

It is interesting to compare the expressions above to experimental results. Such results are often summarized by the empirical Tafel equation [10, 17, 18]:

$$\eta^{s,c} = \frac{2RT}{F} \ln \frac{j}{j_0} \tag{63}$$

with the exchange current density, j_0, directly proportional to the oxygen pressure, p_{O_2}, $j_0 = j_0' p_{O_2}$. The exchange current density and the factor 2 depend on the electrode activity [13]. A direct comparison of the two equations (61) and (63) says that the two expressions lead to the same behavior if the chemical activity of H is given by $a_H^{s,c}(j) = a_H^{s,c}(0)[1 + (j/j_0)^2]$, and $r^{s,c}j$ can be neglected. The polarized nature of the atom and Eq. (44) is relevant in this context. By putting the two equations equal to one another, we can determine $a_H^{s,c}(j)$ [or $a_{H^+ + e^-}^{s,c}(j)$] for the cathode from Tafel plots. The overpotential for hydrogen evolution has also been related to the hydrogen pressure [12]. With the terminology used in this work, we have from [12]

$$\eta^{o,a} = -\frac{RT}{2F} \ln \frac{p_{H_2}^{g,a}(j)}{(p_{H_2}^{g,a})_{j=0}}$$

This equation is obtained by neglecting $r^s j$, and by assuming that there are (different) equilibria across the interface, depending on the current density, $\mu_H^s(j) = \frac{1}{2}\mu_{H_2}^g(j)$.

VI. CELL DIMENSIONS AND PROPERTIES

A. Cell Geometry and Operation

The single fuel cell used in our model study was constructed by Møller-Holst [16]. The carbon backing (part 3 of Fig. 1) has a thickness of 180 μm, and a porosity of 0.4. The tortuosity is taken to be 7 [14]. The carbon backing is made from a porous carbon cloth, impregnated with carbon and Teflon. The interface is made by mixing 65 wt% of 20 wt% Pt on C with 15 wt% Nafion 117 and 20 wt% carbon [16]. The result is the 10 μm catalyst layer, shown in detail on the insert in Fig. 1. The final layer has 13 wt% or 0.1 mg Pt/cm^2 membrane surface. The carbon backing of the two sides are made the same way, and have the same properties. The membrane is standard for the purpose,

Nafion 117 from DuPont, 175 μm thick (part 1 of Fig. 1). The membrane has molecule weight of $M_m = 1.1$ kg/mol, dry density of $\rho_{dry} = 1.64 \times 10^3$ kg/m^3, and swelling factor $s = 0.0126$ [10].

The outer parts of the carbon backing are thermostatted at 70°C and the cell is operated at 1 bar. The hydrogen and oxygen gases are saturated with water at a slightly higher temperature, to maintain the saturation pressure p_w in the cell. Gases are supplied by flows perpendicular to the transport direction with flow rates $F_{H_2} = F_{O_2} = 3.406 \times 10^{-5}$ mol/s, and $F_w^a = F_w^c = 2.984 \times 10^{-6}$ mol/s.

B. Transport Properties and Thermodynamic Data

We have taken a constant water transference number through the membrane, $t_w = 1.2$. Ottøy [19] found this result for a membrane in contact with water vapor, and with a water contents, λ, between 2 and 14 molecules of water per ionic site. Likewise, the diffusion constant of water, scaled to dry membrane, was taken as the constant self diffusion constant, in the absence of pressure gradients, $D_w = 1.2 \times 10^{-10}$ m^2/s [10]. In the presence of pressure gradients, we used $l_{ww} = 1.2 \times 10^{-6}$ s mol^2 (m^3 kg)$^{-1}$) [15].

The thermal conductivity of the membrane was estimated to $\lambda^e = 0.2$ W/K m as the harmonic mean of the conductivity of rubber (60 vol%) and water (40 vol%) [20]. The thermal conductivity of the electrodes were taken to be that of carbon, $\lambda^a = \lambda^c = 10$ W/K m [21]. The excess interface resistance to heat transfer was taken to be 100 times larger than that of the membrane, so that it scales similar to the electric resistance [9].

The electric resistance of the membrane varies largely with the membrane water content and will therefore give a varying electric potential gradient through the membrane. According to Springer et al. [10] we have

$$r^e(30°C) = \frac{1}{0.005139\lambda - 0.00326} \tag{64}$$

$$r^e(T) = \exp\left[-1268\left(\frac{1}{303} - \frac{1}{T}\right)\right] \tag{65}$$

The excess resistance of the two interfaces was found by subtracting the membrane resistance and the resistance of the carbon backing from the total cell resistance [16]. The excess interface resistance of one electrode was then found as half this value, giving $r^{s,a} = r^{s,c} = 7.15 \times 10^{-6}$ ohm m^2 for the 10 μm layer. The resistance of the carbon backing was 2×10^{-4} ohm m.

Thermodynamic data were taken from Ref. 22. The standard Gibbs energies of formation for liquid and vapor water at this temperature and pressure are $g_w^\circ = -237$ and -229 kJ/mol, respectively. Standard entropies are $s_{H_2}^\circ = 131$, $s_{O_2}^\circ = 205$, $s_w^\circ = 189$ J/mol K for the gas and $s_w^\circ = 70$ J/mol K for the liquid.

The standard Gibbs free energies of formation for the pure gases are zero. The transported entropy of electrons was neglected, giving $S_{H^+}^* - t_w S_w = 13.4$ J/K mol [15].

VII. FURTHER RESULTS

A. The Water Concentration Profile

The concentration profile of water in the membrane as a function of current density, was determined from Eq. (16) rewritten as

$$J_w = -D_w \frac{dc_w}{dx} + t_w j \tag{66}$$

Here D_w is the diffusion constant of water and c_w is the water concentration in the membrane. The current density varied between 10^{-3} and 0.7 A/cm². The equation was solved for constant J_w, j, T, and p. The iteration procedure of Springer et al. [10] was applied, to adjust the water activity at the boundaries to the water activity in the gas phase, and to the gas flow rates. We thus assumed equilibrium for water across the membrane surface, $\Delta\mu_w^{s, a} = \Delta\mu_w^{g, a} = 0$ and $\Delta\mu_w^{s, c} = \Delta\mu_w^{g, c} = 0$. The resulting concentration profiles for $dP = 0$ and $dT = 0$ are shown in Fig. 3. The water flux consistent with this calculation was constant within a few percent for current densities chosen.

The figure shows that the concentration profiles for water are linear across the membrane for all current densities. This is due to the constant D_w and t_w. The value of D_w is so small, that we only have a significant contribution to J_w from diffusion when j is very large. As a consequence, the membrane resistance, that is a function of the water content, will vary largely for high current densities. We shall see that this determines the shape of the electric potential profile in the membrane. The results of Fig. 3 raise the question of how back diffusion can be increased. This lead us to investigate the effect of a pressure gradient across the membrane, see below.

From the water concentration profiles, the membrane resistance at any position in the membrane was calculated from Eqs. (64) and (65). The electric potential profile across the membrane was then calculated from Eq. (20) for varying current densities (see below).

B. Electric Potential Profiles and the Polarization Curve

The electric potential profile, calculated for $j = 0$, with $dT = 0$ and $dp = 0$, is shown by horizontal lines connected with jumps over the interfaces in Fig. 4. The electric potential is constant in all bulk phases, since there are no ohmic losses. The importance of the cathode as the place where the potential jump of the cell is generated, is seen. The small, but significant contribution by the

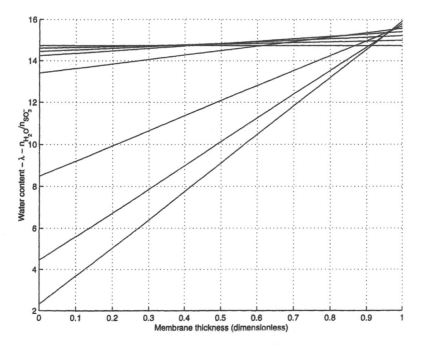

FIG. 3 The calculated water concentration profile through the membrane under fuel cell operation. The current density varies from 1 mA/cm^2 to 600 mA/cm^2. The anode is to the left.

anode to the total potential, means that this interface should not be neglected when improvements are discussed. The sum of the electrode potential jumps is the emf of the cell, as discussed in Sec. V.

Electric potential profiles for increasing values of j are compared in the same figure. The electric potential profile is (almost) constant in the carbon backing, due to the high electric conductivity, except at very high current densities. The positive potential gain in the anode, as well as in the cathode, is visibly reduced by the ohmic resistance that we have used for the interfaces, already for the lowest current density. The nonlinear profile in the electrolyte, especially at high current densities, is due to the changing water content of the membrane. The curve has a higher slope close to the anode, in agreement with Fig. 3.

The relation between the cell potential $\Delta\phi$ and the electric current density j, is the polarization curve (see Fig. 5 below). Such curves have been used extensively to evaluate fuel cell performance. In order to establish a basis for our results, we recalculated the results of Springer et al. [10], using their expressions Eqs. (64) and (65), with the water concentration profiles from Fig. 3. The

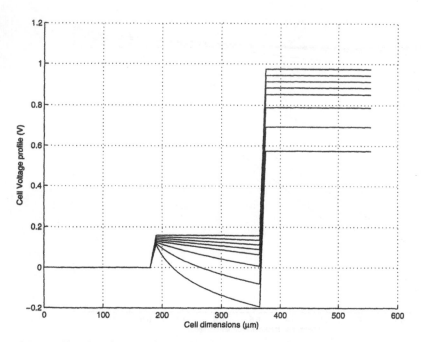

FIG. 4 The electric potential profile through the fuel cell at different current densities. The anode is to the left.

model has later been extended by Springer et al. [11], but we have chosen their first work as a principle reference because of its clearness.

The polarization curve, derived from their expressions, is shown with star symbols in Fig. 5. The curve has three typical phases. There is a rapid potential drop for small current densities, followed by an approximately linear region up to 0.5 A/cm², and an increasing negative slope as the current density increases beyond that value. While the first phase has been explained by the cathode overpotential, the last phase has been explained by the change in the membrane resistance with the water content.

The corresponding polarization curve from our equations is given by the open symbols in Fig. 5. This curve uses the same $\mu_H^{s\,a}$ and $\mu_H^{s\,c}$ that we found in the estimates above, a constant temperature and pressure, and the membrane water content profiles of Fig. 3. We start the curve at 1.09 V. The first phase has a different structure, because we have not used a chemical potential of H that varies with j (i.e., we have not introduced overpotentials). The second phase can be used to determine the constant cell resistance. The third phase of the curve is similar to that of the reference model. The difference between the curves represents the difference of chemical potentials of the polarized H-atom at the membrane–electrode interface. By taking the difference between our

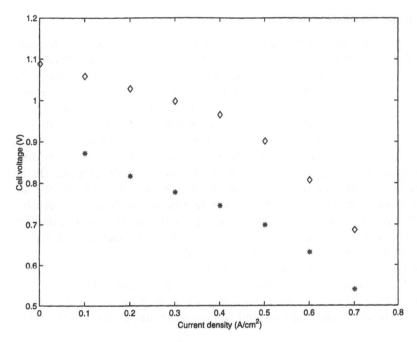

FIG. 5 Polarization curves calculated for different mathematical models of the solid polymer fuel cells. * The model based on Springer et al. [10]. ◇ = Model based on equations given here, without overpotentials.

curve and an experimental polarization curve, we can obtain an estimate for $\mu_{\mathrm{H}}^{\mathrm{s,\,c}}$, when $\mu_{\mathrm{H}}^{\mathrm{s,\,a}}$ is known.

C. Pressure Difference Effects

The fact that diffusion of water in the membrane from the cathode to the anode is low, with the set of data that we have used, leads to a speculation that a positive *pressure difference* across the membrane may be profitable for the membrane resistance: If one can increase the force on water in this direction, one will need a smaller supply of water on the anode side. A calculation using a pressure difference of 1 bar between the electrodes indeed led to a more even distribution of water across the membrane. At very small current densities, there was even a net transport of water from the cathode to the anode. The cell potential was affected by this through $\Delta\mu_{\mathrm{w}} = V_{\mathrm{w}}\,\Delta p$. The difference in chemical potential of water across the membrane lead to a decrease in the emf we calculate of 30 mV. This means that there is a trade-off between reducing the membrane resistance loss, and increasing the chemical potential difference of water across the membrane.

D. Thermal Gradient Effects

In the laboratory, the outer parts of the cell are normally kept at constant temperature. One may ask where it is profitable to maintain a difference in temperature between the two sides. The electric potential profile through the cell is affected by the temperature according to Eqs. (35) and (52). This was not taken into account in the calculation of potential profiles described above, where we assumed that the total cell was thermostatted, and that $\Delta P = 0$.

In order to find the impact of the local temperature on the cell behaviour, we calculated the temperature profile through the cell setting the same terminal temperature of the carbon backing on the two sides. We did not include the overpotentials at the electrodes. The results are presented in Fig. 6. We see that the temperature of the membrane rises, depending on the current density, to about 4 K above the terminal temperature for the highest current density. The rise in surface temperatures is proportional to the current density, as expected from the Peltier effect, see Eqs. (21) and (23).

The higher temperature in the membrane is caused by the Joule heat. The estimated thermal conductivity that we have used, is obviously so low that heat can accumulate. Such heat accumulation may have a bearing on the kinetics of the electrode reactions and the overpotential of the cathode. (The

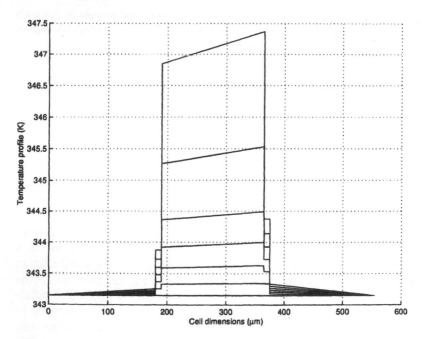

FIG. 6   Temperature profiles in the fuel cell for different current densities. The anode is to the left.

effect on the reversible part of the cell potential is small.) More should be known about the thermal conductivity of the membrane and the membrane surface, to establish what the correct surface conditions are.

The temperature profiles in the bulk phases are linear, consistent with constant thermal conductivity in these phases, and a negligible local Joule heat. The fuel cell process are maintained by an energy flux from the cathode to the anode. A temperature difference of 5 K in either direction between the electrodes, has a negligible impact on this energy flux. The surface temperature is always higher than the electrode bulk temperature. The next step will be to see how the overpotential affects this situation.

VIII. DISCUSSION AND CONCLUSIONS

Irreversible thermodynamics has been used to analyze major events in the solid polymer fuel cell; that is the membrane–electrode interface reactions, membrane transport, and a few operating conditions. From the chemical potential of hydrogen at the electrode surface, we have estimated the membrane–electrode interface potential jumps, and given the emf of the system. We have calculated the electric potential profile through the cell and have shown how it varies with current density and membrane water content for isothermal, isobaric conditions. We have given expressions for the overpotential, and shown how that the drop in electric potential is related to the chemical potential of hydrogen in the interface. Equations that deal with pressure and temperature gradients and their interaction with other intensive variables, have been presented and discussed, so that a basis for more detailed calculations has been laid.

While the equations that are obtained for the overpotential from irreversible thermodynamics are almost the same as those normally used, the premises that are used in their derivation differ. We assume local equilibrium in the interface (for all current densities) and linear flux–force relationships. The overpotential has a reversible and a dissipative term. The Butler–Volmer equation and the Tafel equation, on the other hand, have a nonlinear relation between *one* flux, j, and the overpotential, η^s. The Butler–Volmer model has inherent a dissipative term, as is seen by expansions for small current densities. The model behind the Butler–Volmer equation, the jump of the charged particle across an activation barrier, was however also related to differences in chemical potentials [18].

Our equation for the overpotential can be tested by measuring $\mu_H^s(j)$, independent of the electrochemical reaction. Further progress could be made in this manner. A simultaneous solution of all variables in the heterogeneous system is also lacking. Several aspects remain to be studied; for instance the gas diffusion in the carbon backing. This is, however, outside the scope of a book dealing with membrane surfaces.

ACKNOWLEDGMENTS

P. J. S. Vie is grateful for a grant given by the Norwegian Research Council.
D. Bedeaux was Onsager professor at NTNU when the work was done. S.
Møller-Holst is thanked for critical comments to the manuscript. K. Nisancioglu is thanked for pointing out to us Newman's equivalent forms for the
surface overpotential.

LIST OF SYMBOLS

a   anode
a_i^y activity of i in y
$A^{s,y}$ affinity in y surface reaction
c   cathode
d   differential
d   distance [m]
D_i diffusion constant of i [m²/s]
e^- electron
emf   electromotive force
F   Faraday's constant [96,487 C/mol]
F_i flow of i
g   gas
g_i^y Gibbs energy of i in y [J/mol]
G   Gibbs energy [J]
h_i^y enthalpy of i in y [J/mol]
H   enthalpy [J]
i component
j current density [A/m²]
j_0 exchange current density
J_i^y flux of i in y [mol/m² s]
$J_q'^y$ flux of measurable heat in y
J_e energy flux [J/m² s]
l_{ij} Onsager coefficient for diffusion
L_{ij} Onsager coefficient (basic)
m   membrane
M_m molecular weight [kg/mol]
n_i mass density of i
P_i pressure of i [Pa]
r^y electrical resistivity in y [Ω m]
R   universal gas constant [8.3143 J/mol K]
s   surface
s   swelling factor
s   entropy density

s_i^y entropy of i in y [J/mol K]

S entropy [J/K]

S^* transported entropy [J/mol K]

t_w^y water transference number in y

T^y temperature in y [K]

u energy density

$v^{s,\,y}$ surface reaction rate in y [mol/m^2 s]

V_i molar volume of i [m^3/mol]

w   water, H$_2$O

x coordinate

y phase, example: s, a, g, c or g

α $J_w^a/J_{H_2}^a$

Δ a difference

η^y overpotential in y

λ^y Fourier thermal conductivity in y [W/K m]

μ_i^y chemical potential of i in y

π^y Peltier coefficient in y

ρ density [kg/m^3]

σ^y entropy production in y [J/K m^3 s]

ϕ electrical potential [J/mol]

REFERENCES

1. S. R. de Groot and P. Mazur, *Non-equilibrium Thermodynamics*, North-Holland, Amsterdam, 1962.
2. D. Bedeaux, A. M. Albano, and P. Mazur, Physica A *82*: 221 (1976), and A. M. Albano and D. Bedeaux, Physica A *147*: 407 (1987).
3. D. Bedeaux, in *Advances in Thermodynamics*, Vol. 6. *Flow, Diffusion and Rate Processes*, (Stanislaw Sieniutycz and Peter Salamon, eds.), Taylor and Francis, New York, 1992.
4. J. W. Gibbs, *Collected Works*, Dover, New York, 1961.
5. D. Bedeaux, L. J. F. Hermans, and T. Ytrehus, Physica A *169*: 263 (1990).
6. D. Bedeaux, J. A. M. Smit, L. J. F. Hermans, and T. Ytrehus, Physica A *182*: 388 (1992).
7. D. Bedeaux and S. Kjelstrup Ratkje, J. Electrochem. Soc. *143*: 767 (1996).
8. S. Kjelstrup Ratkje and D. Bedeaux, J. Electrochem. Soc. *143*: 779 (1996).
9. S. Kjelstrup and D. Bedeaux, Physica A *244*: 213 (1997).
10. T. E. Springer, T. A. Zawodzinski, and S. Gottesfeld, J. Electrochem. Soc. *138*: 2334 (1991).
11. T. E. Springer, M. S. Wilson and S. Gottesfeld, J. Electrochem. Soc. *140*: 3513 (1993).
12. G. Jerkiewicz and A. Zalfaghari, J. Electrochem. Soc. *143*: 1240 (1996), ibid. *144*: 3034 (1997).

13. N. J. T. T. Vermeijlen, L. J. J. Janssen, and G. J. Visser, J. Appl. Electrochem. *27*:497 (1997).

14. T. E. Springer, T. A. Zawodzinski, M. S. Wilson, and S. Gottesfeld, J. Electrochem. Soc. *143*:587 (1996).

15. S. Kjelstrup Ratkje, M. Ottøy, R. Halseid, and M. Strømgård, J. Membrane Sci. *107*:219 (1995).

16. S. Møller-Holst, Solid polymer fuel cells. Electrode and membrane performance studies, Ph.D. Thesis No. 49, Institute of Physical Chemistry, Norwegian Institute of Technology, University of Trondheim, Norway, 1996.

17. J. O'M. Bockris and S. Srinivasan, *Fuel Cells: Their Electrochemistry*, McGraw-Hill, New York, 1969.

18. J. S. Newman, *Electrochemical Systems*, 2nd Ed., Prentice-Hall, Englewood Cliffs, New Jersey, 1991.

19. M. Ottøy, Mass and heat transfer in ion-exchange membranes, Ph.D. Thesis No. 50, Institute of Physical Chemistry, Norwegian Institute of Technology, University of Trondheim, Norway, 1996.

20. L. Nummedal, Thermal osmosis in a cation exchange membrane, M.Sc. Thesis, Institute of Physical Chemistry, Norwegian Institute of Technology, University of Trondheim, Norway, 1996.

21. P. Delhaes and F. Carmona, Chem. Phys. Carbon *17*:89 (1981).

22. G. H. Aylward and T. J. V. Findlay, *SI Chemical Data*, 2nd Ed., Wiley, Hong Kong, 1971.

15

Electroosmotic Transport Through Ion-Exchange Membranes

C. RUÍZ BAUZÁ and V. M. BARRAGÁN GARCÍA   Department of Applied Physics I, University Complutense of Madrid, Madrid, Spain

Abstract

The electroosmotic transport through different ion-exchange membranes, separating equal solutions of monovalent electrolytes, was obtained under different experimental conditions. From these measurements the electroosmotic permeability, W, of the membranes has been determined. The effect of the concentration and nature of the solutions, the current density, the unstirred solution layers and the temperature on the value of W is analyzed and discussed.

I. INTRODUCTION

The application of an electric field to a cell of type:

$$\text{Anode} \mid \text{Solution}(c_0) \mid \text{Membrane} \mid \text{Solution}(c_0) \mid \text{Cathode} \qquad (1)$$

causes not only transference of specific ions through the membrane but also transference of liquid existing in its pores. This solvent transport accompanying ion transport is called in a phenomenological way electroosmosis. The magnitude and direction of the total volume flux is determined by the nature of the membrane system, the quantity of water transported by electroconvection, and some other relevant parameters such concentration and stirring rate of the solutions, temperature, etc.

Virtually all types of membranes, in contact with electrolyte solutions and subject to a potential gradient normal to the membrane, exhibit electroosmosis. This phenomenon arises from a nonuniform distribution of ions close to the walls of the pores of the membrane due to (1) the preferential adsorption of one type of ion on the walls of an uncharged membrane, or (2) the existence of charged groups in the structure of the membrane itself.

In the first case, the preferencial adsorption of one species of ion leads to a type of distribution associated with the idea of "electrical double layer" in the area separating the two phases introduced by Helmholtz and Smoluchowski. This comprises the charged surface and a neutralizing excess of counterions in the adjacent solution as it is shown in Fig. 1. The electrical potential in the plane separating the immobile and mobile parts of the double layer is called zeta potential (ζ).

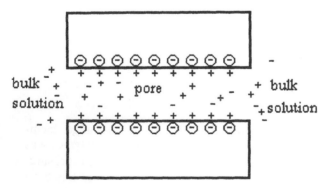

FIG. 1 Sketch of the liquid pore in a cation-exchange membrane.

When an electric field is applied parallel to the walls of the pores, forces are exerted on both part of the double layer. As a consequence, the mobile part of the double layer moves under the influence of the electric field, carrying solvent molecules with it. It can be shown that the electroosmotic velocity, v_E, of the solution at a large distance from the walls of the pores is given by:

$$v_E = \frac{\varepsilon \zeta E}{4\pi\eta} \tag{2}$$

where ε and η are the dielectric constant and viscosity of the solution, respectively, and E is the applied potential gradient. The corresponding volume of solution transported per unit time and per unit area is given, for a current density I, by

$$V = \frac{\varepsilon \zeta I}{4\pi\eta\bar{k}} \tag{3}$$

where $\bar{k}$ is the specific conductance of solution filling the pores of the membrane.

Equations (2) and (3) are ideal and they apply only to uncharged membranes of relatively large pore radius and in contact with very diluted solutions where a double layer of significant magnitude is obtained.

In the second case, the membranes consist generally of sheets of homogeneous or heterogeneous, natural or synthetic, ion-exchange substances. These are characterized by a high concentration of fixed charge and a correspondingly high concentration of counterions, the pore radius being usually much smaller than in those of the first type, often of molecular dimensions. Such ion-exchange membranes approximate to ideal selective systems in which, although there are two ionics species, only one of them, the counterion, can pass across the membrane.

Thus, using very diluted solutions and ion exchange membranes it can be considered that only counterions flux in one direction giving rise to a flux of solvent in that direction. This flux of solvent thus enables counterions to move faster than they would otherwise in the absence of the solvent flux. Therefore, for any given applied potential difference, the net current density, I, flowing will be greater than I' flowing in absence of solvent flux. Schmid [1–4] and Schmid and Schwarz [5–7] have related the convection current density $\Delta I = I - I'$ to the total current density I by means of the equation

$$\frac{I - I'}{I} = \frac{F^2 \bar{X}^2 r^2}{8\eta\bar{k}} \tag{4}$$

where F is the Faraday number, $\bar{X}$, is the fixed charge concentration and r is the radius of the pores.

The total volume flux through the membrane can be expressed as:

$$J_V = \sum_{i=0,+,-} J_i \bar{V}_i \tag{5}$$

where 0, +, and − refer to solvent, cation, and anion, respectively, and $\bar{V}_i$ and J_i are the partial molar volume and the flux of the ith component. The relation between the volume flux, J_V, and the applied current density, I, in the absence of a pressure difference, is called apparent or measured electroosmotic permeability, W,

$$W = \left(\frac{J_V}{I}\right)_{\Delta P = 0} \tag{6}$$

Basing on the equations derived by Bjerrum, Manegold, and Solf [8,9], Schmid developed a theory of electroosmosis using a model of fine pores [1–4]. One of the essential features of this model is the condition that the mean pore diameters have to be so small that the different components of the liquid pore can be considered to distribute homogeneously over the cross-section of the pore. Schmid showed, in the said model, that the electroosmotic permeability is given by:

$$W = \frac{F \bar{X} D_h d}{\bar{k}} \tag{7}$$

where d is the thickness of the membrane, and D_h is the hydraulic permeability defined as the volume of solution transferred under unit pressure difference in unit time through unit area of membrane.

The electroosmotic transport of solvent through the membrane is usually characterized by means of the transport number of the solvent, $\bar{t}_0$. It is defined as the number of solvent moles transferred in the direction of the current by 1 faraday of electricity and it can be calculated by subtracting the contribution from ionic transference to the volume of the solution transferred by 1 faraday $(-\theta F W)$ and dividing into the partial molar volume of the solvent (V_0). Thus:

$$\bar{t}_0 = -\frac{\theta F W + \sum_i V_i \bar{t}_i}{V_0} \tag{8}$$

where $\theta = -1$ for a cationic membrane and $\theta = +1$ for an anionic membrane, $\bar{V}_i$ is the partial molar volume of the ith ionic specie, and $\bar{t}_i$ its corresponding ionic transport number in the membrane phase defined by $\bar{t}_i = FJ_i/I$.

Equation (8) gives the total transport number of the solvent including the solvation shells. The transport number of the free solvent can be calculated by using the solvated ionic volumes instead of the partial molar volumes. The difference between the total transport of solvent and the transport of free solvent is $\sum_i n_i \bar{t}_i$ where n_i is the solvation number of the ith specie.

Usually the electrolyte solutions used are aqueous solutions, that is, the solvent is water. For this reason the water transport number, $\bar{t}_w$, is the one that usually appears in the literature in relation to the electroosmotic transport.

Some authors have tried to connect the water transport number, $\bar{t}_w$, to the cation transport number, $\bar{t}_+$, directly. In this sense, Winger et al. [10] try to interpret the experimental results by means of a very simple model, assuming that a mean number of molecules move with each mobile ionic specie migrating under the action of a potential gradient. According to it, the water transport number is given by:

$$\bar{t}_w = \frac{n_+ \bar{t}_+}{z_+} - \frac{n_- \bar{t}_-}{z_-} \tag{9}$$

where n_+ and n_- are the number of moles of water associated with the cation and anion of valences z_+ and z_- respectively.

Taking into account that $\bar{t}_+ + \bar{t}_- = 1$, Eq. (9) for $z_+ = z_- = 1$ can be written as:

$$\bar{t}_w = (n_+ + n_-)\bar{t}_+ - n_- \tag{10}$$

that expresses that if n_+ and n_- are considered to be constant and independent on the external solution concentration, $\bar{t}_w$ may be a linear function of $\bar{t}_+$.

A more sophisticated treatment dealing with this topic was also presented by Oda and Yawataya [11]. These authors divided the membrane water into (1) hydration water which moved with the migrating ions, (2) free water which was dragged in the direction of movement of counterion but a lower velocity, and (3) fixed water which did not move at all being bound chemically to the fixed charges or trapped some how physically in the membrane.

Taking into account this distribution of water in the membrane phase, the water transport number is expressed by the relation:

$$\bar{t}_w = (n_+ \bar{t}_+ - n_- \bar{t}_-) + \bar{t}_+ \frac{f}{1 + s} \cdot \frac{\bar{u}_w}{\bar{u}_+} \tag{11}$$

where f and s are the number of moles of free water and the equivalent of coions, respectively, per equivalent of fixed charge present in the membrane, and $\bar{u}_w$ and $\bar{u}_+$ are the mobilities of free water and counterion in the membrane. Thus, the third term in Eq. (11) expresses that $[f/(1 + s)]\bar{t}_+$ moles of water per $\bar{t}_+$ moles of migrating cations are transferred with a mobility $\bar{u}_w/\bar{u}_+$. Equation (11) holds some magnitudes which are hardly individually evaluated but it indicates in a qualitatively way the main causes involved.

Kressman et al. [12] found that the plot of $\bar{t}_w$ against $\bar{t}_+$ was nonlinear. Laksminarayanaiah and Brennen [13] considered that the curvature of this plot was ascribed to the number of moles of water per equivalent of counterion, $\bar{m}_w = n_+ + n_-$, in the membrane is not constant.

In our earlier work [14], using weak cationic cellulosic membranes, a linear dependence between $\bar{t}_w$ and $\bar{t}_+$ was not found either. On the other hand, as the evaluation of $\bar{m}_w$ and its variation are difficult, the found behavior could not be quantitatively justified.

The electroosmosis phenomenon has also been studied by a number of investigators especially within the framework of the thermodynamics of irreversible processes [15–17]. Spiegler [16] obtained an equation for the water flux through a membrane due to the interaction among the migrating ions and surrounding water. On the other hand, Sørensen and Koefoed [18] studied the electrokinetic effects in charged tubes solving the linearized Poisson–Boltzmann equation in the tube just as in the classical electrolyte theory of Debye and Hückel. (See also Chap. 17 for non-classical contributions to electroosmosis.)

Electroosmosis reduces the efficiency of electrodialysis since not only ions but also solvent are removed from the solution. In order to keep electroosmotic losses low, membranes should be chosen which combine high ionic mobilities with a high flow resistance.

If the solutions in the membrane system contain a nonelectrolyte solute in addition to the electrolyte, then the nonelectrolyte also is electroosmotically transferred together with the solvent [19]. When aqueous solutions are used, it was observed that the mole ratio of nonelectrolyte to solvent transferred is smaller than the mole ratio in the solutions [19]. This fact has explication since water is transferred not only by electroosmotic convection but also in form of ionic hydration shells.

We have measured the electroosmotic transport through different ion-exchange membranes, separating equal solutions of monovalent electrolytes, under different experimental conditions. From the measurements, the electroosmotic permeability W has been determined. The effect of the concentration and nature of the solutions, the current density, the unstirred solution layers, the temperature, etc., on the value of W has been studied.

II. EXPERIMENTAL

A. Materials

1. Membranes

In the experiments about electroosmosis seven different ion-exchange membranes were used. Two of them are commercial cation-exchange membranes:

Nepton Cation-Exchange 61 AZL 183 membrane and Ionics Cation-Transfer 61 CZL 386 membrane.

Three are commercial anion-exchange membranes:

Ionics Anion-Transfer 204 U 386, 103 QZL 386, and 204 SXZL 386 membranes.

Two are cation-exchange cellulose acetate membranes:

CA300 and CA500 membranes.

The commercial cation-exchange membranes are homogeneous films comprising cross-linked sulfonated copolymers of vinyl compounds. The anion-exchange membranes are homogeneous films comprising cross-linked copolymers of vinyl monomers and containing quaternary ammonium anion exchange groups. Their characteristics referred to a 0.1 mol/L NaCl solution, and specified by the manufacture, are shown in Table 1.

The cellulose acetate membranes CA300 and CA500 were obtained in our laboratory through evaporation, under controlled humidity and temperature conditions, of a solution of 300 and 500 mg, respectively, of cellulose acetate in $60 \ cm^3$ of pure acetone. The fixed charge density of the membranes CA300 and CA500, obtained from membrane potential measurements, was estimated in 2.1×10^{-2} and 3.0×10^{-2} mol/L, respectively [20].

2. Solutions

In the different experiments, electrolyte aqueous solutions of LiCl, NaCl, and KCl (from Merck s.a.) in bidistilled, deionized, and doubly filtered by means of a Milli-Q purification system water were used. Before the solutions were made, the water was degassed.

B. Experimental Device

1. Electroosmotic Flux

The experimental device used in the determination of the electroosmotic flux consists of three different parts: the cell, the thermostatic system, and the auxiliary systems.

The cell consists essentially of two equal cylindrical glass chambers opened in one of its bases and having a volume large enough to ensure that the concentration changes in the solutions during measurements may be considered

TABLE 1 Characteristics of the Studied Commercial Membranes (Provided by the Manufacturer)

Membrane	Selectivity %	Electric resistance ($\Omega \cdot cm^2$)	Capacity (meq/g)
61 AZL 183	98	5.6	3.0
61 CZL 386	94	11	2.7
294 U 386	97	6.0	2.8
103 QZL 386	97	9	2.1
204 SXZL 386	96	11	2.2

negligible. Each chamber is provided with three orifices communicating to the exterior, in one of them the electrode used to inject the current is introduced, in other orifice a capillary tube is introduced to measure the flux, and the third orifice is used as solution inlet and to eliminate the bubbles in the chamber. The membrane was positioned between the chambers by means of two methacrylate disks. The cell was provided with a chain-driven cell magnetic stirrer assembly which permits the stirring of both solutions.

The thermostatic system is a mixed system. On the one hand, the device is contained in a large ambient thermostat which was kept at the previously chosen temperature. Moreover, the cell was immersed in a thermostatic bath which was placed inside the ambient thermostat. A circulating thermostat permit us to maintain constant the chosen temperature of the bath.

The auxiliary systems consists basically of the current source and the electrodes to inject the electric current, capillary tubes of different sections depending on the magnitude of the measured electroosmotic flux, and a Cathetometer Griffin and George with 0.05 mm sensibility to measure the displacement of the meniscus in the capillary tube. Figure 2 shows a sketch of the experimental device used in the determination of the electroosmotic fluxes.

2.   Curves (*I*, *V*)

The cell employed in the (*I*, *V*) curves measurements also consists of two glass chambers opened in one of its bases and between which the membrane holder is placed. Each chamber has a volume of ~ 100 cm^3 and it is provided with

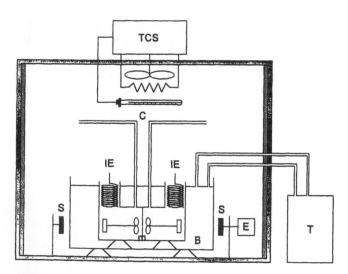

FIG. 2   Sketch of the experimental device used in the determination of the electroosmotic fluxes: m, membrane; S, stirrers; B, bath; T, thermostat; IE, injector electrodes; C, capillary tubes; E, stirrer engine; TCS, ambient temperature control system.

four orifices communicating to the exterior. In one of the orifices the electrode used to measure the potential difference is placed. Other two orifices are used as solution inlet and outlet in the chamber, and in the fourth orifice an electrode to inject the current is introduced.

The inlet and outlet of the solutions in the chambers is realized by means of a circulating system which is used at the same time to stir and homogenize the solutions. The circulation system is provided with two deposits, each having a volume of 1 L, and a Heidolph RUMO 100 peristaltic pump with double pump head working between 20 and 100 rpm and with capacity of rotation reversal. Each half-cell is provided with a circulation assembly where the solution is impelled by means of the peristaltic pump between the deposits and the chambers.

The thermostatic system in this case is only an ambient thermostat similar to the one used in the measurements of the electroosmotic flux.

C. Electroosmosis Measurements

The membrane, prior to be positioned in the electroosmotic cell, was equilibrated with the solution to be used. To this end, it was immersed for a minimum of 24 h in the solution.

When the cell was set up, it was introduced in the thermostatic system. Once the thermal equilibrium state was reached, a constant current density was passed through the membrane during a determinated time which varied according to the applied current density.

The electroosmotic flux was determined by measuring the displacement of the meniscus in the capillary tubes as a function of time. The capillary tubes were kept horizontally and at the same height to prevent pressure differences between the two chambers.

The increase of volume in the cathodic compartment and the decrease of volume in the anodic compartment, when a density current passes through the cation-exchange membrane should be equal. However, a small difference usually existed between the two volumes measured. For this reason, the absolute mean value of both variation was used.

To avoid the possible variation of the initial solution concentrations and to reclaim the electrodes, the polarity of the electrodes was changed, after every measurement, passing the same electric current in the opposite sense and during the same time.

The volume flux, J_V, can be expressed by:

$$J_V = \bar{V}_s \cdot J_1 + \bar{V}_w \cdot J_w \tag{12}$$

where J_1 and J_w are counterion and water fluxes, respectively, per unit membrane area, and $\bar{V}_s$ and $\bar{V}_w$ are the partial molar volumes of the salt and water in a solution of the concentration c.

However, it must be taken into account that the rate of change with time of the volumes in the compartment obtained experimentally, from the displacement with time of the meniscus in the capillary tubes, does not coincide with the volume flux, J_V, given in the previous equation, due to the volume changes measured in the two compartments include the volume change caused by the electrochemical reactions in the Ag|AgCl electrodes:

in the cathode $AgCl + e^- \Leftrightarrow Ag + Cl^-$

in the anode $Ag + Cl^- \Leftrightarrow AgCl + e^-$

The passing of one faraday causes 1 mol of AgCl to disappear and 1 mol of Ag to appear at the cathode while the opposite happens at the anode.

Taking into account these changes of volume, when a current density, I, passes through a cation-exchange membrane of effective area A, the increase of volume per unit time in the cathodic compartment, ΔV_c, and the corresponding decrease in the anodic compartment, ΔV_a, are given by:

$$\Delta V_c = (\bar{V}_s \cdot J_1 + \bar{V}_w \cdot J_w) \cdot A + \frac{(\bar{V}_{Ag} - \bar{V}_{AgCl}) \cdot I \cdot A}{F} \tag{13}$$

$$\Delta V_a = -(\bar{V}_s \cdot J_1 + \bar{V}_w \cdot J_w) \cdot A + \frac{(\bar{V}_{AgCl} - \bar{V}_{Ag}) \cdot I \cdot A}{F} \tag{14}$$

where $\bar{V}_{Ag}$ and $\bar{V}_{AgCl}$ are the partial molar volumes of silver and silver chloride, respectively.

In Fig. 3 an example of the volume changes in the cathodic and anodic compartments, as a function of time, for a cationic-exchange membrane is shown.

Taking into account that $\bar{V}_{AgCl} - \bar{V}_{Ag}, = 15.5 \text{ cm}^3/\text{mol}$, and using the mean value of the two measured volumes we get:

$$J_V(\text{cm/s}) = \frac{|\Delta V_a| + |\Delta V_c|}{2 \cdot A} + 1.6 \times 10^{-4} \cdot I \tag{15}$$

From Eqs. (6) and (15), the electroosmotic permeability can be expressed as:

$$W(\text{ml/C}) = \frac{|\Delta V_a| + |\Delta V_c|}{2 \cdot A \cdot I} + 1.6 \times 10^{-4} \tag{16}$$

In the case of anion-exchange membranes, the flux sense is from the chamber connected to the negative pole of the current source toward the chamber connected to the positive pole. Thus, the meniscus goes forward in the anodic capillary tube and goes backwards in the cathodic one. In this case the electrochemical reactions that occurs in the electrodes are the same, but the volume changes in the cathodic and the anodic compartments have opposite sign that in the former case. From a similar algebra it follows that

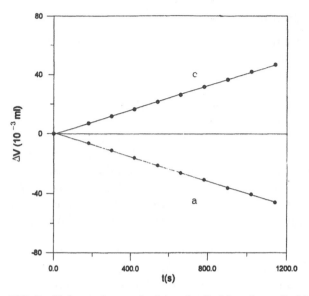

FIG. 3 Volume changes in the cathodic (c) and anodic (a) compartments, as a function of time, for the cation-exchange membrane 61 AZL 183 with a 0.01 N KCl and a current density of 18.9 mA/cm².

for anion-exchange membranes the electroosmotic permeability is given by:

$$W(\text{ml/C}) = -\frac{|\Delta V_a| + |\Delta V_c|}{2 \cdot A \cdot I} + 1.6 \times 10^{-4} \tag{17}$$

According to Eq. (17) the electroosmotic permeability will have negative sign for anionic membranes. Nevertheless, the absolute value of the electroosmotic permeability is taken in the corresponding plots.

D. Current–Voltage Curves

Prior to carrying out the measurements, the membrane was immersed for a minimum of 24 h in the solution. Once the thermal equilibrium state was reached, an electric current was injected by means of a current source and Ag|AgCl electrodes, measuring the potential difference established between the two faces of the membrane when the system was stabilized by using two probe electrodes placed the nearest possible of the membrane to reduce the contribution of the solution. The separation between both probe electrodes was always the same so that this contribution was also the same. This process was repeated for every value of the injected current density.

III. RESULTS AND DISCUSSION

The electroosmotic transport through the ion-exchange membranes used has been determined, following the methodology previously exposed in Sec. II, under different conditions of concentration, current density, stirring rate of the solutions, temperature, etc.

The values of the electroosmotic permeability, W, of the membranes, under different experimental conditions, were determined from the volume changes of the cathodic and anodic compartments by using Eqs. (16) and (17).

In all the cases studied the electroosmotic permeability depends strongly on the external salt concentration, decreasing when the solution concentration increases. These results agree with the ones obtained by other authors [21,22] and can be explained, according to Eq. (7), by the increase of the specific conductance in the membrane phase when the concentration of the external salt solution is increased.

This variation of the electroosmotic permeability with the concentration can be observed in Fig. 4 for membranes 61 AZL 183, 61 CZL 386, and CA300. For this last membrane it is observed that, for concentration greater than 10^{-1} mol/L, the electroosmotic permeability becomes practically zero.

The results obtained for the electroosmotic permeability of membrane CA500 are shown in Table 2. As can be observed W depends strongly on the concentration, but, the more notable aspect in this dependence is that, at

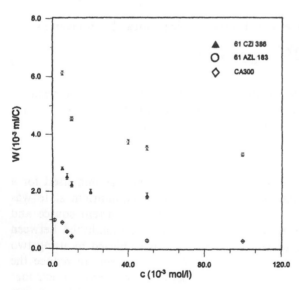

FIG. 4 Electroosmotic permeability as a function of concentration for membranes 61 AZL 183, 61 CZL 386, and CA300.

TABLE 2 Values of the Electroosmotic Permeability of Membrane CA500 as a Function of the Concentration with Different Electrolytes

c_0(mol/L)	$W(10^{-4}$ ml/C)		
	LiCl	NaCl	KCl
1×10^{-3}	—	9.57 ± 0.82	8.75 ± 0.29
2×10^{-3}	33.20 ± 0.06	8.70 ± 0.29	8.05 ± 0.31
5×10^{-3}	11.42 ± 0.06	7.58 ± 0.32	6.70 ± 0.31
1×10^{-2}	8.36 ± 0.15	7.05 ± 0.27	6.12 ± 0.37
2×10^{-2}	7.87 ± 0.12	5.55 ± 0.28	5.16 ± 0.40
5×10^{-2}	6.30 ± 0.30	4.40 ± 0.40	4.04 ± 0.44
7.5×10^{-2}	4.64 ± 0.15	3.54 ± 0.38	3.20 ± 0.40
1×10^{-1}	1.81 ± 0.80	3.20 ± 0.33	2.85 ± 0.34
2.5×10^{-1}	-1.12 ± 0.07	-0.36 ± 0.06	0.76 ± 0.12
5×10^{-1}	-4.00 ± 0.11	-0.76 ± 0.08	-1.72 ± 0.12

higher concentrations, the electroosmotic permeability not only becomes zero but also becomes slightly negative. It indicates that, at high concentrations comparing with the fixed charge density of the membrane, the electroosmotic flux reverses its usual sense and occurs from the cathodic compartment to the anodic compartment.

A similar result was obtained by Demisch and Pusch [23] with asymmetric cellulose acetate membranes. They considered that the strong concentration dependence as well as the sign reversal of W may be interpreted by treating the asymmetric membrane as a two-layer membrane and employing a finely pores model for both layers, leading to the conclusion that both the weak cation-exchange character as well as the asymmetry of the membrane are responsible for the significant sign reversal of the electroosmotic permeability at high concentration. In the case of our membrane CA500, the strong dependence on permeability have been related [20] to a decrease in the ionic selectivity of the membrane when the concentration increases and to the anion's higher mobility relative to the cation in the larger concentrations.

An inspection of Table 2 also indicates that the electroosmotic permeability, at a given concentration, decreases when the atomic number of the cation involved increases, in such a way that:

$$W(\text{LiCl}) > W(\text{NaCl}) > W(\text{KCl})$$

result that was also obtained with the other membranes studied in this work and that is in agreement with the results obtained by other authors [22].

From Eqs. (6) and (12) it is obtained, in the case of a cation-exchange membrane, that the water transport number, $\bar{t}_w = FJ_w/I$, is given by:

$$\bar{t}_w = \frac{1}{\bar{V}_w} (FW - \bar{V}_s \bar{t}_+) \tag{18}$$

On the other hand, the true cation transport $\bar{t}_+$ can be determined [14] by using the measurement of the emf of the concentration cell and the electroosmosis, by means of the following expression $\bar{t}_+ = Fc[W - dE^*/d(\Delta \pi)]$ where $dE^*/d(\Delta \pi)$ is the derivative of the emf with respect to the difference in osmotic pressure among the two external solutions, for a given value c of the concentration.

Known the values of the electroosmotic permeability and the cation transport number in the membrane phase, $\bar{t}_+$ and taking into account that $\bar{V}_w = 18$ ml/mol and that for NaCl and KCl it is

$$\bar{V}_{NaCl} = 16.4 + 2.1 \cdot (c)^{1/2}$$
$$\bar{V}_{KCl} = 26.3 + 3.6 \cdot (c)^{1/2}$$

the values of $\bar{t}_w$, for membrane CA500, were found from Eq. (18).

In Fig. 5 the value obtained for $\bar{t}_w$ as a function of the corresponding $\bar{t}_+$ has been shown. As can be observed, $\bar{t}_w$ increases when $\bar{t}_+$ increases, which is a

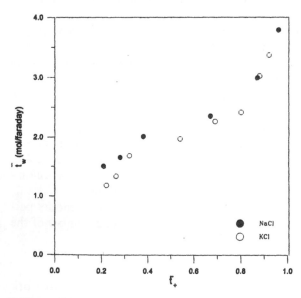

FIG. 5 $\bar{t}_w$ as a function of the corresponding $\bar{t}_+$ for membrane CA500.

natural requirement to make since the greater the electroosmotic transport, the greater the membrane selectivity. On the other hand, as previously mentioned in Sec. I, in neither of the two cases (KCl, NaCl) is a linear dependence between $\bar{t}_w$ and $\bar{t}_+$ found.

A. Dependence of the Electroosmotic Permeability on the Current Density

Special attention has been paid to the study of the dependence of the electroosmotic permeability, W, on the current density, I, although, at least in some aspects, no definite conclusions have been reached. Thus, in some papers [24–26] it was stated that there is no dependence between W and I, whereas in other papers [27–29], a dependence was found, showing the following two characteristic: (1) at sufficiently low values of the current density, the electroosmotic permeability increases when the current density decreases, and the increase is the more appreciable, the lower is the concentration of the solution and (2) at intermediate and high values of the current density, the electroosmotic permeability is practically independent of the current density. Laksminarayanaiah and Subrahmanyan [22,27] have related the existence of a dependence of W on I to the water content of the membrane, in such a way that for water contents of the membranes greater than about 14% there should exist dependence whereas for water content less than 14% no dependence exists. Khedr et al. [29] have tried to relate the anomalous transference of water observed at the lowest values of the current density with the phenomenon of concentration polarization leading to the conclusion that it is not possible to relate these phenomena.

We have determined the electroosmotic permeability, W, of different ionic-exchange membranes as a function of the current density, I, at different values of the concentration and stirring rate of the used electrolyte solutions [30].

In Figs. 6 and 7 the data (I, W) for the cationic membranes 61 AZL 183 and 61 CZL 3867 are shown. These data correspond to different concentrations of KCl solutions and they have been obtained in the absence of stirring. The data (I, W) for the anionic membranes 204 U 386, 103 QZL 386, and 204 SXZL 386, using a 10^{-2} mol/L concentration of KCl and in the absence of stirring, are shown in Fig. 8.

In most cases a dependence was found showing the two characteristics mentioned above, and a third one, that is, the existence of a local maximum in the curves (I, W), at a determined value of the current density. The value of the current density for which this maximum occurs, I_M, depends, for a determined membrane, on the experimental conditions.

The size of the local maximum decreases when the solution concentration increases (as a matter of fact, the maximum is hardly distinguished for the

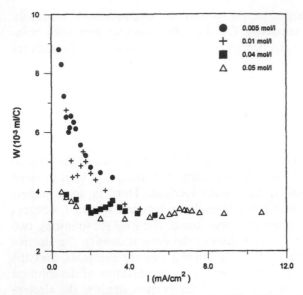

FIG. 6 Data (I, W) for membrane 61 AZL 183 for different concentrations of KCl solutions (from [30]).

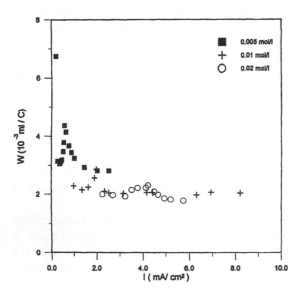

FIG. 7 Data (I, W) for membrane 61 CZL 386 for different concentrations of KCl solutions (from [30]).

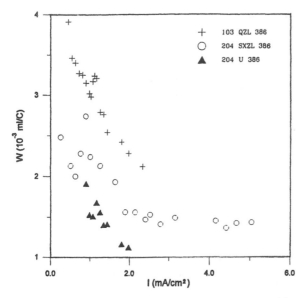

FIG. 8 Data (I, W) for the anionic membranes with a 10^{-2} mol/L concentration of KCl.

highest studied concentrations). Otherwise, the value for the current density at which the local maximum occurs increases when the solution concentration increases. On the other hand, it can be observed in some cases at the lowest concentrations, that the local maximum is found in the region of decreasing of W at the lowest I, in which case the maxima can not be clearly observed in some of these cases.

In Fig. 9, the (I, W) data obtained for the cationic membrane 61 AZL 183 with 0.005 mol/L KCl solution and various stirring rates are shown. As can be seen, the more efficient the stirring, the higher the values of I_M. On the other hand, the local maximum is clearly observed without stirring, but its existence becomes less appreciable, or even undetectable, for the greatest stirring rates. The slopes of the increase and decrease are greater at lower stirring rates. From the previous observations, it is a natural requirement so that the existence of this local maximum is directly related to the concentration polarization phenomenon.

As is well known, the passing of an electric current through an ion-exchange membrane separating two electrolyte aqueous solutions causes, because of the difference between the ionic mobilities of the counterion in the membrane and free solution phases, a depletion in the electrolyte concentration on one side of the membrane and an enrichment on the other side

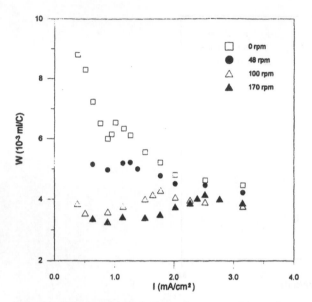

FIG. 9 Data (I, W) for membrane 61 AZl 183 with 0.005 mol/L KCl solution and various stirring rates (from [30]).

(concentration polarization). As a consequence, a concentration gradient is established through each of the layers that adjoin the membrane at the two faces, which are known as Nernst layers or polarization layers. Then, the concentration profile shown in Fig. 10 is established. The value of the current density at which the concentration in the depletion layer/membrane interface becomes zero is known as limiting current density.

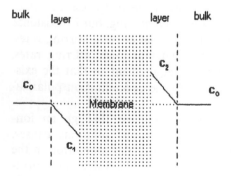

FIG. 10 Sketch of the concentration profile in the studied system.

From the classical theory of polarization [31] the limiting current density can be expressed by:

$$I_L = \frac{F \cdot D \cdot c_0}{\Delta t_+ \delta} \qquad (19)$$

where D is the salt diffusion coefficient, c_0 is the solution concentration corresponding to the bulk phase, δ is the thickness of the polarization layers and $\Delta t_+ = \bar{t}_+ - t_+$ is the difference between the cationic transport numbers in the membrane and in the free solution.

In Figs. 11 and 12 curves (V, I) are shown for membranes 61 AZL 183 and 61 CZL 386, in the absence of stirring and at different concentrations of KCl solutions.

Three characteristic regions can be distinguished on the curves (V, I). A first region in which the behavior is approximately ohmic; a second region, in which the electric current varies very slightly with the voltage (this region is the plateau, and corresponds to the limiting density current); and, finally, a third region, in which the electric current increases sharply with the voltage (overlimiting electric currents) and that is not yet fully understood (see, however, Chap. 17).

The study, from these curves, of the (V, I) data permits to obtain the value of the limiting current density corresponding to the plateau. However, as can be observed, the plateau became progressively less clear and, consequently, the

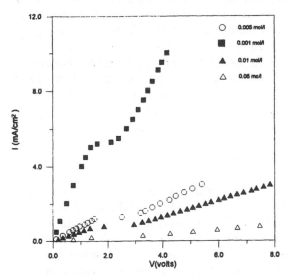

FIG. 11 Curves (V, I) for membrane 61 AZL 183 with different KCl solutions and without stirring (from [30]).

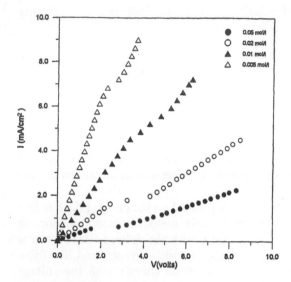

FIG. 12 Curves (V, I) for membrane 61 CZL 386 with different KCl solutions and without stirring (from [30]).

value of I_L less definite, when the solution concentration increases. In this case other standard methods (tangent or Cowan methods) [32] are used to obtain the value of the limiting current density, I_L. The values of I_L thus obtained and the values of I_M for which a local maximum in the curves (I, W) occurs are shown in Table 3 for the studied membranes, in the absence of stirring and with different values of the solution concentrations. Each one of the values of I_L and the corresponding one of I_M (under the same experimental conditions) are very close to each other, the deviation between both values is always lower than 5%. This similarity in the numerical values suggests that the existence of the plateau in the curves (V, I) and the local maximum in the curves (I, W) are closely related, both being a consequence of the concentration polarization. Therefore it may be considered that $I_L \cong I_M$ and, as consequence, the study of the curves (I, W) could be used as an alternative method to estimate the value of the limiting current density.

The displacement of the local maximum in the curves (V, I) toward higher values of the current density when the concentration of the solution and the stirring rate are increased, may be easily explained if one takes into account that $I_L \cong I_M$. In fact, if one considers Eq. (19), an increase of the concentration, c_0, causes I_L, and consequently I_M, to increase. On the other hand, an increase of the stirring rate causes the thickness of the polarization layer, δ, decreases, so, I_L, and consequently I_M, increases.

The thickness of the polarization layer can be obtained, from Eq. (19), when

TABLE 3 Values of I_L, I_M, and their Relative Deviation for all the Commercial Membranes at Different Solution Concentrations

Membrane	c_0(mol/l)	I_L(mA/cm²)	I_M(mA/cm²)	$(|I_M - I_L|/I_L)$ × 100
61 AZL 183	5×10^{-3}	1.07	1.07	0
	10^{-2}	1.64	1.64	0
	4×10^{-2}	3.24	3.28	1.2
	5×10^{-2}	6.62	6.62	0
61 CZL 386	5×10^{-3}	0.55	0.56	1.8
	10^{-2}	1.90	1.90	0
	2×10^{-2}	4.25	4.20	1.2
	5×10^{-2}	6.74	6.74	0
204 U 386	10^{-2}	1.20	1.17	2.6
103 QZL 386	10^{-2}	1.20	1.15	4.3
204 SXZL 386	10^{-2}	0.85	0.89	4.5

I_L has been determined from curves (V, I). Figure 13 shows δ as a function of stirring rate, w, for membrane 61 AZL 183 and different stirring rates. The stirring of solutions in this case was assessed by circulating them by means of a peristaltic pump. The values of δ are of the same order of magnitude as those obtained by other authors [33] for ion-exchange membranes.

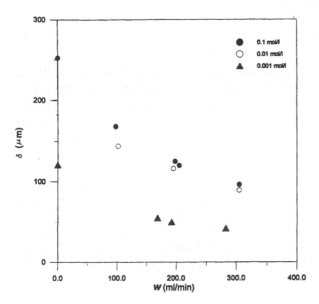

FIG. 13 Thickness of polarization layers vs. stirring rate for membrane 61 AZL 183 with different KCl solutions (from [30]).

B. Effect of Unstirred Solution Layers on the Electroosmotic Permeability

The unstirred solution layers (polarization layers) adjacent to the membrane at the two faces (Fig. 10) act as liquid membranes in series with the original one, and consequently affect the measured transport properties. This influence of the concentration polarization, although it can be controlled and reduced [34–36], can never be completely avoided.

The concentration gradient established through each one of the polarization layers give rise to a concentration difference existing between both sides of the membrane. The effect of this concentration difference is to add an osmotic component to the water flux. Thus, under these conditions, the total water flux through the membrane can be split, to a first approximation, into two contributions, (1) the net electroosmotic flux, J_e, which is proportional to the current density I and would take place even in the absence of a concentration gradient, and (2) the osmotic flux, J_0, due to the different values of the concentration in the solution–membrane two interfaces and which is proportional to the difference $(c_2 - c_1)$. That is:

$$J_V = J_e + J_0 = W_e \cdot I + B \cdot (c_2 - c_1) \tag{20}$$

where W_e is the net electroosmotic permeability and B is a coefficient directly related to the osmotic coefficient [37].

From Eqs. (6) and (20) it gets:

$$W = W_e + \frac{B}{I} \cdot (c_2 - c_1) \tag{21}$$

Equation (21) relates the apparent electroosmotic permeability, W, to the net electroosmotic permeability, W_e, and to a term that represents the contribution due to the polarization layers. It must be taken into account that the apparent electroosmotic permeability can be obtained from the experiments, by using Eq. (6), while the net electroosmotic permeability cannot. Consequently, to calculate the net electroosmotic permeability it is necessary to obtain the contribution of the unstirred layers to the value of W.

For current densities lower than the limiting current density, the concentration difference, $(c_2 - c_1)$, may be calculated by means of the classical concentration polarization theory [31]. In the anodic compartment, the electric current is transported by the positive ions in the direction of solution to membrane. Once the steady state has been reached (for a given value of the current density), the following relationship applies, in a region of solution near the membrane surface:

$$t_+ \cdot \frac{I}{F} + D_+ \cdot \frac{c_0 - c_1}{\delta_1} = \bar{t}_+ \cdot \frac{I}{F} \tag{22}$$

where D_+ is the cation diffusion coefficient. The last equation can be solved for the thickness of the layer δ_1:

$$\delta_1 = \frac{F \cdot D_+ \cdot (c_0 - c_1)}{(\bar{t}_+ - t_+) \cdot I} \tag{23}$$

In the same way, a similar relation can be obtained for the other layer:

$$\delta_2 = \frac{F \cdot D_+ \cdot (c_2 - c_0)}{(\bar{t}_+ - t_+) \cdot I} \tag{24}$$

Taking into account that the temperature and the stirring rate are the same in both chambers, one can presume that $\delta_1 \cong \delta_2 \cong \delta$. In these conditions, it can be assumed that c_0 is the mean value of c_1 and c_2, and from Eqs. (23) and (24) it is obtained that:

$$c_2 - c_1 = \frac{2 \cdot I \cdot \Delta t_+ \cdot \delta}{F \cdot D_+} \tag{25}$$

where $\Delta t_+ = \bar{t}_+ - t_+$. Equation (25) says that, under the experimental conditions considered, the transmembrane concentration difference is proportional to the polarization layer thickness.

From Eqs. (21) and (25) it follows:

$$W = W_e + \frac{2 \cdot B \cdot \Delta t_+ \cdot \delta}{F \cdot D_+} \tag{26}$$

The second term on the r.h.s. of Eq. (26) represents the osmotic contribution, W_{osm}, to the value of the apparent electroosmotic permeability. This term, for a given membrane and solution, is proportional to the layer thickness, δ.

Equation (25) and (26) state that an increase in the thickness of the layer gives rise to increases in both the transmembrane concentration gradient and the apparent electroosmotic permeability of the membrane.

It is well known that the effects of concentration polarization may be reduced by increasing the stirring rate of the solutions in the chambers. This fact may be taken into account, in a quantitative way, by assuming a simple relationship between the thickness of the layer for a determined stirring rate, $\delta(w)$, and this stirring rate, w:

$$\delta(w) = \frac{\delta_0}{\alpha \cdot w + 1} \tag{27}$$

where δ_0 is the layer thickness in absence of stirring and α is a positive adjustment parameter. A dependence similar to the one proposed in Eq. (27) was used in [38] in order to consider the temperature polarization effect in somewhat similar experiments of thermoosmosis and membrane distillation.

Equations (26) and (27) give:

$$W = W_e + \frac{B'}{\alpha \cdot w + 1} \tag{28}$$

where $B' = (2 \cdot \Delta t_+ \cdot B \cdot \delta_0)/(F \cdot D_+)$ is another positive parameter. Equation (28) states that the apparent electroosmotic permeability decreases with the stirring rate. On the other hand, in the absence of stirring ($w = 0$), we have:

$$W_0 = W_e + B' \tag{29}$$

where W_0 is the apparent electroosmotic permeability without stirring.

The obtained values of the apparent electroosmotic permeability as a function of the stirring rate for membrane 61 CZL 386, under different experimental conditions, are shown in Figs. 14 and 15. Figure 14 shows the results (w, W) obtained using KCl solution of different concentrations. Figure 15 refers to the result (w, W) obtained with solutions of the same concentrations (5×10^{-2} mol/L) but with different salts.

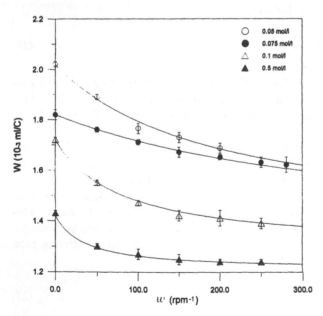

FIG. 14 Apparent electroosmotic permeability as a function of the stirring rate for membrane 61 CZL 386 with different KCl solutions. The experimental points correspond to a current density of 5.4 mA/cm² (from [37]).

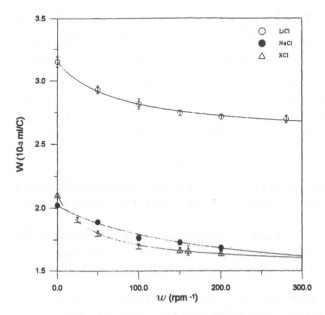

FIG. 15 Apparent electroosmotic permeability as a function of stirring rate for membrane 61 CZL 386 and different electrolytes. The experimental points correspond to a current density of 5.4 mA/cm^2 and a solute concentration of 0.05 mol/L (from [37]).

A visual inspection of Figs. 14 and 15 shows that the apparent electro-osmotic permeability decreases, in all cases, when the stirring rate increases, according to Eq. (28). This behaviour is due to the fact that the higher is the stirring rate, the smaller is the thickness of the polarization layer and, according to Eq. (25), the smaller is the membrane concentration difference as well.

The pair of values (w, W) have been adjusted to Eq. (28) by using a three parameter (W_e, B', and α) nonlinear method. The obtained theoretical curves are shown in Figs. 14 and 15 together with the experimental results corresponding to the different experimental situations studied. The adjustment parameters obtained are shown in Tables 4–6 together with the correlation coefficient. As can be observed, the value of the correlation coefficient is greater than 0.99, in the most unfavorable case, which confirms the accuracy of the assumptions made to obtained Eq. (28). On the other hand, Tables 4–6 show that the net electroosmotic permeability, W_e, decreases when the solution concentration and the cation atomic number increase. This behaviour agrees with the results reported by other authors [22,39]. In the same way parameter B', which is related to the osmotic contribution, decreases when the solution concentration increases and when the membrane selectivity decreases, but no significant dependence on the cation nature is observed. Finally,

TABLE 4 Parameters W_e, B', and α and Correlation Coefficient r for Membrane 61 CZL 386 at Different KCl Concentration for a Current Density of 5.4 mA/cm^2

c_0(mol/L)	5×10^{-2}	7.5×10^{-2}	10^{-1}	5×10^{-1}
W_e (10^{-3} ml/C)	1.37 ± 0.02	1.32 ± 0.05	1.29 ± 0.02	1.21 ± 0.01
B' (10^{-3} ml/C)	0.60 ± 0.02	0.50 ± 0.05	0.43 ± 0.02	0.21 ± 0.01
α (10^{-2}/rpm)	0.54 ± 0.04	0.27 ± 0.04	1.3 ± 0.2	3.0 ± 0.2
r	0.999	0.998	0.998	0.999

parameter α seems to increase both with solution concentration and with the membrane selectivity, and no definite pattern with the cation nature is observed.

Tables 7–9 present the percentage of the osmotic contribution to the apparent electroosmotic permeability value for each one of the stirring rates. As can be observed, the osmotic contribution decreases, in all cases, when the stirring rate increases.

Considering that the quantitative influence of the osmotic contribution to the apparent electroosmotic permeability decreases when the stirring rate

TABLE 5 Parameters W_e, B', and α and Correlation Coefficient r for Membrane 61 CZL 386 at Different Electrolytes for 5×10^{-2} mol/L Concentration and a Current Density of 5.4 mA/cm^2

Electrolyte	LiCl	NaCl	KCl
W_e (10^{-3} ml/C)	2.56 ± 0.03	1.53 ± 0.01	1.37 ± 0.02
B' (10^{-3} ml/C)	0.59 ± 0.03	0.57 ± 0.01	0.60 ± 0.02
α (10^{-2}/rpm)	1.3 ± 0.2	2.2 ± 0.2	0.54 ± 0.04
r	0.997	0.998	0.999

TABLE 6 Parameters W_e, B', and α and Correlation Coefficient r for Membranes 61 CZL 386 and 61 AZL 183 with 0.1 mol/L KCl

Membrane	61 CZL 386	61 AZL 183
W_e (10^{-3} ml/C)	1.26 ± 0.08	1.94 ± 0.03
B' (10^{-3} ml/C)	0.43 ± 0.07	0.89 ± 0.03
α (10^{-2}/rpm)	0.4 ± 0.1	0.66 ± 0.04
r	0.992	0.999

TABLE 7 Osmotic Contribution to the Apparent Electroosmotic Permeability, for Membrane 61 CZL 386, at Different Stirring Rates and KCl Concentrations. The Current Density is 5.4 mA/cm²

	$(W_{osm}/W) \cdot 100$			
w(rpm)	5×10^{-2} (mol/L)	7.5×10^{-2} (mol/L)	1×10^{-1} (mol/L)	5×10^{-1} (mol/L)
0	32.3	27.5	25.0	14.7
50	27.2	25.0	16.8	6.5
100	24.0	23.0	12.7	4.1
150	20.7	21.3	10.3	3.0
200	18.6	19.7	8.5	2.4

increases, one can assume that the apparent electroosmotic permeability, W, corresponding to infinite stirring rate may be equated to the net electroosmotic permeability W_e. These last values and the values of the measured electroosmotic permeability in the absence of stirring appear in Fig. 16 as a function of solution concentration. An inspection of this figure demonstrates that the osmotic contribution is important in all cases, reaching 1/3 of the total value in the most unfavorable case. On the other hand, both the electroosmotic and the osmotic contribution decrease when the concentration increases, being this decrease greater for the osmotic contribution.

TABLE 8 Osmotic Contribution to the Apparent Electroosmotic Permeability, for Membrane 61 CZL 386 and Different 0.05 mol/L Electrolytes, at Different Stirring Rates. The Current Density is 5.4 mA/cm²

	$(W_{osm}/W) \cdot 100$		
w(rpm)	LiCl	NaCl	KCl
0	18.7	27.1	32.2
50	12.2	15.1	27.2
100	9.1	10.5	24.0
150	7.3	7.9	20.7
200	6.0	6.4	18.6

TABLE 9 Osmotic Contribution to the Apparent Electroosmotic Permeability, for Membranes 61 CZL 386 and 61 AZL 183, at Different Stirring Rates. The Current Density is 6.3 mA/cm² and the Concentration of KCl 0.1 mol/L

	$(W_{osm}/W) \cdot 100$	
w(rpm)	61 CZL 386	61 AZL 183
0	25.3	31.3
50	22.1	25.5
100	19.5	21.6
150	17.7	19.0
200	16.2	16.5

C. Dependence of the Electroosmotic Permeability on the Temperature

Little attention has been devoted to the dependence of the electroosmotic permeability on the temperature and references found in the literature are scarce. Most of them state that the electroosmotic permeability increases when the

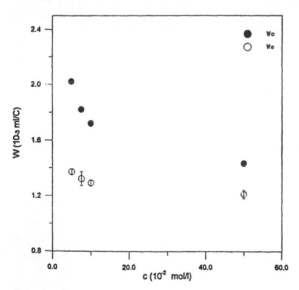

FIG. 16 Electroosmotic permeabilities W_0 and W_e as a function of KCl concentration for membrane 61 CZL 386 and a current density of 5.4 mA/cm² (from [37]).

temperature increases [40–42], but some authors also obtain a light decrease with the temperature [28]. However, in these works the dependence of the water electroosmotic transport on the temperature is not studied in depth, and the manner of this dependence is not very clear.

We have studied the influence of the temperature on the value of the electroosmotic permeability for the cation-exchange membranes 61 AZL 183 and 61 CZL 386. The results obtained show that a clear dependence of the electroosmotic permeability on the temperature, T, exists, in such a way that, as a general trend, at the lowest values of the temperature in the studied range the electroosmotic permeability decreases when the temperature increases, and afterwards the electroosmotic permeability increases with increasing T, presenting the (T, W) data a minimum value at certain value of temperature. Figure 17 shows, as an illustration of the above mentioned behaviour, the results obtained with the two studied commercial cation-exchanged membranes.

The reasons for the dependence of the electroosmotic permeability on the temperature are not clear, probably influenced by various factors. The observed minimum, however, may be due to the dependence of the osmotic contribution (from concentration polarization) to the total volume flux on the temperature. This contribution depends on two factors one of them increasing

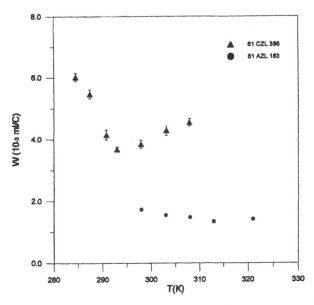

FIG. 17 Electroosmotic permeability as a function of temperature for the two commercial cationic membranes.

with temperature, and another decreasing with it. The balance between these two trends should explain the minimum observed in the (T, W) curves. In addition, the position of the minimum permits us to establish in which temperature range one trend predominates over the other. However, to achieve a better and more complete understanding of the behaviour of W with T, more information about the dependence of the osmotic contribution to the W value is required. Further work is in progress in this direction.

IV. CONCLUSIONS

The electroosmotic permeability depends strongly on the external salt concentration, decreasing when the solution concentration increases. In some cases, at high concentrations, the electroosmotic flux reverses its usual direction.

The electroosmotic permeability, for a given concentration, decreases when the atomic number of the alkali cation involved increases.

The electroosmotic permeability presents a dependence on the current density which shows the following characteristics: (1) at sufficiently low values of the current density, the electroosmotic permeability increases when the current density decreases; (2) at intermediate and high values of the current density, in the studied range, the electroosmotic permeability presents a local maximum; (3) in the range of the highest current densities, the electroosmotic permeability seems to be independent of the current density. The value of the current density, I_M, at which the local maximum in the curves (I, W) is observed, and the value of the limiting current density, I_L, under the same experimental conditions, are very close, so, the determination of I_M can be used as an alternative method to estimate I_L.

Due to the concentration polarization effect, an osmotic contribution to the value of the measured electroosmotic permeability exists. This contribution is important, although it decreases with increasing solution stirring.

The electroosmotic permeability depends on the temperature. At the lowest values of the temperature, in the studied range, the apparent electroosmotic permeability decreases with increasing the temperature up to a certain value of the temperature and afterwards, the opposite behavior occurs, i.e., the electroosmotic permeability increases when the temperature increases. Thus, the curves (T, W) show a minimum at certain value of the temperature.

REFERENCES

1. G. S. Schmid, Z. Elecktrochem. *54*:424 (1950).
2. G. S. Schmid, Z. Elecktrochem. *55*:229 (1951).
3. G. S. Schmid, Z. Elecktrochem. *56*:181 (1952).
4. G. S. Schmid, Chem. Ing. Techn. *37*:616 (1965).
5. G. S. Schmid and H. Z. Schwarz, Eleckrochem. *55*:295 (1951).

6. G. S. Schmid and H. Z. Schwarz, Eleckrochem. *55*:684 (1951).
7. G. S. Schmid and H. Z. Schwarz, Eleckrochem. *56*:35 (1952).
8. N. Bjerrum and E. Manegold, Kolloid-Z. *43*:5 (1927).
9. E. Manegold and K. Solf, Kolloid-Z. *55*:273 (1931).
10. A. G. Winger, R. Ferguson, and R. Kunin, J. Phys. Chem. *60*:556 (1956).
11. Y. Oda and T. Yawataya, Bull. Chem. Soc. Jpn *30*:213 (1957).
12. T. R. E. Kressman, P. A. Stanbridge, and F. L. Tye, Trans. Faraday Soc. *59*:2139 (1963).
13. N. Laksminarayanaiah and K. R. Brennen, Electrochim. Acta *11*:949 (1966).
14. C. Ruíz-Bauzá, C. Rueda, and V. M. Barragán, J. Non Equilib. Thermodyn. *15*:383 (1990).
15. A. J. Staverman, Trans. Faraday Soc. *48*:176 (1952).
16. K. S. Spiegler, Trans. Faraday Soc. *54*:1048 (1958).
17. Y. Kobatake, J. Chem. Phys. *28*:146 (1958).
18. T. S. Sørensen and J. Koefoed, J. Chem. Soc. Faraday Trans. II *70*:665 (1974).
19. J. W. Jarris and F. L. Tye, J. Chem. Phys. *28*:166 (1961).
20. V. M. Barragán, C. Rueda, and C. Ruíz-Bauzá, J. Colloid Interface Sci. *172*:361 (1995).
21. P. Trivijitkasem and F. Ostwold, Electrochim. Acta *25*:171 (1984).
22. N. Laksminarayanaiah, J. Electrochem. Soc. *116*:338 (1969).
23. K. V. Demisch and W. Pusch, J. Colloid Interface Sci. *76*:445 (1980).
24. D. Mackay and P. Meares, Trans. Faraday Soc. *55*:1221 (1959).
25. T. R. E. Kressman, P. A. Stanbridge, and F. L. Tye, Trans. Faraday Soc. *59*:2129 (1963).
26. C. W. Carr, R. MacClintock, and K. Sollner, J. Electrochem. Soc. *109*:251 (1962).
27. N. Laksminarayanaiah and V. Subrahmanyan, J. Phys. Chem. *72*:1253 (1968).
28. J. K. B. George and R. A. Courant, J. Phys. Chem. *71*:246 (1967).
29. A. Khedr, A. Schmitt, and R. Varoqui, J. Colloid Interface Sci. *66*:516 (1978).
30. V. M. Barragán, C. Ruíz-Bauzá, and J. I. Mengual, J. Membrane Sci. *95*:1 (1994).
31. F. Helfferich, *Ion-Exchange*, McGraw-Hill, New York, 1962.
32. J. A. Manzanares, K. Kontturi, S. Mafé, V. M. Aguilella, and J. Pellicer, Acta Chem. Scand. *45*:115 (1991).
33. K. Inenaga and N. Yoshida, J. Membrane Sci. *6*:271 (1980).
34. N. Laksminarayanaiah, *Transport Phenomena in Membranes*, Academic Press, New York, 1969.
35. C. R. House, *Water Transport in Cells and Tissues*, Arnold, London, 1975.
36. P. H. Barry and A. B. Hope, Biophys. J. *9*:760 (1969).
37. V. M. Barragán, C. Ruíz-Bauzá, and J. I. Mengual, J. Colloid Interface Sci. *168*:458 (1994).
38. J. M. Ortíz de Zárate, F. García-López, and J. I. Mengual, J. Membrane Sci. *56*:181 (1991).
39. E. Pfefferkorn, A. Schmitt, and R. Varoqui, J. Membrane Sci. *4*:17 (1978).
40. R. Haase and K. Harff, J. Membrane Sci. *12*:279 (1983).
41. A. Narebska, W. Kujawski, and S. Kotter, J. Membrane Sci. *30*:125 (1987).
42. R. P. Rastogi and K. M. Jha, J. Phys. Chem. *70*:1017 (1966).

16

Anion-Exchange Membranes with Viologen Cross-Links Showing Photovoltaic Effects and with Permselective Properties Determined by Photoirradiation

TOSHIKATSU SATA Department of Applied Chemistry and Chemical
Engineering, Yamaguchi University, Yamaguchi, Japan

Abstract

Anion-exchange membranes having a viologen moiety as anion-exchange groups were prepared by the reaction of copolymer membranes composed of chloromethylstyrene and divinylbenzene and chloromethylated polysulfone with 4,4'-bipyridine. The viologen moiety of the membranes was reduced from a dication to a monocation radical and biradical by photoirradiation in organic solvents and aqueous salt solutions to release electrons. The active wavelength to reduce a viologen moiety of the membranes was below around 450 nm due to polymer effect. The anion-exchange membranes with a viologen moiety generated a photovoltage and photocurrent by photoirradiation after the membranes had been swelled with solvents, clamped between two ITO electrodes, and sealed with adhesive. This is based on the photoreduction of the viologen moiety of the membranes at photoside to release electrons and the electrochemical reduction of a viologen moiety at the dark side. Though the generation of photovoltage and photocurrent was very slow at the first irradiation, the generation speed was rapid once photoirradiation had been carried out due to the existence of the monocation radical. The 50–150 mV of photovoltage was observed at 200 kΩ load resistance which was dependent on membrane species, species of solvent, additives in the photocell, etc. Another property of the anion-exchange membranes was the change in the transport numbers of sulfate, bromide, fluoride and nitrate ions relative to chloride ions in electrodialysis in the presence or absence of photoirradiation. In general, the permeation of anions larger than chloride ions through the membranes decreased in the presence of photoirradiation compared with those without the irradiation. It was concluded that the change in the transport numbers of various anions relative to chloride ions was due to the decrease in the pore size of the membrane because the charge density of the membrane decreased with photoirradiation.

I. INTRODUCTION

Ion-exchange membranes are among the most advanced separation membranes and have been widely used in various industries [1–3]: in electrodialysis processes, diffusion dialysis processes, as separators of electrolysis, solid polymer electrolytes for fuel cell and water electrolysis, etc. Basically, the ion-exchange groups of the membranes, which are the active sites, are the origin of the function of the ion-exchange membranes. Today, sulfonic acid groups and carboxylic acid groups are used as the cation-exchange groups, and anion-exchange groups of the anion-exchange membranes are limited to benzyl trimethylammonium groups and *N*-alkylpyridinium groups. Bipyridinium groups, which act as cross-linking point and have photosensitivity, are interesting as new anion-exchange groups.

Conversion of visible light into electricity is an important research subject in relation to photoenergy conversion and photoinformation. Inorganic semiconductors are already used in the field, such as solar cells, etc. On the other hand, if controlling permeation of a specific ion through the ion-exchange membrane by photoenergy in electrodialysis is possible, it might provide a new application for the ion-exchange membranes, not only the separation of ions, but also photoswitching, etc.

Because aza-aromatic molecules have photoreactivity which is governed by the presence of the nitrogen lone pair of electrons [4], numerous studies on 4,4'-bipyridine and its derivatives and complexes of 2,2'-bipyridine and ruthenium have been made not only for the preparation of materials and methods which utilize photoenergy, such as water splitting to produce hydrogen gas by photoirradiation [5–12] and photoreductive organic synthesis [13,14], but also for electrochemical uses, such as electrochromic displays [15,16], oxygen sensors [17,18] etc. Also various kinds of polymers possessing a viologen moiety have been synthesized, and precise analyses of their properties were reported. These polymers were examined for modified electrodes [19–22], photoassisted hydrogen evolution [23] photochromic materials [24–27], organic synthesis [28–30], photomemory [31], electron transfer membranes [32], etc. The insoluble membranous polymers with a 4,4'-bipyridine moiety are naturally one type of anion-exchange membranes.

The anion-exchange membranes having a 4,4'-bipyridine moiety are attractive for two reasons.

1. Because the membrane releases electrons from a membranes surface by photoirradiation due to photoreduction of a viologen moiety, which means that the dication (MV^{2+}) of the viologen moiety changes into a monocation radical (MV^+) and then the monocation radical becomes biradical (MV^0) (Scheme 1), the membrane becomes an electron donor by collecting the released electron. On the other hand, a viologen moiety of the membrane is easily reduced by chemical reduction. Namely, if the electron released by the photoirradiation is fed to the opposite side of the membrane surface via a suitable load resistance, a kind of photocell can be prepared [33].

2. Because the viologen moiety of the membrane changes from divalent cation to monocation radical, and then the monocation radical to biradical, which is neutral, the charge density of the anion-exchange membrane can be controlled by photoirradiation. Thus, the permselectivity between two anions should change. Although the membrane with a viologen moiety may possibly show other new properties, in this work, these two properties of the membranes are mentioned together with the basic properties of the anion-exchange membrane.

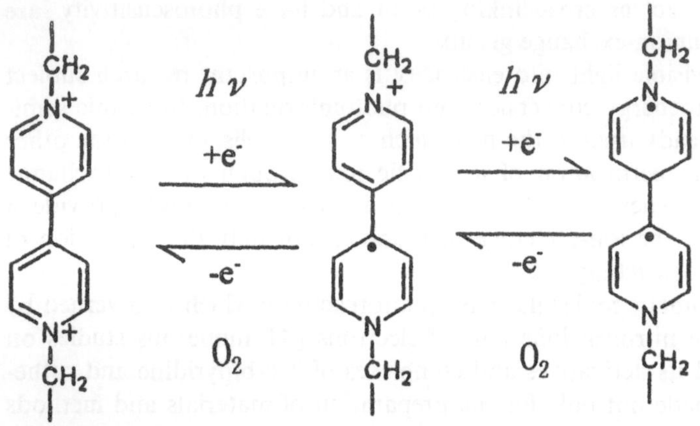

SCHEME 1

II. EXPERIMENTAL

A. Preparation of Ion-Exchange Membranes Containing a Viologen Moiety

As a preliminary experiment, to examine the photoreduction of a viologen moiety in the membrane matrix, methyl viologen was ion-exchanged with cation-exchange membranes, and the membranes were photoirradiated to observe the generation of photovoltage [34]. Anion-exchange membranes having a viologen moiety were then prepared.

The cation-exchange membrane containing methyl viologen (1,1'-dimethyl-4,4'-bipyridinium chloride) was prepared by immersing the cation-exchange membrane of the sulfonic acid form into an aqueous 10% methyl viologen solution and renewing the solution repeatedly until the pH of the solution attained the value of the 10% viologen solution. Because viologen molecules are large compared with inorganic ions, it is not easy to ion-exchange completely between the sulfonic acid groups of the membrane and methyl viologen. The cation-exchange membranes used were NEOSEPTA C66-5T (ion-exchange capacity: 2.45 meq/g-dry Na^+ form membrane; thickness: 170 μm; electrical resistance: 1.6 Ω cm^2, measured in 0.500 N sodium chloride solution at 25.0°C with 1000 cycle AC; transport number: greater than 0.98, measured by electrodialysis of 0.500 N sodium chloride solution at current density of 20 mA/cm^2 at 25.0°C; water content: 0.42, g H_2O/g Na^+ form dry membrane), CH-45T (ion-exchange capacity: 2.11 meq/g-dry Na^+ form membrane; thickness: 160 μm; electrical resistance: 2.3 Ω cm^2, measured in 0.500 N sodium chloride solution at 25.0°C with 1000 cycle AC; transport number: greater than 0.98, measured by electrodialysis of 0.500 N sodium chloride solution at current density of 20 mA/cm^2 at 25.0°C; water content: 0.38, g H$_2$O/g Na$^+$ form dry membrane) produced by Tokuyama Corp. and Nafion 117 (ion-exchange capacity: 0.92 meq/g-dry Na$^+$ form membrane; thickness: 175 μm; electrical resistance: 3.5 Ω cm^2, measured in 0.500 N sodium chloride solution at 25.0°C with 1000 cycle AC; transport number: greater than 0.95, measured by electrodialysis of 0.500 N sodium chloride solution at current density of 20 mA/cm^2 at 25.0°C; water content: 0.22, g H$_2$O/g Na$^+$ form dry membrane) produced by E.I. du Pont de Nemours & Co. Inc.

The anion-exchange membranes having a viologen moiety as anion-exchange groups were prepared by reacting 4,4'-bipyridine with the chloromethyl groups of membranous polymers: copolymer membranes composed of chloromethylstyrene and divinylbenzene and membranes of chloromethylated polysulfone. The copolymer membranes of chloromethylstyrene and divinyl-benzene were prepared by copolymerization of chloromethylstyrene and divinylbenzene by radical polymerization using benzoyl peroxide as an initiator in the presence of an inert polymer (acrylonitrile–butadiene rubber) and backing fabric [a woven cloth made of poly(vinyl chloride)] to impart mechanical strength to the membrane [35]. The ratio of divinylbenzene to total vinyl-monomers (cross-linking degree) was changed: 4.5, 8.0, 10.0, 14.0 and 20.0 (wt%, [0.55 commercial divinylbenzene/(chloromethylstyrene + commercial divinylbenzene)] × 100). Chloromethylated polysulfone was prepared by the reaction of polysulfone, Udel P-1700 (Amoco Corp.), with chloromethyl-methyl ether in the presence of zinc chloride anhydride (solvent: ethylene dichloride) [36]. The Cl-content of the obtained polymer was 6.95% by elemental analysis. The membranous polymers were obtained by casting a 1-methyl-2-pyrrolidone solution (basically, 10%) on a glass plate and evaporating the solvent at 100°C in an air oven.

To introduce a viologen moiety into the obtained membranous polymers having chloromethyl groups, the membranous polymers were immersed in a 5% 4,4'-bipyridine ethyl alcohol solution and heated at 75°C for 120 h. After the reaction, the membranes were thoroughly washed with ethyl alcohol and then 1.0 N hydrochloric acid solution to remove unreacted 4,4'-bipyridine. The reaction was confirmed by measurement of the FTIR-ATR spectra of the anion-exchange membrane prepared from the copolymer membrane of chloromethylstyrene and divinylbenzene and 4,4'-bipyridine and the corresponding copolymer membrane. A characteristic peak was found in the reacted membrane at 1637 cm^{-1} which is attributed to quaternized 4-vinylpyridine groups. This peak is thought to be the stretching vibration of C=N and C=C in the pyridine ring. The viologen moiety was introduced into the membranous copolymers, and the membranes changed into anion-exchange membranes. As an example, Fig. 1 shows a schematic molecular structure of the anion-exchange membrane prepared from chloromethylated polysulfone and 4,4'-bipyridine.

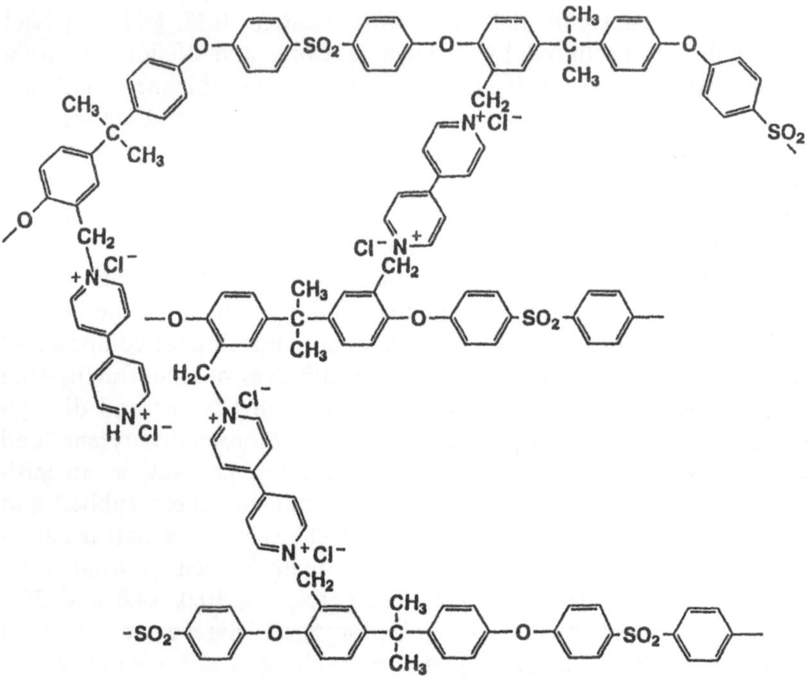

FIG. 1 Schematic molecular structure of anion-exchange membrane having viologen moiety (anion-exchange membrane from chloromethylated polysulfone and 4,4'-bipyridine).

B. Measurements of Electrochemical Properties of Anion-Exchange Membranes Having a Viologen Moiety as Anion-Exchange Groups

Because 4,4'-bipyridine is a bifunctional and bulky amine, the amine was difficult to react completely with the chloromethyl groups of the membranes, and at the same time cross-linking reaction occurred between the chloromethyl groups. Table 1 shows the electrochemical properties of the anion-exchange membranes having a viologen moiety as anion-exchange groups together with those of the membranes of benzyl trimethylammonium groups. In general, the increase in the cross-linkage of the membranes provided the increase in their electrical resistance. The ion-exchange capacity of the membranes with a viologen moiety was lower than that of the membranes reacted with trimethylamine due to the difficulty of the reaction. It is interesting that the ratio of tertiary amino groups to total anion-exchange capacity decreased with increasing content of the divinylbenzene of the membranes. It was reported that the copolymer of chloromethylstyrene and divinylbenzene exists in the

TABLE 1 Characteristics of Anion-Exchange Membranes Prepared in this Work

Name	M-1	M'-1	M-2	M-3	M'-3	M-4	M'-4	M-5	M'-5	M-6[l]
Backing	PVC	PVC	PVC	PVC	PVC	PVC	PVC	PVC	PVC	
Content of divinylbenzene (%)	4.5	4.5	8.0	10.0	10.0	14.0	14.0	20.0	20.0	—
Anion-exchange groups	Vio[a]	BTMA[b]	Vio[a]	Vio[a]	BTMA[b]	Vio[a]	BTMA[b]	Vio[a]	BTMA[b]	Vio[a]
Electrical resistance[c]										
0.500 N NaCl (1)[d]	2.2	0.8	5.5	8.3	1.1	14.4	2.2	25.5	3.5	11.0
1.000 N HCl	1.4	—	3.2	4.6	—	7.6	—	12.0	—	1.1
0.500 N NaCl (2)[e]	7.8	0.8	17.5	25.3	1.1	41.8	2.2	43.6	3.5	5.2
0.500 N TMAC[f]	160.5	—	405.9	670.5	—	999.0	—	1498.6	—	82.5
Transport number[g]	>0.98	>0.98	>0.98	>0.98	>0.98	>0.98	>0.98	>0.98	>0.98	>0.98
Ion-exchange capacity[h]	1.90	2.70	1.59	1.42	2.25	1.20	2.11	0.94	1.56	1.36
Quaternary	1.29	2.70	1.21	1.09	2.25	0.92	2.11	0.83	1.56	1.21
Tertiary[i]	0.61	0	0.38	0.33	0	0.28	0	0.11	0	0.15
Water content[j]	0.20	47.1	0.15	0.11	0.31	0.09	0.27	0.08	0.15	0.16
Thickness (μm)[k]	125	150	121	127	130	121	130	108	120	75

[a] Reacted with 4,4′-bipyridine (viologen moiety).

[b] Reacted with trimethylamine (benzyl trimethylammonium moiety).

[c] In Ω cm^2; measured with 1000-cycle AC at 25.0°C after membranes had been equilibrated with each solution to be measured.

[d] After membranes had been immersed in a 1.0 N hydrochloric acid solution, the membranes were equilibrated with a 0.500 N sodium chloride solution.

[e] After membranes had been immersed in a 0.5 N ammonia solution, the membranes were equilibrated with a 0.500 N sodium chloride solution.

[f] After membranes had been dried under vacuum at 50°C for 4 h, the membranes were equilibrated with a 0.500 N tetramethylammonium chloride ethylene glycol solution.

[g] Measured by electrodialysis of a 0.50 N sodium chloride solution at 25.0°C at the current density of 20 mA/cm^2 for 1 h.

[h] Meq/g-Cl$^-$ form dry membrane.

[i] Meq/g-Cl$^-$ form dry membrane (After the membranes had been equilibrated with the mixed solution composed of 4.0 N sodium chloride and 0.05 N sodium hydroxide (pH 12.17), chloride ions in the membrane were determined after eluting chloride ions with 0.20 N sodium nitrate.)

[j] g-H$_2$O/g-Cl$^-$ form dry membrane, equilibrated with a 0.50 N sodium chloride solution.

[k] After equilibration with a 0.500 N sodium chloride solution.

[l] M-6 membranes of various thickness were prepared, and characteristics of a typical membrane are shown in Table 1.

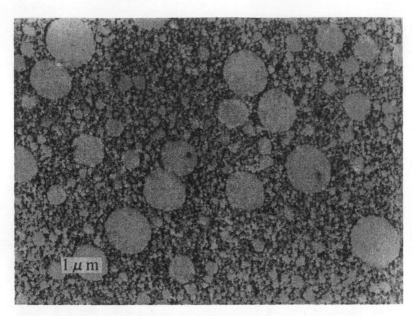

FIG. 2 Scanning transmission electron micrograph of the cross-section of copolymer membrane for M-3 membrane (before reaction with 4,4'-bipyridine).

membrane matrix forming a microdomain as shown in Fig. 2 (scanning transmission electron micrograph of the cross-section of the membrane before introduction of anion-exchange groups) [37–40]. This suggests that the cross-linking by the 4,4'-bipyridine effectively proceeded in the microdomain having a high content of divinylbenzene. Thus, the electrical resistance of the membranes with a viologen moiety steeply increased with increasing cross-linkage of the membrane due to the decrease in ion-exchange capacity and the development of cross-linkage by the diamine (Fig. 3). Because the inert polymer and backing fabric in these membranes are soluble in aprotic solvents, the anion-exchange membranes broke by immersing the membranes into such solvents.

The anion-exchange membranes prepared from the membranes of chloromethylated polysulfone and 4,4'-bipyridine were insoluble in any kind of solvents: dioxane, 1-methyl-2-pyrrolidone, etc., because the membranes were composed of a single polymer cross-linked with the diamine. Also the thickness of the anion-exchange membranes was changed by changing the concentration of the casting solution of chloromethylated polysulfone. Especially, a 14 μm thick membrane was prepared for the measurements of the spectrum change with photoirradiation.

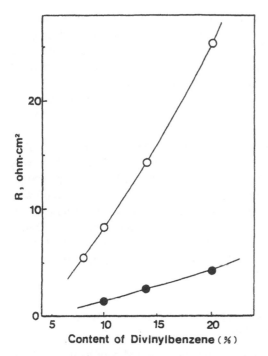

FIG. 3 Comparison of electrical resistance of anion-exchange membranes having a viologen (4,4′-bipyridine) moiety with that of benzyl trimethylammonium groups in anion-exchange membranes with different cross-linkage. ●, reacted with trimethylamine; ○, reacted with 4,4′-bipyridine.

C. Photoreduction of a Viologen Moiety Bonded to Anion-Exchange Membranes

It is well-known that viologen compounds are reduced by photoirradiation as demonstrated by Scheme 1. The viologen moiety of the membranes was also reduced by photoirradiation to release electrons. Absorption spectra of the membranes were measured after the membrane, which had been swelled with ethylene glycol, clamped between two ITO electrodes (Indium-Tin-Oxide electrodes: obtained from Geomatec Co. Ltd., Japan) and sealed with epoxide adhesive, had been irradiated with light (500 W xenon lamp) from one side of the membrane for various periods. Other measurements of absorption spectra of the thin membrane were performed after the membrane had been equilibrated with degassed water or various sodium salt solutions under nitrogen atmosphere using quartz cells after irradiation for various periods. The membrane used was a thin anion-exchange membrane having a viologen moiety (14 μm thick) prepared from chloromethylated polysulfone and 4,4-bipyridine.

In both cases, upon photoirradiation, the color of the membranes changed from pale yellow to deep blue (formation of MV^+) and then became transparent, slightly brown (formation of MV^0), in various organic solvents, water and various aqueous salt solutions. As previously mentioned, because both tertiary amino groups of 4,4'-bipyridine did not react completely with the chloromethyl groups of the membranes, tertiary amino groups remain in the membrane. It was reported that the spectrum of the reduced form of the protonated 4-(N-methyl-pyridinium)-pyridine is identical with that of methyl viologen [41]. Thus, all membranes for photovoltage measurement were equilibrated with an aqueous 1.0 N hydrochloric acid solution before use. In fact, there was a remarkable difference between the absorption spectra of the anion-exchange membrane immersed in hydrochloric acid solution and those of the membrane immersed in ammonia solution after photoirradiation [42]. Measurements of transport numbers of various anions relative to chloride ions and permeability coefficient of urea were also carried out after the membrane had been immersed in 1.0 N hydrochloride acid solution and then equilibrated with mixed salt solutions to be used in electrodialysis.

D. Measurements of Photovoltage and Photocurrent and Change in Electrical Resistance of the Cell

After the cation-exchange membrane with which methyl viologen had been ion-exchanged had swelled with ethylene glycol after drying, or the anion-exchange membrane with a viologen moiety had been equilibrated with water or various organic solvents (after drying completely), the membrane was clamped between two ITO electrodes and completely sealed with epoxide adhesive. The effective membrane area was 7.0 cm^2 (2.15 cm × 3.26 cm) or 4.0 cm^2 (2.0 cm × 2.0 cm) according to the experiment. The cell was assembled under a nitrogen atmosphere using degassed water or organic solvents, because oxygen in the solvent acts as an electron acceptor; a photovoltage was observed immediately after photoirradiation and soon decayed according to the amount of oxygen in the cell. When two ITO electrodes had been separated with any nontransparent film wetted with the solvent and irradiated with light from one side, the generation of an electrical potential was observed because ITO electrodes are a kind of n-type semi-conductor. To decrease the potential due to the ITO electrodes below 1.0 mV, a 200 kΩ load resistance was selected. Figure 4 shows a cell and circuit to measure photovoltage and photocurrent.

Photovoltage and photocurrent were measured by irradiating the cell with a 500 W xenon lamp after the cell had been placed in a dark box. Because the distance between the cell and the lamp was 60 cm, the cell was immersed in a liquid paraffin bath, which was maintained at 30°C. The strength of the light was 300,000 lx, measured by an illuminance meter. Photovoltage and photo-

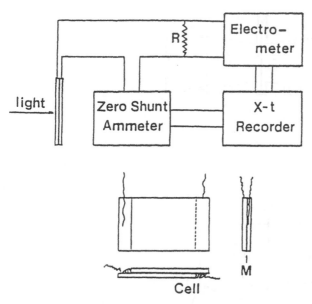

FIG. 4 A cell and circuit to measure photovoltage and photocurrent. M, ion-exchange membrane (the membrane was clamped between two ITO electrodes with Cu wire and sealed with adhesive); R, load resistance (200 kΩ); light: 500 W xenon lamp.

current were recorded on an X-t recorder via an electrometer and zero-shunt ammeter.

Radicals are formed in the membrane and the solvent by photoirradiation; therefore, the electrical resistance of the cell should change due to the irradiation. The change in the electrical resistance during irradiation was measured while the cell was being irradiated from one side of the cell. Both ITO electrodes were connected to an LCR meter using suitable condensers to avoid disturbance by the photovoltage. Measurement was made at constant temperature (30°C).

E. Measurement of Transport Numbers of Various Anions Relative to Chloride Ions in Electrodialysis

A two-compartment cell and four-compartment cell with Ag–AgCl electrodes were used as shown in Fig. 5. The two-compartment cell was used for measurements of mixed sodium sulfate and sodium chloride solution, and the four-compartment cell was for the mixed solutions of sodium bromide and sodium chloride, sodium nitrate and sodium chloride, and sodium fluoride and sodium chloride. The cells were made of glass to allow photoirradiation on the membrane surface. The capacity of each compartment was 115 cm³, and the solu-

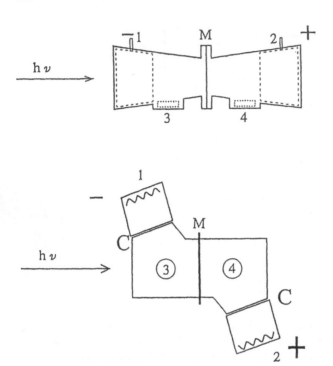

FIG. 5 Electrodialysis cell to measure transport number between anions (two-compartment and four-compartment cell). 1,2: Ag–AgCl electrodes for current supply; 3,4: stirrers; C: cation-exchange membrane (separator); M: anion-exchange membrane to be measured (effective membrane area: 10 cm^2); capacity of each compartment: 115 cm^3; hv: light from 500 W xenon lamp. (Two-compartment cell was used in mixed sodium sulfate and sodium chloride solution, and four-compartment cell was used in measurements of solutions containing bromide, nitrate, fluoride ions together with chloride ions.)

tions were vigorously agitated with stirrers (the effective membrane area was 10 cm^2). The light from a xenon lamp (500 W) was used to irradiate the desalting-side surface of the anion-exchange membrane before and during electrodialysis (the distance between the lamp and the membrane surface was 60 cm.). The cell was immersed in a thermostated water bath maintained at 25.0°C, placed in a dark box.

The measured transport properties of the anion-exchange membranes with a viologen moiety were the transport numbers of various anions relative to chloride ions and the current efficiency with or without photoirradiation. The transport number of anions relative to chloride ions was defined by, $P_{Cl}^A = (t_A/t_{Cl})/(C_{Cl}/c_{Cl})$: t_A and t_{Cl} are the transport numbers of anion A and the chloride ions; C_A is the average of the concentrations of the anion A before and after electrodialysis, and so is C_{Cl} for the chloride ion. P_{Cl}^A is the equivalent of anion A permeated through the membrane when one equivalent of chloride ion permeates through the membrane because a $1:1$ mixed salt solution was used.

The procedure for the electrodialysis was as follows: After an anion-exchange membrane had been placed in the cell, the two-compartments adjacent to the anion-exchange membrane to be measured were filled with 115 cm^3 of the mixed salt solution. In the case of the four-compartment cell, both anolyte and catholyte compartments were filled with the sodium chloride solution of the same sodium concentration as the mixed salt solution (115 cm^3; all solutions were degassed before use). The two middle compartments and the anolyte and catholyte compartments were separated with cation-exchange membranes (NEOSEPTA CM-2 made by Tokuyama Corp.; the transport number of sodium ions in the membrane is greater than 0.99 in the electrodialysis of a 0.50 N sodium chloride solution at a current density of 20 mA/cm^2; electrical resistance is 2.8 Ω cm^2). Electrodialysis was carried out at a current density of 1 mA/cm^2 when the concentration of the mixed salt solution was 0.04 N. When the mixed salt solutions of sodium sulfate and sodium chloride, or sodium bromide and sodium chloride were used, the concentration of the solutions was changed. Thus, the current density was changed: 0.50 N, 10 mA/cm^2; 0.15 N, 3 mA/cm^2; 0.04 N, 1 mA/cm^2; 0.01 N, 1 mA/cm^2.

Electrodialysis was carried out without photoirradiation and then with photoirradiation. To estimate the effect of the irradiation time on the transport properties of the membranes, electrodialysis was carried out after the membrane had been irradiated for a given period. The solutions adjacent to the anion-exchange membrane to be measured were vigorously agitated with stirrers to eliminate the effect of diffusion boundary layers on the transport properties of the membrane. After electrodialysis, the solutions adjacent to the membrane were analyzed by the Mohr method (for Cl$^-$), conventional chelate back titration (for SO$_4^{2-}$), or ion chromatography (TOSOH CCPD, IC-8010, Chromatocorder 21). Thus, the transport numbers of anions relative to chloride ions were calculated from the change in the concentration of each anion. The current efficiency was calculated from the change in the concentrations of the anions in each compartment and from the electricity measured with a coulometer.

According to Scheme 1, the reduction of a viologen moiety of the membranes is reversible. Thus, the reversibility of the change in the transport number of the anions relative to chloride ions in the anion-exchange membranes with a viologen moiety was measured with and then without photoirradiation: after the transport number of the sulfate ions relative to chloride ions had been measured in the presence of photoirradiation, nondegassed solution was added to the cell (the blue color of the membrane was decolorized by oxidation with dissolved oxygen) and electrodialysis was carried out without photoirradiation. Also, the transport number of sulfate ions relative to chloride ions was repeatedly measured with photoirradiation and then without the irradiation after the oxidation of the reduced form in a similar manner.

To estimate the change in the pore size of the anion-exchange membrane with photoirradiation, the permeability coefficient of a neutral solute, urea, was measured using a two-compartment cell under vigorous agitation (1500 rpm) at 25.0°C with or without irradiation. After an aqueous 2 mol/L urea solution had filled the concentrated compartment of the cell (250 cm^3) and pure water the dilute compartment (120 cm^3), dialysis was carried out for 48 h without the irradiation. After filling both compartments with the solution, the membrane surface facing the urea solution was irradiated for 40 min, and dialysis was then carried out for 48 h in the presence of irradiation (degassed solution and pure water were used). The permeated amount of urea was analyzed using HPLC (Hitachi L-6000), and the permeability coefficient of urea (P) was calculated by the following equation: $P = \Delta m / At(C_C - C_D)$: Δm is the permeated amount of urea, A the effective membrane area (20 cm^2), t the diffusion period (s), C_C the average concentration of the concentrated compartment during dialysis and C_D the average concentration of the dilute compartment during dialysis.

III. RESULTS AND DISCUSSION

A. Generation of Photovoltage and Photocurrent

1. Confirmation of Photoreduction of a Viologen Moiety of Anion-Exchange Membranes by Absorption Spectra

Photoreduction of a viologen moiety of anion-exchange membranes was confirmed by measurements of the absorption spectra of a thin anion-exchange membrane (14 μm thick) with photoirradiation. Figure 6 shows the change in the UV–visible spectra of the thin membrane (swelled with ethylene glycol) upon photoirradiation from one surface. Though the membrane has an absorbance at 320 nm before irradiation, absorbances of 406 nm and 615 nm appeared with increasing irradiation time and then decreased with further irradiation. This is due to the formation of the monocation radical and then that of the biradical. The same spectra were also observed in degassed water and various salt solutions, and the appearance of the absorbances was somewhat slow compared with the membrane in ethylene glycol. Thus, to clarify the active wavelength to reduce a viologen moiety of the membrane, 313 nm light from the mercury lamp filtered by a monochromenter was irradiated on the membrane for various periods (Fig. 7). Absorbances at 406 and 615 nm appeared and rapidly increased up to 10 min irradiation and did not increase on further irradiation. Then 435 nm light from mercury lamp filtered by a monochromenter was irradiated on another membrane. The absorbances at 406 and 615 nm increased very slowly and decreased on further irradiation as

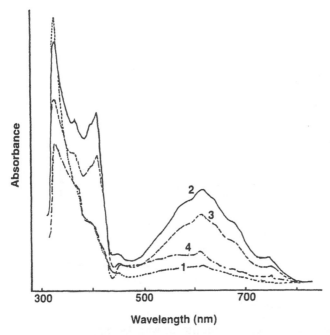

FIG. 6 Change in absorption spectra of a thin membrane (14 μm, similar to the M-6 membrane) with photoirradiation time. Irradiation times for numbered curves: 1, 1 min; 2, 10 min; 3, 60 min; 4, 10 h.

shown in Fig. 8. Furthermore, when irradiated with 313 nm light, followed by 404 nm light, the absorbances at 406 and 615 nm, which appeared with the irradiation of 313 nm, weakened due to the irradiation with 404 nm light. These results imply that 313 nm light caused reduction, $MV^{2+} \rightarrow MV^{+}$ in the membrane, and 404 and 435 nm light caused reduction of both $MV^{2+} \rightarrow MV^{+}$ and $MV^{+} \rightarrow MV^{0}$. However, there is no absorbance peak in the range of 400–450 nm. It was reported that when methyl viologen is adsorbed on cellulose, its λ_{max} shifts to a longer wavelength, and the absorption width becomes broader [43]. In fact, long tailing of the absorbance at 320 nm (before irradiation) was observed in Figs. 6–8. Because the viologen moiety was bonded to the polymer matrix, the absorbance broadened and showed tailing. It is thought that the fact that $MV^{2+} \rightarrow MV^{+}$ reduction occurred with 435 nm light is due to this broadening and tailing of the spectrum (polymer effect). However, when both an interference filter of 610 nm (KL-61) and a cutoff filter (0–58, cutoff below 580 nm) were used, no absorbance was observed during a 5 h irradiation with the xenon lamp.

To further confirm this, a methyl viologen ethylene glycol solution was irradiated with a xenon lamp for 30 min with and without a filter cutoff below

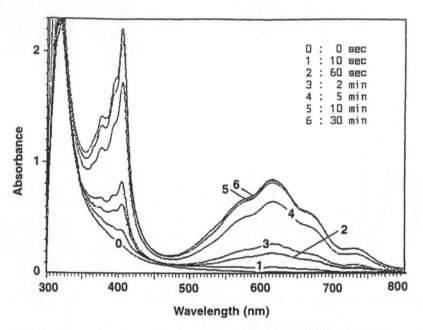

FIG. 7 Change in spectra of anion-exchange membrane with 4,4'-bipyridine moiety on irradiation with 313 nm light of a mercury lamp (filtered by a monochrometer).

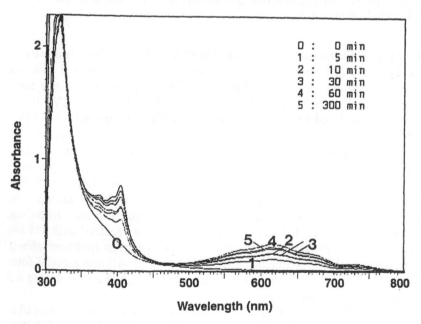

FIG. 8 Change in spectra of anion-exchange membrane with 4,4'-bipyridine moiety on irradiation with 435 nm light of a mercury lamp (filtered by a monochrometer).

400 nm. With the filter, the 261 nm absorbance did not change, and no new absorbance was observed. However, the absorbances of 261 nm decreased, and 401 nm absorbance appeared without the filter. On the other hand, when the anion-exchange membrane with a viologen moiety was irradiated by the lamp with the same filter, 406 and 615 nm absorbances were clearly observed. It is concluded that light below around 450 nm was effective in reducing a viologen moiety bonded to the membrane due to the polymer effect.

2. Generation of Photovoltage and Photocurrent from Cation-Exchange Membranes Ion-Exchanged with Methyl Viologen

It was reported that after Ru(bipy)$_3$ and methyl viologen, which were separately loaded onto perfluorocarbon sulfonic acid membrane (Nafion), are clamped between two ITO electrodes, visible light is irradiated from the Ru(bipy)$_3$ side and photocurrent is observed [44]. Ru(bipy)$_3$ is an electron donor, and methyl viologen acts as an electron acceptor. Because methyl viologen is reduced by photoirradiation and releases an electron, methyl viologen can also act as an electron donor. Accordingly, when methyl viologen molecules exist in both the photoside and the dark side, the electrical potential should be generated on photoirradiation. To confirm this, a cation-exchange membrane, NEOSEPTA C66-5T, on which methyl viologen had ion-exchanged, was used in the photovoltage generation. The membrane was completely dried, swelled with ethylene glycol, clamped between two ITO electrodes and completely sealed. Figure 9 shows the change in the photovoltage with irradiation time. A photovoltage of 155.3 mV (photocurrent: 776.5 nA) was observed immediately after the photoirradiation, decreased over 5 h to 45 mV, drifted up to 49.5 mV, and then gradually decreased. After interruption of the irradiation at 23.5 h, the voltage decreased abruptly and then very slowly. Other cation-exchange membranes with different ion-exchange capacity (NEOSEPTA CH-45T and Nafion 117) were used for the same measurement after methyl viologen had been ion-exchanged with the membranes. Though the maximum value and decrease in the photovoltage were different according to the species of the membranes, similar photovoltage and photocurrent were observed. The irradiation caused methyl viologen (MV^{2+}) at the irradiated side to be reduced to the cation radical and biradical, MV$^+$ and MV^0 (MV^{2+} + e → MV$^+$ is -0.45 V and MV$^+$ + e → MV^0 is -0.88 V), which released an electron. The released electron then reduced methyl viologen on the dark side, because the polarity of the potential was positive on the dark side and negative on the irradiated side. The abrupt decrease in the photovoltage at the initial stage of the irradiation might occur because most of the methyl viologen ion-exchanged near both membrane surfaces was converted to the reduced forms. It is thought that the rate of methyl viologen reduction by the photoirradiation was balanced with the ion-exchange or coupling rate

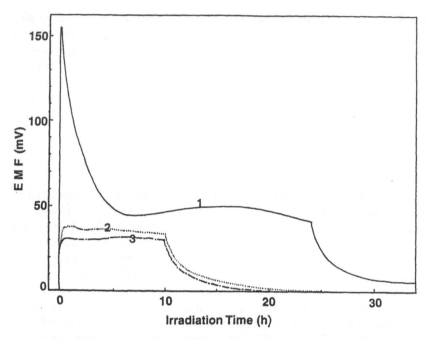

FIG. 9 Change in photovoltage of cation-exchange membrane (NEOSEPTA C66-5T) ion-exchanged with methyl viologen with photoirradiation time. 1, first irradiation; 2, second irradiation, 12 h after the first; 3, third irradiation, 14 h after the second.

between MV^{2+} of the inner side of the membrane and MV^+ or MV^0 formed on the membrane surfaces on both the photoside and the dark side, or with electron hopping speed. The peak in curve 1 after 18 h might be due to the balancing of the formation of the reduced forms with electron transfer in the cell. Curve 2 was measured at 12 h after the measurement of curve 1, and curve 3, 14 h after the curve 2 measurement. An almost constant photovoltage was observed during the irradiation. Because the photovoltage is based on reductions, $MV^{2+} \rightarrow MV^+$ and $MV^+ \rightarrow MV^0$, in both the photoside and the opposite side, it is calculated that about 8.5×10^{-7} eq of methyl viologen was consumed during this potential generation, which is less than 1% of the methyl viologen ion-exchanged in the membrane [34].

Before the above-experiment was performed, 5 wt% methyl viologen in ethylene glycol solution filling a slit (0.5-mm thick) between two ITO electrodes was irradiated with light from one side. A photovoltage of 40.6 mV was instantly generated; it decreased abruptly, attained 4.5 mV after 1.0 h (the color of the solution changed to blue), and no further increase in the voltage was observed during 11 h of photoirradiation. Furthermore, the same methyl viologen solution was impregnated in a porous polysulfone membrane (prepared by the phase inversion method using a 10% polysulfone 1-methyl-2-pyrrolidone solution, 237 μm thick; porosity, 88%), clamped between two ITO electrodes, and photoirradiation was carried out. The value and decay of the photovoltage was almost the same as when the methyl viologen solution was in the slit.

3. Generation of Photovoltage and Photocurrent from Anion-Exchange Membranes with a Viologen Moiety as Anion Exchange Groups

Before the experiments of the generation of photovoltage and photocurrent using anion-exchange membranes having a viologen moiety, an anion-exchange membrane having a benzyl trimethylammonium moiety (M'-2 and M'-3 membranes) and commercial anion-exchange membrane, NEOSEPTA AFN-7 (ion-exchange groups: N-methylpyridinium chloride; ion-exchange capacity: 3.33 meq/g Cl^- form dry membrane; water content: 0.48, g-H_2O/g Cl^- form dry membrane; electrical resistance: 0.5 Ω cm^2, measured in 0.500 N sodium chloride solution using 1000 cycle AC at 25.0°C, produced by Tokuyama Corp.), were used in the measurement of photovoltage generation after swelling with ethylene glycol under the same conditions as the cation-exchange membrane. A photovoltage below 10 mV was observed within a minute after photoirradiation, decreased rapidly and was not generated during further long-term irradiation.

Figure 10 shows a typical example of the change in the photovoltage with irradiation time (the M-2 membrane in Table 1 was used). After the irradiation, the membrane color gradually changed from slightly pale yellow to blue, and the photovoltage increased very slowly and attained 81 mV (photocurrent, 405 nA) after 17-h irradiation (curve 1). When this membrane was irradiated again after the remaining voltage had decreased below 0.5 mV, after interrupting the irradiation, the photovoltage generated immediately upon photoirradiation, showed a maximum value and decreased very slowly during long-term irradiation, as shown in curve 2 of Fig. 10. The anion-exchange membrane prepared from chloromethylated polysulfone and 4,4'-bipyridine (the M-6 membrane) also showed generation of a photovoltage similar to that of the M-2 membrane as shown in Fig. 11, though the generation speed was slightly higher. It should be noted that the voltage (curve 2) was generated instantly, even after a 31-day interruption of the photoirradiation.

To obtain higher photovoltage, the effect of various characteristics of the anion-exchange membranes with a viologen moiety on the photovoltage was examined. Figure 12 shows the relationship of the ion-exchange capacity and the swelling degree of the membranes (prepared from copolymer membranes of chloromethylstyrene and divinylbenzene and 4,4'-bipyridine) by ethylene glycol to the photovoltage. Though the degree of swelling of the membranes

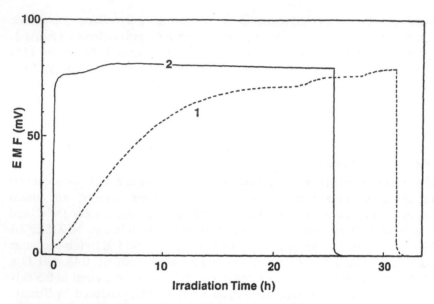

FIG. 10 Change in photovoltage of M-2 membrane with photoirradiation time. 1, first irradiation; 2, second irradiation, 14 h after the first.

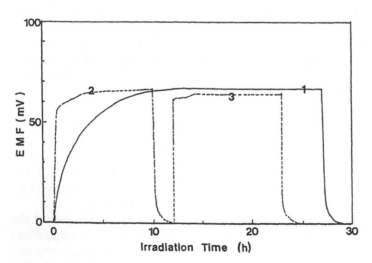

FIG. 11 Change in photovoltage of M-6 membrane with photoirradiation time. 1, first irradiation; 2, second irradiation, measured at 31 days after measurement of the first; 3, third irradiation, measured at 2 h after the second.

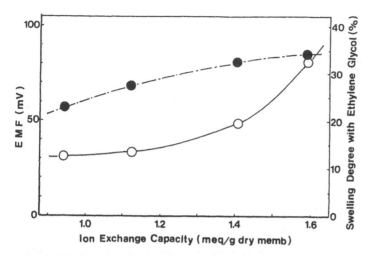

FIG. 12 Effect of ion-exchange capacity of anion-exchange membranes on swelling degree with ethylene glycol and photovoltage. ○, photovoltage; ●, swelling degree with ethylene glycol.

slightly increased with increasing ion-exchange capacity, the photovoltage steeply increased with an increase in the ion-exchange capacity. It is proved that the amount of the viologen moiety in the membranes is important for generating the higher photovoltage.

To examine the effect of the amount of the viologen moiety in the membranes on the photovoltage from another viewpoint, the membranes with different thickness prepared from chloromethylated polysulfone and 4,4'-bipyridine were examined. It is thought that because the photoreduction to release an electron and the reduction by the released electron occur on both surfaces of the membrane, the density of the viologen moiety is important being independent of the membrane thickness (ion-exchange capacity of these membranes: 1.36 meq/g-Cl⁻ dry membrane). Thus, the value of the photovoltage should be the same regardless of the membrane thickness, but then decays quickly in the thin membrane. However, Fig. 13 shows that the photovoltage decreased with decreasing thickness of the membranes. When the thickness was more than about 70 μm, the photovoltage attained almost a constant value. The membranes used are transparent with a slightly pale yellow color, and the active wavelength to reduce the viologen moiety was below around 450 nm. It is thought that the active light penetrated through the membranes below 70 μm thickness and the viologen moiety in the dark side might be reduced by both the released electron and penetrated light. In fact, when the cell was irradiated from the dark side with a halogen lamp (100 W) during generation of the photovoltage by photoirradiation, the voltage rapidly

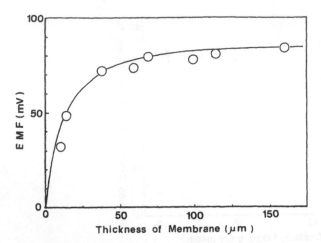

FIG. 13 Effect of thickness of anion-exchange membranes on photovoltage. Membranes were prepared from chloromethylated polysulfone and 4,4'-bipyridine.

decreased. Also, the period to attain the maximum value of the photovoltage became shorter with decreasing membrane thickness.

Figure 14 shows the change in the photovoltage from the M-6 type membranes during the second irradiation (prepared from chloromethylated polysulfone and 4,4'-bipyridine, 115 μm) with and without immersion in the

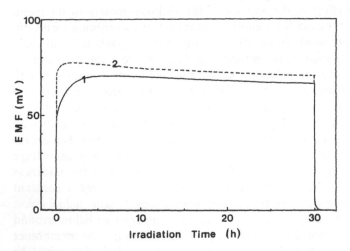

FIG. 14 Comparison of photovoltage of anion-exchange membrane immersed in hydrochloric acid solution with that of the membrane without immersion. 1, without immersion after preparation; 2, with immersion. Membranes (115 μm thick) were prepared from chloromethylated polysulfone and 4,4'-bipyridine.

hydrochloric acid solution. Although the generation speed of the photovoltage was almost the same in both membranes during the first irradiation, it is apparent from Fig. 14 that the membrane equilibrated with the hydrochloric acid solution more rapidly generated a higher photovoltage (The second irradiation was started 48 h after the interruption of the first). This is consistent with the results of the spectrum measurement [41,42].

When a methyl viologen ethylene glycol solution was impregnated in a porous membrane, a stable photovoltage was not observed. Also, high swelling of the membrane with a solvent, ethylene glycol, provided the higher photovoltage (Fig. 12). Thus, a porous anion-exchange membrane with a viologen moiety was prepared: a porous membrane of chloromethylated polysulfone (prepared by phase inversion method) reacted with 4,4′-bipyridine (thickness, 229 μm; the weight of ethylene glycol in the total membrane weight: 87.5% in swelling state.) Figure 15 shows the generation of the photovoltage from the porous anion-exchange membrane. Relatively high and stable photovoltage was observed, and the generation speed of the photovoltage was faster than that of the corresponding thickness of the dense membrane.

To examine the life of the photocell, the generation of the photovoltage with long-term irradiation was carried out using the M-2 membrane (irradiation and interruption were repeated five times: total irradiation time: 68 h; average photovoltage: about 80 mV). In every photoirradiation, except the first, the voltage was instantly generated, increased slightly in the initial stage and decreased slightly with increasing irradiation time. It was calculated from the ion-exchange capacity of the membrane and the discharged electricity

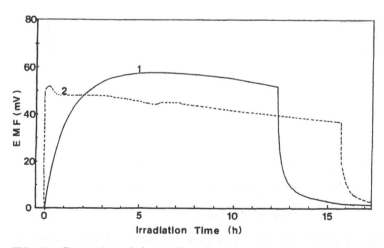

FIG. 15 Generation of photovoltage from porous anion-exchange membrane having a viologen moiety. 1, first irradiation; 2, second irradiation.

that only about 1% of a viologen moiety in the membrane changed to the reduced forms [42].

4.   Addition of Oxidizing or Reducing Agent in the Photo-Cell

Though the viologen moiety bonded to the cross-linked polymer matrix acted as both electron donor and acceptor, the generation of the photovoltage at the first irradiation was very slow. It is expected that quick generation and higher photovoltage would be observed with the addition of other electron acceptors and donors in the cell. Figure 16 shows the change in the photovoltage with the irradiation time when ferric chloride was dissolved in ethylene glycol in which the membrane had been equilibrated (ferric ions were adsorbed in the membrane matrix; the M-2 membrane was used). The high voltage was observed immediately after the photoirradiation, in contrast to the membrane equilibrated with ethylene glycol. When the concentration of ferric chloride was 0.171 mol/L, a potential of 258 mV (photocurrent: 1.29 μA) was initially observed. This suggests that though the speed of the photoreduction of the viologen moiety is very fast, electron capture in the dark side is slow. The highest initial potential occurred at the highest concentration of ferric chloride (curve 1). Two peaks of the potential were observed for lower concentrations of ferric chloride. The first peak might be due to ferric ions adsorbed on the ITO surface, and those in the thin liquid layer between the ITO and the membrane act as electron acceptors in the dark side. After rapid consumption of

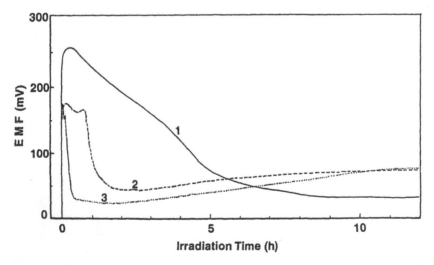

FIG. 16   Change in photovoltage of M-2 membrane with photoirradiation in the presence of ferric ions. Concentration of ferric chloride: 1. 1.71×10^{-1} mol/L; 2. 1.65×10^{-2} mol/L; 3. 8.3×10^{-3} mol/L.

ferric ions on the membrane surface, ferric ions were fed from the membrane matrix; thus, the second potential peak would be observed because the second peak was not observed at the highest ferric concentration. The photovoltage decreased during the photoirradiation, dependent on the concentration of ferric ions, and increased again because the 4,4′-bipyridine moiety began to act as an electron acceptor. In these cases, the membrane changed color from pale yellow to deep blue.

The membrane immersed in the hydrazine solution shows absorbance at 615 nm based on the formation of MV^+. However, the blue-colored membrane was decolorized by a trace amount of oxygen. Similarly, when the membrane was immersed in aqueous trimethylamine, triethanolamine, and other amine solutions, the color of the membrane changed to blue and was decolorized by exposure of the membrane to air. Thus, to obtain the reduced-form membrane, the membrane was equilibrated with the ethylene glycol solution containing triethanolamine (the membrane colored deep blue). When the cell had been assembled with the solvent containing triethanolamine and irradiated with light, a photovoltage of 120 mV was observed immediately after the irradiation, decreased abruptly, increased slightly, and again gradually decreased as shown in curve 1 in Fig. 17. It is thought that the voltage was

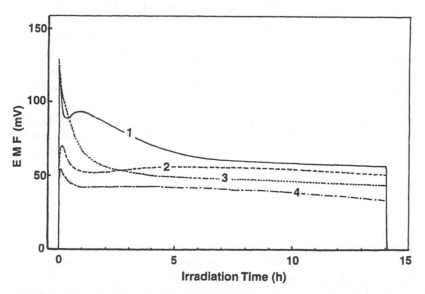

FIG. 17 Change in photovoltage of M-2 membrane after immersion in ethylene glycol containing triethanolamine on photoirradiation. 1, first irradiation; 2, second irradiation, 2 h after the first; 3, third irradiation, 114 h after the second; 4, fourth irradiation, 3 h after the third. The cell was assembled after the membrane had been immersed in a 10.6 wt% triethanolamine ethylene glycol solution for 48 h.

generated from the photoreduction, $MV^+ \rightarrow MV^0$. The second irradiation (curve 2) was performed 2 h after turning off the first, and a small peak of the potential (71 mV) was observed immediately after the irradiation. The third irradiation (curve 3) was carried out 114 h after turning off the second irradiation, and the 129 mV potential was again observed. This suggests that MV^0 formed on the membrane surface coupled with MV^+ of the inner part of the membrane during the interruption period. The fourth irradiation (curve 4) was carried out 3 h after turning off the third. The behavior of the potential in the fourth (maximum value: 55.5 mV) is similar to that of the second. This proves that the $MV^0 \rightarrow MV^+ + e$ reaction between the membrane surfaces and the inner part of the membrane occurs relatively rapidly. The electron transfer might be a hopping mechanism [45] and mediated by ethylene glycol and triethanolamine.

The presence of an oxidizing agent in the cell provided rapid generation of a high photovoltage, and the presence of a reducing agent such as triethanolamine also caused high and rapid generation of a photovoltage. The former acts as an electron acceptor in the dark side, and the latter forms cation radicals (MV^+) on the membrane matrix before the irradiation.

5. Effect of Solvent Species on Photovoltage Generation

The generation of the photovoltage was examined after the anion-exchange membranes with a viologen moiety had been swelled with a solvent such as ethylene glycol, because the membranes swelled well with ethylene glycol (dry membrane did not generate the appreciable photovoltage by the photoirradiation). Upon photoirradiation, radicals are formed in the cross-linked polymer matrix, and the released electron from the viologen moiety of the matrix should migrate to the electrodes. Accordingly, the charge transfer was postulated to proceed by a hopping mechanism [45] and was mediated by radicals formed from ethylene glycol and chloride anion radicals because the viologen moiety is fixed on a cross-linked polymer matrix and exists in the membrane matrix forming microdomains (Fig. 2). Because others have reported that the photoreduction of the methyl viologen leads to the formation of the N,N'-dihydro radical cation in acidified aqueous and alcoholic solutions during flash photolysis experiments [46] and also abstracts hydrogen from 2-butyl alcohol to form radicals [47], such radical might be formed in the solvent and mediate the charge transfer. Thus, the $-OH$ groups of the ethylene glycol are thought to play an important role in easily forming radicals and contribute to the charge transfer; therefore, the effect of the number of $-OH$ groups of ethylene glycol on the photovoltage was examined using ethylene glycol, diethylene glycol, and triethylene glycol [48].

Figure 18 shows the generation of the photovoltage and the change in electrical resistance of the cell (M-2 membrane: to estimate the change in electrical conductivity due to the formation of radicals, the membrane area in the cell

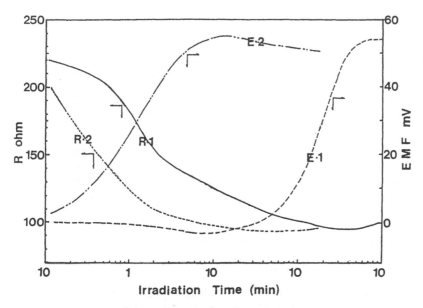

FIG. 18 Change in photovoltage and electrical resistance of the cell with M-2 membrane swelled with diethylene glycol. E-1, photovoltage during the first irradiation; E-2, photovoltage during the second irradiation; R-1, electrical resistance of the cell during the first irradiation; R-2, electrical resistance of the cell during the second irradiation.

was decided as 4.0 cm^2 from this experiment) when diethylene glycol was used as the solvent. During the first irradiation, the maximum voltage was observed about 16 h (960 min) after the irradiation (curve E-1), and the electrical resistance of the cell continued to decrease from the beginning of the irradiation (curve R-1), which means the increasing formation of radicals in the cell. However, during the second irradiation, the photovoltage attained a maximum about 10 min after the irradiation (curve E-2). The electrical resistance was low before the irradiation due to the existence of radicals formed during the first irradiation and then further decreased (curve R-2). Thus, it is reasonable that the generation of the photovoltage in the second irradiation became rapid.

Figure 19 shows the relationship of the photovoltage and swelling degree of the M-2 membrane to the species of polyethylene glycol (swelling degree = $[W_{EG} - W_{dry}]/W_{dry}] \times 100$; W_{EG}: weight of swelled membrane; W_{dry}: weight of dry membrane). Though the M-2 membrane was doubly cross-linked by both divinylbenzene and the 4,4'-bipyridine, the membrane swelled well with ethylene glycols having a higher molecular weight (the water content of the M-2 membrane was 15% in Table 1) due to the good affinity of polyethylene glycol for the membrane matrix. The value of the photovoltage was almost the same

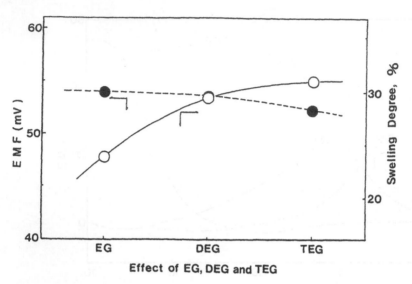

FIG. 19 Relationship of photovoltage and swelling degree of the M-2 membrane to the polyethylene glycol series. ○, swelling degree; ●, photovoltage.

(from 52 to 54 mV) and independent of the molecular weight of the polyethylene glycol, which means that the number of −OH groups was directly unrelated to the value of the photovoltage in the range of this work.

Figure 20 shows the change in the electrical resistance of the cell during the irradiation, which is dependent on the molecular weight. The electrical resistance of 0.50 N tetramethylammonium chloride solutions of ethylene glycol, diethylene glycol, and triethylene glycol increased: 367.3, 819.6 and 1283.5 Ω cm, respectively, measured at 25.0°C (by 1000-cycle, AC). However, the resistance of the cells with diethylene glycol and triethylene glycol decreased upon photoirradiation and then slightly increased during long-term irradiation. This suggests that the formation of radicals was limited by the decreasing number of −OH groups from some irradiation time. Though the photovoltage was independent of the number of −OH groups, the −OH groups of the ethylene glycols are thought to be related to the formation of the radicals.

To further confirm the effect of the −OH groups on the photovoltage, dimethoxyethane and diethoxyethane were used as the solvent (the M-6 membrane was used). The maximum value of the voltage was only 9.9 and 6.3 mV in dimethoxyethane and diethoxyethane, respectively, though the membrane in the cell was blue (formation of MV^+). The electrical resistance of the cell decreased upon photo-irradiation, showed a minimum (705 Ω in dimethoxyethane and 39,085 Ω in diethoxyethane) and increased during the irradiation. Because the −OH groups of polyethylene glycol provide ionic conductivity to the cell and high swelling of the membranes, glycerol was used as the solvent

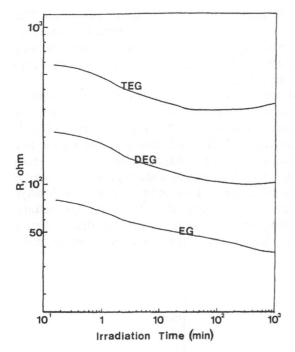

FIG. 20 Change in electrical resistance of the cell during photoirradiation with ethylene glycols (M-2 membrane was used). EG, ethylene glycol; DEG, diethylene glycol; TEG, triethylene glycol.

for the M-6 membrane (swelling degree of the M-6 membrane with glycerol was 21.4%). The photovoltage was generated very slowly during the first irradiation (the photovoltage attained a maximum value 38 h after the irradiation) and showed a maximum value of 28.9 mV. The electrical resistance of the cell decreased from 286.0 to 135.5 Ω. Though the photovoltage from the M-6 membrane swelled with glycerol was high and the electrical resistance was low compared with those of dimethoxyethane and diethoxyethane, the photovoltage was relatively low. This might be due to less swelling of the membrane and the high viscosity of glycerol. It is concluded that the $-OH$ groups of the solvent apparently contribute to the charge transfer in the system.

Because ethylene glycols produced good swelling of the anion-exchange membranes with a viologen moiety, there is the possibility that ethylene glycol changes to ethylene glycol derivatives, i.e., dimer, trimer, and ethylene glycol derivatives with chlorines due to coexistence with viologen radicals and chloride anion radicals. To examine this, ethylene glycol in the membrane, which had been used in the photovoltage generation, was analyzed by GC–MS after extraction from the membrane. A trace amount of a new compound was detected by the GC–MS which showed m/z 73 as a main fragment ion. This spectrum is similar to that of 1,3-dioxolane or its derivatives; therefore, 1,3-dioxolane or related compounds may have formed during the photoirradiation. Though the reaction mechanism is not clear, this is evidence that ethylene glycol is involved in the charge transfer.

The possibility of other solvents without —OH groups was then examined. First, 1,3-dioxolane was used as the solvent for the M-6 membrane to observe the photovoltage generation (swelling degree: 65.6%). The E-1 curve of Fig. 21 shows the change in the photovoltage with irradiation time during the first irradiation. The maximum value of the photovoltage reached 146.5 mV about 6 h after the irradiation. Thus, a high voltage and a short period to reach the maximum voltage were observed (the same M-6 membrane swelled with ethylene glycol: the period to attain the maximum, 16 h; the maximum voltage, 93.1 mV). In particular, a shoulder appeared about 6 min after the irradiation in curve 1 of Fig. 21. The viologen moiety of the surface parts of the mem-

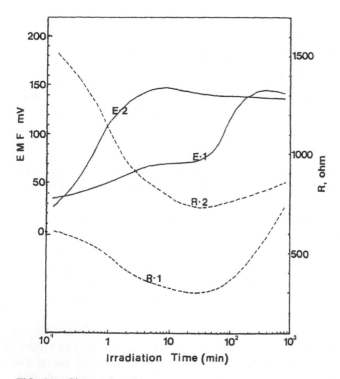

FIG. 21 Change in photovoltage and electrical resistance of the cell with M-6 membrane swelled with 1,3-dioxolane. E-1, photovoltage during the first irradiation; E-2, photovoltage during the second irradiation; R-1, electrical resistance of the cell during the first irradiation; R-2, electrical resistance of the cell during the second irradiation.

brane was believed to be rapidly reduced, and then the cross-linking of the membrane retarded the charge transfer from the membrane surfaces to the interior of the membrane. During the second irradiation (E-2 curve), a photo-voltage of 147.0 mV was observed about 7 min after the irradiation and slightly decreased with increasing irradiation time. A solvent without $-OH$ groups was also effective for the generation of the high photovoltage.

Although the electrical resistance before the irradiation was high (644 Ω: R-1 curve), which is about 200 times that of ethylene glycol, the resistance abruptly decreased upon irradiation, showed a minimum value, and then increased, which means that most of the viologen moiety of the membrane would be rapidly changed into $MV^{2+} \rightarrow MV^+ \rightarrow MV^0$. In fact, the membrane rapidly turned blue and then became transparent and slightly brown. The resistance during the second irradiation (R-2 curve in Fig. 21) started to decrease from a high value (1639 Ω), showed a minimum (739 Ω), and then increased. It is thought that because the second irradiation was performed after the interruption of the first irradiation, the concentration of radicals in the cell decreased due to the coupling among MV^{2+}, MV^+, MV^0, chloride anion radicals, and radicals formed from the solvent during the interruption. Measurements of the photovoltage generation were repeated, and the maximum values were 134.5 and 129.0 mV, respectively; the resistance increased with increasing repetition and attained 1957 Ω before the fourth irradiation.

It is well-known that the hydrogen of methylene groups neighboring an oxygen is easily attracted and radicals are formed due to the electron acceptive properties of the oxygen. In fact, it was reported that the synthesis of a block copolymer in aqueous media was performed using Mn^{3+} salts in combination with reducing agents such as glycerol, ethylene glycol and ethoxyacetic acid [49]. The reaction between Mn^{3+} and methylol provides the free radicals. The hydrogen of the methylene groups bonded to oxygen in ethylene glycol is thought to become involved in the radical formation, which contributes to the charge transfer in the cell. Accordingly, it is possible that the hydrogen of a methylene group between the two oxygens of 1,3-dioxolane is easily attracted and radicals are formed. To examine this, dioxane, 1,4-dioxane and 1,3-dioxane were used as the solvent for the M-6 membrane. Although the swelling degree of the M-6 membrane with 1,4-dioxane was relatively low (swelling degree, 14.4%), the M-6 membrane significantly swelled with 1,3-dioxane (65.6%). Though the photovoltage of the M-6 membrane swelled with 1,4-dioxane was extremely low (maximum, 4.8 mV), the voltage of the membrane swelled with 1,3-dioxane was high (93 mV). The behavior of the photovoltage generation and the change in the electrical resistance of the cell were similar to those with 1,3-dioxolane. Tetrahydropyran was also examined in connection with dimethoxyethane and diethoxyethane; the voltage was 3.2 mV with a 4.0% swelling degree. These results also support the belief that the hydrogen of the methylene group between the two oxygens is easily attracted and radicals are formed. However, the electrical resistance of the cell containing solvents without —OH groups was high compared with those having —OH groups due to a lack of ionic conductivity.

The M-6 membrane significantly swelled with 1-methyl-2-pyrrolidone (swelling degree, 147.4%), and a photovoltage of 142.8 mV was observed. The behavior of the photovoltage generation and the change in the electrical resistance of the cell were similar to the results with 1,3-dioxolane and 1,3-dioxane. In fact, the formation of MV$^+$ in the membrane was rapid compared with the membrane swelled with ethylene glycol, which was confirmed by the absorption spectrum. In general, the solvents which significantly swelled the membrane tended to induce a high photovoltage. Figure 22 shows the relationship

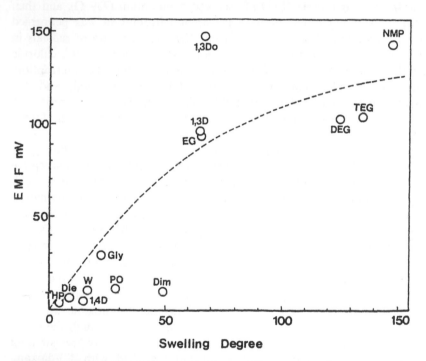

FIG. 22 Relationship of photovoltage to swelling degree using various solvents (M-6 membrane was used). THP, tetrahydropyran; Die, diethoxyethane; W, water; 1,4D, 1,4-dioxane; PO, propylene carbonate; Gly, glycerol; Dim, dimethoxyethane; EG, ethylene glycol; 1,3D, 1,3-dioxane; 1,3-Do, 1,3-dioxolane; DEG, diethylene glycol; TEG, triethylene glycol; NMP, 1-methyl-2-pyrrolidone. The maximum photovoltage was used (the voltage during the second irradiation was higher than that during the first). The membrane was swelled at room temperature or at elevated temperature to quickly attain equilibrium.

of the photovoltage to the swelling of the M-6 membrane with various solvents (though water and propylene carbonate generated a photovoltage, gas was evolved in the cell during photoirradiation, and the voltage became unstable). There were several exceptions: the low photovoltage of dimethoxyethane and diethoxyethane, etc., and the extremely high photovoltage of 1,3-dioxolane. To further examine this, ethylene glycol containing trioxane (1.10 mol/L), which has three methylene groups between oxygens, was used as the solvent for the M-6 membrane. The photovoltage of the cell with trioxane was high, and its electrical resistance was low compared to those without trioxane, as shown in Fig. 23. The addition of trioxane to 1,4-dioxane was also examined with the M-6 membrane; the voltage of the cell with trioxane was three

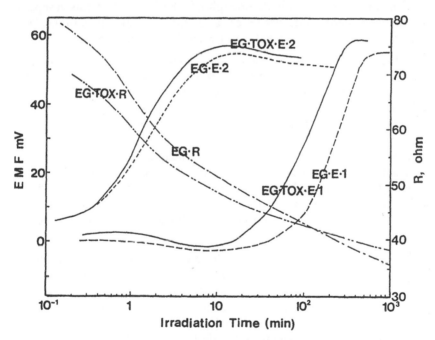

FIG. 23 Change in photovoltage and electrical resistance of the cell with M-2 membrane swelled with ethylene glycol and ethylene glycol containing trioxane. EG-E-1, photovoltage of the membrane swelled with ethylene glycol during the first irradiation; EG-E-2, photovoltage of the membrane swelled with ethylene glycol during the second irradiation; EG-TOX-E-1, photovoltage of the membrane swelled with ethylene glycol containing trioxane during the first irradiation; EG-TOX-E-2, photovoltage of the membrane swelled with ethylene glycol containing trioxane during the second irradiation; EG-R, electrical resistance of the cell with ethylene glycol during the first irradiation; EG-TOX-R, electrical resistance of the cell swelled with ethylene glycol containing trioxane during the first irradiation.

times that without trioxane, and the resistance was also lower. It is concluded that the solvents with the hydrogens which are easily attracted provide the high photovoltage with rapid generation of the photovoltage due to their contribution to the charge transfer.

6.   Effect of a Separator in the Cell on the Photovoltage

It was reported that when the viologen moiety in the polymers is reduced to MV^+ upon photoirradiation, counteranions are oxidized into anion radicals and remain near the MV^+ radicals [50,51]. Others reported that when a polymer having a viologen moiety is used in an electrochromic display, counteranions move to the electrode to maintain electroneutrality [52]. Because a potential gradient (photovoltage) exists, anions and anion radicals should migrate to the positive side (dark side), and protons attracted from the solvent should move to the cathode side (photoside). To confirm this, a separator, an anion-exchange membrane or a cation-exchange membrane, was inserted between the two M-6 membranes swelled with ethylene glycol:

1.   A perfluorocarbon $—SO_3H$-type cation-exchange membrane (Nafion, produced by E.I. du Pont de Nemours & Co.: 51 μm thick; ion-exchange capacity: 0.92 meq/g-Na^+ dry membrane; electrical resistance: 0.86 Ω cm^2 in 0.500 N sodium chloride solution; used after swelling the membrane with ethylene glycol) was sandwiched between the same two M-6 membranes.

2.   A chloride ion-form anion-exchange membrane with benzyl trimethylammonium groups (NEOSEPTA AM-1, produced by Tokuyama Corp.: 125 μm; ion-exchange capacity: 2.25 meq/g-Cl^- form dry membrane; electrical resistance: 1.1 Ω cm^2 in 0.500 N sodium chloride solution; used after swelling with ethylene glycol) was sandwiched between the same two M-6 membranes.

Figure 24 shows the change in the photovoltage of the cell with a cation-exchange membrane or an anion-exchange membrane when the irradiation and interruption were repeated ten times. Although the values of the voltage were almost the same during the first irradiation in both cases (two membranes without the separator: 105.7 mV), the voltage of the cell with the cation-exchange membrane significantly decreased with an increase in the repetitions of the irradiation and interruption. On the other hand, the voltage of the cell with the anion-exchange membrane did not remarkably decrease. In particular, though the voltage was generated immediately after the irradiation in the cells without the ion-exchange membrane separator and with the anion-exchange membrane separator once the photoirradiation had been done (due to existence of MV^+), the generation speed of the photovoltage of the cell with the cation-exchange membrane was very slow (during the second, third, etc.) as shown in Fig. 25. It is well-known that the permeation of hydrogen ions cannot be blocked with the anion-exchange membrane in the presence of a

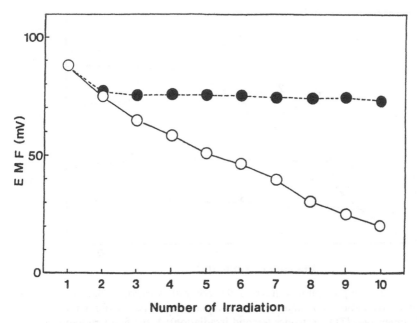

FIG. 24   Change in photovoltage of the cell having an ion-exchange membrane separator with increasing repetitions of irradiation and interruption. ●, anion-exchange membrane was sandwiched between the M-6 membranes. ○, cation-exchange membrane was sandwiched between the M-6 membranes.

concentration gradient or an electrical field [53]. It is thought that because the anion-exchange membrane cannot block the permeation of the hydrogen ions through the membrane and chloride ions and chloride anion radicals can easily permeate through the membrane, the anion-exchange membrane separator did not affect the generation of the photovoltage.

In the cell with a cation-exchange membrane, because the color of the membrane changed to deep blue during the photoirradiation and did not appreciably discolor during the interruption, MV^+ was formed and retained in the cell. Although the abnormal behavior of the voltage of the cell with the cation-exchange membrane is not clear, the following reason is considered. The cation-exchange membrane blocks the permeation of chloride ions and chloride anion radicals to the dark side (positive side); therefore, the concentration of chloride ions on both the photoside and the dark side cannot change. Thus, chloride anion radicals increase on the photoside and might couple with the formed MV^+ and MV^0 during the interruption. The amount of MV^+ and MV^0 on the photoside is thought to decrease during the inter-

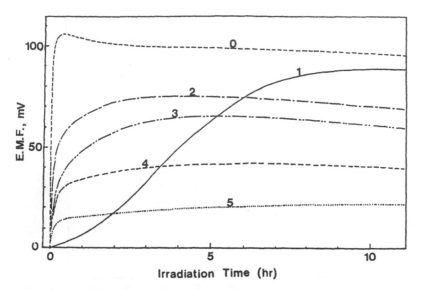

FIG. 25 Relationship of photovoltage of the cell with a cation-exchange membrane separator to irradiation time and number of repetitions. 0, two M-6 membranes were placed between two ITO electrodes (second irradiation); 1, the first irradiation when a cation-exchange membrane was sandwiched between two M-6 membranes; 2, the second irradiation after 6.5 h on curve 1; 3, the third irradiation after 12.5 h on curve 2; 4, the seventh irradiation of the cell with cation-exchange membrane; 5, the tenth irradiation of the same cell.

ruption period, and the generation of the voltage then becomes slow after the interruption.

On the other hand, it is possible that electrons passed through the load resistance were accepted mainly by chloride ions to become chloride anion radicals on the dark side, and then MV^{2+} on the dark side was indirectly reduced or via solvent radicals to become MV^+ and MV^0. During the interruption, chloride ions existing on the dark side, which are not fed from the photoside, might be changed into chloride anion radicals by the electron transfer from MV^+ and MV^0 formed on the dark side. Therefore, chloride ions on the dark side, as one of the electron acceptors, might decrease during the interruption (corresponding to the decrease in the anode active material in a battery).

Because chloride ions on the dark side are thought to play an important role, nonion-exchanged chloride ions were added in the cell (prior to this, the anion-exchange membrane had been equilibrated in a 1.0 N hydrochloride acid solution, and the membrane was used in the measurement after being completely rinsed with pure water to remove excess chloride ions). When the

M-6 membrane had been equilibrated with a mixed solution composed of 25 parts ethylene glycol and 1 part water which contained 0.461 mol/L hydrochloric acid, the maximum photovoltage was 117.4 mV. On the other hand, when the membrane had been equilibrated with a mixed ethylene glycol (25 parts) and water (1 part) solution, the voltage was 81.1 mV. However, the swelling degree of the membrane was 77.4% and 56.7%, respectively. As previously mentioned, the highly swelled membrane provided a higher voltage. Thus, after the membrane had been equilibrated with ethylene glycol containing 1.29 N sodium chloride (near-saturation of sodium chloride in ethylene glycol), the photovoltage was measured. The value was 105.4 mV, and the swelling degree of the membrane was 58.6%. On the other hand, when the same membrane was equilibrated with ethylene glycol, the value was 93.1 mV (the swelling degree was 65.1%). Although the swelling degree of the membrane decreased upon adding sodium chloride to the solvent, the voltage was high. The same measurement was made after adding calcium chloride anhydride to ethylene glycol (0.116 N), and a higher photovoltage (115.5 mV) was observed (swelling degree, 63.0%). Chloride ions, which were not ion-exchanged with the anion-exchange groups, provided a higher photovoltage. Furthermore, the M-6 membrane swelled with the mixed ethylene glycol and water solvent containing hydrobromic acid (0.344 N) showed very slow generation of the photovoltage and attained 59.1 mV 50 h (swelling degree, 69.7%) after the beginning of the irradiation. These results suggest that chloride ions are important as one of the electron acceptors in this photocell.

B. Change in Transport Numbers of Various Anions Relative to Chloride Ions in Electrodialysis

Many studies on the ion-exchange membranes having permselectivity for a specific ion have been reported: monovalent ion permselective [54], nitrate ion permselective [55,56], etc. When anion exchange membranes having a viologen moiety were used in electrodialysis in the presence of photoirradiation, it is expected from the formation of radicals in the membranes that the pore size of the anion-exchange membrane would change due to the change in the charge density of the membrane (due to shrinking of the membrane), and that the transport numbers of various anions relative to chloride ions change. In fact, it was confirmed from absorption spectra that when anion-exchange membranes with viologen moiety which were immersed in water and various aqueous sodium salt solutions were irradiated by a xenon lamp, radicals, MV^+, and MV^0, were formed on the membranes [57].

First, to find a stable condition for forming the radicals in the membrane in aqueous salt solutions, the photoirradiation on the membrane surface was carried out for various periods before electrodialysis, and then electrodialysis was performed (the M-3 membrane was used). Figure 26 shows the change in

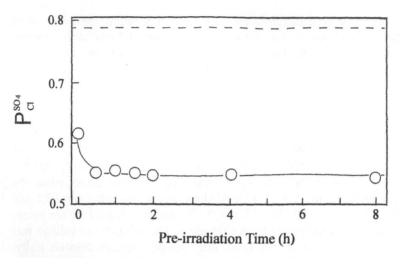

FIG. 26 Effect of preirradiation time on $P_{Cl}^{SO_4}$ of the anion-exchange membrane with a viologen moiety (M-3 membrane) (see p. 554 for a definition) dotted line, without photoirradiation; ○, with photoirradiation. (After the anion-exchange membrane had been installed in the cell and each compartment had been filled with mixed salt solution of sodium chloride and sodium sulfate (0.04 N as sodium ion concentration), light from a xenon lamp irradiated the desalting side of the membrane surface for a given period and then electrodialysis was carried out in the presence of photoirradiation.)

the transport number of sulfate ions relative to chloride ions with the irradiation time before electrodialysis (preirradiation time). Namely, after the anion-exchange membrane had been placed in the cell, the desalting side of the membrane was irradiated from a xenon lamp for a given period (the membrane colored in blue: formation of MV$^+$), and electrodialysis was carried out for 1 h in the presence of photoirradiation. The dotted line in Fig. 26 shows the transport number of the sulfate ions relative to chloride ions of the M-3 membrane in the absence of irradiation ($P_{Cl}^{SO_4}$: 0.78). When the membrane was not irradiated before electrodialysis (irradiated only during electrodialysis), the relative transport number decreased from 0.78 to 0.62. The value attained an almost constant value ($P_{Cl}^{SO_4}$: 0.52) when the preirradiation time was more than 30 min. Though the color of the membrane was blue during electrodialysis, MV^0 might be formed on the membrane surface of the photoside. It is not clear whether the change in the relative transport number was based on the formation of MV$^+$ or that of MV^0, because it was difficult to confirm the formation of MV^0 on the membrane surface. From Fig. 26, the irradiation time before electrodialysis (preirradiation time) was then set at 40 min in subsequent measurements.

After the transport number of sulfate ions relative to chloride ions had been measured, the colored membrane was decolorated by exposure to air or by filling the cell with nondegassed mixed salt solution (due to oxidation of a reduced viologen moiety) because the change from MV^{2+} to MV^+ and from MV^+ to MV^0 is reversible. The transport number of sulfate ions relative to chloride ions in the decolorated membrane was the same as the value without photoirradiation ($P_{Cl}^{SO_4} = 0.78$). When the coloration and decoloration of the membrane were repeated several times, the same reversible change in the transport number of sulfate ions relative to chloride ions was observed in the measurement of electrodialysis.

Figure 27 shows the change in $P_{Cl}^{SO_4}$ with the concentration of the mixed salt solution of sodium sulfate and sodium chloride with or without photoirradiation on the M-3 membrane. The behavior of $P_{Cl}^{SO_4}$ of the anion-exchange membrane with a viologen moiety was different from that of the membrane with a benzyl trimethylammonium moiety (the M'-3 membrane), though the content of divinylbenzene was the same. The $P_{Cl}^{SO_4}$ of the anion-exchange membrane with a viologen moiety was relatively low compared with that of the membrane with benzyl trimethylammonium groups. It is thought that because sulfate ions are larger than chloride ions, sulfate ions encounter difficulty in permeating through the membrane due to the development of cross-linkage

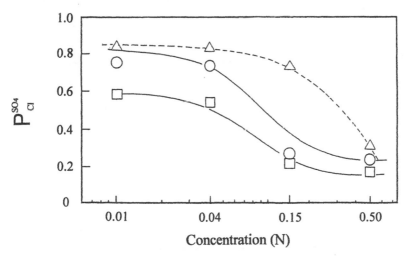

FIG. 27 Effect of concentration of the mixed salt solution on $P_{Cl}^{SO_4}$ of the anion-exchange membrane with a viologen moiety (M-3 membrane) and the membrane with benzyl trimethylammonium moiety (M'-3 membrane). ○, without photoirradiation; □, with photoirradiation during electrodialysis (preirradiation time, 40 min); △, anion-exchange membrane with benzyl trimethylammonium moiety as anion-exchange groups without the irradiation.

with the 4,4′-bipyridine (Stokes radii of sulfate and chloride ions are 2.31 Å and 1.21 Å [58], respectively). On the other hand, the $P_{Cl}^{SO_4}$ of the membrane with a viologen moiety in the presence of the irradiation was lower than that of the membrane without the irradiation over the entire concentration range, especially, in the lower concentration range. The effect of the irradiation on the decrease in $P_{Cl}^{SO_4}$ became weak in the higher concentration range. Because the ion-exchange membrane shrinks in a solution of high-salt concentration, the membrane shrinkage due to the decrease in the charge density with photoirradiation might be slight, and then the decrease in $P_{Cl}^{SO_4}$ due to photoirradiation might be weak in the higher concentration range.

Figure 28 shows the change in $P_{Cl}^{SO_4}$ with the content of divinylbenzene (cross-linking agent) of the anion-exchange membranes with or without photoirradiation (the M-1, M-2 and M-3 membranes were used). Because the ion-exchange capacity of the membranes increased with decreasing divinylbenzene content (Table 1), the viologen moiety of the membrane increased, and the membrane shrinkage due to the decrease in the charge density (photoreduction) of the membrane should then become remarkable. In fact, $P_{Cl}^{SO_4}$ decreased with decreasing divinylbenzene content upon irradiation. On the other hand, it is reasonable that the $P_{Cl}^{SO_4}$ of the anion-exchange membrane decreased with increasing divinylbenzene content in the absence of irradiation due to the bulkiness of sulfate ions (sieving effect). The behavior of $P_{Cl}^{SO_4}$ was reversed upon irradiation.

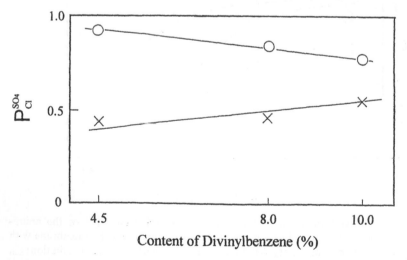

FIG. 28 Effect of divinylbenzene content of the anion-exchange membranes with a viologen moiety on $P_{Cl}^{SO_4}$ (M-1, M-2 and M-3 membranes). ○, without photoirradiation; ×, with photoirradiation during electrodialysis (preirradiation time, 40 min).

Upon photoirradiation, the viologen moiety of the membrane is reduced to MV^+, and then to MV^0 with further irradiation. Electrons are released from the membrane. It was reported that the reduction potentials of poly(benzyl viologen) in an aqueous solution are -0.37 V and -0.88 V vs. SCE from cyclic voltammogram measurement [59]. Although the reduction potentials were not measured for the viologen moiety of the membranes, similar potentials are expected. The membrane is in contact with a large amount of water containing a trace amount of H^+, OH^-, and sodium salts. The reduction potential for the couple $2H_2O + 2e = 2OH^- + H_2$ is -0.828 V, so that the first reduction potential of the viologen cannot reduce the water molecules. Upon immersion of a membrane of surface area 30 cm^2 containing protonated viologen moiety (cross-linking degree: 10%) in degassed 0.10 N sodium chloride solution (50 cm^3) and irradiated for 8 h, the pH decreased slightly compared with a nonphotoirradiated solution. In radiolysis of water, a hydrated electron is formed [60] which reacts with H_3O^+: $H_3O + e \rightarrow H\cdot + H_2O$ [61]. Although the electron released from a viologen moiety of the membrane by photoreduction might behave like the hydrated electron, the detailed behavior has not been clarified.

As previously mentioned and as Table 1 also shows, all of the chloromethyl groups of the copolymer membranes did not react with the 4,4'-bipyridine. It is well-known that benzyl chloride groups are photosensitive and that benzyl chloride groups are cross-linked by UV-irradiation [62]. It is possible for the remaining chloromethyl groups to be involved in a cross-linking reaction during photoirradiation. If the cross-linking reaction occurred, the permeation of bulky anions, sulfate ions, should decrease. Thus, after the copolymer membrane had reacted with 1,4-diazabicyclo-[2,2,2]-octane (Dabco), which is a bifunctional amine having a structure similar to 4,4'-bipyridine, the transport number of sulfate ions relative to chloride ions was measured changing the concentration of the mixed salt solution (from 0.01 N to 0.50 N) in the presence or absence of the irradiation [The anion-exchange membrane having a Dabco moiety was prepared from the copolymer membrane whose divinylbenzene content was 4.5% (copolymer membrane for the M-1 membrane) and Dabco: the copolymer membrane reacted with a 5% Dabco ethyl alcohol solution at 60°C for 168 h; it was then washed with ethyl alcohol and with pure water. The electrical resistance of the membrane was 4.5 Ω cm^2 (measured in 0.500 N sodium chloride solution at 25.0°C using 1000-cycle AC) and the ion-exchange capacity was 2.34 meq/g Cl$^-$ form dry membrane. Because the ion-exchange capacity of the membrane was 2.70 meq/g-Cl$^-$ form dry membrane in the reaction of the same copolymer membrane with trimethylamine (M'-1), unreacted chloromethyl groups remained in the Dabco membrane]. There was no difference between the $P_{Cl}^{SO_4}$ of the Dabco membrane with photoirradiation and that without irradiation. It is concluded that the remaining chloromethyl groups in the membrane were not involved in the cross-linking reaction, or that the cross-linking reaction did not occur so as to affect the $P_{Cl}^{SO_4}$.

Figure 29 shows the change in P_{Cl}^{Br} with the irradiation time before electrodialysis (the photoirradiation was continued during electrodialysis), which was measured in the same manner as previously described. The dotted line is the P_{Cl}^{Br} of the anion-exchange membrane with a viologen moiety in the absence of photoirradiation. Because bromide ions are, in general, selectively ion-exchanged with the anion-exchange membrane compared to chloride ions [63], bromide ions permeate selectively through the membrane. However, the P_{Cl}^{Br} decreased with increasing preirradiation time up to about 1 h, and then attained a constant value. The preirradiation time to decrease P_{Cl}^{Br}, which was the time to form radicals, MV^+ and MV^0, in the membrane matrix to an extent to decrease P_{Cl}^{Br}, was almost the same as that in the case of the mixed sodium sulfate and sodium chloride solution. Thus, the preirradiation time was also set at 40 min, and the effect of the concentration of the mixed salt solution on P_{Cl}^{Br} was observed (Fig. 30). The P_{Cl}^{Br} decreased in the concentration range higher than around 0.04 N in the presence of the irradiation compared with that of the membrane without the irradiation.

However, at a concentration of around 0.01 N, the P_{Cl}^{Br} of the membrane with the irradiation was higher than that of the membrane without the irradia-

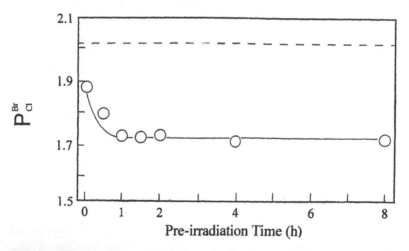

FIG. 29 Effect of preirradiation time on P_{Cl}^{Br} of the anion-exchange membranes with a viologen moiety (M-3 membrane). dotted line, without photoirradiation; ○, with photoirradiation. (After the anion-exchange membrane had been installed in the cell and each compartment had been filled with mixed salt solution of sodium chloride and sodium bromide (0.04 N as sodium ion concentration), light from a xenon lamp irradiated the desalting side of the membrane surface for a given period and then electrodialysis was carried out in the presence of photoirradiation.)

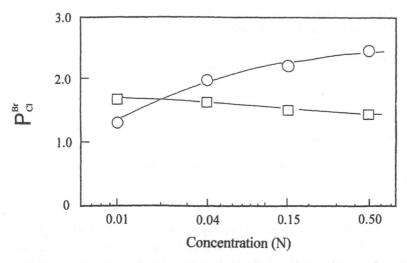

FIG. 30 Effect of the concentration of the mixed salt solution on P_{Cl}^{Br} of the anion-exchange membranes with a viologen moiety (M-3 membrane). $\bigcirc$, without photoirradiation; $\square$, with photoirradiation during electrodialysis (preirradiation time, 40 min).

tion. It is well-known that bromide ions are hydrophobic relative to chloride ions (Gibbs hydration energies of bromide ions and chloride ions are 303 kJ/mol and 317 kJ/mol, respectively) [58]. Substantially, because bromide ions can permeate selectively through the anion-exchange membrane, the effect of the shrinkage of the membrane due to the irradiation on P_{Cl}^{Br} would become weak in the dilute concentration range of the mixed salt solution, in which the swelling of the membrane is the highest. At the same time, the decrease in the charge density of the membrane with the irradiation makes the membrane hydrophobic, which increases the affinity of the bromide ions for the membrane. The ionic radius of the bromide ions is not very different from that of the chloride ions. The effect of the irradiation on P_{Cl}^{Br} is thought to be reversed in the case of bromide ions at a low concentration, because the selective ion-exchange of bromide ions with the membrane might be superior to a sieving effect due to the decrease in the charge density of the membrane. This is the reverse of the results with sulfate ions and chloride ions because sulfate ions are hydrophilic (Gibbs hydration energy: 1000 kJ/mol) and are larger than chloride ions [58].

Table 2 shows the relative transport numbers of nitrate and fluoride ions relative to the chloride ions of the membrane with or without photoirradiation (concentration of the solution was 0.04 N). Apparently, both P_{Cl}^{F} and $P_{Cl}^{NO_3}$ decreased with irradiation compared with those of the membrane without the irradiation. The Stokes radii of the anions used in this work are in the order:

TABLE 2 Transport Numbers of Nitrate and Fluoride Ions Relative to Chloride Ions in the M-3 Membrane

	With photoirradiation	Without photoirradiation
$P_{Cl}^{NO_3}$	1.11	1.41
P_{Cl}^{F}	0.16	0.20

Electrodialysis was carried out at a current density of 1 mA/cm² at 25.0°C for 1 h using a 1:1 mixed salt solution (0.04 N as sodium ion concentration) with and without photoirradiation (preirradiation time, 40 min; irradiation of the desalting side of the membrane during electrodialysis).

sulfate ions (2.31 Å) > fluoride ions (1.66 Å) > nitrate ions (1.29 Å) > chloride ions (1.21 Å) > bromide ions (1.18 Å) [58]. Chloride ions are small. Accordingly, anions measured in this work should be difficult to permeate through the membrane relative to chloride ions in the presence of photoirradiation because the pore size of the membrane becomes smaller. To confirm this, the permeability coefficient of a neutral molecule, urea, through the anion-exchange membrane with a viologen moiety (M-3 membrane: Cl⁻ form) was measured in the presence or absence of photoirradiation. The coefficients, which decreased with irradiation, are listed in Table 3. The pore size of the anion-exchange membrane with a viologen moiety apparently decreased with photoirradiation. It is concluded that the cationic charge density of anion-exchange membranes can be controlled by photoirradiation by introducing a viologen moiety as anion-exchange groups. Consequently, the transport numbers of various anions, sulfate, fluoride, nitrate, and bromide ions (in higher concentration ranges), relative to the chloride ions decreased.

Finally, when the transport numbers of various anions relative to chloride ions were measured, the current efficiency of all anion-exchange membranes was measured in the presence or absence of photoirradiation. If all of the

TABLE 3 Permeability Coefficient of Urea with and Without Irradiation Through the M-3 Membrane

	With photoirradiation	Without photoirradiation
Permeability coefficient	1.08	1.43

Dialysis was carried out using a two-compartment cell (2 mol/L urea/Mem./pure water) for 48 h at 25.0°C using a M-3 membrane with or without photoirradiation on the concentrated side of the membrane surface.

viologen moieties of the anion-exchange membranes change into biradicals, MV^0, the membranes become neutral and the current efficiency should be that of a neutral membrane (the same value as the solution transport number for chloride ions which in 0.05 N sodium chloride solution is 0.612 [64]). However, the current efficiency of all membranes was greater than 98% both in the presence and absence of the irradiation.

IV. CONCLUSIONS

The anion-exchange membranes having a viologen moiety showed interesting properties in the presence of photoirradiation, because the dication of the viologen moiety reversibly changed to monocation radical and biradical.

Consequently, the anion-exchange membranes, which had been swelled with a solvent, generated photovoltage and photocurrent in the presence of photoirradiation on one surface of the membrane by assembling a photocell containing the membrane. The value of the photovoltage was affected by the membrane species, additives to the photocell and species of solvents. At 200 k Ω load resistance, 50–150 mV of photovoltage was observed. Especially, solvents having methylene groups between two oxygens, such as 1,3-dioxolane, 1,3-dioxane, etc., and solvents which swelled well the membrane, such as 1-methyl-2-pyrrolidone, produced a high photovoltage. It is apparent from the measurements of the photocell having a cation exchange or anion exchange membrane separator that chloride ions in the cell play an important role to charge transfer in the cell.

Because the valence of the anion-exchange membranes having a viologen moiety changes by photoirradiation, the pore size of the membranes changed due to the shrinkage of the membranes with irradiation. Thus, the transport numbers of various anions relative to chloride ions changed in the presence of photoirradiation. In general, anions larger than chloride ions encountered difficulty in permeating through the membrane in the presence of photoirradiation. The change in the transport numbers between anions was reversible between the reduction of the viologen moiety and the oxidation of the reduced forms.

REFERENCES

1. A. Eisenberg and H. L. Yeager (eds.), *Perfluorinated Ionomer Membranes*, ACS Symposium Series, No. 180, 1982.
2. D. S. Flett (ed.), *Ion Exchange Membranes*, Ellis Horwood, Ltd. Chichester, 1983.
3. T. Sata, *Macromolecules* (J. Kohovec, ed.) VSP, Utrecht, The Netherlands, 1992, p. 451.
4. P. Beak and W. R. Messer, *Organic Photochemistry* (O. L. Chapman, ed.) Marcel Dekker, New York, 1969, Vol. 2., p. 117.

5. I. Willner, J. Yang, C. Loane, J. W. Otvas, and M. Calvin, J. Phys. Chem. *85*: 3277 (1981).
6. A. Slama-Schwok, O. Ottolenghi, and D. Avnir, Nature *355*: 240 (1992).
7. S. B. Ungashe, W. L. Wilson, H. E. Katz, G. R. Scheller, and T. M. Putvinski, J. Am. Chem. Soc. *114*: 8718 (1992).
8. L. A. Vermeuleny, J. L. Snover, L. S. Sapochak, and M. E. Thompson, J. Am. Chem. Soc. *115*: 11767 (1993).
9. R. E. Sassoon, S. Gershuni, and S. Rabini, J. Phys. Chem. *96*: 4692 (1992).
10. J. K. Hurst, D. H. D. Thompson, and J. S. Connolly, J. Am. Chem. Soc. *109*: 507 (1987).
11. I. Willner and Y. Eichen, J. Am. Chem. Soc. *107*: 6862 (1987).
12. P. K. Datta and M. Borja, J. Chem. Soc., Chem. Commun. 1565 (1993).
13. T. Endo, Y. Saotome, and M. Okamura, J. Am. Chem. Soc. *106*: 1124 (1984).
14. R. Sato, Y. Kobayashi, Y. Tomiya, H. Takeuchi, and M. Takeishi, Polymer J. *25*: 655 (1993).
15. M. Yamana and T. Kawata, Nippon Kagaku Zasshi, 941 (1977).
16. H. Miyata, Y. Sugahara, K. Kuroda, and C. Kato, J. Chem. Soc., Faraday Trans., I. *83*: 1851 (1987).
17. C. Stradowski, J. Applied Polym. Sci. *41*: 2511 (1990).
18. B. Maiti and S. Schlick, Chem. Mater. *4*: 458 (1992).
19. H. Akahoshi, S. Toshima, and K. Itaya, J. Phys. Chem. *85*: 818 (1981).
20. H. Chang, M. Osawa, T. Matsue, and I. Uchida, J. Chem. Soc., Chem. Commun. 611 (1991).
21. A. Walcarius, L. Lamberts, and E. G. Derquane, Electrochim. Acta *38*: 2257 (1993).
22. T. Saita, T. Iyoda, and T. Shimidzu, Bull. Chem. Soc. Japan *66*: 2054 (1993).
23. H. D. Abruña and A. J. Bard, J. Am. Chem. Soc. *103*: 6898 (1981).
24. M. S. Simon and P. T. Moore, J. Polym. Sci., Polym. Chem. Ed. *13*: 1 (1975).
25. H. Kamogawa, T. Masui, and S. Amemiya, J. Polym. Sci., Polym. Chem. Ed. *22*: 383 (1984).
26. H. Kamogawa and S. Amemiya, J. Polym. Sci., Polym. Chem. Ed. *23*: 2413 (1985).
27. W. Xu and G. Wan, J. Macromol. Sci. Pure Appl. Chem. *A30*: 373 (1993).
28. M. Furue, S. Yamanaka, L. Phat, and S. Nozakura, J. Polym. Sci., Polym. Chem. Ed. *19*: 2635 (1981).
29. F. Liu, X. Yu, and S. Li, Eur. Polym. J. *30*: 289 (1994).
30. F. Liu, X. Yu, and S. Li, Eur. Polym. J. *30*: 689 (1994).
31. H. Kamogawa, K. Kikushima, and M. Nanasawa, J. Polym. Sci., Polym. Chem. Ed. *27*: 393 (1989).
32. K. Ageishi, T. Endo, and O. Okawara, Macromolecules *16*: 884 (1983).
33. T. Sata, J. Membrane Sci. *118*: 121 (1996).
34. T. Sata, J. Colloid Interface Sci. *181*: 275 (1996).
35. T. Sata, K. Teshima, and T. Yamguchi, J. Polym. Sci., Polym. Chem. Ed. *34*: 1475 (1996).
36. P. Zschocke and D. Quellmatz, J. Membrane Sci. *22*: 325 (1985).
37. K. Takata, K. Kusumoto, T. Sata, and Y. Mizutani, J. Macromol. Sci. *A24*: 645 (1987).

38. J. Ceynowa, Polymer, *19*: 73 (1978).
39. T. D. Gierke and W. Y. Hsu, *Perfluorinated Ionomer Membranes*, ACS Symposium Series No. 180, p. 283, 1982.
40. T. Kawahara, H. Ihara, and Y. Mizutani, J. Appl. Polym. Sci. *33*: 1343 (1987).
41. L. Hammarström, M. Almgren, J. Lind, G. Merényi, T. Norrby, and B. Akermark, J. Phys. Chem. *97*: 10083 (1993).
42. T. Sata and K. Matsusaki, J. Polym. Sci., Polym. Chem. Ed., *34*: 2123 (1996).
43. M. Kaneko and A. Yamada, Makromol. Chem. *182*: 1111 (1981).
44. G. Yao, T. Onikubo, and M. Kaneko, Electrochim. Acta *38*: 1093 (1993).
45. A. Walcarius, L. Lamberts, and E. G. Derouane, Electrochim. Acta *38*: 2267 (1993).
46. F. Elisei, U. Mazzucato, H. Gorner, and D. Schulte-Frohlinde, J. Photochem. Photobiol. *50A*: 209 (1989).
47. M. Furue, S. Yamanaka, L. Phat, and S. Nozakura, J. Polym. Sci., Polym. Chem. Ed. *19*: 2635 (1981).
48. T. Sata, J. Colloid Interface Sci. *186*: 160 (1997).
49. I. Cakmak, Angwew. Makromol. Chem. *224*(1): 49 (1995).
50. H. Kamogawa, K. Kikushima, and M. Nanasawa, J. Polym. Sci., Polym. Chem. Ed. *27*: 393 (1989).
51. L. A. Vermeulen, J. L. Snover, L. S. Sapochak, and M. E. Thompson, J. Am. Chem. Soc. *115*: 11767 (1993).
52. W. Xu and G. Wan, J. Macromol. Sci., Pure Appl. Chem. *A30*: 373 (1993).
53. T. Sata, F. Kishimoto, and S. Ogura, J. Chem. Soc., Chem. Commun. 1159 (1993).
54. T. Sata, J. Membrane Sci. *93*: 117 (1994).
55. T. Sata, T. Yamaguchi, and K. Matsusaki, J. Chem. Soc., Chem. Commun. 1153 (1995).
56. T. Sata, T. Yamaguchi, K. Kawamura, and K. Matsusaki, J. Chem. Soc., Faraday Trans. *93*: 457 (1997).
57. T. Sata, Y. Matsuo, T. Yamaguchi, and K. Matsusaki, J. Chem. Soc., Faraday Trans. *93*: 2553 (1997).
58. H. Ohotaki, *Hydration of Ions*, Kyoritsu Shuppan Co., Ltd., Tokyo, 1992, p. 20.
59. H. D. Abruña and A. J. Bard, J. Am. Chem. Soc. *103*: 6898 (1981).
60. W. H. Hamill, J. Chem. Phys. *49*: 2446 (1968).
61. Z. Kuri, *Radiation Chemistry*, Kyoritsu Shuppan, Tokyo, 1979, p. 57.
62. K. Tanigaki, M. Suzuki, Y. Saotome, and Y. Ohnoshi, J. Electrochem. Soc. *132*: 1678 (1985).
63. I. Inoue, T. Tanaka, and T. Yamabe, Nippon Kagakukai Shi *83*: 1161 (1962).
64. Kagaku Binran, Kiso-hen, (*Handbook of Chemistry, Basic Volume*), 4th Ed., The Chemical Society of Japan, Tokyo, 1993, p. 455.

17

Electroconvective Mechanisms in Concentration Polarization at Electrodialysis Membranes

I. RUBINSTEIN and B. ZALTZMAN   Department of Environmental Physics and Energy Research, Blaustein Institute for Desert Research, Ben-Gurion University of the Negev, Sede Boqer Campus, Israel

Abstract

Electroconvection is reviewed as a mechanisms of mixing in the diffusion layer, responsible for the overlimiting conductance in the course of concentration polarization at a cation-exchange electrodialysis membrane. Two types of electroconvection in strong electrolytes may be distinguished: bulk electroconvection, due to the action of the electric field upon the residual space charge of a locally quasi-electroneutral electrolyte with nonuniform concentration, and convection induced by electroosmotic slip of either equilibrium (first) or nonequilibrium (second) kind. Theories of electroosmotic slip of both kinds are reviewed and the derivation of a correct slip condition for nonequilibrium electroosmosis, relevant for a developed concentration polarization, is outlined. The following two onset mechanisms for electroconvection of all three above mentioned types are discussed: the onset due to hydrodynamic instability of the quiescent concentration polarization at a homogeneous electrodialysis membrane and the thresholdless onset due to possible short-scale conductive inhomogeneities of the membrane surface. As for the former, both bulk electroconvection and electroosmosis of the second kind yield instability, while this is not the case, for a realistic low molecular electrolyte, for electroosmosis of the first kind. So far, there is no definitive information as to whether the bulk electroconvective instability may develop into a fully-fledged convection, capable of providing a mixing of the diffusion layer at a cation-exchange membrane, sufficient to account for the overlimiting conductance through it. On the other hand, recent calculations show that this is the case for convection induced by electroosmosis of the second kind, through any one of the aforementioned onset mechanisms.

I. INTRODUCTION

In this chapter we review electroconvection in strong electrolytes. This term pertains to a complex of phenomena which were invoked and described theoretically to a certain degree, to explain the overlimiting conductance through cation-exchange electrodialysis membranes (see Chap. 15).

The use of the term electroconvection, in relation to strong electrolytes, is not very conventional. Traditionally, by electroconvection was meant the flow of nematic liquid crystals [1–3] or that of a liquid dielectric caused by the action of the electric field on the macroscopic space charge formed by ions of the appropriate sign, injected in a low quantity into the fluid [4–6]. As opposed to this, we are about to address electroconvection in a liquid abundant with charge carriers of both signs. In such a liquid, near the equilibrium, the space charge is confined to diffuse electric double layer, of thickness of the order of a Debye length, at the membrane–solution interface.

The following two types of electroconvection in strong electrolyte may be distinguished. The first is the common electroosmosis, either classical, of the first kind, or of the second kind, according to the terminology in Ref. 7. The term electroosmosis of the first kind, relates to electrolyte slip resulting from the action of tangential electric and concentration gradient fields upon the space charge of a quasiequilibrium diffuse double layer. Electroosmosis of the second kind, invoked by Dukhin et al. [7–9], results from the similar action upon the extended space charge of a double layer far from equilibrium, developing at a permselective interface in the course of concentration polarization under the passage of a normal electric current [10,11].

Another phenomenon is the recently described bulk electroconvection due to the volume electric forces acting on a macroscopic scale in a locally quasi-electroneutral electrolyte [12,13]. In this chapter we shall review both afore-mentioned types of electroconvection in the context of concentration polarization in electrodialysis, or, more specifically, at a cation-exchange electrodialysis membrane.

Concentration polarization (CP) is an electrochemical and membranological nickname for a complex of effects. These are related to the formation of electrolyte concentration gradients resulting from the passage of an electric current through a solution adjacent to an ion-selective interface. This phenomenon forms a basic element of charge transfer from electrolyte solutions to ion-exchange membranes. The specific aspect of concentration polarization we address here concerns the stationary voltage–current (VC) curves of highly permselective cation-exchange membranes (C membranes) employed in electrodialysis which typically are of general form depicted schematically in Fig. 1. The following three regions are distinguishable in such a typical curve. The low current Ohmic region I is followed by a plateau (region II) of a much lower slope. Inflection of the VC curve at the plateau is followed by region III,

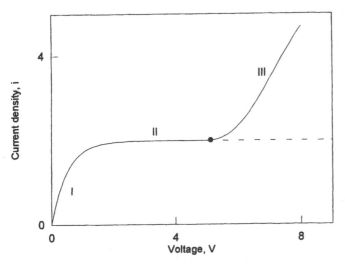

FIG. 1 Sketch of a typical voltage current curve of a cation-exchange membrane. The black spot marks the onset of noise.

in which the slope of the VC curve is somewhat lower than in region I. Inflection of the VC curve (transition to region III) is preceded by the appearance of a low-frequency excess electric noise. The noise amplitude increases with the distance above the threshold and may reach up to a few percent of the appropriate mean values.

The classical theory of concentration polarization at ion-selective interfaces predicts a true saturation of the VC curves, characterized by the limiting current (the dashed line in Fig. 1) [14.i,15]. Let us recapitulate this theory briefly. Consider an unstirred layer of thickness δ of a univalent electrolyte adjacent to an ideally permselective homogeneous interface (e.g., a cation-exchange membrane). Let us direct the axis $\tilde{y}$ normally to this interface, with the origin at the membrane–solution interface and $\tilde{y} = -\delta$ coinciding with the outer (bulk) edge of the unstirred layer. Let us assume local electroneutrality and neglect the electroosmotic flow. With these assumptions, stationary ionic transport across the unstirred layer will be described by the following boundary value problem:

$$-D\left(\frac{d\tilde{c}}{d\tilde{y}} + \frac{F}{RT}\,\tilde{c}\,\frac{d\tilde{\phi}}{d\tilde{y}}\right) = -\tilde{j} = -\frac{\tilde{i}}{F}, \tag{1}$$

$$\frac{d\tilde{c}}{d\tilde{y}} - \frac{F}{RT}\,\tilde{c}\,\frac{d\tilde{\phi}}{d\tilde{y}} = 0, \tag{2}$$

$$\tilde{c}(-\delta) = c_0, \quad \tilde{\phi}(-\delta) = 0, \quad \tilde{\phi}(0) = -\tilde{V} \tag{3}$$

Here, $\tilde{y}$, $\tilde{c}$, $\tilde{\phi}$, $\tilde{j}$, $\tilde{i}$ and $\tilde{V}$ are, respectively, the dimensional coordinate, ionic concentration, electric potential, cation flux, electric current density, and voltage drop across the unstirred layer, whereas c_0 is bulk concentration, F is the Faraday constant, R is the universal gas constant, T is the absolute temperature, and D is cation diffusivity.

Equations (1) and (2) are the stationary Nernst–Planck equations for electrodiffusional transfer of cations and anions, respectively.

Integration of (1)–(3) yields

$$\tilde{c} = c_0[1 - (\tilde{j}/2Dc_0)(\tilde{y} + \delta)] \tag{4}$$

$$\tilde{\phi} = (RT/F)\ln[1 - (\tilde{j}/2Dc_0)(\tilde{y} + \delta)] \tag{5}$$

$$\tilde{i} = (2FDc_0/\delta)(1 - e^{-\tilde{V}R/RT}) \tag{6}$$

For $\tilde{V} \to \infty$, Eq. (6) predicts

$$\tilde{i} \to \tilde{i}^{\text{lim}} = 2Dc_0\,F/\delta \tag{7}$$

It has been shown conclusively by several authors that no such mechanisms as loss of permselectivity at high voltage or the appearance of additional charge carriers ("water splitting") are responsible for the discrepancy between the behavior prescribed by Eqs. (6) and (7) and the observed overlimiting properties of the C membranes [16–20]*. (Herein, we use the terms underlimiting and overlimiting in relation to the features in the current ranges corresponding to the regions I, II, and III of the VC curve, respectively).

Eventually, a fair amount of indications has been accumulated, suggesting that the overlimiting behavior of the C membranes is associated with some kind of convective mixing that develops spontaneously in the depleted diffusion layer at the advanced stage of CP [16,21–23]. This has been finally confirmed by a straightforward experimental finding: if the surface of the cation-exchange membrane facing the diluate is coated by a gel, a plateau is reached at saturation, and the excess electric noise disappears [24].

It was suggested that gravitational convection, brought about by the density gradients due to concentration polarization, may destroy the unstirred layer [21,22]. It should however be remembered that gravitational instability of a laminar sublayer at a smooth solid–liquid interface in a well mixed bulk flow may occur only upon the fulfillment of quite general hydrodynamic conditions. Whatever is the nature of the bulk flow, laminar or turbulent, natural or forced, gravitational instability will destroy an already existing diffusion layer only if the dimensionless Rayleigh number, Ra, related to this layer, is above a certain critical value. The Rayleigh number is defined as

$$Ra = g\rho'\delta^3/\nu D \tag{8}$$

where g is the gravitational acceleration, ρ' the relative density drop across the layer, and ν the kinematic viscosity of the fluid. Let us consider an unstirred layer of 200 μm or less. When a current is passed through a membrane so that polarization creates a heavier layer on top of a lighter one, the critical Rayleigh number is larger than 1000. For a 0.01 N NaCl solution Ra $\sim$ 11.6 and for 0.1 N $-$ Ra $\sim$ 116, that is at least an order of magnitude below the instability threshold.

Electroconvection was suggested as an alternative mixing mechanism drawing together the phenomena related to the voltage–current curves of cation-exchange membranes [7,12,13,25–30]. Below we review this mechanism in the following order.

In Sec. II we present the equations governing electroconvection. We do this separately for bulk electroconvection and electroosmosis of both kinds. In reality, bulk electroconvection and electroosmosis are always superimposed. In fact, both results from the action of the same Coulomb forces on different length scales (macroscopic and Debye length, respectively).

In Sec. III, we shall outline the scenarios for onset of electroconvection, as driven by any of the aforementioned mechanisms. These scenarios concern the

---

* As opposed to most anion-exchange membranes which intensely "split water" in the course of concentration polarization due to a particular catalytic surface reaction [18–20].

onset due to either inhomogeneity of the membrane or instability of quiescent conduction through (concentration polarization at) a homogeneous membrane.

Finally, in Sec. IV we present some preliminary results of numerical computations of nonlinear electroconvection, developing from both onset mechanisms for electroosmosis of the second kind.

II. ELECTROCONVECTIVE MECHANISMS

A. Bulk Electroconvection

Let us consider a domain in a univalent electrolyte characterized by a typical single length scale L, macroscopic but still sufficiently small for all inertial effects of fluid motion to be negligible.

We shall write down the usual equations of convective electrodiffusion for the ionic species, the Poisson equation for the electric potential (without the a priori assumption of local electroneutrality) and the Stokes momentum equation, with a volume electric force in it, bilinear in the electric field intensity and space charge density. The electric term is being kept in the Stokes equation, in spite of our a priori knowledge of the fact that on a macroscopic length scale not too far from equilibrium local electroneutrality holds with a very high accuracy. Indeed, a straightforward dimensional analysis shows that upon a natural scaling a very small parameter (squared dimensionless Debye length) appears in the dimensionless Poisson equation, which implies local stoichiometric electroneutrality. Nevertheless, the typical circulation velocity of fluid, induced by the electric force, is such that the Péclet number in the dimensionless transport equation, evaluated near the equilibrium, turns out to be universally of order unity. This implies that the contribution of electroconvection to the ionic transport in a locally electroneutral liquid system is universally comparable with the contribution of electrodiffusion.

In accordance with the outline above let us write down the Nernst–Planck equations of stationary convective electrodiffusion as

$$\tilde{v}\tilde{\nabla}\tilde{c}_+ = \tilde{\nabla}[D\tilde{\nabla}\tilde{c}_+ + (DF/RT)\tilde{c}_+\,\tilde{\nabla}\tilde{\phi}] \tag{9}$$
$$\tilde{v}\tilde{\nabla}\tilde{c}_- = \tilde{\nabla}[D\tilde{\nabla}\tilde{c}_- - (DF/RT)\tilde{c}_-\,\tilde{\nabla}\tilde{\phi}] \tag{10}$$

Here $\tilde{v}$ is convection velocity, $\tilde{c}_+$ and $\tilde{c}_-$ are the cation and anion concentrations, respectively, and $\tilde{\nabla}$ is the dimensional ∇ operator; for simplicity, ionic diffusivity D has been assumed equal for both ions.

Furthermore, the Poisson equation reads

$$d\varepsilon_0\,\tilde{\Delta}\tilde{\phi} = -\tilde{\rho} \tag{11}$$
$$\tilde{\rho} = F(\tilde{c}_+ - \tilde{c}_-) \tag{12}$$

Here d is the dielectric constant (assumed concentration and electric field independent) and ε_0 is the dielectric permeability of the vacuum, $\tilde{\rho}$ is the space charge density, and $\tilde{\Delta}$ is the dimensional Laplacian. Finally, the Stokes equation and the incompressibility condition read, respectively,

$$-\tilde{\nabla}\tilde{p} - \tilde{\rho}\tilde{\nabla}\tilde{\phi} + \eta\tilde{\Delta}\tilde{v} = 0 \qquad (13)$$

$$\tilde{\nabla}\cdot\tilde{v} = 0 \qquad (14)$$

Here $\tilde{p}$ is the pressure and η is the dynamic viscosity.

Let c_0 be some given typical ionic concentration (e.g., bulk electrolyte concentration). Let us introduce the following dimensionless variables:

$$\mathbf{x} = \frac{\tilde{\mathbf{x}}}{L} \qquad (15)$$

$$c_{\pm} = \frac{\tilde{c}_{\pm}}{c_0} \qquad (16)$$

$$\phi = \frac{F\tilde{\phi}}{RT} \qquad (17)$$

$$\mathbf{v} = \frac{\tilde{v}}{v_0} \qquad (18)$$

$$p = \frac{\tilde{p}}{p_0} \qquad (19)$$

Here $\mathbf{x}$, $\tilde{\mathbf{x}}$ stand for the dimensionless and dimensional position vectors.

Generally, untilded notations stand for the dimensionless counterparts of the appropriate dimensional (tilded) variables. As scales for the space variables, concentration c_0, and the electric potential we chose, as is usual in electrodiffusion, the typical macroscopic length L, typical concentration c_0, and the thermal potential RT/F. On the other hand, there is no a priori pressure and velocity scales present in the system. These are to be inferred from the momentum Eq. (13) or its derivatives. Thus we shall identify v_0 with the typical rotational flow velocity that is to be evaluated from the vorticity equation. Substitution of Eq. (11) into Eq. (13) yields

$$-\tilde{\nabla}\tilde{p} + d\varepsilon_0\,\tilde{\Delta}\tilde{\phi}\tilde{\nabla}\tilde{\phi} + \eta\tilde{\Delta}\tilde{v} = 0 \qquad (20)$$

Taking the curl of Eq. (20) yields the vorticity equation in the form

$$d\varepsilon_0\,\mathrm{curl}(\tilde{\Delta}\tilde{\phi}\tilde{\nabla}\tilde{\phi}) + \eta\tilde{\Delta}\,\mathrm{curl}\tilde{v} = 0 \qquad (21)$$

The term balance in (21) yields for v_0

$$v_0 = \frac{d\varepsilon_0 1}{L\eta}\left(\frac{RT}{F}\right)^2 \qquad (22)$$

The balance of the first and second term in (20) yield in turn for p_0

$$p_0 = \frac{d}{4\pi}\left(\frac{RT}{F}\right)^2 \qquad (23)$$

Let us note that the above scaling is unique, corresponding to the fluid motion induced by the nonpotential component of the electric volume force acting in the fluid, with the potential part of this force balanced by pressure, as expressed by Eq. (23). Substitution of Eqs. (14)–(17), (22), and (23) into Eqs. (9)–(14) yields the governing equations in terms of dimensionless variables in the form

$$Pe \mathbf{v} \nabla c_+ = \nabla(\nabla c_+ + c_+ \nabla\phi) \tag{24}$$

$$Pe \mathbf{v} \nabla c_- = \nabla(\nabla c_- - c_- \nabla\phi) \tag{25}$$

$$\varepsilon^2 \Delta\phi = c_- - c_+ \tag{26}$$

$$-\nabla p + \Delta\phi \nabla\phi + \Delta\mathbf{v} = 0 \tag{27}$$

$$\Delta \cdot \mathbf{v} = 0 \tag{28}$$

Here Pe is the dimensionless Péclet number, given by the expression

$$Pe = \frac{v_0 L}{D} = \left(\frac{RT}{F}\right)^2 \frac{d\varepsilon_0}{\eta D} \tag{29}$$

whereas ε is the dimensionless Debye length

$$\varepsilon = \frac{r_0}{L} \tag{30}$$

where r_0 is the dimensional Debye length, defined as

$$r_0 = \frac{(d\varepsilon_0 RT)^{1/2}}{F c_0^{1/2}} \tag{31}$$

For L in the range

$$10^{-6} < L < 2 \times 10^{-5} \text{ m},$$

and c_0 in the range

$$1 < c_0 < 10^3 \text{ mol/m}^3$$

equations (30) and (31) yield ε in the range

$$5 \times 10^{-12} < \varepsilon^2 < 2 \times 10^{-6} \tag{32}$$

The extreme smallness of ε for any reasonable macroscopic ionic system motivates the commonly employed approximation of local stoichiometric electroneutrality whose essence we briefly recall below. This approximation amounts to formally setting ε equal to zero in Eq. (26), that is, assuming the space charge density in the Poisson equation equal to zero, i.e., replacing the Poisson equation by the algebraic electroneutrality condition

$$c_+ = c_- = c$$

everywhere in the bulk of the electrolyte, except for the boundary (double) layers of typical thickness r_0. Of course, this does not imply that the respective electric field, as determined from the Nernst–Planck equations and the electroneutrality condition will be solenoidal*. What the stoichiometric local electroneutrality condition does imply, is that the dimensionless space charge, equal to the divergence of the electric field times ε^2, is small compared to the local ionic concentrations. On the other hand, the need to keep the electric force term (also proportional to the space charge density) in the Stokes equation (27), can be judged upon only through evaluating the respective Péclet number in (24) and (25). If the latter is not too small, then the effect of convection due to the electric force should not be neglected. In this connection, it is observed first from Eq. (29) that the electroconvectional Pe is independent of the typical concentration c_0 and the length scale L. Second, for $T = 300$ K and $d = 80$, $\eta = 10^{-3}$ kg/s $\cdot$ m, $D = 10^{-9}$ m^2/s, typical for an aqueous low molecular electrolyte, Eq. (29) yields

$$\text{Pe} \sim 0.5 \tag{33}$$

that is, in accordance with the statement in the beginning of this subsection, the transport effect of electroconvection, evaluated near the equilibrium, is expected to be comparable with that of electrodiffusion, independently of the size and concentration of an ionic system, characterized by a single macroscopic length scale. Naturally, this effect is to increase, when the system is being driven further from equilibrium, e.g., by applying a higher voltage to it. Finally, by employing the known relation

$$D\eta = kT/6\pi a \tag{34}$$

---

* In locally electroneutral ionic systems under direct electric current some nonsolenoidality (space charge) is imminent, irrespectively of the ionic diffusivities being equal or different for different ionic species, in order to provide for solenoidality of the electric current, that is, to preclude a further charge accumulation due to conductivity variation. The one-dimensional concentration polarization of Sec. I provides a prototypical example of this situation. The respective weak macroscopic space charge occurring on the scale of the entire diffusion layer (microns to tens of μm), is not to be confused with the strong short scale space charge of the nonequilibrium double layer at the interface. The width of the latter increases with the decrease of the interface concentration in the course of concentration polarization, and may reach up to a few hundred angstroms. This development is at the basis of electroosmosis of the second kind discussed below in Sec. II.B.3. However, for this extended microscopic scale to begin to overlap with the macroscopic diffusion layer length scale discussed in this paper, unrealistically high voltages are necessary, well above the dielectric breakdown threshold [11]. With differing diffusivities, macroscopic nonsolenoidality of the electric field may occur even without the electric current as a feature of the diffusion potential, which is formed to maintain the local electroneutrality. For a discussion of the local electroneutrality approximation as an outer asymptotic limit of the full electrodiffusional formulation viewed as a singular perturbation problem, see Ref. 11, Chapters 1, 4, and 5.

(a combination of the Einstein's relation with the Stokes formula), where a is the viscous ionic radius, Eq. (29) may be rewritten as

$$Pe = 6\pi(r_0^2 a/\lambda^3) \tag{35}$$

Here

$$\lambda = 1/(Nc_0)^{1/3} \tag{36}$$

is the average interionic distance (N is the Avogadro number).

Thus, summarizing, the set of equations for stoichiometrically locally electroneutral electroconvection is

$$Pe\mathbf{v}\nabla c = \nabla(\nabla c + c\nabla\phi) \tag{37}$$

$$Pe\mathbf{v}\nabla c = \nabla(\nabla c - c\nabla\phi) \tag{38}$$

$$-\nabla p + \Delta\phi\nabla\phi + \Delta\mathbf{v} = 0 \tag{39}$$

$$\nabla\cdot\mathbf{v} = 0 \tag{40}$$

The above consideration does not imply, of course, that electroconvection actually occurs in any macroscopic liquid ionic system with a nonsolenoidal electric field. It just defines a framework in which bulk electroconvection, whenever occurring, is to be treated. In Sec. III we outline two situations of this type, those of bulk electroconvective instabilities at a homogeneous membrane and thresholdless bulk electroconvection at an inhomogeneous membrane.

B. Electroosmotic Slip

In this subsection we review the theory of electroosmotic slip. Thus in Sec. II.B.1 we reproduce the standard crude calculation of the electroosmotic slip velocity, followed in Sec. II.B.2 by a rederivation of the Dukhin and Derjaguin's expression for the electroosmotic slip at a flat solid–liquid interface with a quasi-equilibrium double layer. This derivation shows how the account for polarization of the double layer by the tangential electric field, yields an expression for the slip velocity which is essentially different from that commonly obtained by disregarding polarization. The difference lies in the proportionality factor (electroosmotic factor) relating the slip velocity to the intensity of the tangential electric field. In the first case this factor tends to a finite value upon an infinite increase of the potential drop between the nonslip surface at the interface and the bulk (ζ-potential), in the other case the slip velocity is proportional to ζ-potential. A review of these issues is followed in Sec. II.B.3 by developing a modified theory of electroosmotic slip of the second kind. Both the term and the topic deserve elaboration. As already mentioned in the Introduction, the term electroconvective phenomena of the second kind was invoked by Dukhin and his collaborators to designate the electroosmotic effects due to the extended space charge of the strongly nonequilibrium diffuse electric double layer, developing at a permselective interface in the course of concentration polarization. Ironically, in his theory of this phenomenon [7], Dukhin disregarded the very same effects of double layer polarization, he accounted for in his and Derjaguin's theory of quasi-equilibrium electrokinetic phenomena and which resulted in the aforementioned formula for the electro-osmotic slip of the first kind [31]. This inconsistency has been removed through an accurate asymptotic analysis of polarization of the nonequilibrium double layer by the tangential components of the external gradients, yielding a correct condition for electroosmotic slip of the second kind [30.i]. According to this condition, electroosmotic slip velocity is proportional to the tangential derivative of the logarithm of normal component of current density through the membrane, with the applied voltage squared as the proportionality factor.

1. Classical Expression for Electroosmotic Slip (Helmholtz–Smoluchowski Formula)

The standard classical calculation of electroosmotic slip velocity proceeds as follows [14.ii]. Consider the diffuse part of a two-dimensional double electric layer

$$\{-\infty < \tilde{x} < \infty, \quad -\infty < \tilde{y} < 0\}$$

adjacent to a flat membrane at $\tilde{y} = 0$. Let us assume the electric potential $\tilde{\phi}(\tilde{y})$ in the double layer to be independent of the externally applied tangential electric field $\bar{E}i$ (Assumption I). Here i is the unit vector in $\tilde{x}$ direction. Let us assume furthermore that there is no lateral pressure variation in the double layer (Assumption II). Thus, the only forces acting in the double layer are the Coulombic electric force and the viscous drag. As long as fluid inertia may be neglected, these two forces balance. By the Poisson's law and in accordance with Assumption I, we have for the charge density ρ in the double layer

$$\tilde{\rho} = -d\varepsilon_0 \tilde{\phi}_{\tilde{y}\tilde{y}} \tag{41}$$

Furthermore, according to the Assumption II the force balance in the double layer (for the $\tilde{x}$-force component) reads

$$-d\varepsilon_0 \tilde{\phi}_{\tilde{y}\tilde{y}} \tilde{E} + \eta \tilde{u}_{\tilde{y}\tilde{y}} = 0 \tag{42}$$

Here $\tilde{u}$ is the tangential component of the fluid velocity $\tilde{v}_c = \tilde{u}(\tilde{x}, \tilde{y})i + \tilde{w}(\tilde{x}, \tilde{y})j$.

Two integrations of Eq. (42) from $y = 0$ to $y = -\infty$ yield, assuming nonslip at $y = 0$ and boundedness of ϕ at infinity,

$$\tilde{u}(-\infty) = -\frac{d\varepsilon_0 \tilde{\zeta}}{\eta} \tilde{E}, \quad \zeta \overset{\text{def}}{=} \tilde{\phi}(0) - \tilde{\phi}(-\infty) \tag{43a,b}$$

This is the classical Helmholtz–Smoluchowski formula for the electroosmotic slip velocity. As we just saw, this formula follows directly from Assumptions I and II independently of the properties of the solid surface at $y = 0$ or the structure of the double layer.

2. Effect of Polarization of a Quasi-Equilibrium Double Layer upon the Electroosmotic Slip Velocity (Dukhin–Derjaguin Formula)

Below we outline the major steps of the relevant boundary layer analysis. For details of this analysis in terms of a matched asymptotic expansions, the reader is referred to Ref. 30.i. The small boundary layer parameter in these expansions, is the previously defined dimensionless Debye length.

Mechanical equilibrium across the double layer implies, to the leading order in ε,

$$p_z = \varepsilon^{-2}\phi_{zz}\phi_z \tag{44a}$$

where z is the boundary layer variable, defined as

$$z = \frac{y}{\varepsilon} \tag{44b}$$

and y–dimensionless distance from the membrane. Integration of Eq. (44a) across the double layer yields, to the leading order in ε, for the hydrostatic pressure in the double layer

$$p(x, z) = \tfrac{1}{2}(\phi_z)^2\varepsilon^{-2} \tag{45}$$

Equation (45) implies a strong lateral dependence of the hydrostatic pressure through the respective dependence of the electric potential (in contradiction to Assumption II of the classical calculation).

Substitution of Eq. (45) into Stokes equation for the tangential velocity u yields

$$-\tfrac{1}{2}[(\phi_z)^2]_x + \phi_x\phi_{zz} + u_{zz} = 0 \tag{46}$$

This equation is valid irrespectively of the magnitude of the electric current passed through the membrane, i.e., quasi-equilibrium or nonequilibrium structure of the double layer. The latter pertains to the properties of electric potential $\varphi(x,z)$ in the double layer, as prescribed by the Nernst–Planck–Poisson equations for the ionic concentrations and the electric potential, in accordance with the range of the electric current crossing the double layer. For a quasi-equilibrium double layer, with the current below the limiting value, the ionic concentrations within the boundary layer obey, to the leading order in ε, the Boltzmann relations

$$c_{\pm} = \bar{c}e^{\mp\phi\pm\bar{\phi}} \tag{47}$$

Here $\bar{c}(x)$ and $\bar{\phi}(x)$ are, respectively, the electrolyte concentration and the electric potential at the outer edge of the boundary (electric double) layer. As a result, the Nernst–Planck–Poisson equations are reduced, to the same order, to the Poisson–Boltzmann equation

$$\phi_{zz} = \bar{c}(e^{\phi - \bar{\phi}} - e^{-\phi + \bar{\phi}}) \tag{48}$$

for the electric potential in the double layer.

Away from quasiequilibrium, with $I \to I^{\text{lim}}$ and $\bar{c} \to 0$, upon $\varepsilon \to 0$, $\bar{\phi} \to -\infty$ and $c_{\pm} \to 0$ in a part of the boundary layer. This, together with unboundedness of ϕ, yield in the r.h.s. of Eq. (48) indeterminacies of the type infinity times zero. As a result, Eq. (48) becomes unsuitable for calculation of the electric potential and the need arises for some additional analysis in this case.

On the other hand, as long as quasiequilibrium holds, integration of Eq. (48) yields

$$\phi(x, z) = \bar{\phi}(x) + 2 \ln \frac{e^{\zeta/2} + 1 + (e^{\zeta/2} - 1)e^{-[2\bar{c}(x)z]^{1/2}}}{e^{\zeta/2} + 1 - (e^{\zeta/2} - 1)e^{-[2\bar{c}(x)z]^{1/2}}} \tag{49}$$

Here, ζ is the dimensionless counterpart of $\bar{\zeta}$, that is the potential drop between the inner and the outer edges of the diffuse part of the double layer. Substitution of Eq. (49) into Eq. (46) and a subsequent integration with the relevant boundary conditions yields the following modified version of the classical expression for the electroosmotic slip velocity, generally valid for a quasiequilibrium double layer at an arbitrary solid surface

$$u_s = 2\bar{\mu}_x^- \frac{\ln \dfrac{A + 1}{2}}{A + 1} + 2\bar{\mu}_x^+ \frac{1}{1 + 1/A} \ln \frac{1 + 1/A}{2} \tag{50a}$$

Here

$$\bar{\mu}^{\pm} = \ln \bar{c} \pm \bar{\phi} \tag{50b}$$

are the interface values of the bulk electrochemical potentials and

$$A = \exp(\zeta(x)/2) \tag{50c}$$

Expressions of this kind for the electroosmotic slip velocity have been first derived by Dukhin and Derjaguin in Ref. 31.

A distinguishing feature of Eq. (50) is that

$$u_s \to 2 \ln(2)\mu_x^{\pm} \quad \text{when } \zeta \to \pm\infty \tag{51}$$

that is the coefficient at the $\mu_x^{\pm}$ (electroosmotic factor) tends to a maximal upper limit upon the increase of ζ. This feature is closely related to such nonlinear ionic equilibrium phenomena as counterion condensation and electric field and force saturation in electrolyte solutions [11, p. 23].

Different quasi-equilibrium systems are distinguished by the way ζ and $\bar{\mu}^{\pm}$ are specified through the boundary conditions at the solid–liquid interface.

Thus for a conducting solid, impermeable for both cations and anions, $\bar{c}$ and $\bar{\phi}$, entering $\mu_x^{\pm}$ in Eq. (51), are fully determined by the bulk solution only, independently of the double layer and the bulk solid. In particular, $\bar{\phi}_x$ and $\bar{c}_x$ in (51) could be in principle imposed independently of each other.

This is not the case for a permselective membrane maintained at a specified electric potential. In this case, the electrochemical potential of the membrane is essentially constant, and, due to the local equilibrium across the double layer, so is $\bar{\mu}(x)$. As a result Eq. (51) is reduced to

$$u_s = 4\bar{\phi}_x \frac{\ln \dfrac{A+1}{2}}{A+1} \tag{52}$$

3. Electroosmosis of the Second Kind

In this case Eq. (46) is still valid but this time $\bar{c} = 0$, $\bar{\phi} \to \infty$ which makes Eq. (47) inapplicable for calculation of ϕ in the double layer and thus of u_s. This reflects a fundamental structural change which occurs in the system as it moves away from quasiequilibrium upon $I \to I^{\lim}$.

Generally, quasi-equilibrium is typified by the division of the system into a locally quasi-electroneutral bulk and a quasi-equilibrium boundary layer (diffuse electric double layer). This picture breaks down upon $I \to I^{\lim}$, as reflected, in particular, in the inconsistency of the local electroneutrality approximation which appears in the basic CP solution Eqs. (4)–(6) in this limit. Indeed, in terms of dimensionless variables, this solution assumes the form:

$$c = 1 - \frac{i}{2}(y+1) \quad -1 < y < 0 \tag{53}$$

$$\phi = \ln\left(1 - \frac{i}{2}(y+1)\right) \tag{54}$$

$$i = 2(1 - e^{-V}) \tag{55a}$$

$$V \overset{\text{def}}{=} \phi(-1) - \phi(0) \tag{55b}$$

According to Eq. (54),

$$\phi_{yy}(0) = \frac{I^2}{4} \frac{1}{\left(1 - \dfrac{I}{2}\right)^2} \to \infty, \quad \text{when } I \to I^{\lim} = 2 \tag{56}$$

This implies that for any finite ε, however small, setting the l.h.s. of the Poisson Eq. (26) equal to zero, becomes inconsistent. This was the motivation behind the study of the space charge of the nonequilibrium electric double layer which develops in the course of concentration polarization when the interface concentration approaches zero and, accordingly, the local Debye length tends to infinity [10]. This study essentially consisted of a numerical solution of the counterpart of the basic model problem (1)–(3) but without use of local electroneutrality. In dimensionless form:

$$(c_{+y} + c_{+} \phi_y)_y = 0 \quad -1 < y < 0 \tag{57}$$

$$(c_{-y} - c_{-} \phi_y)_y = 0 \quad -1 < y < 0 \tag{58}$$

$$\varepsilon^2 \phi_{yy} = c_{-} - c_{+} \tag{59}$$

$$c_{+}(-1) = c_{-}(-1) = 1, \quad \phi(-1) = 0 \tag{60}$$

$$c_{+}(0) = N, \quad (c_{-y} - c_{-} \phi_y)|_{y=0} = 0, \quad \phi(0) = -\ln N - V \tag{61}$$

Here N is the fixed charge concentration in the membrane, assumed equal to that of cations.

In Figs. 2a and b we present schematically the ionic concentrations and space charge density profiles obtained in Ref. 10 (and in a number of studies that followed, [11,32,33]) for a sequence of applied voltage V.

The respective results may be summarized as follows. For $0 < V = O(1)$ ($I < I^{\text{lim}}$), local electroneutrality holds in the entire system except for the boundary layer (B) of the order of thickness ε at the right edge of the region. In the respective electroneutral region (N) a linear ionic concentration profile holds in accordance with Eq. (53). The maximal negative slope of the concentration profile in these conditions is 1 (which corresponds to $I = I^{\text{lim}} = 2$). This picture remains essentially valid up to $V = O(|\ln \varepsilon|)$ ($I \leq I^{\text{lim}}$). For $O(|\ln \varepsilon|) < V < O(\varepsilon^{-1})$ ($I \approx I^{\text{lim}}$), the following three regions may be distinguished. An electroneutral region (N) with a linear concentration profile with the slope approximately -1. This region borders on the right with the extended, $O(\varepsilon^{2/3})$ to $O(1)$ thick diffuse space charge region (C), followed by the quasi-equilibrium, $O(\varepsilon)$ thick, boundary layer (B) at the right edge. Upon a further increase of voltage up to $O(\varepsilon^{-1})$ the extended space charge region (C) reaches a finite size $O(1)$ and so does the current increment over the limiting value $[0 < I-I^{\text{lim}} = O(1)]$.

The main, and perhaps the only importance of this observation of development, in the course concentration polarization, of a nonequilibrium electric double layer with the extended space charge region, lied in its contribution to the discovery of the so called electrokinetic phenomena of the second kind by Dukhin and his colleagues [7–9] (see also references in [7]).

Derivation of the respective slip condition amounts to carrying out an analysis of polarization of the nonequilibrium double layer by the external fields similar to that of Sec. II.B.2. An account for polarization is the more necessary, since a large potential drops between the membrane surface and the bulk is concerned, that is, namely those conditions for which, saturation of the electroosmotic factor occurred for the quasi-equilibrium electroosmotic slip

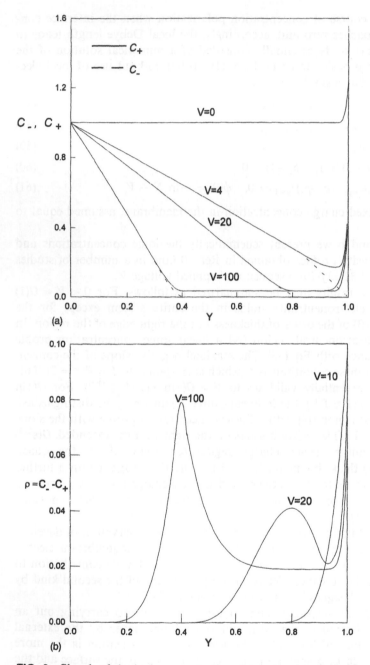

(a)

(b)

FIG. 2 Sketch of the ionic concentrations (a) and space charge density (b) profiles in the diffusion layer and nonequilibrium diffuse double layer ($\varepsilon = 10^{-2}$).

[see Eq. (51)]. The original theory of the electrokinetic phenomena of the second kind reproduced the classical derivation of Sec. II.B.1 for the nonequilibrium double layer with the extended space charge zone [7]. Nevertheless, a major step towards developing a correct nonequilibrium electroosmotic slip condition has been already made by a member of Dukhin's team, A. V. Listovnichy, through his developing of an elegant asymptotic theory of the nonequilibrium double layer [34]. This theory has been heavily used in Ref. 30.i to derive the following expression for the electroosmotic slip velocity at a flat permselective membrane with an applied voltage V ($V > O(|\ln \varepsilon|)$), taking into account polarization of the nonquasi-equilibrium double layer by the external fields,

$$
u_s = -\frac{1}{8} V^2 \left. \frac{\dfrac{\partial^2 c}{\partial x \partial y}}{\dfrac{\partial c}{\partial y}} \right|_{y=0}
\tag{62}
$$

Noticeable is the complete absence of the electric field from Eq. (62). This is not very surprising in itself, considering the fact that the membrane is maintained at high constant potential $-\ln N - V$, so that, to the leading order, the lateral electric potential variations are not expected to represent a major driving force for the flow. On the other hand, as shown below (Sec. III.C and III.D) this greatly simplifies the computations of the resulting bulk flow, compared to other mechanisms of electroconvection considered in this chapter.

III. ELECTROCONVECTIVE ONSET MECHANISMS

In this section we review the two possible scenarios for the onset of electroconvection of any of the aforementioned types.

A. Electroconvection Due to Conductive Inhomogeneity of Membrane Surface

The first thresholdless onset, occurring simultaneously with switching on any voltage, however small, is related to the conductive inhomogeneity of the membrane surface. Such an inhomogeneity results in the lateral concentration and electric potential gradients, and, simultaneously, in the nonconservative character of the bulk electric force (that is, in the product $\Delta\phi\nabla\phi$ not being a gradient of any scalar). The first two result in electroosmotically induced bulk flow, the third in bulk electroconvection. Conductive inhomogeneity, on the microns scale, of allegedly homogeneous ion-exchange membranes has been invoked to explain their variable polarizability under the passage of a direct electric current, and, in particular, the lower-than-theoretical values of the limiting current [13,24,35,36]. To be sure, such an inhomogeneity has never been observed directly, although some recent studies on modification of membrane surface [37] may also point to its existence. On the other hand, for the so-called heterogeneous membranes, composed of ion-exchange granules of μm-size imbedded in a nonconducting polymer matrix, electric inhomogeneity is self evident and is bound to result in electroconvection of either bulk type or electroosmotically driven. The onset of bulk electroconvection due to membrane inhomogeneity was studied by an integral method applied to the leading order calculations in terms of the expansion in powers of the Péclet number [12,13]. In these studies, the not unexpected conclusion was reached that, for a two-dimensional setup (periodic array of permselective spots imbedded in a nonconductive matrix) a pair of vortices arises at each conductive spot at the membrane surface. The size of vortices was of the order of half the center to center distance between the spots. Thus, for the spot size, spot center to center distance and thickness of the diffusion layer ratio of the order of 1:10:100 (assumed as to account for the observed discrepancies between the measured and theoretical limiting current and the typical frequencies of excess electric noise) the question arose: how could such small vortices mix up such a big diffusion layer as would be necessary to account for the overlimiting phenomena. Of course, no answer to this question could be provided by the onset analysis of the aforementioned type. One hypothetical answer concerned the alleged growth of vortices with voltage due to their pairing [38]. This hypothesis has been recently confirmed by the calculations of nonlinear convection driven by electroosmosis of the second kind [30.ii] outlined in the next section.

B.   Electroconvective Instabilities in Concentration Polarization

Linear hydrodynamic stability of the concentration polarization solution Eqs. (53)–(55b) for a homogeneous permselective interface has been studied in a number of papers for all aforementioned mechanisms [25–29,30.i,39,40].

1.   Bulk Electroconvective Instability

Study of this type of instability has been initiated by Grigin [25]. In his paper Grigin used the lowest order Galerkin approximation to study the critical perturbation mode for unrealistic boundary conditions [25,26]. The main importance of this pioneering work lied in the very claim of possibility of bulk electroconvective instability. Grigin's papers were followed by an independent study by Bruinsma and Alexander in which they investigated the bulk electroconvective instability in a very narrow polarization cell of finite thickness for galvanostatic conditions [27] which likely amounted, in terms of concentration polarization in a flat layer, to consideration of some very particular perturbation mode. A systematic numerical study of linear bulk electroconvective instability in an electrolyte layer flanked by cation-selective surfaces has been carried out in Refs. 28 and 29 for galvano- and potentiostatic conditions, respectively. In Fig. 3 we reproduce a typical marginal stability curve in the perturbation mode wave number–current plane for galvanostatic operation (the region above the curve corresponds to instability).

So far we have been unable to come up with a reliable and efficient numerical solution for nonlinear bulk electroconvection. In this sense, we do not know whether the aforementioned bulk electroconvective instability may actually develop into an efficient mixing mechanism on a macroscopic (diffusion layer) scale. Based on heuristic energy balance arguments, Bruinsma and Alexander claim in Ref. 27 that it cannot. Some physical insight into the physical mechanism of bulk electroconvective instability on its linear and nonlinear aspects may be gained from the one-dimensional loop models [28,29].

2. Electroosmotic Instability of the First Kind

Stability of the quiescent CP solution Eqs. (53)–(55b) with respect to electroosmosis of the first kind (with a constant electroosmotic factor) has been studied numerically in [39]; and, independently, by an elegant analytic analysis of marginal stability for the limiting electroosmotic factor (51) in [40]. Both studies conform in the conclusion that electroosmotic instability of the first kind could in principle occur, but not for any realistic low molecular aqueous ionic system. This conclusion followed from the fact that, according to both studies, an electroosmotic factor at least one order of magnitude greater than the maximal limiting value 2ln2 of Eq. (51), is required for this

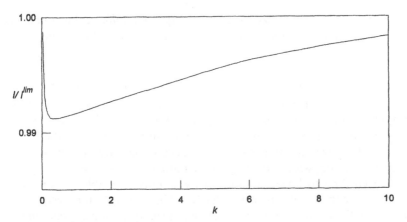

FIG. 3 Marginal stability curve for bulk electroconvection in galvanostatic conditions (k = dimensionless wavevector).

type of instability to occur, unless the coion diffusivity is lower than 1×10^{-6} cm^2/s (e.g., polycoion in an aqueous medium). Once more, some physical insight into the physical mechanism behind this, not very realistic, instability may be gained from the respective loop model [30.i].

3. Electroosmotic Instability of the Second Kind

Stability of the quiescent concentration polarization solution Eqs. (53)–(55b) with respect to electroosmosis of the second kind [with a correct slip condition Eq. (62)] has been studied in [30.i]. Somewhat paradoxically, the respective mathematical problem is the simplest among those considered in this chapter and allows for an analytical treatment. This results from the fact that for the high voltage conditions, appropriate for electroosmosis of the second kind, the boundary value problem for ionic concentration and fluid velocity is decoupled from that for electric potential. The relevant time dependent nonlinear problem for concentration and velocity reads (the diffusion layer occupies this time the interval $0 < y < 1$ with $y = 1$, corresponding to the solution–membrane interface).

$$c_t + (\mathbf{v} \, grad)_c = \Delta c, \quad \mathbf{v} = u\underline{i} + w\underline{j}, \quad -\infty < x < \infty, \quad 0 < y < 1 \qquad (63a,b)$$

$$-grad \, p + \Delta \mathbf{v} = 0 \qquad (64)$$

$$div \, \mathbf{v} = 0 \qquad (65)$$

$$c(x, 0) = 1, \quad c(x, 1) = 0 \qquad (66a,b)$$

$$u_y |_{y=0} = w |_{y=0} = w |_{y=1} = 0 \qquad (67)$$

$$u |_{y=1} = -\frac{V^2}{8} \frac{c_{xy}}{c_y} \bigg|_{y=1} \qquad (68)$$

Analytical solution of the linearized version of Eqs. (63)–(68), in the course of the linear stability analysis of the relevant limiting quiescent CP solution

$$c_0(y) = 1 - y, \quad \mathbf{v} = 0 \qquad (69a,b)$$

yields the marginal stability curve presented in Fig. 4. Here once more the unstable region lies above the curve and $a \overset{def}{=} V^2/8$. As opposed to the bulk electroconvective marginal stability curve (Figs. 3), this time there is no finite critical wave number (corresponding to the minimum in the threshold current dependence on the wave number). Rather, in this case, the threshold value of a decreases monotonically with k, tending to the finite limit $a \to \underline{a} = 4$ $(V \to \underline{V} = \sqrt{32})$. Thus, according to linear stability analysis, most unstable are the perturbation modes with infinitesimal wavelength. This suggests the need for a search for a nonlinear wave number selection principle. Some preliminary information in this respect is provided by the nonlinear convection computations described in the following section.

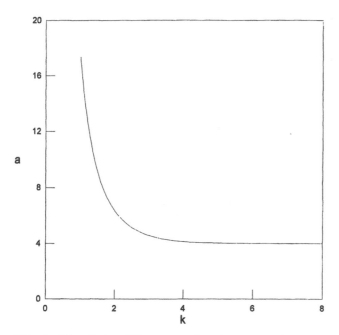

FIG. 4 Marginal stability curve for electroosmotic instability of the second kind, $a = V^2/8$, $k =$ dimensionless wavevector.

IV. NONLINEAR CONVECTION DRIVEN BY ELECTROOSMOSIS OF THE SECOND KIND

In this section we present some results of a numerical solution of the full nonlinear system Eqs. (63)–(68). As mentioned previously, this is the only type of nonlinear electroconvection we have been able to investigate numerically so far. We report here the results concerning convection due to both short scale macroscopic conductive inhomogeneity of the membrane surface and electroosmotic instability. We begin with the latter as a direct continuation of discussion of previous Sec. III.B.3.

A. Nonlinear Stage of Electroosmotic Instability of the Second Kind

The time dependent system Eqs. (63)–(68) was solved by finite differences until stabilization at steady state in the domain $\{0 < x < H, \ 0 < y < 0.5\}$ (membrane–solution interface, this time, at $y = 0$, the outer edge of the diffusion layer at $y = 0.5$), for various H and V. Boundary conditions at $x = 0$, H were those of symmetry.

In Figs. 5a,b and 6a,b we present the calculated families of flow streamlines and concentration level lines for $V = \underline{V} + 2$ and $H = 0.5$, 10, respectively. The

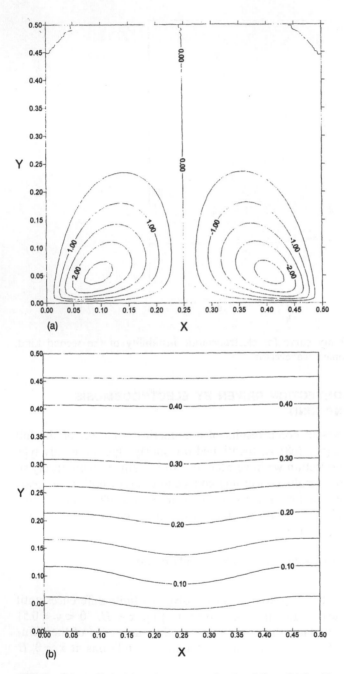

FIG. 5   Streamlines (a) and concentration level lines (b) for $H = 0.5$, $V = 7.657$ ($\underline{V} + 2$).

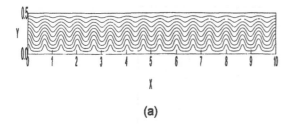

(a)

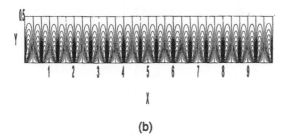

(b)

FIG. 6 Streamlines (a) and concentration level lines (b) for $H = 10$, $V = 7.657$.

qualitative image emerging from the calculations for different H may be summarized as followed. Vortices form in pairs; their size depends on H; a maximal size of H exists for a given number of vortex pairs per box; upon the increase of H above this size, an additional vortex pair appears; the maximal vortex size, corresponding to the maximal box size, roughly matches the size of vortices which emerge for an infinite layer ($H \to \infty$); this size, that is the half width of the periodicity cell formed in an infinite layer, is of order of the width of the diffusion layer; this may suggest the criteria for nonlinear mode selection, we mentioned previously. Finally, in Fig. 7 we present the calculated average current density vs. voltage curve for the "infinite" layer ($0 < x < 10$, $0 < y < 0.5$). Let us note the nearly linear shape of the overlimiting part of this I/V (VC) curve.

B. Nonlinear Convection Due to Conductive Inhomogeneity of Membrane Surface

This is the only system for which we have so far a definitive information concerning the effect of nonlinear interaction of small-scale electroconvective eddies (vortex pairing) and its possible role upon the mixing of the diffusion layer. The two model problems treated in relation to this concerned the equations (63)–(65) in the region $\{-5 < x < 5, \; 0 < y < 4\}$ (membrane–solution interface at $y = 0$), both with boundary conditions (66a)–(67) at the outer edge

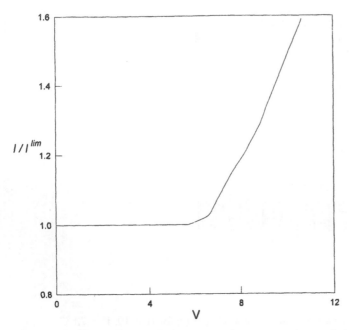

FIG. 7 Overlimiting average current–voltage curve for an infinite solution layer of thickness 0.5 at a homogeneous membrane.

of the diffusion layer at $y = 4$, and symmetry conditions at the lateral edges $x = \pm 5$ [30.ii]. The difference between the two models lay in the distribution of the conductive spots at the membrane surface. In the first, "periodic", model the conductive spots of width 0.2 were placed in the centers of 10 "periodicity" cells of unit width. At the conductive part of each periodicity cell the slip condition Eq. (68) was applied, to the nonslip condition at the insulating part. The second "nonperiodic" model, aimed at investigating the effect of long scale modulations in the distribution of short scale inhomogeneities, differed from the periodic one by skipping the conductive spot in the central periodicity cell. Some results of computations are presented in Figs. 8–12.

Thus in Figs. 8 and 9 we present the families of flow streamlines and concentration level lines, for a sequence of voltages. A rapid growth of vortices through their pairing is observed for voltages above $V = 4$. The respective voltage–current curve is presented in Fig. 10 (continuous line), with, again, a nearly linear overlimiting current increase with voltage for $V > 5$. In Figs. 11 and 12 we present the respective curves for the periodic case. Also in this case, vortex pairing is observed above $V = 5$, resulting in mixing of the diffusion layer and a nearly linear increase of current with voltage. This time, vortex pairing is likely to occur through instability of small "seed" vortices. This is

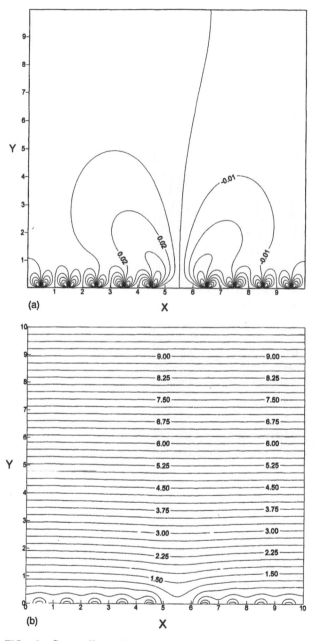

(a)

(b)

FIG. 8 Streamlines (a) and concentration level lines (b) for a "heterogeneous nonperiodic" membrane for $V = 2$.

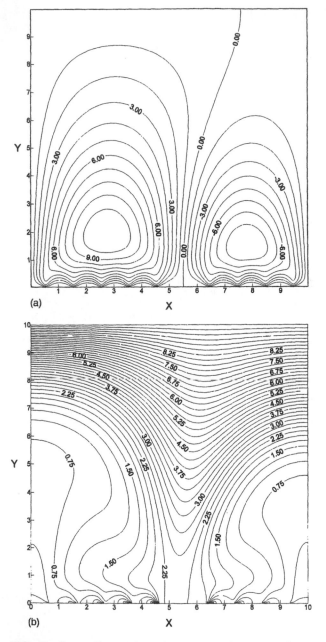

FIG. 9 Streamlines (a) and concentration level lines (b) for a "heterogeneous nonperiodic" membrane for $V = 10$.

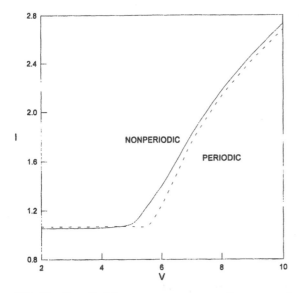

FIG. 10 Overlimiting average current–voltage curve for heterogeneous "periodic" and "nonperiodic" membrane. ——— "nonperiodic", – – – – "periodic".

reflected in a sharper transition in the VC curve from the "plateau" to the "overlimiting" current growth regime than in nonperiodic case. On the practical side, this seems to suggest that introduction of long scale disturbances into the distribution of microscopic inhomogeneities on the membrane surface may facilitate the onset of overlimiting conductance through a cation-exchange membrane. For higher voltages, the slopes of both curves asymptotically level off and, upon the decrease of the scale of inhomogeneity, approach the slope of a homogeneous membrane (see Fig. 7). In this respect, vortex pairing may be merely viewed as a particular scenario for realization of instability of the quiescent concentration polarization at a cation-exchange membrane, irrespectively of homogeneity of inhomogeneity of the latter, with the excess electric noise related to the slow process of readjustment of vortices.

V. CONCLUSIONS

Convection due to electroosmotic slip of the second kind, adequately described by the boundary condition Eq. (62), provides a unique, so far, model system for which definitive results have been obtained, concerning the possible role of nonlinear electroconvection in concentration polarization at a cation-exchange electrodialysis membrane. These results suggest that this type of electroconvection provides a mechanism capable of explaining self-consistently the

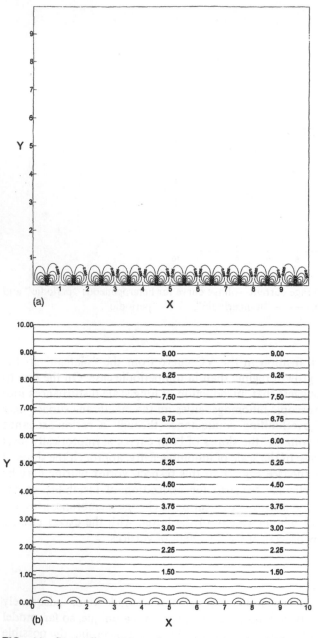

(a)

(b)

FIG. 11 Streamlines (a) and concentration level lines (b) for a "heterogeneous periodic" membrane for $V = 2$.

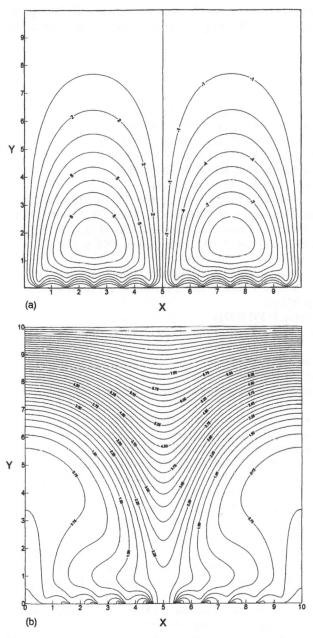

FIG. 12 Streamlines (a) and concentration level lines (b) for a "heterogeneous periodic" membrane for $V = 10$.

overlimiting phenomena at a cation-exchange membrane, including the growth of the current above the limiting value and the appearance of the excess electric noise.

REFERENCES

1. S. Nasumo, Europhys. Lett. 14:779 (1991).
2. L. Rehberg, F. Horner, and G. Hartung, J. Stat. Phys. 64:1017 (1991).
3. I. Rehberg and B. L. Winkler, Phys. Rev. A 43:1940 (1991).
4. J. M. Schneider and P. K. Watson, Phys. Fluids 19:1948 (1970).
5. A. Castellanos and M. G. Velarde, Phys. Fluids 24:1784 (1981).
6. A. T. Perez and A. Castellanos, Phys. Rev. A 40:5844 (1989).
7. S. S. Dukhin, Adv. Colloid Interface Sci 35:173 (1991).
8. S. S. Dukhin and N. A. Mishchuk, Kolloidn. Zh. 51:659 (1989) (in Russian).
9. S. S. Dukhin, N. A. Mishchuk, and P. B. Takhistov, Kolloidn. Zh. 51:616 (1989).
10. I. Rubinstein and L. Shtilman, J. Chem. Soc., Faraday Trans. II 75:231 (1979).
11. I. Rubinstein, *Electrodiffusion of Ions*, SIAM, Philadelphia, 1990, p. 170.
12. I. Rubinstein, Physics of Fluids A 3:2301 (1991).
13. I. Rubinstein and F. Maletzki, J. Chem. Soc., Faraday Trans. II 87:2079 (1991).
14. V. G. Levich, *Physicochemical Hydrodynamics*, Prentice-Hall, Englewood Cliffs, New Jersey, p. 242(i), p. 473 (ii).
15. K. S. Spiegler, Desalination 9:367 (1971).
16. M. Block and J. A. Kitchener, J. Electrochem. Soc. 113:947 (1966).
17. V. J. Frillete, J. Phys. Chem. 61:168 (1957).
18. R. Simons, Desalination 29:41 (1979).
19. R. Simons, Nature 280:824 (1979).
20. I. Rubinstein, A. Warshawsky, L. Schechtman, and O. Kedem, Desalination 51:55 (1984).
21. S. Reich, B. Gavish, and S. Lifson, Desalination 24:295 (1978).
22. S. Lifson, B. Gavish, and S. Reich, in *Physicochemical Hydrodynamics II*, (D. B. Spalding, ed.), Advance Publications Ltd., London, 1977, p. 141.
23. Q. Li, Y. Fang, and M. Green, J. Colloid Interface Sci. 91:412 (1983).
24. F. Maletzki, H. W. Rossler, and E. Staude, J. Membrane Sci. 71:105 (1992).
25. A. P. Grigin, Electrokhimia 21:52 (1985) (in Russian).
26. A. P. Grigin, Electrokhimia 28:307 (1992) (in Russian).
27. R. Bruinsma and S. Alexander, J. Chem. Phys. 92:3074 (1990).
28. I. Rubinstein, T. Zaltzman, and B. Zaltzman, Physics of Fluids 7:1467 (1995).
29. T. Zaltzman, Physics of Fluids 8:936 (1996).
30. I. Rubinstein and B. Zaltzman, Electroosmotically induced flows at a cation-exchange membrane. i. Electroosmotic slip of the second kind and hydrodynamic instability in concentration polarization at electrodialysis membranes. ii. Nonlinear convection due to electroosmosis of the second kind at a homogeneous and heterogeneous electrodialysis membrane (unpublished).
31. S. S. Dukhin and B. V. Derjaguin, *Electrophoresis*, Nauka, Moscow (1976), p. 132 (in Russian).
32. V. V. Nikonenko, V. I. Zabolotsky, and N. P. Gnusin, Elektrokhimia 25:301 (1989) (in Russian).

33. J. A. Manzanares, W. D. Murphy, S. Mafé, and H. Reiss, J. Phys. Chem. 97: 8524 (1993).
34. A. V. Listovnichy, Electrokhimia 51: 1651 (1989).
35. V. K. Indusekhar and P. Meares, in *Physicochemical Hydrodynamics II*, (D. B. Spalding, ed.), Advance Publications Ltd., London, 1977, p. 1031.
36. I. Rubinstein, E. Staude, and O. Kedem, Desalination 69: 101 (1988).
37. Ch. Müller, Entwicklung von Elektrokonvectoren an Kationenaustauschermembranen zur kationenselektiven Separation, Ph.D. Thesis, University of Essen, Germany, 1996 (in German).
38. I. Rubinstein, B. Zaltzman, and O. Kedem, J. Membrane Sci. 125: 17 (1997).
39. T. Zaltzman, Electrodiffusion and viscous flow dynamics, Ph.D. Thesis, Ben Gurion University of the Negev, Israel, 1996.
40. E. K. Zholkovskij, M. A. Vorotynsev, and E. Staude, J. Colloid Interface Sci. 181: 28 (1996).

18

Interfacial Electrodynamics of Membranes and Polymer Films

TORBEN SMITH SØRENSEN* Physical Chemistry, Modelling &
Thermodynamics/DTH, Nørager Plads 3, DK 2720 Vanløse (Copenhagen),
Denmark

* Also affiliated with The Danish National Museum, Department of Conservation, Brede, Denmark,
as a senior scientist.

Abstract

The basic principles behind the interfacial electrodynamics of membranes and polymer films in the Nernst–Planck–Maxwell approximation
are stated. Formulae for the complex permittivity and the impedance of
heterogeneous biphase systems are derived and discussed in relation to
measurements on membranes and on polymer films. The classical
Maxwell–Wagner–Sillars (MWS) approach is only valid as a limiting
case of high frequencies (or high concentrations at not too low
frequencies) where the local current density is everywhere proportional
to the local electric field and where the layers of polarization are
restricted to infinitely thin boundary layers. This leads to the "principle
of generalized conductivity" and formulae in which complex conductivities may be replaced by complex permittivities and vice versa. In other
cases, it is necessary to account for a nonequilibrium electric double
layer of the order of the Debye length, the electrodynamics of which
layer can be understood (to a good approximation) by a combination of
the Maxwell equations in the quasi-static limit (the equation of Poisson)
with the electrodiffusion equations of Nernst, Planck and Smoluchowski.
This dynamic electric double layer leads to an additional impedance, the
excess impedance, over and above the MWS impedance. The problem of
how to separate, in dielectric measurements of ion conducting amorphous polymer films, the contribution at low frequencies of the electric
interfacial polarization from other low frequency dielectric contributions
stemming from glass transition relaxations or even more slow "reptation
modes" is discussed in relation to specific examples of dielectric studies
of various polymers. Performing such a separation, the temperature
dependence of the ionic diffusion coefficients in the polymers may also be
found, throwing light on the "free volume" structure of the amorphous
polymers under study.

I. INTRODUCTION

The study of the two closely connected areas of dielectric spectroscopy (DS)
and impedance spectroscopy (IS) of heterogeneous media have presented challenges to the researchers ever since J. C. Maxwell initiated the field in his
"Treatise of Electricity and Magnetism" [1]. Those studies were followed up
by studies of Wagner [2,3] and Sillars [4]. In the following I shall name the
approach of these three authors as the MWS approach, for short. IS was used

early to study biotissue. Höber [5–7] studied suspended red blood cells and made the first estimate of the capacity of their cell membranes. The Belgian radio engineer Philippson studied packed blood cells, muscle and liver cells and resting vs. germinating potatoes [8]. The foundations of the use of IS as an important tool in biophysics were laid by Fricke and Morse [9] who already in 1925 estimated the thickness and the internal, relative permittivity of the cell membrane to 3.3 nm and 3, respectively, measuring impedance of blood in the extended frequency range 800 Hz–4.5 MHz. These early, as well as later, advances in the application to biophysics until 1968 have been summarized neatly by Cole [10]. A later valuable source of information on IS and its applications, especially to solid materials and systems, is the monograph edited by Macdonald [11]. Buck and his school have used IS to characterize membranes [12,13]. The Australian school of Coster, Chilcott and others have recently reviewed the application of IS to characterize cells of *Chara corallina* [14], bipolar (water-splitting) membranes [15] and interfaces, membranes and ultrastructures [16].

The theory of dielectrics has been reviewed by, e.g., Fröhlich [17] and Böttcher [18]. Application of DS (and of anelastic mechanical spectroscopy) to polymeric solids has been extensively discussed in the monograph by McCrum, Read and Williams [19]. DS of heterogeneous media (emulsions have been treated by Hanai [20] and by Clausse [21]. The Ukrainian school of Dukhin and coworkers have also made extensive studies of DS in disperse systems [22,23], and recently Zholkovskij (also from this school) has proposed elegant solutions for the impedance of multilayer systems in the limit of thick layers compared to the Debye length [24–26].

In the latest years, I have myself been involved with the formulation of models for situations where the size of the microheterogeneities is *not* much larger than the Debye length [27–29], and with the application of such models to actual measurements. With Danish colleagues [30–33], desalination membranes of the phase inversion type (especially cellulose acetate membranes) have been investigated by IS using also data obtained earlier for such membranes by means of emf studies, see Chapter 10 and the references herein. With Spanish colleagues from Valencia, Madrid and Castellón [34–37], DS of thick films of amorphous polymers containing conducting, ionic impurities has been analyzed in terms of more or less overlapping relaxations due to dielectric relaxations of the polymer chains, ionic conductivity and interfacial, nonelectroneutral polarization. The present chapter deals with these two abovementioned topics. It is my hope that this chapter together with the chapters of Coster and Chilcott [38] and that of Zholkovskij [39] may complement each other, so that a platform is made for the readers to grasp the essentials in the recent evolution of concepts within IS/DS of heterogeneous media.

In Sec. II, the theoretical foundations for the rest of the chapter are laid. The simplifying approximations behind the MWS approach and behind the "principle of generalized conductivity" are made clear and illustrated by means of an example (Sec. II.A). To proceed further, one needs to solve more general electrodiffusion equations at least in the Nernst–Planck–Smoluchowski approximation. The linearized Nernst–Planck equations for any geometry are presented in Sec. II.B and general solutions are given in one-dimensional (1D) geometry. The concept of *excess impedance* is introduced in general terms to be specialized later in specific situations. The excess impedance is the impedance over and above the MWS impedance. Single (solid or liquid) films placed between blocking electrodes and with dissolved electrolytes of arbitrary charge type are considered in Sec. II.C, and in Sec. II.D the paper of Trukhan [40] is examined. This paper is important as probably the first work in which a simplified Nernst–Planck–Maxwell electrodynamics is explicitly proposed. The work of Trukhan is a major step forwards from the MWS theories and it will be discussed in some detail to clarify some strange features in the original derivation of this theory.

In Sec. II.E the very simplest (though not very realistic) example of excess impedance of a single (leaky) interface between two ion conducting media with different permittivities is discussed as an introduction to more complicated cases. Such a case is treated in Sec. II.F wherein the formalism is generalized to lamellar membranes consisting of two different phases in identical bilayers with leaky interfaces. The limits of validity of equivalent circuit (RC) approaches are tested against the more fundamental approach involving excess impedance.

In Sec. III, the application of the Trukhan theory for spherical geometry to the capacitance part of the impedance of desalination membranes of the phase inversion type is discussed. A "hybrid model" is used in the form of a parallel equivalent RC circuit where the resistance (R) is calculated as a function of the salt concentration in the membrane in Donnan equilibrium with the external electrolyte solution, and the capacitance (C) as a function of concentration is calculated for the assembly of water rich and ion filled "alveoles" in the membrane by means of the Trukhan theory for spherical geometry, suitably modified to take into account the effect of alveole "concentration". It is tested to which degree this approach is working for actual IS measurements on desalination membranes, especially cellulose acetate membranes.

In Sec. IV, the application of the concept of excess impedance to dielectric measurements on quite thick films consisting of different kinds of amorphous polymers containing traces of ionic impurities is studied. The reader is equipped in Sec. IV.A with some basic notions concerning "free volume" transport theories in such polymers, the nature of the "glass–rubber" relaxation and other relaxations and the significance of "micro-brownian motions" of the chain segments.

In Sec. IV.B some earlier dielectric data of Furukawa et al. [41] for copolymers of vinylidene cyanide and vinyl acetate, characteristic for their very high static permittivity are revisited. The equivalent circuit approach of these authors and their use of an "unphysical" network element, the constant phase element, is criticized. Especially, it is criticized that their model is in conflict with the second law of thermodynamics at very low frequencies, see the concluding Sec. V. This is not the case with the excess impedance model. In Sec. IV.C and D, dielectric measurements on two specific acrylic polymers with side chains of somewhat complicated nature are studied. The aim is everywhere to separate the various relaxations from each other, especially the low frequency contribution from some glass–rubber and from some very "slow modes" (perhaps the so-called "reptation" modes) from the low frequency contribution from interfacial, excess impedance. From the former relaxations, interesting information about the polymer "soft material" structure may be obtained. From the latter, information about the temperature dependence of the ionic diffusion coefficients is obtained—and from this once again information of the "free volume" structure of the polymer.

Finally, in the conclusion, Sec. V, I shall summarize what has been obtained, what is still wanting, and what is the relation between the present chapter and the complementary chapters of Coster and Chilcott (Chapter 19, [38]) and of Zholkovskij (Chapter 20, [39]).

II. THEORETICAL CONSIDERATIONS

A. The MWS Procedure and the "Principle of Generalized Conductivity"

The MWS procedure for the calculation of the impedance (complex conductivity) or the complex capacitance (complex permittivity) of heterogeneous media rests basically on the following three assumptions [21]:

1. The heterogeneous medium consists of *homogeneous* sybsystems (phases) which are *isotropic* and have *linear* constitutive relations, e.g., between the local electric displacement (**D**) and the local electric field (**E**) or between the local current density ($\mathbf{J_q}$) and the electric field. Shortly, the medium is an assembly of LHI media. In this case we can write (ε = permittivity; σ = specific conductivity):

$$\mathbf{D} = \varepsilon \mathbf{E} \tag{1}$$

$$\mathbf{J_q} = \sigma \mathbf{E} \tag{2}$$

2. The solutions to the Maxwell equations can be treated in the *quasi-stationary* approximation: The equations may be solved in each instant as a stationary problem, and the stationary fields thus found may be used as an approximation of their actual time dependent values. This amounts to neglecting the propagation of electromagnetic waves, which is permitted

when the wavelength is large compared to the dimensions of the sample under study.

3. The *bulk phases* of which the system consist is assumed not to contain any charge density. All excess charge is assumed to be displaced to an infinitely thin layer at the interfaces between the homogeneous subsystems.

If we assume all the fields to vary sinusoidally with an angular frequency ω and introduce all the fields as phasors in the form ($i \equiv \sqrt{-1}$)

$$X(r, t) = X^*(r) \cdot \exp(i\omega t) \tag{3}$$

we obtain from the Maxwell equations:

$$\nabla \times H = J_q + i\omega D \equiv J_{tot} \tag{4}$$
$$\nabla \times E = -i\omega B \tag{5}$$

H is the magnetic field and B the magnetic induction. J_{tot} is the *total current density* of Maxwell. B being a divergence free field, it can be regarded as the curl of a vector potential A:

$$B = \nabla \times A \tag{6}$$

From (5) and (6) we obtain:

$$\nabla \times (E + i\omega A) = 0 \tag{7}$$

In the quasi-stationary approximation (2), we have $\omega |A| \ll E$ and the electric field is irrotational:

$$\nabla \times E \approx 0 \tag{8}$$

Because of the LHI assumption (1), D and J_q in (4) can be expressed through (1) and (2) where the permittivity now in general has to be taken as complex and frequency dependent quantity $\varepsilon^*(\omega)$:

$$\nabla \times H = \{\sigma + i\omega\varepsilon^*(\omega)\}E \equiv \sigma^*_{eff}(\omega)E = J_{tot} \tag{9}$$

The middle relation is a definition of the complex and frequency dependent *effective conductivity*, $\sigma^*_{eff}(\omega)$. Defining the complex *effective permittivity* as

$$\varepsilon^*_{eff}(\omega) \equiv \varepsilon^*(\omega) - i\sigma/\omega \tag{10}$$

as opposed to the "true" (purely dielectric) complex permittivity $\varepsilon^*(\omega)$, we may write Eq. (9) in the alternative form:

$$J_{tot} = i\omega\varepsilon^*_{eff}(\omega)E \tag{11}$$

Comparing Eqs. (9)–(11) the following connection is seen to hold true:

$$\sigma^*_{eff}(\omega) = i\omega\varepsilon^*_{eff}(\omega) \tag{12}$$

At the surfaces between two different media, 1 and 2, the **D** field satisfies the following boundary condition in the direction normal to the interface:

$$(\mathbf{D}_2 - \mathbf{D}_1) \cdot \mathbf{n} = S_q \qquad (13)$$

where **n** is the unit normal to the interface in the direction $1 \to 2$ and S_q is the phasor corresponding to the local charge density on the interface, the existence of which is allowed according to assumption (3) above. From the interfacial conservation of charge one obtains:

$$(\mathbf{J}_{q, 1} - \mathbf{J}_{q, 2}) \cdot \mathbf{n} = i\omega S_q \qquad (14)$$

Eqs. (13) and (14) may be combined into the boundary condition:

$$(\mathbf{J}_{tot, 1} - \mathbf{J}_{tot, 2}) \cdot \mathbf{n} = 0 \qquad (15)$$

Equation (15) expresses that the total current of Maxwell is conserved during a transition from one phase to another phase. Using the definitions of the effective, complex permittivity and the effective, complex conductivity defined in Eqs. (10) and (12), the interfacial conservation equation may be written in two alternative ways:

$$(\sigma^*_{eff, 1}(\omega)\mathbf{E}_1 - \sigma^*_{eff, 2}(\omega)\mathbf{E}_2) \cdot \mathbf{n} = 0 \qquad (16)$$
$$(\varepsilon^*_{eff, 1}(\omega)\mathbf{E}_1 - \varepsilon^*_{eff, 2}(\omega)\mathbf{E}_2) \cdot \mathbf{n} = 0 \qquad (17)$$

The tangential b.c. for the electric field is

$$(\mathbf{E}_1 - \mathbf{E}_2) \cdot \mathbf{t} = 0 \qquad (18)$$

where **t** is any unit vector in the local tangential plane between the two interfaces. Equations (4)–(7) and (9)–(18) are *general* (for LHI systems) but if we further assume quasi-stationarity (2) and therefore adopt the approximation (8), the electric field is also *irrotational* and may be described by a negative gradient in a scalar electric potential (ψ). Furthermore, when there is *no space charge* according to assumption (3) we have from one of the Maxwell equations that the **E** field is also free of divergence:

$$\nabla \cdot \mathbf{D} = \nabla \cdot \mathbf{E} = 0 \qquad (19)$$

The set of equations to be solved is then the following:

$$\nabla \times \mathbf{E} = 0; \quad \nabla \cdot \mathbf{E} = 0; \quad (a_1\mathbf{E}_1 - a_2\mathbf{E}_2) \cdot \mathbf{n} = 0; \quad (\mathbf{E}_1 - \mathbf{E}_2) \cdot \mathbf{t} = 0 \qquad (20)$$

with

$$a_p = \sigma^*_{eff, p}(\omega) \quad \text{or} \quad \varepsilon^*_{eff, p}(\omega) \quad (p = 1, 2) \qquad (21)$$

As it happens, exactly the same set of Eqs. (20) has to be fulfilled in any *stationary* problem of *electric conduction* of current in heterogeneous media (with $a_p = \sigma_p$ and $\mathbf{E}$ being a stationary field distribution rather than a phasor). The set of equation (20) has also to be solved in any *electrostatic* problem in heterogeneous media (with $a_p = \varepsilon_{s,\,p}$ = the *static* permittivity in medium p).

Thus, the "principle of generalized conductivity" may be formulated in the following manner: Given that the above assumptions (1)–(3) hold, the solutions for a given geometry and constellation of subsystems are *formally identical* for any problem of stationary conduction, electrostatics or stationary, periodic variation of fields using the values of the "generalized conductivity coefficients" (a_p) described above.

To illustrate the machinery at work in a simple example, consider a one-dimensional situation with two layers ($p = 1$ and 2) in contact. The widths of the layers may be taken as L_1 and L_2 and the cross-sectional area is A. We need only to solve one problem, e.g., derive a formula for the total conductance of the bilayer with a stationary current:

$$\sigma_{bi} A/(L_1 + L_2) = [\{L_1/[A\sigma_1]\} + \{L_2/[A\sigma_2]\}]^{-1} \tag{22}$$

Introducing the volume fractions of the two phases (Φ_1 and Φ_2) we may write instead:

$$\sigma_{bi} = [\{\Phi_1/\sigma_1\} + \{\Phi_2/\sigma_2\}]^{-1} \tag{23}$$

In the case of two dielectric *isolators* we might solve the corresponding electrostatic problem to find the total capacitance of the bilayer (expressed as the static permittivity for the system as a whole $\varepsilon_{s,\,bi}$). However, the expression wanted is immediately written from Eq. (23) substituting σ_{bi} by $\varepsilon_{s,\,bi}$:

$$\varepsilon_{s,\,bi} = [\{\Phi_1/\varepsilon_{s,\,1}\} + \{\Phi_2/\varepsilon_{s,\,2}\}]^{-1} \tag{24}$$

In the case of *periodic variations* of the fields and with each layer having conductance as well as capacitance, we have immediately from the assumptions (1)–(3):

$$\varepsilon^*_{eff,\,bi}(\omega) = [\{\Phi_1/\varepsilon^*_{eff,\,1}(\omega)\} + \{\Phi_2/\varepsilon^*_{eff,\,2}(\omega)\}]^{-1} \tag{25}$$

In the latter case there may be dispersion with frequency because of internal, dielectric losses in the two layers. Expressions such as (23)–(25) are typical MWS expressions. In Eq. (25) all the $\varepsilon^*_{eff}(\omega)$ may be replaced by $\sigma^*_{eff}(\omega)$, and the formula still holds true.

Before we finish the present section we might point out the following *general* observation (independent of the assumptions (1)–(3) above): The total current of Maxwell most generally defined by

$$\mathbf{J}_{tot} \equiv \mathbf{J}_q + \partial\mathbf{D}/\partial t \tag{26}$$

is not only conserved in the passage from one medium to another. It is *always* conserved, also in *nonelectroneutral* media. This follows easily from the

Maxwell equation

$$\nabla \cdot \mathbf{D} = \rho_q \tag{27}$$

applying the operator $\partial()/\partial t$ on both sides and subtracting it from the charge conservation equation:

$$\partial\rho_q/\partial t = -\nabla \cdot \mathbf{J}_q \tag{28}$$

The symbol ρ_q is used for the local space charge density. It follows that

$$\nabla \cdot \mathbf{J}_{tot} = 0 \tag{29}$$

which means that the total current has neither accumulation nor sources in the various bulk phases. It also passes unaltered to other phases and indeed it pops up in the external (metal) wiring of any experiment practically as 100% galvanic current. That is, the total current is the *measurable* one in any experiment, a fact that we shall use later on. Also, it is seen from Eqs. (9) and (11) that the effective, complex conductivity and permittivity are the ones really *measurable* in a measuring cell, in contrast to the "intrinsic" quantities σ and $\varepsilon^*(\omega)$ which refer to purely galvanic conductivity and purely dieletric permittivity (with dielectric loss), respectively.

B. The Linearized Electrodiffusion Equations and Their Solutions in One Dimension

In the present chapter, we want to go beyond the MWS theory and the "principle of generalized conductivity". We maintain the assumption (2) from the beginning of the last subsection (the quasistationarity assumption). However, in assumption (1) it is no longer correct that the local current density is everywhere proportional to the local electric field. It has to be recognized that concentration differences in the charge carriers can also produce electric fields without currents ("diffusion potential differences", see Chapter 10, [42]) and that such differences may produce currents without electric fields. Furthermore, electric fields exist near the phase boundaries—even at equilibrium—caused by electric double layers built up either of fixed charges and their counterions or of oriented layers of dipoles near the phase boundaries.

As mentioned in the introduction, the theory of Trukhan [40] was a great step forward from the MWS approach. He used the simplest extension possible—that of Nernst, Planck and Smoluchowski. According to the concepts of these authors, the local (molar) flux of ionic species no. k is given as

$$\mathbf{J}_k = -D_k\{\nabla c_k - (z_k F/RT)c_k \mathbf{E}\} \tag{30}$$

where D_k is the diffusion coefficient, c_k is the local concentration, z_k the charge of the kth ion measured in units of the elementary charge, F is the Faraday constant and R the gas constant. The local galvanic current density is then given by:

$$\mathbf{J}_q = -F \sum_k D_k z_k \nabla c_k + (F^2/RT)\left\{\sum_k z_k^2 c_k D_k\right\}\mathbf{E} \tag{31}$$

From Eq. (31) it is seen that the specific conductivity in the Nernst–Planck (NP) approximation is given by:

$$\sigma = (F^2/RT)\left\{\sum_k z_k^2 c_k D_k\right\} \tag{32}$$

The conservation of ionic species no. k ($\partial c_k/\partial t = -\nabla \cdot \mathbf{J}_k$) and the assumption of space (and concentration) independent diffusion coefficients lead to the partial differential equations:

$$\begin{aligned}(1/D_k)\partial c_k/\partial t &= \nabla^2 c_k - (z_k F/RT)\nabla \cdot (c_k \mathbf{E}) \\ &= \nabla^2 c_k - (z_k F/RT)c_k \nabla \cdot \mathbf{E} - (z_k F/RT)\mathbf{E} \cdot \nabla c_k \end{aligned} \tag{33}$$

Small perturbations of all quantities from their equilibrium values are introduced in terms of complex phasors. Thus, Eq. (3) should be generalized to the form:

$$\mathbf{X}(\mathbf{r}, t) = \mathbf{X}_{eq}(\mathbf{r}) + \mathbf{X}^*(\mathbf{r}) \cdot \exp(i\omega t) \tag{34}$$

The factorization of the perturbations into a sinusoidal time variation and a spatially dependent, complex "amplitude" (quantities with an asterisk) will be correct for the *linearized* partial differential equations since they are first order with respect to time. The equilibrium quantities (eq) are valid for the unperturbed situations. For the ionic fluxes ($\mathbf{J}_k$), the galvanic current density ($\mathbf{J}_q$) and the total (Maxwell) current density ($\mathbf{J}_{tot}$) there is no equilibrium value $\mathbf{X}_{eq}(\mathbf{r})$, of course. Furthermore, in 1D geometry $\mathbf{J}_{tot}^*$ is independent of the single space variable (x) and also independent of which chemical phase is considered.

In contrast, the electric field ($\mathbf{E}$), the electric potential (ψ), the space charge $\rho_q(\mathbf{r})$ and the molar concentrations (c_k) may have space dependent equilibrium values. Far from any interfaces we have $\mathbf{E}_{eq}(\mathbf{r}) \approx 0$, $\rho_{q, eq}(\mathbf{r}) \approx 0$, whereas $\psi_{eq}(\mathbf{r})$ and $c_{k, eq}(\mathbf{r})$ are constant, but near to the interfaces there may be equilibrium electric double layers even in the unperturbed situation. In the linearisation we regard $\mathbf{E}(\mathbf{r}, t)$ and $\rho(\mathbf{r}, t)$ to be a small quantities and not only $\mathbf{E}^*(\mathbf{r})$ and $\rho_q^*(\mathbf{r})$, i.e., the fields from the permanent electric double layers and dipole layers should be small. In practice, this means linearizable (Gouy-Chapman) double layers, see the discussion in Ref. 27, Sec. 2.

Thus, dropping the term proportional with $\mathbf{E} \cdot \nabla c_k$ in (33) as a "second-order quantity" one obtains:

$$(1/D_k)\partial c_k/\partial t \approx \nabla^2 c_k - (z_k F/RT)c_k \nabla \cdot \mathbf{E} \tag{35}$$

From the Maxwell equation (27) one has:

$$\nabla \cdot \mathbf{D} = \nabla \cdot \mathbf{D}_{\text{eq}} + (\nabla \cdot \mathbf{D}^*)\exp(i\omega t)$$
$$= \rho_{\text{q, eq}} + \rho_{\text{q}}^* \exp(i\omega t) \approx \varepsilon_s \nabla \cdot \mathbf{E}_{\text{eq}} + \varepsilon^*(\omega)(\nabla \cdot \mathbf{E}^*)\exp(i\omega t) \qquad (36)$$

The last approximation is valid if the space dependence, or concentration dependence, of ε_s and $\varepsilon^*(\omega)$ may be neglected. With this further approximation we have the following two Poisson equations:

$$\nabla \cdot \mathbf{E}_{\text{eq}} = \rho_{\text{q, eq}}/\varepsilon_s; \quad \nabla \cdot \mathbf{E}^* = \rho_{\text{q}}^*/\varepsilon^*(\omega) \qquad (37)$$

In the first equation, the static permittivity should be used, in the second the complex permittivity. Inserting Eq. (37) into (35), using that the equilibrium distributions also satisfy Eq. (35) with the l.h.s. $= 0$ and neglecting second-order terms (also the $c_k^* \rho_{\text{q, eq}}/\varepsilon_s$ term), the small signal equations may be written

$$(i\omega/D_k)c_k^* \approx \nabla^2 c_k^* - (z_k F/RT)c_{k, \text{eq}}(\rho_{\text{q}}^*/\varepsilon^*(\omega)) \qquad (38)$$

Inserting $\rho_{\text{q}}^* = F \sum_k z_n c_n^*$ into Eq. (38) and rearranging, one has finally the following system of homogeneous, second-order differential equations:

$$\nabla^2 c_k^* = \kappa^2 \sum_n K_{\text{kn}} c_n^* \qquad (39)$$

$$K_{\text{kn}} = (i\omega/D_k \kappa^2)\delta_{\text{kn}} + (z_n/z_k)\alpha_k[\varepsilon_s/\varepsilon^*(\omega)] \qquad (40)$$

In (40), δ_{kn} is the Kronecker symbol, κ is the *inverse Debye length* and α_k the *ionic strength fraction* of the kth ion:

$$\kappa^2 \equiv (F^2/RT\varepsilon) \sum_k z_k^2 c_{k, \text{eq}} \qquad (41)$$

$$\alpha_k \equiv (z_k^2 c_{k, \text{eq}}) \Big/ \sum_p z_p^2 c_{p, \text{eq}} \qquad (42)$$

The solution of Eq. (39) for any geometry is greatly simplified, if the equations are *diagonalized*. The equations then decouple into "electrodiffusion normal modes" and the general solutions for the complex concentration amplitudes are simply the *eigenfunctions* of the Laplacian in the geometry given. Being a trivial eigenvalue problem we shall not go into the details, but just state the form of the general solution in 1D geometry for a binary electrolyte of arbitrary charge type. There are two eigenvalues to Eq. (39) in that case which are called λ_1^2 and λ_2^2, respectively, where the λs have the same dimension as κ (length^{-1}). The dimensionless eigenvalues are given by:

$$\beta_1^2 \equiv \lambda_1^2/\kappa^2 = (1/2)\{1 + i(d_1^2 + d_2^2) + \sqrt{\Delta}\} \qquad (43)$$

$$\beta_2^2 \equiv \lambda_2^2/\kappa^2 = (1/2)\{1 + i(d_1^2 + d_2^2) - \sqrt{\Delta}\} \qquad (44)$$

$$d_k \equiv \sqrt{[\omega/(D_k \kappa^2)]} \quad (k = 1, 2) \qquad (45)$$

$$\Delta \equiv 1 - [d_1^2 - d_2^2]^2 + 2i\{d_1^2(1 - 2\alpha_2[\varepsilon_s/\varepsilon^*]) - d_2^2(1 - 2\alpha_1[\varepsilon_s/\varepsilon^*])\} \qquad (46)$$

For a $1:1$ (or $z:z$) electrolyte, the ion strength fractions are $1/2$ and the imaginary term in Eq. (46) for the discriminant vanishes if we may put $\varepsilon^* = \varepsilon_s$ (no "intrinsic" dielectric dispersion in the frequency range considered). If we further have $D_1 = D_2 = D$, the two last terms in Eq. (46) vanish and $\Delta = 1$. In that special case we have:

$$\lambda_1 = \sqrt{(\kappa^2 + i\omega/D)} \equiv \gamma; \quad \lambda_2 = \sqrt{(i\omega/D)} \equiv \delta \tag{47}$$

The "γ-polarization" is related to the dynamic, electric double layers at the interfaces. The length $1/\gamma$ is a generalized Debye length, and it has the Debye length as an upper limit at small frequencies. The length $1/\delta$ is a Nernst polarization layer thickness, and it is unlimited, when the frequency tends to zero. It should be stressed, however, that this clean cut separation is only true in the case $D_1 = D_2$. (The γ/δ separation can be proved in any mixture of electrolytes with a common D, see Sec. II.E).

The 1D eigenfunctions of the Laplacian are $\sinh(x)$ and $\cosh(x)$ or, alternatively, $\exp(x)$ and $\exp(-x)$. The general expressions for the concentration perturbations in a binary electrolyte may be written:

$$c_1^*(x) = A_1 \cosh(\lambda_1 x) + A_2 \cosh(\lambda_2 x) + B_1 \sinh(\lambda_1 x) + B_2 \sinh(\lambda_2 x) \tag{48}$$

$$\begin{aligned} c_2^*(x) = w_1 A_1 \cosh(\lambda_1 x) + w_2 A_2 \cosh(\lambda_2 x) \\ + w_1 B_1 \sinh(\lambda_1 x) + w_2 B_2 \sinh(\lambda_2 x) \end{aligned} \tag{49}$$

Their "lengths" being without importance, the eigenvectors have been chosen as $(1, w_1)$ and $(1, w_2)$, respectively, with

$$w_k = \begin{cases} ([\varepsilon_s/\varepsilon^*]\alpha_1 + id_1^2 - \beta_k^2)/[\varepsilon_s/\varepsilon^*]\alpha_2 & \text{(50a)} \\ [\varepsilon_s/\varepsilon^*]\alpha_1/([\varepsilon_s/\varepsilon^*]\alpha_2 + id_2^2 - \beta_k^2) & \text{(50b)} \end{cases} \quad (k = 1, 2)$$

where the two expressions for w_k are equivalent. (See footnote below.)

The coefficients A_1, B_1, A_2, and B_2 in Eqs. (48) and (49) are "arbitrary" constants to be fixed by the boundary conditions and/or conditions of symmetry,

---

Unfortunately, there have appeared some misprints in connection with the expressions (43) and (44) in previous papers. In [34], Eqs. (A21a) and (A21b) the expressions for the βs are correctly stated, but in Eqs. (B22) the expression in terms of the dimensionless frequency (Ω) should have β_k^2 on the l.h.s. instead of β_k. It was checked, however, that this misprint did not occur in the computer programme for the numerical calculations in that paper. In [29], the misprint was repeated in Eq. (9), but the later expressions (65a) and (65b) are correct and the ones used in the computer programme for the infinite lamellar membrane studied in that paper. The formulae given here in the text differ from the formulae of previous papers by the factor $\varepsilon_s/\varepsilon^*$ multiplying the ionic strength fractions (α_k) everywhere. This is a result of the more careful analysis to the problem given in the present chapter, see Eqs. (37)–(40) in the text. Previously, it was tacitly assumed that $\varepsilon^* = \varepsilon_s$ at the low frequencies where interfacial polarization is important. However, this is not an exact assumption in the cases in which slow, collective, dielectric normal modes exist in polymeric "solvents", see Sec. IV.

if any. From (48) and (49) one obtains for the charge density amplitude, ρ_q^*:

$$\rho_q^*(x)/F = P_1 A_1 \cosh(\lambda_1 x) + P_2 A_2 \cosh(\lambda_2 x)$$
$$+ P_1 B_1 \sinh(\lambda_1 x) + P_2 B_2 \sinh(\lambda_2 x) \tag{51}$$

$$P_1 \equiv z_1 + z_2 w_1 = (z_1/\alpha_1)[\varepsilon^*/\varepsilon_s](\beta_1^2 - id_1^2) \tag{52}$$

$$P_2 \equiv z_1 + z_2 w_2 = (z_1/\alpha_1)[\varepsilon^*/\varepsilon_s](\beta_2^2 - id_1^2) \tag{53}$$

Notice that in the special case $D_1 = D_2$ we have $P_2 = 0$. This corresponds to the fact that only the γ-polarization has any effects on the charge density and on quantities derived from it in this special case, cf. for example Eqs. (27), (29), (31), (32) and (36) in [27].

The amplitude in the galvanic current density may be found by integration of the continuity equation for electric charge:

$$dJ_q^*/dx = -i\omega\rho^* \tag{54}$$

The result is

$$J_q^*(x) = \iota - (i\omega/\lambda_1)P_1 A_1 \sinh(\lambda_1 x) - (i\omega/\lambda_2)P_2 A_2 \sinh(\lambda_2 x)$$
$$- (i\omega/\lambda_1)P_1 B_1 \cosh(\lambda_1 x) - (i\omega/\lambda_2)P_2 B_2 \cosh(\lambda_2 x) \tag{55}$$

where ι (iota) is an integration constant. On the other hand, the field strength amplitude may be found from an integration of the Poisson equation (37, right):

$$E^*(x) = \eta + F/(\varepsilon^*\lambda_1)P_1 A_1 \sinh(\lambda_1 x) + F/(\varepsilon^*\lambda_2)P_2 A_2 \sinh(\lambda_2 x)$$
$$+ F/(\varepsilon^*\lambda_1)P_1 B_1 \cosh(\lambda_1 x) + F/(\varepsilon^*\lambda_2)P_2 B_2 \cosh(\lambda_2 x) \tag{56}$$

Again, η is an integration constant. The complex amplitude of the *total current* of Maxwell is given by:

$$J_{\text{tot}}^* = J_q^* + i\omega\varepsilon^* E^* = \iota + i\omega\varepsilon^*\eta \tag{57}$$

It is seen that the total current may be a function of frequency through $\varepsilon^*(\omega)$, but it is *not* a function of x. For the ion flux amplitudes we have (eliminating second-order terms):

$$J_k^*(x)/D_i = -dc_k^*/dx + (z_k F/RT)c_{k,\,\text{eq}} E^* \quad (k = 1, 2) \tag{58}$$

From Eqs. (58), (48), (49) and (56) an alternative expression for the amplitude in the galvanic current is:

$$J_q^*(x) = \sum_i z_i F J_i^*(x)$$
$$= \sigma\eta + F \sum_k [A_k \sinh(\lambda_k x)\{(\sigma/\varepsilon^*\lambda_k)P_k - z_2 D_2 P_k \lambda_k - z_1 D_1 \lambda_k\}]$$
$$+ F \sum_k [B_k \cosh(\lambda_k x)\{(\sigma/\varepsilon^*\lambda_k)P_k - z_2 D_2 P_k \lambda_k - z_1 D_1 \lambda_k\}] \tag{59}$$

The quantity σ is the bulk (galvanic) conductivity, see Eq. (32). After tedious transformations (59) can be shown to be equivalent to (55). Thus, one obtains for the integration constant $\imath$:

$$\imath = \sigma\eta \tag{60}$$

Thus we have

$$J^*_{tot} = \imath + i\omega\varepsilon^*\eta = (\sigma + i\omega\varepsilon^*)\eta$$

so that the two integration constants may both be expressed through the fundamental amplitude J^*_{tot} which is the current amplitude available to external control:

$$\eta = J^*_{tot}/(\sigma + i\omega\varepsilon^*); \quad \imath = J^*_{tot}\sigma/(\sigma + i\omega\varepsilon^*) \tag{61}$$

The amplitude of the electric potential perturbation is found by integration of the electric field strength:

$$\begin{aligned}
\psi^*(x) = \Psi &- [J^*_{tot}/(\sigma + i\omega\varepsilon^*)]x \\
&- (F/\varepsilon^*) \sum_k [P_k A_k \cosh(\lambda_k x)/\lambda_k^2] \\
&- (F/\varepsilon^*) \sum_k [P_k B_k \sinh(\lambda_k x)/\lambda_k^2]
\end{aligned} \tag{62}$$

In (62), Ψ is an integration constant which is really arbitrary, since only potential differences have physical significance. The A- and B-coefficients are proportional to J^*_{tot} dependent on the precise nature of the boundary conditions and/or the symmetry of the system. Since the impedance is defined as the complex potential drop divided by the complex total current, it is evident from (62) that the impedance (per unit area) of a homogeneous film (of width L) of the system is found as:

$$Z^*_{film} = Z^*_{MWS,\,film} + Z^*_{ex,\,film} \tag{63}$$

$$Z^*_{MWS,\,film} \equiv L/(\sigma + j\omega\varepsilon^*_{diel}) \tag{64}$$

$$\begin{aligned}
Z^*_{ex,\,film} \equiv (F/\varepsilon^*) \sum_k [P_k(A_k/J^*_{tot})\cosh(\lambda_k x)/\lambda_k^2] \\
+ (F/\varepsilon^*) \sum_k [P_k(B_k/J^*_{tot})\sinh(\lambda_k x)/\lambda_k^2]
\end{aligned} \tag{65}$$

The MWS contribution is the Maxwell–Wagner–Sillars contribution (assuming proportionality between J_{tot} and E and bulk properties everywhere in the film) whereas the term $Z^*_{ex,\,film}$ is the *excess impedance* of the film. This term is caused by the surface polarization caused by the two electrodiffusion normal modes at the film boundaries. In order to proceed further, boundary and symmetry conditions have to be incorporated to determine the constants (A_k/J^*_{tot}) and (B_k/J^*_{tot}) in (65).

C.   A Single Film with an Arbitrary Binary Electrolyte Between Blocking Electrodes

In this section a planar, homogeneous and isotropic membrane or film is considered. The dielectric constitutive relations are assumed linear. Thus, the medium is an LHI medium in the sense of Sec. II.A except for the feature that Eq. (31) is valid for the current density rather than the linear equation (2). An arbitrary binary (strong) electrolyte is dissolved in the film. If there is ion pairing or nondissociation, for example because of a low permittivity in the medium, we consider only the concentrations of fully dissociated ions.

The film is placed between electrodes at $x = -L/2$ and $x = L/2$ which are blocking for the galvanic (but not for the total) current. Thus, the ionic species are conserved in the film. From this and (48) and (49) follows that the A-coefficients have to be zero, since the hyberbolic sine is antisymmetric around the mid point of the membrane (zero integral of the concentration perturbation) whereas the hyperbolic cosine is symmetric around $x = 0$. The two "arbitrary constants" (B_1/J^*_{tot}) and (B_2/J^*_{tot}) remaining in the expression (65) for the excess impedance are found by the two conditions that the ionic fluxes at $x = L/2$ are both zero (the similar conditions for $x = -L/2$ are equivalent because of the system symmetry):

$$J^*_1(L/2) = 0; \qquad J^*_2(L/2) = 0 \tag{66}$$

Introducing (58), (48), (49) and (56) into the above two equations one obtains a 2×2 matrix equation for the B-coefficients. A lot of tedious transformations are necessary to transform this matrix equation and the expression for the excess impedance into a form containing a minimum of dimensionless variables. For details, see Ref. 34, Appendix B. Here, I shall only state the final result specializing, for simplicity, to the case where $\varepsilon^* = \varepsilon_s$ as was indeed assumed in [34]. The dimensionless excess impedance of the film is defined by

$$\zeta_{ex, film} \equiv Z^*_{ex, film} \kappa^3 \varepsilon_s (D_1 D_2)^{1/2} \tag{67}$$

with the dimensionless angular frequency given by:

$$\Omega \equiv \kappa^{-2}(D_1 D_2)^{-1/2}\omega \tag{68}$$

Furthermore, the square root of the diffusion coefficient ratio (d) is defined by

$$d \equiv \sqrt{(D_2/D_1)} \tag{69}$$

and the parameter M by

$$M \equiv [dz_2^2 v_2 + d^{-1}z_1^2 v_1]/[z_2^2 v_2 + z_1^2 v_1] \tag{70}$$

where v_1 and v_2 are the stoichiometric coefficients of the two ions in the binary electrolyte. Now, the expression for the excess impedance can be expressed as

$$\zeta_{ex, film} = (4\alpha_1 \sqrt{\Delta i\Omega})^{-1}\{Nd/[M + i\Omega]\} \tag{71}$$

with

$$N \equiv [H_1 + \sqrt{\Delta}][H_2 + \sqrt{\Delta}][H_3 + \sqrt{\Delta}]\beta_1^{-1} \tanh(\beta_1 \kappa L/2)$$
$$- [H_1 - \sqrt{\Delta}][H_2 - \sqrt{\Delta}][H_3 - \sqrt{\Delta}]\beta_2^{-1} \tanh(\beta_2 \kappa L/2) \tag{72}$$

$$H_1 \equiv 1 - 2\alpha_2 + i\Omega(d - d^{-1}) \tag{73}$$

$$H_2 \equiv 1 - i\Omega(d - d^{-1}) \tag{74}$$

$$H_3 \equiv 2d^{-1}(\alpha_2 d + \alpha_1 d^{-1}) - 1 - i\Omega(d - d^{-1}) \tag{75}$$

$$\Delta = 1 - [d - d^{-1}]^2 \Omega^2 + 2i\Omega[d(1 - 2\alpha_2) - d^{-1}(1 - 2\alpha_1)] \tag{76}$$

$$\beta_k^2 = (1/2)\{1 + i\Omega(d + d^{-1}) + (-1)^{k+1}\sqrt{\Delta}\} \quad (k = 1, 2) \tag{77}$$

The dimensionless MWS impedance of the film may be written as:

$$\zeta_{\text{MWS, film}} = \kappa L/[M + i\Omega] \tag{78}$$

The *total* dimensionless impedance of the film is given as

$$\zeta_{\text{film}} = \zeta_{\text{MWS, film}} + \zeta_{\text{ex, film}} \tag{79}$$

Even if the linear constitutive relation $J_q = \sigma E$ (2) is *not* valid with $\sigma = $ the galvanic conductivity (32) since the galvanic current is driven by concentration gradients as well as by the electric field, see Eq. (31), we may define a local, operational complex, galvanic conductivity $\sigma_{\text{galv}}^*(x)$ in the film as:

$$\sigma_{\text{galv}}^*(\omega, x) \equiv J_q^*(x)/E^*(x) \tag{80}$$

Instead of Eq. (9) one obtains:

$$J_{\text{tot}}^* = \{\sigma_{\text{galv}}^*(\omega, x) + i\omega\varepsilon^*(\omega)\}E^*(x) \equiv \sigma_{\text{eff}}^*(\omega, x)E^*(x) \tag{81}$$

In contrast to the case in Sec. II.A, the effective complex conductivity σ_{eff}^* (ω, x) is now space dependent in such a way as to counteract the space dependence of $E(x)$. Integration of Eq. (81) through the film yields (remember that Z_{film}^* (ω) is the impedance of one unit of area):

$$J_{\text{tot}}^* = -(1/L) \int_{-L/2}^{L/2} \sigma_{\text{eff}}^*(\omega, x)(d\psi^*(x)/dx)\, dx \equiv -\{\Delta\psi^*/L\}/Z_{\text{film}}^*(\omega) \tag{82}$$

In analogy with Eq. (10) we define:

$$\varepsilon_{\text{eff}}^*(\omega, x) \equiv \varepsilon^*(\omega) - i\sigma_{\text{galv}}^*(\omega, x)/\omega \tag{83}$$

Comparing the definitions (81) and (82) we obtain the *local* version of Eq. (12):

$$\sigma_{\text{eff}}^*(\omega, x) = i\omega\varepsilon_{\text{eff}}^*(\omega, x) \tag{84}$$

Thus, Eq. (82) can also be written:

$$J_{\text{tot}}^* = -(i\omega/L) \int_{-L/2}^{L/2} \varepsilon_{\text{eff}}^*(\omega, x)(d\psi^*(x)/dx)\, dx$$
$$\equiv -i\omega\{\Delta\psi^*/L\}\varepsilon_{\text{eff, mean}}^*(\omega) \tag{85}$$

Comparing Eqs. (82) and (85) it is seen that the *mean, effective complex permittivity* taken over the film is related to the impedance of one unit of area of the film as follows:

$$\varepsilon^*_{\text{eff, mean}}(\omega) = 1/[i\omega Z^*_{\text{film}}(\omega)] \tag{86}$$

This quantity is the one measured in dielectric spectroscopy experiments with the film placed between condensor plates in oscillating electric fields. In terms of the dimensionless variables of the special model treated here we have:

$$\varepsilon^*_{\text{eff, mean}} = \kappa L[i\Omega\zeta_{\text{film}}] \tag{87}$$

A special approximation to $\varepsilon^*_{\text{eff, mean}}$ with ζ_{film} given by Eqs. (71)–(79) may be made for "thick films" (compared to the Debye length) which will be of value later (in Sec. IV). We assume that:

$$\kappa L \gg 1 \tag{88}$$

In this case one may put

$$\tanh(\beta\kappa L/2) \approx 1 + \{2i\sin(\beta''\kappa L/2)/\exp(\beta'\kappa L/2)\} \approx 1 \quad \text{with} \quad (\beta = \beta' + i\beta'') \tag{89}$$

Further simplification may be obtained in the case of a symmetrical electrolyte $(z_1 = -z_2 = z)$ with equal diffusion coefficients $(D_1 = D_2)$. One then obtains

$$\Delta = 1; \quad H_1 = 0; \quad H_2 = H_3 = 1; \quad M = 1; \quad N = 4/\beta_1;$$
$$\beta_1 = (1 + i\Omega)^{1/2}; \quad \beta_1 = (i\Omega)^{1/2} \tag{90}$$

we arrive at the relatively simple formula:

$$\varepsilon^*_{\text{eff, mean}}/\varepsilon_s = (1 + i\Omega)/\text{Denominator};$$
$$\text{Denominator} = (2/\kappa L)(1 + i\Omega)^{-1/2} + i\Omega \tag{91}$$

Using the usual decomposition

$$\varepsilon^*_{\text{eff, mean}} = \varepsilon' - i\varepsilon'' \tag{92}$$

we have to the leading orders of $(1/\kappa L)$ and up to the 2nd power in Ω, see [36]:

$$\varepsilon'/\varepsilon_s \approx [(2/\kappa L) + \Omega^2]/\text{Denominator} \tag{93}$$
$$\varepsilon''/\varepsilon_s \approx [\Omega]/\text{Denominator} \tag{94}$$
$$\text{Denominator} = (2/\kappa L)^2 + \Omega^2 \tag{95}$$

From Eq. (91) it is seen that the low frequency and high frequency limits of $\varepsilon^*_{\text{eff, mean}}/\varepsilon_s$ are given by:

$$\varepsilon^*_{\text{eff, mean}}/\varepsilon_s \rightarrow \kappa L/2 \quad \text{for} \quad \Omega \rightarrow 0 \tag{96}$$
$$\varepsilon^*_{\text{eff, mean}}/\varepsilon_s \rightarrow 1 \quad \text{for} \quad \Omega \rightarrow \infty \tag{97}$$

The former expression is an expression of the *equilibrium macropolarization* of the film. The ions are in Boltzmann quasi-equilibrium in the slowly varying electric field, and the film acts as a giant capacitor because of the interfacial polarization. The latter expression is only correct if there is no *intrinsic*, dielectric dispersion in the medium. In the case of such dispersion, the static permittivity is exactly defined as the *low frequency* limit of ε'. On the other hand, Eq. (96) shows that this limit may be hard to find, if there are ionic impurities in the sample. Even if the further approximations (93)–(95) should only be expected to be valid for small values of Ω, these formulae are seen to yield correct high as well as low frequency limits for ε' and ε''. The latter should go to zero at low as well as high frequencies. Furthermore, at high frequencies the efficient dielectric loss obtained from (94) and (95) is given by the approximation:

$$\varepsilon''/\varepsilon_s \approx 1/\Omega = \kappa^2 D/\omega = \sigma/\omega \quad \text{(high } \omega) \tag{98}$$

(D is the common diffusion coefficient). Thus, the MWS approximation is valid at high frequencies, cf. Eq. (78). This is as it should be, since the MWS approach is a high frequency limit. In the special case of a common D it is seen from Eq. (47), that the dynamic layers of polarization in connection with the γ-polarization as well as the δ-polarization shrink to zero thickness when $\omega \to \infty$ in accordance with the requirement 3) for the validity of the MWS approach mentioned in Sec. II.A. It is also seen from Eq. (47) that the absolute magnitudes of γ and δ may be made large even at lower frequencies if a high κ is chosen. The MWS is also a high concentration limit. For different diffusivities, the βs also become proportional to $\sqrt{(i\Omega)}$ at high Ω, and the approximation (89) is valid either for high κL or for high frequency or both. It is then seen, that the excess impedance given by Eq. (71) is small compared to the MWS impedance, Eq. (78), for high κL as well as for high frequencies.

As an illustration, Fig. 1 shows the calculated dispersion in $\varepsilon^*_{\text{eff, mean}}$ for a film with $\kappa L = 32$ and common D. The MWS approach (crosses) cannot capture the macropolarization (limiting value 16) shown by $\varepsilon'/\varepsilon_s$ at low Ω. Furthermore, the effective dielectric loss ε'' shows a maximum at intermediate frequencies which is missed by the MWS theory which predicts a dielectric loss increasing to infinity when the frequency goes to zero. Since the dielectric loss is proportional to the dissipation in each cycle [17] this feature is in contradiction with the second law of thermodynamics. At very low frequencies, quasi-equilibrium with the E-field of the ions in the sample is reached and the dissipation vanishes. In Fig. 1, the fully drawn curves (without crosses) are the values calculated from the exact formulae (with the hyperbolic tangents slightly different from 1). The rectangles are calculated from the large κL formula Eq. (91), where the hyperbolic tangents have been set to unity. There is no visible difference between the results of the two formulae. The diamonds correspond to the further approximation in (93)–(95). This approximation is perfect

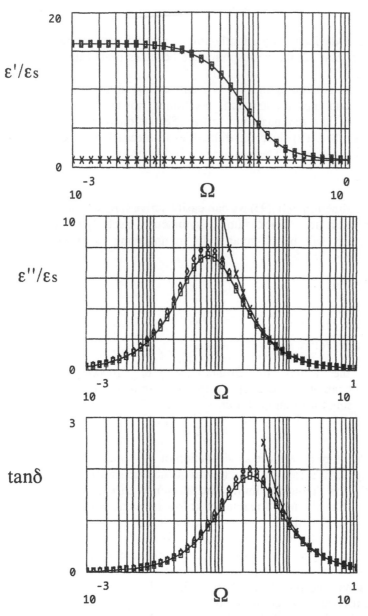

FIG. 1 The two components of the relative complex permittivity and the loss tangent as a function of the dimensionless frequency (Ω) for a conducting film of dimensionless thickness $\kappa L = 32$ in the case of a symmetrical electrolyte and equal cation and anion diffusion coefficients ($d = 1$). The fully drawn curves (without crosses) are calculated from the exact formulae (with tanh slightly different from 1). The rectangles are calculated from the large κL formula Eq. (91). The diamonds correspond to the further approximation Eqs. (93)–(95). The full lines with crosses represent the MWS theory.

in the limits and deviates only slightly for ε'' around the maximum. If κL becomes greater than 32, the correspondence becomes practically perfect for all frequencies.

The last of the subfigures in Fig. 1 is interesting, showing that the *loss tangent* (tan δ) also has a maximum, positioned however at considerably higher frequencies than the maximum in the effective dielectric loss. This will show useful later (Sec. IV) since the difficulties in measuring at very low frequencies may be substantial. The loss tangent is defined as:

$$\tan \delta \equiv \varepsilon''/\varepsilon' \tag{99}$$

Using the approximation (93)–(95) we can easily derive simple formulae for the two maxima—valid for "thick films", symmetric electrolytes and equal diffusivities—which will be of great help in analyzing experimental data (Sec. IV):

$$\Omega(\max \varepsilon'') \approx 2/\kappa L \tag{100}$$

$$\varepsilon''(\max)/\varepsilon_s \approx \kappa L/4 \tag{101}$$

$$\Omega(\max \tan \delta) \approx (2/\kappa L)^{1/2} \tag{102}$$

$$\tan \delta(\max) \approx (\kappa L/8)^{1/2} \tag{103}$$

For $\kappa L = 32$ the values are $\Omega(\max \varepsilon'') \approx 1/16$, $\varepsilon''(\max)/\varepsilon_s \approx 8$, $\Omega(\max \tan \delta) \approx 1/4$ and $\tan \delta(\max) \approx 2$ which are all near to the correct values as seen in Fig. 1. Using the decomposition

$$\zeta_{\text{film}} = \zeta' - i\zeta'' \tag{104}$$

the dimensionless film impedance as a function of the dimensionless frequency is shown in Fig. 2. It is seen that the low frequency resistance is visibly lower than the MWS low frequency limit. The reactance part ζ'' behaves qualitatively different than the MWS reactance at low frequencies with a steep rise. This is due to the dynamical, interfacial capacitance (macropolarization) at low frequencies. It is also worth mentioning that the "impedance relaxation" takes place at much higher frequencies (reactance maximum at $\Omega = 1$) than the "dielectric relaxation" in Fig. 1 (dielectric loss maximum at $\Omega = 1/16$). Thus, although the same information is obtained from IS and DS, the ranges frequencies to be used may be very different.

Figure 3 shows the so-called "Cole–Cole plots" corresponding to Figs. 1 and 2, respectively. The "dielectric Cole–Cole plot" is close to a semicircle with center on the ε'-axis. The arc is transcurred counterclockwise as the frequency increases. The MWS theory (crosses) predicts just a vertical line in the high frequency limit. The reason why the dielectric Cole–Cole plot cannot be a perfect semicircle is that $\varepsilon'/\varepsilon_s$ has to tend to the limit $1 > 0$ for $\Omega \to \infty$. This also depresses the maximum of the arc somewhat compared to a perfect semi-

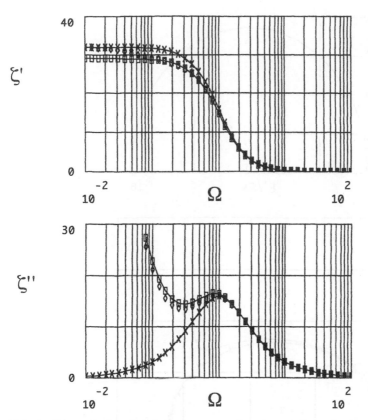

FIG. 2 Dimensionless film impedance as a function of dimensionless frequency in the same case as in Fig. 1. The symbols also represent the same.

circle. As κL increases it becomes more and more difficult to see the difference from a true semicircle with radius $(\kappa L/2)$ and center $(\kappa L/2, 0)$. The "impedance Cole–Cole plot" is distorted from the perfect MWS semicircle at low frequencies, where a vertical asymptote is reflecting the polarization capacitance.

Figure 4 compares the dielectric Cole–Cole plot and the tan δ dispersion for a film with $\kappa L = 32$ for a symmetric electrolyte with equal diffusion coefficients (crosses) with a symmetric electrolyte where one ion diffuses 100 times faster than the other ($d = 10$ or $d = 1/10$, rectangles). In the latter case there are two partially overlapping arcs in the Cole–Cole plot, one for each ion. These two arcs are inscribed in the arc for the electrolyte with equal diffusivities in the sense that the high frequency and low frequency behavior of the two electrolytes coincide. This is easy to understand: The macropolarization at very low frequencies is an equilibrium thermodynamic phenomenon and

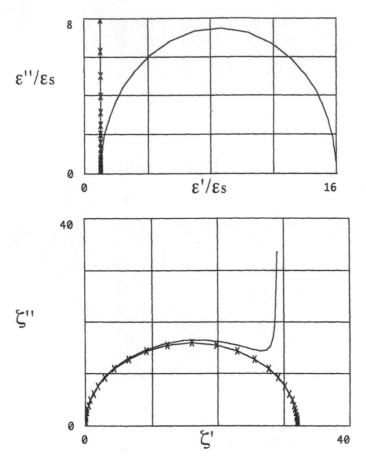

FIG. 3 Permittivity and impedance Cole–Cole plots for the same film as in Fig. 1. Full curves: Exact theory. Curves with crosses: MWS.

cannot depend on diffusion coefficients. At very high frequencies, the MWS theory is valid (very thin electrical boundary layers), and this theory only "knows of" a conductivity, not individual ion diffusion coefficients. The low frequency arc (corresponding to the slow ion) is dominated by a much greater high frequency arc (fast ion). For $\kappa L = 1$, the two arcs are of equal size, but as κL grows to values much greater than unity, the "slow arc" becomes a shoulder on the "fast arc" and finally disappears. In the plot of tan δ in Fig. 4, the "slow peak" is made more visible using a logarithmic scale for tan δ.

For very thick films, the approximate formulae (102) and (103) are even more useful than one should first think for the following reason: if the two

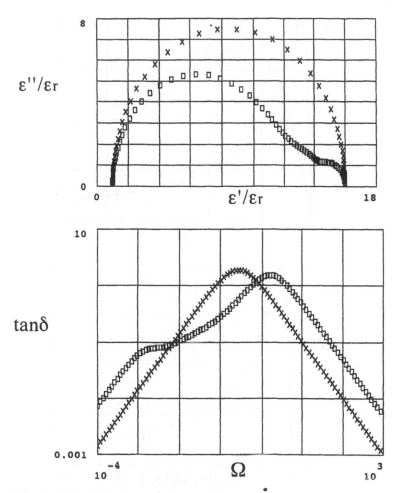

FIG. 4 Cole–Cole plot and the logarithm of the loss tangent as the function of the dimensionless frequency for $\kappa L = 32$ and a symmetrical electrolyte. The rectangles correspond to $d = \sqrt{(1/100)}$ and the crosses to $d = 1$.

diffusion coefficients are not too similar, it is possible to make a *general scaling* of the tan δ vs. Ω curve, so that the dispersion curves for different diffusivities *coincide* with that for equal diffusivities [36]. As an example, I show in Fig. 5 the tan δ dispersion curves for a film of thickness $\kappa L = 3200$ in the case of equal D's (crosses) and in the case of one ion diffusing 100 times faster than the other ($d = 1/10$ or $d = 10$). In the latter case, coinciding curves are obtained if tan δ is multiplied by 1.13 and Ω by $1.75d$ (where d should be taken as the lower value = 1/10). A lot of high values of κL and of d-values have been tried,

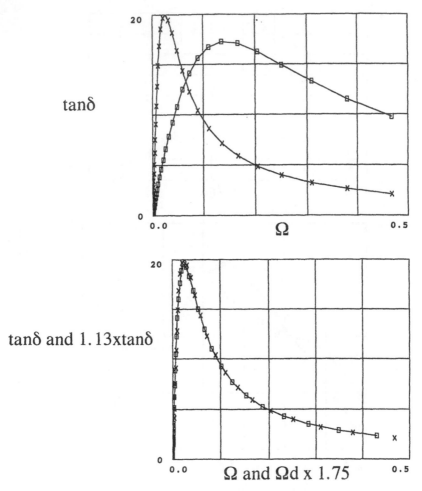

FIG. 5 The loss tangent as a function of the dimensionless frequency for $\kappa L = 3200$. The rectangles correspond to $d = 1/10$ and the crosses to $d = 1$. It is seen, that when the loss tangent for $d = 1/10$ is multiplied by 1.13 and plotted against 1.75 Ωd, the loss tangent curve for $d = 1/10$ coincides with the loss tangent curve for $d = 1$ plotted against Ω.

and the scaling factors are always 1.13 and 1.75d(low). Since we have that

$$\Omega \, d(\text{low}) = \omega \kappa^{-2} (D_{\text{slow}} D_{\text{fast}})^{-1/2} (D_{\text{slow}}/D_{\text{fast}}) = \omega/(\kappa^2 D_{\text{fast}}) \tag{105}$$

it is clear that by comparison of the frequency and the height of the maximum of experimental dispersion curves with the model given here, one is able to determine the diffusion coefficient of the *fast* ion, only. Of course there is a transition zone, when d comes nearer to 1, in which the scaling factors have to move towards unity, too. However, even at $d = 0.3$ the above mentioned scaling works pretty well, see Fig. 8 in [36].

I shall finish this section showing a single example of a 2:1 electrolyte ($z_1 = 2$, $z_2 = -1$, $BaCl_2$ for example). In Fig. 6, the dielectric relaxation of such an electrolyte in a very thin film ($\kappa L = 1$) is shown. The doubly charged

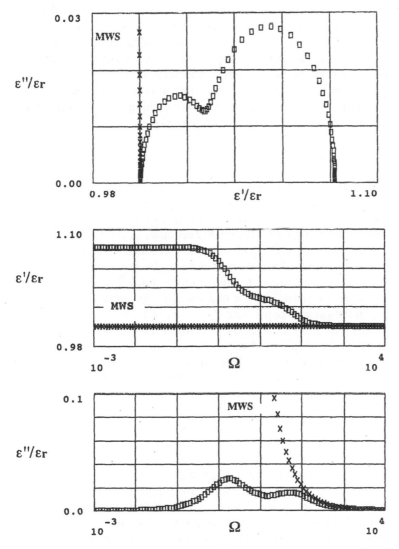

FIG. 6 Cole–Cole plot and dielectric dispersion of a 2:1 electrolyte in a film with $\kappa L = 1$. The doubly charged cation diffuses 36 times more slowly than the anion. The crosses represent MWS (which theory cannot distinguish charge types).

cation (1) is assumed to diffuse 36 times more slowly than the anion (2), $d = 6$. The relaxation is again in two "steps" one for the slow ion and one for the fast. The "slow arc" in the Cole–Cole plot is somewhat greater than the "fast arc" in contrast to a $1:1$ electrolyte in a membrane with $\kappa L = 1$. Thus, the double charge of the slow ion seems to make greater the dielectric loss caused by this ion. This is confirmed by changing to $d = 1/6$ instead of 6. These two cases are no longer symmetric for an asymmetric electrolyte. Now, it is the doubly charged cation which is the fast ion. The result is that the small arc and the grand arc in the dielectric Cole–Cole plot change position. Thus, the "dominance" follows the ion with the higher absolute charge. Increasing the magnitude of κL, the same thing happens as was seen for $1:1$ electrolytes: The "slow arc" diminishes in size and the "fast arc" increases in size. For very thick films, information can only be obtained concerning the diffusion of the *fast* ion, irrespective of its charge. For details, see [34].

D. Trukhan Theories Revisited

For a $1:1$ electrolyte, the formalism given in Sec. II.C should in principle be the same as the one given for 1D geometry in the paper of Trukhan [40]. However, the original derivation of Trukhan is not so easy to follow. Firstly, there is a sign error in the paper of Trukhan. Secondly, Trukhan operates with much more "arbitrary constants" and boundary conditions than considered here, and many of the intermediary steps leading to the end result are omitted. Therefore, we discuss a corrected derivation following the Trukhan procedure as closely as possible. Comfortably, the end result is the same as in the paper of Trukhan and in the present paper with $z_1 = -z_2 = 1$.

Readers not interested in following the control of the present theory against the derivation of Trukhan are invited to bypass the first part of this subsection. However, they should skim the second part, since it summarizes the Trukhan theory for spherical geometry which will be of use in Sec. III.

Equations (39) and (40) in Sec. II.B (taken in one dimension only) are the same as Eqs. (9) and (10) in [40], if $z_1 = -z_2 = 1$ (and $\alpha_1 = \alpha_2 = 1/2$). The expressions (43) and (44) for the eigenvalues also reduce to Trukhan's expressions below Eq. (13) in [40] in that special case. However, there is a sign error in the eigenvectors. The (unnumbered) expressions for the B-coefficients in terms of the A-coefficients in column 2 of page 2561 in [40] should be multiplied by -1 at the r.h.s. This is both evident by comparison with the expressions in the main text of the present paper, and by following Trukhan's own procedure of substituting his Eq. (13) into his Eqs. (9) and (10). The error continues in Trukhan's Eq. (15) for the perturbation in the anion concentration, where the r.h.s. should be multiplied by -1. The error has also consequences for Trukhan's Eqs. (16) and (17) for the electric field and potential, so that the equations in [40] are not the same as the equations given here. For example, Eq. (56) above may be written as (for an $1:1$ electrolyte):

$$E^*(x) = \eta + (2F/\varepsilon)B_1[(\lambda_1^2 - jd_1^2\kappa^2)/(\lambda_1\kappa^2)]\cosh(\lambda_1 x)$$
$$+ (2F/\varepsilon)B_2[(\lambda_2^2 - jd_1^2\kappa^2)/(\lambda_2 \kappa^2)]\cosh(\lambda_2 x) \tag{106}$$

Apart from differences in nomenclature (and other electric units), this is clearly the same as Eq. (16) in [40] except for the change of sign in the last two terms. This is of importance in the boundary conditions Eq. (66) above or the topmost (unnumbered) equations in the second column of p. 2562 in [40], where also the sign error in the concentration perturbations is important. Strangely enough, the final result Trukhan's Eq. (22) is correct, so the errors pointed out here seem to be misprints in the paper.

The detailed derivation of the final formula is not shown in the paper of Trukhan, and it is somewhat obscured by the need to find simultaneously eight different arbitrary constants by eight boundary conditions. However, the main difference with our approach seems to be the following:

Instead of fixing the constant η in Eq. (106) ($-C_2$ in the nomenclature of Trukhan) by requiring the total current to be constant *everywhere*, as we have done above, Trukhan determines this constant by means of the boundary conditions. Let us try to follow this procedure. Afterwards we discuss its rationality. We now need *three* boundary conditions at for example $x = L/2$ to determine the three "arbitrary" constants B_1, B_2 and η. As the two first boundary conditions we take, as before, the zero flux conditions for the cation and the anion, also used in the paper of Trukhan. As the third b.c. we use the electric field condition

$$\varepsilon E^*(L/2) = \varepsilon_{\text{right}} E^*_{\text{right}}(L/2) = J^*_{\text{tot}}/(i\omega) \tag{107}$$

where the index "right" stands for the right of the two (non-conductive) dielectric slabs between which the conductive film is sandwiched in the theory of Trukhan. The following matrix equation is obtained:

$$\mathbf{Qb} = \mathbf{J} \tag{108}$$

$$\mathbf{Q} \equiv \begin{bmatrix} (\beta_1^2 - id_1^2)/\lambda_1 & (\beta_2^2 - id_1^2)/\lambda_2 & -1 \\ -id_1^2/\lambda_1 & -id_1^2/\lambda_2 & -1 \\ (\beta_1^2 - id_1^2)/\lambda_1 & (\beta_2^2 - id_1^2)/\lambda_2 & \\ -(\beta_1/\kappa)[2(\beta_1^2 - id_1^2) - 1] & -(\beta_2/\kappa)[2(\beta_2^2 - id_1^2) - 1] & -1 \end{bmatrix} \tag{109}$$

$$\mathbf{b} \equiv \begin{bmatrix} (2FB_1/\varepsilon)\cosh(\lambda_1 L/2) \\ (2FB_2/\varepsilon)\cosh(\lambda_2 L/2) \\ -\eta \end{bmatrix} \tag{110}$$

$$\mathbf{J} \equiv \begin{bmatrix} J^*_{\text{tot}}/(i\omega\varepsilon) \\ 0 \\ 0 \end{bmatrix} \tag{111}$$

Solving this equation by the rule of Cramer we obtain:

$$B_1/J_{tot}^* = [\kappa/\{2F\beta_1 \cosh(\lambda_1 L/2)i\omega\sqrt{\Delta}\}][1 - (\beta_2^2 - id_1^2)] \tag{112}$$

$$B_2/J_{tot}^* = -[\kappa/\{2F\beta_2 \cosh(\lambda_2 L/2)i\omega\sqrt{\Delta}\}][1 - (\beta_1^2 - id_1^2)] \tag{113}$$

$$\eta = [J_{tot}^*/(i\omega\varepsilon)][id_1^2/\sqrt{\Delta}]$$
$$\times \{[1 - (\beta_2^2 - id_1^2)]/\beta_1^2 - [1 - (\beta_1^2 - id_1^2)]/\beta_2^2\} \tag{114}$$

Thus, we obtain apparently a quite complicated expression for η. The second factor may be simplified, however, using the characteristic equation which is (for a 1:1 electrolyte):

$$\beta_k^4 - [1 + i(d_1^2 + d_2^2)]\beta_k^2 - d_1^2 d_2^2 + (i/2)(d_1^2 + d_2^2) = 0 \qquad (k = 1, 2) \tag{115}$$

One obtains

$$[1 - (\beta_2^2 - id_1^2)]/\beta_1^2 - [1 - (\beta_1^2 - id_1^2)]/\beta_2^2 = id_2^2(\beta_1^2 - \beta_2^2)/(\beta_1^2\beta_2^2)$$
$$= id_2^2\sqrt{\Delta}/(\beta_1^2\beta_2^2)$$

and

$$\eta = -[J_{tot}^*/(i\omega\varepsilon)][d_1^2 d_2^2/(\beta_1^2\beta_2^2)] \tag{116}$$

We have

$$J_{tot}^*/\eta = -i\omega\varepsilon(\beta_1^2\beta_2^2)/d_1^2 d_2^2$$
$$= i\omega\varepsilon\{d_1^2 d_2^2 - (i/2)(d_1^2 + d_2^2)\}/d_1^2 d_2^2 = i\omega\varepsilon + (\kappa^2/2)\varepsilon(D_1 + D_2)$$

or

$$\eta = J_{tot}^*/[i\omega\varepsilon + \sigma] \tag{117}$$

Thus, we regain the same equation which we have derived earlier without using any boundary conditions. Thus, the procedure of Trukhan is correct, but unnecessarily complicated. With the value of η fixed to the value in Eq. (117), only two boundary conditions are necessary, for example the two zero flux conditions. This implies the condition of zero galvanic current at the interface, which is *identical* to the electric field expression, when Eq. (117) is satisfied. The only reason why it is possible to solve the three b.c. above is, that η is allowed to vary freely. Then it is fixed by the b.c. to the value it should have in any case.

The electric potential distribution in the film is given by

$$\psi^*(x) = \Psi - \eta x - (2F/\varepsilon\kappa^2)B_1[(\beta_1^2 - id_1^2)/(\beta_1^2)]\sinh(\lambda_1 x)$$
$$- (2F/\varepsilon\kappa^2)B_2[(\beta_2^2 - id_1^2)/(\beta_2^2)]\sinh(\lambda_2 x) \tag{118}$$

and the contribution to the impedance from the conducting film is given by:

$$Z_{\text{film}} = (\eta/J_{\text{tot}}^*)L + [2/(\varepsilon\kappa \cdot i\omega \cdot \sqrt{\Delta})]$$
$$\times [(\beta_1^2 - id_1^2)(1 - \{\beta_2^2 - id_1^2\})/(\beta_1^3)]\tanh(\lambda_1 L/2)$$
$$+ [2/(\varepsilon\kappa \cdot i\omega \cdot \sqrt{\Delta})][(\beta_2^2 - id_1^2)(1 - \{\beta_1^2 - id_1^2\})/(\beta_2^3)]\tanh(\lambda_2 L/2))$$

(119)

Once more, the characteristic equation (115) is used to simplify the formula. From this we have

$$\beta_1^2 + \beta_2^2 = 1 + i(d_1^2 + d_2^2)$$ (120)

$$Z_{\text{film}}^* = (\eta/J_{\text{tot}}^*)L + [2/(\varepsilon\kappa \cdot i\omega\sqrt{\Delta})]\{[(\beta_1^2 - id_1^2)(\beta_1^2 - id_2^2)/(\beta_1^3)]$$
$$\times \tanh(\lambda_1 L/2) + [(\beta_2^2 - id_1^2)(\beta_2^2 - id_2^2)/(\beta_2^3)]\tanh(\lambda_2 L/2)\}$$ (121)

The first term on the r.h.s. of Eq. (121) is the Maxwell–Wagner–Sillars impedance and the sum of the tanh-terms is the excess impedance. When Eq. (116) is inserted for η/J_{tot}^*, when the impedances of the two sandwiching dielectrica are added and when the result is transformed to the complex dielectric constant of the total system, we obtain exactly the Eq. (22) in Trukhan's paper, which is therefore completely correct for a 1:1 electrolyte. It has also been controlled that Trukhan's Eq. (22)—having a somewhat different appearance than the equations given in the preceding section—gives the same numerical results. The theory presented in Sec. II.C is a generalization of the Trukhan formalism to electrolytes of any charge type, and the exposition in terms of the excess impedance is more rational and readily amenable to generalizations in various directions.

In the paper of Trukhan another case was also treated: A conducting, spherical particle surrounded by an electrically insulating, dielectric medium. Trukhan treated only the case of 1:1 electrolytes inside the spherical particle and equal diffusion coefficient (D) of the two ions. In this case, the perturbation Eqs. (39) and (40) in Sec. II.B degenerates to two decoupled modes corresponding to the eigenvalues γ and δ, see Eq. (47). The γ-polarization corresponds to the difference between the two ion concentrations (the deviation from electroneutrality) and this is the only important one for the calculation of the instantaneous dipole moment of the sphere in an oscillating electric field. Thus, one has for the charge distribution inside the sphere, see Eq. (35) in [40]:

$$\nabla^2 \rho_q^* = \gamma^2 \rho_q^*$$ (122)

The complex parameter γ is a dynamic generalization of the inverse Debye length κ. The eigenfunction of the Laplacian satisfying the requirements that the volume integral of ρ_q^* be always zero and that ρ_q^* be regular at the center of the sphere can be shown to be given by

$$\rho_q^*(r, \theta) = \{Q \cdot \cos \theta / \gamma r\}[\cosh(\gamma r) - \{\sinh(\gamma r)/\gamma r\}] \tag{123}$$

where (r, θ) are the distance from the center and the azimuthal angle (relative to the applied external electric field far from the sphere, $\mathbf{E}_o^*$) of the radius vector to the point considered. Eq. (123) may be inserted into the equation of Poisson (37). Q is an "arbitrary" constant. The solution of this partial differential equation in terms of the perturbation of the electric potential inside the sphere (1) is then found as:

$$\psi_1^*(r, \theta) = B \cdot r \cdot \cos \theta - [Q/\varepsilon_1^* \gamma^2][\cos \theta / \gamma r]\{\cosh(\gamma r) - \{\sinh(\gamma r)/\gamma r\}\} \tag{124}$$

ε_1^* is the complex permittivity of the sphere material and B a new "arbitrary" constant. Trukhan has replaced ε_1^* by its static value $\varepsilon_{s,1}$. It has been used that the potential is regular at $r = 0$. Using the b.c. that the galvanic current density is zero everywhere at the surface of the sphere $(r = a)$ a relation between B and Q in (124) is produced, so that Q may be eliminated, for example.

The external (2) potential distribution is a spherical harmonic function and should produce the oscillating field far from the sphere:

$$\psi_2^*(r, \theta) = (Ar^{-2} - E_o^* r)\cos \theta \tag{125}$$

The conditions that the potential be continuous at any point of the surface of the sphere and that the normal component of the **D**-fields are also continuous at the surface determines A and B in terms of E_o^*. Especially for A one has:

$$A = a^3 E_o^* \{\varepsilon_1^* - \varepsilon_2^* + \varepsilon_1^* \beta^*\}/\{\varepsilon_1^* + 2\varepsilon_2^* - 2\varepsilon_1^* \beta^*\} \tag{126}$$

$$\beta^* = (\varepsilon_2^*/\varepsilon_1^*)(\kappa/\gamma)^2 \frac{[3 + (\gamma a)^2]\tanh(\gamma a)}{[2 + (\gamma a)^2]\tanh(\gamma a) - 2\gamma a} \tag{127}$$

There seems to be a misprint in Trukhan's expression for B. Instead of the formula in [40] p. 2566 one should have (translated to the present nomenclature):

$$B = \{3i\omega(\varepsilon_2^*/\varepsilon_1^*)E_o^*/\gamma^2 D\}[2\varepsilon_1^* \beta^* - 2\varepsilon_2^* - \varepsilon_1^*]^{-1} \tag{128}$$

This has no importance, however, since only A is used furtheron in Trukhan's paper. It is immediately seen from Eq. (125) that A represents the instant dipole moment of the conducting sphere seen from outside:

$$\mathbf{P}^* = \varepsilon_2^* a^3 \mathbf{E}_o^* \{\varepsilon_1^* - \varepsilon_2^* + \varepsilon_1^* \beta^*\}/\{\varepsilon_1^* + 2\varepsilon_2^* - 2\varepsilon_1^* \beta^*\} \tag{129}$$

In the case of a *very dilute*, random dispersion of equally sized, conducting spherical inclusions in a dielectric medium, the effective, complex permittivity of the whole medium can then be calculated by a formula derived by Maxwell (N = number of inclusions per unit volume):

$$\varepsilon_{eff}^* = \varepsilon_2^* + 4\pi N(P^*/E_o^*) \tag{130}$$

Thus we have

$$\varepsilon_{eff}^* = \varepsilon_2^*\{1 + 3\Phi[\varepsilon_1^* - \varepsilon_2^* + \varepsilon_1^*\beta^*]/[\varepsilon_1^* + 2\varepsilon_2^* - 2\varepsilon_1^*\beta^*]\} \tag{131}$$

where Φ is the volume fraction of spheres. The formula is only valid for $\Phi \ll 1$. The range of validity may be extended by Brüggemann integration, see Sec. III.A.

E. The Excess Impedance of a Very Simple Case with One Leaky Interface

The specific examples treated above have all been cases with no electric and ionic currents through the interfaces—blocking interfaces. In order to treat leaky interfaces it is expedient to consider first a very simple—though somewhat unrealistic example [27]. I shall calculate the excess impedance of an isolated interface between two dielectric and conducting media. It will be assumed that the two media contain any mixture of ions, which may even react with each other. However, for simplicity, we consider all the ion diffusion coefficients to be equal ($= D$). A chemical source term

$$\sigma_k(x, t) = \sigma_k^*(x)\exp(i\omega t) \tag{132}$$

is added for each ionic component on the r.h.s. of Eq. (33). Instead of Eq. (38) is obtained:

$$(i\omega/D)c_k^* = \nabla^2 c_k^* - (z_k F/RT)c_{k, eq}(\rho_q^*/\varepsilon^*) + \sigma_k^*(x) \tag{133}$$

Multiplying each of the equations by $z_k F$ and summing over all ions ("$z_k F$ summation") yields:

$$(i\omega/D)\rho_q^* = \nabla^2\rho_q^* - \kappa^2(\varepsilon_s^*/\varepsilon^*)\rho_q^* \tag{134}$$

The perturbed electrochemical reaction equilibria have no influence since no net charge is produced in the reactions. The general solution of this decoupled differential equation for the perturbed charge density is

$$\rho_q^*(x) = A \cosh(\gamma^* x) + B \sinh(\gamma^* x) \tag{135}$$

with γ^* defined by:

$$\gamma^* \equiv \kappa[(\varepsilon_s^*/\varepsilon^*) + (i\omega/D\kappa^2)]^{1/2}; \quad \mathrm{Re}(\gamma^*) > 0 \tag{136}$$

With the interface placed at $x = 0$, separating two semiinfinite regions, the solution should be proportional to $\exp(-\gamma x)$ in the right region (+) and to $\exp(\gamma x)$ in the left region (−). Thus, only one "arbitrary" constant is needed for each phase:

$$\rho_q^*(x) = A_\pm[\cosh(\gamma^*x) \mp \sinh(\gamma^*x)] \tag{137}$$

From Eq. (137), the galvanic current density amplitude can be calculated by integration of $i\omega\rho_q^*$ with respect to x, and the electric field and potential can be calculated integrating ρ_q^*/ε^* one and two times with respect to x.

Following exactly the same procedure as in Sec. II.B we calculate for the impedance (for a unit area) between a point at $x = -L_1$ in phase 1 and a point at $x = +L_2$ in phase 2:

$$Z_{12}^* = -\Delta\psi_{12}^*/J_{tot}^* = Z_{MWS,12}^* + Z_{ex,12}^* \tag{138}$$

$$Z_{MWS,12}^* = \{L_1/(\varepsilon_1^* D^{(1)}\gamma_1^{*2})\} + \{L_2/(\varepsilon_2^* D^{(2)}\gamma_2^{*2})\} \tag{139}$$

$$Z_{ex,12}^* = \{A_-F/(J_{tot}^* \varepsilon_1^*\gamma_1^{*2})\}[1 - \exp(-\gamma_1^* L_1)]$$
$$- \{A_+F/(J_{tot}^* \varepsilon_2^* \gamma_2^{*2})\}[1 - \exp(-\gamma_2^* L_2)] \tag{140}$$

The common diffusion coefficient in phase 1 is $D^{(1)}$ and in phase 2, $D^{(2)}$. These two values may be different, of course. With the electrodes far from the interface, $\mathrm{Re}(\gamma^*L) \gg 1$, the excess impedance takes the simpler form:

$$Z_{ex}^* = \{A_-F/(J_{tot}^* \varepsilon_1^* \gamma_1^{*2})\} - \{A_+F/(J_{tot}^* \varepsilon_2^* \gamma_2^{*2})\} \tag{141}$$

To determinate the two "arbitrary constants" we need two independent boundary conditions. The continuity of the galvanic current and the continuity of the **D**-field at the interface show up to be one and the same condition, see [27], Eqs. (41)–(43). This common condition will only eliminate one of the As above.

Another relation is found from the *local Nernst equilibrium* of the ion's at the interface. The most simple special case which is still nontrivial, is the one where the Nernst distribution coefficients of all the ions have the common value K. In general, we write:

$$c_{2,k}^*(x = 0_+) = K_k c_{1,k}^*(x = 0_-) \tag{142}$$

Taking all Ks equal and performing a "$z_k F$ summation" one obtains:

$$\rho_2^*(x = 0_+) = K\rho_1^*(x = 0_-) \tag{143}$$

Using Eq. (137) we have another relation between A_+ and A_-, i.e., $A_+ = KA_-$. The final expression for the excess impedance in this simple case—passing to the minimum number of the most natural and symmetric dimensionless variables—is given by Eq. (55) in [27], where the complex permittivities for simplicity were assumed to have their static values:

$$\zeta_{ex} = F\{\Omega, (p \cdot d), (p/K)\} \tag{144}$$

$$\zeta_{ex} \equiv Z_{ex}^*[D^{(1)}D^{(2)}\varepsilon_{s,1}\varepsilon_{s,2}]^{1/2}[\kappa_1\kappa_2]^{3/2} \tag{145}$$

$$F\{\Omega, (p \cdot d), (p/K)\} \equiv (1/i\Omega)[f_1^{-2} - f_2^{-2}]^2/[(p/K)^{1/2}f_1^{-1} + (K/p)^{1/2}f_2^{-1}] \tag{146}$$

$$\Omega \equiv \omega/[\kappa_1\kappa_2(D^{(1)}D^{(2)})^{1/2}] \tag{147}$$

$$p \equiv \kappa_2/\kappa_1 = (K\varepsilon_{s,\,1}/\varepsilon_{s,\,2})^{1/2} \tag{148}$$

$$d \equiv (D^{(2)}/D^{(1)})^{1/2} \tag{149}$$

$$f_1(\Omega) \equiv [1 + i(p \cdot d)\Omega]^{1/2} = \gamma_1/\kappa_1;$$
$$f_2(\Omega) \equiv [1 + i(p \cdot d)^{-1}\Omega]^{1/2} = \gamma_2/\kappa_2 \tag{150}$$

The number of mapping parameters for the excess impedance is reduced to three: $p \cdot d$, p/K and the dimensionless frequency Ω. Going back to dimensions the expression for the excess impedance

$$Z_{ex}^* = \kappa_1^{-3}[D^{(1)}D^{(2)}]^{-1/2} \cdot p^{-3/2}[\varepsilon_{s,\,1}\varepsilon_{s,\,2}]^{-1/2}F\{\Omega, (p \cdot d), (p/K)\} \tag{151}$$

may be compared to the MWS impedance between the electrodes and the surface:

$$Z_{MWS}^* = \kappa_1^{-2}\{L_1/[\varepsilon_{s,\,1}D^{(1)}f_1^2] + L_2/[\varepsilon_{s,\,2}D^{(2)}p^2f_2^2]\} \tag{152}$$

It is seen that the MWS impedance is dominating for large values of the inverse Debye lengths (large concentrations) and for large values of the distances L_1 and L_2. A closer inspection also shows that the MWS impedance is dominating at high frequencies [27]. Thus, it appears that the MWS impedance is a valid approximation at high frequencies as well as at electrolyte concentrations and/or electrode separation. To observe clearly the excess impedance phenomenon, the electrolyte concentration should be low and the voltage electrodes should be placed close to the interface, but far enough to avoid the "tails" of the dynamic double layers.

In Fig. 7, a typical example of an excess impedance spectrum is shown ($pd = 6$ and $p/K = 9$, $Re(L\gamma) \gg 1$). It should be noticed that the excess impedance exhibits negative resistances in an intermediate range of frequencies. The situation will not be unstable, however, since the excess impedance has to be added to a MWS impedance, normally of much greater magnitude. It is also seen that two regions exist with negative excess capacitance, i.e., positive values of $Im(\zeta_{ex})$. These negative excess capacitances are also normally overcompensated by the MWS contribution.

The dimensionless version of Eq. (152) expresses ζ_{MWS} in terms of the dimensionless parameters Ω, $(d \cdot e)$, p, $L_1\kappa_1$ and L_2/L_1:

$$\zeta_{MWS} = L_1\kappa_1p^{1/2}\{(d \cdot e \cdot p)/f_1^2 + (L_2/L_1) \cdot (d \cdot e \cdot p)^{-1}/f_2^2\} \tag{153}$$

$$e \equiv [\varepsilon_{s,\,2}/\varepsilon_{s,\,1}]^{1/2} \tag{154}$$

In reality there are not so many independent variables, however, since we have that the salt concentration in phase 2 is K times the salt concentration in phase 1:

$$p \equiv \kappa_2/\kappa_1 = (\sqrt{K})/e \tag{155}$$

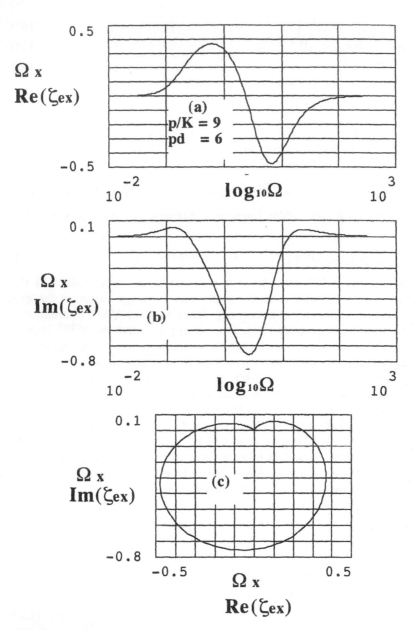

FIG. 7 A numerical calculation showing different representations of the excess imped-ance for an isolated "leaky" interface between two conductive, dielectric media. The diffusion coefficients of the two ions are equal in one and the same medium, but differ-ent in two media. The Nernst distribution coefficients between the two phases are equal for the two ions.

Furthermore:

$$(d/e^2) = (K/e^2) \cdot (d/K) = (p/K) \cdot (pd) \tag{156}$$

Thus, given $(p \cdot d)$, (p/K) and e, the parameter d is calculated from Eq. (156) and the parameter p from $(pd)/d$. Therefore, the dimensionless MWS impedance requires three more parameter (e, $L_1\kappa_1$ and L_2/L_1) than is required for the calculation of the excess impedance.

Figure 8 shows the dispersion of the total impedance (curves) compared to the MWS impedance (crosses) in a case with $L_1\kappa_1 = L_2\kappa_2 = 3$, $L_2/L_1 = 1$; $p/K = 9$, $pd = 6$, $e = 1/3$ (K = 1/9; $p = 1$; $d = 6$). The excess impedance produces only a minor correction to the MWS impedance even in this case where the voltage electrodes are only separated three Debye lengths from the interface. The MWS impedance exhibits two partially overlapping arcs in the Cole–Cole plot with the dimensionless frequencies at the top point around $1/pd = 1/6$ and $pd = 6$, respectively. The effect of the excess impedance is roughly to wipe out some of the difference between these two arcs. In addition, the low frequency peak in the reactance is displaced somewhat towards higher frequencies. Comparing Fig. 8 to Fig. 2, it is seen that the very large capacitance at low frequencies has disappeared. This, of course, reflects the difference between electric polarization against an impenetrable wall and against a "leaky interface". In the latter case, no charge separation can survive at very low frequencies.

The above model of a leaky interface is admittedly oversimplified. If we want to proceed one step further on, we might relieve the condition that all the ion distribution coefficients be equal to a common value (K), maintaining the identity of the diffusion coefficients of all ions in the same solution. The latter condition simplifies considerably the diagonalization of the differential equations. Indeed, one obtains immediately (by summation and by $z_k F$ summation) of the linearized Eq. (38):

$$\nabla^2 c_{\text{tot}}^* \approx \delta^2 c_{\text{tot}}^* \tag{157}$$

$$\nabla^2 \rho_{\text{q}}^* \approx \gamma^* \rho_{\text{q}}^* \tag{158}$$

where c_{tot}^* is the complex amplitude of the total concentration of ions, δ is the "inverse Nernst length" and γ^* a "generalized inverse Debye length":

$$\delta \equiv \sqrt{(i\omega/D)}; \qquad \gamma^* \equiv \sqrt{\{(\varepsilon_{\text{s}}/\varepsilon^*)\kappa^2 + (i\omega/D)\}} \tag{159}$$

Thus, the expression for the total ion concentration and the expression for the space charge density may be found immediately for N ions with the same diffusion coefficient. For binary electrolytes this is enough to find the two ion concentration profiles. When the Nernst distribution coefficients for the ions are different, the final expression for the excess impedance becomes very complicated, however. The two b.c. that the galvanic current is conserved and Eq.

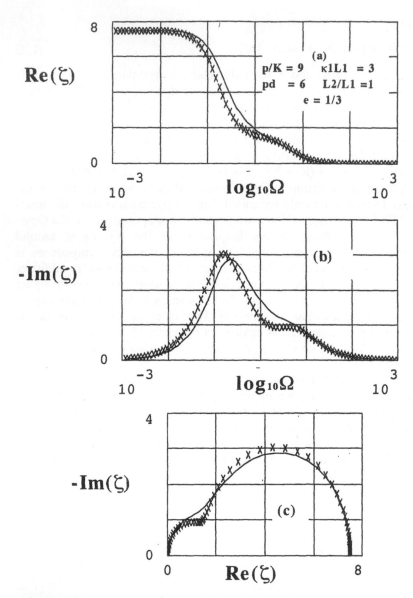

FIG. 8 A numerical example showing the dispersion of the total impedance between two voltage electrodes placed outside the dynamical, electric double layers on each side of the same "leaky," interface as in Fig. 7. The MWS results are given as crosses. The effect of the excess impedance is to wipe out the difference between the two relaxations corresponding to each phase. The ratio between the characteristic frequencies of the two relaxations is predicted by the MWS theory to be the same as the ratio between the diffusion coefficients (= 36).

(143) are now replaced by individual conservation conditions for the ion fluxes and individual local Nernst distributions for the ions. For N ions one has $2N$ conditions to determine $2N$ "arbitrary constants".

Furthermore, it is important to realize, that the difference in Ks introduces a further restriction in the applicability of the final formula for the excess impedance. It was mentioned in connection with the general differential equations for the concentration perturbations (39) and (40) that any *equilibrium* electric double layers at the interfaces should be linearizable. A difference between the Nernst distribution coefficients of the ions introduces an equilibrium, electric potential difference between the ions. In the next section two formulae for this potential difference will be derived (for a 1:1 and a 2:1 electrolyte). Here, it suffices to say that the Ks of the ions should not differ too much from each other for the equilibrium electric double layers to be linearizable.

Finally, it must be said that the case with exactly equal diffusion coefficients for all ions is a somewhat "pathological case". The "Nernst length" (δ^{-1}) goes to infinity when the frequency goes to zero. Thus, it will eventually surpass any realistic physical dimension in a realistic system. In reality, the diffusion coefficients are always somewhat different, and the eigenvalue "inverse lengths" will rather be more complicated versions of "generalized inverse Debye lengths" see, e.g., (43) and (44). These generalized Debye lengths do *not* go to infinity at very low frequency, but rather to the equilibrium Debye length. Therefore, for all the reasons mentioned above, we shall not discuss the special case of equal diffusion coefficients and different Ks. Instead, we shall in the next subsection pass directly to the case of a lamellar membrane containing a binary electrolyte with different Ds in each lamellar phase and with different Ks for the two ions. The dynamical double layers from two subsequent interfaces may be overlapping each other in this model. As a preparation for this study, an intermediate case of a lamellar membrane with overlapping double layers—but with the restrictive condition of "same Ds/same Ks"—was studied in [28]. A very strong deviation from MWS behavior of the effective complex permittivity was found in this study, except at high frequencies or high values of κL. This finding stimulated the more profound investigation in the recent theoretical study to be discussed in the next subsection [29].

F. Lamellar Bilayer Membrane with Leaky Interfaces

An "infinite" lamellar membrane consisting of a repetition of identical bilayers is considered. The bilayer is built up of one layer of chemical phase no. 1 and thickness L_1 and another layer of phase no. 2 and thickness L_2. Both phases are assumed to be dielectrics, conductive to some degree because of the presence of a binary electrolyte of any charge type. Any intrinsic dielectric dispersion is neglected in this subsection, however, so that the permittivity can be set equal to the static permittivity at all frequencies. There are four different diffusion coefficients (for the two ions in the two phases) and two different Nernst distribution coefficients, one for each kind of ion. The detailed derivation of the excess impedance and a comprehensive discussion of examples of calculations have been given in Ref. [29]. Therefore, here I shall limit myself to an outline of the basic principles, assumptions and formulae and some discussion of the results.

In general, one has to adopt the concentration perturbation profiles given by (48) and (49) with different values of the "arbitrary constants" $A_k^{(p)}$ and $B_k^{(p)}$ ($k = 1, 2$) for each phase p ($= 1, 2$). However, if we consider one lamella (of type 1, say) in an infinite array of bilayers, it is surrounded to both sides by lamellae of type 2, and the situation looks perfectly symmetric from the midpoint of the lamella in focus. The same is true for the other lamella. Only in a finite array of bilayers there can be any asymmetry between the two interfaces. Thus, we would expect to have *ion conservation* in each lamella: If some ions are added from the left lamella, the same amount of ions is given off to the right lamella. Therefore, we have (x is the distance from the midpoint in each lamella):

$$\int_{-L_1/2}^{L_1/2} c_k^{(1)*}(x)\, dx = 0 \quad (k = 1, 2) \tag{160a}$$

$$\int_{-L_2/2}^{L_2/2} c_k^{(2)*}(x)\, dx = 0 \quad (k = 1, 2) \tag{160b}$$

Only the sinh solutions in Eqs. (48) and (49) can satisfy these conditions since they are antisymmetric around the midpoint of the lamella. Thus, we restrict the form of the concentration dependence to the following expressions:

$$c_1^{(1)*}(x) = B_1^{(1)} \sinh(\kappa_1 \beta_1^{(1)} x) + B_2^{(1)} \sinh(\kappa_1 \beta_2^{(1)} x)$$
$$(-L_1/2 \le x \le L_1/2) \tag{161}$$

$$c_2^{(1)*}(x) = w_1^{(1)} B_1^{(1)} \sinh(\kappa_1 \beta_1^{(1)} x) + w_2^{(1)} B_2^{(1)} \sinh(\kappa_1 \beta_2^{(1)} x) \tag{162}$$

$$c_1^{(2)*}(x) = B_1^{(2)} \sinh(\kappa_2 \beta_1^{(2)} x) + B_2^{(2)} \sinh(\kappa_2 \beta_2^{(2)} x)$$
$$(-L_2/2 \le x \le L_2/2) \tag{163}$$

$$c_2^{(2)*}(x) = w_1^{(2)} B_1^{(2)} \sinh(\kappa_2 \beta_1^{(2)} x) + w_2^{(2)} B_2^{(2)} \sinh(\kappa_2 \beta_2^{(2)} x) \tag{164}$$

We adopt the convention to write the ion number as a subscript and the phase number as a superscript between parenthesis (to distinguish the phase number from powers). The only exceptions from this will be made for basic characteristics of the two phases, where the phase number will be written as a subscript. Thus κ_1, ε_1, σ_1 and L_1 signify the inverse Debye length, the static permittivity, the specific conductivity and the thickness of a lamella of type 1.

The argument used to restrict the solutions to the ones given in Eqs. (161)–(164) is not free of ambiguity. We might just as well have selected a sequence such as |phase 2|phase 1|phase 2| to be the "central unit" in the infinite array. Since the situation looks the same to the left of the leftmost interface as it does to the right of the rightmost interface there is ion conservation in each triple layer as a whole but not in each lamella. Then we need both the A and the B coefficients and more boundary conditions than used in the present paper (see the section "Boundary conditions and other restrictions"). Similarly we might take as a central unit |phase 1|phase 2|phase 1|phase 2|phase 1| and indeed any block with an uneven number of lamellae. Contributions from such normal modes might very well be of importance for very low frequencies where the concentration perturbations extend over several lamellae. At the present stage of analysis, however, it would intolerably complicate the calculations to include such "multilamellar" normal modes. Furthermore, in [28] the same restriction was used for a lamellar membrane as the one used here with the further restrictions of identical diffusion coefficients and Nernst distribution coefficients of the two ions. In the present section and in [29], the study is generalized to unequal diffusion coefficients and Nernst distribution coefficients, but it is chosen not to complicate the analysis with the "multilamellar" normal modes.

There are four "arbitrary constants" $B_1^{(1)}$, $B_2^{(1)}$, $B_1^{(2)}$ and $B_2^{(2)}$ which can be eliminated by four independent boundary conditions. These boundary conditions are (a) the continuity of the fluxes of the two ionic species through the interface and (b) the local Nernst distribution equilibrium of the two ions at the interface.

The ion fluxes entering in the conditions (a) are given by the Nernst–Planck equations, and in the linearized form these may be written as

$$J_k^{(n)*}(x) = D_k^{(n)}[-(dc_k^{(n)*}/dx) + \varepsilon_n(\alpha_k^{(n)}/z_k F)\kappa_n^2 E^{(n)*}] \tag{165}$$

where the x-derivative of the concentration perturbation amplitudes can be found from (161)–(164) and

$$J_k^{(n)}(x, t) = J_k^{(n)*}(x) e^{i\omega t} \tag{166}$$

We need only to consider an interface of the type 1|2 since the interface of type 2|1 yields identical boundary conditions because of the symmetry adopted. Thus, we have the boundary conditions (a):

$$J_k^{(1)*}(L_1/2) = J_k^{(2)*}(-L_2/2) \quad (k = 1, 2) \tag{167}$$

1. Restrictions on the Input Parameters

With respect to the local equilibrium of the ions at the interface (b) it is important to realize that the electric potential is the same at contact, so that the equality of the electrochemical potentials of the ions on the two sides amounts to an equality of the chemical potentials, i.e., a Nernst distribution equilibrium for the ideal electrolytes considered. Any difference between the two Nernst distribution coefficients leads to the generation of a difference in electric potential between the two "bulk electrolytes" far from the interfaces. (There may be not be any "bulk electrolyte" present physically in narrow lamellae, but a "would be" bulk concentration can nevertheless be defined). The identity of the electrochemical potentials of the ions in the "bulk electrolytes" and the requirement that the equilibrium electric double layer be linearizable leads to other restrictions which we shall consider afterwards, but first we state the local equilibrium conditions (b):

$$c_k^{(2)*}(-L_2/2) = K_k\, c_k^{(1)*}(L_1/2) \quad (k = 1, 2) \tag{168}$$

In these equations, K_1 and K_2 are the Nernst distribution constants for the two ions at constant electric potential. Since the bulk solution has to be electroneutral, an electric potential between the bulk solutions has to arise if $K_1 \neq K_2$. The identity of the electrochemical potentials for the ions in the bulk phases with the salt concentrations $c_s^{(1)}$ and $c_s^{(2)}$ leads to the following equations for the bulk salt equilibrium and the bulk, electric potential difference:

$$(\mu_k^{0(2)}/RT) - (\mu_k^{0(1)}/RT) + \ln[(c_{k,\,\mathrm{bulk}}^{(2)})/(c_{k,\,\mathrm{bulk}}^{(1)})]$$
$$+ z_k F\, \Delta\psi_{\mathrm{eq,\,bulk}}/RT = 0 \quad (k = 1, 2) \tag{169}$$

These equations may also be written

$$-\ln K_k + \ln K_s + z_k F\, \Delta\psi_{\mathrm{eq,\,bulk}}/RT = 0 \quad (k = 1, 2) \tag{170}$$

using the usual relation between an equilibrium constant and the difference in standard chemical potentials ($\mu_k^{0(n)}$) for the ions and using the definition of the Nernst distribution coefficient for the whole salt between the electroneutral bulk solutions:

$$K_s = c_s^{(2)}/c_s^{(1)} = c_{1,\,\mathrm{bulk}}^{(2)}/c_{1,\,\mathrm{bulk}}^{(1)} = c_{2,\,\mathrm{bulk}}^{(2)}/c_{2,\,\mathrm{bulk}}^{(1)} \tag{171}$$

Eliminating the equilibrium electric potential difference $\Delta\psi_{\mathrm{eq,\,bulk}}$ from the two Eqs. (170) and using formal electroneutrality of the salt (ν_1 and ν_2 are the stoichiometric coefficients)

$$\nu_1 z_1 + \nu_2 z_2 = 0 \tag{172}$$

we obtain:

$$K_s = K_1^{(\nu_1/\nu)} K_2^{(\nu_2/\nu)} \quad (\nu = \nu_1 + \nu_2) \tag{173}$$

On the other hand, subtracting the two Eqs. (170) we obtain for the equilibrium potential difference:

$$F\, \Delta\psi_{\mathrm{eq,\,bulk}}/RT = (\psi_{\mathrm{eq,\,bulk}}^{(2)} - \psi_{\mathrm{eq,\,bulk}}^{(1)})/RT$$
$$= [1/(z_1 - z_2)]\ln(K_1/K_2) \tag{174}$$

Thus, when the two Nernst distribution coefficients for the ions are different there is a nonzero potential difference between the two bulk phases at equilibrium.

Now, the present model is based on a linearization not only of the dynamic, electric double layers, but also of the initial equilibrium double layers present, see especially the discussion in [27], Sec. 2, and [29], Appendix A. For a Gouy–Chapman linearization to be valid we should have the approximation

$$\exp(\pm |z_{max}| F | \psi_{eq,\,interface} - \psi_{eq,\,bulk} |/RT)$$
$$\approx 1 \pm |z_{max}| F | \psi_{eq,\,interface} - \psi_{eq,\,bulk} |/RT$$

where z_{max} is the maximum value of the ionic valencies. We have very crudely that

$$| \psi_{eq,\,interface} - \psi_{eq,\,bulk} | \approx | \Delta \psi_{eq,\,bulk} |/2$$

Thus, the criterion is

$$\exp(\pm F | z_{max} \Delta \psi_{eq,\,bulk} |/2RT) \approx 1 \pm F | z_{max} \Delta \psi_{eq,\,bulk} |/2RT \qquad (175)$$

For $F | z_{max} \Delta \psi_{eq,\,bulk} |/2RT < 0.4$, the deviation between the two sides of the approximation (175) is less than 10% which is quite acceptable for a linearization to be made. Using Eq. (174) we see that we should have

$$| \ln(K_1/K_2) | < 0.8 | z_1 - z_2 |/| z_{max} | \qquad (176)$$

For a symmetric ($z:z$) electrolyte we have:

$$1/5 < K_2/K_1 < 5 \qquad (177)$$

For a 2:1 electrolyte:

$$1/3 < K_2/K_1 < 3 \qquad (178)$$

These are the limits inside which we have to stay to be sure that the linear theory is approximately correct.

Of great importance is also the fact that the ratio between the inverse Debye lengths, which are expressed through the bulk concentrations in Eq. (41) and the ratio between the permittivities of the two lamellae cannot be chosen independently for a given salt distribution coefficient. Introducing the dimensionless quantities p and e given by Eqs. (155) and (154), respectively, we see that

$$p = (\varepsilon_1/\varepsilon_2)^{1/2}[\{(v_1 z_1^2 + v_2 z_2^2)c_s^{(2)}\}/\{(v_1 z_1^2 + v_2 z_2^2)c_s^{(2)}\}]^{1/2} = (1/e)\sqrt{K_s} \qquad (179)$$

Because of the bulk electroneutrality, the ionic strength fractions are also restricted to simple, fixed fractions dependent on the type of electrolyte only.

Symmetric electrolytes: $\qquad \alpha_1^{(n)} = \alpha_2^{(n)} = 1/2 \qquad (180)$

$$(n = 1, 2)$$

2:1 electrolytes: $\qquad \alpha_1^{(n)} = 2/3; \quad \alpha_2^{(n)} = 1/3 \qquad (181)$

2. Boundary Conditions in Terms of Dimensionless Variables

Returning now to the boundary conditions (167) and (168), we may write these conditions in matrix form. After introduction of dimensionless variables and with considerable algebraic manipulation, see [29], one finally obtains:

$$
\begin{bmatrix}
F_{11}/p & F_{12}/p & D_1^{(21)}F_{13} & D_1^{(21)}F_{14} \\
F_{21}/p & F_{22}/p & D_2^{(21)}F_{23} & D_2^{(21)}F_{24} \\
K_1 \text{th}_{11} & K_1 \text{th}_{12} & \text{th}_{21} & \text{th}_{22} \\
w_1^{(1)} K_2 \text{th}_{11} & w_2^{(1)} K_2 \text{th}_{12} & w_1^{(2)} \text{th}_{21} & w_2^{(2)} \text{th}_{22}
\end{bmatrix}
\begin{bmatrix}
X_1^{(1)} \\
X_2^{(1)} \\
X_1^{(2)} \\
X_2^{(2)}
\end{bmatrix}
=
\begin{bmatrix}
G_1 \\
G_2 \\
0 \\
0
\end{bmatrix}
\tag{182}
$$

We have introduced the (geometric) mean diffusion coefficient

$$
D_m \equiv [D_1^{(1)} D_1^{(2)} D_2^{(1)} D_2^{(2)}]^{1/4}
\tag{183}
$$

the dimensionless (and symmetrizised) angular frequency

$$
\Omega \equiv \omega/(\kappa_1 \kappa_2 D_m)
\tag{184}
$$

and the functions of Ω:

$$
F_{1k} \equiv (\alpha_1^{(1)}/z_1) P_k^{(1)}(1/\beta_k^{(1)}) - \beta_k^{(1)} \quad (k = 1, 2)
\tag{185}
$$

$$
F_{1(k+2)} \equiv \beta_k^{(2)} - (\alpha_1^{(2)}/z_1) P_k^{(2)}(1/\beta_k^{(2)}) \quad (k = 1, 2)
\tag{186}
$$

$$
F_{2k} \equiv (\alpha_2^{(1)}/z_2) P_k^{(1)}(1/\beta_k^{(1)}) - w_k^{(1)} \beta_k^{(1)} \quad (k = 1, 2)
\tag{187}
$$

$$
F_{2(k+2)} \equiv w_k^{(2)} \beta_k^{(2)} - (\alpha_2^{(2)}/z_2) P_k^{(2)}(1/\beta_k^{(2)}) \quad (k = 1, 2)
\tag{188}
$$

$$
G_k \equiv (\alpha_k^{(2)}/z_k) D_k^{(21)}[p/(ps_2 + i\Omega)]
$$
$$
- (\alpha_k^{(1)}/z_k)[1/(ps_1 + ip\Omega)] \quad (k = 1, 2)
\tag{189}
$$

In the above functions and in the matrix Eq. (182) we have introduced the dimensionless diffusion parameters

$$
D_k^{(21)} \equiv D_k^{(2)}/D_k^{(1)} \quad (k = 1, 2)
\tag{190}
$$

and the parameters

$$
s_n \equiv [D_1^{(nm)} z_1^2 v_1 + D_2^{(nm)} z_2^2 v_2]/[z_1^2 v_1 + z_2^2 v_2] \quad (n = 1, 2)
\tag{191}
$$

with

$$
D_k^{(nm)} \equiv D_k^{(n)}/D_m \quad (k = 1, 2; n = 1, 2)
\tag{192}
$$

Furthermore we have:

$$
[\beta_1^{(n)}]^2 = (1/2)\{1 + i([d_1^{(n)}]^2 + [d_2^{(n)}]^2) + \sqrt{\Delta^{(n)}}\}
\tag{193a}
$$

$$
[\beta_2^{(n)}]^2 = (1/2)\{1 + i([d_1^{(n)}]^2 + [d_2^{(n)}]^2) - \sqrt{\Delta^{(n)}}\}
\tag{193b}
$$

$$
\Delta^{(n)} = 1 - \{[d_1^{(n)}]^2 - [d_2^{(n)}]^2\}^2
$$
$$
+ 2i\{[d_1^{(n)}]^2(1 - 2\alpha_2^{(n)}) - [d_2^{(n)}]^2(1 - 2\alpha_1^{(n)})\}
\tag{194}
$$

$$
[d_k^{(1)}]^2 = p\Omega/D_k^{(1m)}
\tag{195}
$$

$$
[d_k^{(1)}]^2 = (1/p)\Omega/D_k^{(2m)}
\tag{196}
$$

In the matrix Eq. (182), the four "unknowns" are defined in terms of the "arbitrary" constants as follows:

$$\begin{bmatrix} X_1^{(1)} \\ X_2^{(1)} \\ X_1^{(2)} \\ X_2^{(2)} \end{bmatrix} \equiv \begin{bmatrix} \kappa_2 B_1^{(1)} \text{ch}_{11} \\ \kappa_2 B_2^{(1)} \text{ch}_{12} \\ \kappa_1 B_1^{(2)} \text{ch}_{21} \\ \kappa_1 B_2^{(2)} \text{ch}_{22} \end{bmatrix} \cdot (D_m F/J_{tot}^*) \tag{197}$$

We also use the following abbreviations:

$$\text{sh}_{nk} \equiv \sinh(\kappa_n \beta_k^{(n)} L_n/2); \quad \text{ch}_{nk} \equiv \cosh(\kappa_n \beta_k^{(n)} L_n/2);$$
$$\text{th}_{nk} \equiv \tanh(\kappa_n \beta_k^{(n)} L_n/2) \tag{198}$$

3. Dimensionless Impedance and Complex Permittivity

The calculation of the excess impedance and of the MWS impedance of one of the bilayers proceed exactly as we have seen before. In dimensional form one has:

$$Z_{\text{bi, MWS}} \equiv L_1/(\sigma_1 + i\omega\varepsilon_1) + L_2/(\sigma_2 + i\omega\varepsilon_2) \tag{199}$$

$$Z_{\text{bi, ex}} \equiv [2F/(J_{tot}^* \varepsilon_1 \kappa_1^2)] \sum_k [P_k^{(1)} B_k^{(1)} \text{sh}_{1k}/(\beta_k^{(1)})^2]$$
$$+ [2F/(J_{tot}^* \varepsilon_2 \kappa_2^2)] \sum_k [P_k^{(2)} B_k^{(2)} \text{sh}_{2k}/(\beta_k^{(2)})^2] \tag{200}$$

A (symmetrized) dimensionless impedance is now introduced

$$\zeta_{\text{bi}} \equiv (\kappa_1 \kappa_2)^{3/2} (\varepsilon_1 \varepsilon_2)^{1/2} D_m Z_{\text{bi}} = \zeta_{\text{bi, MWS}} + \zeta_{\text{bi, ex}} \tag{201}$$

and one obtains finally:

$$\zeta_{\text{bi, MWS}} = (ep^{3/2})[(\kappa_1 L_1)/(s_1 + ip\Omega)]$$
$$+ (ep^{3/2})^{-1}[(\kappa_2 L_2)/(s_2 + i\Omega/p)] \tag{202}$$

$$\zeta_{\text{bi, ex}} = 2(ep^{1/2})\left\{\sum_k [P_k^{(1)} X_k^{(1)} \text{th}_{1k}/(\beta_k^{(1)})^2]\right\}$$
$$+ 2(ep^{1/2})^{-1}\left\{\sum_k [P_k^{(2)} X_k^{(2)} \text{th}_{2k}/(\beta_k^{(2)})^2]\right\} \tag{203}$$

The four coefficients $X_k^{(n)}$ are found as solution to the simultaneous linear equations Eq. (182).

Now, consider a membrane considering of a large number (N) of bilayers so that we can neglect end effects. The observed ("effective") complex permittivity (ε^*) is then given as

$$\varepsilon_{\text{eff}}^* = (\text{total thickness})/(i\omega Z_{\text{total}})$$
$$= N(L_1 + L_2)/(i\omega N Z_{\text{bi}}) = (L_1 + L_2)/(i\omega Z_{\text{bi}}) \tag{204}$$

which is independent of the thickness of the multilayer membrane as it should be as an intrinsic property of the heterogeneous medium. Introducing the dimensionless bilayer impedance and the dimensionless angular frequency we obtain:

Reduced permittivity

$$
\begin{aligned}
\varepsilon_{red}^* &\equiv \varepsilon_{eff}^*/\sqrt{(\varepsilon_1\varepsilon_2)} \\
&= [p^{1/2}\kappa_1 L_1 + p^{-1/2}\kappa_2 L_2]/(i\zeta_{bi}\,\Omega) \\
&= (\kappa_1 L_1)(\sqrt{p})[1 + (L_2/L_1)]/(i\zeta_{bi}\,\Omega)
\end{aligned}
\tag{205}
$$

We may compare this reduced permittivity with the reduced permittivity obtained from the MWS approach:

$$
\varepsilon_{red,\,MWS}^* = \varepsilon_{MWS}^*/\sqrt{(\varepsilon_1\varepsilon_2)} = (\kappa_1 L_1)(\sqrt{p})[1 + (L_2/L_1)]/(i\zeta_{MWS}\,\Omega)
\tag{206}
$$

To perform a calculation we have to proceed in the following way:

1. Select the type of electrolyte (1:1, 2:1, etc). This fixes the parameters: z_1, z_2, v_1, v_2, $\alpha_1^{(1)}$, $\alpha_1^{(2)}$, $\alpha_2^{(1)}$, $\alpha_2^{(2)}$.
2. Choose the Nernst distribution coefficient for the salt (K_s) and the Nernst distribution coefficient ratio for the two ions (K_2/K_1). Then, K_1 and K_2 follow from Eq. (173). The ratio K_2/K_1 has to stay inside the ranges determined by the type of electrolyte for the linearization to be valid.
3. Choose $e = \sqrt{(\varepsilon_2/\varepsilon_1)}$. Then $p = \kappa_2/\kappa_1$ follows from Eq. (179).
4. Choose $\kappa_1 L_1$ and L_2/L_1. Since p is known, $\kappa_2 L_2$ can be calculated.
5. Choose $D_1^{(1m)}$ ($= D_1^{(1)}/D_m$), $D_2^{(1m)}$ and $D_1^{(2m)}$. Calculate the remaining diffusion ratio $D_2^{(2m)}$ from the relation:

$$
D_1^{(1m)}D_2^{(1m)}D_1^{(2m)}D_2^{(2m)} = 1
\tag{207}
$$

6. Select a range of dimensionless angular frequencies (Ω).
7. Calculate $X_1^{(1)}$, $X_2^{(1)}$, $X_1^{(2)}$ and $X_2^{(2)}$ from the linear equations Eq. (182) for each Ω.
8. Calculate the dimensionless MWS impedance for each bilayer $\zeta_{bi,\,MWS}$ from Eq. (202) and the dimensionless excess impedance $\zeta_{bi,\,ex}$ from Eq. (203) and add them to the total impedance of a bilayer.
9. Calculate the reduced, complex permittivity of the lamellar membrane from Eq. (205).

In summary, we need the following input for the calculation (electrolyte type; K_s; K_2/K_1; e; $\kappa_1 L_1$; L_2/L_1; $D_1^{(1m)}$; $D_2^{(1m)}$; $D_1^{(2m)}$; Ω). Once having calculated ε_{red}^* in a range of Ω we need ε_1 and ε_2 (and not only e) to interpret physically the result in terms of absolute permittivity. Furthermore, we need D_m, κ_1 and κ_2 to interpret the frequency Ω in terms of the angular frequency ω. Thus, we need all the four diffusion coefficients, the two (ion free) permittivities and the (bulk) electrolyte concentration in one of the phases to interpret physically the spectrum. For the interpretation of the impedance spectrum the same information is needed.

4. A Lamellar Membrane with Two Distinct Impedance Relaxations, One for Each Layer

In the present section I shall present some sample calculations for $1:1$ electrolytes. The real and the complex component of the permittivity and the dimensionless bilayer impedance are denoted by a prime and a double prime, respectively, and these components are defined by:

$$\varepsilon_{\text{eff}}^* = \varepsilon' - i\varepsilon''; \qquad \zeta_{\text{bi}} = \zeta_{\text{bi}}' - i\zeta_{\text{bi}}'' \tag{208}$$

In the present series of calculations the common input parameters are given as:

$$K_s = 1/9; \qquad e = 1/3; \qquad L_2/L_1 = 1 \tag{209}$$

In addition, the following choices of parameters have been selected in succession:

$$\kappa_1 L_1 = 10; \ K_2/K_1 = 1; \ D_1^{(1m)} = 1/6; \ D_2^{(1m)} = 1/6; \ D_1^{(2m)} = 6 \tag{210a}$$

$$\kappa_1 L_1 = 10; \ K_2/K_1 = 1/3; \ D_1^{(1m)} = 1/6; \ D_2^{(1m)} = 1/6; \ D_1^{(2m)} = 6 \tag{210b}$$

$$\kappa_1 L_1 = 10; \ K_2/K_1 = 1; \ D_1^{(1m)} = 1/12; \ D_2^{(1m)} = 1/3; \ D_1^{(2m)} = 3 \tag{210c}$$

$$\kappa_1 L_1 = 10; \ K_2/K_1 = 1/3; \ D_1^{(1m)} = 1/12; \ D_2^{(1m)} = 1/3; \ D_1^{(2m)} = 3 \tag{210d}$$

$$\kappa_1 L_1 = 1; \ K_2/K_1 = 1/3; \ D_1^{(1m)} = 1/12; \ D_2^{(1m)} = 1/3; \ D_1^{(2m)} = 3 \tag{210e}$$

The diffusion coefficients have in all the cases Eqs. (210a–e) been chosen such that the ratio between the geometric mean value of the diffusion coefficient in phase 2 (with low permittivity, $\varepsilon_2 = \varepsilon_1/9$) and the geometric mean of the diffusion coefficients in phase 1 (with high permittivity) is equal to 36. In the first four cases, the thickness of each of the layers is 10 times the Debye length whereas in the last case, the thickness is equal to the Debye length. (As it happens, $\kappa_1 L_1 = \kappa_2 L_2$ in all the above cases since $p = \kappa_2/\kappa_1 = \sqrt{K_s/e} = 1$).

In the first case, Eq. (210a), the two ions have equal Nernst distribution coefficients and equal diffusion coefficients in each phase. Figure 9 shows the real and imaginary component of the reduced permittivity as a function of the dimensionless angular frequency (Ω). The imaginary component has been multiplied by Ω to show more clearly the limiting behavior of $\varepsilon_{\text{red}}''$ at low and high frequencies. A "dielectric Cole–Cole plot" of $\varepsilon_{\text{red}}''$ vs. $\varepsilon_{\text{red}}'$ is also shown. This plot exhibits a vertical asymptote at low frequencies (caused by conductivity and surface polarisation). This asymptote to a considerable degree deforms the semicircular relaxation at higher frequencies. The curves without symbols are calculated from the model above, whereas the (xxxx) curves are calculated by means of simple Maxwell–Wagner–Sillars (MWS) theory.

The model values of the low frequency limit of $\varepsilon_{\text{red}}'$ in Fig. 9 are displaced towards smaller values compared to the MWS limiting value. This is so because the macrodipole formed by the surface polarization charges in the

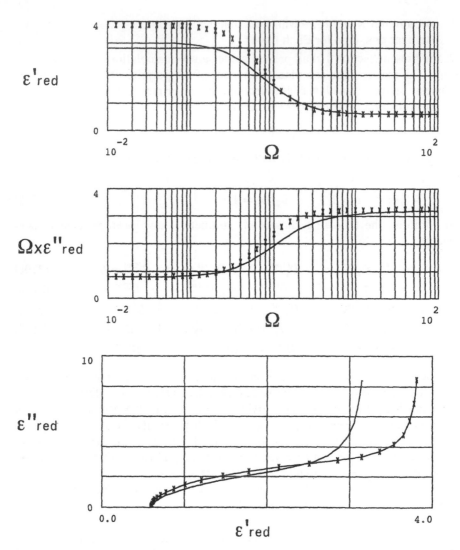

FIG. 9 Upper and middle figure: Dispersion of the reduced, complex permittivity of a lamellar membrane as a function of the dimensionless angular frequency Ω. Lower figure: Dielectric "Cole–Cole plots" showing a MWS semi-circle (xxx) perturbed by the vertical conductivity asymptote at low frequencies and by the excess impedance (full line). The case corresponds to Eq. (210a) with equal ion diffusion coefficients in each phase and equal Nernst distribution coefficients. The diffusion is more rapid in phase 2 with the lower permittivity. The Maxwell–Wagner–Sillars (MWS) values yield higher results for the low frequency plateau in the real part of the complex permittivity (higher dipole moment).

present model is smeared out in contrast to the assumption of sharply localized surface charges in the MWS calculation, see Sec. II.A. Since $\sigma_2/\sigma_1 = 4$, the
MWS value of the low frequency limit of ε'_{red} is calculated to be ~ 3.87 but the
model value is rather ~ 3.2. The high frequency limits of ε'_{red} ($=0.6$) and of ε''_{red}
($=0$) are the same for the model and for the MWS calculation. This is so since
the (complex) "extension" of the "dynamical double layer" in phase k is
$(\kappa_k \beta_k)^{-1}$ which is proportional to $1/\omega$ at high frequencies. Thus, at high frequencies the extension of the dynamical double layers shrinks to zero, and the
assumption of localized surface charges made in the MWS model becomes
exact.

The value of $\Omega \cdot \varepsilon''_{red}$ for the model coincides exactly with the MWS limits
at low as well as at high frequencies. The low frequency limit is 0.8 and the
high frequency limit 3.25. Thus, the frequency dependence of ε''_{red} is as Ω^{-1} for
low as well as for high frequencies, but the coefficient is different in the two
ranges. Only at intermediate frequencies the frequency dependence is more
complicated and $\Omega \cdot \varepsilon''_{red}$ deviates from $\Omega \cdot \varepsilon''_{red, MWS}$.

Figure 10 shows for the example Eq. (210a) a Cole–Cole plot of the negative, imaginary part of the total dimensionless impedance of a bilayer vs. the
real part. The plot is read from low frequencies to the right (dimensionless DC

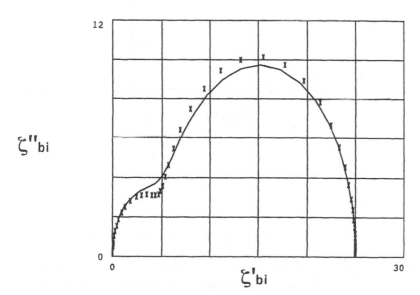

FIG. 10 Impedance Cole–Cole plots showing two partially overlapping semi-circles,
one for each kind of layer. The case corresponds to Eq. (210a). The effect of the excess
impedance (full line) with $\kappa_1 L_1 = \kappa_2 L_2 = 10$ is partially to wipe out the distinction
between the two relaxations compared to the MWS values (xxx).

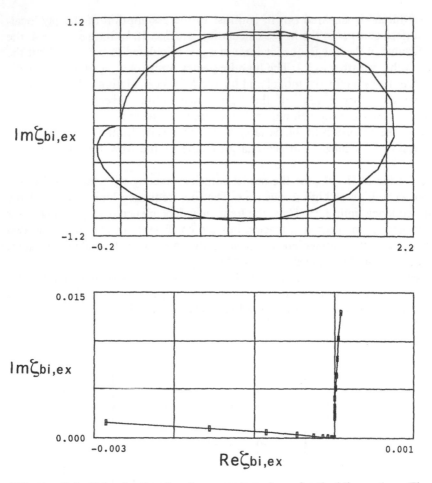

FIG. 11 Cole–Cole plot showing the excess impedance for the bilayer alone. The case corresponds to Eq. (210a). The magnification (lower subfigure) shows the behavior in the neighbourhood of (0,0). The low frequency asymptote is upward vertical and starting from (0,0) at zero frequency. The high frequency asymptote is always a straight line with slope -1 ending in (0,0).

membrane resistance = 25) to high frequencies to the left with zero resistance. (The surface polarization condenser is short-circuiting at high frequency). Two partially overlapping semicircular arcs are seen, one for each lamella. The effect of the excess impedance is to a certain degree to blur out the distinction between the two arcs.

The plot in Fig. 10 is identical to the plot shown in Fig. 9 in [28] since the input data are the same. The latter figure was calculated by the much simpler formalism resulting when it is assumed that $K_1 = K_2 = K_s$ and $D_1^{(nm)} = D_2^{(nm)}$

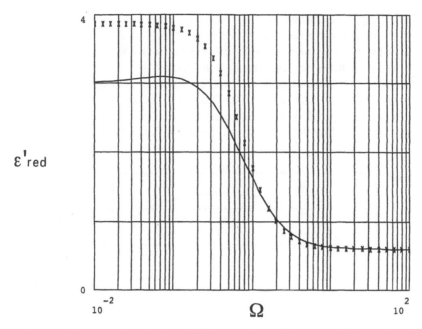

FIG. 12 The case given by Eq. (210b): equal ion diffusion coefficients in each phase, but $K_2/K_1 = 1/3$. A maximum at intermediate frequencies in the real part of the complex permittivity is seen. MWS values (xxx).

($n = 1, 2$) from the start. The example Eq. (210a) therefore constitutes a control of the more complicated and general formalism derived in this paper. The plot in Fig. 10 is also practically identical to the plot in Fig. 5 of [27]—if the resistance and reactance in that figure is divided by 500, since there were 500 bilayers in this example. In this calculation the input was the same but the additional simplifying assumption was made that all the dynamical electric double layers of the interfaces in the stack of bilayers were nonoverlapping. This seems to be a very good approximation when $\kappa_1 L_1 = \kappa_2 L_2 = 10$. In fact, the excess impedance corresponds to Fig. 7 in Sec. II.E in the present work.

The imaginary part of the dimensionless excess bilayer impedance has been plotted vs. the real part in Fig. 11. The point on the closed curve moves clockwise from (0,0) with increasing frequency. The curve runs through the first, fourth, third and second quadrant in turn, ending up again in (0,0). The result is a "lemon-shaped" figure. The magnification around (0,0) shows that the low frequency results start vertically upwards, and that the high frequency asymptote is a line with slope -1 through (0,0). Weighing with Ω, the "apple-shaped" curve of Fig. 7 appears.

In the example Eq. (210b), the diffusion coefficients are still equal for the two ions in one and the same phase. However, now the ratio K_2/K_1 is $1/3$

rather than unity. The changes brought about by such a deviation from equality of the ion distribution coefficients are most clearly seen in the real part of the effective permittivity at intermediate frequencies and in the excess impedance at low frequencies. In the former, a maximum is seen (Fig. 12). In the latter, a constant negative contribution to the excess impedance is seen in the low frequency limit, so that the "Cole–Cole plot" is similar to the "peeled lemon" shown in Fig. 13. The magnification shows, that the high frequency asymptote is still the line through zero in the second quadrant with slope -1.

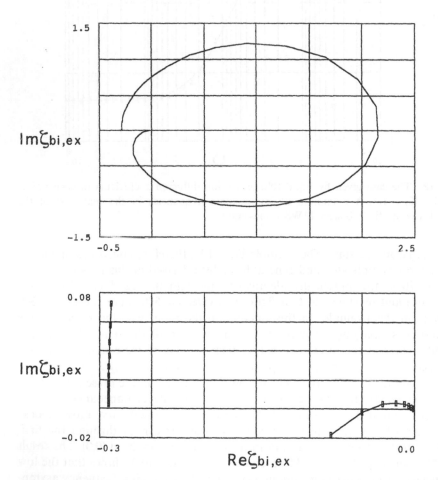

FIG. 13 Cole–Cole plot for the excess impedance taken apart in the case Eq. (210b). The same conditions as in Fig. 12. Because the Ks are different, the low frequency vertical asymptote does not start in (0,0), but in a different point on the real axis. The magnification shows that the high frequency asymptote is still a straight line with slope -1 ending in (0,0).

Weighing with Ω, the usual "apple curve" (starting and ending in the origin) reappears. However, a close inspection shows that the Ω-weighed "Cole–Cole plot" starts with a horizontal low frequency asymptote towards the left bending upwards and crossing the high frequency branch in the second quadrant, see Fig. 5 in [29]. It should be noticed that the negative excess impedance at zero frequency has as a consequence that the DC resistance of a bilayer is a little less than predicted by the MWS theory.

In the example Eq. (210c), the diffusion coefficients are different but the Ks equal. One ion diffuses four times more rapidly than the other in both phases. This case is very similar to the case Eq. (210a). The excess impedance "lemon" is a little smaller but closed (starts and ends in the origin). There is no maximum in ε''_{red} at intermediate frequencies. In example Eq. (210d) the diffusion coefficients as well as the Ks are different. The results are very similar to the case Eq. (210b): Maximum in ε''_{red} and constant, negative excess impedance at low frequencies.

In the example Eq. (210e) the parameters are as in Eq. (210d) except for the widths of the lamellae which have the same size as the Debye length in the case Eq. (210e). Figure 14 shows that the effect of excess impedance is to wipe out completely the difference between the two arcs (corresponding to each kind of lamella) in the impedance Cole–Cole plot. The DC resistance is strongly reduced by the surface polarization, too.

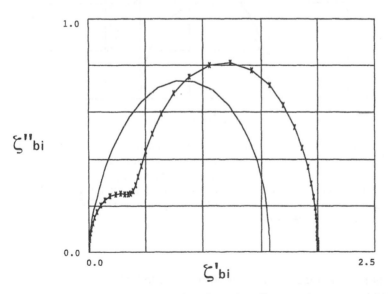

FIG. 14 Dielectric Cole–Cole plots for a lamellar membrane corresponding to case Eq. (210e) with $K_2/K_1 = 1/3$ and $\kappa_1 L_1 = \kappa_2 L_2 = 1$. The MWS values (xxx) are completely wrong in this case.

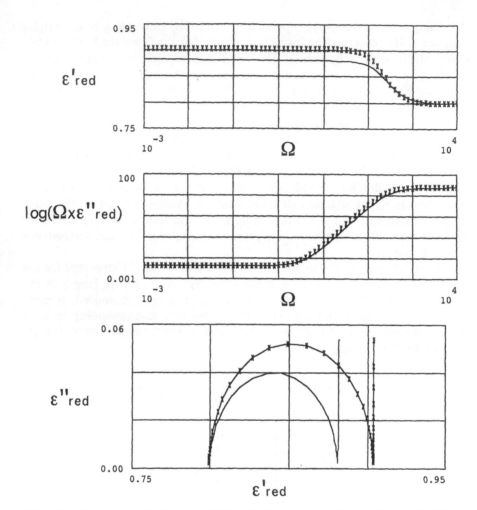

FIG. 15 Upper and middle figure: Dielectric dispersion for the model, lamellar "dense cellulose acetate" membrane with NaCl electrolyte. Lower figure: Dielectric Cole–Cole plots. MWS values (xxx). With excess impedance included and $\kappa_1 L_1 = 10$ (full line). In both cases there is complete separation between the vertical, low frequency conductivity asymptote and the semicircle of dielectric relaxation, but the MWS Cole–Cole plot differs substantially from the real Cole–Cole plot.

5. A Lamellar "Cellulose Acetate" Membrane with NaCl Electrolyte

As the final numerical example in this section, I shall consider a lamellar model of a dense cellulose acetate (CA) membrane imbibed with NaCl electrolyte. In reality, cellulose acetate membranes are phase inversion systems with water rich "alveoles" dispersed in a low conductivity/low permittivity continuous phase, see Sec. III. The lamellar structure is simpler to model without additional simplifications, however. It is therefore of interest to compare the more advanced approach given here with the more traditional approach treating membrane impedance as a parallel connection of a "geometric capacitance" and a membrane resistance. The parameters chosen correspond to the data found by a combination of emf measurements, see [42] and references given there, and hybrid models using the Trukhan theory for spherical geometry–see Sec. III and Sec. II.D. Here, the parameters will just be given without discussion (phase 1 is the water rich phase with volume fraction Φ, phase 2 is the phase with little water, ε_r is a relative permittivity, ion $1 = Na^+$ and ion $2 = Cl^-$):

$$K_s = 0.033; \quad K_1/K_2 = 1/3; \quad \varepsilon_{r,1} = 30;$$
$$\varepsilon_{r,2} = 15.7; \quad \Phi = L_1/(L_1 + L_2) = 0.20$$
$$D_1^{(1)} = 1.32 \times 10^{-9} \text{ m}^2/\text{s}; \quad D_2^{(1)} = 2.00 \times 10^{-9} \text{ m}^2/\text{s} \tag{211}$$
$$D_1^{(2)} = 1.85 \times 10^{-13} \text{ m}^2/\text{s}; \quad D_2^{(2)} = 7.40 \times 10^{-13} \text{ m}^2/\text{s}$$

In terms of the dimensionless parameters used in the present model one obtains from Eq. (211) the following dimensionless input values:

$$K_s = 0.033; \quad K_1/K_2 = 1/3; \quad L_2/L_1 = 4; \quad e = 0.723$$
$$D_1^{(1m)} = 53.9; \quad D_2^{(1m)} = 81.6; \quad D_1^{(2m)} = 7.55 \times 10^{-3} \tag{212}$$

In addition to these parameters, we have to select the value $\kappa_1 L_1$. Choosing $\kappa_1 L_1 = 10$, we obtain the curves shown in Figs. 15 and 16. In Fig. 15 it is seen that the dielectric relaxation is first taking place at quite high dimensionless frequencies. The low frequency values of ε'_{red} exhibit significant deviation from the MWS values (xxx). The MWS values for $\Omega \cdot \varepsilon''_{red}$ are correct for low as well as for high frequencies and the deviations inbetween are greater than apparent in the double logarithmic dispersion plot, which is apparent in the dielectric Cole–Cole plot. Thus, using the MWS theory to characterize a dense CA membrane would be quite erroneous. The vertical low frequency, conductivity asymptote is much more sharply separated from the semicircle of dielectric relaxation than in the examples in the previous section, because of the very low overall conductivity of the system treated here.

The upper Cole–Cole plot for the bilayer impedance in Fig. 16 seems to follow an almost perfect semicircle. The impedance Cole–Cole plot is very close to the plot calculated by the MWS procedure (crosses) in contrast to the dielectric Cole–Cole plot. The real DC dimensionless resistance ≈ 5940 is in this case somewhat *higher* than the value ≈ 5860 calculated from the MWS theory. The magnification of the high frequency region shows that there *is* another semicircle (corresponding to the aqueous phase) in analogy with the

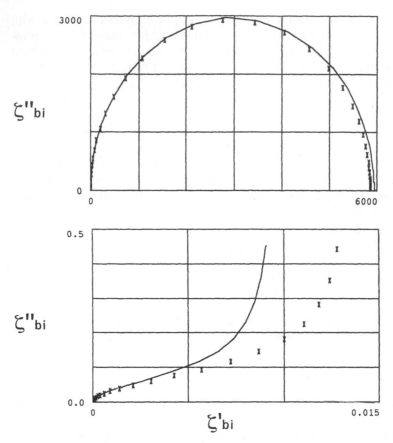

FIG. 16 The same conditions as in Fig. 15. Impedance Cole–Cole plots. Upper figure: Low frequency, semicircular relaxation corresponding to diffusional relaxation in the layer rich in cellulose acetate (=the "grand arc"). Lower figure: Magnification of the high frequency relaxation (the "petit arc") partially masked by the high frequency "tail" of the "grand arc". This relaxation corresponds to diffusional relaxation in the aqueous microphase. Total impedance at $\kappa_1 L_1 = 10$ (full line), MWS (xxx). The DC resistance (right point on the abscissa in the upper curve) is slightly lower than the MWS value.

examples in Figs. 10 and 14. However, this semicircle is very small and difficult to distinguish from the grand arc. Thus, the impedance plot is completely dominated by the phase with low conductivity as might be expected.

When the calculations are repeated for several values of $\kappa_1 L_1$ one obtains the values given in Table 1 for "big" impedance relaxation and the dielectric relaxation, and (in the cases possible) estimations of $\zeta''_{bi, max}$ and Ω_{max} for the "small" impedance relaxation. It is plausible that the "small" impedance

TABLE 1 Parameters Calculated for the Lamellar "Cellulose Acetate" Membrane

$\kappa_1 L_1$	Big impedance semicircle				Small impedance semicircle		Dielectric semicircle			
	$\zeta'_{bi}(L)$	$\zeta'_{bi,MWS}(L)$	$\zeta''_{bi,max}$	Ω_{max}	$\zeta''_{bi,max}$	Ω_{max}	$\varepsilon'_{red}(L)$	$\varepsilon'_{red}(H)$	$\varepsilon''_{red,max}$	Ω_{max}
1	623.0	586.1	310	0.00501	—	—	0.8064	0.7993	0.00340	3160
5	3011	2930	1503	0.00501	≈ 0.015	≈ 900	0.8596	0.7993	0.0292	398
10	5943	5861	2970	0.00501	≈ 0.05	≈ 450	0.8808	0.7993	0.0397	251
20	11,800	11,720	5890	0.00501	≈ 0.2	≈ 200	0.8921	0.7993	0.0459	251
50	29,390	29,300	14,668	0.00501	—	—	0.8990	0.7993	0.0497	251
100	58,700	58,610	29,300	0.00501	—	—	0.9014	0.7993	0.0509	251

L and H stands for low and high frequency, respectively. The value of $\varepsilon'_{red}(L)$ is taken at the frequency where ε''_{red} is most close to zero (corresponding to the rightmost point of the dielectric semicircle).

relaxation is the same as the dielectric relaxation observed and that the deviations in characteristic frequencies seen are due to uncertainty in estimation of the parameters for the former relaxation.

To have the sharpest distinction between the relaxation in the two phases we should have $\kappa_1 L_1 \gg 1$. The dielectric relaxation has in this case a dimensionless characteristic frequency equal to 251 and the "big" impedance relaxation has always a characteristic frequency equal to 0.00501. The ratio is $\sim 5 \times 10^4$. The inverse relaxation time for diffusion relaxation in a phase is proportional to some mean diffusion time divided by the square of the layer thickness. The geometric mean diffusion coefficients in the two phases bear a ratio $= 66.3/0.0151$ but this has to be multiplied by 16 since the CA rich layer is 4 times more thick than the aqueous layer. The ratio is then $\sim 7 \times 10^4$ which is comparable to the frequency ratio 5×10^4. Thus, the dielectric relaxation and the (almost invisible) impedance relaxation is related to the polarization in the water layer whereas the grand impedance arc is related to the polarization in the CA rich layer with low conductivity.

The model membrane can now be used to test the "equivalent circuit method" for finding the capacitance (and the effective permittivity) of the membrane. An equivalent circuit consisting of a pure resistor of resistance R in parallel with a pure capacitor of capacitance C relaxes with time constant $\tau = RC$. If the resistor and the capacitor are each made up of n bilayer resistors and capacitors of cross-sectional area A connected in series (with resistance and capacitance for each unit of area equal to R_{bi} and C_{bi}) the total resistance $R = n \cdot R_{bi}/A$ and the total capacitance is $C = A \cdot C_{bi}/n$ and the relaxation time is also given as $\tau = R_{bi} C_{bi}$. From the definition (201) one obtains:

$$
\begin{aligned}
R_{bi}(\text{ohm} \cdot \text{m}^2) &= (\kappa_1 \kappa_2)^{-3/2} (\varepsilon_1 \varepsilon_2)^{-1/2} D_m^{-1} \zeta'_{bi}(L) \\
&= (\kappa_1 \kappa_2)^{-3/2} \varepsilon_0^{-1} (15.7 \times 30)^{-1/2} D_m^{-1} \zeta'_{bi}(L) \\
&= (\kappa_1 \kappa_2)^{-3/2} \zeta'_{bi}(L)/(4.71 \times 10^{-21})
\end{aligned}
\tag{213}
$$

The time constant is found as the inverse of the angular frequency corresponding to the maximum of ζ''_{bi}, the "top point" in the grand impedance semicircle, i.e., $\tau = (1/\omega_{max})$ where ω_{max} is found from Ω_{max}. Then, C_{bi} (farad/m^2) is calculated from $C_{bi} = \tau/R_{bi}$ and the equivalent circuit value of the effective relative (static) permittivity of the membrane from $\varepsilon_r(\text{eqv}) = C_{bi} (L_1 + L_2)/\varepsilon_0$. Examples of such calculations for $\kappa_1 L_1 = 1$ and different salt concentrations are shown in Table 2.

The value calculated for $\varepsilon_r(\text{eqv})$ by the equivalent circuit method is constant in all cases at the fixed value of $\kappa_1 L_1 = 1$ as seen in Table 2. Similar tables may be made for other values of $\kappa_1 L_1$, and the value of $\varepsilon_r(\text{eqv})$ is always found to be independent of concentration. The values of $\varepsilon_r(\text{eqv})$ may be expressed as reduced permittivities $\varepsilon_{red}(\text{eqv})$ by division by $\sqrt{(15.7 \cdot 30)}$ and compared to

TABLE 2 Equivalent Circuit Calculations from the Big Impedance Semicircle Taking $\kappa_1 L_1 = 1$

c_s (mol/L)	κ_1 (m^{-1})	κ_2 (m^{-1})	$(L_1 + L_2)$ (nm)	ω_{max} (Hz)	R_{bi} (ohm·m^2)	C_{bi} (farad·m^{-2})	ε_r(eqv)
10^{-4}	3.65×10^8	9.18×10^7	13.69	4.11×10^3	2.16×10^{-2}	1.127×10^{-2}	17.44
10^{-3}	1.155×10^9	2.90×10^8	4.33	4.11×10^4	6.82×10^{-4}	3.57×10^{-2}	17.43
10^{-2}	3.65×10^9	9.18×10^8	1.369	4.11×10^5	2.16×10^{-5}	1.127×10^{-1}	17.43
10^{-1}	1.155×10^{10}	2.90×10^9	0.433	4.11×10^6	6.82×10^{-7}	3.57×10^{-1}	17.43

The value of $\Omega_{max} = 0.00501$ and the value of $\zeta'_{bi}(L) = 623$ in all cases.

TABLE 3 Equivalent Circuit Parameters and Comparison of $\varepsilon_{red}(eqv)$ with $\varepsilon'_{red}(L)$

$\kappa_1 L_1$	$(L_1 + L_2)$ (nm) (at 10^{-4} mol/L)	R_{bi} (ohm·m^2) (at 10^{-4} mol/L)	C_{bi} (farad·m^{-2}) (at 10^{-4} mol/L)	$\varepsilon_r(eqv)$	$\varepsilon_{red}(eqv)$	$\varepsilon'_{red}(L)$
					(at all concentrations)	
1	13.69	2.16×10^{-2}	1.127×10^{-2}	17.43	0.803	0.806
5	68.4	1.042×10^{-1}	2.33×10^{-3}	18.03	0.831	0.860
10	136.9	2.056×10^{-1}	1.182×10^{-3}	18.28	0.842	0.881
20	274	4.08×10^{-1}	5.95×10^{-4}	18.40	0.848	0.892
50	684	1.017×10^{0}	2.39×10^{-4}	18.48	0.851	0.899
100	1369	2.031×10^{0}	1.196×10^{-4}	18.50	0.853	0.901

The maximum dimensionless frequency is $\Omega_{max} = 0.00501$ in all cases. At a salt concentration c_s (mol/L) the values of $(L_1 + L_2)$ has to be multiplied by $(10^{-4}/c_s)^{1/2}$, the values of R_{bi} by $(10^{-4}/c_s)^{3/2}$ and the values of C_{bi} by $(c_s/10^{-4})^{1/2}$ (at fixed $\kappa_1 L_1$).

the directly "observed" values of $\varepsilon'_{red}(L)$ from Table 1. The calculations are summarized in Table 3.

It is apparent from Table 3 that the value of $\varepsilon_{red}(eqv)$ and of $\varepsilon'_{red}(L)$ are quite identical at $\kappa_1 L_1 = 1$. When $\kappa_1 L_1$ increases, both values increase asymptotically towards an upper limit which is higher for $\varepsilon'_{red}(L)$ than for $\varepsilon'_{red}(eqv)$. As identical to the MWS value, the value of the high frequency limit $\varepsilon'_{red}(H)$ is 0.799 in all cases—independent of concentration and $\kappa_1 L_1$, i.e., independent of the concentration and the dimensions of the layer, see Table 1 and Eq. (25). It is noteworthy that $\varepsilon'_{red}(eqv)$ has nothing to do with $\varepsilon'_{red}(H)$ even if the frequency at the maximum of the big impedance semicircle is many orders of magnitudes higher than the characteristic frequency for the dielectric relaxation. Nevertheless, the values of $\varepsilon'_{red}(eqv)$ *are* lower than $\varepsilon'_{red}(L)$ at fixed $\kappa_1 L_1$, and this might well reflect that $\varepsilon'_{red}(eqv)$ is in reality a kind of "mixture" between $\varepsilon'_{red}(L)$ and $\varepsilon'_{red}(H)$.

III. HYBRID MODELS FOR THE CHARACTERIZATION OF PHASE INVERSION MEMBRANES

A. RC Models Based on Donnan Equilibrium and Trukhan Theory for Spherical Geometry

As mentioned in Sec. II.F, the lamellar model is a poor model for cellulose acetate membranes. In reality, CA-membranes consist of two phases, one rich in water and one rich in CA. Like many other synthetic membranes they are cast on glass or on a support layer from a solution of polymer (CA) in solvent (acetone) with the possible admixture of a nonsolvent "swelling agent" (for example formamide), and—after a certain time of solvent evaporation—exposed to a cold water bath with possible added electrolyte. The water precipitates in a so-called "phase inversion process" leaving (on solidification) an alveolar or "foamy" structure of small water alveoles separated by "lamellae" of the phase rich in polymer. The size of the alveoles is determined by the supersaturation obtained before precipitation sets in, and this in turn depends on the concentration profile of the precipitant (water), i.e., on the relative rates with which the precipitant is diffusing into the membrane and solvent out. The latter relative rates also determine the final composition of the membrane as a point on the polymer–precipitant axis of the triangular solvent–polymer–precipitant phase diagram [43,44].

Long time evaporation of the solvent into air at a certain humidity before exposure to the quenching bath leads to a uniform microalveolar structure (dense membrane) whereas quenching after short time of evaporation leads to asymmetric membranes with a dense skin layer at the water-membrane interface and with increasing alveolar size in the direction away from this interface [44]. The alveolar structure of many membranes may be seen directly on SEM micrographs [44,45] and indirectly by the *increase in membrane capacitance* (observed by electric impedance spectroscopy) *with increasing electrolyte concentration*. This fact has been, at least partially, explained [30–33] using the model of Trukhan—see [40] and Sec. II.D—for an isolated, electrolyte containing, spherical alveole embedded in an infinite dielectric nonconductor, extending the range of validity of the Trukhan formula to higher volume fractions of alveoles by means of a Brüggemann integration [46], see Appendix A in [30].

The structure of a continuous phase with little water and low conductivity and alveoles of a water rich phase containing most of the ions has also been found in a number of ion exchange membranes by means of a variety of techniques (electron microprobe/X-ray spectroscopy, small angle X-ray and neutron scattering spectroscopy, ESR and Mössbauer spectroscopy) [47].

The model used previously [30–33] to explain the rise in the apparent permittivity (capacitance) of dense as well as asymmetric CA membranes with increasing concentration of electrolyte was based on the following assumptions:

1. The membrane may be considered to be a pure capacitor (representative of the alveolar phase) in parallel with a pure resistance (representative of the continuous phase).
2. The apparent permittivity of the capacitor may be calculated (at not too high electrolyte concentrations) by the Brüggemann integrated, low frequency limit of the Trukhan formula Eq. (131) for spherical geometry assuming equal ion diffusion coefficients in the alveolar phase. (Any intrinsic dielectric dispersion of the polymer chains or the water is neglected).

Thus, it is assumed that the ions are always in quasi-equilibrium with the oscillating electric field in each alveole.

3. The conductance of the parallel resistance may be calculated by the Nernst–Planck–Donnan expression with the choice of parameters (ion diffusion coefficients, Nernst distribution coefficients of ions and fixed charge of the membrane) restricted by the combinations of the same parameters deduced from emf studies of concentration cells with CA membranes as separators, see [42] and references therein.

Assumption (1) may be criticized on the grounds that the ascription of the resistance and the capacitance to a resistor and a capacitor in parallel appears quite ad hoc—although it is in the vein of the traditional "equivalent circuit" approach of electrochemists. We call the model presented here a "hybrid model" because it possesses some traits of a purely phenomenological equivalent circuit model, but at the same time it uses specific physical models for the description of the conductance and the capacitance involved.

Assumptions (2) and (3) may be criticized for the assumption of nonconducting alveolar walls in the Trukhan model of assumption (2) at the same time that a certain (low) conduction *is* ascribed to the lamellar phase in assumption (3). Another objection is that the two ion diffusion coefficients in the alveolar phase are usually *not* identical as assumed by Trukhan (in the spherical case). However, with the further assumption of quasi-equilibrium, the diffusion coefficients are of no importance.

For these reasons we studied the lamellar model in Sec. II.F. The price paid is a less realistic geometry, but the gain is that no "equivalent circuit" assumption is involved, that one can assume that the interfaces between the water rich and the CA rich phases are "leaky" and that one can assume that there is diffusion (with different Ds) and conduction in both phases. To generalize the lamellar model to alveoles dispersed in a continuous phase is not an easy task, however. Thus, in the present section we study the hybrid Trukhan–Brüggemann–Donnan model of phase inversion membranes.

1. Brüggemann Integration of the Trukhan Formula for Spherical Geometry and Low Frequency

The low frequency limits of Eqs. (127) and (131) are given by (1 is the alveolar phase and 2 the continuous phase; s means "static"; a is the alveole radius):

$$\beta' \equiv \{[3 + (\kappa a)^2]\tanh(\kappa a)\}/\{[2 + (\kappa a)^2]\tanh(\kappa a) - 2\kappa a\} \tag{214}$$

$$\varepsilon_{s,\,eff}/\varepsilon_{s,\,2} - 1 = 3\Phi[\varepsilon_{s,\,1} - \varepsilon_{s,\,2}(1 - \beta')]/[\varepsilon_{s,\,1} + 2\varepsilon_{s,\,2}(1 - \beta')] \tag{215}$$

Equation (215) is restricted to very low values of the volume fraction of alveoles ($\Phi \ll 1$). At higher volume fractions, it is necessary in some manner to take into account the interaction between the polarization of neighbouring alveoles. The simplest way to do this is the approximation made by Brüggemann [46].

The general idea is the following: The alveoles are introduced randomly in a large amount of the continuous phase. First $\varepsilon_{s,\,2}$ is inserted in Eq. (215) and $\varepsilon_{s,\,eff}$ is calculated. In the next step, $\varepsilon_{s,\,eff}$ is used as the "external" static permittivity instead of $\varepsilon_{s,\,2}$ and a new $\varepsilon_{s,\,eff}$ is calculated from Eq. (215). In this way an approximative value of $\varepsilon_{s,\,eff}$ at higher volume fractions may be calculated by "Brüggemann integration". The final result is (see [20] or Appendix A in [30] for details):

$$\{(\varepsilon_{s,\,1}/\varepsilon_{s,\,2}) - \eta(1 - \beta')\}/\{(\varepsilon_{s,\,1}/\varepsilon_{s,\,2}) - (1 - \beta')\} = (1 - \Phi)(\eta)^{1/3} \tag{216}$$

$$\eta = \varepsilon_{s,\,eff}/\varepsilon_{s,\,2} \tag{217}$$

The value of η (and then $\varepsilon_{s,\,eff}$) can be found from Eq. (216) with a few iterations knowing $\varepsilon_{s,\,1}/\varepsilon_{s,\,2}$, Φ and κa. The first guess of η on the r.h.s. of Eq. (216) may be taken as the uncorrected Trukhan value, for example. The Brüggemann method should be valid up to volume fractions of randomly distributed spheres as high as 0.5. For example, Eq. (216) is in accordance with experimental results for water-in-oil emulsions, see Fig. 46, p. 427, in the paper of Hanai [20].

When the effective static permittivity has been calculated, the membrane capacitance (C_m) is calculated from

$$C_m = (A\varepsilon_{s,\,eff}/L) \tag{218}$$

where A is the cross-sectional area and L the width of the membrane.

2. Conductance of the Membrane by Nernst–Planck–Donnan Theory

The membrane may have a fixed charge and/or the individual ion distribution coefficients may differ. In cellulose acetate membranes there is a small, but significant, fixed charge from dissociated glucuronic acid groups formed by oxidation of the primary alcohol groups in the original cellulose material [48]. The equilibrium distribution of ions (membrane/external solution) is then determined by finding the single, real and positive root to a "Donnan polynomial", the structure of which is determined by the valencies of the ions in the mixture. This is explained in Chapter 10 of the present book and in the references cited therein [42]. In many synthetic membranes, it is necessary to account for the presence of fast H^+ ions (or OH^- ions depending on the pH) in addition to the ions of the electrolyte under study. In the paper of Malmgren-Hansen, Sørensen, Jensen and Hennenberg [30] the impedance of dense cellulose acetate membranes was studied at varying NaCl concentrations mostly at pH $= 5$ (fixed by addition of HCl). Combining the Donnan distribution of ions with the Nernst–Planck equations, one obtains the simplest possible expression for the specific conductivity (σ) of the membrane. In the case mentioned, one has for the conductance (G_m) of the membrane (the fixed charge equivalent concentration, c_q, has been assumed nonvanishing):

$$G_m = 1/R_m = (A/L)\sigma = (A/L)D_{Cl}c_q(F^2/RT)$$
$$\times \{(c_{m,\,Cl}/c_q) + (D_{Na}/D_{Cl})(c_{m,\,Na}/c_q) + (D_H/D_{Cl})(c_{m,\,H}/c_q)\} \quad (219)$$

The concentration $c_{m,\,Cl}$ is the overall molar concentration in the membrane of the chloride ions, and so on. The concentration c_q is the molar concentration of (negative) glucuronic acid groups. Equation (219) is written so to express the conductance as far as possible in terms of parameters already estimated from emf measurements. The concentration ratios in Eq. (219) can be calculated from (see [30], Appendix B):

$$(c_{m,\,Cl}/c_q) = (K_{NaCl}/c_q)c_{Cl}\,\xi^{-1}; \quad (c_{m,\,Na}/c_q) = (K_{NaCl}/c_q)c_{Na}\,\xi \qquad (220a)$$
$$(c_{m,\,H}/c_q) = 1 + (c_{m,\,Cl}/c_q) - (c_{m,\,Na}/c_q)(\text{electroneutrality}) \qquad (220b)$$

K_{NaCl} is the Nernst distribution coefficient for NaCl (membrane/external). The parameter combination (K_{NaCl}/c_q) is evaluable from emf experiments. The concentrations c_{Na} and c_{Cl} are concentrations in the *external* solution. The Donnan parameter (ξ) is the positive root to a Donnan polynomial—being of second order since the maximum difference between the valencies of the ions is 2:

$$[1 + (c_H/c_{Na})(K_{HCl}/K_{NaCl})^2]\xi^2 - [1/c^*]\xi - [1 + (c_H/c_{Na})] = 0 \qquad (221)$$
$$c^* \equiv c_{Na}(K_{NaCl}/c_q) \qquad (222)$$

Since (K_{NaCl}/c_q), $(K_{HCl}/K_{NaCl})^2$, (D_{Na}/D_{Cl}) and D_H/D_{Cl} can be found fitting the model to emf experiments, the membrane conductivity can be fitted to data adjusting the parameter combination $D_{Cl}c_q$, see Eq. (219).

3. Hybrid RC Model of Membrane

The impedance data are fitted to the "Cole–Cole expression"

$$Z_m^* = R_m/[1 + (i\omega\tau)^\alpha]; \quad \tau \equiv R_m C_m; \quad \alpha \le 1 \qquad (223)$$

In a "Cole–Cole plot" of $-\mathrm{Im}(Z^*)$ vs. $\mathrm{Re}(Z^*)$, (223) represents a "sunken semicircle". If $\alpha = 1$, the center of this semicircle is situated on the $\mathrm{Re}(Z^*)$ − axis, but for $\alpha < 1$ the center is below. The case $\alpha = 1$ is the case of a resistor R_m in parallel with a capacitor C_m. There is no really good theory concerning the α-exponent, but presumably it has something to do with a distribution over different values of the time constant (τ). Values of α less than 1 are commonplace in heterogeneous materials, synthetic as well as biologic [10]. The mean time constant (and from this the "geometric capacitance" C_m) is found from the frequency at the "top point" of the semicircle, where $\omega\tau = 1$. It is most easy to fit the Cole–Cole semicircle using the *admittance*:

$$Y_m^* \equiv 1/Z_m^* \qquad (224)$$

One obtains:

$$\text{Re}(Y_m) = G_m\{1 + (\omega\tau)^\alpha \cos(\alpha\pi/2)\}; \quad \text{Im}(Y_m) = G_m(\omega\tau)^\alpha \cos(\alpha\pi/2) \tag{225}$$

Plotting the logarithm of $\text{Im}(Y_m)$ vs. the logarithm of ω, the slope is α. The intercept is

$$\ln G_m + \alpha \ln \tau + \ln \cos(\alpha\pi/2)$$

G_m is the low frequency limit of $\text{Re}(Y_m)$ and τ may thus be found from the intercept. It is clear that τ is independent of the membrane thickness or area, since the factor A/L cancels in the product $R_m C_m$.

B. Experimental Studies of Desalination Membranes, Mostly of Cellulose Acetate (CA)

1. Impedance of Dense and Asymmetric CA Membranes and a Two-Layer Composite Membrane

In 1989 [30], I published the results of impedance measurements on a number of dense and asymmetric cellulose acetate (CA) membranes together with three colleagues, two Danish and one Belgian. The membranes were cast by ourselves. The method used was four electrode impedance spectroscopy (two current electrodes and two voltage electrodes). The measurements were performed using a Solartron 1250 Frequency Response Analyzer in combination with an external potentiostat designed to maintain a prescribed voltage oscillation by regulating the current. Two potentiostats were used: A Solartron 1286 Electrochemical Interface (input impedance > 10 GΩ) and a potentiostat made by our order in a small Danish electronics firm (Ring Instruments, input impedance > 1 TΩ). Three types of reference (voltage) electrodes were used: Gold plated net of stainless steel or "tip electrodes" made of Pt or Ag with AgCl$^-$ coating. The current electrodes were circular silver plates coated with AgCl. The measuring cells had rapid circulation of electrolyte on both sides, laterally along the membrane surfaces to prevent polarization layers just outside these surfaces. The equipment is shown schematically in Fig. 17. Using the same membrane specimen, the measurements were reproducible to within ±7% (except at very low salt concentrations) using any combination of the above mentioned equipment. The frequency range covered was from 1 mHz to 25–65 kHz, the upper limit being determined by the potentiostat (65 kHz for 1286, 25 kHz for the Ring). In total, 150 impedance spectrograms were measured using 10 different membranes.

The temperature was 25.0°C and pH in most experiments adjusted to 5.0 using HCl. The main electrolyte was NaCl, and the concentration was the same at both sides. Mostly, only one semicircle was found in the Cole–Cole plots for dense (symmetric) as well as for asymmetric CA membranes. The

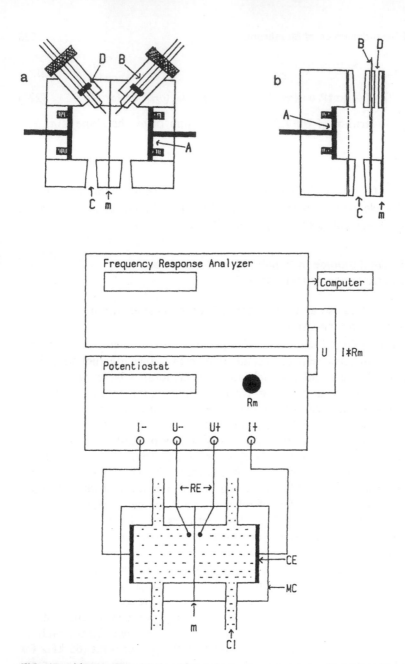

FIG. 17 Above: Two kinds of four-electrode measuring cells both with circular plate Ag/AgCl current electrodes (A). Membrane at "m". To the left, tip voltage electrodes ("B", Pt or Ag/AgCl). To the right, gold plated net reference electrode at "B". "D" = inlet for electrolyte recirculation between net electrode and membrane. Only one half cell shown. Below: Sketch of the measuring principle and the experimental set-up. The current signal is measured as a voltage over a calibration resistance (called R_m in the figure, but this is *not* the membrane resistance). *Source*: Ref. 30.

latter have a dense "skin layer" at one membrane face and a porous layer with gradually increasing size of the alveoles towards the other membrane face. For the dense membranes, the parameter α was close to or equal to unity at low electrolyte concentrations, showing some decrease with increasing electrolyte concentrations. For asymmetric membranes, the value of α was generally lower because the degree of heterogeneity (and the dispersion of time constants) is greater. The "geometric" membrane capacitance was generally of the order of some nanofarads. In two experiments with a dense membrane, a quite unstable second, low frequency arc appeared at very low electrolyte concentration (10^{-4} mol/L NaCl and 10^{-5} mol/L HCl) with a giant capacitance of the order of some millifarads. The latter is probably due to electric macropolarization of the entire membrane (and not only polarization in the alveoles). The value of α for this second arc seems very low (0.60–0.67).

(a) *Dense CA Membranes.* In Fig. 18 a sample Cole–Cole plot for a dense membrane is shown. It is seen that the tangents to the curve in the two end points are not completely vertical. Thus, we have a "sunken semicircle" with $\alpha = 0.944$. The resistance in the low frequency end (rightmost point on the real axis) is the sum of the membrane resistance and the electrolyte resistances between the voltage electrodes and the membrane surfaces. The latter resistance is the resistance corresponding to the leftmost point on the real axis. The experiments were subtracted "blind experiments" without membrane but with the same electrolyte, however. Thus, the membrane resistance is the indicated 31.6 kΩ. From the frequency in the top point, a "geometric" capacitance of 2.45 nF is calculated.

Varying the bathing concentration of NaCl, the values of R_m and C_m vary, too. In Figs. 19 and 20 these variations are shown. Figure 19 shows that the resistance increases with decreasing NaCl concentration down to a concentration of ~ 0.005 mol/L. At lower concentrations, the resistance increases again. It must be remembered that the HCl concentration is constant (10^{-5} mol/L). At low NaCl concentrations, the Donnan exclusion of coions (Cl^- ions) is strong, and a great proportion of the counterions become protons at low concentrations of Na^+, also for the reason that the hydrated Na^+ ion is excluded from the dense parts of the CA membrane to a much greater extent than the proton. Furthermore, the proton diffuses much faster in the CA matrix than the Na^+ ion. This is the reason for the decrease of the resistance at very low NaCl concentrations. The resistance of the various dense membranes cast by us varied considerably, but from the ones with the maximum resistance a value

$$D_{Cl} c_q = 7.5 \times 10^{-13} \ (meqv/L)(m^2/s)$$

was estimated from Eq. (219). Using estimations of c_q from various sources, the diffusion coefficient of Cl^- lies in the range $(0.8–3) \times 10^{-12} \ m^2/s$.

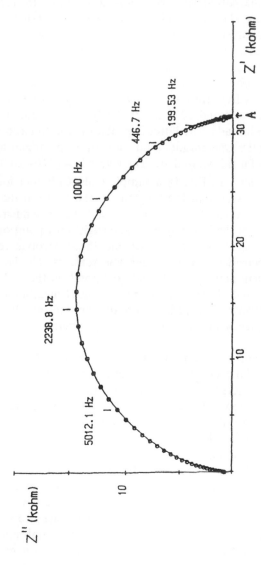

FIG. 18 Cole–Cole impedance plot for a dense cellulose acetate membrane soaked in 0.001 mol/L NaCl. Membrane DC resistance $R_m = 31.6$ kΩ and membrane capacitance $C_m = 2.45$ nF. The parameter $\alpha = 0.944$. Temperaure 25.0°C. *Source:* Ref. 30.

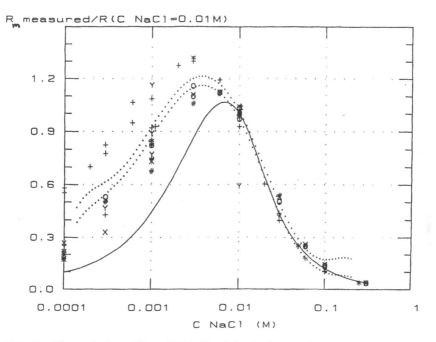

FIG. 19 The variation of R_m with NaCl concentration at temperature 25.0°C for many dense CA membranes with considerable variation from membrane to membrane of the resistance in 0.01 mol/L NaCl. Therefore, the values have been scaled with this resistance to have less scattering. The dotted curves are the limits of the uncertainty belts of fitted least square polynomial values. The solid curve is calculated from the Nernst–Planck–Donnan formulae Eqs. (219–222) with $c_q/K_{12} = 0.029$ eqv/L, $(K_{HCl}/K_{NaCl})^2 = 9.5$, $D_{Na}/D_{Cl} = 0.25$ and $D_H/D_{Cl} = 10$. *Source*: Ref. 30.

Figure 20 shows that the geometric capacitance increases (in an accelerating way) with increasing external NaCl concentration. To some extent this is explained by the Trukhan polarization of alveoles: With increasing ionic strength, the Debye length shrinks. Then the dynamical double layers (of opposite charge) shrink at opposite poles of the alveole in the field direction, producing a greater dipole moment. However, this tendency should saturate with increasing concentration and should not escalate as in the figure. When the double layers are of practically no extension, the dipole moment cannot increase more. The correction involved in the Brüggemann formula does not change this fact in any qualitative way.

Figure 21 shows how the capacitance data—reformulated as effective permittivity using $L = 33 \mu$ and $A = 4.91$ cm²—for dense membranes (inside the uncertainty belt given by the two solid curves) can be approximately fitted to the Trukhan–Brüggemann formula Eq. (216) using various combinations of

Capacity (nF)

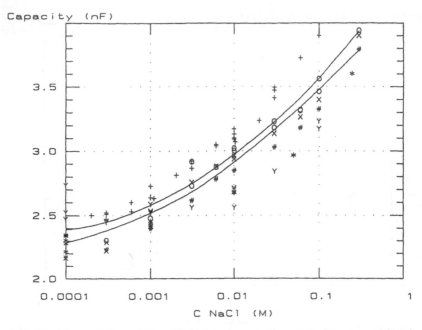

FIG. 20 The variation of C_m with NaCl concentration at temperature 25.0°C for many dense CA membranes. The uncertainty belt of the smoothed polynomial values are shown. (The values shown here are not scaled like the R_m values). *Source*: Ref. 30.

the parameters. The radius of the alveoles has been set to $a = 7$ nm in all cases. There is a considerable covariance between the rest of the parameters: the two permittivities and the volume fraction of the water rich phase, which is not easy to determine with precision, due to the increasing difficulties in evaporating water from the smaller cavities.

Some help may here be found noting that the effective, relative permittivity of the membrane practically free of ions is ~ 18. This corresponds to ~ 2.4 nF. A Taylor expansion of the expression for β' in Eq. (214) reveals that $\beta' \to (\kappa a)^2/5 \to 0$ when the ion concentration tends towards zero. The "ion free" version of Eq. (216) is therefore (subscript r stands for *relative*, static permittivity):

$$(1 - \Phi) = (18/\varepsilon_{r,2})^{-1/3}\{(\varepsilon_{r,1}/\varepsilon_{r,2}) - (18/\varepsilon_{r,2})\}/\{(\varepsilon_{r,1}/\varepsilon_{r,2}) - 1\} \qquad (226)$$

Thus, introducing a value for the relative permittivity of the continuous phase ($\varepsilon_{r,2}$) and a value for the relative permittivity of the alveolar phase ($\varepsilon_{r,1}$) we may calculate the corresponding volume fraction of the alveolar (water rich) phase. In case of large alveoles which are almost free of CA chains we may put $\varepsilon_{r,1} = 78.3$ at 25°C. For small alveoles partially penetrated by CA chains, the water is much more restricted and we might have $\varepsilon_{r,1} = 30$ or

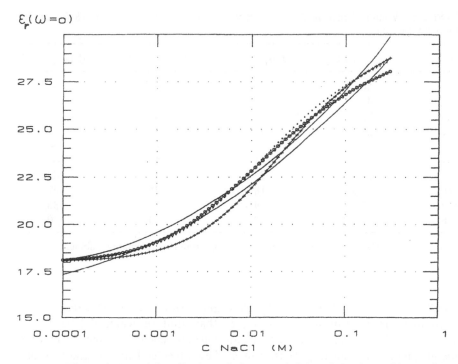

FIG. 21 The variation of the effective, relative permittivity of the dense CA membrane (calculated from C_m) with NaCl concentration—inside the polynomial uncertainty belt delimited by the solid curves—compared to various Trukhan–Brüggemann fits at a constant radius of the alveoles, $a = 7.0$ nm. Dots: $\varepsilon_{s,1} = 30.0$, $\varepsilon_{s,2} = 15.7$, $\Phi = 0.20$; OOO: $\varepsilon_{s,1} = 19.0$, $\varepsilon_{s,2} = 17.8$, $\Phi = 0.16$; $+ + +$: $\varepsilon_{s,1} = 78.3$, $\varepsilon_{s,2} = 6.05$, $\Phi = 0.42$. *Source*: Ref. 30.

perhaps even $\varepsilon_{r,1} = 25$ or 20. For these four choices of $\varepsilon_{r,1}$ and various values of $\varepsilon_{r,2}$, the values of Φ are shown in Table 4.

Various methods of the determination of water content lead to values between 0.083 and 0.17 for Φ, with the higher values being more likely, see the discussion in [32] p. 207. Even if "inextractable" water should bring up the volume fraction of the alveolar phase to 0.20, a quick glance on Table 4 shows that $\varepsilon_{r,2}$ (the relative permittivity of the "water poor" continuous phase) is then limited to the range 12–18. Published values of ε_r for dry cellulose esters are in the range 2–6 (see [48] p. 44). This must mean that even the "water poor" continuous phase has some admixture of water, increasing the relative permittivity.

(b) Asymmetric CA Membranes. In Fig. 22, the effective relative, static permittivities for an asymmetric CA membrane is shown as a function of the

TABLE 4 Volume Fraction (%) of Alveoles Corresponding to $\varepsilon_{r,\,eff} = 18$ for an Ion Free CA Membrane

$\varepsilon_{r,\,2}$	$\Phi\ (\varepsilon_{r,\,1} = 78.3)$	$\Phi\ (\varepsilon_{r,\,1} = 30)$	$\Phi\ (\varepsilon_{r,\,1} = 25)$	$\Phi\ (\varepsilon_{r,\,1} = 20)$
3	56	—	—	—
6	42	65	—	—
10	28	51	62	—
12	21	42	53	—
13	17	37	48	—
14	14	31	42	—
15	10.4	25	34	62
16	6.9	18	25	52
17	3.5	9.4	14	35
18	0	0	0	0

Volume fractions above 65% have been excluded (Brüggemann approximation dubious).

NaCl concentration ($L = 55\ \mu$). The first impression is that these relative permittivities are enormous—much higher than that of water (78.3)! This is explainable by the large size of the microheterogeneities (alveoles) in those membranes. The electric polarization in these alveoles leads to giant dipoles. The charge displacement length is the higher the higher the concentration, since the dynamical electric double layers then crowd up at opposite interfaces in the direction of the field. Therefore, a dramatic increase in the effective permittivity with increasing salt concentration is seen. There is no difference between the results before heat treatment of the membrane ($\bigcirc$) and after (15X). Heat treatment only has an effect on the skin layer. But the dielectric properties are exclusively determined by the "foamy" part of the membrane, which is the main part. The sample calculations using the Trukhan–Brüggemann theory shows that this theory (as mentioned before) has difficulties in explaining the sharp rise in the effective permittivity. Rather, the theory predicts a leveling out at high concentrations, when a given value of the alveolar radius (a) is used. In Fig. 22 the model radii have been chosen as 0.1, 0.2 and 0.3 μ. These radii correspond well to the electron micrographs in Figs. 6d and 6e in [45].

One explanation of the behavior observed might be that the membrane is a "fractal structure" of all different sizes of alveoles. When we start with very low electrolyte concentration (low κ), the values of κa become significant for the biggest alveoles. When the polarization in these alveoles saturates with increasing κ, smaller alveoles begin to contribute and so on. The smaller the alveoles the more there are (perhaps to a certain limit). This explains the accelerating rise in the effective permittivity. Another reason might be that the

$\varepsilon_r(\omega=0)$

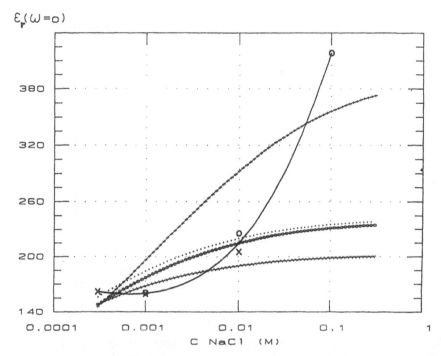

C NaCl (M)

FIG. 22 Very large effective, relative permittivities of an asymmetric CA membrane as a function of the NaCl concentration at 25.0°C. Curve with positive curvature: experimental points, ○ before annealing, X after annealing. The curves with downward curvature are calculated from Trukhan–Brüggemann theory with the fixed value $\varepsilon_{s,1} = 78.3$ and different sets of the other parameters. Dots: $\varepsilon_{s,2} = 50.0$, $a = 0.2$ μm, $\Phi = 0.41$; $+++$: $\varepsilon_{s,2} = 50.0$, $a = 0.1$ μm, $\Phi = 0.50$; ○○○: $\varepsilon_{s,2} = 30.0$, $a = 0.2$ μm, $\Phi = 0.50$; Y: $\varepsilon_{s,2} = 25.3$, $a = 0.3$ μm, $\Phi = 0.50$. Source: Ref. 30.

increase in salt concentration causes an increasing "contamination" of the surroundings of an alveole with ions. Thus, the effective sizes of the alveoles increases with concentration, and so their dipole moments.

Figure 23 shows the membrane resistance R_m as a function of the concentration for the same asymmetric membrane. Heat treatment (also called "annealing") of the membrane definitively increases the membrane resistance as seen in the figure. The membrane was "annealed" in water at 75°C in 2 min. Such a thermal curing is used in the membrane technology to close partially the narrow pores in the skin layer and to strike a compromise between high salt rejection and not too low water permeability, see Figs. 3–6 in [48]. The skin layer has a thickness of 1 μ or below but since it is dense, the main part of the resistance is found in this layer.

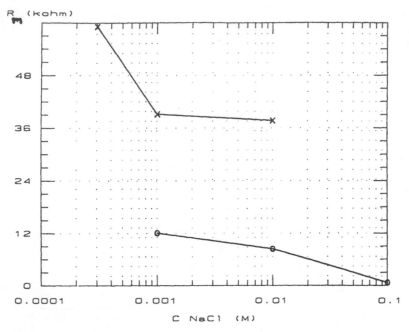

FIG. 23 The resistance of the same asymmetric membrane as in Fig. 22 as a function of NaCl concentration at 25.0°C, ○ before annealing, X after annealing. *Source*: Ref. 30.

(c) *Two-Layer Composite Membrane.* Finally, a commercial (Fluid Systems) composite membrane was investigated. This membrane is designed for one-step reverse osmosis desalination of sea water. (In contrast, CA membranes can only be used for one-step desalination of brackish water). The skin layer of the composite membrane was most probably polyether/urea and the support layer polysulfone. Figure 24 shows a Cole–Cole impedance plot with two partially overlapping "sunken semicircles" at a NaCl concentration of 0.001 mol/L and pH = 5. The parameters fitted for this and other experiments are shown in Table 5.

It should be noticed that the membrane does not seem to attain perfect equilibrium with the bath in all measurements, compare the first and the last measurement, both at a concentration 0.001 mol/L. The arc with subscript 1 is the high frequency arc (grand arc) and the one with subscript 2 the low frequency arc (petit arc). The grand arc has a capacitance about 0.4 nF and the petit arc a capacitance about 20 nF, i.e., $C_2/C_1 \approx 50$. As a first approximation we assume that the two capacitances represent the overall polarization in each layer treated as a capacitor, and that the effective permittivities in the two layers are the same. Then the thickness of layer 2 should be 1/50 of the thick-

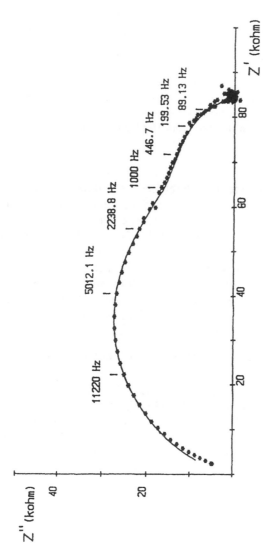

FIG. 24 Cole–Cole impedance plot for a two-layer composite membrane for sea water desalination. Electrolyte: 0.001 mol/L NaCl at pH = 5 (adjusted with HCl). The solid curve is a series combination of two RC circuits. The pameters of the Cole–Cole expressions are: $R_1 = 66$ kΩ, $C_1 = 0.37$ nF, $\alpha_1 = 0.85$; $R_2 = 18.3$ kΩ, $C_1 = 27$ nF, $\alpha_2 = 0.88$. *Source*: Ref. 30.

TABLE 5 Best Fits for Cole–Cole Plots of a Two-Layer Composite Sea Water Desalination Membrane

Sequence (1 first)	c_{NaCl} (mol/L)	R_1 (kΩ)	C_1 (nF)	α_1	R_2 (kΩ)	C_2 (nF)	α_2	C_2/C_1
3	0.0003	109	0.37	0.84	45	20	0.87	54
1	0.001	42	0.37	0.68	26.5	11	0.85	30
4	0.001	66	0.37	0.85	18.3	27	0.88	73
2	0.01	4.75	0.47	0.76	2.6	16	0.78	34

The concentration of HCl $= 10^{-5}$ in all experiments. Membrane thickness 120 μ.
Source: Ref. 30.

ness of layer 1. With a total membrane thickness equal to 120 μ, layer 2 should be 2.3 μ in width. According to [49], p. 665, the thickness of the skin layer should be about 0.2–0.5 μ in typical composite membranes, however. This could be so, were $\varepsilon_{eff, 2}/\varepsilon_{eff, 1} = 0.083$ to 0.21. That might be the case, if the skin layer (2) were a hydrophobic layer with very low permittivity and the polysulfone layer (1) a layer with high effective permittivity, due to either alveoles or high, orientable dipole moments. Both might be the case. In Fig. 15d in [49] an electron micrograph is shown of a polysulfone supporting layer presumably very like the one in the membrane investigated here. The largest alveoles appearing in the micrograph have a size about 1 μ.

2. Impedance of Dense CA Membranes in NaCl and KCl Solutions and Different pH

In 1994 [33], Plesner, Malmgren-Hansen and Sørensen published another study using dense CA membranes only. This time, however, NaCl as well as KCl solutions were used and pH was varied from 1 to 6. The measuring cells were as in the 1989 study (the type with tip electrodes as voltage electrodes, Pt or Ag/AgCl). The Solartron 1250 + potentiostat was replaced by a Schlumberger SI 1260 Impedance/Gain-Phase Analyzer with a frequency range of 1 μHz to 32 MHz. The much broader range of frequencies and the fact that no external potentiostat is necessary with this equipment is a major advantage compared with the earlier equipment.

The reason why measurements with NaCl and KCl were compared is to be found in a statement by Wiggins and van Ryn [50] that KCl (and CsCl) behaved quite differently from other salts (like NaCl) with respect to their distribution between membrane and bathing solution. These authors used copolyoxamide/cellulose acetate membranes as model systems for biological membranes with reference to their mixed hydrophobic/hydrophilic surface properties. At low external concentrations, KCl and CsCl should have apparent distribution coefficients (membrane/external) much larger than unity, decreasing with increasing external concentration. Other alkali metal salts have apparent distribution coefficients less than unity at low concentrations. Based on these results, and on an interpretation of the properties that they surmised were conferred by K^+ on the water inside the membrane, qualitative models for the mechanisms of active transport of ions, for Na–K–ATPase and Ca–ATPase from the sarcoplasmic reticulum have been proposed, see the papers by Wiggins et al. cited in [33]. We were puzzled by these findings, since we had only observed small quantitative differences between the behavior of NaCl and KCl in emf experiments with concentration cells with CA membranes as a separator, see Chapter 10 and references therein [42]. Thus, we decided to carry out very precise measurements of impedance with NaCl and KCl at various pH. Even if these experiments turned out negatively with respect to the postulated differences between the K^+ and the Na^+ ions (there are no qualitative differences) the experiments were most useful for an increased understanding of alkali chlorides in dense CA membranes.

(a) *Membrane Resistance as a Function of Salt Concentration and pH.* Figure 25 shows the membrane resistance as a function of the concentration of NaCl at the pH values 6, 5, 4, 3, 2 and 1. The data points represent averages of repeated measurements on the same dense CA membrane or averages of measurements on different membrane species. Except at the two lowest pH values, the curves have the same "bell shape" as discussed earlier. However, the resistance data were much more uniform between the samples than in the 1989 study, and it was not necessary to scale the values such as was done in Fig. 19. Furthermore, the theoretical resistance curves (solid curves) are fitting much better than in Fig. 19 at the lower NaCl concentrations. This is due to the realization of *two* new features:

1. The titration of the fixed charge (COO$^-$ groups) by the H^+ ions was explicitly taken into account in the Donnan equilibrium. This leads to a third-order Donnan polynomial instead of the second-order polynomial (221), for details see [33]:

$$(K_{HCl}/K_{NaCl})[1 + (c_H/c_{Na})(K_{HCl}/K_{NaCl})^2][c_H/K_a^*]\xi^3$$
$$+ [1 + (c_H/c_{Na})(K_{HCl}/K_{NaCl})^2]\xi^2$$
$$- [\{c_q^0/(K_{NaCl}\,c_{Na})\} + \{(K_{HCl}/K_{NaCl})(c_{Cl}/c_{Na})c_H/K_a^*\}]\xi - (c_{Cl}/c_{Na}) = 0$$
$$(227)$$

The root ξ to be used is the (only) real and positive root of (227). The new parameters are the completely dissociated equivalent concentration of negative charges (c_q^0) and the modified *dissociation constant* for the glucuronic acid (K_a is the acid strength constant in the membraneous ambience):

$$K_a^* = K_a/K_{HCl} \qquad (228)$$

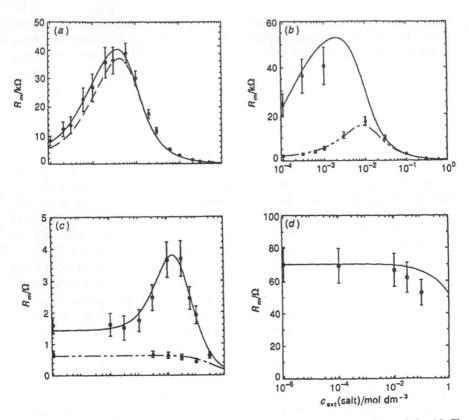

FIG. 25 Resistance of dense cellulose acetate membranes as a function of the NaCl concentration at 25°C and at various pH values (addition of HCl): (a) pH = 5. (b) pH = 6 (upper curve); pH = 4 (lower curve). (c) pH = 3 (upper curve); pH = 2 (lower curve). (d) pH = 1. The data points represent the average of unscaled resistances taken from 187 individual impedance spectra on many membrane samples. The curves are calculated from the Nernst–Planck–Donnan theory taking account of the dissociation of the glucuronic acid groups. All curves were calculated using the same "global" values of the parameters using $D_H/D_{Cl} = 40$ (see the text), except the full curve in (a) where $D_H/D_{Cl} = 29$. The other parameters are as given in Table 6. The, fully dissociated, fixed (negative) charge is $c_q^o = 7 \times 10^{-4}$ eqv/L total membrane volume. *Source*: Ref. 33.

2. It was realized that the ratio of diffusion constants $D_H/D_{Cl} = 10$ which had been used in the fitting of all earlier emf experiments could never explain the impedance behavior at the lower values of pH. The ratio rather have to be ~ 40. The emf measurements were performed at pH values 4–6 and most measurements were done at pH = 5. With $D_H/D_{Cl} = 10$ or $D_H/D_{Cl} =$

40, the fit could be made equally well adjusting the parameter K_{HCl}/K_{NaCl}, see the discussion in Chapter 10 [42]. Concentration cell emf data with HCl were also measured, but because the transference number of the proton is very close to unity, it is not easy to distinguish if the ratio is 10 or 40.

Thus, it can now be stated, that the proton diffuses 40 times more rapidly than the Cl^- ion in dense CA membranes. Since $D_{Na}/D_{Cl} = 0.25$ from the emf measurements (unaffected by the choice of the ratio 10 or 40), the proton diffuses 160 times faster than the Na^+ ion in dense cellulose acetate!

Figure 26 shows the same dependence on the salt concentration of the membrane resistance for the averages over many membranes membrane speci-

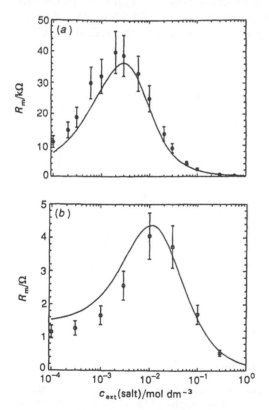

FIG. 26 Resistance of dense cellulose acetate membranes in equilibrium with KCl/HCl solutions as a function of the KCl concentration at 25°C. (a) pH = 5. (b) pH = 3. The data points are pooled from many experiments as in Fig. 25. The parameters are as given in Table 6. $c_q^o = 7 \times 10^{-4}$ eqv/L. *Source*: Ref. 33.

men at pH = 5 and 3. However, now the electrolyte is KCl rather than NaCl. Compared to the NaCl data, there are only small and insignificant differences as also shown in the Fig. 27 with measurements on a single membrane specimen at pH 5. This finding contradicts the postulates of Wiggins and van Ryn [50], that the K^+ ions should behave specially.

In [33] the derivation of the expression for R_m was also performed in a more refined way than in [30], taking explicitly into account the distribution of the ions between the alveolar phase and the continuous phase and that all the diffusion resistance is in the continuous phase. However, with simple redefinitions of the symbols, the result is as before.

In Table 6, the parameters fitted globally to all the data of R_m vs. c_{Na} and pH (using a nonlinear bivariate, least squares analysis) are shown together with the standard deviations of these parameters.

(b)　*The Capacitance as a Function of Concentration.* Figure 28 shows how the capacitance grows with increasing concentration of KCl at pH = 5 and 3. Only data up to 0.1 mol/L were used in fitting the theoretical Trukhan–

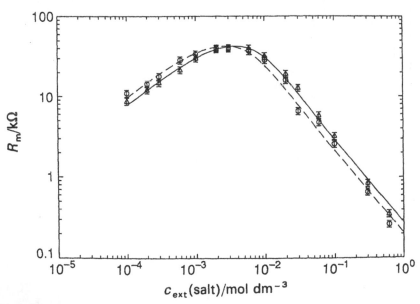

FIG. 27 Comparison of membrane resistance values for a single, dense CA membrane in NaCl (△) and (○) solutions at pH = 5. The lengths of the error bars are 2 × SD. The curves are the best fitting curves of the improved Nernst–Planck–Donnan theory, NaCl (——) and KCl (- - -). For NaCl: $K_{NaCl} = 0.031$; $(K_{HCl}/K_{NaCl})^2 = 0.74$; $D_{Na}/D_{Cl} = 0.25$. For KCl: $K_{KCl} = 0.041$; $(K_{HCl}/K_{KCl})^2 = 0.52$; $D_K/D_{Cl} = 0.25$. Common parameters: $D_H/D_{Cl} = 40$ and $c_q^o = 7 \times 10^{-4}$ eqv/L. *Source*: Ref. 33.

TABLE 6 Parameter Values ($\pm$SD) Obtained Considering all Membrane Resistance Data

Electrolyte	K_{NaCl}	K_{HCl}	K_a (mol/L)	D_{Cl} (m^2/s)	D_{Na}/D_{Cl}	D_H/D_{Cl}
NaCl/HCl	[0.034]	0.037 ± 0.009	$(6.3 \pm 0.2) \times 10^{-5}$	$(1.70 \pm 0.13) \times 10^{-12}$	[0.25]	40 ± 5
KCl/HCl	0.043 ± 0.002	[0.037]	$[6.3 \times 10^{-5}]$	$[1.70 \times 10^{-12}]$	[0.28]	[40]

A value in square bracket has been set to that value: literature value for K_{NaCl}; fit to emf data for D_{Na}/D_{Cl} or D_H/D_{Cl}; transfer of parameters from NaCl to KCl measurements. K_a is based on total membrane volume; the value based on pore volume is 3.7×10^{-4} ($\Phi = 0.17$).

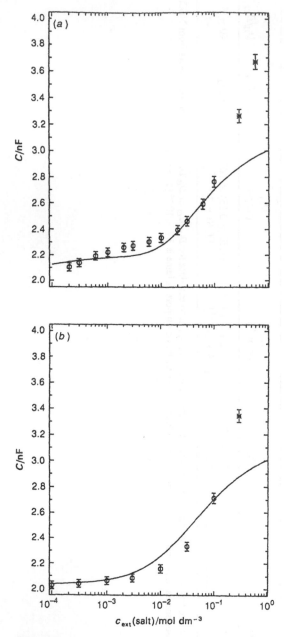

FIG. 28 The "geometric" membrane capacitance, C_m, for dense CA membranes in equilibrium with KCl/HCl solutions at 25°C as a function of KCl concentration at (a) pH = 5 and (b) pH = 3. The curves represent Trukhan–Brüggemann fits to the data with KCl concentrations less than 0.1 mol/L. Parameters, see Table 7. *Source*: Ref. 33.

TABLE 7 Parameter Values ($\pm$ SD) obtained Considering all Membrane Capacitance Data

Electrolyte	Alveole radius (a) (nm)	Relative permittivity	
		matrix, $\varepsilon_{r,\,2}$	alveole, $\varepsilon_{r,\,2}$
NaCl/HCl	5.5 ± 1.0	14.8 ± 1.0	17.9 ± 7.5
KCl/HCl	7.5 ± 1.0	13.9 ± 1.0	19.9 ± 7.2

Brüggemann curves (solid curves). It is seen that the uncertainty is very small compared to the earlier study (Fig. 20). Furthermore, there is little influence of pH, and the corresponding curves for NaCl (not shown here) show that there is also little influence of whether the cation is K^+ or Na^+. These two findings are as they should be, if (1) any electric double layer in the alveoles with a fixed charge variable with pH can be linearized away in the equations of perturbance as described in Sec. II.B; (2) the diffusion of the ions in the alveoles is so fast that the ions are in Boltzmann quasi-equilibrium with the oscillating field, in order for the different diffusion coefficients of the ions *in the alveoles* to be of no importance.

Table 7 shows the best fits (up to 0.1 mol/L) for the parameters of the Trukhan–Brüggemann formula: the alveole radius (a) and the two relative permittivities. It should be noticed that in Table 2 of Ref. 33, the quantity "a" was erroneously called the "alveole diameter". The numbers stated were the radii. The value of the effective permittivity of the "ion free" membrane corresponding to (2.10 $\pm$ 0.05) nF corresponds to an effective permittivity of 15.9. The two values of the volume fraction calculated from the permittivities given in Table 7 by means of Eq. (226)—with "18" replaced by "15.9"—are $\Phi = 0.37$ (from the NaCl data) and $\Phi = 0.36$ (from the KCl data). This is considerably more than the 0.17 estimated by Demisch and Pusch [51].

IV. INTERFACIAL POLARIZATION, CONDUCTIVITY AND SLOW DIELECTRIC MODES IN POLYMER FILMS

Until now we have neglected any "intrinsic" dielectric dispersion of the membrane material. Since many membranes are made of polymers and since many polymers (with dipole moments in the backbone or in the side chains) are known to have dielectric relaxations in a broad range of frequencies [19], this is a quite crude assumption. In order to analyze the interplay between intrinsic dielectric dispersion, the influence of conductivity and the influence of interfacial polarisation, I have recently in collaboration with Spanish colleagues (Ricardo Diaz-Calleja from Valencia Polytechnics, Evaristo Riande and Julio

Guzman from Polymer Institute, Madrid, Vicente Compañ and Andreu
Andrio from the University of Castellón) studied the dielectric dispersion of
"dry" films made of some selected, amorphous polymers containing traces of
conductive ions. These studies proved to be a very good illustration of the
theoretic principles put forward in the Sec. II.A–C. Furthermore, dielectric
spectroscopy of such polymer films may evolve into an important, nondestructive tool for the penetration of the human mind into the physical structure of
"soft materials".

Since it is notorious that many electrochemists and membrane scientists
neglect intrinsic dielectric relaxation, and since the field of polymer relaxations
is a world apart inside physics, I have found it expedient to start this with a
short survey of some of the most important features of amorphous polymers.
This might be a help to the unarmed reader (and a nuisance to the "know-
all"!).

A. Free Volume Theory, Glass–Rubber Relaxation and Diffusion

One of the most important characteristics, in physics as well as in technology,
of amorphous polymers is the so-called "glass transition". The "glass transition temperature" (T_g)—below which temperature the material becomes hard
and brittle—is not a thermodynamic transition temperature, but a dynamic
one, depending for example of the rate of cooling or heating or the frequency
of deformation. For example for poly(n-butyl)methacrylate, the value of T_g
found by differential scanning calorimetry (DSC) changed from 16.6 to 22.3°C
when the rate of heating varied from 0.5 to 20°C/min. ([52] Table 1)

Indeed, it is much more precise to talk about a "glass–rubber relaxation"—
easily visible as quite dominant dispersions with frequency of, e.g., the complex
Young's modulus or the complex permittivity. The position of the "loss
peaks" is a function of the temperature. Alternatively, one may work at a fixed
frequency ("isochronous" measurements) and measure the complex moduli as
a function of temperature. The maxima of the loss or the loss tangent indicate
the "dynamic transitions". Changing the frequency, the "transition
temperature" (loss peak maximum) changes. Viscoelastic and dielectric relaxations in polymers may often be treated in a parallel way [19], although
dielectric relaxations are not found in all amorphous polymers but only in
polymers with favorably oriented dipoles. Important source books of information on polymer relaxations are still the, not very recent, monographs by
McCrum, Read and Williams [19], Ferry [53] and de Gennes [54]. The information in this section is mainly a summary of the first two of these monographs.

In amorphous polymers, the relaxations are often classified as α-, β-, γ-
relaxations and sometimes δ-relaxations in the order of *decreasing* peak temperature in isochronous maps (or in the order of *increasing* peak frequency in

isothermal measurements). [It should be noticed that this classification of the polymer scientists has nothing to do with the α-, β-, γ-classification used in the subsequent chapter by Coster and Chilcott [38]. They use the classification introduced by Schwan [55] in the description of biological systems and artificial membranes permeated by ionic solutions].

The broad α-peak is related to the glass–rubber transition which is connected with the "freezing" or "thawing" of the "micro-Brownian motions" of entire segments of the polymer backbone. Below the transition temperature, the segments are locked by their interaction with neighboring chain segments. The corresponding loss peak is broad because there are so many different "modes" when these interactions are "thawing", in the statistical mechanical sense of the word. The activation energies involved may also be quite large, since the interactions are summed up of contributions over long segments of the polymers. However, the α-relaxation is strongly *non-Arrhenius* in character. Usually, the so-called Vogel relation applies [56] (A, B and T_0 are material constants; f is the frequency):

$$\ln(f_{max,\, \alpha}/Hz) = \ln A - [B/(T - T_0)]; \quad T > T_0 \tag{229}$$

In contrast, the "subglass transitions" (β-, γ- $\cdots$) are transitions with time constants following the exponential law of Arrhenius. They are connected with more rapid motions of limited spatial extension (rotations and librations) in the side chains and in the local part of the backbone.

The concept of "free volume" is important not only for describing rate processes in liquids [57–60] but certainly also in glassy polymers—glasses being sub-cooled liquids. In such polymers, the concept may be used to explain the non-Arrhenius character of the glass–rubber relaxation [53]. Furthermore, "free volume" theories have been most useful in describing diffusive transport processes, such as gas permeation, in polymeric membranes [61,62]; see also the chapter by Petropoulus, Sanopoulo and Papadokostaki in the present monograph [63].

According to Glasstone, Laidler and Eyring [57], the free volume may be regarded as the volume in which each molecule in a liquid moves in an average potential field due to its neighbors. This volume is more or less easily redistributed during time and is the controlling factor for transport processes like viscosity and self-diffusion in liquids or glassy/rubbery polymers. A simpler, more operational, definition was given in the theory of Cohen and Turnbull [59,60]: The free volume (v_f) is that part of the excess volume (= total volume minus volume occupied by the repulsive cores of the molecules) which may be redistributed without change in energy. The main points of their theory may be formulated as follows: the translational friction coefficient of the liquid is to some approximation dependent only on the temperature through the so-called *fractional free volume*, and since the relaxation times for viscosity, for self diffusion and for diffusion of foreign molecules in the liquid are all proportional to the *translational friction coefficient*, the same is true for these coefficients. More specifically, we write for the logarithm of the relaxation time relative to the relaxation time of a reference state:

$$\ln(\tau/\tau_{ref}) \approx \gamma_f v_m^*[(1/v_{fm}) - (1/v_{fm}^{ref})] \tag{230}$$

In this expression, the subscript m stands for either the liquid molecule or (in polymers) the chain segment involved in the relaxation process. γ_f is a constant between 0.5 and 1 accounting for the overlap of free volume, v_m^* is the *minimum hole volume* to be created by redistribution of free volume for the molecule or segment to change place in the relaxation at hand, and v_{fm} is the average free volume per molecule or segment. We introduce the *fractional free volume*

$$\phi = v_{fm}/v_m \tag{231}$$

where v_m is the (total) average volume per molecule or segment and write:

$$\ln(\tau/\tau_{ref}) \approx \gamma_f(v_m^*/v_m)[(1/\phi) - (1/\phi_{ref})] \tag{232}$$

We consider a temperature T_o, lower than T as well as T_{ref}, and having the property that at T_o the free volume would be reduced to zero, were the glassy state not formed. We have then approximately (at constant pressure) that

$$\phi = \alpha_f(T - T_o) \qquad (T \geq T_o) \tag{233}$$

where α_f would be the true thermal expansion coefficient if all expansion were in the form of Cohen-Turnbull free volume. Introducing Eq. (233) in (232) we obtain for the temperature dependence of any relaxation time which is dependent on free volume only:

$$\ln \tau \approx \text{constant} + B/(T - T_o) \qquad (T > T_o) \tag{234}$$
$$B = \gamma_f v_m^*/[\alpha_f v_m] \tag{235}$$

Using the latter equation we can also reformulate Eq. (232):

$$(1/\tau) \approx A \exp(-B\alpha_f/\phi) \tag{236}$$
$$A = (1/\tau_{ref})\exp(+B\alpha_f/\phi_{ref}) \qquad (\text{for any } T_{ref} > T_o) \tag{237}$$

Clearly, the Vogel expression (229) conforms to Eqs. (234)–(237), and both the Vogel temperature and the B parameter may now be interpreted physically. The Vogel temperature is the temperature were the free volume (which can be redistributed without use of energy) is zero in a hypothetical state where the glass transition does not take place. Furthermore, the relaxation times tend towards infinity when $T \to T_o$ from above. Below T_o there cannot be any relaxation. The coefficient B is the activation energy (in degrees Kelvin) of the relaxation at very high temperatures ($T \gg T_o$), and it is also proportional to the critical volume v_m^* for accommodating the molecule or segment relaxing.

The expression of Doolittle [58] for the viscosity in terms of fractional free volume, found to represent with high accuracy viscosities of ordinary liquids of low molecular weight, is also of the same type. Cohen and Turnbull used their theory for self-diffusion in hard sphere fluids, but the same relation has been used for real diffusion of foreign molecules in polymers [64,65]. Indeed, the concept of fractional free volume has been found to be very useful in the study of diffusive transport processes [61,62].

In accordance with Eq. (236) we write for the maximum frequency of the glass–rubber relaxation and for a diffusion coefficient:

$$f_\alpha \approx A_\alpha \exp(-B_\alpha \alpha_f/\phi) \tag{238}$$

$$D \approx A_{diff} \exp(-B_{diff} \alpha_f/\phi) \tag{239}$$

$$B_\alpha = \gamma_\alpha v^*_{m,\,\alpha}/[\alpha_f v_m] \tag{240}$$

$$B_{diff} = \gamma_{diff} v^*_{m,\,diff}/[\alpha_f v_m] \tag{241}$$

Assuming that the overlap factors are approximately the same in the two cases $(\gamma_\alpha \approx \gamma_{diff})$ we have

$$B_\alpha/B_{diff} \approx v^*_{m,\,\alpha}/v^*_{m,\,diff} \tag{242}$$

since the total volume for the polymer segment active in the redistribution of free volume (v_m) is the same in the two processes. The ratio between the two B-coefficients in the Vogel equations for the glass–rubber relaxation and the diffusion coefficient should therefore be equal to the ratio between the critical void volume for the two processes.

B. Vinylidene Cyanide/Vinyl Acetate Copolymer

A publication by Furukawa et al. from 1986 [41] aroused my curiosity few years ago. These authors studied the very large dielectric relaxations in an alternate 1:1 copolymer of vinylidene cyanide and vinyl acetate (VDCN/VAc). This amorphous polymer is interesting by possessing a larger static permittivity than water and by being piezoelectric. However, for our purpose the study is interesting, because the authors attempted a separation between dielectric relaxation, conductivity and space charge accumulation at the electrodes. The complex permittivity $\varepsilon^*(\omega)$ was described by means of an effective permittivity as in Eq. (10) combined *in series* with an "electrode polarization permittivity":

$$\varepsilon^*_{HN,\,eff}(\omega) = \varepsilon(\infty) + \Delta\varepsilon/[1 + (i\omega\tau)^b]^a - i\sigma/\omega \tag{243}$$

$$1/\varepsilon^*_{eff} = (1/\varepsilon^*_{HN,\,eff}) + (1/\varepsilon^*_{el}) \tag{244}$$

$$\varepsilon^*_{el} = \varepsilon^o_{el}(i\omega)^{-m} \tag{245}$$

The first two terms on the r.h.s. of (243) represent the so-called *Havriliak–Negami* (HN) empirical relation [66]. The third term is the contribution from the conductivity. The HN relation is popular among researchers in the field of dielectric relaxation of polymers, since it is able to fit approximately the behavior of a broad range of polymers, choosing the constants $\varepsilon(\infty)$, $\Delta\varepsilon$, τ, a and b appropriately. As far as I know, there is not much physical content in the expression, however. The static (intrinsic) permittivity is given by $\varepsilon(\infty) + \Delta\varepsilon$ where $\Delta\varepsilon$ is the "relaxation strength". The electrode polarization permittivity (245) has been set to the form of a "constant phase element". Such a hypothetical circuit element is much used by impedance electrochemists, see for example [11], pp. 90–95.

Furukawa et al. made dielectric measurements on 10 μm thick films between two thin gold layers in a frequency range from 0.01 Hz to 10 kHz at temperatures 170, 175, 180, 185, 190, 195°C. The authors used a special technique of measuring with a composite sinusoidal wave containing eight frequencies in ratio 2 measuring the frequency spectrum over two decades at a time with an accuracy of 0.1% in tan δ. The sample was annealed at 200°C for 1 h, and the spectra were taken from high to low temperatures after 30 min for reaching thermal equilibrium after each new temperature.

The parameter m was chosen to be 0.2 and the other seven parameters in (243) and (245) were fitted at each temperature. In the paper of Furukawa et al., however, the fitted parameters were only incompletely stated. Therefore, I have magnified the Figs. 2, 3 in their paper, read the experimental points and refitted the data anew. The parameters of the best fits found are given in Table 8. In the brackets, alternative fits are given for some temperatures being also

TABLE 8 Reffitted Furukawa Parameters for the Dielectric Dispersion of Poly-VDCN/VAc

Temp. (°C)	$\varepsilon_r(\infty)$	$\Delta\varepsilon_r$	τ (s)	a	b	σ ($\Omega^{-1}\,m^{-1}$)	$\varepsilon_{el}^0/\varepsilon_0$	m
170	4	90	500	0.43	0.72	3.1×10^{-10}	9.0×10^4	0.2
	[5]	[99]	[160]	[0.56]	[0.76]	$[5.0 \times 10^{-10}]$	$[7.0 \times 10^4]$	[0.2]
175	5	122	2.5	0.55	0.78	1.8×10^{-9}	9.0×10^4	0.2
	[5]	[122]	[2.5]	[0.57]	[0.77]	$[2.0 \times 10^{-9}]$	$[9.0 \times 10^4]$	[0.2]
180	5	127	0.1	0.58	0.78	7.9×10^{-9}	1.1×10^5	0.2
185	5	125	1.1×10^{-2}	0.60	0.79	2.0×10^{-8}	1.2×10^5	0.05
	[5]	[125]	$[1.13 \times 10^{-2}]$	[0.59]	[0.79]	$[2.5 \times 10^{-8}]$	$[1.3 \times 10^5]$	[0.2]
190	5	117	3.1×10^{-3}	0.62	0.80	5.0×10^{-8}	1.5×10^5	0.2
	[5]	[117]	$[2.0 \times 10^{-3}]$	[0.60]	[0.80]	$[6.3 \times 10^{-8}]$	$[1.5 \times 10^5]$	[0.2]
195	5	109	5.3×10^{-4}	0.65	0.80	1.0×10^{-7}	1.4×10^5	0.2
	[5]	[109]	$[5.0 \times 10^{-4}]$	[0.61]	[0.81]	$[1.58 \times 10^{-7}]$	$[1.7 \times 10^5]$	[0.2]

The unbracketed parameter values are the best fitting. The bracketed values are also acceptable. However, at 185°C tan δ is better fitted at low frequencies with $m = 0.05$ than with $m = 0.2$. The parameters indicated in [41] are the following: $\varepsilon_r(\infty) = 5$, $\Delta\varepsilon_r = 122$, $\tau = 3.1$ ms, $a = 0.6$, $b = 0.8$, $\sigma = 6.9 \times 10^{-8}$, $\varepsilon_{el}^0/\varepsilon_0 = 1.5 \times 10^5$ (at 190°C); $\tau = 160$ s, $\varepsilon_{el}^0/\varepsilon_0 = 7 \times 10^4$ (at 170°C); $\Delta\varepsilon_r = 125$ (at 180°C).

acceptable. There is considerable covariance in the parameter determination. The value of $m = 0.05$ for 185°C deviate strongly from $m = 0.2$, but the fit to the tan δ values at low frequencies is far better than can be obtained from any fit with $m = 0.2$. Of course, there is nothing "sacrosanct" with the value $m = 0.2$.

A detailed view of the dielectric dispersion at the temperature 185°C is given in Fig. 29. It is seen, that the effective permittivity is given by the intrinsic Havriliak–Negami (HN, $+ + +$) dispersion above 0.3 Hz for ε_r', above 30 Hz for ε_r'' and above 300 Hz for tan δ. Below 300 Hz tan δ starts to deviate because of the conductivity. The same is true for ε_r'' below 30 Hz. The latter quantity is given by its MWS expression in a wide range of frequencies, with the slope approximately equal to -1 in the doubly logarithmic plot vs. frequency. The steep rise in ε_r' below 0.3 Hz is caused by the interfacial polarization and by nothing else, since the MWS theory has a constant ε_r'. The low frequency peak in tan δ centered around 0.1 Hz is the result of the varying relative importance of the "σ effect" on ε_r'' and the effect of interfacial polarization on ε_r'. The curve with tan δ multiplied by 20 shows that there is a broad peak centered around 300 Hz, probably the glass–rubber relaxation.

In Fig. 30 the calculated values of the real component of $\varepsilon_{r,\,eff}^*$ are shown for the six temperatures. In this and the following figures, the calculations have been extended down to 0.001 Hz, even if the measurements did only reach down to 0.01 Hz. Thus, one has to be cautious with the extrapolated values in the range 0.0001–0.01 Hz although they might show the tendency. The $+ + +$ curves represent the intrinsic dielectric dispersion as calculated by the HN relation. It is evident, that interfacial polarization is of importance below the frequencies 0.01, 0.03, 0.1, 0.3, 1 and 2 Hz for the temperatures 170, 175, 180, 185, 190 and 195°C, respectively.

Figure 31 shows the corresponding dielectric losses at the same temperatures. The deviations from the HN dispersion starts below the frequencies 30, 30, 30, 30, 1 and 3 Hz for the six temperatures from 170 to 195°C. These frequencies are much higher than the frequencies where ε_r' starts to deviate. Thus, there is a relatively wide intermediate frequency range in which only the conductivity is of importance for the deviation. In this region, the plot of log ε_r'' vs. log(frequency) is approximately a straight line with slope -1. A very good estimate of σ may be found from the intercept of this line with log $f = 0$. At the three highest temperatures there is evidence for a maximum in ε_r'' between 0.001 and 0.01 Hz although the precise positions and heights of these maxima cannot be inferred from such extrapolations.

Figures 32 shows what happens when the measured values of ε_r'' are corrected for the conductivity in the following way:

$$\varepsilon_r''(\text{corr}) \equiv \varepsilon_r'' - \sigma/(\varepsilon_0 \omega) \tag{246}$$

The corrected curves now follow the HN values ($+ + +$) down to about

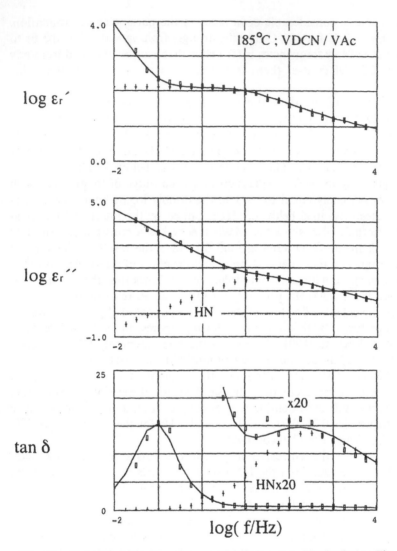

FIG. 29 The dielectric dispersion at 185°C for poly-VDCN/VAc. The (+ + + +) curves represent the intrinsic dielectric dispersion of the polymer given by the Havriliak–Negami expression. The rectangles are measured data and the full curves represent the combination of HN, conductivity and interfacial polarization. Two dielectric loss peaks are clearly seen in the tan δ data. The low frequency peak is due to conductance + interfacial polarization, the high frequency peak (magnified twentyfold) is the glass–rubber relaxation.

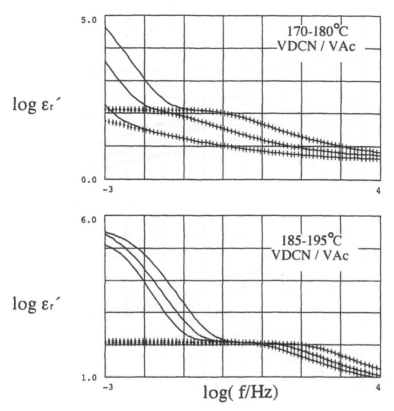

FIG. 30 Calculated values of the real component of the effective permittivity as a function of frequency at temperatures from 180 to 195°C for poly-VDCN/VAc. The intrinsic dispersions (given by the HN expression) are shown as the (+ + + +) curves, the total effective permittivities as the full line curves. The steep rises of ε_r' at low frequencies are a consequence of the interfacial polarization (described by the "constant phase element").

the frequencies were ε_r' starts to deviate, i.e., down to about the frequencies where interfacial polarization becomes important After a transition, the values of ε_r'' (corr) follow approximately straight lines in the log–log plots but with slopes much steeper that in a MWS dependence. The correct thing is to say, however, that the values of ε_r''(corr) are only meaningful as long as interfacial polarization is *not* of importance. Should the contribution from interfacial polarization be negligible in the frequency range studied, another kind of problems will appear. Since ε_r'' rises to very high values when the frequency goes towards zero, ε_r''(corr) will be a "small difference between large numbers" (SDLN). In data with experimental scattering, the values of ε_r''(corr) will loose

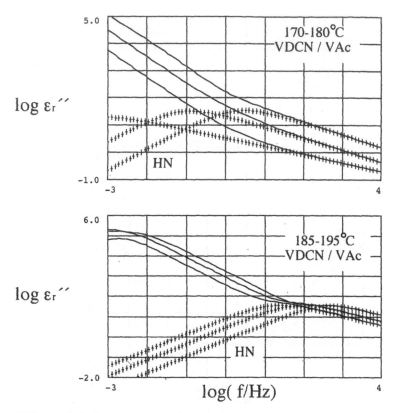

FIG. 31 Calculated values of the effective dielectric loss as a function of frequency at temperatures from 180 to 195°C for poly-VDCN/VAc. The intrinsic dispersions (given by the HN expression) are shown as the $(+ + + +)$ curves, the total dielectric loss as the full line curves. The linear part of the curves with slope -1 at intermediate to low frequencies in the doubly logarithmic plots is determined by the membrane conductance. At the higher temperatures, the extrapolations to very low frequencies indicate a maximum in the dielectric loss. This is a result of interfacial polarization.

physical meaning because of "SDLN effects" below frequencies where the standard errors of the measured ε_r'' become comparable to $\varepsilon_r''(\text{corr})$.

In the discussion above, I have assumed that the intrinsic dielectric dispersion is known, e.g., by measurements on the ion free polymer. This is very difficult, however, since traces of ions almost invariably are left over from the preparation. Especially for a polymer with such large static permittivity as the VDCN/VAc copolymer studied here, it would be very difficult to keep out ionic impurities. Therefore, the reality is that the measured dielectric dispersions have always contributions from interfacial polarization + conductivity at very low frequencies and from conductivity alone at intermediate frequencies.

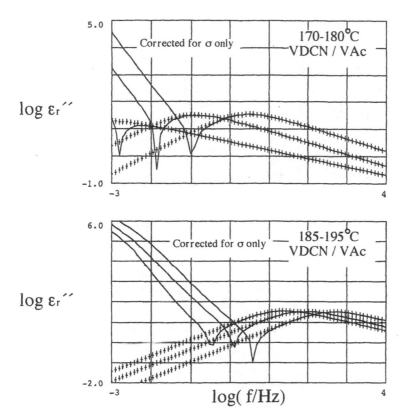

FIG. 32 Calculated values of the dielectric loss corrected for the conductivity for poly-VDCN/VAc at 180–195°C. The corrected curves (full line) follow the intrinsic polymer dispersion (+ + + +) down to frequencies where interfacial polarization becomes of importance. Below these frequencies, the corrected curves have no meaning.

Thus, it is a good question how one can deduce an intrinsic dielectric relaxation (such as a HN expression with given parameters) from experimental data in an impeccable way. In connection with the parameter estimation in Table 8 we saw that many different sets of parameters may be fitted to the same data. Only the value of σ is relatively well determined, if the log–log line with slope -1 extends over an appreciable range of frequencies. The truth is that we cannot know much about the intrinsic dielectric dispersion below the frequency where interfacial polarization effects commence to influence the data.

Fortunately, the opposite is *not* true. It *is* very often possible to estimate quite well the effects of the combined conductivity and interfacial polarization. Figure 33 shows the loss tangent as a function of frequency for the raw dielectric data (upper curve) and for the intrinsic HN dielectric relaxation (lower

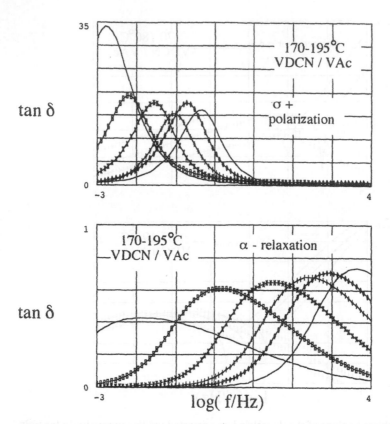

FIG. 33 Calculated values of the loss tangent for poly-VDCN/VAc at 180–195°C. The upper curves are the peaks corresponding to conductance + polarization. The loss tangent is here calculated as the combination of HN dispersion, conductance and polarization. The lower curves are the peaks corresponding to the α-relaxation (glass–rubber) calculated from the HN contribution alone. At the lower temperatures, there is a considerable overlap of the σ + polarization peak and the α-peak, and since the former is dominating, the latter may be hard to get.

curve). The loss tangents of the former values are much greater than the loss tangents of the latter. Thus, the loss tangent peaks corresponding to σ + polarization are relatively unaffected by the intrinsic dielectric relaxation. Comparing with Fig. 30, it is seen that the σ + polarization peaks in tan δ are situated at frequencies where the intrinsic dielectric dispersion has not yet commenced, so that the intrinsic permittivity may be set equal to the static permittivity. Therefore, the methods outlined in Sec. II.C may be used here. In particular, the diffusion coefficients of the ions present may be estimated from the heights and frequencies of the maxima in the loss tangents at low frequencies, see Fig. 5.

On the other hand, the lower figure in Fig. 33 indicates that it may well be difficult to reveal an α-relaxation (glass–rubber) peak masked by a much greater σ + polarization peak. This is the case especially at the lowest temperature (170°C). Overlapping sub-glass peaks are even more difficult to reveal, being usually smaller than the α-peak.

Table 9 lists the data for the σ + polarization and for the α-loss tangent peaks and for the peaks in ε_r'' for the α-relaxation. From the σ + polarization maxima, the values of κL and one diffusion coefficient are estimated assuming for simplicity that the electrolyte is binary and symmetric. The diffusion coefficient is either the common diffusion coefficient (D) in the case that the ionic mobilities are approximately equal or the diffusion coefficient of the faster ion in the case where this ion diffuses 9 or more times faster than the slower ion, see the discussion in connection with the general scaling in Fig. 5. The formulae used for the calculation of κL and $\kappa^2 D$ are the good approximations (102), (103) together with the definition of Ω in Eqs. (68) and (105). The values obtained for κL, κ and D or D_{fast} are listed in Table 10. It is seen that even if the film width is several thousand times greater than the Debye length there are very large macropolarization effects at very low frequencies which cannot be explained by the MWS approach. Thus, the MWS approach is not generally valid in situations where the structural elements of a system have sizes much greater than the Debye length, a statement which is sometimes met [39]. Rather, the MWS approach is correct in the limit of high frequencies (a limit which moves towards lower frequencies when κL is increased!).

For an ideal 1:1 electrolyte one should have the following expressions for the static permittivity and the salt concentration in the cases $D_1 = D_2 = D$ and

TABLE 9 The Maxima of the tan δ Peaks (α and σ) and the ε_r'' Peak (α only) for Poly-VDCN/VAc

Temp. (°C)	tan δ_{max} (α)	log $f_{max, \delta}$ (α) log (Hz)	log $\varepsilon_{r, max}''$ (α)	log $f_{max, \varepsilon''}$ (α) log (Hz)	tan δ_{max} (σ)	log $f_{max, \delta}$ (σ)
170	0.428	−1.87	(1.29)	(−3.05)	(34.1)	(−2.82)
175	0.609	0.12	1.52	−0.90	19.3	−2.24
180	0.648	1.53	1.54	0.50	17.8	−1.58
185	0.682	2.40	1.56	1.39	15.4	−1.03
190	0.708	2.91	1.53	1.93	17.8	−0.73
195	0.736	3.62	1.52	2.69	16.3	−0.35

The values in parentheses are uncertain (extrapolations to low frequencies).

TABLE 10 Calculated Diffusion Coefficients and Inverse Debye Lengths for $D_1 = D_2$ and for $D_1 \gg D_2$ for Poly-VDCN/VAc

Temp. (°C)	$D_1 = D_2 = D$			$D_{fast} \gg D_{slow}$		
	κL	$10^{-8}\,\kappa$ (m^{-1})	$10^{16}\,D$ $(m^2\,s^{-1})$	κL	$10^{-8}\,\kappa$	$10^{16}\,D_{fast}$
170	(9300)	(9.30)	(0.0075)	(11900)	(11.9)	(0.0091)
175	2980	2.98	0.157	3805	3.81	0.191
180	2535	2.54	0.911	3235	3.24	1.111
185	1900	1.90	5.01	2420	2.42	6.09
190	2530	2.53	6.50	3235	3.24	7.86
195	2120	2.12	20.4	2714	2.71	24.6

The values in parentheses are uncertain (extrapolations). Film thickness $L = 10^{-5}$ m.

$D_{fast} \gg D_{slow}$, respectively:

$$\varepsilon_s/\varepsilon_o = (\sigma/\varepsilon_o)/(D\kappa^2_{common}) \quad \text{or} \quad (2\sigma/\varepsilon_o)/(D_{fast}\,\kappa^2_{fast}) \tag{247}$$

$$c_{salt}(mol/L) = RT\varepsilon_s\,\kappa^2_{common}/[2000 \cdot F^2] \quad \text{or} \quad RT\varepsilon_s\,\kappa^2_{fast}/[2000 \cdot F^2] \tag{248}$$

In Table 11 these quantities are calculated and the calculated values of $\varepsilon_s/\varepsilon_o$ are compared to the Havriliak–Negami values (the sum of the 2nd and 3rd column in Table 8). At least, the compared values are of the same order of magnitude and for the highest three temperatures the correspondence is quite good. The great deviation of the value at 170°C may point to the danger connected with extrapolation to low frequencies of fits based on the

TABLE 11 Calculated Values of the Static Permittivity and the Electrolyte Concentrations in Poly-VDCN/VAc for the Cases $D_1 = D_2 = D$ (common) and $D_{fast} \gg D_{slow}$ (fast)

Temp. (°C)	$(\varepsilon_s/\varepsilon_o)_{common}$	$(\varepsilon_s/\varepsilon_o)_{fast}$	$(\varepsilon_s/\varepsilon_o)_{HN}$	c_{salt} (common) (mol/L)	c_{salt} (fast) (mol/L)
170	(54)	(55)	94	(0.14)	(0.23)
175	146	147	127	0.020	0.033
180	152	153	132	0.015	0.025
185	125	127	130	0.0085	0.014
190	136	137	122	0.014	0.024
195	123	125	114	0.0095	0.016

The values in parentheses are uncertain (extrapolations). The HN static permittivities are given as the sums of the 2nd and the 3rd columns in Table 8. The static permittivities used in Eq. (248) are the HN static permittivities.

"unphysical" constant phase element. However, also at 175°C and 180°C there are some deviation. Three sources of errors can be identified:

1. There might be deviations from ideality.
2. The intrinsic dielectric dispersion is neglected in the film polarization theory and Fig. 33 shows that especially for the lowest temperatures there is considerably overlap between the α-relaxation and the conductivity/polarization relaxation.
3. The static permittivity of the HN dispersion is a parameter which cannot be determined unambiguously from experimental data with so much contribution from conductivity and interfacial polarization as seen here. The ambiguity is the most for the lowest temperatures (with most overlap).

The calculated salt concentrations in Table 11 are of the order of magnitude of 0.01 mol/L. This is a quite high level for uncontrolled ionic "impurities". It illustrates the difficulties connected with freeing a polymer of such a high permittivity for ions.

In Fig. 34 (upper subplot), the logarithm of some characteristic frequencies for the *glass–rubber* relaxation is plotted vs. $1/(T - T_0)$ according to the Vogel relation Eq. (229). The "Vogel temperature" $T_0 = 427$ K has been determined such that the correlation coefficient (r) of the least square fit is as close as possible to unity for $\ln(1/\tau)$ where the relaxation times τ are the Havriliak–Negami relaxation times listed in Table 8 (the ones not in square brackets). However, the plots of the logarithms of the frequencies of maximum tan δ and ε'' are also excellently linear using the same T_0. The same is true for the logarithm of the diffusion coefficient. This plot is shown for D_{fast} in the lower regression of Figure 34, the regression for the case of a common diffusion coefficient being just parallelly shifted relative to the line shown. It is remarkable that even the data for $f_{max,\,\varepsilon''}$ and D_{fast} for 170°C—which were considered highly uncertain because of the extrapolation of the empirical fitting relations to low frequencies—lie perfectly on the regression lines (rightmost points). For these two quantities the regression line shown were based only upon the other five temperatures! The regression lines obtained are the following:

$$\ln(1/\tau) = \ln A_\tau - B_\tau/[T - T_0] = 16.02 - 359.0/[T - 427];$$
$$r = -0.99937 \text{ (6 points)} \quad (249)$$

$$\ln(f_{max,\,\delta}) = \ln A_\delta - B_\delta/[T - T_0] = 16.16 - 332.1/[T - 427];$$
$$r = -0.99916 \text{ (6 points)} \quad (250)$$

$$\ln(f_{max,\,\varepsilon''}) = \ln A_\varepsilon - B_\varepsilon/[T - T_0] = 14.42 - 348.9/[T - 427];$$
$$r = -0.9978 \text{ (5 points)} \quad (251)$$

$$\ln(D_{fast}) = \ln A_{diff} - B_{diff}/[T - T_0] = -28.73 - 206.6/[T - 427];$$
$$r = -0.9915 \text{ (5 points)} \quad (252)$$

$(1/\tau, f_{max,\,\delta}$ and $f_{max,\,\varepsilon''}$ measured in s^{-1}; D_{fast} measured in $m^2\,s^{-1}$).

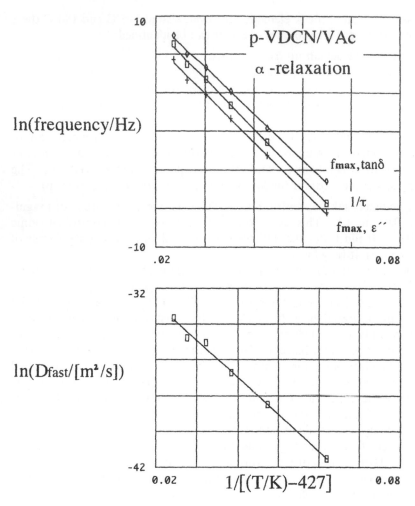

FIG. 34 "Vogel plots" for the α-relaxation (glass–rubber) and the diffusion coefficient of the faster ion in poly-VDCN/VAc for temperatures between 180 and 195°C. The "Vogel temperature" is 427 K in both cases.

The "activation energies" (at infinite temperature) for the glass–rubber relaxation (B, measured in K) are quite similar calculated by the three methods in Eqs. (249)–(251). However, whereas τ in the HN expression is a somewhat mystical "average" relaxation time without any physical basis, and dependent on the choice of the exponents a and b in Eq. (243), the two frequency maxima are at least easily identifiable. The maxima of tan δ lie always at somewhat higher frequencies than the maxima of the intrinsic dielectric loss.

This may be of value in cases where the maxima of the dielectric loss are positioned below the experimental range of frequencies, or when the intrinsic dielectric dispersion at low frequencies is difficult to estimate because of conductance and polarization.

The usual Arrhenius activation energy (E^*), the negative slope of ln(frequency) vs. $1/T$, varies with the temperature for the glass–rubber relaxation. It is easily seen that one has:

$$E^*(T)/R = [T/(T - T_o)]^2 B \tag{253}$$

Thus, at the mean temperature of the measurements (182°C), $E^*(455$ K)$/R \approx 92,000$ K which is a very high activation energy even for a glass–rubber relaxation. This is surely a reflection of the strongly cohesive polar forces in this polymer.

Following the free volume expression (242) it is seen that the critical void volume necessary for the polymer segment displacement in the glass–rubber relaxation (α) is ~ 1.7 times the critical void volume for the diffusion of the faster of the ions:

$$v^*_{m,\,\alpha}/v^*_{m,\,\text{diff}} = B_\alpha/B_{\text{diff}} \approx 350/207 = 1.69 \tag{254}$$

Thus, the "fast ion" (if any) must possess a certain "bulkiness"; it cannot be a fast diffusing proton, for example.

Taking the glass transition temperature of poly-VDCN/VAc to be 182°C (455 K), as estimated by DSC by Furukawa et al., and using the relation (233) one obtains for the (scaled) *fractional free volume* at the glass temperature:

$$\phi(\text{glass})/(B_\alpha \alpha_f) = (455 - 427)/350 = 0.080 \tag{255}$$

The value 0.080 is unusually high for an amorphous polymer, since Ferry [53, p. 288] states that it is in the range 0.025 ± 0.005 for the majority of amorphous polymers. (Ferry calls the quantity on the l.h.s. of (255) for the "fractional free volume at the glass temperature" and the quantity $B_\alpha \alpha_f$ in the present treatment is called B in the nomenclature of Ferry). It is perhaps understandable, since the copolymer studied by Furukawa et al. is very unusual with strong polar interactions and a very high glass temperature. Although its diffuse X-ray diffraction pattern indicates that it is probably amorphous or very poorly crystalline, the discussion in the paper of Furukawa et al. points to strong collective interaction phenomena of the dipoles with concerted rotation in clusters of four to five monomers (perhaps a situation in some sense similar to the situation in liquid water?).

C. Poly[4-(Acryloxy)phenyl-(4-Chlorophenyl)Methanone]

In this subsection and in the next, some results of dielectric studies on two acrylic acid based polymers are discussed. The repeating units of each of the two polymers are shown in Fig. 35. The investigation of the polymer poly[4-acryloxy)phenyl-(4-chlorophenyl)methanone] = poly-APCM was performed by T. S. Sørensen, V. Compañ and R. Diaz-Calleja [36].

The polymer was synthesized in the Instituto de Polímeros, Consejo Superior de Investigaciones Científicas, Madrid. The procedure was explained in detail in [67]. Of interest in the present connection is the information that during the different steps of the synthesis of the monomer the following electrolytes were used (in chronological order): NaOH, Bu$_4$NCl, AlCl$_3$, HCl, NaOH, HCl, NaOH, Bu$_4$NCl. In the final step, tetrabutylammonium chloride is reacted with (4-chlorophenyl)(4-hydroxyphenyl)methanone and acryloyl

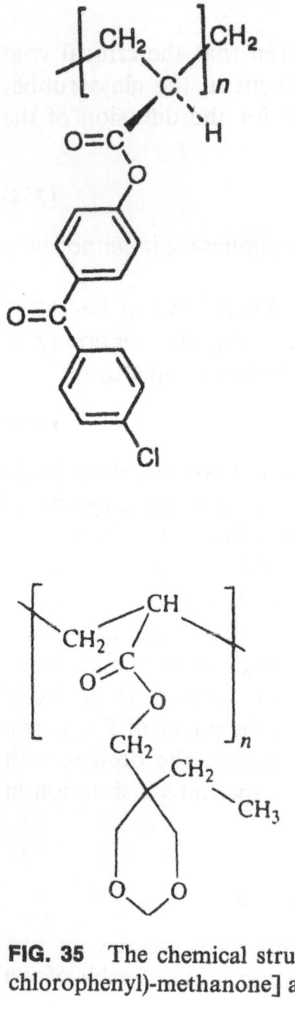

FIG. 35 The chemical structure of the repetition units of poly [4-acryloxy)phenyl)(4-chlorophenyl)-methanone] and poly [5-ethyl-1,3-dioxane-5-yl)methyl acrylate].

chloride in an emulsion with water, NaOH and dichloromethane. After reaction, the organic phase was separated by chromatography over basic alumina beads (using dichloromethane as eluent) and recrystallized from toluene–hexane. The 4-(acryloxy)phenyl-(4-chlorophenyl)methanone thus obtained was then polymerized in toluene solution using the nonionic initiator AIBN ($=2,2'$-azo-bisisobutyronitrile) and the polymer was finally precipitated with methanol and dried.

The contamination level of ionic impurities as estimated by the present dielectric studies is $\sim 5 \times 10^{-6}$ mol/L, a very low level indeed, but nevertheless of great importance for the effective permittivity at low frequencies as we shall see. Looking at the final steps of the synthesis, the likely candidates as free charge carriers are Bu_4N^+, Cl^-, Na^+, OH^- and perhaps Al^{3+}, whereas H^+ is quite unlikely. It is possible that the primary contamination stems from very small amounts of Bu_4N^+ interdispersed in the polymer network and various small counterions (Cl^-, OH^-) and even smaller amounts of coions as for example Na^+ which account for the erratic fluctuations in the "efficient" salt concentrations calculated later on.

The dielectric measurements were performed using a ceramic parallel plate condenser with a gap width $L = 0.257$ mm and a surface area $A = 380$ mm^2. The polymer was molten between the condenser plates and the gap width was measured after cooling and solidification. The measurements were taken using the capacitance measuring apparatus TA DEA 2970. The experiments proceeded from 40°C to $+ 140$°C in the frequency range from 0.01 Hz to 100 kHz. The rate of heating between two measuring temperatures was 1°C/min and measurements were performed under isothermal conditions with temperature steps of 5°C. The sample was equilibrated for ~ 20 min. at each temperature.

A β-relaxation of the polymer was observed by thermomechanical analysis (TMA) with a loss peak centring around -76°C at 10 Hz [67]. By differential scanning calorimetry using a DSC7 calorimeter at a heating rate of 20°C/min, an α-transition (glass–rubber) was observed at an onset temperature equal to $+78$°C. Thus, the glass-transition temperature is ≥ 78°C. In the investigation reported here, the focus is on the α-relaxation (glass–rubber) which seems partially to overlap with conduction and interfacial polarization phenomena at higher temperatures (120–140°C).

The low frequency conductivity/polarization peak in the loss tangent was analyzed in the same way as indicated in the previous subsection with the difference, however, that our measured experimental data for the effective permittivity were analyzed *directly* (without fitting these data to an artificial combination of a Havriliak–Negami equation, a conductivity term and a "constant phase element"). The data for tan δ around the maximum were smoothed by a least square polynomial in order to determine the peak height and the frequency of the maximum with greater precision. The conductivities (σ) are estimated from the intercepts of best-fitting straight lines (with slope

-1) to the doubly logarithmic plots of log ε'' vs. log(frequency), see Fig. 36. The data for the conductivity/polarization peaks and for the conductivities are given in Table 12 together with the calculated values of κL and the diffusion coefficient in the two cases $D_1 = D_2 = D$ and $D_{fast} \gg D_{slow}$. Comparing with Table 10 it is seen that the diffusion coefficients are about 100 times higher than in poly-VDCN/VAc. Probably, the strong dipoles in the latter polymer bind the ions strongly and thereby retard the diffusion of the latter.

In Table 13, the values of the electrolyte concentrations, calculated by means of Eq. (248), are shown. Comparing with Table 11 it is seen that the concentrations are about ten thousand times smaller in poly-APCM than in poly-VDCN/VAc, surely a result of the much lower permittivity in the former polymer than in the latter (the Born free energy of charging is much higher then). The static permittivities calculated by means of Eq. (247) are also shown. They show a clear decreasing tendency with increasing temperature as would be expected.

In Fig. 37, the isothermal spectra of the experimental values of the two components of the effective permittivity ε' and ε'' are given. The latter values have been subtracted the estimated conductivity contribution, see Eq. (246). It is evident from both subfigures that there is a high frequency relaxation and

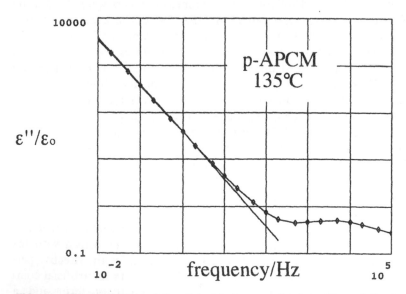

FIG. 36 The logarithm of the dielectric loss vs. the logarithm of the frequency for poly-APCM is a straight line with slope -1 at low and intermediary frequencies. Experimental points (rectangles) are very slightly below the line at the lowest frequencies. Temperature: 135°C. The straight line correspond to a specific conductivity $\sigma = 2.11 \times 10^{-9} \, \Omega^{-1} \, m^{-1}$. *Source*: Ref. 36.

TABLE 12 The Maxima of the σ/Polarization tan δ Peaks and the Conductivities for Poly-APCM

Temp. (°C)	tan δ_{max}	f_{max} (Hz)	$10^9 \, \sigma$ ($\Omega^{-1} \, m^{-1}$)	$D_1 = D_2 = D$		$D_{fast} \gg D_{slow}$	
				κL	$10^{14} \, D$ ($m^2 \, s^{-1}$)	κL	$10^{14} \, D_{fast}$ ($m^2 \, s^{-1}$)
120	20.7	0.0105	0.334	3430	1.53	4380	1.86
125	20.3	0.0282	0.668	3297	4.37	4210	5.30
130	20.9	0.0479	1.224	3490	6.80	4460	8.25
135	22.8	0.0794	2.11	4160	8.69	5310	10.54
140	24.1	0.158	3.62	4650	14.7	5930	17.8

$L = 2.57 \times 10^{-4}$ m.

most probably there is also a low frequency relaxation, although ε'' (corr) exhibits much "noise" at the lower frequencies. For this reason, the data for ε'' (corr) are only shown down to 1 Hz. For the highest temperature (140°C) the maximum of the low frequency peak is about 20 Hz. Looking at the data for ε', it does not seem likely that there should be any influence of interfacial polarisation at that high frequencies. If any such influence of polarization on ε' it should be below 1 Hz, judging from the upper subfigure of Fig. 37. Therefore, the low frequency peak seems to be a real one. To be more specific, the permittivities are plotted in a logarithmic scale at 140°C in Fig. 38 showing their decomposition into intrinsic dielectric dispersion (equal to the effective permittivities above 2 kHz), MWS dispersion (equal to the effective permittivities above 0.5 Hz for ε' and above 0.01 Hz for ε'') and interfacial polarization (the steep rise in ε' below 0.5 Hz).

TABLE 13 The Electrolyte Concentrations and the Calculated Static Permittivities (Poly-APCM)

Temp. (°C)	$D_1 = D_2 = D$		$D_{fast} \gg D_{slow}$	
	$10^6 \, c_{salt}$ (mol/L)	$\varepsilon_s/\varepsilon_o$	$10^6 \, c_{salt}$ (mol/L)	$\varepsilon_s/\varepsilon_o$
120	3.83	13.8	6.31	14.0
125	2.72	10.5	4.48	10.6
130	3.24	11.0	5.34	11.1
135	4.43	10.5	7.31	10.6
140	4.54	8.51	7.49	8.61

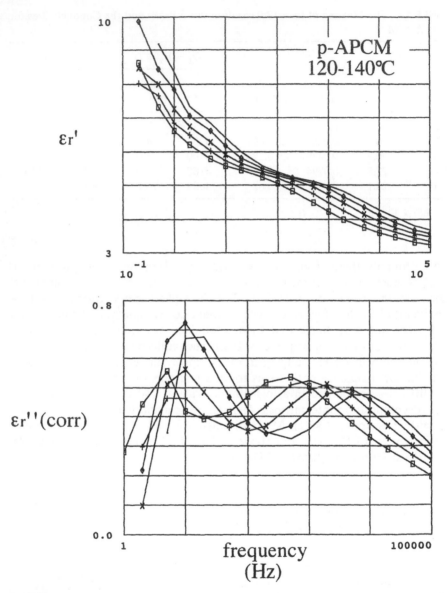

FIG. 37 The real and imaginary part of the complex permittivity for poly-APCM at intermediate to high frequencies after correction of the latter for conductivity effects. Temperatures: 120°C (rectangles), 125°C (+), 130°C (x), 135°C (diamonds), 140°C (line). In both sets of curves two relaxation steps are clearly revealed. *Source*: Ref. 36.

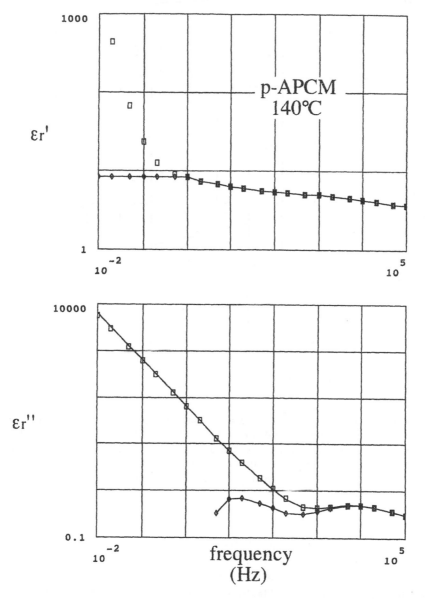

FIG. 38 Figure showing the contribution of the relaxations of the ion-free poly-APCM and of the conductivity to the components of the total experimental relative, complex permittivity. The experimental data are shown as rectangles. The relaxations of the ion free polymer as diamonds, and the Maxwell–Wagner–Sillars values (polymer relaxations + conductivity) as a solid curve. The MWS-values fit for the dielectric loss in the whole range of measured frequencies (Magnification shows that the MWS values are slightly too high at the lowest frequencies, however). The real part of the relative permittivity is highly influenced by the interfacial polarization below ~0.5 Hz. Temperature: 140°C. *Source: Ref. 36.*

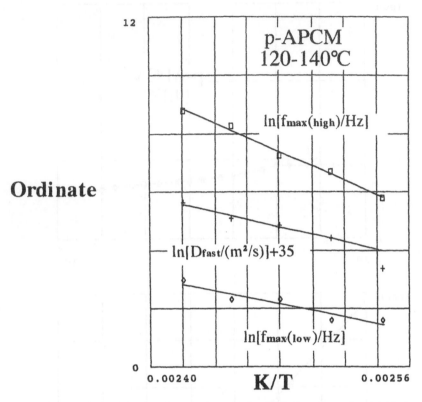

FIG. 39 Arrhenius plot of the maxima of the high frequency (rectangles) and low frequency (diamonds) peaks of the dielectric loss and of the diffusion coefficient of the faster ion. The point corresponding to the diffusion coefficient at 120°C has been excluded from the regression. The diffusion process and the "slow" relaxation have approximately the same activation energy. The activation energy for the high frequency relaxation is higher.

In Fig. 39, Arrhenius plots are shown for the low frequency as well as high frequency relaxation of the polymer. The high frequency Arrhenius plot is perfectly linear ($r = -0.9959$) with an activation energy $E^*/R \approx 24{,}500$ K, a value more typical for an α-relaxation than for a β-relaxation. If it is an α-relaxation, however, the Vogel temperature T_0 has to be much lower than the temperatures of the measurements for the Arrhenius plot to be linear. Because of the "noise", the Arrhenius plot of the low frequency relaxation is of a more poor quality. However, one obtains an activation energy $E^*/R \approx 11{,}200$ K with a correlation coefficient $r = -0.943$.

The Arrhenius plot for the calculated diffusion coefficient (of the fast ion) is also shown in Fig. 39. If one point is excluded (120°C), the plot is also perfectly linear ($r = -0.9909$) and the activation energy is $E \neq /R \approx 12,800$ K, quite close to the activation energy found for the low frequency relaxation.

The analysis of these findings in terms of the usual patterns found in such polymers [19] does not seem easy. Usually in isothermal spectra, the α-relaxation (glass–rubber) is found at the lowest frequencies and they have a high mean activation energy—being usually highly non-Arrhenius, however. The β-relaxation (involving more local motions of the side chains) are found at higher frequencies. They follow the Arrhenius law with a lower activation energy and they are sometimes found to merge together with the α-relaxation at the higher temperatures, see the next subsection. A "bold conjecture" might be that poly-APCM is special by having a very long and bulky side chain, almost an "oligomer" in itself. Interaction with neighboring side chains or backbones may produce a "quasi-glass–rubber relaxation" with smaller activation energies. These micro Brownian motions might be critical for the creation of holes for the ion diffusion as well. Hence the similarity of the activation energies of the diffusion process and the low frequency relaxation.

D. Poly[(5-Ethyl-1,3-Dioxane-5-yl)Methyl Acrylate]

The last study on which I want to report in this chapter is a dielectric investigation of poly[(5-ethyl-1,3-dioxan-5-yl)methyl acrylate = poly-EDMA. The repetition unit was shown in Fig. 35. Details are found in the paper of T. S. Sørensen, R. Diaz-Calleja, E. Riande, J. Guzman and A. Andrio [37].

1. Experimental

The polymer was synthesized in three steps [37]:

1. Synthesis of 5-hydroxymethyl-5-ethyl-1,3 dioxane (HED) by reaction of 2-ethyl-2-hydroxymethylpropane-1,3-diol with *para*-formaldehyde in toluene solution with toluene-*p*-sulfonic acid as catalyst.
2. Synthesis of (5-ethyl-1,3-dioxane-5-yl)methyl acrylate (EDMA) by reaction of HED with acryloyl chloride in chloroform solution. In this process, the side product triethylammonium chloride was removed by filtration and the EDMA was distilled under vacuum.
3. Radical polymerization of EDMA in benzene solution at 50°C using AIBN as initiator. The polymer was precipitated several times in *n*-hexane and finally purified by freeze drying from benzene solutions. Impurities in the solvents and precipitants used are usually metallic salts of Al, Pb, Sn, Zn, etc. The proportion of each of these impurities is in most cases less than 10^{-5} wt%. A more likely candidate for the ionic impurity found in the dielectric measurements is a trace of the triethylammonium chloride from step (2).

The dielectric measurements were performed at the Polytechnic University of Valencia using a ceramic parallel-plate condenser with a gap width $L = 0.4$

mm and a surface area $A = 380$ mm^2. The polymer was molded as a circular disc and placed between the electrodes. After this, the assembly was heated to a temperature 20°C above the glass transition temperature ($T_g \approx 36$°C) and was pressed using a force equal to 250 N in order to avoid irregular air gaps and voids of air between the electrodes and in order to maintain a uniform thickness of the sample.

The capacitance measuring apparatus was the same TA DEA 2970 as used for the study reported in the preceding subsection with a frequency range from 0.01 Hz to 100 kHz. In the apparatus there is a built-in automatic device that discharges the condenser for protection when the condenser charge is extremely high. This occasionally affects the measured values of the real part of the permittivity at very low frequencies and high temperatures. However, these discharges are easily discernible as jumps in the measurements, and when these were seen, the measurements were discarded.

Experiments were carried out for each frequency (isochronous measurements) from low (-135°C) to high temperature at 1°C/min until room temperature. From room temperature to temperatures well above T_g, measurements were carried out in the isothermal mode at 5°C steps equilibrating the sample about 20 min at each temperature. Successive runs of isothermal measurements at the same frequencies were reproducible (within $\sim 4\%$ relative uncertainty) which fact reveals the stability of the properties of the sample.

Mechanical measurements of the complex Young modulus (for simple extension with lateral contraction, E^*) were carried out at the Polytechnic University of Valencia by means of a DMTA-Mark II apparatus in the same range of temperatures as the dielectric experiments. Measurements were made from low temperatures to room temperature in the multiplexing mode using 0.3, 1, 3, 10 and 30 Hz at 1°C/min and from room temperature to higher temperatures in steps of 5°C with about 15 min between two successive measurements.

A glass–rubber "transition temperature" of the present amorphous polymer was determined as 36°C by Differential Scanning Calorimetry (DSC) at a heating rate of 20°C/min. A peak in the *mechanical* loss modulus of the polymer (E'') was also seen at 35°C at 3 Hz using the above apparatus. A subglass peak in E'' (β-relaxation) was observed at -70°C, similarly at 3 Hz mechanical vibration frequency. Such "transition temperature" are kinetic properties (not thermodynamic) and depend on the frequency (or heating rate). This is clearly seen in the thermomechanical isochronous map, Fig. 40b, where the subglass peak in E'' moves from -80°C to -50°C when the frequency moves from 0.3 Hz to 30 Hz, and the glass–rubber peak similarly moves from 30°C to 40°C. The downward steps in the real part of Young's modulus (E') move correspondingly, see Fig. 40a.

The same features are seen in the isochronous maps for the dielectric properties of poly-EDMA, see Fig. 41. The maxima of the dielectric losses are

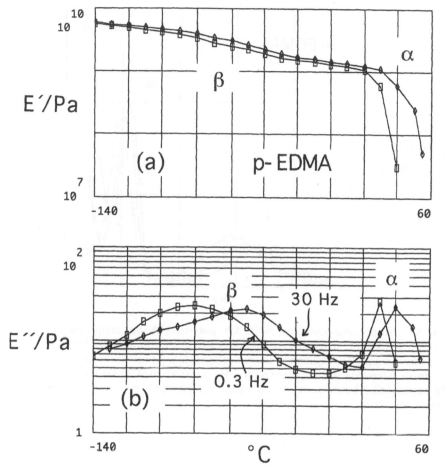

FIG. 40 Isochronous thermomechanical measurements (of the complex Young's modulus) on poly-EDMA for temperatures between $-140°C$ and $+60°C$. Two relaxations (α and β) are seen. The position of the relaxations shifts somewhat towards higher temperatures, increasing the frequency from 0.3 Hz to 30 Hz. *Source*: Ref. 37.

positioned approximately at the temperatures where the given frequency is the frequency of maximum loss for the relaxation in question in an *isothermal* loss spectrum. Whereas in the *isochronous* plots the succession of the α-, β-, γ-relaxation is from high to low temperature, the succession in *isothermal* plots is from low to high frequencies.

2. α- and β-Relaxation

Figure 42 shows Arrhenius plots of the frequencies of maximum dielectric loss for the α- and the β-relaxation of poly-EDMA. The α-relaxation (glass–rubber)

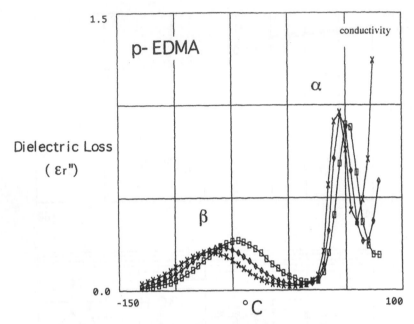

FIG. 41 Isochronous dielectric maps for poly-EDMA for temperatures between −140°C and +60°C. The same relaxations (α and β) are seen as in the thermomechanical measurements. The position of the relaxations shifts somewhat towards higher temperatures, increasing the frequency from 5 Hz (crosses), over 20 Hz (diamonds) to 100 Hz (rectangles). The steep rise at the highest temperatures is caused by conductance. *Source*: Ref. 37.

is clearly non-Arrhenius. The β-relaxation is Arrhenius neglecting some systematic deviations of the experimental values at the lowest and highest temperatures. The following expressions are found:

$$\ln[f_{\max, \alpha}/\text{Hz}] = \ln A_\alpha - B_\alpha/[T - T_0] = 31.55 - 2608/[T - 228]; \qquad (256)$$
$$r = -0.99003$$

(39 datapoints from two independent experimental runs; T_0 chosen with

max. abs(r))

$$\ln[f_{\max, \beta}/\text{Hz}] = 29.93 - 5778/T; \quad r = -0.9986 \text{ (16 datapoints)} \qquad (257)$$

It is seen from Fig. 42 that the two relaxations seem to come close together at a temperature about 100°C, although the extrapolation to this temperature is somewhat uncertain because of lack of data in the high temperature region. The points of highest temperature shown for the β-relaxation probably deviate

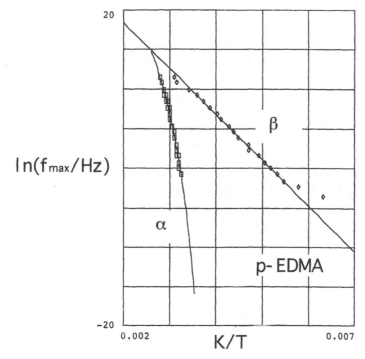

FIG. 42 Arrhenius plots for the α- and β-relaxations of poly-EDMA. The α-relaxation (glass–rubber) is strongly non-Arrhenius, following a Vogel relation (full line curve). The linear regression line for the β-relaxation is obtained neglecting four deviating points. *Source*: Ref. 37.

from the Arrhenius line because the maxima are distorted before their complete absorption in the ostensible α-peak, and with the α-relaxation there is a considerable covariance between the choice of the B and T_0 parameters in the Vogel expression, and the specific choice affects the extrapolation.

It has been observed in many other cases and stressed especially by Williams [56,68–72] that the *dielectric* α-relaxation and the β-relaxation seem to merge to an $\alpha\beta$-relaxation above a certain temperature and that the α and the β-processes cannot cross in the frequency domain. According to Williams these processes are coupled at high temperatures since they both involve motions of the same dipolar group [68,70]. However, the *mechanical* measurements of, for example, the shear loss module $G''(\omega)$ exhibit a similar merging of the α- and the β-relaxation, see [52], Fig. 2. One possible explanation of this phenomenon might be that the motions involved in the β-relaxation are the "minimum motions" involved also in the long range chain conformational changes corresponding to the α-relaxation. If the α-relaxation corresponds to some kind of "broken zip fastener" rearrangements involving shorter or longer sequences of the chains interacting cooperatively with neighbouring chains, then at high temperatures—when there are many unlocked loops in the "broken zipper",—the restrictions of the motions of the β-relaxations are the only remaining "bottlenecks".

It should be mentioned that the phenomenological situation with respect to these features is not yet completely clarified. The group of Donth, for example, maintain that there must be a "minimal cooperativity" in such a way that there cannot be a smooth transition from the α-relaxation to the $\alpha\beta$-relaxation [52,73,74]. At least a small number of monomer units must be involved to have an α-relaxation. Therefore, the α-relaxation should vanish shortly before it would have merged with the β-relaxation at high temperatures. Bartenev *et al.* [75] have very recently stressed that there are *two* mechanical β-relaxations in poly(methyl-methacrylate), poly-MMA, corresponding to the rotation of the CH_2 group and the rotation of the more bulky $C(CH_3)COOCH_3$ group in the polymer backbone. The former one seems to be the one approaching the non-Arrhenius α-relaxation at high temperatures whereas plots of $\ln f_{max}$ for the latter one is crossing the α-relaxation in a plot vs. $1/T$ (at much lower frequencies), see [75], Fig. 1. This seems to be in favor of the "broken zipper model" since the $\beta(CH_2)$ relaxation is likely to be the high temperature "bottleneck" mode for the zipper.

From the data and extrapolations made in Fig. 42, it is unfortunately not possible to clarify if (a) the α- and the β-relaxations merge to a single $\alpha\beta$-relaxation (as described by Williams), if (b) the α-relaxation vanishes shortly before merging with the β-relaxation because of the concept of "minimal cooperativity" advocated by the group of Donth, or (c) if the α-relaxation and the β-relaxation crosses each other in the $\ln f$ vs. $1/T$ plot as the case is with the $\beta(C(CH_3)COOCH_3)$-relaxation in the mechanical study of poly-MMA of Bartenev et al.

The activation energy found for the β-relaxation in the present study is $E^*/R = 5780$ K or $E^* = 48.0$ kJ/mol. For poly-MMA, Bartenev et al. found 30 kJ/mol for the $\beta(CH_2)$ relaxation and 69 kJ/mol for the $\beta(C(CH_3)COOCH_3)$-relaxation. The value found for poly-EDMA is midway between these values. Another clue is the limiting frequency at high temperatures. For the β-relaxation of poly-EDMA this is $\exp(29.93) = 9.96 \times 10^{12}$ Hz. This value is about 10 times higher than the limiting value of 1×10^{12} Hz stated by Bartenev et al. for the $\beta(CH_2)$ relaxation in poly-MMA. It is usual to have considerable shifts in frequencies between dielectric and mechanical measurements, however. For the $\beta(C(CH_3)COOCH_3)$-relaxation, Bartenev et al. found the much lower limiting frequency 2×10^9 Hz. The great magnitude of the limiting frequency for the β-relaxation found for poly-EDMA makes it likely that the relaxation observed is indeed a $\beta(CH_2)$ relaxation and not for example a $\beta(CHCOOCH_2, C_2H_5,$ dioxane$)$ relaxation. If this is true, it is most likely that the α- and the β-relaxation for poly-EDMA merges in Fig. 42 without crossing. However, if the β-relaxation found here corresponds to hindered rotations in the side chain (for example around the $O-CH_2$ bond) without any relation to the chain backbone, the β-relaxation might be crossing rather than merging with the α-relaxation.

Final conclusions are also made difficult by the present unclear state of the art. Bartenev *et al.* seem to be at variance with previous authors in their observation of two β-relaxations for poly-MMA. In addition, in [19] Table 8.2 the activation energy of the (unique) β-relaxation is listed as found for various authors. In dielectric studies it varies from 79 to 96 kJ/mol. In mechanical studies some authors find 71–75 kJ/mol others 121–125 kJ/mol. The latter two groups might be an indication of the existence of two different relaxations, but all the activation energies listed are far higher than the 30–32 kJ/mol which Bartenev et al. states as the "universal" activation energy for the $\beta(CH_2)$ relaxation "observed in all linear polymers containing CH_2 groups in the chain", [75], pp. 839–840. In the similar tables in [19] for other polymers containing CH_2 groups in the chain, no indication of any "universal" activation energy is found.

The activation energy 48 kJ/mol found here for the β-relaxation of poly-EDMA (an alkyl acrylate polymer) is lower than the values found for poly-MMA and various alkyl methacrylate polymers, [19] Table 8.2). For polymethyl acrylate, however, some authors have found a dielectric β-relaxation with activation energy 31–40 kJ/mol, and others a dielectric β-relaxation with activation energy 58–63 kJ/mol, see [19] Sec. 8.9b. The activation energy 48 kJ/mol found in the present study is well inside this range.

3. The Low Frequency tan δ Peak and Ion Diffusion

The loss tangent peaks found at low frequencies at nine temperatures in the dielectric data of poly-EDMA were analyzed in terms of the film-polarization model just like the data of the preceding two polymers (Sec. IV.B and C). The results are given in Tables 14 and 15.

It is seen that the trace concentrations of the ionic impurities are of the same order of magnitude in poly-EDMA as in poly-APCM (cf. Tables 13 and 15). It is likely that in the former case, the fast ion is chloride and the slow ion a triethylammonium ion somewhat entangled in the network of polymer chains. In the poly-APCM case, the fast anion might be Cl^- or OH^- and the slow cation is likely to be a tetrabuthylammonium ion. The diffusion coefficients are considerably higher in poly-EDMA than in poly-APCM in spite of the higher temperatures in the poly-APCM measurements (compare Tables 12 and 14). This cannot be explained by the greater "entanglement" of the tetrabuthylammonium ion than that of the triethylammonium ion, since it is the diffusion coefficient of the fast ion which is the important one. However, the

TABLE 14 The Maxima of the σ/Polarization tan δ Peaks and the Conductivities for Poly-EDMA

Temp. (°C)	tan δ_{max}	f_{max} (Hz)	$10^9\,\sigma$ ($\Omega^{-1}\,m^{-1}$)	$D_1 = D_2 = D$		$D_{fast} \gg D_{slow}$	
				κL	$10^{13}\,D$ ($m^2\,s^{-1}$)	κL	$10^{13}\,D_{fast}$ ($m^2\,s^{-1}$)
75	26	0.0178	0.61	5408	0.318	6905	0.386
80	26	0.0224	1.00	5408	0.400	6905	0.486
85	24	0.0501	1.60	4608	1.14	5884	1.38
90	23	0.0631	2.6	4232	1.63	5404	1.98
95	23	0.1584	3.8	4232	4.09	5404	4.96
100	25.5	0.224	6.1	5202	4.24	6642	5.15
105	26.5	0.282	9.2	5618	4.76	7174	5.77
110	26	0.316	16.0	5408	5.65	6905	6.85
115	29	0.631	30.0	6728	8.13	8591	9.86

$L = 4 \times 10^{-4}$ m.

differences in the void structures of the two amorphous polymers may also be important: poly-EDMA has much more "bulky" side chains than poly-APCM and this may create wider temporary, local "diffusion channels" in the former than in the latter.

The values of the static permittivities in Table 15, calculated by means of Eq. (247), are quite erratic, although they are of the right order of magnitude.

TABLE 15 The Electrolyte Concentrations and the Calculated Static Permittivities (Poly-EDMA)

Temp. (°C)	$D_1 = D_2 = D$		$D_{fast} \gg D_{slow}$		Best estimates $\varepsilon_s/\varepsilon_0$
	$10^6\,c_{salt}$ (mol/L)	$\varepsilon_s/\varepsilon_0$	$10^6\,c_{salt}$ (mol/L)	$\varepsilon_s/\varepsilon_0$	
75	2.98	11.9	4.91	12.0	11 ± 1
80	3.94	15.4	6.49	15.6	
85	2.25	12.0	3.70	12.1	
90	2.59	16.1	4.27	16.3	11 ± 1
95	1.53	9.4	2.52	9.5	
100	2.39	9.6	3.95	9.7	11.5 ± 1
105	3.26	11.1	5.38	11.2	
110	4.85	17.5	7.99	17.7	12 ± 1
115	6.40	14.7	10.6	14.9	9.2 ± 0.5

Best estimates of $\varepsilon_s/\varepsilon_0$ are found from the experimental values of ε_r' at low frequencies disregarding the interfacial polarization.

Better values can be estimated from the measured values of ε', see later. These estimated, best values are shown for some temperatures in Table 15.

Figure 43 shows a "Vogel plot" of the logarithm of the diffusion coefficients of the fast ion in poly-EDMA. The application of the same "Vogel temperature" as in the case of the glass–rubber relaxation yields a quite satisfactory straightening out of the plot, although there appears to be some systematic deviation in the neighborhood of 95°C. The regression line is given by:

$$\ln[D_{fast}/m^2\ s^{-1}] = \ln A_{diff} - B_{diff}/[T - T_o]$$
$$= -17.36 - 1616/[T - 228]; \quad r = -0.971 \qquad (258)$$

4. Interpretation in Terms of "Free Volume" Theory

Comparing Eq. (256) with Eq. (258) one observes that the ratio of the critical void volumes for the glass–rubber relaxation and for diffusion is given by:

$$v^*_{m,\,\alpha}/v^*_{m,\,diff} = B_\alpha/B_{diff} \approx 2608/1616 = 1.61\ \text{(poly-EDMA)} \qquad (259)$$

This figure is interestingly close to the figure 1.69 found in Eq. (254) for poly-VDCN/VAc in spite of the great differences between the latter polymer and poly-EDMA (reflected in the fact that the B coefficients of poly-EDMA are almost an order of magnitude greater than the B coefficients of poly-VDCN/VAc.

Compañ et al. [64] have investigated the permeability of oxygen through poly(cyclohexyl acrylate) = poly-CHA as a function of temperature from mea-

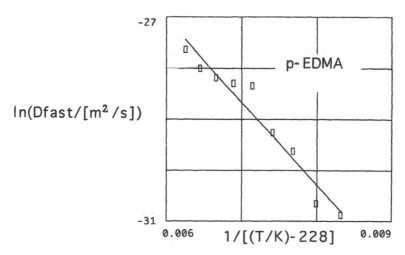

FIG. 43 Vogel plot for the faster ion diffusion coefficient in poly-EDMA using the same Vogel temperature (228 K) as found for the α-relaxation. *Source:* Ref. 37.

surements of the stationary reduction current in an electrochemical per-
meometer using an oxygen electrode. The diffusion coefficient was also found
at each temperature using the transients and the time-lag method. Fig. 4 in
[64] shows that $-\ln D_{O_2}$ and the logarithms of the relaxation times associated
with the mechanical as well as with the dielectric dispersion for the glass–
rubber relaxation are all given by straight line "Vogel plots" with a common
$T_o = 248$ K. The values $B_\alpha \approx 1300$ K and $B_{diff} \approx 392$ K were found. Thus, in
that case we have:

$$v^*_{m,\,\alpha}/v^*_{m,\,diff} = B_\alpha/B_{diff} \approx 1300/392 = 3.32 \text{ (poly-CHA)} \tag{260}$$

This value is much higher than found for the fast ion in poly-VDCN/VAc and
poly-EDMA. Perhaps it would be expected that the fast anion in the latter
two polymers is considerably smaller than the oxygen molecule, so that,
$v^*_{m,\,\alpha}/v^*_{m,\,diff}$ for poly-CHA should be *less* than ~ 1.6. This tendency should even
be reinforced by the fact that the side chain of poly-EDMA is much more
bulky than the side chain of poly-CHA so that $v^*_{m,\,\alpha}(\text{p-CHA})/v^*_{m,\,\alpha}(\text{p-EDMA})$
should be expected to be less than unity.

At the glass temperature ($\sim 36°$C) we have for poly-EDMA:

$$\phi(\text{glass})/(B_\alpha\,\alpha_f) = (T_g - T_o)/B_\alpha = 81/2608 = 0.031 \text{ (poly-EDMA)} \tag{261}$$

The value 0.031 is almost within the range 0.025 ± 0.005 found for many
amorphous polymers according to Ferry [53, p. 288]. The quantity is called
the "fractional free volume" at the glass temperature, since $B_\alpha\,\alpha_f$ is often close
to unity. In poly-CHA the somewhat higher value 0.038 was found [64].

5. Detection of a "Slow Mode" and Its Possible Interpretation

Finally, we would like to see which intrinsic dielectric relaxations are possibly
hiding behind the conductivity and the interfacial polarization. For this end,
the experimental values of ε'' are corrected for the conductivity contribution.
Figure 44 shows isothermal spectra at temperatures 45, 60 and 75°C. At 45°C
one loss peak has a frequency maximum at ≈ 20 Hz. This is within the uncertainty of the value 14 Hz calculated from the Vogel expression (256) for the
α-relaxation. The other peak has a maximum at frequencies greater than 100
kHz. Therefore the peak maximum cannot be observed, but the left side of the
peak is clearly visible at high frequencies. According to the regression Eq. (257)
for the β-relaxation, the frequency maximum should be ≈ 129 kHz. Thus, the
high frequency relaxation is surely the β-relaxation. The rise in ε'_r seen below
0.6 Hz should be ascribed to surface polarization. In that case, the *static* value
(for $\omega \to 0$) of the relative permittivity for the polymer would be 11 ± 1 at
45°C.

At the temperature 60°C, the Vogel value of the maximum frequency for the
α-relaxation is found to be ≈ 850 Hz which corresponds well with the ≈ 1000
Hz observed in the figure. The maximum frequency for the β-relaxation is

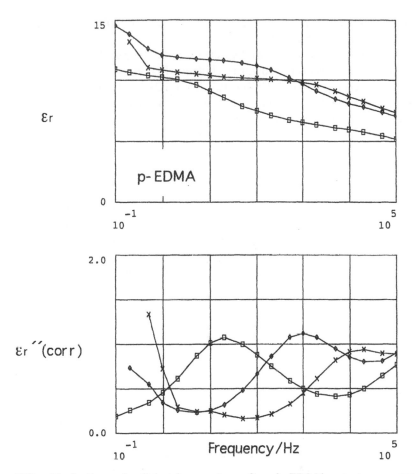

FIG. 44 Isothermal, dielectric spectra of poly-EDMA at temperatures 45°C (rectangles), 60°C (diamonds) and 75°C (crosses). The α and β-relaxations are seen in both components of the complex permittivity at the lower two temperatures. They are moving towards higher frequencies with increasing temperatures. *Source: Ref. 37.*

found from the (extrapolated) regression Eq. (257) to be ≈ 293 kHz, far above the maximum value of 100 kHz observed. However, the left side tail of the β-relaxation is still clearly seen at high frequencies since the activation energy of this relaxation is far less than that of the α-relaxation. There is a nice plateau in the values of ε_r' between 1 Hz and 10 Hz. The rise in ε_r' below 1 Hz is due to surface polarization and the rise in $\varepsilon_r''(corr)$ due to the effect of "small difference between large numbers" (called SDLN-effect for brevity). The static value of the relative permittivity seems to be 12 ± 1 at 60°C. At 75°C the β-relaxation has disappeared to the right.

Figure 45 shows similar isothermal spectra for 90, 100 and 110°C. Now, the α-relaxation is disappearing towards higher frequencies and a "slow relaxation" is emerging beyond the "noise" (from SDLN and interfacial polarization effects) at the lowest frequencies. In the raw experimental data this relaxation is completely masked by conductance.

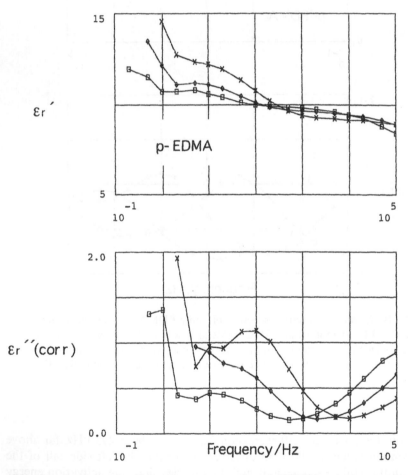

FIG. 45 Isothermal, dielectric spectra of poly-EDMA at temperatures 90°C (rectangles), 100°C (diamonds) and 110°C (crosses). The α-relaxation is moving towards higher frequencies with increasing temperature. Another "slow relaxation" is emerging out of the "noise" from SDLN-effects and interfacial polarization at low frequencies. *Source*: Ref. 37.

The "slow relaxation" is seen even more clearly in isochronous maps of $\varepsilon''(\text{corr})$ vs. temperature, see Fig. 46. We call the relaxation found at high temperatures (or low frequencies) for the "X-relaxation". In the isochronous maps, the X-relaxation is dominant over the α-relaxation at low frequencies (lower subfigure) whereas the inverse is true at higher frequencies (upper subfigure). In Fig. 46 it is seen that the X-peak is really a "twin peak". This is more and more clearly revealed as the X-peak grows larger when the fixed frequency is lowered.

The slow relaxation X-peak observed exhibits a maximum dielectric loss. These maxima are approximately positioned at 10 Hz, 50 Hz, 100 Hz, 200 Hz, 700 Hz and 1500 Hz for the temperatures 90°C, 100°C, 110°C, 115°C, 130°C and 140°C. The temperature dependence from 90 to 140°C is quite perfectly Arrhenius:

$$\ln(f_{\text{max, x}}) = 42.82 - 14620(1/T), \quad r = -0.9945 \ (90°\text{C to } 140°\text{C}) \tag{262}$$

The mean activation energy is 14,620 K. We can compare this with the mean activation energy for the α-relaxation extrapolated to the same range of temperatures. In general, the "local activation energy" at the temperature T is given by $E^{\neq}(T)/R = -d\ln(f_{\text{max}})/d(1/T)$ and from the Vogel relation with $T_0 = 228$ K and $B = 2608$ K one obtains from Eq. (253) and at a mean temperature 115°C (in the range 90–140°C):

$$E_{\alpha}^{\neq}(115°\text{C})/R = 15,340 \text{ K} \tag{263}$$

This mean activation energy is very close to the mean activation energy 14,620 K found for the slow relaxation. This might be an indication that the same inter- or intramolecular interactions are involved in the α-relaxation and the slow relaxation.

Thus, there are many indications of a quite complex dielectric relaxation pattern of the polymer studied here. The correction for conductivity has clearly revealed a high temperature relaxation with larger relaxation times than the α-relaxation. This relaxation has a similar mean activation energy as the α-relaxation extrapolated to the same range of temperatures. In the modified Rouse theory for undiluted polymers (entropic bead-spring model of the normal modes of the generalized micro-Brownian motions of the polymer (see [53], Chapters 9 and 10 and [19], Sec. 5.3) the relaxation times of all the normal modes are proportional to the *translational friction coefficient* for the monomer (ζ_0) in the "solvent" constituted by the surrounding polymer chains. When this theory is used for the glass–rubber relaxation, the first three normal modes (with the most long relaxation times) are often ignored and the discrete summation over the other normal modes is replaced by the integration over a continuous spectrum, see [19] pp. 156–159. If the slow relaxation observed here is just the sum of the "discarded" modes (two modes as indicated by the

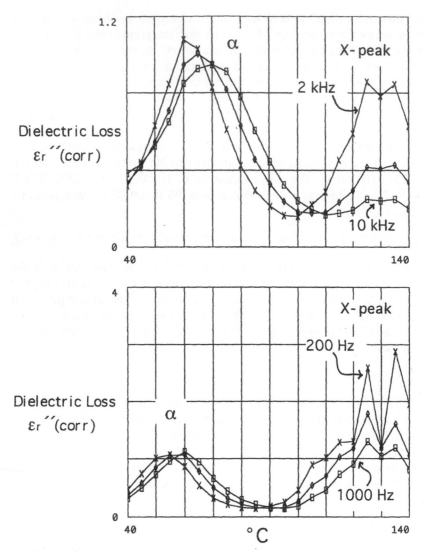

FIG. 46 Isochronous plots of the dielectric loss corrected for conductivity. An α-relaxation peak and a high temperature "X-peak" is seen. At high frequencies, the α-peak is large and the X-peak small. For decreasing frequencies, the α-peak diminishes and the X-peak grows up, revealing a more and more pronounced bimodal nature. *Source*: Ref. 37.

twin peak?) this will explain that the "local activation energy" for this process is the same as for the α-relaxation, since the basic activation energy is the one for $1/\zeta_0$.

For uncross-linked, amorphous polymers of high molecular weight, there is much evidence that topological "entanglements" (where the polymer chains loop around each other in their long-range contour) restrict the cooperative micro-Brownian motions of the glass–rubber relaxation, see [53], Chapter 10, Sec. C1. This explains the M-independence of the glass–rubber transition in such polymers, since the micro-Brownian motions only involve chain segments confined between two entanglements. The entanglement concept also explains that at still lower frequencies than the glass–rubber relaxation (α-relaxation) the *mechanical* relaxation spectra of polymers, complex Young modulus $E^*(\omega)$ or shear modulus $G^*(\omega)$-exhibit another relaxation which is strongly dependent on molecular weight (M). The relaxation time of this absorption scales as $\approx M^{3.4}$ for chains in which M is larger than a critical value M_{cr}, see Ref. 53, Chapter 10, Sec. C1. This relaxation involves motions of the chain as a whole and various theories have been proposed to explain it. For example the entanglement theory of Bueche [76,77] predicting a power 3.5 and an $M_{cr} \approx$ two times the mean molecular weight between two entanglements, or the "tube model" of de Gennes [54,78], Doi and Edwards [79] and Graessley [80] where the entanglements are described as a "virtual tube", from which the easiest escape of the polymer molecule in focus is by snakelike "reptation" along its own contour. Clearly, this reptation gives rise to very long relaxation times.

On the other hand, the Rouse theory has also been used in the connection with entanglement coupling of high molecular weight, amorphous polymers. In that case, a common enhancement factor Q_e has been inserted in the expressions for the normal mode relaxation times. This factor represents the enhancement of the friction by the entanglement constraints. Since the relaxation times are still proportional to ζ_0, the activation energy of micro-Brownian motions with entanglement constraints would still be the same as for the α-relaxation. However, this model does not furnish us with the correct frequency dependence of the *mechanical*, shear storage modulus (G') in the limit of low frequencies, see [53], Chapter 10, Sec. C3.

In the *dielectric* spectra, the slow relaxation connected with the motion of the whole chain relative to the confinements of the entanglements should also be visible in some cases. The theory for polymer melts (or rubbers) has been reviewed [81,82]. As we have seen, one problem is that the peak in the dielectric loss ε'' corresponding to this "normal mode process" is quite often completely masked by conductivity and surface polarization phenomena. However, the "tube evaporation by reptation" model of Doi and Edwards [79] also produce a sum of relaxation terms with the longest relaxation time corresponding to the so-called "reptation" process of de Gennes. Once more, all the relaxation times are proportional to ζ_0, see [53], Chapter 10, Eqs. (54) and (57a). This model is valid for mechanical relaxations, but probably dielectric relaxations can be treated similarly.

Finally, it should be mentioned that neither the high frequency splitting of the α-peak into a twin peak nor the slow relaxation can be the results of nonequilibrium "ageing" phenomena, since both phenomena occur above the glass transition temperature ($\approx 36°C$), and Beiner et al. have shown in a mechanical relaxation study of a number of poly(alkyl methacrylates) [83] that keeping the polymers 10 min above the glass transition temperatures is enough for a complete elimination of the "memory" of the thermal history of the polymer.

The EDMA polymer treated in this paper seems to be an interesting target for more detailed dielectric and mechanical investigations in the future because of the many complex features exhibited. For example, it would be interesting to study samples with different and well defined mean molar masses (M) of the polymer in order to investigate the M-dependence of the different relaxation peaks observed, especially to see if the relaxation times of the slow "X-relaxation" scales as $M^{3.4}$ as has been found experimentally for other polymers.

V. CONCLUSIONS

In the present chapter I have treated cases of impedance and dielectric spectroscopy of membranes and polymer films in which it is important to consider the constitutive relations of the electrodiffusion of the ions and dynamical, electric double layers near to impenetrable "walls" or penetrable interfaces. After having introduced the classical methods of Maxwell, Wagner and Sillars and of the "principle of generalized conductivity" and after having discussed the limitations of these procedures, various theoretical models were discussed based upon the linearized Nernst–Planck equations. Not only the perturbing signals are linearized but also the permanent equilibrium electric double layers should be linear. On the one side this is a limitation, on the other this linearization makes unimportant (in the first approximation) the presence of double layers due to fixed charges or fixed dipole layers.

As illustrations of the applicability of the theoretical approach (which is far more involved than the MWS approach) the *Nernst–Planckian electrodynamics* of films or membranes between blocking electrodes containing binary electrolytes of arbitrary charge type were investigated in details and practical methods were devised to calculate ion concentrations and ion diffusion coefficients from the characteristics of the low frequency maximum in the loss tangent tan δ. Investigations of "leaky" interfaces and lamellar films were also studied in some details, but in this field there is still much to do in the future. The present treatment will be a good starting point for that. The relation to the similar theory of Trukhan for planar and spherical geometry [40] was also carefully discussed.

In Sec. III, the Trukhan theory of impenetrable, ion filled "alveoles" dispersed in a dielectric, nonconductive matrix was used (in a reinforced Brüggemann integrated form) to describe the concentration dependence of the C-component in a "hybrid" RC model for the impedance of cellulose acetate and other desalination membranes. The R-component was described by a Nernst–Planck–Donnan treatment using the methods and data obtained in connection with the treatment of emf measurements of concentration cells with membrane separators, see Chapter 10 in the present volume.

In Sec. IV, the Nernst–Planckian electrodynamics of polymer films with ion "impurities" was discussed. It is interesting to try to separate the conductivity effects, the interfacial polarization and the intrinsic relaxations of the polymer itself. In the literature much confusion prevails due to the overlapping of glass–rubber relaxation with the "ion impurity relaxation". Small amounts of ions seem to be present even in polymers which are very apolar due to the preparation or due to contamination in the measuring process, and they have a profound influence on the effective permittivity at low frequencies. As has been shown, this disadvantage may be turned into a benefit since one may study the temperature dependence of the glass–rubber relaxation, the subglass relaxations and the diffusion of ions in the polymer in one stroke by means of a swift and nondestructive measuring technique. Especially the glass–rubber relaxation (α-relaxation) and the diffusion of ions (or gases) are connected *via* the "free volume theory". Therefore, the main connections of this important theory was covered in Sec. IVA.

As a "training example" an extensive treatment was given of some experimental, dielectric data of Furukawa et al. [41] on copolymer films of polyvinylidene cyanide/vinyl acetate. This is a highly polar polymer with a relatively high contamination of ions. The use of an empirical Havriliak–Negami expression for the intrinsic dielectric dispersion combined with an empirical "constant phase element" for the description of the interfacial polarization is characteristic for this study. It is indeed seen, that the constant phase element *does* describe the maximum in tan δ and even the maximum in the dielectric loss ε'' quite well at moderately low frequencies. However, the opportunity of obtaining useful information on ion concentrations and diffusion coefficients is missed using such a technique. Furthermore, the constant phase element, described by Eq. (245), has basically a fundamental flaw in common with the MWS approach: It violates the second law of thermodynamics when the frequency goes to zero. Ultimately, the dielectric loss ε'' predicted by the constant phase element goes towards infinity in that limit. Since the dielectric loss is proportional to the dissipation in a cycle of inversion of the electric field [17], this feature is quite unphysical. Between blocking electrodes, the ions will ultimately be in quasi-equilibrium (Boltzmann equilibrium) with the slowly varying electric field, when the frequency is low enough for diffusional redistribution of the ions to take place.

Two other, much more apolar, polymers of the polyacrylic acid type with bulky side chains have also been studied. In these polymers the ions are really only present in trace amounts, but their relative influence in the low frequency regime are not less than in poly-VDCN/VAc. Both acrylic polymers show signs of a more slow relaxation than the α-relaxation. Especially the EDMA polymer shows an interesting and complex dielectric behavior. A slow, sometimes clearly bimodal, relaxation is exhibited which seems linked to the most fundamental micro-Brownian motions, where especially the snakelike motion of the polymer chain along its countour (the "reptation" mode of de Gennes [54]) is a very likely candidate.

The next two chapters, Chapter 19 [38] by Coster and Chillcott and Chapter 20 by Zholkovski [39], are complementary to the present chapter in developing other aspects of this rich subject. Chapter 19 discusses MWS and Nernst–Planck–Poisson studies of membranes in aqueous/ionic ambience, especially biological membranes. A somewhat broader framework of irreversible thermodynamics, than the simple Nernst–Planck equations used here, is presented although the studies are until now restricted to the somewhat artificial restriction that the pressure and osmotic pressure perturbations always counterbalance. Intriguing reports concerning frequency bands with negative membrane capacitances are given. In the present chapter, I have shown that the effects of even trace impurities of ions may be very large over broad ranges of frequency, so it is undoubtedly correct when Coster and Chillcott postulate that intrinsic dielectric dispersion in membranes soaked in aqueous electrolytes may often be completely neglected.

In Chapter 20, the MWS approach is developed. Using the central concept of the "chemical capacity", elegant and comprehensive methods are devised for the treatment of lamellar membranes. The definite advantage is, that the treatment is phenomenological and model independent. The prize paid is that *electric* polarization at the interfaces is neglected, the Debye length being much smaller than the characteristic dimensions of the membrane substructures. An important caveat in this connection is, however, that this criterion is not always sufficient for the application of the MWS procedure. It has been shown here, that the MWS approach basically renders correct results in the limit of high frequencies. In cases of films between blocking interfaces, the film thickness may be many thousand times the Debye length with the effects of electropolarization having an *increasing* significance at low frequencies (macropolarization). It is correct, however, that the upper frequency limit, where these interfacial polarization phenomena cease to be of importance, is depressed more and more the thicker is the film compared to the Debye length.

REFERENCES

1. J. C. Maxwell, *A Treatise of Electricity and Magnetism*, Dover, New York, 1954, Articles 310–314 (originally Clarendon Press, 1891).
2. K. W. Wagner, Arch. Elektrotech. *2*: 371 (1914).
3. K. W. Wagner, Arch. Elektrotech. *3*: 67 (1914).
4. R. W. Sillars, Proc. Inst. Electr. Eng. London *80*: 378 (1937).
5. R. Höber, Arch. ges. Physiol. *133*: 237 (1910).
6. R. Höber, Arch. ges. Physiol. *148*: 189 (1912).
7. R. Höber, Arch. ges. Physiol. *150*: 15 (1913).
8. M. Philipson, Bull. Acad. roy. Belgique. Cl. Sci. *7*: 387 (1921).
9. H. Fricke and S. Morse, J. Gen. Physiol. *9*: 153 (1925).
10. K. S. Cole, *Membranes, Ions and Impulses*, University of California Press, Berkeley, 1968.
11. J. R. Macdonald (Ed.), *Impedance Spectroscopy. Emphasizing Solid Materials and Systems*, John Wiley & Sons, New York, 1987.
12. R. P. Buck, *Electroanalytical Chemistry of Membranes*, CRC Publishing Co., West Palm Beach, Florida 1976.
13. R. P. Buck, M. B. Madaras, and R. Mackel, J. Electroanal. Chem. *362*: 33 (1993).
14. T. C. Chilcott and H. G. L. Coster, Aust. J. Plant Physiol. *21*: 147 (1994).
15. T. C. Chilcott, H. G. L. Coster, and E. P. George, J. Membrane Sci. *100*: 77 (1995).
16. H. G. L. Coster, T. C. Chilcott, and A. C. F. Coster, Bioelectrochem. Bioenergetics *40*: 79 (1996).
17. H. Fröhlich, *Theory of Dielectrics. Dielectric Constant and Dielectric Loss*, 2nd Ed., Clarendon Press, Oxford, 1958.
18. C. J. F. Böttcher, *Theory of Electric Polarization. Vol I. Dielectrics in Static Fields*, 2nd Ed. (revised by O. C. van Belle, P. Bordewijk, and A. Rip), Elsevier, 1973.
19. N. G. McCrum, B. E. Read, and G. Williams, *Anelastic and Dielectric Effects in Polymeric Solids*, Dover, New York, 1991 (originally John Wiley & Sons, 1967).
20. T. Hanai, in *Emulsion Science*, Academic Press, San Diego, 1968, Chapter 5.
21. M. Clausse, in *Encyclopedia of Emulsion Technology. Vol. 1* (P. Becher, ed.), Marcel Dekker, New York, 1983, pp. 481–715.
22. S. S. Dukhin, in *Surface and Colloid Science. Vol. 3* (E. Matijevic, ed.), Wiley-Interscience, New York, 1971, pp. 83–165.
23. S. S. Dukhin and V. N. Shilov, *Dielectric Phenomena and the Double Layer in Disperse Systems and Polyelectrolytes*, Wiley, New York, 1974.
24. E. K. Zholkovskij, Colloid Journal of the USSR *51*: 457 (1989).
25. E. K. Zholkovskij, J. Colloid Interface Sci. *169*: 267 (1995).
26. E. K. Zholkovskij, V. N. Shilov, and V. I. Koval'chuk, J. Colloid Interface Sci. *184*: 414 (1996).
27. T. S. Sørensen, J. Colloid Interface Sci. *168*: 437 (1994).
28. T. S. Sørensen and V. Compañ, J. Colloid Interface Sci. *178*: 186 (1996).
29. T. S. Sørensen, J. Chem. Soc., Faraday Trans. *93*: 4327 (1997).
30. B. Malmgren-Hansen, T. S. Sørensen, B. Jensen, and M. Hennenberg, J. Colloid Interface Sci. *130*: 359 (1989).
31. T. S. Sørensen, J. B. Jensen, and B. Malmgren-Hansen, Desalination *80*: 293 (1991).

32. T. S. Sørensen, in *Capillarity Today. Lecture Notes in Physics, Vol. 386* (G. Petré and A. Sanfeld, eds.) Springer, Berlin, 1991, pp. 188–213.

33. I. W. Plesner, B. Malmgren-Hansen, and T. S. Sørensen, J. Chem. Soc., Faraday Trans. *90*:2381 (1994).

34. T. S. Sørensen and V. Compañ, J. Chem. Soc., Faraday Trans. *91*:4235 (1995).

35. V. Compañ, T. S. Sørensen, R. Diaz-Calleja, and E. Riande, J. Appl. Phys. *79*:1 (1996).

36. T. S. Sørensen, V. Compañ, and R. Diaz-Calleja, J. Chem. Soc., Faraday Trans. *92*:1947 (1996).

37. T. S. Sørensen, R. Diaz-Calleja, E. Riande, J. Guzman, and A. Andrio, J. Chem. Soc., Faraday Trans. *93*:2399 (1997).

38. H. G. L. Coster and T. C. Chilcott, in *Surface Chemistry and Electrochemistry of Membranes* (T. S. Sørensen, ed.), Marcel Dekker, New York, 1998, Chapter 19.

39. E. K. Zholkovskij, in *Surface Chemistry and Electrochemistry of Membranes* (T. S. Sørensen, ed.), Marcel Dekker, New York, 1998, Chapter 20.

40. E. M. Trukhan, Soviet Physics Solid State *4*:2560 (1963).

41. T. Furukawa, M. Date, K. Nakajima, T. Kosaka, and I. Seo, Jpn. J. Appl. Phys. *25*:1178 (1986).

42. T. S. Sørensen and S. Rivera, in *Surface Chemistry and Electrochemistry of Membranes* (T. S. Sørensen, ed.), Marcel Dekker, New York, 1998, Chapter 10.

43. H. Strathmann, P. Scheible, and R. W. Baker, J. Appl. Polym. Sci. *15*:811 (1971).

44. H. Strathmann and K. Kock, Desalination *21*:241 (1977).

45. W. Pusch, J. Membrane Sci. *21*:325 (1982).

46. D. A. G. Brüggemann, Ann. Phys. (Leipzig) *24*:636 (1935).

47. M. Pinéri, in *Coulombic Interactions in Macromolecular Systems* (A. Eisenberg and F. E. Bailey, eds.), ACS Symposium Series 302, American Chemical Society, Washington DC, 1986, pp. 159–175.

48. U. Merten (Ed.) *Desalination by Reverse Osmosis*, The M.I.T. Press, Cambridge, Massachusetts, 1966.

49. W. Pusch and A. Walch, Angew. Chem. Int. Ed. Engl. *21*:660 (1982).

50. P. M. Wiggins and R. T. van Ryn, J. Macromol. Sci., A: Chem. *23*:875 (1986).

51. H. U. Demisch and W. Pusch, J. Electrochem. Soc.: Electrochem. Sci. Technol. *123*:370 (1976).

52. M. Beiner, F. Garwe, E. Hempel, J. Schawe, K. Schröter, A. Schönhals, and E. Donth, Physica A. *201*:72 (1993).

53. J. D. Ferry, *Viscoelastic Properties of Polymers*, 3rd Ed., Wiley-Interscience, New York, 1980.

54. P. G. de Gennes, *Scaling Concepts in Polymer Physics*, Cornell University Press, 1985.

55. H. P. Schwan, in *Advances in Biological and Medical Physics, Vol. 5*, Academic Press, New York, 1957, pp. 147–209.

56. G. Williams, in *Material Science and Technology Series, Vol. 12. Structure and Properties of Polymers*, (E. L. Thomas, ed.) VCH, London, 1993, Chapter 11.

57. S. Glasstone, K. J. Laidler, and H. Eyring, *The Theory of Rate Processes*, McGraw-Hill, New York, 1941.

58. A. K. Doolittle and D. B. Doolittle, J. Appl. Phys. *28*:901 (1957).

59. M. H. Cohen and D. Turnbull, J. Chem. Phys. *31*:1164 (1959).

60. D. Turnbull and M. H. Cohen, J. Chem. Phys. *34*: 120 (1961).
61. S. A. Stern and H. L. Frisch, Annu. Rev. Mater. Sci. *11*: 523 (1981).
62. M. H. Y. Mulder, *Basic Principles of Membrane Technology*, Kluwer Academic, Dordrecht, 1991.
63. J. H. Petropoulus, M. Sanopoulo, and K. G. Papadokostaki, in *Surface Chemistry and Electrochemistry of Membranes* (T. S. Sørensen, ed.), Marcel Dekker, New York, 1998, Chapter 5.
64. V. Compañ, E. Riande, J. San Román, and R. Diaz-Calleja, Polymer *34*: 3843 (1993).
65. R. Diaz-Calleja, E. Riande, and J. San Román, Macromolecules *25*: 2875 (1992).
66. S. Havriliak and S. Negami, J. Polym. Sci. *C14*: 99 (1966).
67. R. C. Nunes, R. Diaz-Calleja, M. Pinto, E. Saiz, and E. Riande, J. Phys. Chem. *99*: 12962 (1995).
68. G. Williams and D. C. Watts, in *NMR, Basic Principles and Progress, Vol. 4: NMR of Polymers*, Springer, Heidelberg, 1971, p. 271.
69. G. Williams, Spec. Period. Rep. Dielectr. Relat. Mol. Processes *2*: 151 (1975).
70. G. Williams, Adv. Polymer Sci. *33*: 60 (1979).
71. G. Williams, in *Comprehensive Polymer Science* (G. Allen and J. C. Bevington, eds.), Pergamon, Oxford, 1989, Vol. 2, Chapter 7, p. 601.
72. G. Williams, in *Keynote Lectures in Selected Topics of Polymer Science*, (E. Riande, ed.), Consejo Superior de Investigaciones Científicas, Madrid, 1995, Chapter 1, pp. 8–9.
73. M. Beiner, F. Garwe, K. Schröter, and E. Donth, Polymer *35*: 4127 (1994).
74. E. Donth, M. Beiner, S. Reissig, J. Korus, F. Garwe, S. Vieweg, S. Kahle, E. Hempel, and K. Schröter, Macromolecules *29*: 6589 (1996).
75. G. M. Bartenev, G. M. Sinitsyna, A. G. Barteneva, and N. Yu. Lomovskaya, Polymer Sci. A *38*: 839 (1996). (Transl. from Vysokomol Soedin. A *38*: 1302 (1996)).
76. F. Bueche, J. Chem. Phys. *20*: 1959 (1952).
77. F. Bueche, *Physical Properties of Polymers*, Interscience, New York, 1962.
78. P. G. de Gennes, J. Chem. Phys. *55*: 572 (1971).
79. M. Doi and S. F. Edwards, J. Chem. Soc. Faraday Trans. 2 *74*: 1789, 1802 (1978).
80. W. W. Graessley, J. Polym. Sci. Polym. Phys. Ed. *18*: 27 (1980).
81. K. Adachi and T. Kotaka, Macromolecules *21*: 157 (1988).
82. D. Boese and F. Kremer, Macromolecules *23*: 829 (1990).
83. M. Beiner, F. Garwe, K. Schröter and E. Donth, Colloid Polym. Sci. *272*: 1439 (1994).

19

The Characterization of Membranes and Membrane Surfaces Using Impedance Spectroscopy

HANS G. L. COSTER and TERRY C. CHILCOTT UNESCO Centre for Membrane Science and Technology, and Department of Biophysics, School of Physics, University of New South Wales, Sydney, New South Wales, Australia

Abstract

Experimental measurements of the electrical characteristics of cellular and synthetic membranes have been used widely in investigations of membrane structure, function and the relationship between these. In cellular as well as synthetic membranes, the electrical response time of the system is limited by diffusion time constants as well as dielectric charging time constants of the membrane and its substructure. Such systems display characteristic dispersions with frequency of the capacitance and conductance. The diffusion limited processes can be analyzed in terms of generalized Nernst–Planck–Poisson equations for electrodiffusion. A review is presented of the various mechanisms and membrane attributes that contribute to the dispersion of the impedance. The expected impedance dispersions are compared to experimental measurements for a variety of systems and illustrate the scope of the impedance spectroscopy technique in the study of membrane systems.

I. INTRODUCTION

Impedance measurements have been used to characterize membranes for many decades. Indeed, impedance measurements provided the first direct evidence for the existence of membranes surrounding living cells [1], although their existence was suggested by the slow exchange of ions between the cell interior and the surrounding medium [2]. These impedance measurements provided the first good estimate of the thickness of the membrane surrounding living cells [3]; some 30 years before these membranes could be imaged using electron microscopy [4]!

Similarly, impedance measurements on artificial lipid bilayer membranes provided the first estimates of their thickness and remarkable insulating properties [5–7].

Impedance measurement have been also utilized very extensively in the study of tissue membranes [8–16]. More recently, these techniques have been applied increasingly to study and monitor synthetic membranes used in industrial separation processes [17–37] and in fundamental studies of membrane-based sensors [38–42].

The functional properties of membranes and solid–aqueous systems in general, are closely connected to the electrochemical processes that occur within the interfacial regions between the membrane surface and the bulk electrolyte [43–46]. The electrochemistry of these interfaces, which are of the order of molecular dimensions, remains largely unresolved mainly because conventional techniques for studying such processes are disruptive. Impedance spectroscopy may provide a unique approach for the study of these "structures" which persist only in the undisturbed system.

In this review we have deliberately emphasized impedance studies of double layers and unstirred layers [47] which are sometimes considered to be a nuisance, but which in fact feature strongly in membrane transport processes and form an integral part of new devices such as membrane-based biosensors.

II. FUNDAMENTALS

Impedance measurements are made by injecting an alternating current (AC) $\tilde{I}$ of known angular frequency, ω and (preferably) small amplitude I_0 into the system via current electrodes (located at $x = \pm L/2$ in Fig. 1a), and measuring the amplitude V_0 and phase difference ϕ of the concomitant electrical potential difference that develops across the sample under study. The potential difference may also be measured using separate electrodes situated between the current electrodes (at $x = \pm l/2$ in Fig. 1a). Of course these AC signals will be, more often than not, offset by other residual steady-state signals ($\bar{I}$ and $\bar{V}$) generated by the sample. Then the measurements of current and electrical potential will be, respectively

$$I = \bar{I} + \tilde{I} \quad \text{and} \quad V = \bar{V} + \tilde{V} \tag{1}$$

The DC contributions $\bar{I}$ and $\bar{V}$ can be subtracted from Eq. (1) using either analogue offset adjustments to the amplifiers used for the measurements or by computational techniques applied to the digitized data.

The identities $e^{j\theta} \equiv \cos\theta + j\sin\theta$ and $j \equiv \sqrt{-1}$ enables us to express the AC variables for electrical potential difference and current as phasors;

$$\tilde{V} = V_0 e^{j(\omega t + \phi)} \quad \text{and} \quad \tilde{I} = I_0 e^{j\omega t} \tag{2}$$

where t denotes time. The ratio of these two AC variables defines the impedance

$$Z \equiv \frac{\tilde{V}}{\tilde{I}} = \frac{V_0}{I_0} e^{j\phi} = |Z| e^{j\angle Z} \tag{3}$$

With the identities Eq. (1) impedance can be expressed in Cartesian coordinates so;

$$Z = R + jX = \frac{V_0}{I_0}\{\cos\phi + j\sin\phi\} \tag{4}$$

where R is the resistance and X is the reactance.

Note that in the definition of impedance [Eq. (3)], the time dependent term $e^{j\omega t}$ in each of the expressions for the AC electric potential and current [Eq. (2)] cancel leading to the time-independent relationship Eq. (4). In impedance analysis this cancellation always occurs resulting in time-independent amplitudes and phase angles for all the AC variables involved in such relationships. Although all AC variables include the $e^{j\omega t}$ term it is customary to take this as

(a)

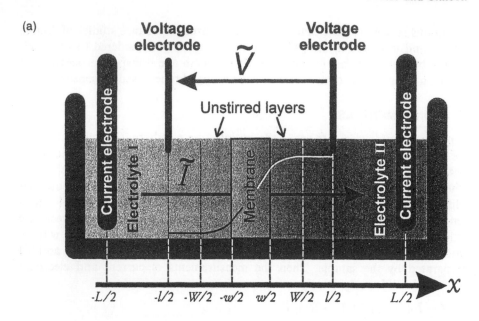

(b)

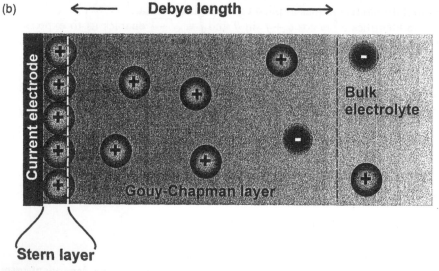

FIG. 1 Four-terminal configuration for measuring the impedance of aqueous systems. a. The electrode configuration. Current electrodes are used to inject an AC current $\tilde{I}$ into the electrolytes on either side of the membrane. Separate (voltage) electrodes are sometimes used to sense the AC electrical potential difference, $\tilde{V}$, that develops across the "system". For this configuration the "system" includes electrolyte I ($-l/2 < x <$ $-W/2$), unstirred layer I ($-W/2 < x < -w/2$), the membrane ($-w/2 < x < w/2$),

understood and for simplicity all the expressions involving time-dependent quantities refer to those dependencies that are *not* associated with $e^{j\omega t}$, that is, those that are *not* periodic. Here, notations $\bar{E}$ and $\tilde{E}$ refer to, respectively, DC and AC components of the general variable E.

The phasor representation of AC variables [Eq. (2)] has a further benefit when considering variations with time because, upon differentiating any AC variable $\tilde{E}$ (whose amplitudes and phase are constant in t) with respect to time, one obtains the general relationship;

$$\frac{\partial \tilde{E}}{\partial t} = j\omega \tilde{E} \tag{5}$$

where the $j\omega$ term arises directly from differentiating the $e^{j\omega t}$ term which is understood to be included in the definition of the AC variable $\tilde{E}$ [cf. Eq. (2)].

A. Physical Interpretation of Impedance

We will restrict ourselves to systems in which the electrochemical potential varies only in one dimension and the fluxes and current density are uniform in that direction. Whilst this restricts us to systems with planar geometry, large thin membranes usually approximate a one-dimensional system in that the current and fluxes, etc. are essentially normal to the surface. The radius of curvature of the latter is often large compared with the thickness of the membrane.[a] Thus for a sample of material of planar geometry and cross-sectional

---

[a] This is true even for the membrane surrounding a living cell which typically have radii of only $\sim 5~\mu m$. Such radii remain large compared to the thickness of the plasma membrane which is ~ 5–8 nm. For synthetic, hollow fibre membranes this may not always be true.

---

unstirred layer II ($w/2 < x < W/2$) and electrolyte II ($W/2 < x < l/2$). If the current electrodes are also used to sense $\tilde{V}$ then the system includes the electrode–electrolyte double layer (Fig. 1b), the impedance of which can exceed that for the rest of the system and is also strongly frequency dependent. This is especially so at low frequencies (see below). Therefore two terminal impedance measurements are best confined to high frequencies. b. Electrode–electrolyte double layer. At the interface with an electrolyte electron conduction is replaced by ionic conduction. Electrodes made from inert noble metals such as gold, do not readily react chemically with ions in the solution and hence are blocking electrodes. A consequence of using blocking electrodes is that cations are absorbed to the surface via "image" forces. The layer at the metal–electrolyte interface, so formed, is called the Stern layer. Further from the Stern layer the anions and cations in the electrolyte form a "diffuse layer" (Gouy–Chapman layer). The layer of charges at the surface and the diffuse layer in the solution together constitute what is termed the "double-layer'. Since the ionic current is zero, the impedance of this layer is large at low frequencies. At higher frequencies the impedance of the double decreases as the displacement current increases.

area A, such as depicted in Fig. (1), the current density and electric field are;

$$J \equiv \frac{\bar{I}}{A} \quad \text{and} \quad \bar{E}(x) \equiv -\frac{\partial \bar{V}(x)}{\partial x}$$

respectively, for DC conditions and

$$J = \bar{J} + \tilde{J} \equiv \frac{\bar{I} + \tilde{I}}{A} \quad \text{and} \quad E(x) = \bar{E}(x) + \tilde{E}(x) \equiv -\frac{\partial \bar{V}(x)}{\partial x} - \frac{\partial \tilde{V}(x)}{\partial x}$$

respectively, upon introducing the AC contributions $\tilde{J}$ and $\tilde{E}$. Subtracting the DC terms $\bar{J}$ and $\bar{E}$, then yields expressions for these contributions

$$\tilde{J} = \frac{\tilde{I}}{A} \quad \text{and} \quad \tilde{E}(x) = -\frac{\partial \tilde{V}(x)}{\partial x} \tag{6}$$

Similarly, Poisson's equation[b] applies for DC as well as for DC plus AC conditions and this yields:

$$\frac{\partial \mathbf{D}(x)}{\partial x} \equiv \bar{\rho}(x) \quad \text{and} \quad \frac{\partial(\bar{\mathbf{D}}(x) + \tilde{\mathbf{D}}(x))}{\partial x} \equiv \bar{\rho}(x) + \tilde{\rho}(x)$$

respectively, where $\rho(x)$ denotes the density of electric charge at position x and $\mathbf{D}(x)$ denotes the electric displacement vector (or electric flux density vector) at that position[c]. Subtraction yields the AC density of electric charge

$$\tilde{\rho}(x) = \frac{\partial \tilde{\mathbf{D}}(x)}{\partial x} \tag{7}$$

In the electrolyte the current is comprised of an ionic contribution J_{ionic} as well as the displacement current $\partial \mathbf{D}(x)/\partial t$. The total current is then

$$J \equiv J_{ionic} + \frac{\partial \mathbf{D}(x)}{\partial t}$$

---

[b] Note that Poisson's equation is the differential form of Gauss's Law which takes the integral form

$$\iint_S \mathbf{D} \cdot dS = \iiint_V \rho \, dV.$$

This holds irrespective of the nature of the spatial distribution of either the charge ρ or permittivity, ε, *within* the volume V. The local external electric field, E, on the surface, S, can be determined from the electric displacement vector via the relation $\mathbf{D} = \varepsilon E$.

[c] For isotropic dielectrics the electric flux density $\mathbf{D}$ is defined as εE and is a vector dependent on only the electric charge ρ and position, but unlike E, is independent of the media.

which upon differentiating becomes

$$\frac{\partial J}{\partial x} = \frac{\partial J_{ionic}}{\partial x} + \frac{\partial \rho(x)}{\partial t}$$

with the Poisson equation. The continuity equation[d] describing the conservation of electric charge requires that $\partial J/\partial x = 0$ which for DC conditions alone yields

$$\frac{\partial \bar{J}_{ionic}}{\partial x} = 0 \quad \text{since} \quad \frac{\partial \overline{D}(x)}{\partial t} = 0$$

and for DC plus AC conditions yields

$$\frac{\partial \tilde{J}_{ionic}}{\partial x} + j\omega \frac{\partial \tilde{D}(x)}{\partial x} = 0$$

after substituting the above conditions for DC and Eq. (5). For isotropic dielectrics $\tilde{D}(x) \equiv \varepsilon(x)\tilde{E}(x)$, when we obtained a more commonly used form for the continuity equation

$$\frac{\partial \tilde{J}_{ionic}}{\partial x} + j\omega\varepsilon(x) \frac{\partial \tilde{E}(x)}{\partial x} = 0 \tag{8}$$

The definition of conductivity is

$$\sigma(x) \equiv \frac{\tilde{J}_{ionic}(x)}{\tilde{E}(x)} \tag{9}$$

and integration of Eq. (8) gives

$$\tilde{J} = \{\sigma(x) + j\omega\varepsilon(x)\}\tilde{E}(x) = \frac{\tilde{I}}{A} \tag{10}$$

in which the total AC current density $\tilde{J}$ is the constant of integration equal to the applied AC current divided by the area A over which it was injected [see Eq. (6)]. Rearrangement of Eq. (10) provides a definition for the complex conductivity at the position x;

$$\sigma^*(x) \equiv \frac{\tilde{J}}{\tilde{E}(x)} = \sigma(x) + j\omega\varepsilon(x) \tag{11}$$

which approaches the definition of conductivity (9) as $\omega \Rightarrow 0$, i.e., as $\tilde{J} \Rightarrow \tilde{J}_{ionic}$.

---

[d] The integral form of the continuity equation is

$$\iint_S J \cdot dS = -\frac{\partial}{\partial t} \iiint_V \rho \, dV$$

which states that the net influx of charge across the surface S is equal to the rate of increase of charge in the volume V.

The average field in a sample of length l is $\tilde{E}_{av} = \tilde{V}/l$. This and Eq. (11) then give an expression for the average complex conductivity σ^*_{av} of the sample of length l and area A.

$$\sigma^*_{av} = \sigma_{av}(\omega) + j\omega\varepsilon_{av}(\omega) = \frac{\tilde{J}}{\tilde{E}_{av}} = \frac{l}{A}\left\{\frac{I_0}{V_0}\cos\phi - j\frac{I_0}{V_0}\sin\phi\right\} \tag{12}$$

in which the replacements $\sigma(x) \leftarrow \sigma_{av}(\omega)$ and $\varepsilon(x) \leftarrow \varepsilon_{av}(\omega)$ acknowledge that spatial variations in the conductivity and dielectric permittivity within the volume $A \times l$ now manifest as dispersions with frequency ω. The nature of these manifestations are measurable since ω is known and the complex conductivity can be seen in Eq. (12) to be a function of V_0, I_0 and ϕ, the measurable parameters which define impedance, that is Eq. (3). In fact, direct comparison of Eqs. (12) and (4) show that

$$Z = \frac{l}{A\sigma^*_{av}} \tag{13}$$

The origin of the $j\omega\varepsilon_{av}(\omega)$ term in Eq. (12) can be seen to arise directly from the Poisson and charge continuity equations. Thus the impedance, as well as providing a direct measure of charge carrying capacity in terms of the conductivity $\sigma(x)$ [Eq. (9)], also provides a measure of the charge storing capacity in terms of the dielectric permittivity $\varepsilon(x)$ [Eq. (7)].

Note that whilst $\sigma^*(x)$ may be spatially dependent it is not dependent on frequency, whereas $\sigma^*_{av}(\omega)$ becomes dependent on frequency whenever $\sigma^*(x)$ varies within the volume $l \times A$. In a homogeneous system these variables will be the same, i.e., $\sigma^*_{av}(\omega) = \sigma^*(x)$ and, hence, constant in x and ω. Although, such is clearly not the case in general, the one variable σ^* is often used to represent either $\sigma^*(x)$ or $\sigma^*_{av}(\omega)$ with their dependencies being taken from the text or the context of the equations in which they are used. This is because both $\sigma^*(x)$ or $\sigma^*_{av}(\omega)$ are defined in the same way, cf. Eqs. (11) and (12). Such a convention is also applied to the real and imaginary parts of σ^*. That is, σ is generally used to denote either $\sigma(x)$ or $\sigma(\omega)$ and ε is generally used to denote either $\varepsilon(x)$ or $\varepsilon(\omega)$. Such also applies to the following definitions.

An alternative way of expressing the impedance is in terms of the admittance which is the reciprocal of impedance. Thus;

$$Y \equiv \frac{1}{Z} = G + j\omega C = \frac{A}{l}\{\sigma + j\omega\varepsilon\} \tag{14}$$

where G is the conductance and C the capacitance. Dividing Eq. (14) by the area A yields the admittance per unit area

$$y \equiv \frac{Y}{A} = g + j\omega c \tag{15}$$

where g is the conductance for a unit area and c the capacitance per unit area.

Dividing Eq. (15) by $j\omega$ yields an expression for the complex capacitance:

$$C^* \equiv \frac{Y}{j\omega} = \frac{A}{l} \left\{ \varepsilon + \frac{\sigma}{j\omega} \right\} \tag{16}$$

which leads to the definition of complex relative permittivity (or complex dielectric constant)

$$\varepsilon^* \equiv \varepsilon' - j\varepsilon'' \equiv \frac{\varepsilon}{\varepsilon_0} - j \frac{\sigma}{\varepsilon_0 \omega} \tag{17}$$

where ε_0 is the dielectric permittivity of free space.

III. THE IMPEDANCE OF MEMBRANE AND MEMBRANE SURFACES

The determination of the impedance of a membrane immersed in an electrolyte, even a homogeneous planar dielectric membrane, introduces complications not only in measurement but also in the definition of what constitutes the impedance of the membrane. This becomes evident by reference to Fig. 1a. Here we consider a planar membrane consisting of a sheet of homogeneous material, immersed in an electrolyte. To measure the impedance of this system requires the use of electrodes in contact with the electrolyte. Current is injected via the current electrodes. To determine the impedance requires the measurement of the potential difference (and phase) of the potential developed across the sample. However, the "sample" in this case includes not only the membrane but also the solution in contact and the electrode–solution interface impedances which are in series with it.

A further complication arises if the potential developed is measured using the same electrodes used to inject the current, for then we must also include the impedance of the ionic double layer (Fig. 1b) which is present between the electrodes and the aqueous solution. The effect arising from the latter can be very large and is complicated by the fact that the impedance of the electrode–solution double layer is strongly frequency dependent at low frequencies.

Some simplification becomes possible by the use of so called *four terminal* measurements, e.g., see Refs. 48 and 49. In this method (see Fig. 1a) the potential difference developed across the sample is measured using a separate pair of electrodes, at $x = \pm l/2$, connected to an electronic measuring device (not shown) with a very high input impedance. The latter ensures that the current flowing in these voltage electrodes is very small, thus eliminating any significant effects of the electrode–solution impedance at these electrodes. A further advantage of the four terminal method is that the voltage electrodes may be placed arbitrarily close to the membrane. The impedance determined in this matter then refers to the impedance of the sample between these two voltage electrodes. The latter will include, of course, not only that of the membrane but also the slabs of electrolyte on both sides of the membrane between the membrane surface and the plane containing the voltage electrodes. The membrane impedance we so define, and measure, will depend on the distance of the voltage electrodes from the membrane surface.

The electrical impedance of some membranes is very high compared to that of the aqueous solutions in which they are immersed. In those situations the impedance of the slabs of electrolyte between the membrane surface and the voltage electrodes may contribute little to the total impedance measured. The membrane impedance can then be unequivocally specified. This is the case for artificial bimolecular lipid membranes. In practice this situation may present some other problems in that the impedance of the amplifiers connected to the voltage electrodes will need to have input impedances even higher than that of the membrane and this might introduce problems of noise and resolution.

More commonly, the impedance of the electrolyte in series with the membrane cannot be ignored. In order to use impedance measurements to characterize the membrane or membrane transport processes, will require attention to the electrodiffusion processes in these regions external to the membrane. Further, it should be recognized that in the regions close to the membrane surface, both in the external solution as well as in the membrane interior, the ionic profiles may vary rapidly with position, even in an intrinsically homogeneous membrane. The ionic profiles in the aqueous solution near the membrane surface modify the operational characteristics of the membrane. Impedance spectroscopy provides a means of probing the systems as a whole and is not restricted, as so many other technologies are, to determining the properties of the isolated membrane. Further analysis of impedance spectra provides a means of characterizing the various individual regions in and near to the membrane.

A. Impedance Dispersion in Membrane Systems

In ionic systems electric current is carried by ions which move by diffusion under the influence of concentration gradients as well as by electric fields. The one-dimensional electrodiffusion of ions is described by the Nernst–Planck and Poisson equations. For a homogeneous, isotropic material the equation for the current density, J_m, of an ion species "m" is;

$$J_m = -z_m q D_m \frac{\partial C_m}{\partial x} + \frac{z_m^2 q^2 D_m C_m E}{kT} + v_\text{W} z_m q C_m \quad \text{with} \quad \frac{\partial E}{\partial x} = \frac{q}{\varepsilon} \sum_m z_m C_m$$

$$(18)$$

where q is the absolute value of the electronic charge, ε the dielectric permittivity and z_m, C_m and D_m are, respectively, the valency, concentration and diffusion constant of the ion species m. The term involving the bulk velocity of water v_W needs to be included when water fluxes are present.

In the aqueous solution the diffusion constants D_m and the steady state electric field E will in general not be the same as those in the membrane. Further, within the membrane these parameters will vary with the substructure of the membrane. In the external solution, at large distances from the membrane surface, bulk stirring effects may "wash-out" any gradients in ion concentrations. However, closer in there will remain "unstirred" layers in which the ion profiles are determined by the electrodiffusion equations. Moreover, particularly in the external solutions, it becomes necessary to consider also osmotic effects which produce bulk flow that might be coupled to the electrodiffusion; these include electroosmotic and streaming potential effects.

Under these conditions, the continuity equation for a molecular species m is

$$\frac{\partial J_m}{\partial x} + z_m q \frac{\partial C_m}{\partial t} = z_m q s_m \tag{19}$$

where the source–sink term, s_m, is zero in the absence of chemical reactions involving either the production or utilization of this species.

B. The AC Nernst–Planck–Poisson Equations

The processes described above contribute to the impedance and the dispersion of the impedance with frequency. Formal procedures for evaluating these various effects exist and are given in the Appendices. Here, we will provide only a brief overview, the starting point for which is the Nernst–Planck equations for the steady-state AC electrodiffusion of ions.

For simplicity we will consider a membrane system permeated by a univalent–univalent electrolyte. The DC concentrations of the anions and cations are denoted by $\bar{N}$ and $\bar{P}$, respectively and we denote AC perturbations of the cation and anion concentrations by lower case characters $\tilde{n}$ and $\tilde{p}$, respectively, so that $C_N = \bar{N} + \tilde{n}$ and $C_P = \bar{P} + \tilde{p}$. To deduce the AC components of the currents, we use the "substraction" procedure that we used in Sec. I to derive, for instance, the AC version of the Poisson equation. In effect we substituted $\bar{E} + \tilde{E}$ for the total electric field and $\bar{p} + \tilde{p}$ for the charge density into the Poisson equation and found that all the terms involving DC variables $\bar{E}$ and $\bar{p}$ cancelled leaving terms containing only the AC variables $\tilde{E}$ and $\tilde{p}$. This yielded Eq. (7) and since $\tilde{p}$ is simply $q(\tilde{p} - \tilde{n})$, we obtain a more specific expression for the AC Poisson equation;

$$\frac{\partial \tilde{E}}{\partial x} = \frac{q}{\varepsilon} (\tilde{p} - \tilde{n}) \tag{20}$$

To obtain an expression for the DC and AC components of the current we replace C_P by $\bar{P} + \tilde{p}$ and C_N by $\bar{N} + \tilde{n}$ in Eqs. (18) and (19). However, in this instance the procedure produces additional terms which do not cancel. Those terms involving the product of two small AC variables, e.g., $\tilde{E}\tilde{p}$ and $\tilde{E}\tilde{n}$, make a negligible contribution to the total current and can be neglected. However those terms involving the product of a DC and only one small AC variable, e.g., $\bar{P}\tilde{E}$ and $\tilde{p}\bar{E}$, are larger by an order of magnitude and cannot be neglected. The AC perturbations of the currents $\tilde{J}_N$ and $\tilde{J}_P$ are then given by the following AC Nernst–Planck equation for the total AC current density in the absence of osmotic and electroosmotic effects ($v_W = 0$)

$$
\tilde{J} = -q\left(D_P \frac{\partial \tilde{p}}{\partial x} - D_N \frac{\partial \tilde{n}}{\partial x}\right) + \frac{q^2}{kT}(D_P \tilde{p} + D_N \tilde{n})\bar{E}
$$

$$
+ \left(\frac{q^2}{kT}(D_P \bar{P} + D_N \bar{N}) + j\omega\varepsilon\right)\tilde{E} \tag{21}
$$

Osmotic effects arise as a consequence of the bulk flow of water ($v_W \neq 0$) induced by concentration differences between the bulk solutions or established by the AC flows of ions themselves [see Eq. (B2) in Appendix B]. Coupling between water and ionic fluxes (electroosmotic effects) can also occur. These additional effects give arise to additional terms to those shown in Eq. (20).

Spatial variations in the diffusion constants and permittivity due to any substructure in the membrane will also lead to a dispersion of the impedance with frequency as a result of interfacial polarization effects at the boundaries of substructural layers.

Finally, time dependent molecular re-orientation of dipoles may produce a further dispersion in the impedance. Such dispersions have been reported [62, 89] for essentially dry "glassy" polymer-films at quite low frequencies (0.1–1 Hz). However, for membrane systems permeated by ionic solutions, dispersions arising from double layers, unstirred layers and interfacial polarisation effects between the solution (of very high dielectric permittivity) and the membrane will dominate at these low frequencies and many decades above that. An overview of the principal dispersions[e] of interest which occur in membranes permeated by ionic solution is given in Fig. 2.

Below we examine in a little more detail the dispersion with frequency of the impedance which originates from the membrane structure and these membrane processes.

C. The α-Dispersion

The dispersion of the impedance[e] at very low frequencies is dominated by effects which arise as a result of diffusion limited perturbations of the ionic

---

[e] It should be noted that the definitions of α-, β- and γ- dispersions are not universal. The nomenclature used here is essentially that originally promoted by Schwan [9] in 1959 and is relevant to biological systems and artificial membranes permeated by ionic solutions.

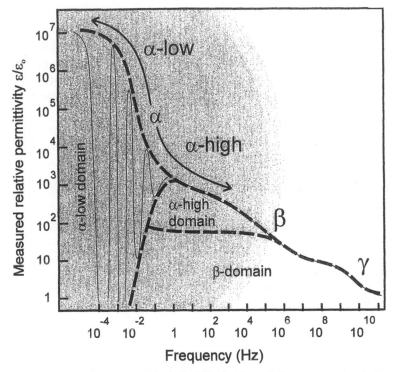

FIG. 2 Characteristic α-, β- and γ-dispersions of the measured relative permittivity. The α-dispersion may be subdivided into "α-low" and "α-high" dispersions that manifest as "domains" in the permittivity–frequency plane. The "α-low domain" is the largest and sometimes includes negative values of permittivity. The "α-low" dispersions have their origin in diffusion polarization effects occurring in the electrolytes, unstirred layers, membrane interfaces, etc. The diffusion currents are usually out of phase with the field driven current and depending on the degree of coupling to water flow, can manifest as either a positive or negative "pseudo" permittivity, usually of very large magnitude. The "α-high" dispersion can, for example, originate from intrinsic fixed charge structures that modulate the phase of the diffusion currents and manifest a positive permittivity dependent on the dimensions of that region. At sufficiently high frequencies the α-dispersions diminish, revealing β-dispersions which derive from interfacial polarization effects between substructural elements with different dielectric permittivity and/or conductance properties. At even higher frequencies these dispersions also diminish, revealing γ-dispersions which arise from electric field re-orientations of molecular dipoles.

concentration profiles in the solution external to the membrane as well as within the membrane.

At the lowest frequencies, this dispersion is dominated by osmotic polarization effects in the unstirred regions and electroosmotic effects in the membrane which arise when the solvent is not stationary (i.e., $v_W \neq 0$, see Appendix D). The former also includes effects originating at the electrodes used to inject the current.

We may, in a somewhat arbitrary way, divide the α-dispersion into two subregions. The impedance dispersion will manifest itself in dispersions of the overall capacitance and conductance of the system.

1. Polarization Effects due to Current Injected by Blocking Electrodes

In general electrodes used in actual measurements are "blocking" electrodes, that is, the electrode does not provide a source or sink for the ions carrying current in the solution. This has a number of ramifications [50–52]. Even without a membrane, that is the electrolyte solution only, the limiting values of conductance (per unit area) and capacitance (per unit area) for DC conditions is given by (see Appendix C):

$$g(\omega = 0) = 0 \quad \text{and} \quad c(\omega = 0) = \frac{\varepsilon}{l\delta} \tag{22}$$

where l is the distance between the voltage electrodes and δ is given by:

$$\delta \approx \frac{2\lambda}{l} e^{-[L-1]/2\lambda} \ll 1 \tag{23}$$

Here L is the distance between the current electrodes and λ is the Debye length for the solution.

The capacitance and conductance at high frequencies are simply

$$c(\omega > 0) = \frac{\varepsilon}{l} \quad \text{and} \quad g(\omega > 0) = \frac{\sigma}{l} \tag{24}$$

and thus the capacitance (or the operational permittivity) of the solution on its own will appear to rise from $\varepsilon/l\delta$ to ε/l as $\omega \to 0$ and the conductance will appear to decrease from σ/l to zero as $\omega \to 0$.

Equation (22) applies to a system in which the diffusion constants for the anions and cations are equal. An even more marked dispersion occurs at higher frequencies when the diffusion constants differ (e.g., see Refs 53 and 54). The capacitance similarly increases with increasing electrode separation. However, although larger, this dispersion moves to lower frequencies with increased electrode separations as shown in Fig. 3. Whilst this effect can be very large, the capacitance approaches the dielectric value ε/l at moderately

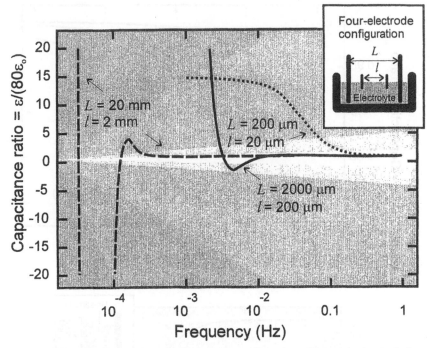

FIG. 3 "α-low" dispersions originating in an electrolyte. Theoretical calculations [54] of the capacitance of a 1 M/m³ electrolyte (expressed as its ratio to the dielectric geometrical capacitance) as a function of frequency and electrode spacings $L - l$ (see inset). The magnitude of the dispersion increases as the differences between the diffusion constant for anions and cations increases (not shown); only a small difference ($D_N = 10^{-9}$ m²/s and $D_P = 1.001 \times 10^{-9}$ m²/s) produces dispersions which move to lower frequencies only as $L - l$ increases. For the larger spacings the capacitance is many orders of magnitude larger than the dielectric geometrical capacitance and characteristically increases in magnitude and changes sign several times as the frequency decreases.

low frequencies, typically <0.01 Hz for practical electrode separations of the order of millimetres.

An interesting outcome of the electrode polarization effects is that under certain conditions the operational capacitance can become negative ($\delta < 0$) at low frequencies (less than 0.1–1 Hz). An example of the type of dispersion in the capacitance that can be expected is shown in Fig. 3, for typical values of the various parameters encountered in practical systems (see caption to Fig. 3). The effect is dependent on electrode separation (increases with increasing electrode separation), but the frequency range of the dispersion also moves to lower frequencies with increased electrode separations. This highlights the problems that can arise when one is tempted to move the voltage and current

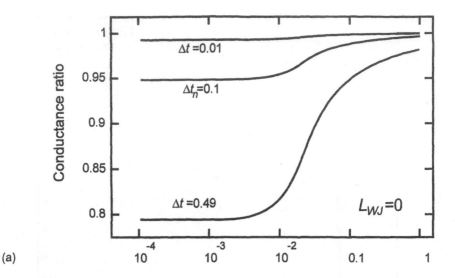

(a)

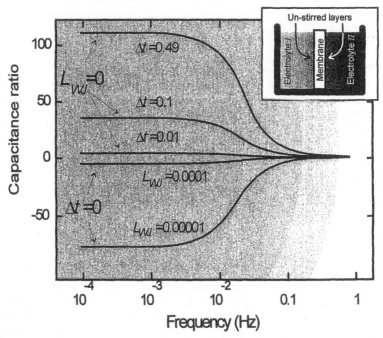

(b)

FIG. 4 The effect of unstirred layers on measurements of the impedance of a membrane. Barry [82] and Smith [79] independently derived expressions for the impedance of unstirred layers in series with a homogeneous membrane of conductance g_m and capacitance c_m. For very small ionic transport number differences, Δt, between the membrane and the electrolyte (for definition see Appendix D), the total conductance of

electrodes closer to the membrane surface in order to reduce contributions from the external solution. The ramification would be that while the dispersion resulting from the injection of current via the blocking electrodes decreases with decreasing electrode separation, the dispersion will also move to higher frequencies and could overlap with other dispersions reflecting membrane transport processes or even those arising from interfacial polarizations due to the presence of membrane substructure. An example of the expected dispersion due to current injection via blocking electrodes is shown in Fig. 3.

2. Diffusion Polarization in Unstirred Layers

In the presence of a membrane, layers of the external solution close to the membrane surface will remain unstirred, even if the bulk solution is deliberately stirred by mechanical means.

Electroosmotic effects arise from the coupling between ion flow and the water flux. Osmotic polarization layers will be established in "unstirred" layers when, for instance, the relative magnitudes of the currents carried by anions and cations in the membrane are different from those relative magnitudes in the external aqueous solutions; that is, the transport numbers for cations and anions in the membrane are different from those in the external solution. The AC perturbations in the osmotic gradients so established, will produce bulk AC water fluxes which will in turn further perturb the ionic fluxes.

An AC field at low frequencies will establish AC ionic concentrations and gradients which will generally be different for cations and anions. The extent of the AC polarization effect is directly related to the differences in the transport numbers, Δt, of the anions and cations in the membrane and the external solution. This has several consequences.

Firstly, the diffusion currents can be significant larger in magnitude to the (AC) field currents and since the diffusion currents involve the establishment of

---

the series combination, expressed as the ratio to g_m shows a strong dispersion (a) at low frequencies which increases as Δt increases. Similarly the capacitance, expressed as a ratio to c_m (the intrinsic geometrical–dielectric membrane capacitance) displays an even stronger dispersion with frequency (b); at low frequencies the total capacitance is several orders of magnitude larger than c_m (capacitance ratio $\gg 1$). Because these capacitances do not have a dielectric geometrical origin, they can be classified as α-dispersions. Smith's derivation also accounted for coupling between the water and the ionic current (that is, $L_{WJ} > 0$) which can be seen to result in negative capacitance ratios that become more negative as L_{WJ} increases. Unstirred layers thus introduce "α-low" dispersions (shaded regions) which diminish at high frequencies. (parameters used: $g_m = 1$ S/m^2, $c_m = 0.01$ F/m^2,   diffusion constants for anions and cations $= 2 \times 10^{-9}$ m^2/s, the electrolyte concentration $= 0.1$ M/m^3, width of unstirred layers $= 100$ μm, hydraulic permeability $= 10^{-13}$ m/Ns).

AC ionic concentrations (and their gradients), they will generally be out of phase (lag) the AC field ($\tilde{E}$). This yields low frequency impedances corresponding to those of very large capacitors; operationally the system behaves as though the permittivity is greatly enhanced over its high frequency "dielectric" value. These layers also lower the conductance of the system. An example of the effects predicted due to this type of diffusion polarisation effect in the unstirred layers is given in Fig. 4a.

Secondly, the AC polarization effects produce osmotically driven water flows which can couple to the ionic fluxes (coupling coefficient denoted by L_{WJ} in Fig. 4) to yield operationally negative capacitances. An example of the calculated effects due to electroosmotic coupling is provided in Fig. 4b.

Generally both these effects occur at very low frequencies since at higher frequencies the time available in each half cycle of the AC field is insufficient to cause significant AC perturbations to the ionic concentrations. The AC diffusion currents then become negligible compared to the AC field-driven currents. It should be noted that these effects diminish and move to lower frequencies as the membrane conductance, g_m, decreases (see Fig. 5).

Very low frequency α-dispersions of the type illustrated above have been observed in impedance measurements on biological systems. In some cases, the

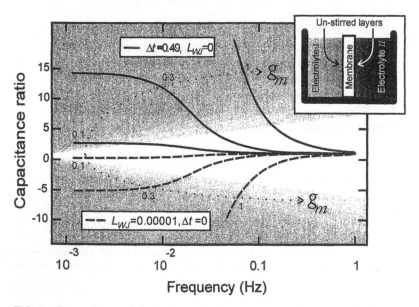

FIG. 5 Dependence of the "α-low" dispersions originating in unstirred layers on membrane conductance g_m. The capacitance dispersions [79] due to diffusion polarization effects in unstirred layers diminish as g_m decreases (see previous figure caption for details).

capacitance of cell membranes at very low frequencies can have values well in excess of the dielectric capacitance and in some instances values that are negative. In both cases the capacitance also disperses monotonically back to the dielectric values at higher frequencies (see example in Fig. 6). In some instances the membrane capacitance becomes alternatively positive and negative as the

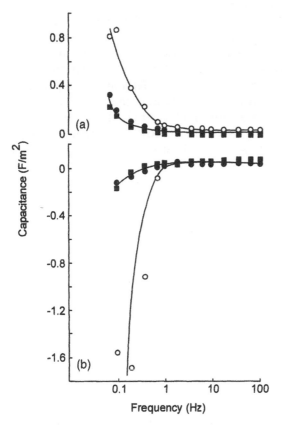

FIG. 6 Examples of positive and negative α-dispersions in the membranes of *Chara*. Cells of *Chara* have two membranes; an outer membrane (plasmalemma) and an inner membrane (tonoplast) which separates the central vacuole from the cytoplasm. The impedance of the two membranes can be measured separately and simultaneously using microelectrodes inserted in the cell's cytoplasm and its vacuole. Such measurements [80] have revealed two distinct types of capacitance dispersion for both the inner (○) and outer (■) membrane and the series combination (●). The experiments most often revealed positive capacitances at low frequencies which were too large to be attributable to the dielectric geometrical capacitance of the membrane or substructure within these membranes (a). Less frequent were the negative capacitances (b) which were even larger in magnitude. (Re-drawn from Ref. 80.)

frequency varies in this low frequency region [55,56]. This behavior is strongly correlated to other ion transport effects. A dramatic example of this can be seen in the α-dispersion of the impedance of the membrane of *Chara corallina* which varies with position along the surface of these giant cylindrical cells, as can be seen in Fig. 7. The variations in the impedance spectra are correlated with acid and alkaline banding developed in these cells when they exposed to light [55,56]. The measured dispersion of the capacitance in the acidic and alkaline regions are vastly different at low frequencies but both approach the same dielectric geometrical values at high frequencies (see also Fig. 8). In this instance, the pH-dependence of the α-dispersion can be interpreted in terms of the degree to which pH influences the ionization of intrinsic proteins in the cell membrane. The details of the impedance spectra in *Chara* and its dependence on pH, suggests that the plasmalemma of these cells may contain protein modules which behave like bipolar (or double fixed charge) membrane modules. The latter have interesting impedance spectra which reflect both dif-fusion polarization effects as well as ion profile structures which are voltage dependent. We briefly examine these below.

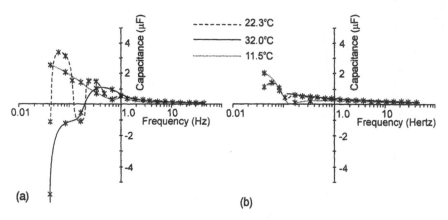

FIG. 7 The dependence of "α-low" dispersions in the acidic and alkaline regions of a *Chara* cell on temperature. In the presence of light, long (∼30 mm) cells of *Chara corallina* develop acidic and alkaline regions that alternate along the cylindrical surface of the cell. Measurements [55] of the membrane impedance in these regions have revealed positive and negative capacitances of magnitude too large to be attributable to dielectric geometrical capacitances from the cell. These "α-low" dispersions are shown to be more pronounced for alkaline conditions (a) than for acidic conditions (b). Not only are the "α-low" dispersions dependent on pH but their character is modulated by the temperature. For instance, in the alkaline region the "α-low" dispersion can be seen to be distinctively positive at very low temperatures or distinctively negative at high temperatures. At room temperature both these characteristics are observed. (Re-drawn from Ref. 55.)

3. Double Fixed Charge or Bipolar Membrane

The α-dispersions that have been described so far originated from regions peripheral to the membrane. They are characterized by large capacitances which cannot be attributed to a dielectric geometrical origin. Furthermore, these capacitances are sometimes negative or alternate between positive and negative values at different frequencies. Since these dispersions occur at very low frequencies it is convenient to classify them as α-low dispersions in order to distinguish them from other α-dispersions which also do not have a dielectric geometrical basis but which are *not* associated with negative capacitances. This latter type of α-dispersion generally occurs at somewhat higher frequencies which might overlap with β-dispersions described below. Such α-high dispersions have been observed in membranes in which one half contains fixed charges with sign opposite to that of the fixed charges in the other half [37,57]. Membranes containing such juxtaposed regions of fixed charges of opposite sign are referred to as "bipolar" membranes or in the context of cellular membranes as "double fixed charge membranes" (DFCM). In DFCM membranes only those ions with charge opposite in sign to that of the fixed charges readily permeate the separate halves of the membrane. This results in the concentration of cations being enhanced in one half but depleted in the other, and vice versa for anions. A consequence of these counterion distributions is the formation of a layer at the centre of the membrane in which the concentration of both anions and cations are depleted [58]. This depletion layer and the external regions on either side, although possessing different ionic selectivity and conduction properties, nonetheless, have the same dielectric permittivity ε. Hence at sufficiently high frequencies the capacitance of the membrane will be ε/w where w is the width of the membrane. At very low frequencies, however, there will be sufficient time for ions in the regions external to the depletion layer to be perturbed by the applied AC electric field used for impedance measurements. Because the concentration of ions is high in these regions the conductance will be also high. This means that most of the applied electric field will appear across the central layer which is depleted of ions (and hence has a low conductance at these low frequencies [59]). The capacitance of the membrane at these frequencies [60,61] would be then ε/λ_d where λ_d is the width of the depletion layer. Since $\lambda_d < w$ then the membrane capacitance will be larger at low frequencies than at high frequencies, thereby giving rise to a dispersion (see Fig. 8). This dispersion originates from geometrical properties of a structure that develops in the membrane as a consequence of the presence of fixed charges. It is therefore dependent on, for instance, the pH which influence the concentration of fixed charges. It is also dependent on the diffusion constants of the ions in the membrane. These factors, combined, determine the frequency range over which the applied AC electric potential shifts from appearing across the membrane as a whole to appearing essentially across the depletion layer only [60,61,37]. It is therefore an α-dispersion but, since it derives from an

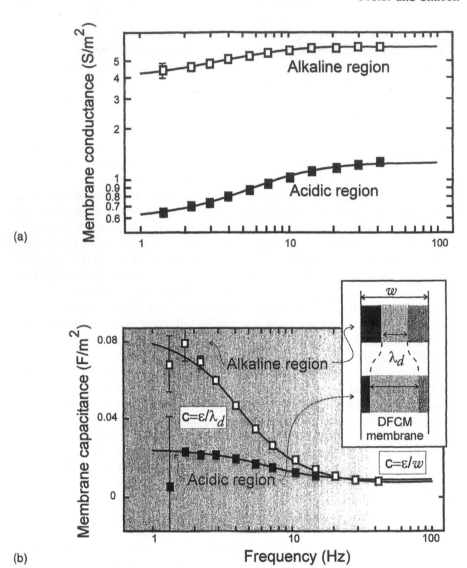

FIG. 8 Impedance of the membranes of *Chara corallina* and the bipolar membrane. Conductance (a) and capacitance (b) dispersions from the membrane of the giant aquatic plant cells of *Chara corallina* [56]. The impedance dispersions differ significantly in acidic (■) and alkaline (□) regions (bands) that form along the cell's cylindrical surface. The differences in the capacitance dispersions are very pronounced at low frequencies but the capacitances approach the same dielectric geometrical values ($= \varepsilon/w$) for the membrane at high frequencies. The curves are theoretical plots of the impedance of a shunted double fixed charge (bipolar) membrane [61]. The fixed charges in the bipolar membrane establish a "depletion" layer of low conductance

intrinsic dimension of the membrane, it cannot like the other α-dispersions, become negative.

D. The β-Dispersion (Interfacial Polarizations)

If the system is not homogeneous but contains a substructure in which the dielectric and/or conductance properties of the substructural elements are different, a β-dispersion[f] will arise in the impedance due to interfacial polarization at the substructural element interfaces. This dispersion provides a means of detecting and characterizing that substructure at a level of resolution that can in some cases be better than that discernible under electron microscopy. However, the dispersion due to interfacial polarization can often overlap with the α-dispersion described above and this can complicate the analysis. An example of a method used to separate these contributions in dry polymer membranes is given by Sørensen et al. [62,89] and is also applicable to membranes permeated by ionic solutions. Notwithstanding that complication, impedance spectroscopy has been widely used to characterize such substructural elements or monitor changes due to adsorption of molecules into the substructure [42,46,63–70,83–85].

For frequencies above the α-dispersion, the capacitance and conductance of the membrane can be expressed in terms of a conductance element g_1 in parallel with a capacitance element c_1. Thus,

$$Z(\omega) = \frac{1}{g_1 + j\omega c_1} \tag{25}$$

---

[f] Here again we wish to draw your attention to the fact that the classification of α-, β- and γ-dispersions is arbitrary. The nomenclature used here is essentially that originally promoted by Schwan [9] in 1959 and is relevant to biological systems and artificial membranes permeated by ionic solutions.

(width λ_d) sandwiched by layers of high conductance (see inset). The theory predicts that the capacitance of the membrane decreases from approximately ε/λ_d to ε/w as the frequency increases over the indicated range. The different dispersions can be explained if the acidic and alkaline conditions in the different regions induce the indicated changes in λ_d through the dependency of this parameter on fixed charge concentration. The fixed charges arise from ionized acidic and basic amino acids in the protein membrane modules which are known to be strongly dependent on pH. (Parameters used: diffusion constant 2.2×10^{-17} m^2/s, $\varepsilon = 7.3\varepsilon_0$, $w = 8 \times 10^{-9}$ m, alkaline region: $\lambda_d = 4.6 \times 10^{-10}$ m, fixed charge concentration $= 840$ M/m^3, shunt conductance $= 7.8$ S/m^2, acid region: $\lambda_d = 1.2 \times 10^{-9}$ m, fixed charge concentration $= 200$ M/m^3, shunt conductance $= 1.2$ S/m^2).

If the membrane consists of a homogeneous slab of material the g_1 and c_1 are independent of frequency. Nonetheless, however, the impedance will disperse with frequency as shown in Fig. 9. Inspection of Eq. (25) reveals that the dispersion becomes most pronounced for frequencies greater than g_1/c_1. At the frequency given by;

$$\omega_1 = \frac{g_1}{c_1} \tag{26}$$

the impedance measurement will provide the most accurate simultaneous estimates of both the conductance and capacitance. This frequency defines the "natural" or characteristic frequency or inverse time constant of this homogeneous system.

1. Maxwell Wagner Dispersion

Consider now a system composed of a sandwich of substructural layers, in which each layer has different dielectric and conductance properties. The total impedance of this membrane is given by;

$$Z_k(\omega) = \sum_{i=1}^{k} \frac{1}{g_i + j\omega c_i} \tag{27}$$

where the subscripts "i" identifies the conductances and capacitances of each of the layers in the membrane. The dispersion described by Eq. (27) comprises k superimposed dispersions of the type described by Eq. (25), each of which commence near their respective "characteristic" frequencies, that is,

$$\omega_i \equiv \frac{g_i}{c_i} \tag{28}$$

If these characteristic frequencies are sufficiently different and the magnitudes of the impedance dispersions at these frequencies are sufficiently large, each of the dispersions in the impedance can be readily discerned in the overall impedance dispersion.

2. Importance of Dispersions of Conductance and Capacitance

Often the magnitudes of the one or more of the dispersions is too small to allow it to be readily seen in the impedance–frequency plane. However, if the phase angle can be also accurately, and independently determined, the capacitance and conductance for the whole membrane can be determined directly as

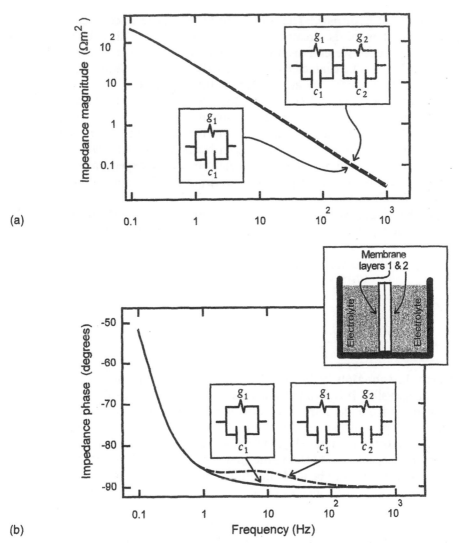

FIG. 9 Interfacial polarization: dispersions of the impedance magnitude and phase. Dispersions of the impedance magnitude (a) and phase (b) in a system comprised of a single electrically homogeneous layer (———) and for those of a system comprised of a sandwich of two electrically distinct homogeneous layers (– – –). The dispersions in impedance are almost identical although the phase (b) in the frequency range of 1–100 Hz shows differences of several degrees. The electrical equivalent circuit representing the first layer is shown in the inset and consists of a resistor (of conductance $g_1 = 0.003$ S/m²) in parallel with a capacitor (of capacitance $c_1 = 0.006$ F/m²). The two-layer system consists of this layer in series with a second layer of significantly higher conductance and capacitance ($g_2 = 4.347$ S/m² and $c_2 = 0.0586$ F/m²).

a function of frequency.[s] The dispersion in the capacitance often provides a clear indication of the presence of substructural layer. This is best illustrated by a simple example of a membrane containing two layers, as depicted in the inset to Fig. 9. The characteristic frequencies for the two layers in this system are approximately 0.1 Hz and 10 Hz. In the impedance–frequency plane, the dispersion due to the presence of the second layer cannot be discerned within the resolution of the thickness of the plots drawn in Fig. 9a. When plotted in the conductance–frequency (Fig. 10a) and the capacitance–frequency domain (Fig. 10b) the addition of the second layer becomes dramatically obvious. Thus effectively the presence of the second slab requires independent and accurate measurement of the phase [71]; the precision required for the phase can be gauged from Fig. 9b.

In the simple two-layered system referred to thus far, the overall parallel conductance $g(\omega)$ and capacitance $c(\omega)$ at a particular ω is given by:

$$g(\omega) = \frac{g_1 g_2 (g_1 + g_2) + \omega^2 (c_1 g_2^2 + c_2 g_1^2)}{(g_1 + g_2)^2 \omega^2 (c_1 + c_2)^2} \tag{29}$$

and

$$c(\omega) = \frac{\omega^2 c_1 c_2 (c_1 + c_2) + (c_1 g_2^2 + c_2 g_1^2)}{(g_1 + g_2)^2 \omega^2 (c_1 + c_2)^2} \tag{30}$$

where the subscripts "1" and "2" identify the frequency independent properties of each slab. It is thus possible to deduce the dielectric substructure (c_1, c_2, g_1 and g_2) from the impedance dispersion. Synthetic separation membranes often have a substructure consisting of a tight skin layer containing sub-μm pores supported on a base layer which is more porous and has large channels. Impedance spectroscopy allows the characterization of the substructural layers of such membranes to be made in situ [17,36], see Fig. 11 (although it requires high precision measurements of both phase and impedance magnitude [71]).

For membranes with large numbers of substructural layers, the dispersions extend over a wider range of frequencies and the form of the dispersion curves become dependent on the number of layers (k). In contrast, the dispersions of the impedance magnitude are largely unaltered by the number of layers (cf. Fig. 9 and 10). Thus, dispersions of the conductance and capacitance, at frequencies beyond the α-dispersion, provide an immediate indication of the pres-

---

[s] The capacitance and conductance for a specified circuit containing capacitors and conductances in parallel can, of course, in principle also be deduced from the variation of the total impedance with frequency, without any information concerning the variation of phase with frequency. However, if the phase is known for each measurement at the various frequencies, the capacitance and conductance at that frequency can be then determined directly, independently of any model or equivalent circuit of the system.

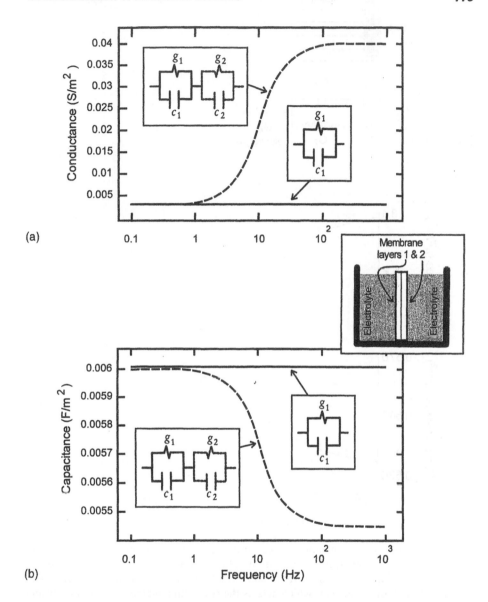

FIG. 10 Interfacial polarization: dispersions of the conductance and capacitance. For the systems described in the previous figure, there is no dispersion of the total conductance (a) nor of the total capacitance (b) of the single layer (———). In contrast, the dispersions in conductance and capacitance for the two-layered system (– – –) are very obvious, especially that of the total conductance which approaches the value for the series layer (i.e., $g_2 = 4.347$ S/m^2) at high frequencies. The conductance and capacitance as a function of frequency immediately reveal whether the system is homogeneous and the extent of heterogeneity, which is not readily discernible in the impedance plot (based on Ref. 71).

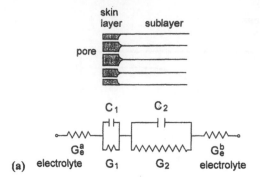

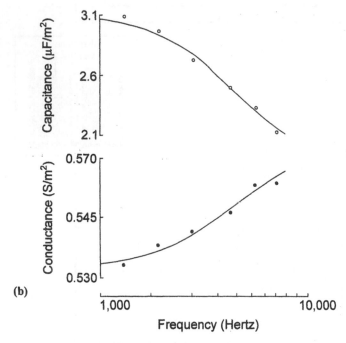

FIG. 11 Ultrafiltration membrane and dispersions of the conductance and capacitance. A simple equivalent circuit for an ultrafiltration membrane and electrolyte system. Such ultrafiltration membranes contain a thin skin layer with low porosity and a much thicker, open sublayer which acts as the supporting matrix. The skin layer and the sublayer can be considered to be electrically distinct regions [17]. The conductance and capacitance of the former are represented by G_1 and C_1, respectively, and those of the latter by G_2 and C_2, respectively. The total conductance attributable to the electrolyte is $G_e = G_e^a G_e^b / (G_e^a + G_e^b)$ and was measured separately in the absence of the membrane.

Capacitance and conductance dispersions for an ultrafiltration membrane (PM30) in a 0.2 mM KCl electrolyte. The continuous lines are theoretical curves from the equivalent circuit shown in previous figure (a). The parameter values used were $C_1 = 0.2$ mF/m², $C_2 = 2$ μF/m², $G_1 = 6$ S/m² and $G_2 = 0.58$ S/m². (Re-drawn from Ref. 17.)

ence of substructure within the system. An example of this for bimolecular lipid membranes is shown in Fig. 12.

E. The γ-Dispersion

Molecular dipole re-orientation gives rise to a net polarization which manifests as an enhanced permittivity. Thermal agitation causes a relaxation of the polarisation and this results in a dispersion of the dielectric permittivity with frequency. The characteristic frequencies of these dispersions decrease with increasing molecular size (and mass). Typically, for water and protein they are, respectively, 20,000 MHz and 1 MHz. In this review we concerned ourselves with impedance dispersions which relate to diffusion limited transport processes and interfacial polarizations arising from substructural layers. In systems permeated by ionic solutions, these typically manifest dispersions below 100 kHz. Polymer scientists working with dry materials (including dry membranes) observe dispersions at low frequencies which are referred to as γ-dispersions.[h] In systems permeated by ionic solutions the total impedance, however, is dominated by the ionic conduction pathways. We refer readers to other sources for more comprehensive descriptions of polar relaxation and the γ-dispersion [52,72–74,83–85].

IV. IMPORTANCE OF IMPEDANCE SPECTROSCOPY TO STUDIES OF MEMBRANES AND MEMBRANE SURFACES IN THE FUTURE

We have principally focused our review on biological systems and have shown how impedance spectroscopy can probe membranes at the molecular resolution, provide useful insights into the function of membrane-proteins that transport and pump ions, and characterise the interfaces that membranes form with electrolytes including the unstirred layers that arise from membrane function. Of all of these, least is known about the chemical and physical processes occurring at membrane interfaces and unstirred layers, as these regions cannot be studied in isolation.

Future studies of such surface phenomena via impedance spectroscopy rely on further development of electrodiffusion models to explain the origin of the various types of low frequency dispersion as well as on minimizing the degree to which impedance measurements interfere with the processes giving rise to these dispersions. Adherence to the latter essentially rules out the use of potentiostat and voltage clamp methodologies which inherently override intrinsic feedback processes of the systems under study.

---

[h] The nomenclature used here for the γ-dispersion is essentially that originally promoted by Schwan [9] in 1959 and is relevant to biological systems and artificial membranes permeated by ionic solutions.

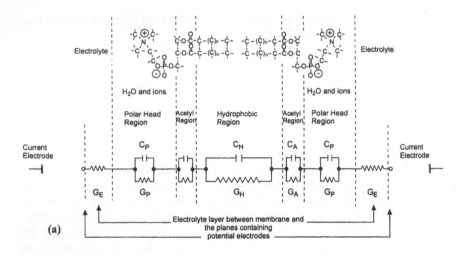

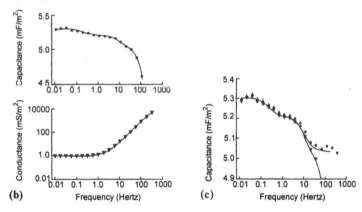

FIG. 12 Phosphatidylcholine bilayer membrane and dispersions in the conductance and capacitance. (a) An equivalent circuit for a biomolecular lipid membrane (BLM) of phosphatidylcholine (lecithin) [81]. Such BLMs were formed from a saturated solution of egg phosphatidylcholine in n-tetradecane or n-decane solvent over a 1.2 mm diameter hole in a polycarbonate septum dividing a cell containing KCl solution. Each region of the bilayer is associated with a chemically distinct portion of the phosphatidylcholine molecule. The hydrocarbon region is associated with the acyl chains which has a low permittivity $\varepsilon_H = 2.13\,\varepsilon_0$. Partitioning of ions into such a medium is energetically extremely unfavourable. Water readily penetrates the flexible polar-head region and to a lesser extent the more rigid acetyl regions. A likely permittivity for these regions is $\varepsilon_P = \varepsilon_A = 20\,\varepsilon_0 - 50\,\varepsilon_0$. Partitioning of ions into the polar-head region would be favorable but less so for the more rigid acetyl region. These electrical properties form the basis of estimating the values for the components (that is, the conductances

The low frequency α-dispersions in biological membranes can be related to electrodiffusion processes in simple electrolytes, e.g. [54], and diffusion polarizations in unstirred layers that form next to membranes [79,82]. However, in many biological membranes, active ion transport processes further complicate the analysis. In such systems, distinctive periodic variations in the measured capacitance of the membrane have been observed [50,80]. The variations are large in magnitude often extending into the negative capacitance ("inductive") domain (see Fig. 2). The membrane potential in such cells also show distinctive periodic fluctuations [86] probably related to positive feedback processes associated with active transport and the observed "inductive" behavior. Interference between the AC signal used for impedance measurements and the fluctuations in membrane potential probably underlie this type of α-dispersion.

The corollary to this is that knowledge gained about the α-dispersion can become the means of observing, evaluating and understanding the chemical and physical phenomena occurring in membranes and over membrane surfaces.

V. APPENDICES

A. The Generalized Nernst–Planck Equations

The movement of molecules is controlled by the spatial variation of the thermodynamic potentials. These thermodynamic potentials include both energy and entropy terms which, together, determine how the system approaches

---

G_H, G_A, G_P and G_E and capacitances C_H, C_A and C_P) that form the equivalent circuit for the bilayer. The electrolyte, in this instance, can be represented by a single conductance element G_E. (Redrawn from Ref 81.) (b) Experimental data [81] for the dispersion in capacitance (a) and conductance (b) for a BLM formed in 1 mM KCl. The points shown represent the experimental measurements, including error bars which are only large enough to be discernible in the plot of capacitance on an expanded scale (c). For the latter two curves and data point are shown; one (●) for the total capacitance and the other (▼) for the BLM alone after subtraction of the value for G_E measured in the absence of the BLM. In each case the continuous lines are theoretical curves of the dispersions predicted from the equivalent circuit for such a BLM shown in the previous figure. This fit of the data to the model yielded the following values for the capacitances and conductances of the substructural layers of the BLM: $C_H = 5.35 \pm 0.05$, $C_A = 390 \pm 50$ and $C_P = 275 \pm 100$ mF/m^{-2} and $G_H = 0.75 \pm 0.35$, $G_A = 470 \pm 100$ and $G_P = 16,500 \pm 650$ mS/m^{-2} (subscript H ≡ acyl chain hydrocarbon region, A ≡ Acetyl oxygen region and P ≡ polar head region). (Redrawn from Ref. 81.)

equilibrium. In a mixture of molecules the relevant thermodynamic potential is the electrochemical potential, μ. The thermodynamic potential for a molecular species is comprised of electrical, chemical, mechanical and entropy contributions and is given by:

$$\mu_m = z_m q \Psi + \mu_m^o + v_m P + kT \ln X_m \tag{A1}$$

where:

X_m is the mole fraction[i] of the molecular species m,
q is the electronic charge, z_m is the valency and Ψ the electric potential,
μ_m^o the standard chemical potential at position x for the standard (reference) concentration of species m, C_o (usually 1 mole of Molec/L),
$P \equiv P_{abs} - P_o$ where P_{abs} is the absolute pressure and P_o is the pressure in the standard state to which μ_m^o refers,
v_m the partial molecular volume for m,
k is the Boltzmann constant and T the absolute temperature.

For a very dilute solution of a univalent cation at concentration C_P, the expression (A1) can be written as:

$$\mu_P = q \Psi + \mu_P^o + v_P P + kT \ln \frac{C_P}{C_o} \tag{A2}$$

Similarly for univalent anions at concentration C_N, the electrochemical potential is given by:

$$\mu_N = - q \Psi + \mu_N^o + v_N P + kT \ln \frac{C_N}{C_o} \tag{A3}$$

The solvent which is often water and is usually in abundance needs also to be considered. The chemical potential for water is given by:

$$\mu_W = \mu_W^o + v_W P + kT \ln(\gamma_W X_W) \tag{A4}$$

where γ_W is the activity coefficient[j] which needs to be introduced for nonideal solutions. When the solutes are at a very low concentration so that the mole

---

[i] For systems without ideal mixing, the mole fraction X_m should be replaced with $X_m \gamma_m$ where γ_m is the activity coefficient which has a value <1.
[j] For typographical convenience we will not expressly include the activity coefficient, γ_W, that is, we have set $\gamma_W = 1$. For low concentrations of solutes, that is, when $X_W \approx 1$, clearly γ_W will be <1. The activity coefficient for water can, however, be readily introduced in the expressions that follow.

fraction of water is close to unity, this expression can be simplified to:

$$\mu_W \approx \mu_W^o + v_W \mathbf{P} - kTX_s = \mu_W^o + \{\mathbf{P} + kTC_s\}/C_W \tag{A5}$$

where C_W is the concentration of water (~ 55.5 moles/L) and X_s refers to the mole fraction of the solute of concentration

$$C_S = C_P + C_N$$

for the dilute solution under consideration. The term kTC_s can be recognized as the van't Hoff expression for the osmotic pressure.

For the membrane systems we are considering, there will be regions in which the dielectric permittivities are different. This has important implications for the standard chemical potential (energy), μ^o. The latter will then contain a contribution due to the electrostatic self energy (or Born [75] energy). It can be readily shown that for a univalent cation or univalent anion of radius r, in a medium with dielectric constant ε, this contribution to the standard chemical potential is given by:

$$\mu_{Born}^o = \frac{q^2}{8\pi r \varepsilon} \tag{A6}$$

For two points far removed from the interface between regions with different dielectric permittivities, the difference in the standard chemical potentials from this dielectric effect is then:

$$\Delta \mu_{Born}^o = \frac{q^2}{8\pi r}\left[\frac{1}{\varepsilon_2} - \frac{1}{\varepsilon_1}\right] \tag{A7}$$

where ε_1 and ε_2 are the dielectric permittivities of the juxtaposed regions. For a membrane immersed in electrolyte, Neumcke and Lauger [76] used "image charge" techniques to derive expressions for the spatial variations in μ_{Born}^o. Their expressions revealed, as might be expected, that spatial variations were most pronounced near the membrane–electrolyte interfaces but diminish in the bulk electrolyte and towards the centre of the membrane. Further, the difference in chemical potentials at these extreme locations was found to be approximately Eq. (7) even for very thin membranes. The analysis of Neumcke and Lauger is strictly valid for only dilute solutions. In real solutions, Debye shielding of ions modifies the "image charge" calculations and hence expression for $\Delta\mu_{Born}^o$ [24].

In a system which is not in equilibrium, the random motion and collisions of molecules in the presence of gradients in the electrochemical potential, produce macroscopic fluxes of molecules which can be expressed in terms of a "drift" velocity of the molecules. The fluxes can be described in terms of generalized thermodynamic forces which are the (negative) gradients of the relative thermodynamic potential [77,87,88]. The resulting flux may be described in terms of a "mobility" which is the drift velocity of a molecule, relative to the solvent, under a unit gradient in its electrochemical potential. Thus for a molecular species m

$$v_m - v_W = -u_m \nabla \mu_m \tag{A8}$$

where v_m is the velocity of the species m and v_W is the bulk velocity of water (which may, for instance, be moving under the influence of an osmotic gradient). ∇ refers to the gradient and for a one-dimensional system equates to $\hat{\imath}(\partial/\partial x)$.

The product of velocity and concentration define the flux Φ (volume flow per unit area) which with Eq. (A8) becomes

$$\Phi_m = C_m v_m = -C_m u_m \nabla \mu_m + C_m v_W \tag{A9}$$

It should be noted that flux is a vector but for convenience we have omitted to notate this as so. Water can also move down its chemical potential gradient producing a flux,

$$\Phi_W = C_W v_W = -C_W u_W \nabla \mu_W \tag{A10}$$

The flux of a solute is immediately effected, as can be seen from Eq. (A8) by the presence of osmotic (solute concentration) gradients which produces flows of the solvent (water). Further interactions can also take place and these may be described by coupling coefficients between the fluxes of materials and the gradients in the chemical potentials of other molecular species. Within the framework of the thermodynamics of irreversible processes this is introduced via coupling between fluxes and nonconjugated forces. For a system containing cations, anions and water, the expressions for the fluxes may be generalized to give the following phenomenological relationships,

$$\begin{pmatrix} \Phi_W \\ \Phi_P \\ \Phi_N \end{pmatrix} = -\begin{pmatrix} C_W u_W & L_{WP} & L_{WN} \\ L_{PW} & C_P u_P & L_{PN} \\ L_{NW} & L_{NP} & C_N u_N \end{pmatrix}\begin{pmatrix} \nabla \mu_W \\ \nabla \mu_P \\ \nabla \mu_N \end{pmatrix} + v_W\begin{pmatrix} 0 \\ C_P \\ C_N \end{pmatrix} \tag{A11}$$

where the elements in this 3×3 matrix are called the kinetic coupling coefficients. The latter contains "self"-coefficients which are related to the diffusion constants of the molecular species which couple fluxes to conjugated "forces", as well as "cross-coefficients" which describe the coupling between the fluxes of the different species.

The current densities for cations and anions are, respectively,

$$J_P = q\Phi_P \quad \text{and} \quad J_N = -q\Phi_N \tag{A12}$$

For systems not far removed from equilibrium, the Onsager's relationships for the phenomenological Eq. (A11) are;

$$L_{PW} = L_{WP} \quad \text{and} \quad L_{NW} = L_{WN} \tag{A13}$$

The direct coupling between the fluxes of cations and anions in dilute solutions is very small and hence

$$L_{PN} = L_{NP} = 0 \tag{A14}$$

Substituting these relationships as well as Eqs. (A2), (A3), (A4), (A12), (A13) and (A14) into Eq. (A11) yields

$$\begin{pmatrix} \Phi_W \\ J_P \\ J_N \end{pmatrix} = - \begin{pmatrix} u_W C_W & L_{WP} & L_{WN} \\ qL_{WP} & qu_P C_P & 0 \\ -qL_{WN} & 0 & -qu_N C_N \end{pmatrix}$$
$$\times \begin{pmatrix} \nabla\mu_W^o + \{\nabla P - kT\nabla C_S\}/C_W \\ \nabla\mu_P^o - qE + kT\nabla C_P/C_P \\ \nabla\mu_N^o + qE + kT\nabla C_N/C_N \end{pmatrix} + v_W \begin{pmatrix} 0 \\ qC_P \\ -qC_N \end{pmatrix} \tag{A15}$$

which is a generalized form for the Nernst–Planck equations for a simple aqueous system in which ion–ion coupling is not as significant as electro-osmotic coupling.

Further simplifications can be made if we assume that μ_W^o is spatially constant and a pressure P is applied to the system to offset the osmotic pressure, $kT\nabla C_S$. For this situation the chemical potential gradient for water $\Delta\mu_W^o$ is then zero. Assuming further that $\Delta\mu_N^o = \Delta\mu_P^o = 0$, then, on substituting the Einstein relationship between the mobility and the diffusion constants;

$$u_W = \frac{D_W}{kT}, \quad u_P = \frac{D_P}{kT} \quad \text{and} \quad u_N = \frac{D_N}{kT} \tag{A16}$$

Eqs. (A15) then reduce to the more familiar form of the Nernst–Planck equation given earlier [Eq. (18)].

B. The AC Nernst–Planck–Poisson and Continuity Equations

If we denote AC perturbations of cations and anions by lower-case characters $\tilde{p}$ and $\tilde{n}$, respectively, that of the electric field inducing these perturbations by $\tilde{E}$, then the AC perturbations of the Nernst–Planck currents, i.e., $\tilde{\Phi}_W$, $\tilde{J}_P$ and $\tilde{J}_N$, are obtained by substituting

$$C_P = \bar{P} + \tilde{p}, \quad C_N = \bar{N} + \tilde{n} \quad \text{and} \quad E = \bar{E} + \tilde{E} \tag{B1}$$

in Eq. (A15) and collecting 1st order AC perturbations and neglecting 2nd order small terms. The AC generalized Nernst–Planck equations become;

$$
\begin{pmatrix} \tilde{\Phi}_W \\ \tilde{J}_P \\ \tilde{J}_N \end{pmatrix} = - \begin{pmatrix} u_W C_W & L_{WP} & L_{WN} \\ q L_{WP} & q u_P \bar{P} & 0 \\ -q L_{WN} & 0 & -q u_N \bar{N} \end{pmatrix}
$$
$$
\times \begin{pmatrix} \{\nabla \tilde{P} - kT\nabla \tilde{c}_S\}/C_W \\ -q\tilde{E} - \{q\bar{E}\tilde{p} - kT\nabla \tilde{p}\}/\bar{P} \\ q\tilde{E} + \{q\bar{E}\tilde{n} + kT\nabla \tilde{n}\}/\bar{N} \end{pmatrix} + \bar{v}_W \begin{pmatrix} 0 \\ q\tilde{p} \\ -q\tilde{n} \end{pmatrix} + \tilde{v}_W \begin{pmatrix} 0 \\ q\bar{P} \\ -q\bar{N} \end{pmatrix} \quad (\text{B2})
$$

where it has been assumed $\nabla \mu_P^o = \nabla \mu_N^o = \nabla \mu_W^o = 0$ and that the source–sink terms for water, cations and anions are unaffected by the perturbations. Note that terms involving the DC concentrations $\bar{N}$ and $\bar{P}$ and the DC field $\bar{E}$ feature as prominently as the AC variables in these expressions. The AC continuity equations for these three species [cf. Eq. (19)] are then given by,

$$
\nabla \cdot \tilde{\Phi}_W = 0, \quad \nabla \cdot \tilde{J}_P + qj\omega\tilde{p} = 0 \quad \text{and} \quad \nabla \cdot \tilde{J}_N - qj\omega\tilde{n} = 0 \quad (\text{B3})
$$

Charge conservation requires that the total AC current $\tilde{J}$ and the field $\tilde{E}$ satisfy the AC forms of the charge conservation [Eq. (8)] and Poisson equation [Eq. (21)], i.e.,

$$
\nabla \cdot \tilde{J} = \nabla \cdot \{\tilde{J}_P + \tilde{J}_N + j\omega\varepsilon\tilde{E}\} = 0 \quad (\text{B4})
$$
$$
\nabla \cdot \tilde{E} = \tilde{\rho}/\varepsilon = q(\tilde{p} - \tilde{n})/\varepsilon \quad (\text{B5})
$$

If the water is stationary ($\bar{v}_W = \tilde{v}_W = 0$) and the perturbed pressure gradient always counterbalances that of the osmotic gradient ($\tilde{P} - kT\tilde{c}_S = 0$) then integration of Eq. (B4) and substitution of (B2) yields the total AC current density [Eq. (20)]. Analytical solutions of these equations are found in the following appendix and are used to derive an expression for the impedance of an electrolyte.

C. Impedance of an Electrolyte Using a Four-Electrode Configuration

Here we consider an ideal electrolyte where $D_P = D_N = D$. At positions remote from interfaces it can be assumed $\nabla \mu_P^o = \nabla \mu_N^o = \nabla \mu_W^o = 0$, $\bar{E} = 0$ and $v_W = 0$. Equations (B2)–(B5) show that the AC charge density $\tilde{\rho}$ must satisfy the following conditions;

$$
\nabla^2 \tilde{\rho} - \kappa^2 \tilde{\rho} = 0 \quad \text{where} \quad \kappa^2 \equiv \frac{\sigma + j\omega\varepsilon}{\omega D} \quad \text{and} \quad \sigma \equiv \frac{q^2 D(\bar{P} + \bar{N})}{kT} \quad (\text{C1})
$$

The solution of this equation yields

$$
\tilde{\rho} = \rho_c \sinh \kappa x \quad \text{where} \quad \rho_c \text{ is constant in } x \quad (\text{C2})
$$

for the symmetrical electrode configuration depicted in Fig. 1. Integrating the AC Poisson Eq. (B5) twice gives, respectively, the AC field $\tilde{E}$ and potential difference $\tilde{V}$;

$$\tilde{E} = \frac{\rho_c}{\varepsilon\kappa}\cosh\kappa x + E_c \quad \text{where} \quad E_c \text{ is constant in } x \tag{C3}$$

$$\tilde{V} = \Psi\left(-\frac{l}{2}\right) - \Psi\left(\frac{l}{2}\right) = l\left\{\frac{2\rho_c}{\varepsilon\kappa^2}\sinh\frac{\kappa l}{2} + E_c\right\} \tag{C4}$$

where $x = \pm l/2$ are the positions of the voltage electrodes. Equation (B2) and the AC Poisson equation gives the total ionic current as

$$\tilde{J}_P + \tilde{J}_N = -qD\nabla(\tilde{p} - \tilde{n}) + \sigma\tilde{E} = -(\sigma + j\omega\varepsilon)\frac{\nabla^2\tilde{E}}{\kappa^2} + \sigma\tilde{E}$$

and Eq. (8) gives the total current as

$$\tilde{J} = \tilde{J}_P + \tilde{J}_N + j\omega\varepsilon\tilde{E} = (\sigma + j\omega\varepsilon)\left\{\tilde{E} - \frac{\nabla^2\tilde{E}}{\kappa^2}\right\} = (\sigma + j\omega\varepsilon)E_c \tag{C5}$$

which, as expected, is constant in x. The ionic current will be zero at the blocking current electrodes located at $x = \pm L/2$. This boundary condition and Eqs. (C1) and (C3) yields

$$E_c = \frac{j\omega\rho_c}{\sigma\kappa}\cosh\frac{\kappa L}{2} \tag{C6}$$

This and Eq. (C4) defines the admittance, y, per unit area;

$$y = \frac{\tilde{J}}{\tilde{V}} = \frac{\sigma + j\omega\varepsilon}{l\left\{1 + \dfrac{\sigma\delta}{j\omega\varepsilon}\right\}} \quad \text{where} \quad \delta \equiv \frac{2\sinh\dfrac{\kappa l}{2}}{\kappa l\cosh\dfrac{\kappa L}{2}} \tag{C7}$$

The conductance and capacitance (per unit area) are, respectively, σ/l and ε/l, at high frequencies. For DC ($\omega = 0$), the conductance and capacitance are, respectively, 0 and $\varepsilon/l\delta$.

D.   Origin of Concentration Polarization in Unstirred Layers

Here we consider a system consisting of a semipermeable membrane separating electrolytes of different concentration C_I and C_{II}. We assume that no external pressure, **P**, is applied to counter osmotic pressures in the system. It is further assumed that $\nabla\mu_P^o = \nabla\mu_N^o = \nabla\mu_W^o = 0$, $E = 0$, and $L_{WP} = L_{WN} \equiv L_{WJ}$.

With these simplifications and noting that $C_S \approx 2C$, Eq. (A15) becomes;

$$\begin{pmatrix} \Phi_W \\ J_P \\ J_N \end{pmatrix} = -\begin{pmatrix} u_W C_W & L_{WJ} & L_{WJ} \\ qL_{WJ} & qu_P C_P & 0 \\ -qL_{WJ} & 0 & -qu_N C_N \end{pmatrix}\begin{pmatrix} -2kT\nabla C/C_W \\ kT\nabla C_P/C_P \\ kT\nabla C_N/C_N \end{pmatrix} + v_W\begin{pmatrix} 0 \\ qC_P \\ -qC_N \end{pmatrix}$$

(D1)

When applied to the membrane, these generalized Nernst–Planck equations reveal that there will be a water flux given by;

$$\Phi_W = v_W C_W = L_P kT\{C(w/2) - C(-w/2)\}\{1 - \sigma_r\}$$

(D2)

where we have introduced the more familiar hydraulic constants such as the hydraulic conductivity L_p and the reflection coefficient σ_r both of which are simply related to the phenomenological coupling coefficient, L_{WJ}^m, the mobility u_W^m and the membrane width w. Here we use the superscript m to indicate that the variable refers to the membrane. Thus,

$$L_p = \frac{2u_W^m}{w}, \quad \sigma_r = \frac{2L_{WJ}^m}{C_{Av} u_W^m} \quad \text{where} \quad C_{Av} \equiv \{C(w/2) + C(-w/2)\}/2$$

(D3)

Since in the membrane, the mobility of anions is different from that of cations, anions will carry a different fraction of the total ionic current to that of cations. These fractions are called transport numbers and according to Eq. (D1) are given by:

$$t_P^m \equiv \frac{J_P}{J_P + J_N} = \frac{C_W u_P^m - 2u_W^m C_{Av}}{C_W(u_P^m - u_N^m)} \quad \text{and} \quad t_N^m \equiv \frac{J_N}{J_P + J_N} = \frac{C_W u_N^m - 2u_W^m C_{Av}}{C_W(u_N^m - u_P^m)}$$

(D4)

respectively, for the cations and anions.

Note that in the instance of a cation exchange membrane, $u_P^m \gg u_N^m$ and hence $t_P^m \gg t_N^m$, indicating, as expected, that cations will carry the larger fraction of the total current. This contrasts with what happens in the electrolyte where, since $u_P \approx u_N$, the transport numbers in the electrolyte, t_P and t_N, will be very similar in magnitude. A water flux will bring cations and anions to the membrane boundary in equal numbers but only one species (cations in this example) will move readily through the membrane to accumulate on the other side. The extent of accumulation at one boundary and depletion at the opposite boundary, can be formulated if we apply Eq. (D1) and the continuity Eq. (19) to the electrolyte where we assume that L_{WJ} is negligible. This yields;

$$\frac{\partial C}{\partial t} = D\frac{\partial^2 C}{\partial x^2} - \frac{\partial C}{\partial x} v_W$$

(D5)

which for $C = C_P = C_N$ are the convection equations [78] for an electrolyte. Solutions to these equations and many other variations thereof are contained in the comprehensive review by Barry and Diamond [47] of unstirred layers. They show that analytical solutions to Eq. (D5) exist for the steady state and when v_W is constant. For locations $|x| \geq W$ it is assumed that stirring of the electrolytes maintains the electrolyte concentrations at their respective bulk values of C_I and C_{II}. Integrating Eq. (D5) for the ionic species whose transport number is negligible, yields the spatial distributions of the concentration in the unstirred layers on either side of the membrane,

$$C(x) = C_I e^{-\vartheta(2x - W)} \quad \text{and} \quad C(x) = C_{II} e^{\vartheta(2x - W)} \quad \text{where} \quad \vartheta \equiv \frac{v_W}{2D} \qquad \text{(D6)}$$

This reveals that the concentration at the membrane–electrolyte boundaries will be different from their bulk electrolyte values with,

$$C(-w/2) = C_I e^{\vartheta(W - w)} < C_I \quad \text{and} \quad C(w/2) = C_{II} e^{-\vartheta(W - w)} < C_{II} \qquad \text{(D7)}$$

The concentration difference across the membrane will therefore be less than $C_{II} - C_I$, the difference in concentration between the bulk phases outside the unstirred layers.

LIST OF SYMBOLS

Note that variables notated, for example, as $\bar{E}$ and $\tilde{E}$ refer to the respective DC and AC contributions of the generalized variable E.

A [m^2]	cross-sectional area of current electrodes
C [Molec./m^3]	concentration of the electrolyte
C_{Av} [Molec./m^3]	average concentration of the electrolyte in the membrane
C_I, C_{II} [Molec./m^3]	concentration of bulk electrolyte on either side of the membrane
C_m [Molec./m^3]	concentration of species m
C_o [Molec./m^3]	standard (reference) concentration
C_S [Molec./m^3]	total concentration of solute $(C_P + C_N)$
$\tilde{c}_S$ [Molec./m^3]	total AC concentration of solute $(\tilde{p} + \tilde{n})$
C_W [Molec./m^3]	concentration of water
c_i [F/m^2]	capacitance per unit area of region i
$c(\omega)$ [F/m^2]	measured or total capacitance per unit area
C_i [F]	capacitance of region i
$C(\omega)$ [F]	measured or total capacitance
C^* [F]	complex capacitance
D [m^2/s]	diffusion constant for ions when $D_P = D_N$

D_m [m²/s]	diffusion constant of species m
$\mathbf{D}$ [C/m²]	electric displacement vector or electric flux density vector
E [V/m]	electric field
E_c [V/m]	integration constant in x
g_i [S/m²]	conductance per unit area of region i
$g(\omega)$ [S/m²]	measured or total conductance per unit area
G_i [S]	conductance of region i
$G(\omega)$ [S]	measured or total conductance
i (subscript)	identifies properties of electrically distinct regions (layers) generally $i \leftarrow 1, 2, \ldots$ etc., but for an electrically distinct membrane $i \leftarrow m$)
$\hat{i}$ [m]	unit vector along the x-axis
I [A]	total current injected by current electrodes
j	$\sqrt{-1}$
J [A]	total current density injected by current electrodes
J_{ionic} [A/m²]	ionic current density
J_m [A/m²]	current density of species m
$k = 1.38 \times 10^{-23}$ J	Boltzmann constant
$\pm l$ [m]	location of voltage electrodes from the centre of the experimental chamber
$\pm L$ [m]	location of current electrodes from the centre of the experimental chamber
$L_{m1, m2}$	kinetic coupling coefficient of the flux of species m_1 to that of m_2
L_{WJ}	kinetic coupling coefficient of water to the ionic flux (J_{ionic}/q)
L_p [m/N/s]	hydraulic conductivity or permeability
m (subscript)	identifies parameters specific to a species (water: $m \leftarrow W$, cations: $m \leftarrow P$ and anions: $m \leftarrow N$)
m (superscript)	identifies parameters specific to the membrane
$\bar{N}, \tilde{n}$ [Molec./m³]	Concentration of anions for, respectively, DC and AC
$\mathbf{P}$ [N/m²]	pressure difference from the pressure $\mathbf{P_O}$ in the standard state
$\mathbf{P_O}$ [N/m²]	the pressure $\mathbf{P_O}$ in the standard state
$\mathbf{P_{abs}}$ [N/m²]	the absolute pressure
$\bar{P}, \tilde{p}$ [Molec/m³]	Concentration of cations for, respectively, DC and AC
$q = 1.6 \times 10^{-19}$ C	magnitude of the electronic charge
r [m]	radius of an ion
R [Ω]	resistance
t [s]	time
t_P, t_P^m	transport number for cations in, respectively, the electrolyte and membrane

t_N, t_N^m	transport number for anions in, respectively, the electrolyte and membrane
Δt_P, Δt_N	transport number difference between the electrolyte and membrane for, respectively, cation and anions
T [K]	absolute temperature
u_m [m/N/s]	mobility of species m
v_m [m/s]	velocity of species m
V_m	the partial molecular volume for species m
V [V]	electric potential difference measured between voltage electrodes
w [m]	width of membrane
$\pm W$ [m]	extent of the unstirred layer from the centre of the membrane
x [m]	distance from the centre of the experimental chamber
X [Ω]	reactance
X_m	mole fraction of the molecular species m
$y(\omega)$ [S/m^2]	measured or total admittance per unit area
$Y(\omega)$ [S]	measured or total admittance
z_m	valency of species m
$Z(\omega)$	measured or total impedance
γ_m	activity coefficient for species m
γ_W	activity coefficient for water
δ	characteristic ratio of a four-terminal measurement of an ideal electrolyte (Appendix C)
ε^*	complex relative dielectric permittivity
$\varepsilon(x)$ [F/m]	dielectric permittivity at position x
$\varepsilon(\omega)$ [F/m]	measured or total dielectric permittivity
ε_i [F/m]	dielectric permittivity of region i
$\varepsilon_0 = 8.84 \times 10^{-12}$ F/m	dielectric permittivity of free space
∇ [m^{-1}]	$\hat{i}(\partial/\partial x)$ for a system of one dimension
ϕ	phase (between current and voltage)
Φ_m [Molec./m^2/s]	molecular flux of species m for respectively, AC and DC
κ [m$^-$]	reciprocal complex Debye length
λ [m]	Debye length ($= 1/\kappa$ when $\omega = 0$)
λ_d [m]	width of the depletion layer in double fixed charge (bipolar) membrane
ρ [C/m^3]	charge density
ρ_c [C/m^3]	constant in x
$\sigma(\omega)$ [S/m]	measured or total conductivity
$\sigma(x)$ [S/m]	conductivity at position x
σ_i [S/m]	conductivity of region i
σ^* [S/m]	complex conductivity

σ_r	reflection coefficient
μ_m^o [J]	standard chemical potential,
μ_{Born}^o [J]	Born energy, energy of an ion of radius r in dielectric permittivity ε
μ_m [J]	the thermodynamic potential of species m
ϑ [m^{-1}]	reciprocal characteristic length of an unstirred layer
ω [rad/s]	angular frequency ($=2\pi f$ where f is the frequency in Hertz)
Ψ [V]	the electric potential

REFERENCES

1. R. Hober, Arch. Ges. Physiol. *133*: 237 (1910).
2. E. Overton, Vjschr. Naturf. Ges. Zurich *44*: 88 (1899).
3. H. Fricke and S. Morse, J. Gen. Physiol. *9*: 153 (1925).
4. J. D. Robertson, Prog. Biophys. *10*: 343 (1960).
5. T. Hanai, D. A. Haydon, and J. L. Taylor, Proc. R. Soc. London Ser. A *281*: 337 (1964).
6. H. G. L. Coster and R. Simons, Biochim. Biophys. Acta *203*: 17 (1970).
7. H. G. L. Coster and J. R. Smith, Biochim. Biophys. Acta *373*: 151 (1974).
8. C. Clausen, S. A. Lewis, and J. M. Diamond, Biophys. J. *26*: 291 (1979).
9. H. P. Schwan, in *Advances in Biological and Medical Physics, Vol 5*, Academic Press, New York, 1957, pp. 147–209.
10. H. P. Schwan and S. Takashima, in *Encyclopedia of Applied Physics*, VCH, Weinheim, 1992, Vol. 5, pp. 177–200.
11. E. Gheorghiu, J. Phys. A *27*: 3883 (1994).
12. T. C. Chilcott and H. G. L. Coster, J. Plant Physiol. *18*: 191 (1991).
13. T. C. Chilcott, H. G. L. Coster, V. R. Franceschi, and W. J. Lucas, C. R. Acad. Sci. *319*: 17 (1996).
14. R. P. Henderson and J. G. Webster, IEEE Trans. Biomed. Eng. *BME-25*: 250 (1978).
15. E. Gheorghiu, Bioelectrochem. Bioenerg. *40*: 133 (1996).
16. A. M. Woodward, A. Jones, X.-z. Zhang, J. Rowland, and D. B. Kell, Bioelectrochem. Bioenerg. *40*: 99 (1996).
17. H. G. L. Coster, K. J. Kim, K. Dalan, J. R. Smith, and C. J. D. Fell, J. Membrane Sci. *66*: 19 (1992).
18. F. F. Zha, H. G. L. Coster, and A. J. Fane, J. Membrane Sci. *93*: 255 (1994).
19. J. Benavente, Solid State Ionics *97*: 339 (1997).
20. K. Ledjeff, F. Hahlendorf, V. Peinecke, and A. Heinzel, Electrochimica Acta *40*: 315 (1995).
21. J. Benavente, J. M. Garcia, J. G. de la Campa, and J. de Abajo, J. Membrane Sci. *114*: 51 (1996).
22. F. J. R. Nieto and R. I. Tucceri, J. Electroan. Chem. *416*: 1 (1996).
23. L. E. Bromberg, J. Membrane Sci. *62*: 145 (1991).
24. T. S. Sørensen, J. B. Jensen and B. Malmgren-Hansen, Desalination *80*: 265 (1991).

25. R. P. Buck, Electrochimica Acta *35*:1609 (1990).
26. L. Kavan and K. Dobihofer, Werkstoff und Korrosion *42*:309 (1991).
27. R. D. Armstrong and W. G. Proud, J. Electroanal. Chem. *295*:163 (1990).
28. K. Uosaki, K. Okazaki, and H. Kita, J. Electroanal. Chem. *287*:163 (1990).
29. J. R. Macdonald, Electrochimica Acta *35*:1483 (1990).
30. J. Bobacka, M. Grzeszczuk, and A. Ivaska, Electrochimica Acta *37*:1759 (1992).
31. S. Fletcher, J. Electroanal. Chem. *337*:127 (1992).
32. T. E. Springer, T. A. Zawadzinski, M. S. Wilson, and S. Gottesfeld, J. Electrochem. Soc. *143*:587 (1996).
33. C. Deslouis, M. M. Musiani, B. Tribollet, and M. A. Vorotyntsev, J. Electrochem. Soc. *142*:6 (1995).
34. C. Moreno, M. Valiente, J. Electroanalytical Chem. *422*:191 (1997).
35. M. Ikematsu, M. Iseki, Y. Sugiyama, and A. Mizukami, J. Electroanal. Chem. *403*:61 (1996).
36. L. E. Bromberg, J. Membrane Sci. *62*:145 (1991).
37. S. Mafe and P. Ramirez, Acta Polymer *48*:234 (1997).
38. D. Gao, J. Z. Li, R-Q. Yu, and G-D. Zheng, Anal. Chem. *66*:2245 (1994).
39. P. D. van der Wal, E. J. R. Sudholter, B. A. Boukamp, H. J. M. Bouwmeester, and D. N. Reinhoudt, J. Electroanal. Chem. *317*:153 (1991).
40. F. Lisdat and W. Moritz, Thin Solid Films *248*:126 (1994).
41. E. Lindner, E. Graf, Z. Niegreisz, K. Toth, E. Pungor, and R. P. Buck Anal. Chem. *60*:295 (1988).
42. C. Steinem, A. Jansfoff, H.-J. Galla, and M. Sieber, Bioelectrochem. Bioenerg. *42*:213 (1997).
43. J. R. MacDonald and J. R. Garber, J. Electrochem. Soc. Electrochem. Sci. Technol. *124*:1022 (1977).
44. J. B. Bates, J. C. Wang, and Y. T. Chu, Solid State Ionics *18/19*:1045 (1986).
45. C. Deslousis, M. Musiani and B. Triballet, J. Phys. Chem. *100*:8994 (1996).
46. B. Lindhol-Sethson, Langmuir *12*:3305 (1996).
47. P. H. Barry and J. M. Diamond, Physiol. Rev. Am. Physiol. Soc. *64*:763 872 (1984).
48. D. J. Bell, H. G. L. Coster and J. R. Smith, J. Phys. E. *8*:66–70 (1974).
49. M. Schafer, E. Gersing, B. Schultheiss, and M. M. Gebhard., in *Proceedings of International Conference on Electrical Bio-impedance* (E. Gersig and M. Schaefer, eds.), ICPRBI, University of Heidelberg, pp. 32–35 (1995).
50. H. P. Schwan and C. D. Ferris, Rev. Sci. Instrum. *39*:481 (1968).
51. H. P. Schwan, Ann. Biomed. Eng. *20*:269 (1992).
52. T. S. Sørensen, J. Colloid Interface Sci. *168*:437 (1994).
53. J. R. Macdonald, J. Electroanal. Chem. *32*:317 (1971).
54. M. Eberl, Electrodiffusion in electrolytes and membranes, Ph.D. Thesis, University of NSW (1993).
55. T. C. Chilcott,. H. G L. Coster, K. Ogata, and J. R. Smith, Aust. J. Plant Physiol. *10*:353 (1983).
56. T. C. Chilcott and H. G. L. Coster, in *Plant Membrane Transport* (J. Dainty and E. Maree, eds), Elsevier, Amsterdam, 1989.
57. R. Simons, J. Membrane Biol. *16*:175 (1974).
58. A. Mauro, Biophys. J. *2*:179 (1962).

59. H. G. L. Coster, Biophys. J. 5:669 (1965).
60. H. G. L. Coster, Biophys. J. 13:118 (1973).
61. T. C. Chilcott, H. G. L. Coster, and E. P. George, J. Membrane Sci. 100:77 (1995).
62. T. S. Sørensen, V. Compañ and R. Diaz-Calleja, Faraday Trans. 92:1947 (1996).
63. H.-T. Kim, J.-K. Park, and K-H. Lee, J. Membrane Sci. 115:207 (1996).
64. R. Erbach, B. Hoffmann, and A. Vogel, Sensors and Actuators B 4:379 (1991).
65. C. Schyberg, C. Plossu, D. Barbier, N. Jaffrezic-Renault, C. Martelet, H. Maupas, E. Souteyrand, M.-H. Charles, T. Delair, and B. Mandrand, Sensors and Actuators B, 26/27:457 (1995).
66. R. G. Ashcroft, H. G. L. Coster, and J. R. Smith, Biochim. Biophys. Acta 469:13 (1977).
67. R. G. Ashcroft, H. G. L. Coster, and J. R. Smith, Biochim. Biophys. Acta 730:231 (1983).
68. R. Erbach, B. Hoffmann and A. Vogel, Sensors and Actuators B 4:379 (1991).
69. H. Yamada, H. Shiku, T. Matsue, and I. Uchida, J. Phys. Chem. 97:9547 (1993).
70. L. Ding, J. Li, and E. Wang, J. Electroanal. Chem. 416:105 (1996).
71. H. G. L. Coster, T. C. Chilcott, and A. C. F. Coster, Bioelectrochem. Bioenerg. 40:79 (1996).
72. P. Debye, in Polar Molecules, Catalog Co., New York, 1929.
73. J. L. Oncley, in Proteins, Amino Acids and Peptide (E. J. Cohen and J. T. Edsall, eds.), Reinhold, New York, 1943.
74. S. Takashima, In Physical Principles and Techniques of Protein Chemistry, Part A, Academic Press, New York 1969.
75. M. Born, Z. Physik, 1:45 (1920).
76. B. Neumcke and P. Lauger, Biophys. J. 9:1160 (1969).
77. H. G. L. Coster, Thermodynamics of Life Processes, UNSW Press, Sydney, 1981.
78. J. Dainty, Adv. Bot. Res. 1:279 (1966).
79. J. R. Smith, Electrical characteristics of biological membranes in different environments, Ph.D. Thesis, University of NSW, Sydney (1977).
80. H. G. L. Coster and J. R. Smith, Aust. J. Plant Physiol. 4:667 (1977).
81. R. G. Ashcroft, H. G. L. Coster, and J. R. Smith, Biochim. Biophys. Acta 643:191 (1983).
82. P. H. Barry, J. Membrane Biol. 34:243 (1977).
83. B. Malmgren-Hansen, T. S. Sørensen, J. B. Jensen, and M. Hennenberg, J. Colloid Interface Sci. 130:359 (1989).
84. T. S. Sørensen, in Capillarity Today (G. Petre and A. Sanfeld, eds. Springer, Berlin 1991, pp. 164–221.
85. I. W. Plesner, B. Malmgren-Hansen, and T. S. Sørensen, J. Chem. Soc. Faraday Trans. 90:2381 (1994).
86. K. Ogata, T. C. Chilcott, and H. G. L. Coster, Aust. J. Plant Physiol. 10:339 (1983).
87. S. R. De Groot, Thermodynamics of Irreversible Processes, North Holland Pub. Co., Amsterdam, 1963.
88. A. Katchalsky and P. F. Curran, Non-equilibrium Thermodynamics in Biophysics, Harvard University Press, Cambridge, 1965.
89. T. S. Sørensen, R. Diaz-Calleja, E. Riande, J. Guzman, and A. Andrio, J. Chem. Soc. Faraday Trans. 91:4235 (1997).

20

Impedance of Multilayer Membrane Systems

EMILIJ K. ZHOLKOVSKIJ Institute of Bio-Colloid Chemistry of Ukrainian Academy of Sciences, Kiev, Ukraine

Abstract

Impedance of membrane systems is considered within a wide frequency range. Two types of impedance dispersion are discussed to be predictable in frame of the phenomenological approaches. They are the Maxwell and the low-frequency dispersion attributed to the substantially different frequency ranges, however. Classic results concerned with Maxwell's dispersion type are stated as applied to a multilayer membrane characterized by specific conductivities and permittivities of the constituent layers. The restrictions of a phenomenological approach are discussed to single out those membranes in which a sole macroscopic electrodynamics description is possible. A new theoretical approach based on the irreversible thermodynamics is proposed in order to describe the low-frequency dispersion. The property of a medium to accumulate a substance is described in the theory by introducing a special thermostatic coefficient. It is referred to as the chemical capacity being the proportionality coefficient between the amount of the substance accumulated and the change of the chemical potential. The chemical capacity is applied to various models of the media showing that its magnitude substantially depends on the medium sorption properties. In the general problem formulation the chemical capacity is set for each constituent phase as a phenomenological coefficient. The approach enables one to predict the impedance response in purely phenomenological characteristics of the constituent parts of the membrane system. No model of the charge carrier transport is used in the theory. Impedance of both an elementary membrane cell and a multilayer membrane is predicted by using the new approach. Theoretical results presented in literature are shown to be particular cases of the theoretical predictions. Equivalent electric circuits are proposed to simulate impedance behavior. Some methods of data interpretation in impedance spectroscopy are suggested. Experimental data from the literature are analyzed to obtain the chemical capacity of the membranes under consideration. It is shown which conclusions can be made by dealing with the chemical capacity as a function of some parameters.

I. INTRODUCTION

A membrane system employed in a liquid phase technology can be often considered as a multilayer electric conductor having either ionic or mixed (electronic and ionic) type of conductance. The system includes at least the membrane itself and two adjacent electrolyte solutions. In the presence of electric current the system is additionally completed by electrodes. The membranes themselves often consist of two [1–4] or even more [5] layers to provide them with certain properties. There is a necessity to characterize the constituent homogeneous parts of the membrane systems. In many cases one has to do it in a nondestructive way because this is often technically impossible to single out the component layer of interest.

Impedance Spectroscopy (IS) is a powerful nondestructive method used to study properties of heterogeneous conductors. It amounts to measuring the frequency dependency of the system response (electric voltage difference) to a harmonic external signal (electric current). The results of the measurements are performed with the help of the frequency dependency of the impedance. It is a complex value whose modules is the ratio between the voltage and current amplitudes. Its argument is the phase difference. In the case of a slight external signal and a linear response the impedance does not depend on the signal (current) amplitude but depends on the frequency and on the heterogeneous system morphology. Therefore the interpretation of IS data can yield valuable information about constituent phase characteristics.

Electric current passage across a heterogeneous conductor gives rise to the polarization (appearance of a polarization electric charge in the system). The phase of the polarization charge oscillation lags the alternating current phase because of the polarization has nonzero relaxation time. The polarization charge results in an additional portion of the voltage having the same phase as the charge. The heterogeneous conductor polarization is associated with a property by which the constituent phases differ. One can single out the electrical (specific conductivity, permittivity) and selective (transport numbers of the charge carriers) properties.

When two contacting phases have different specific conductivities/permittivities, a free electric charge is formed to provide continuity of the electric current [6]. The electric charge is distributed between the both phases. Due to the diffusion, the charge is localized in some regions having nonzero thickness within each phase (Debye screening length). Hereafter this type of polarization is referred to as Maxwell polarization.* Accordingly, we are to deal with Maxwell's impedance dispersion, relaxation times and frequency range.

Another mechanism of polarization exists when the electric current crosses the interface between two media with different transport numbers of the same species. The diffusion of the free charge carriers occurs within the bulks of each phase. Under certain conditions the diffusion gives rise to the electric charge separation. Finally, the electric field originating in diffusion may appear within each medium. This type of the polarization we shall refer to as the concentration polarization.

Relaxation times of the Maxwell and the concentration polarization can be roughly evaluated as the characteristic diffusion times attributed to Debye length and thickness of the constituent layer, respectively. As a rule, the synthetic membrane systems consist of the layers being much thicker than the Debye length. Hence the relaxation time of the concentration polarization is much longer than the Maxwell relaxation time. Hereafter, we refer to the impedance dispersion caused by the concentration polarization relaxation as the low-frequency dispersion.

---

* Strictly speaking the Maxwell theory deals with the vanishingly thin charge region. However when the Debye screening length is much smaller than the characteristic dimensions of the contacting phases one can use the Maxwell approach as an approximation.

There are two features characteristic for the situation in which the layers are much thicker than the Debye length: (1) the Maxwell and the low-frequency impedance dispersions can be considered separately because their frequency ranges do not intersect; and (b) both the Maxwell and the low-frequency impedance dispersions can be described in frames of purely phenomenological approaches. The latter enables each layer to be considered as a homogeneous phase which is characterized by a set of coefficients. All these coefficients can be phenomenologically defined using no specific model of the electric current transfer.

The phenomenological approach becomes especially valuable when preliminary unknown systems are studied. It is the case when an appropriate model cannot be developed before the interpretation of IS data. It is the phenomenological theory which enables one to interpret IS data without a model. The model is chosen at the next stage of the study to describe the behavior of the phenomenological characteristics already obtained.

As applied to Maxwell's dispersion such a phenomenological method is widely known to be based on the macroscopic electrodynamics [6–9]. As to the low-frequency dispersion it was mainly analyzed earlier in the frame of various models. However in our previous papers [10–12] the low-frequency dispersion was shown to be predictable in phenomenological terms as well. A version of the Irreversible Thermodynamics was used to describe impedance behavior in Refs. 10–12.

This chapter is concerned with phenomenological description of the impedance behavior in the wide frequency range which comprises both Maxwell's and the low-frequency dispersion. This treatise is based on the classic results of Maxwell [6], Wagner [7,8] and Volger [9] and on our theoretical approach stated in Refs. 10–12. Our method is generalized here to obtain new results associated with systems of practical interest.

II. IMPEDANCE, ADMITTANCE AND COMPLEX PERMITTIVITY

Prior to state the theory we define some values conventionally employed in this field of research. Let us consider a function A performing a harmonic dependency on time

$$A = A_0 \sin(\omega\tau + \theta) \tag{1}$$

The complex value

$$\dot{A}_0 = A_0 \exp(i\theta) \tag{2}$$

where $i = \sqrt{-1}$, is referred to as its complex amplitude. Hence one can rewrite Eq. (1)

$$A = \mathrm{Im}\lfloor \dot{A} \exp(i\omega\tau) \rfloor \tag{3}$$

The impedance is the ratio between the complex amplitudes of the harmonic voltage and current attributed to two terminals of an electric circuit

$$\dot{z} = \frac{\dot{U}_0}{\dot{I}_0} = z \exp(i\theta) = \mathrm{Re}\,\dot{z} + i\,\mathrm{Im}\,\dot{z} \tag{4}$$

The reciprocal value is referred to as admittance

$$\dot{y} = \frac{1}{\dot{z}} = y\exp(-i\theta) = \mathrm{Re}\,\dot{y} + i\,\mathrm{Im}\,\dot{y}$$

$$= \frac{\mathrm{Re}\,\dot{z}}{\mathrm{Re}^2\,\dot{z} + \mathrm{Im}^2\,\dot{z}} - i\,\frac{\mathrm{Im}\,\dot{z}}{\mathrm{Re}^2\,\dot{z} + \mathrm{Im}^2\,\dot{z}} \tag{5}$$

An alternative way to represent results is to use the terms of complex capacity

$$\dot{c} = \frac{\dot{y}}{i\omega} = \mathrm{Re}\,\dot{c} + i\,\mathrm{Im}\,\dot{c} = \frac{1}{\omega}\,\mathrm{Im}\,\dot{y} - i\cdot\frac{1}{\omega}\,\mathrm{Re}\,\dot{y} \tag{6}$$

where ω is an applied frequency.

All systems considered in this work are a plane parallel electrochemical cells containing a membrane. It can be considered as a plane electric capacitor. It is convenient to use the value of the complex permittivity. The latter enables one to exclude geometric factor. When the area of the plates is S and a the distance between them d one can define the complex permittivity as

$$\dot{\varepsilon} = \frac{d}{S\varepsilon_0}\,\dot{c} = \mathrm{Re}\,\dot{\varepsilon} + i\,\mathrm{Im}\,\dot{\varepsilon} = \varepsilon' - i\left(\frac{d}{\omega S\varepsilon_0}\,\mathrm{Re}\,\dot{y}(0) + \varepsilon''\right) \tag{7}$$

where ε_0 is a vacuum permittivity; $\dot{y}(0) = \lim_{\omega\to 0}(\dot{y})$. Values ε' and ε'' are usually referred to as the permittivity (proper) and the (net) dielectric loss, respectively.

Both the real and imaginary parts of Eqs. (4)–(7) are always understood to be functions of the applied frequency. One can also deal with the imaginary vs. the real part.

III. MAXWELL DISPERSION OF MULTILAYER MEMBRANE IMPEDANCE

A. General Relationships for Multilayer System

Now we consider the Maxwell's dispersion of the impedance of the multilayer system shown in Fig. 1. Each layer is characterized by a specific conductivity $(\sigma^{(k)})$ and a permittivity $(\varepsilon^{(k)})$. Following Refs. 6–9 an obvious equivalent circuit is presented in Fig. 1.

$$g^{(k)} = \frac{S}{d^{(k)}}\,\sigma^{(k)} \tag{8}$$

$$c^{(k)} = \frac{S}{d^{(k)}} \varepsilon_0 \varepsilon^{(k)} \tag{9}$$

A trivial procedure yields the impedance of the parallelings which are connected in series

$$\dot{z} = \frac{1}{S} \sum_k \frac{d^{(k)}}{\sigma^{(k)} + i\omega\varepsilon_0 \varepsilon^{(k)}} = \sum_k \frac{1/g_k}{1 + i\omega\tau_*^{(k)}} \tag{10}$$

where Maxwell's relaxation time $\tau_*^{(k)}$ does not depend on the layer dimensions. In Sec. II.D we discuss applicability of the circuit in Fig. 1 and Eq. (10).

$$\tau_*^{(k)} = \frac{c^{(k)}}{g^{(k)}} = \frac{\varepsilon_0 \varepsilon^{(k)}}{\sigma^{(k)}} \tag{11}$$

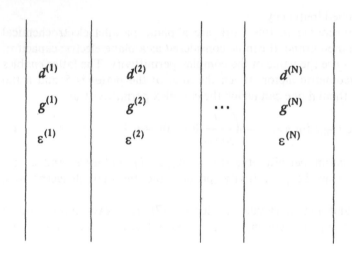

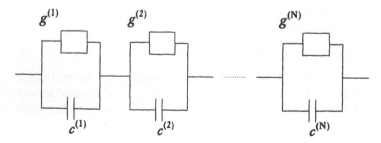

FIG. 1 Multilayer membrane and its equivalent electric circuit in Maxwell frequency range.

This is also possible to write

$$\text{Re } \dot{z} = \sum_k \frac{1/g^{(k)}}{1 + (\omega\tau_*^{(k)})^2} \tag{12}$$

$$\text{Im } \dot{z} = -\sum_k \frac{1/g^{(k)}}{1 + (\omega\tau_*^{(k)})^2}(\omega\tau_*^{(k)}) \tag{13}$$

From Eqs. (4)–(7) and (12) and (13) any of the above defined characteristics can be found. We tabulate their low and high frequency limits (Table 1) ($p^{(k)} = d^{(k)}/d$—volume fraction of a layer).

Both the impedance imaginary part and the dielectric loss go to zero at high and low frequencies (Table 1). Hence, they depend on the frequency with extremum. The admittance imaginary part is an increasing function of fre-

TABLE 1 High and Low Limits of the Functions Describing Multilayer System Impedance ($p^{(k)}$ is Volume Fraction of Layer No. × k)

	$\omega \to 0$	$\omega \to \infty$
Impedance real part Re $\dot{z}$	$\dfrac{d}{S}\sum_k p^{(k)}/\sigma^{(k)}$	0
Impedance imaginary part Im $\dot{z}$	0	0
Admittance real part Re $\dot{y}$	$\dfrac{S}{d} \times \dfrac{1}{\sum_k p^{(k)}/\sigma^{(k)}}$	$\dfrac{S}{d} \times \dfrac{\sum_k p^{(k)}\sigma^{(k)}/(\varepsilon^{(k)})^2}{\left(\sum_k p^{(k)}/\varepsilon^{(k)}\right)^2}$
Admittance imaginary part Im $\dot{y}$	0	∞
Permittivity (proper) ε'	$\dfrac{\sum_k p^{(k)}\varepsilon^{(k)}/(\sigma^{(k)})^2}{\left(\sum_k p^{(k)}/\sigma^{(k)}\right)^2}$	$\dfrac{1}{\sum_k p^{(k)}/\varepsilon^{(k)}}$
Dielectric loss (net) ε''	0	0

quency. It is also possible to prove that

$$\text{Re } \dot{z}(0) \geq \text{Re } \dot{z}(\infty); \quad \text{Re } \dot{y}(0) \leq \text{Re } \dot{y}(\infty); \quad \varepsilon'(0) \geq \varepsilon'(\infty) \tag{14}$$

Both the permittivity proper and the real part of the impedance are decreasing functions of frequency. On the contrary, the real part of the admittance is an increasing functions of frequency.

B. Monolayer System

The impedance dispersion occurs due to the finite time needed to charge the interface membrane–electrode. It follows from Eqs. (12) and (13) in this special case

$$\text{Re } \dot{z} = \frac{1/g}{1 + (\omega\tau_*)^2}; \quad \text{Im } \dot{z} = -\frac{1/g}{1 + (\omega\tau_*)^2}(\omega\tau_*)$$

$$\left[\frac{1}{2g} - \text{Re } \dot{z}\right]^2 + \text{Im}^2 \, \dot{z} = \left(\frac{1}{2g}\right)^2 \tag{15}$$

By combining Eqs. (5), (7) and (15) one can obtain trivial results for both the admittance ($\text{Re } \dot{y} = g$; $\text{Im } \dot{y} = \omega c$) and the complex permittivity ($\varepsilon' = \varepsilon$; $\varepsilon'' = 0$).

The plots illustrating the behavior of the real and imaginary parts of the impedance are shown in Figs. 2a and b. The maxima correspond to the frequency $\omega_* = 1/\tau_*$.

C. Bilayer System

The impedance of bilayer system is given by the following relations

$$\text{Re } \dot{z} = \frac{1/g^{(1)}}{1 + (\omega\tau_*^{(1)})^2} + \frac{1/g^{(2)}}{1 + (\omega\tau_*^{(2)})^2}$$

$$-\text{Im } \dot{z} = \frac{1/g^{(1)}}{1 + (\omega\tau_*^{(1)})^2}\,\omega\tau_*^{(1)} + \frac{1/g^{(2)}}{1 + (\omega\tau_*^{(2)})^2}\,\omega\tau_*^{(2)} \tag{16}$$

Two well expressed maxima occur in Fig. 3a when the relaxation times substantially differ.

The complex permittivity depends on a single relaxation time

$$\bar{\tau}_* = \frac{p^{(2)}\varepsilon^{(1)} + p^{(1)}\varepsilon^{(2)}}{p^{(2)}\sigma^{(1)} + p^{(1)}\sigma^{(2)}} \tag{17}$$

Combining Eqs. (16) and (4)–(7) yields the following expressions for the per-

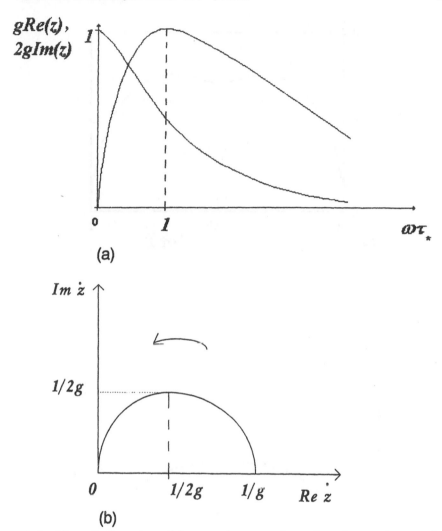

FIG. 2 Maxwell dispersion of the monolayer membrane impedance. (a) Normalized real and imaginary part vs. normalized frequency. (b) Semicircle diagram. Imaginary part vs. real part.

mittivity and (net) dielectric loss

$$\varepsilon' = \frac{\varepsilon'(0) + \omega^2 \bar{\tau}_*^2 \, \varepsilon'(\infty)}{1 + \omega^2 \bar{\tau}_*^2} \tag{18}$$

$$\varepsilon'' = \frac{2\varepsilon''_{max} \, \omega \bar{\tau}_*}{1 + \omega^2 \bar{\tau}_*^2} \tag{19}$$

$$\left\{ \frac{\varepsilon' - [\varepsilon'(\infty) + \varepsilon'(0)]/2}{[\varepsilon'(0) - \varepsilon'(\infty)]/2} \right\}^2 + \left[\cdot \frac{\varepsilon''}{\varepsilon''_{max}} \right]^2 = 1 \tag{20}$$

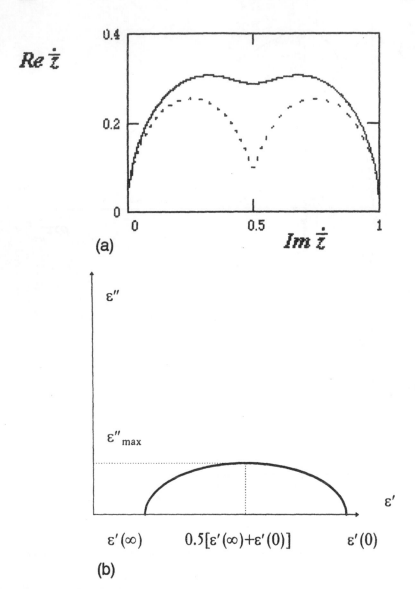

FIG. 3 Maxwell dispersion of the bilayer membrane impedance. (a) Normalized real part of impedance vs. its normalized imaginary part. Re $\hat{\bar{z}}$ = Re $\dot{z}$/Re$\dot{z}(0)$; Im $\hat{\bar{z}}$ = Im $\dot{z}$/Re $\dot{z}(0)$; $g_1 = g_2$; $\tau_*^{(1)}/\tau_*^{(2)} = 10$ (solid line); $\tau_*^{(1)}/\tau_*^{(2)} = 100$ (dotted line). (b) Semielliptic diagram. Permittivity vs. (net) dielectric loss.

The limiting values of the parameters in Eqs. (18)–(20) coincide with the bilayer versions of the expressions presented in Table 1 (Row 5)

$$\varepsilon'(0) = p^{(1)}\varepsilon^{(1)}\left(\frac{\sigma^{(2)}}{p^{(2)}\sigma^{(1)} + p^{(1)}\sigma^{(2)}}\right)^2 + p^{(2)}\varepsilon^{(2)}\left(\frac{\sigma^{(1)}}{p^{(2)}\sigma^{(1)} + p^{(1)}\sigma^{(2)}}\right)^2$$

$$\varepsilon'(\infty) = \frac{\varepsilon^{(1)}\varepsilon^{(2)}}{p^{(2)}\varepsilon^{(1)} + p^{(1)}\varepsilon^{(2)}} \tag{21}$$

The maximum magnitude of the (net) dielectric loss takes the form

$$\begin{aligned}
\varepsilon''_{max} &= \frac{\dot{y}^2(0)(\tau^{(1)} - \tau^{(2)})^2}{2(\varepsilon^{(1)}/p^{(1)} + \varepsilon^{(2)}/p^{(2)})} \\
&= \frac{p^{(1)}p^{(2)}}{2(\varepsilon^{(1)}p^{(2)} + \varepsilon^{(2)}p^{(1)})}\left(\frac{\sigma^{(1)}\varepsilon^{(1)} - \sigma^{(2)}\varepsilon^{(1)}}{\sigma^{(1)}p^{(2)} + \sigma^{(2)}p^{(1)}}\right)^2
\end{aligned} \tag{22}$$

The semielliptic curve is presented as a Cole–Cole diagram (Fig. 3b) corresponding Eq. (20). The maximum value of the dielectric loss is achieved when the applied frequency $\omega = 1/\bar{\tau}_*$.

D. Applicability of the Phenomenological Theory of the Maxwell Dispersion

Presented above classic theoretical results [6–9] hold for any model of the electric current transfer. This valuable feature is associated with two a priori assumptions enabling one to use the equivalent circuit with the ideal frequency independent elements (Fig. 1), namely: (1) the electric charge is supposed to belong only in vanishingly thin regions close to the interfaces; and (2) only migration electric current and displacement electric current is taken into account.

Restrictions of a phenomenological approach often can not be evaluated within its own frame. To do that, one can additionally suppose the electric current to be transferred by charged species simultaneously involved in the thermal (diffusion) motion. The diffusion can result in two consequences: (1) the electric charge is localized in regions having nonzero thickness; and (2) the diffusion fluxes contribute additionally to the electric current. These factors become ignorable under two conditions to be simultaneously satisfied: (1) the space charge regions are much thinner than the membrane layers; and (2) concentration gradients do not occur in the residual electroneutral bulk.

The width of the space charge region can roughly be estimated as a characteristic diffusion length attributed to the Maxwell's relaxation time [Eq. (11)].

$$l^{(k)} \cong (\tau^{(k)}D)^{1/2} \tag{23}$$

While writing Eq. (23) we supposed for simplicity the carriers to have a common diffusion coefficient D. Under this condition the specific conductivity can be represented as follows

$$\sigma = \frac{DF^2}{RT} \sum_i Z_i^2 C_i \qquad (24)$$

where F, R, T are Faraday constant, the gas constant and the absolute temperature, respectively; C_i is the concentration of the corresponding species in the bulk, Z_i is their charge expressed in Faraday units. By combining Eqs. (11), (23) and (24) we have

$$l^{(k)} \cong \left(\frac{\varepsilon_0 \varepsilon^{(k)} RT}{F^2 \sum_i Z_i^2 C_i^{(k)}} \right)^{1/2} = l_D^{(k)} \qquad (25)$$

Thus the polarization charge is localized in the region with the thickness having order of the Debye length $l_D^{(k)}$ attributed to the corresponding layer. Hence, the first abovementioned conditions is satisfied when

$$\frac{l_D^{(k)}}{d^{(k)}} \ll 1 \qquad (26)$$

A violation of condition (26) means that the equivalent circuit (Fig. 1) should be corrected by introducing additional frequency dependent elements to simulate the contribution of the charged regions. Under condition (26) one can also ignore a contribution of the equilibrium electric charge which is localized in the region with the same order of thickness ($l_D^{(k)}$).

The rough estimate presented above shows the results from Eqs. (8)–(21) to be a zero-order term in the expansion by parameter $l_D^{(k)}/d^{(k)}$. The next term in the same expansion was considered in Refs. 13–20 for the simplest models. Unlike the purely phenomenological zero-order term, all the next terms should depend on a model choice including details of the interface region structure.

Thus, the classic approach [6–9] yields the more reliable result the less is the value of the parameter in question. The Debye length is shown to belong within 0.1 to 0.3 nm for ion exchange materials with concentration of the main carriers $1-5 \times 10^3$ mol/m³. Hence Maxwell's approach can be definitely used in the case of the ion-exchange electrodialysis membrane which normally have thickness of order 0.1 mm. There are doubts regarding applicability of the theory to some types of bilayer membranes having active layer of order 10^2 nm. Due to some additional mechanisms of the ion exclusion the concentration of carriers can be, in principle, even less than in electrolyte solution where Debye length is 10 nm (aqueous 1:1 electrolyte solution with concentration 1 mol/m³). The latter can result in the parameter value to be comparable with unity. In such a situation the model approach developed in Refs. 21 and 22 might be used since it is not based on the mentioned above expansion.

One might and that even rather thick membranes can deviate from the behavior predicted by the Maxwell theory when there is internal heterogeneity of the layers. The internal heterogeneity can result in the dispersion of the local parameters (conductivity and permittivity) within the Maxwell frequency range.

The second condition (absence of the concentration gradients in the bulk) restricts the applied frequency as follows.

$$\omega \gg \frac{D}{(d^{(k)})^2} \tag{27}$$

The concentration gradients under condition (27) have only time to evolve in a very thin region compared to the width of each layer. Condition (27) is automatically satisfied when the membrane conforms to condition (26) and when the applied frequency belongs to the Maxwell range (between 10^6 Hz the active skin layer with strong ion exclusion- and 10^{10} Hz-ion-exchange membranes).

When applied frequency becomes comparable with right-hand side of inequality (27) the theory discussed above does not hold any more because of diffusion fluxes appeared in the layer bulks. The low frequency impedance dispersion occurring in this regime can be described in other but also phenomenological terms. It is this theory with which the next section deals.

IV. LOW-FREQUENCY DISPERSION OF IMPEDANCE

We are going to deal with the impedance dispersion occurring under applied frequencies much lower then the reciprocal of the Maxwell relaxation time [Eq. (11)]. There are some intriguing features of this dispersion type. The system behaves as an electric circuit containing capacitors. At the same time the frequencies are so low that the displacement current, usually responsible for the capacitive effects, takes a negligible value. The system equivalent capacity of this type takes a huge value at extremely low frequencies and decreases gradually with frequency increase.

To simulate this type of behavior Barker [23] suggested to use the transmission line model where both the great capacity and the system resistance were modelled as distributed elements. In the paper of Brumleve and Buck [24] this approach was mathematically argued and generalized. In the later works of Buck et al. the capacitive impedance response was predicted applying to various electrochemical systems [25–27].

In the papers referred to above the results were obtained by consideration of specific media. These were either binary or supported electrolyte solutions. Some results were derived as applied to other types of media (polymer films with mixed conductivity [28,29]). However the authors always used models of the media to predict the impedance. That is why in these papers both the equivalent capacitance and resistance were represented as combinations of parameters involved in the particular models employed.

The phenomenological approach was used by Albery et al. [29]. The authors described the conductive elements of the transmission line in terms of phenomenological characteristics of the current transferring media. The expressions for impedance derived in [29] enable one to extract from the IS data those transport characteristics of the charge carriers which can describe an arbitrary type of conductor used in the cells (provided that only two types of the carriers participate in the process). At the same time the relationship between the value of the transmission line capacity and the medium properties was not considered in Ref. 29. In fact, the capacity was used in [25] as an unknown element intended to simulate a certain type of the impedance behavior.

In our previous papers [10,11] the multilayer membrane impedance for the same case of two species was predicted solely in phenomenological terms by using Irreversible Thermodynamics. The key element of that theory is associated with an equilibrium thermodynamic (thermostatic) factor introduced to describe each layer. Generalizing the results of [10,11] in the present section we are going to show this parameter to be of a deep thermodynamic sense. It reflects the property of a medium to accumulate a substance. It is the parameter which is responsible for capacitive behavior of the impedance of the membrane system.

The multilayer systems in consideration are supposed to be fulfilling condition (26). This fact as well as the low value of the applied frequency enable us to use the following simplifications:

1. The quasi-electroneutrality has time to establish almost in the whole bulk of each layer. The electroneutrality condition is violated only in the thin region of width l_D adjacent to the corresponding interface.
2. Quasi-equilibrium condition can be used as applied to the species which belong to the electroneutral bulks of neighboring layers close to the interface.
3. The principle of local equilibrium can be used to characterize each point of the system by equilibrium values (chemical and electrochemical potentials) which can change from point to point under irreversible conditions.
4. Local fluxes of the species are expressed through a superposition of corresponding gradients with time independent kinetic coefficients.
5. The displacement current contribution is negligible.

The above mentioned simplifications make it possible to use the irreversible thermodynamic approach with some modifications.

A. Impedance of the Elementary Membrane Cell

1. Elementary Membrane Cell

Now we consider the simplest membrane system to comprehend why the impedance dispersion exists in spite of the negligible value of the displacement current. The system under consideration contains a membrane and two adjacent compartments filled by the same media (Fig. 4). One should also take into account that the electric current crosses the external surfaces of the system. The system behavior depends on the proportion in which the species transfer the current across these surfaces. To define completely the system one has to introduce a couple of electrodes to be the external bounds of the system. For simplicity we deal with reversible electrodes. Faraday's law is supposed to be fulfilled in the charge carrier transport across the electrodes

$$J_{1,2}^e = \frac{I t_{1,2}^e}{FZ_{1,2}} \tag{28}$$

Hereafter we deal with the system having two types of the charge carriers where $J_{1,2}^e$ are their fluxes across the electrodes and $t_{1,2}^e$ their electrodic migration transport numbers. The transmembrane fluxes $J_{1,2}$ are expressed with the help of irreversible thermodynamic relationship

$$J_{1,2} = \frac{g t_{1,2}}{(FZ_{1,2})^2} \Delta\mu_{1,2} \tag{29}$$

where g is the electric conductivity and $t_{1,2}$ the membrane migration transport numbers of the corresponding species, $\Delta\mu_{1,2}$ are the differences between the corresponding electrochemical potentials attributed to the compartments (Fig. 4). Widely used Eq. (29) is not the most general because it ignores the cross-

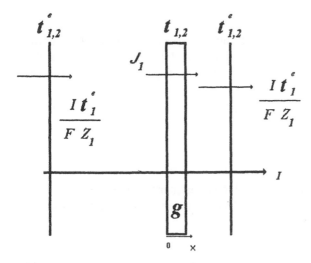

FIG. 4 Elementary membrane cell.

terms, i.e., that an electrochemical potential difference of the 2nd species affects the flux of the 1st species and vice versa. In Ref. 11 it is shown that to use Eq. (29) is the same as to neglect the interionic friction coefficient in the Spiegler's representation of transport equations [30]. There is a number of the experimental results demonstrating ignorable value of the Spiegler interionic friction coefficients (see, for example [31,32]).

Two simplifying assumptions are made. Firstly the conductivity of each compartment is supposed to be much greater than the conductivity of the membrane. It enables one to ignore the changes in the electrochemical potential of each of the carriers within each of the compartments. The second simplification is that transmembrane transport is described by just one single value of the flux corresponding to each species $J_{1,2}$. However in the nonstationary regime the fluxes attributed to external surfaces of membrane can differ due to the accumulation of the species within the membrane body. The thinner membrane the less this difference. We refer as "thin" membrane to those whose thickness is enabling one to ignore the changes of the fluxes within the membrane. Other membranes will be referred to as "thick". We initially consider the more comprehensible situation with a "thin" membrane. Then is Sec. III.A.5 we are to analyze the case of "thick" membrane.

2. Balance Equations

When the electric current is directed according to Fig. 4 one can write the following balance

$$\frac{\partial v''_{1,2}}{\partial \tau} = J_{1,2} - \frac{It^e_{1,2}}{FZ_{1,2}} = -\frac{\partial v'_{1,2}}{\partial \tau} \tag{30}$$

where $v_{1,2}$ are the amounts of the 1st and 2nd species, respectively; τ is time; (') and ('') denote the values attributed to the 1st and 2nd compartments, respectively. Directions of the fluxes is shown in Fig. 4 for the first (positive) species to illustrate balance (30).

Since the displacement current is negligible, one can write the expression for the current in the form

$$I = F(J_1 Z_1 + J_2 Z_2) \tag{31}$$

The species are withdrawn from each compartment and delivered there in a certain proportion to maintain the electroneutrality. One can introduce a value of a substance amount

$$\frac{dv_1}{|Z_2|} = \frac{dv_2}{|Z_1|} = dv_s \tag{32}$$

Combining Eqs. (29)–(32) and using $t_1 + t_2 = t_1^e + t_2^e = 1$ one can obtain that

$$\frac{\partial v_s''}{\partial \tau} = \frac{g t_1 t_2}{(F Z_1 Z_2)^2} \Delta \mu_s + \frac{I(t_1 - t_1^e)}{F |Z_1 Z_2|} = -\frac{\partial v_s'}{\partial \tau} \tag{33}$$

where the value of a coupled chemical potential is introduced by the following definition

$$\mu_s = \mu_1 |Z_2| + \mu_2 |Z_1| \tag{34}$$

3. Chemical Capacity

The thermodynamic quasi-equilibrium is supposed to hold within each compartment in any moment. Hence one can represent the differential of the free energy as follows

$$d\Psi = \mu_1 dv_1 + \mu_2 dv_2 \tag{35}$$

This form is valid under the electroneutrality condition (32) which can be combined with Eqs. (34) and (35) to have

$$d\Psi = \mu_s dv_s \tag{36}$$

Thus, the coupled chemical potential is a function only of the substance amount (at constant volume and temperature) only. This circumstance enables us to introduce the following definition

$$c_{ch} = \frac{1}{(\partial \mu_s / \partial v_s)_{T, V}} \tag{37}$$

We refer to this phenomenological coefficient as a chemical capacity characterization media of any origin in thermodynamic equilibrium. It is also calculable in the frame of particular models (Sec. III.C). The chemical capacity may be transformed to an intensive value defining

$$\alpha_{ch} = \frac{c_{ch}}{V} = \frac{1}{(\partial \mu_s / \partial C_s)_{T, V}} \tag{38}$$

where $C_s = v_s/V$ is a substance concentration.

The chemical capacity can be directly measured when the substance is transferred in a reversible way. We consider the medium in contact with two electrodes reversible with respect to the different species. The electrodes fully block transport of another carrier ("asymmetric cell" [26]). This configuration is often used to study membranes with the mixed conductance [33–35]. An electrode coated by such a membrane is assumed to be reversible for one sort of the species (electrons). The interface membrane–solution serves as the other reversible electrode permeable for the ions. The substance amount inside the "asymmetric cell" can be changed in a reversible way by applying an infinitely small current. In any moment the system is in the thermodynamic equilibrium. One can equate the free energy change and the necessary work to transfer a portion dQ of electric charge against electromotive force of the cell E. With account of Eq. (32) we write

$$d\Psi = EdQ = E|Z_1Z_2|Fdv_s \tag{39}$$

Combining Eqs. (36), (37) and (39) yields the following relationship

$$c_{ch} = \frac{F|Z_1Z_2|}{\partial E/\partial v_s} \tag{40}$$

Thus, to measure the chemical capacity of a layer one should place it in the "asymmetric cell" to observe then the change of the cell electromotive force per 1 mol of the substance amount change.

Now we consider two phenomena resulting in low frequency impedance dispersion. They are electrodialysis effect and concentration voltage.

4. Electrodialysis Effect

The electrodialysis effect is stemming from the fact that the current passage across the membrane gives rise to change of the species amounts $(v_{1,2})$ in the compartments. The introduced value of the chemical capacity yields the following reduction of Eqs. (33)

$$\frac{\partial \Delta \mu_s}{\partial \tau} \frac{c''_{ch} c'_{ch}}{c''_{ch} + c'_{ch}} + \frac{gt_1t_2}{(FZ_1Z_2)^2} \Delta \mu_s = -\frac{I(t_1 - t_1^e)}{F|Z_1Z_2|} \tag{41}$$

Equation (41) enables one to predict the time evolution of the coupled chemical potential difference. The changes of the coupled chemical potential in the adjacent compartments $(\delta \mu'_s, \delta \mu''_s; \delta \mu'_s - \delta \mu''_s = \Delta \mu_s)$ take the form

$$\delta \mu'_s = \frac{c''_{ch}}{c''_{ch} + c'_{ch}} \Delta \mu_s; \qquad \delta \mu''_s = -\frac{c'_{ch}}{c''_{ch} + c'_{ch}} \Delta \mu_s \tag{42}$$

Thus, the electric current results in a redistribution of the substance amount between the compartments when the electrodic and membrane transport numbers differ [right-hand side of Eq. (41)]. The relaxation time is obtained from Eq. (41)

$$\tau_* = \frac{c''_{ch} c'_{ch}}{c''_{ch} + c'_{ch}} \cdot \frac{(FZ_1Z_2)^2}{gt_1t_2} \tag{43}$$

When the applied current is a step-function of time ($I = 0$, as $\tau < 0$; $I = I_0$, as $\tau \geq 0$) the coupled chemical potential difference increases with this delay to go to the steady state value

$$\Delta \mu_s(\tau) = -F|Z_1Z_2| \frac{I_0(t_1 - t_1^e)}{gt_1t_2} [1 - \exp(-\tau/\tau_*)] \tag{44}$$

5. Concentration Voltage

To obtain the electric voltage difference between the electrodes one should divide the difference between the electrochemical potentials of the electrons in the electrodes with the Faraday constant. To derive the corresponding expression one has to consider the equilibrium of the electrodic reactions, i.e., to equate sums of electrochemical potentials of the final and initial substances with account of the proportion (28). Then Eqs. (29), (31) and (34) should be combined. We do not present here this extended derivation but limit ourselves to write the rather simple final result:

$$\Delta\Phi = \frac{I}{g} + (t_1 - t_1^e) \cdot \frac{\Delta\mu_s}{FZ_1Z_2} \tag{45}$$

The first term in right-hand side of Eq. (45) is the Ohm's voltage difference. The concentration voltage is associated with the second term to exist even when current is zero. Concentration voltage as well as the electrodialysis effect exist whenever the electrode and membrane transport numbers differ. Equation (45) is supposed as a momentary established relation since we deal with much longer relaxation times than Maxwell's value.

6. Electric Impedance and Equivalent Circuit of an Elementary Cell with a "Thin" Membrane

Now we consider the electrodialysis effect caused by an electric current which varies periodically. One can rewrite differential Eq. (41) in terms of the complex amplitudes to obtain the following solution

$$\Delta\dot{\mu}_s = \frac{\dot{I}(t_1 - t_1^e)/FZ_1Z_2}{\dfrac{gt_1t_2}{(FZ_1Z_2)^2} + i\omega c_{ch}} \tag{46}$$

where $c_{ch} = c'_{ch} c''_{ch}/(c'_{ch} + c''_{ch})$. Equation (46) shows the phase of the coupled chemical potential difference to lag the current phase. In this way the delay in the concentration redistribution [Eq. (44)] manifests itself here. Accordingly Eq. (45) the voltage phase lags the current phase as in an electric circuit containing capacitors. The expression for the impedance is derived by combining Eqs. (4), (45) and (46).

$$\dot{z} = \frac{\Delta\dot{\Phi}}{\dot{I}} = \frac{1}{g} + \frac{1}{g_L + i\omega c_L} \tag{47}$$

The additional electric capacity and conductivity which appears in Eq. (47) are expressed through the chemical capacity and membrane conductivity.

$$g_L = \frac{t_1t_2}{(t_1 - t_1^e)^2} g \qquad c_L = \frac{(FZ_1Z_2)^2}{(t_1 - t_1^e)^2} c_{ch} \tag{48}$$

The electrical equivalent circuit is presented in Fig. 5a.

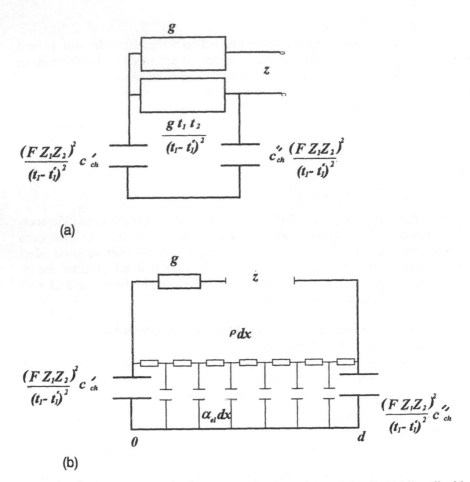

FIG. 5 Equivalent electric circuits of the elementary membrane cell. (a) The cell with "thin" membrane. (b) Transmission line for the cell with "thick" membrane.

7. Impedance of a Cell with a "Thick Membrane". Transmission Line Model

The fluxes attributed to the external membrane surfaces can differ from each other. In the above statement the transmembrane fluxes were considered to differ from the fluxes attributed to the electrodes due to the substance accumulation in the compartments. The accumulation was described with the help of the compartment chemical capacity. The substance can be accumulated in the membrane body too. Hence the membrane can be characterized by its own chemical capacity. The analysis in previous sections holds when the membrane chemical capacity is much smaller than that of the compartments. The term "thin" denotes the membranes having ignorable chemical capacities. In contrary the "thick" membranes have nonzero chemical capacity.

The "thick" membrane is described by using a continuous approach. The continuous version of Eq. (29) can be written by substitute of the specific conductivity for the integral conductivity. Gradients are substituted for the finite differences as well. One obtains:

$$J_{1,2} = -\frac{\sigma t_{1,2}}{(FZ_{1,2})^2} \frac{\partial(\mu_{1,2})}{\partial x} \tag{49}$$

where x is a coordinate (Fig. 4). Equation (49) yields the total voltage to be expressed by Eq. (45) as before. We rewrite the equation as follows

$$\Delta\Phi = \frac{I}{g} + (t_1 - t_1^e) \cdot \frac{\delta\mu_s' + \delta\mu_s''}{FZ_1Z_2} \tag{50}$$

The conservation law for the species is represented by using the definition of the specific chemical capacity (38) and the continuity of the electric current given by Eq. (31).

$$\alpha_{ch} \frac{\partial \delta\mu_s}{\partial t} = -\frac{\partial}{\partial x}\left(\frac{J_1}{Z_2}\right) = \frac{\partial}{\partial x}\left(\frac{J_2}{Z_1}\right) \tag{51}$$

Using Eqs. (31), (32), (34) and (49) yields

$$\frac{J_1}{Z_2} = -\frac{\sigma t_1 t_2}{(FZ_1Z_2)^2} \frac{\partial}{\partial x} \delta\mu_s + \frac{It_1}{FZ_1Z_2} \tag{52}$$

Substitution of Eq. (52) into Eq. (51) results in the diffusion equation to be written in term of the complex amplitudes as follows

$$i\omega\alpha_{ch} = \frac{\sigma t_1 t_2}{(FZ_1Z_2)^2} \frac{d^2}{dx^2} \delta\mu_s \tag{53}$$

Boundary conditions of the interface quasi-equilibrium are employed (Fig. 4).

$$\delta\mu_s(0) = \delta\mu_s'; \qquad \delta\mu_s(d) = \delta\mu_s'' \tag{54}$$

The solution of (53) with account of boundary conditions (54) depends on the values $\delta\mu_s'$ and $\delta\mu_s''$. To find them the species conservation law for the adjacent compartments is employed

$$i\omega c_{ch}' \delta\mu_s' = \frac{\sigma t_1 t_2}{(FZ_1Z_2)^2} \frac{d}{dx} \delta\mu_s(0) - \frac{I(t_1 - t_1^e)}{F|Z_1Z_2|}$$

$$i\omega c_{ch}' \delta\mu_s'' = -\frac{\sigma t_1 t_2}{(FZ_1Z_2)^2} \frac{d}{dx} \delta\mu_s(d) + \frac{I(t_1 - t_1^e)}{F|Z_1Z_2|} \tag{55}$$

where d is the membrane thickness. Then the values $\delta\mu'_s$ and $\delta\mu''_s$ are substituted in Eq. (50). The latter yields an expression for the system impedance

$$\dot{z} = \frac{\Delta\Phi}{\dot{I}} = \frac{1}{g} + \frac{1 + \lambda(i\omega/4\omega_*)^{-1/2}\tanh[(i\omega/4\omega_*)^{1/2}]}{\dfrac{gt_1t_2}{(t_1 - t_1^e)^2}\{(i\omega/\omega_*)^{1/2}\coth[(i\omega/\omega_*)^{1/2}] + \lambda\} + i\omega c_{el}} \tag{56}$$

where $\lambda = c_{ch}^m/(c'_{ch} + c''_{ch})$; c_{ch}^m is the membrane chemical capacity. The characteristic frequency of the impedance dispersion is expressed as

$$\omega_* = \frac{gt_1t_2}{(FZ_1Z_2)^2 c_{ch}^m} = \frac{\sigma t_1 t_2}{(FZ_1Z_2)^2 d^2 \alpha_{ch}^m} \tag{57}$$

Expression (56) is transformed into (47) and (48) when $\lambda \to 0$; $\omega/\omega_* \to 0$ (it depends on the applied frequency whether a membrane is "thin"). $\lambda \to \infty$ when the electrodes are in an immediate contact with the membrane to enable the following reduction of Eq. (56)

$$\dot{z} = \frac{1}{g} + \frac{(t_1 - t_1^e)^2}{gt_1t_2}(i\omega/4\omega_*)^{-1/2}\tanh[(i\omega/4\omega_*)^{1/2}] \tag{58}$$

Equivalent electric circuit is represented in Fig. 5b corresponding to Eq. (56). The circuit includes a so-called transmission line model. A transmission line of this type is characterised by specific resistivity of a wire (ρ) and specific electric capacity (α_{el}) between these wire and a common wire. It is widely accepted to use the model shown in Fig. 5b. The distributed parameters simulated here by means of frequency independent elements whose values are obtained by multiplying the specific values on the differential of length dx. The distribution of the electric current and voltage is described with the help of the so-called telegraph equations

$$i\omega\alpha_{el} \cdot \dot{u} = \frac{1}{\rho}\frac{d^2\dot{u}}{dx^2} \tag{59}$$

$$\dot{I} = -\frac{1}{\rho}\frac{d\dot{u}}{dx} \tag{60}$$

where $\dot{I}$, $\dot{u}$ are complex amplitudes of an electric current and voltage difference attributed to the distributed resistance and capacitance, respectively (Fig. 5b).

Let us show the circuit in Fig. 5b to yield an adequate simulation of the membrane system behavior. One can analyze the procedure which results in obtaining the circuit impedance. This procedure comprises solution of the telegraph equation (59) with boundary conditions

$$\dot{u}(0) = \dot{u}'; \qquad \dot{u}(d) = \dot{u}'' \tag{61}$$

The next step is to find values $\dot{u}'$ and $\dot{u}''$ by using Kirchhoff's second law combined with Eq. (60)

$$i\omega c'_{el} \cdot \dot{u}' = \frac{1}{\rho}\frac{d}{dx}\dot{u}(0) - \dot{I}; \qquad i\omega c''_{el} \cdot \dot{u}'' = -\frac{1}{\rho}\frac{d}{dx}\dot{u}(d) + \dot{I} \tag{62}$$

Finally the impedance can be found as follows

$$\dot{z} = \frac{1}{g} + \frac{\dot{u}' - \dot{u}''}{\dot{I}} \tag{63}$$

This procedure fully coincides with the way to find the impedance of the membrane system described above. The similarity is easily established between Eqs. (53) and (58); (54) and (61); (55) and (62); (50) and (63). The complete coincidence occurs when

$$\alpha_{el} = \frac{(FZ_1Z_2)^2}{(t_1 - t_1^e)^2}\,\alpha_{ch}; \qquad \rho = \frac{(t_1 - t_1^e)^2}{\sigma t_1 t_2} \tag{64}$$

To consider the "symmetric cell" [25] one has to set $t_1^e = 0$ in Eq. (58)

$$\dot{z} = \frac{1}{g} + \frac{t_1}{g t_2}\,(i\omega/4\omega_*)^{-1/2}\,\tanh[(i\omega/4\omega_*)^{1/2}] \tag{65}$$

This formula can be shown to have the same structure as those stated in Refs. [25,26,29]. However the result (65) is more general. It is valid for the arbitrary charged species. Only explicitly defined phenomenological characteristics are employed to express parameter ω_* [Eq. (57)].

To obtain the equivalent circuit for the transmission line from that given in Fig. 5b one has to disconnect the zero capacities corresponding to the compartments. It is possible to ground the middle point of the upper wire to obtain a series connection of the two equal, shortened transmission lines having length $d/2$ [the potential of the middle point evidently coincides with the potential of the common wire ("ground")]. The impedance is given by multiplying the shortened transmission line impedance by 2. It is the same as to divide each conductivity by 2 and capacity by the same coefficient 2. The final structure of the equivalent circuit is presented in Fig. 6. The values of the distributed elements follow from Eqs. (64) with account of the coefficient 2.

$$\rho = \frac{2t_1}{\sigma t_2}; \qquad \alpha_{el} = \frac{(FZ_1Z_2)^2}{2t_1^2}\,\alpha_{ch} \tag{66}$$

An interesting particular case occurs when one electrode is in immediate contact with the membrane $(c_{ch}' \to 0)$ and other one is separated from the membrane by a very highly concentrated and ideally agitated solution $(c_{ch}'' \to \infty)$.

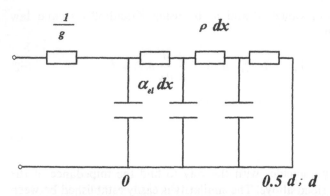

FIG. 6 Shorted transmission line model. Length 0.5 d corresponds to the "symmetric" cell. Length d corresponds to the system whose impedance is given by Eq. (68).

$$\lambda = \frac{c_{ch}^m}{c_{ch}' + c_{ch}''} \to 0; \qquad c_{ch} = \frac{c_{ch}' \cdot c_{ch}''}{c_{ch}' + c_{ch}''} \to 0 \tag{67}$$

According to Eq. (67) the following reduction of Eq. (56) becomes possible

$$\dot{z} = \frac{1}{g} + \frac{(t_1 - t_1^e)^2}{g t_1 t_2} (i\omega/\omega_*)^{-1/2} \tanh[(i\omega/\omega_*)^{1/2}] \tag{68}$$

The equivalent circuit is obtained from that shown in Fig. 5b. to be the shortened transmission line shown in Fig. 6. Its length is d and distributed elements are given by relations (64).

B. Multilayer Membranes

1. General Case

The system discussed above is characterized by the distributed electric capacitance and resistance only as far as it contains a "thick" membrane. All other component parts were considered in Sec. III. A simplifying them to be represented in equivalent circuit as discrete elements. In a general case all parts should be characterized by the distributed parameters. A rather general case was considered in Ref. 11. A multilayer membrane impedance was predicted for the case of $1:1$ electrolyte solution. We generalize here the result of Ref. 11 for any values of the carrier charges.

A multilayer system is considered. It is in contact with two media having infinitely high chemical capacities (Fig. 7) to keep zero the whole coupled chemical potential drop.

$$\sum_{k=1}^{N} \Delta\mu_s^{(k)} = 0 \tag{69}$$

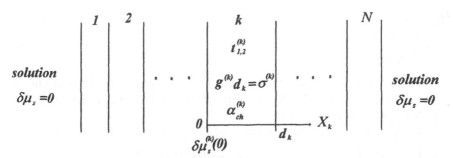

FIG. 7 Multilayer membrane between two media with infinitely high chemical capacities.

were superscripts denote the number of the corresponding layer. All interfaces in the system (Fig. 7) are considered to be quasi-equilibrium. The voltage difference between external surfaces of the multilayer system (Fig. 7) can be presented as the sum of the terms attributed to each constituent layer. With the help of Eqs. (45) and (69) it is shown to take the form

$$\Delta\Phi = I \sum_{k=1}^{N} \frac{1}{g^{(k)}} + \frac{1}{F|Z_1 Z_2|} \sum_{k=2}^{N} (t_1^{(k-1)} - t_1^{(k)}) \cdot \delta\mu_s^{(k)}(0) \tag{70}$$

While deriving Eqs. (69) and (70) we have used the obvious equality:

$$t_1^{(k)} + t_2^{(k)} = 1 \tag{71}$$

Continuity of the fluxes at the internal interfaces yields the following expression

$$g^{(k+1)}t_1^{(k+1)}t_2^{(k+1)} \frac{\partial}{\partial x^{(k+1)}} \delta\mu_s^{(k+1)}(d^{(k+1)}) - g^{(k)}t_1^{(k)}t_2^{(k)} \frac{\partial}{\partial x^{(k)}} \delta\mu_s^{(k)}(0)$$

$$= I(t_1^{(k+1)} - t_1^{(k)})F|Z_1 Z_2| \tag{72}$$

The general solution of Eq. (53) written for the each layer yields functions which depends on the coordinates linked to each layer (Fig. 7). These functions are substituted into Eq. (72). We represent the final expression in the form

$$\dot{z} = \sum_{k=1}^{N} \frac{1}{g^{(k)}} + \sum_{k=2}^{N} (t_1^{(k-1)} - t_1^{(k)})G^{(k)} \tag{73}$$

Constants $G^{(k)}$ are the solutions of the equation set

$$G^{(k+1)} \frac{r^{(k)}}{\sinh r^{(k)}} g^{(k)}t_1^{(k)}t_2^{(k)} - G^{(k)}[g^{(k)}t_1^{(k)}t_2^{(k)}r^{(k)} \coth r^{(k)}$$

$$+ g^{(k-1)}t_1^{(k-1)}t_2^{(k-1)}r^{(k-1)} \coth r^{(k-1)}]$$

$$+ G^{(k-1)} \frac{r^{(k-1)}}{\sinh r^{(k-1)}} g^{(k-1)}t_1^{(k-1)}t_2^{(k-1)} = t_1^{(k-1)} - t_1^{(k)} \tag{74}$$

where

$$r^{(k)} = \sqrt{\frac{i\omega}{\omega_*^{(k)}}} \tag{75}$$

The results of Eqs. (53) and (54) from Ref. 11 can be represented exactly in the same form as Eqs. (74) and (75). The dependency on the species charges occurs only in $\omega_*^{(k)}$ according to Eqn. (57).

The high frequency asymptotic ($\omega \gg \omega_*^{(k)}$) follows from of Eqs. (73)–(75)

$$\mathrm{Re}\left(\dot{z} - \sum_{k=1}^{N} \frac{1}{g^{(k)}} \right) = -\mathrm{Im}\,\dot{z} = (\omega)^{-1/2} \sum_{k=2}^{N} \frac{(t_1^{(k)} - t_1^{(k-1)})^2}{\xi^{(k)} + \xi^{(k-1)}} \tag{76}$$

$$\xi^{(k)} = (2g^{(k)} t_1^{(k)} t_2^{(k)} c_{\mathrm{ch}}^{(k)})^{1/2} F \,|\, Z_1 Z_2 | = (2\sigma^{(k)} t_1^{(k)} t_2^{(k)} \alpha_{\mathrm{ch}}^{(k)})^{1/2} F \,|\, Z_1 Z_2 | \tag{77}$$

The right-hand side of Eq. (76) and (77) depend only on the specific characteristics.

The zero frequency limit of the impedance is given by the following relations

$$\mathrm{Re}\,\dot{z}(0) - \sum_{k=1}^{N} \frac{1}{g^{(k)}} = \frac{\displaystyle\sum_{n,k=1}^{N} \frac{(t_1^{(k)} - t_1^{(n)})^2}{g^{(k)} g^{(n)} t_1^{(k)} t_2^{(k)} t_1^{(n)} t_2^{(n)}}}{2 \displaystyle\sum_{k=1}^{N} \frac{1}{g^{(k)} t_1^{(k)} t_2^{(k)}}} \tag{78}$$

$$\mathrm{Im}\,\dot{z}(0) = 0$$

2. Bilayer Membrane

Expression for impedance (73) contains only one term in the sum. The final result is represented by using Eq. (74) in the form

$$\dot{z} = \frac{1}{g^{(1)}} + \frac{1}{g^{(2)}} + \frac{(t_1^{(2)} - t_1^{(1)})^2}{(g^{(2)} t_1^{(2)} t_2^{(2)} r^{(2)} \coth r^{(2)} + g^{(1)} t_1^{(1)} t_2^{(1)} r^{(1)} \coth r^{(1)})} \tag{79}$$

The equivalent electric circuit is shown to be a parallel connection of two shortened transmission lines attributed to each of the constituent layers, (Fig. 8). This paralleling is connected in series with sum of the layer resistivities (Fig. 8). The distributed electric capacities and resistivities are given by the following relationships

$$\alpha_{\mathrm{el}}^{(1,\,2)} = \frac{(FZ_1 Z_2)^2}{(t_1^{(2)} - t_1^{(1)})^2}\, \alpha_{\mathrm{ch}}^{(1,\,2)}; \qquad \rho^{(1,\,2)} = \frac{(t_1^{(2)} - t_1^{(1)})^2}{\sigma^{(1,\,2)} t_1^{(1,\,2)} t_2^{(1,\,2)}} \tag{80}$$

This is of interest to obtain low frequency limit of the permittivity (real part). With the help of Eqs. (4)–(7), (75), (78) and (79) one can derive:

$$\varepsilon'(0) = \left[\frac{\mathrm{Re}\,\dot{z}(0) - \mathrm{Re}\,\dot{z}(\infty)}{(t_1^{(1)} - t_1^{(2)}) \mathrm{Re}\,\dot{z}(0)}\, FZ_1 Z_2 \right]^2 \frac{d^2 \langle \alpha_{\mathrm{ch}} \rangle}{\varepsilon_0} \tag{81}$$

$$\langle \alpha_{\mathrm{ch}} \rangle = \alpha_{\mathrm{ch}}^{(1)} p^{(1)} + \alpha_{\mathrm{ch}}^{(2)} p^{(2)} \tag{82}$$

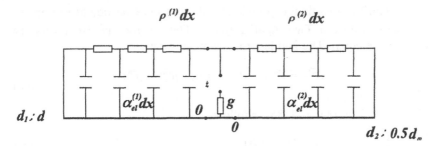

FIG. 8 Equivalent electric circuit of the bilayer membrane.

The high and low frequency limits of the impedance are presented in Eq. (81) to be obtained either from Eq. (79) or from Eqs. (76)–(78)

$$\mathrm{Re}\,\dot{z}(\infty) = \frac{1}{g^{(1)}} + \frac{1}{g^{(2)}}$$

$$\mathrm{Re}\,\dot{z}(0) - \mathrm{Re}\,\dot{z}(\infty) = \frac{(t_1^{(2)} - t_1^{(1)})^2}{g^{(2)}t_1^{(2)}t_2^{(2)} + g^{(1)}t_1^{(1)}t_2^{(1)}}$$

(83)

The permittivity Eq. (81) has a remarkable feature. When the volume fractions are constant the permittivity is proportional to the squared thickness of the system which results in an extremely high values for "thick" systems—some times in millions times greater than that of water (Sec. III.C). With frequency increase the dielectric permeability decreases till it reaches the low frequency limit of Maxwell's dispersion [Eq. (21)]. The circuit in Fig. 8 simulates this behavior.

3. Three-Layer System

The expression for the impedance as applied to this system is derived from Eq. (73) and takes the form:

$$\dot{z} = \sum_{k=1}^{3} \frac{1}{g^{(k)}} + G^{2}(t_1^{(1)} - t_1^{(2)}) + G^{(3)}(t_1^{(2)} - t_1^{(3)})$$

(84)

The coefficients are obtained from the set of equations which follows from (74)

$$-G^{(2)}(g^{(2)}t_1^{(2)}t_2^{(2)}r^{(2)}\coth r^{(2)} + g^{(1)}t_1^{(1)}t_2^{(1)}r^{(1)}\coth r^{(1)})$$

$$+ G^{(3)}g^{(2)}t_1^{(2)}t_2^{(2)}\frac{r^{(2)}}{\sinh r^{(2)}} = t_1^{(2)} - t_1^{(1)}$$

(85)

$$G^{(2)}g^{(2)}t_1^{(2)}t_2^{(2)}\frac{r_2}{\sinh r_2} - G^{(3)}(g^{(2)}t_1^{(2)}t_2^{(2)}r^{(2)}\coth r^{(2)}$$

$$+ g^{(2)}t_1^{(3)}t_2^{(3)}r^{(1)}\coth r^{(1)}) = t_1^{(3)} - t_1^{(2)}$$

Instead of a complicated final expression we discuss some particular examples.

(a) *Membrane Between Two Equal Layers.* The 1st and the 3rd layers are considered to be equal. The 2nd layer is the membrane.

$$t_{1,2}^{(1)} = t_{1,2}^{(3)} = t_{1,2}; \quad t_{1,2}^{(2)} = t_{1,2}^m; \quad g^{1,3} = g; \quad g^{(2)} = g^m;$$

$$r^{(1,3)} = r; \quad r^{(2)} = r^m$$
(86)

One can rewrite Eqs. (84) and (85) as follows

$$\dot{z} = \frac{2}{g} + \frac{1}{g^m} + (t_1 - t_1^m)[G^{(2)} - G^{(3)}]$$
(87)

$$(G^{(2)} - G^{(3)})(g^m t_1^m t_2^m r^m \coth 0.5r^m + gt_1 t_2 r \coth r) = 2(t_1^m - t_1)$$
(88)

The final expression for the impedance takes the form

$$\dot{z} = \frac{2}{g} + \frac{1}{g^m} + \frac{2(t_1^m - t_1)^2}{g^m t_1^m t_2^m r^m \coth 0.5r^m + gt_1 t_2 r \coth r}$$
(89)

The general structure of the equivalent circuit coincides with that presented in Fig. 8 to simulate behavior of the bilayer membrane. The comparison of Eqs. (89) and (79) enables us to find values of the elements. The first layer of the "equivalent" bilayer membrane corresponds to the external layers. It has the same thickness as each of them. The second one corresponds to the inner layer ("membrane"). Its thickness is a half of that of the inner layer. The specific conductivities and chemical capacities attributed to both layers of the "equivalent" bilayer membrane are in two times less than the same characteristics the actual layers.

Expression (89) as well as the equivalent circuit (Fig. 8) may be used to describe impedance of the membrane immersed in an electrolyte solution. It is often reasonable to suppose that applied frequency is much higher than the characteristic frequency attributed to rather thick solution layers. In this case one can simplify formula (89) to the following

$$\dot{z} = \frac{2}{g} + \frac{1}{g^m} + \frac{2(t_1 - t_1^m)^2}{\dfrac{\sqrt{i\omega\sigma t_1 t_2 \alpha_{ch}}}{|Z_1 Z_2|F} + g^m t_1^m t_2^m r^m \coth 0.5r^m}$$
(90)

(b) *Symmetric Cell.* The formula for this case (56) as well as the corresponding equivalent circuit (Fig. 6) were presented in the Sec. III.B. Now we only show that it can be derived by using Eqs. (84) and (85). The 1st and 3rd layers have to be considered as external surfaces of the cell. One can prove that this situation corresponds to the following case

$$t_1^{(1)} = t_1^{(3)} = 0; \quad t_2^{(1)} = t_2^{(3)} = 1; \quad t_{1,2}^{(2)} = t_{1,2};$$

$$g_{1,3} = 0; \quad g_2 = g; \quad r_{1,3} \to 0; \quad r_2 = \sqrt{\frac{i\omega}{\omega_*}}$$
(91)

Substitution of (91) into (84) and (85) yields finally (56).

An interesting result one can obtain deriving of the permittivity in the low frequency limit. With the help of Eqs. (4)–(7) and (65) one can obtain this:

$$\varepsilon'(0) = \frac{(FZ_1 Z_2)^2 d^2}{12\varepsilon_0} \alpha_{ch} \tag{92}$$

(c) *Asymmetric Cell.* The case considered here is also associated with the membrane in immediate contact with electrodes. In contrast with the previous case the electrodes have opposite properties being reversible with respect to the different species. They also fully block transport of the other species. In the terms used in deriving Eqs. (84) and (85) one can set the following

$$t_1^{(1)} = t_2^{(3)} = 0; \quad t_2^{(1)} = t_1^{(3)} = 1; \quad t_{1,2}^{(2)} = t_{1,2};$$

$$g_{1,3} = 0; \quad g_2 = g; \quad r_2 = \sqrt{\frac{i\omega}{\omega_*}}; \quad r_{1,3} \to 0 \tag{93}$$

Under these condition Eq. (84) is transformed into

$$\dot{z} = \frac{1}{g} - G_2 t_1 - G_3 t_2 \tag{94}$$

Equation set (85) takes the form

$$-gt_1 t_2 r \left(G_2 \coth r - \frac{G_3}{\sinh r} \right) = t_1$$

$$-gt_1 t_2 r \left(G_3 \coth r - \frac{G_2}{\sinh r} \right) = t_2 \tag{95}$$

By combining Eqs. (94) and (95) one can derive the following result

$$\dot{z} = \frac{1}{g} + \frac{1}{2gt_1 t_2 \sqrt{i\omega/\omega_*}} [\coth \sqrt{i\omega/\omega_*} + (t_1 - t_2)^2 \tanh \sqrt{i\omega/4\omega_*}] \tag{96}$$

This result comprises the expressions obtained earlier by Buck and Albery [27,29] for 1:1 electrolyte solution. Expression (96) describes any type of conductors with two charge carriers provided that the values of conductivity, migration transport number and chemical capacity are known.

The membrane resistance in the equivalent circuit is connected in series with the shortened and opened transmission lines (Fig. 9). The shortened line elements take the form

$$\alpha_{el}^{sh} = \frac{2(FZ_1 Z_2)^2}{(t_1 - t_2)^2} \alpha_{ch}; \quad \rho^{sh} = \frac{(t_1 - t_2)^2}{2\sigma t_1 t_2} \tag{97}$$

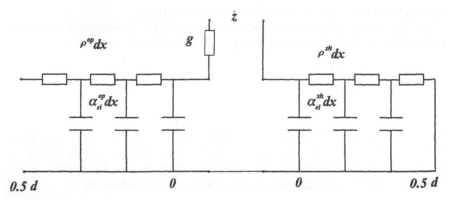

FIG. 9 Equivalent electric circuit of the "asymmetric cell".

The opened one is characterized by

$$\alpha_{el}^{op} = 2(FZ_1Z_2)^2\alpha_{ch}; \quad \rho^{op} = \frac{1}{2\sigma t_1 t_2} \tag{98}$$

It is obvious from the circuit in Fig. 9. that the low frequency limit of the capacity includes only capacities situated in the closed transmission line.

$$c_{el}(0) = \frac{1}{\lim_{\omega \to 0} \text{Re}(\dot{z} \cdot i\omega)} = 2(FZ_1Z_2)^2\alpha_{ch} \cdot \frac{d}{2} = (FZ_1Z_2)^2 c_{ch} \tag{99}$$

The latter expression in Eq. (99) can be obtained with the help of Eq. (40) as well. Equation (40) was derived as applied to the quasi-equilibrium infinity slow charging of the battery formed by the asymmetric cell. It is the regime which corresponds to the infinitely low applied frequency. As matter of the fact the zero frequency limit of the electric capacity can be expressed as

$$c_{el} = \frac{\partial q}{\partial E} = F|Z_1Z_2|\frac{\partial v_s}{dE} \tag{100}$$

By combining Eqs. (40) and (100) one can obtain Eq. (99). The low frequency limit of the permittivity is easily obtained from Eq. (99) to take the form

$$\varepsilon'(0) = \frac{(FZ_1Z_2)^2 d^2\alpha_{ch}}{\varepsilon_0} \tag{101}$$

C. Model Approach and Evaluation of the Low Frequency Dispersion Parameters

In the previous section we defined out a set of the constituent layer phenomenological characteristics used to predict low-frequency impedance dispersion, namely the layer conductivity, the migration transport numbers of the species and the chemical capacity. There are also some parameters of dispersion curves like characteristic frequency (relaxation time), the (low frequency limit of the) permittivity, etc. They occur to be stable combinations of the layer characteristics. Now we evaluate the values by using the simplest microscopic model.

1. Chemical Capacity

In the model we deal with a medium containing two charged species. Each of the species can be either in a free or in fixed state. The free species can be involved into the transport processes. On the contrary the fixed species do not contribute to the fluxes—forming the fixed charges. The electroneutrality condition is supposed to hold locally

$$FC_1|Z_1| + q = FC_2|Z_2| \tag{102}$$

where q is a fixed electric charge density. We equate concentrations of each species $C_{1,2}$ and their activities expressing the electrochemical potentials as follows

$$\mu_{1,2}^e = \mu_{1,2}^0 + RT \ln(C_{1,2}) + FZ_{1,2}\Phi \tag{103}$$

where $\mu_{1,2}^0$ is the standard chemical potential. Hereafter, we suppose that $\mu_1^0 = \mu_2^0 = \mu_{solution}^0$. The latter value is the standard chemical potential of each of the ions in the free solution. The free species concentrations within the medium phase can be represented in the form

$$C_{1,2} = C_s|Z_{2,1}|\gamma^{Z_{1,2}} \tag{104}$$

A physical sense can be assigned to the values on the right-hand side of Eqn. (104). Let us consider an electrolyte solution equilibrated with the medium. The species are supposed to be the ions presented in both the medium and the solution. The concentration C_s corresponds to the binary electrolyte concentration in the equilibrium solution. The other parameter can be represented in the form $\gamma = \exp(-\phi_D)$; ϕ_D is the dimensionless Donnan potential [36]. Such a solution can be absent in reality to attribute the concentration to the so-called virtual solution introduced by Kedem and Katchalsky [37–39]. Accordingly we refer to the concentration as a virtual.

By combining Eqs. (103), (104) and (34) one can express the differential of the coupled chemical potential as follows

$$d\mu_s = RT(|Z_1| + |Z_2|)d[\ln(C_s)] \tag{105}$$

Substitution of (104) enables the electroneutrality Eq. (102) to take the form:

$$\gamma^{Z_1} + \frac{q}{FC_s|Z_1Z_2|} = \gamma^{Z_2} \tag{106}$$

In the case of a constant fixed charge one can write.

$$dv_s = V \frac{dC_1}{|Z_2|} = V\left(\gamma^{Z_1} + C_s \frac{d}{dC_s}\gamma^{Z_1}\right)dC_s \tag{107}$$

Substitution of Eqs. (107) and (106) into definition (37) yields

$$c_{ch} = \frac{VC_s}{RT} \cdot \frac{\gamma^{Z_1+Z_2}}{|Z_1|\gamma^{Z_1} + |Z_2|\gamma^{Z_2}} \tag{108}$$

To obtain from (108) a final expression one has to solve Eq. (106) with regard to γ.

When the system is characterized by a high value of the fixed charge density $(|q|/FC_s|Z_1Z_2| \gg 1)$ one can suppose that

$$\gamma^{Z_1} \ll \gamma^{Z_2}, q > 0, \gamma < 1, Z_1 > 0 \quad \text{and} \quad Z_2 < 0 \tag{109}$$

Equation (106) can be solved in this case to yield the simplified version of formula (108)

$$c_{ch} = |Z_1|^{1/|Z_2|} \cdot |Z_2|^{(1/|Z_2|)-1} \cdot \frac{V}{RT} \cdot \left(\frac{F}{q}\right)^{1/|Z_2|} C_s^{1+(1/|Z_2|)} \tag{110}$$

Another particular case to be considered is $|q|/FC_s|Z_1Z_2| \ll 1$. Substitution of $\gamma = \exp(-\phi_D)$ into (108) using Taylor series up to second-order term of ϕ_D yields

$$c_{ch} = \frac{VC_s}{RT(|Z_1|+|Z_2|)}\left(1 + \frac{\phi_D^2}{2}Z_1Z_2\right) \tag{111}$$

The zero-order term in this expression exhibits the chemical capacity of a binary electrolyte solution.

$$c_{ch} = \frac{VC_s}{RT(|Z_1|+|Z_2|)} \tag{112}$$

Equation (111) can be rewritten in term of the fixed charge density as well

$$c_{ch} = \frac{VC_s}{RT(|Z_1|+|Z_2|)}\left(1 + \frac{q^2}{2F^2C_s^2Z_1Z_2(Z_1-Z_2)^2}\right) \tag{113}$$

It is possible to solve Eq. (106) in the case $Z_1 = -Z_2 = Z$ to have

$$c_{ch} = \frac{VC_s}{2RT|Z|\sqrt{1 + \left(\frac{q}{2FC_sZ^2}\right)^2}} \tag{114}$$

The fixed group density can also change. We focus on a situation where all the fixed charge is formed by binding the coins no. 1 which then become coions to the bound charge. We consider the case where $Z_1 = -Z_2 = Z$ and a high value of the fixed charge density. Equations (105) and (106) yield in this approximation the concentration of coions

$$C_1 = \frac{C_s^2 F |Z|^3}{q} \tag{115}$$

Binding is described with the help of an equilibrium constant K

$$KC_1 = \frac{q}{|Z|F} \tag{116}$$

By combining Eqs. (115), (116) and an appropriate version of Eq. (104) we derive this

$$dv_s = V\sqrt{K}\left(1 - \frac{1}{K}\right) dC_s = V\left(\frac{q}{C_s F|Z|^2} - \frac{C_s F|Z|^2}{q}\right) dC_s \tag{117}$$

Taking into account Eqs. (105) and (37) we derive

$$c_{ch} = \frac{VC_s}{2RT|Z|} \sqrt{K}\left(1 - \frac{1}{K}\right) = \frac{Vq}{RTF|Z|^3} \tag{118}$$

The chemical capacity obtained from Eqs. (110) for $Z_1 = -Z_2 = Z$ is

$$c_{ch} = \frac{VC_s^2 F|Z|}{RTq} \tag{119}$$

The ratio between the chemical capacities given by expressions (118) and (119) is $C_s^2 F^2 \, Z^4/q^2$. It takes on the value 10^{-4} when concentration of the fixed charged groups in 100 times greater than the virtual concentration C_s. This rather usual case shows the chemical capacity to be very sensitive value to the mechanism of the fixed charge formation.

2. Conductivity and Transport Numbers

The Nernst–Planck conductivity and the transport numbers have the following forms

$$g = \frac{S}{d}(D_1 C_1 Z_1^2 + D_2 C_2 Z_2^2)\frac{F^2}{RT}; \quad t_{1,2} = \frac{D_{1,2} C_{1,2} Z_{1,2}^2}{D_1 C_1 Z_1^2 + D_2 C_2 Z_2^2} \tag{120}$$

Substitution of (108) enables us to represent the values through the virtual concentration.

$$g = \frac{S}{d}(D_1 \gamma^{Z_1}|Z_1| + D_2 \gamma^{Z,2}|Z_2|)\frac{F^2}{RT} C_s|Z_1 Z_2|$$

$$t_{1,2} = \frac{D_{1,2}|Z_{1,2}|\gamma^{Z_{1,2}}}{D_1 \gamma^{Z_1}|Z_1| + D_2 \gamma^{Z,2}|Z_2|} \tag{121}$$

A stable characteristic appears in various relationships to have the sense of a diffusion permeability

$$\chi = \frac{g t_1 t_2}{(FZ_1 Z_2)^2} = \frac{S}{d} \cdot \frac{C_s}{RT} \cdot \frac{D_1 D_2 \gamma^{Z_1 + Z_2}}{D_1 \gamma^{Z_1} |Z_1| + D_2 \gamma^{Z,2} |Z_2|} \tag{122}$$

3. Characteristic Frequency

The substitution of Eqs. (108) and (122) into (57) yields

$$\omega_* = \frac{1}{d^2} \cdot \frac{D_1 D_2 (\gamma^{Z_1} |Z_1| + \gamma^{Z,2} |Z_2|)}{D_1 \gamma^{Z_1} |Z_1| + D_2 \gamma^{Z,2} |Z_2|} \tag{123}$$

This formula holds when the fixed charge is constant. When the diffusion coefficients are equal ($D_1 = D_2 = D$) we have the well known expression for the characteristics diffusion frequency

$$\omega_* = D/d^2 \tag{124}$$

Almost the same expression can be obtained for the case of a symmetric electrolyte provided that there is no fixed charge ($\gamma = 1$). The only difference is that $D = 2D_1 D_2/(D_1 + D_2)$. In the case of the high fixed charge one has to insert in Eq. (124) $D = D_1$ (diffusion coefficient of coions).

When the fixed charge is formed due to the binding coions [Eqs. (115)–(118)] the characteristic frequency is shown to be lower. By using (115)–(118) one can obtain this

$$\omega_* = \frac{D_1}{d^2} \cdot \left(\frac{Z^2 F C_s}{q} \right)^2 \tag{125}$$

The same factor has been presented below Eq. (119) to describe the ratio between the chemical capacities predicted for two versions of the fixed charge origin. This factor makes the characteristic frequency much lower than in the case of the constant fixed charge.

4. Low Frequency Limit of Dielectric Permittivity

We compare the value of the low frequency limit of the permittivity with the permittivity of the medium. For membrane in the "asymmetric cell" we have

$$\frac{\varepsilon'(0)}{\varepsilon} = (\kappa d)^2 \frac{|Z_1 Z_2|}{|Z_1| + |Z_2|} \cdot \frac{\gamma^{Z_1 + Z_2}}{|Z_1| + |Z_2| \gamma^{Z_2}} \tag{126}$$

where the reciprocal Debye length is attributed to the virtual concentration

$$\kappa^2 = \frac{F^2 C_s |Z_1 Z_2|}{\varepsilon \varepsilon_0 RT} (|Z_1| + |Z_2|) \tag{127}$$

When the cell is filled by $1:1$ electrolyte solution ($\gamma = 1$; $|Z_{1,2}| = 1$) the ratio (126) takes value $(\kappa d/2)^2$. The systems in consideration have much more thickness than the Debye length. Hence the low frequency limit of the permittivity substantially exceeds the value observed within Maxwell's frequency range. For the aqueous electrolyte solution layer ($C_s = 1$ mol/m^3; $d = 10^{-5}$ m) the low frequency limit reaches value $\varepsilon'(0) \cong 2.5 \times 10^7$. Such a huge permittivity was predicted by Dukhin and Shilov [40] as applied to the systems containing particles incorporated in a medium.

When $Z_1 = -Z_2 = Z$ (114) and (101) yield:

$$\frac{\varepsilon'(0)}{\varepsilon} = \frac{|Z|(\kappa d)^2}{4\sqrt{1 + \left(\dfrac{q}{2FC_s Z^2}\right)^2}} \tag{128}$$

In case of the binding coions we deal even with the higher dielectric permeability limit.

5. High Frequency Impedance Asymptotic

The parameter in the high frequency asymptotic (76) has the form

$$\xi = (FZ_1 Z_2)^2 \frac{C_s \gamma^{Z_1 + Z_2}}{RT}$$
$$\times \left[\frac{2D_1 D_2}{(D_1 \gamma^{Z_1} |Z_1| + D_2 \gamma^{Z,2} |Z_2|)(|Z_1| \gamma^{Z_1} + |Z_2| \gamma^{Z_2})} \right]^{1/2} \tag{129}$$

In the case of the zero fixed charge we have

$$\xi = (FZ_1 Z_2)^2 \frac{C_s}{RT} \left[\frac{2D_1 D_2}{(D_1 |Z_1| + D_2 |Z_2|)(|Z_1| + |Z_2|)} \right]^{1/2} \tag{130}$$

For the symmetric case $Z_1 = -Z_2 = Z$ one can derive this

$$\xi = F^2 |Z|^3 \frac{C_s}{RT}$$
$$\times \left[\frac{2D_1 D_2}{(D_1 + D_2)\left(\left(\dfrac{q}{2FC_s Z^2}\right)^2 + 1\right) + (D_2 - D_1)\dfrac{q}{2FC_s Z^2}\sqrt{\left(\dfrac{q}{2FC_s Z^2}\right)^2 + 1}} \right]^{1/2} \tag{131}$$

For a high fixed charge density one can use the following approximation of Eq. (131)

$$\xi = 2F^3 |Z|^5 \frac{C_s^2}{RTq} D_1^{1/2} \tag{132}$$

Thus in the media with high fixed charge density the parameter takes smaller value than in electrolyte solution.

Thus, when there is an interface between an electrolyte solution and a media with high and constant fixed charged density (ion exchange material, for example) one can ignore those term ζ situated in the denominator of the last expression (76) which are attributed to the ion-exchange phase. For the system solution–membrane–solution the sum in (76) is reduced as follows

$$\text{Re}\left(\dot{z} - \sum_{k=1}^{3} \frac{1}{g^{(k)}}\right) = -\text{Im } \dot{z} = 2(\omega)^{-1/2} \frac{(t_1^{(2)} - t_1^{(1)})^2}{\zeta^{(1)}} \tag{133}$$

Where the value $\zeta^{(1)}$ is given by the relation for the zero fixed charge case [Eq. (130)]. This result is transformed into formula (9) in Ref. 41 in the particular case of the $1:1$ electrolyte.

When charge is formed exclusively by binding of coions, the parameter is shown to coincide by order with the value predicted for zero fixed charge.

V. DISCUSSION AND CONCLUSIONS

Having considered various approaches of IS data interpretation Stoynov [42], has single out two main directions. The first one has been called "theoretical" because it is connected with a model assumed a priori. The second one deals with equivalent circuits with further parameter identification. It has been called "structural". The phenomenological theories discussed here make possible to unite these approaches. Both the structure and the elements of the equivalent circuits are theoretically predicted without model suppositions.

Equivalent circuit elements are determined by carrying out IS measurements in a sufficiently wide frequency range. Then one can obtain the characteristics of the constituent layers involved in theoretical predictions of the values of the elements. The equivalent circuit in Fig. 1 is successfully used in Maxwell's region. For example, in Ref. 43 it enables the authors to obtain information even about the layer morphology.

The systems in consideration are chosen to exhibit Maxwell's and the low-frequency dispersion within the frequency ranges which are far from each other. At the same time the low frequency limit of Maxwell's impedance dispersion coincides with the high frequency limit of the low-frequency impedance dispersion. This common resistance always appears in the low-frequency circuits to be connected in series with a residual circuit. In Maxwell's frequency range the common resistance is split into the resistances of the component layers which are connected in parallel with corresponding capacitors (Fig. 1). The capacitors do not contribute to the impedance in the low-frequency range.

One can obtain a hybrid circuit from a low-frequency circuit by substituting in the latter the appropriate Maxwell circuit (Fig. 1) for the resistance which simulates the high frequency limit of the impedance. Such an example is presented in Fig. 10. The corresponding discrete capacitors are expressed with

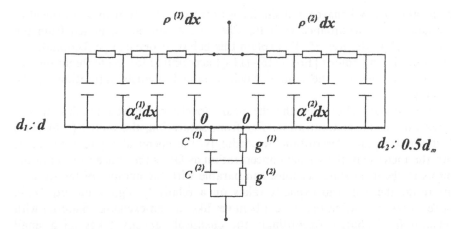

FIG. 10 Hybrid equivalent electric circuit of the bilayer membrane.

help of relation (9). The distributed elements are given by Eqs. (80). All elements in the circuit (Fig. 10) are determined by a procedure of fitting IS data. Then one can obtain all layer characteristics presented in Eqs. (9) and (80).

Another way of interpretation is associated with direct use of the dispersion curves. For example, it is possible to extract the membrane transport numbers from the high frequency impedance asymptotic (76). It can be done when the membrane is in contact with the already characterized media having large values—compared to that of the membrane—of the parameter ξ defined in Eq. (77). An example of that is an ion exchange membrane which is immersed in electrolyte solution. All solution characteristics in Eq. (130) are supposed to be known. The membrane transport number is the only unknown value in the right-hand side of Eq. (133). Hence it can be extracted from the slope of the plot Im $\dot{z}$ vs. $\omega^{-1/2}$. This attempt was made in Ref. 41 in the case of 1:1 electrolyte. Equation (130) enables us to study the systems with arbitrary charged species.

A homogeneous membrane can be fully characterized when it belongs to the "symmetric" or "asymmetric" cell. It is discussed in Ref. 29 how to extract their conductivity and transport numbers from the dispersion curves. We focus on the chemical capacity introduced here. This values does not depend on irreversible characteristics like the species mobilities, diffusion coefficients, transport numbers, etc. We consider finally two examples illustrating the chemical capacity can yield valuable information.

The first example is concerned with the "asymmetric cell". The low frequency limits of its equivalent electric capacity [Eq. (99)] and dielectric permeability [Eq (101)] do not contain unknown irreversible transport characteristics. In Ref. 35 the measured zero frequency limit of the "asymmetric cell" is obtained to be a function of ΔE with a maximum. The chemical capacity behaves in a similar way since it is proportional to the electric capacity in accordance with Eq. (99), i.e., it can be calculated from the results given in the Ref. 35. To explain this behavior one can perfectionate the model of binding coions [Eqs. (116)–(118)] accounting for the finite number of the binding sites for the coions. Such a model predicts saturation of the binding.

Let us initially show that the chemical capacity can have a maximum with increasing virtual concentration. Far from saturation, the model (116)–(118) yields an adequate description. Accordingly, the chemical capacity increases with the increase in the virtual concentration as far as the concentration of the coions in the fixed state becomes comparable with the number of the sites. In this range the chemical capacity takes on a relatively high value Eq. (118). Close to the saturation the system behaves like an ion-exchange material with constant fixed charge. Accordingly the chemical capacity takes on a small value. Hence one can hope to observe a maximum.

For simplicity we consider case $Z_1 = -Z_2 = 1$. The new version of Eq. (116) has the form

$$\bar{K} C_1 \left(C_0 - \frac{q}{F} \right) = \frac{q}{F} \tag{134}$$

where C_0 = a concentration of the sites. Eq. (134) is transformed in (116) when $q/F \ll C_0$ and $\bar{K} C_0 = K$. By using electroneutrality equation (102), the approximation of high value of the fixed charge density and definition of the chemical capacity (37) one can obtain

$$c_{ch} = \frac{V C_0}{RT} \cdot \left(\frac{\tilde{C}_s^2 + 2}{\sqrt{1 + \frac{4}{\tilde{C}_s^2}}} - \tilde{C}_s^2 \right) \tag{135}$$

where the dimensionless virtual concentration $\tilde{C}_s = C_s / \sqrt{C_0/\bar{K}}$.

The virtual concentration is a monotonous function of the cell electromotive force ΔE. By combining Eqs. (36), (40) and (105) we derive this for $Z_1 = -Z_2 = 1$

$$C_s = C_s(0) \exp\left(\frac{\Delta E F}{2RT} \right) \tag{136}$$

where $C_s(0)$ is an initial virtual concentration. The curve plotted in Fig. 11 in accordance with Eqs. (135) and (136) contains maximum as the plots in Ref. 35. These plots can be used to determine some important parameters of the model. In particular the maximum enables the concentration of the sites (C_0) to be found by using the curves presented in Ref. 35 (low frequency electric capacity vs. the electromotive force). It is possible to obtain from (135) and (99)

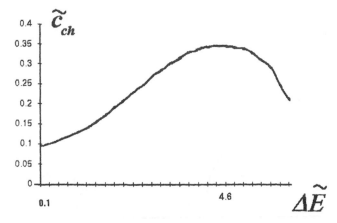

FIG. 11 Dimensionless chemical capacity vs. dimensionless electromotive force of the "asymmetric cell".

that

$$C_0 = \frac{c_{ch}^{max} RT}{0.343d} = 2.91 \frac{c_{el}^{max} RT}{(FZ_1Z_2)^2 d} \tag{137}$$

By applying this expression to the plot with the highest position of the maximum (Fig. 12 from Ref. 35) one can obtain $C_0 \sim 250$ mol/m³.

The second example deals with the chemical capacity extracted from the "symmetric cell" impedance. In this case the chemical capacity is obtained with the help of a complex procedure which comprises determination of the transport numbers as well. Let us consider the curve in Fig. 12 which exhibits the impedance imaginary part vs. its real part according to Eq. (65). One can find the characteristic frequency as well as the low and high frequency limits of the impedance real part. Trivial numerical analysis of the function in the right-hand side of Eq. (65) yields the frequency ω' corresponding to the maximum $\omega' = 10.161\omega_*$. At the same time it follows from Eq. (65) that

$$\text{Re } \dot{z}(0) = \text{Re } \dot{z}(\infty) + \frac{t_1}{t_2 g}; \quad \text{Re } \dot{z}(\infty) = \frac{1}{g} \tag{138}$$

Combining expressions (138) and (57) yields

$$c_{ch} = \frac{10.161}{(FZ_1Z_2)^2} \cdot \frac{\text{Re } \dot{z}(0) - \text{Re } \dot{z}(\infty)}{[\text{Re } \dot{z}(0)]^2 \omega'} \tag{139}$$

One can apply formula (139) to the results obtained with the "symmetric cell" in Ref. 44. For the membrane used there (thickness 33×10^{-6} m) the evaluated specific chemical capacity takes on a value of the order $\alpha_{ch} \cong$

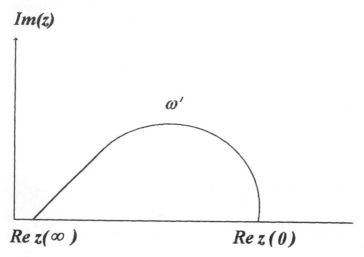

FIG. 12 Low-frequency dispersion of the "asymmetric cell" impedance. Real part of impedance vs. its imaginary part.

5×10^{-6} mol^2 J^{-1} m^{-3}. This value is much smaller than that calculated for adjacent 10^3 mol/m^3 electrolyte solution (0.2 mol^2 J^{-1} m^{-3}). It is also much smaller than the maximal specific chemical capacity evaluated above by using results of the Ref. 35. The latter is of order 3×10^{-2} mol^2 J^{-1} m^{-3}. In contrast to Ref. 35 the value of the chemical capacity in Ref. 44 is a monotonous function of the electromotive force of the third electrode intended to control the properties of the membrane. This conclusion can be made from the plots presented in Fig. 4 from Ref. 44.

The two examples discussed show that the information extracted from IS data in terms of the chemical capacity enables one to figure out in what way the fixed charge is formed. The first example is associated with a fixed charge formed exclusively by binding of coions. The second example corresponds to a constant fixed charge.

ACKNOWLEDGMENT

Financial support in the frame of INCO- COPERNICUS PROJECT N°IC15-CT96-0826 is gratefully acknowledged.

LIST OF SYMBOLS

$C_{1,2}$ concentration of species
C_s concentration of substance
c, c_{el} electric capacity

c_{ch} chemical capacity
D effective diffusion coefficient
$D_{1,2}$ diffusion coefficient of species
$d^{(k)}$ thickness of kth layer
E electromotive force
F Faraday constant
g electric conductivity
$g^{(k)}$ electric conductivity of kth layer
I electric current
i imaginary unit
$J_{1,2}$ fluxes of species
K equilibrium constant
l_D Debye length
N number of layers
$p^{(k)}$ volume fraction of kth layer
q fixed charge density
R gas constant
$r^{(k)}$ complex root of the diffusion equation
S membrane square
T absolute temperature
$t^{(k)}_{1,2}$ transport number of in kth layer
V volume
x coordinate
$\dot{y}$ admittance
$Z_{1,2}$ charge of the species in Faraday units
$\dot{z}$ impedance
α_{ch} specific chemical capacity
α_{el} distributed electric capacity
$\gamma_{1,2}$ distribution coefficient
Δ a difference attributed to membrane
δ deviation from equilibrium magnitude
$\dot{\varepsilon}$ complex permittivity
ε_0 vacuum permittivity
$\varepsilon^{(k)}$ permittivity of kth layer
ε' relative permittivity
ε'' net dielectric loss
θ phase difference
κ reciprocal Debye length
$\mu_{1,2}$ electrochemical potentials
μ_s coupled chemical potential
$\nu_{1,2}$ amounts of the species
ν_s amount of substance
ρ specific value of distributed resistance

$\sigma^{(k)}$ specific conductivity of kth layer

τ time

τ_* relaxation time

Φ electric potential

ϕ_D Donnan potential

Ψ free energy

ω applied frequency

ω_* characteristic frequency

REFERENCES

1. S. B. Sash and H. K. Lonsdale, J. Appl. Polym. Sci. *15*:797 (1971).
2. R. Y. M. Huang, C. J. Gao, and J. J. Kim, J. Appl. Polym. Sci. *28*:3062 (1983).
3. K. Nagasubramanian, F. R. Chlanda, and J. Kang-Jen-Liu, J. Membrane Sci. *2*:109 (1977).
4. F. J. Sata, J. Colloid Polym. Sci. *256*:62 (1978).
5. G. Gittens, P. Hitchcock, and G. Wakley, Dessalination *12*:315 (1973).
6. J. C. Maxwell, *A Treatise on Electricity and Magnetism*, Volume 1, Clarendon Press, Oxford, 1881, second ed., p. 435.
7. K. W. Wagner, Arch. Electrotech. *2*:371 (1914).
8. K. W. Wagner, Arch. Electrotech. *3*:67 (1914).
9. J. Volger, Progress in Semiconductors *4*:205 (1960).
10. E. K. Zholkovskij, Colloid Journal of the USSR *51*:457 (1989).
11. E. K. Zholkovskij, J. Colloid Interface Sci. *169*:267 (1995).
12. E. K. Zholkovskij, V. N. Shilov, and V. I. Koval'chuk, J. Colloid Interface Sci. *184*:414 (1996).
13. E. M. Trukhan, Soviet Physics of Solid State *4*:2560 (1963).
14. B. Malmgren-Hansen, T. S. Sorensen, B. Jensen, and M. Hannenberg, J. Colloid Interface Sci. *130*:359 (1989).
15. T. S. Sørensen, J. B. Jensen, and B. Malmgren-Hansen, Desalination *80*:293 (1991).
16. T. S. Sørensen, in *Capillarity Today, Lecture Notes in Physics*, No. 386 (G. Petre and A. Sanfeld, eds.), Springer, Berlin, 1991.
17. I. W. Plesner, B. Malmgren-Hansen, and T. S. Sørensen, J. Chem. Soc. Faraday Trans. *90*:2381 (1994).
18. T. S. Sørensen, J. Colloid Interface Sci. *168*:437 (1994).
19. T. S. Sørensen and V. Compañ, J. Colloid Interface Sci. *178*:186 (1996).
20. T. S. Sørensen, J. Chem. Soc. Faraday Trans. *93*:4327 (1997).
21. H. G. L. Coster, Biophys. J. *13*:118 (1973).
22. T. C. Chilcott, H. G. L. Coster, and E. P. George, J. Membrane Sci. *100*:77 (1995).
23. G. C. Barker, J. Electroanal. Chem. *41*:201 (1973).
24. T. R. Brumleve, R. P. Buck, J. Electroanal. Chem. *126*:73 (1981).
25. R. P. Buck, J. Phys. Chem. *93*:6212 (1989).
26. D. R. Franceschetti, J. R. Macdonald, and R. P. Buck, J. Electrochem. Soc. *138*:1368 (1991).
27. R. P. Buck, M. B. Madaras, and R. Mackel, J. Electroanal. Chem. *362*:33 (1993).

28. M. A. Vorotintsev, L. I. Daikhin, and M. D. Levi, J. Electroanal. Chem. *364*:37 (1994).
29. W. J. Albery, C. M. Eliott, and A. R. Mount, J. Electroanal. Chem. *288*:15 (1994).
30. K. S. Spiegler, Trans Faraday Soc. *54*:1408 (1958).
31. P. Meares, in *Charged Gels and Membranes, Vol. 3*, (E. Selegny, ed.) Reidel, Dordrecht, 1976.
32. A. Narebska, S. Koter, and W. Kuyavsky, J. Membrane Sci. *25*:153 (1985).
33. I. Rubinstein, E. Sabatani, and J. Rishpon, J. Electrochem. Soc. *134*:3078 (1987).
34. P. G. Pickup, J. Chem. Soc. Faraday Trans. *86*:3631 (1990).
35. X. Ren and P. G. Pickup, J. Phys Chem. *97*:5356 (1993).
36. F. Helfrich, *Ion Exchange*, McGraw-Hill, Englewood Clifs, New Jersey, 1962.
37. O. Kedem and A. Katchalsky, Trans. Faraday Soc. *59*:1918 (1963).
38. O. Kedem and A. Katchalsky, Trans. Faraday Soc. *59*:1931 (1963).
39. O. Kedem and A. Katchalsky, Trans. Faraday Soc. *59*:1941 (1963).
40. S. S. Dukhin and V. N. Shilov, *Dielectric Phenomena and the Double Layer in Disperse Systems and Polyelectrolytes*, Wiley, New York, 1974.
41. J. R. Segal, J. Theor. Biol. *14*:11 (1967).
42. Z. Stoynov, Electrochim. Acta *35*:1393 (1989).
43. F. F. Zha, H. G. L. Coster, and A. G. Fane, J. Membrane Sci. *93*:255 (1994).
44. C. Deslouis, M. Musiani, and B. Tribollet, J. Phys. Chem. *98*:2936 (1994).

M. A. Vannice, J. E. Benson, and M. D. Boudart, J. Electroanal. Chem. 568, 7 (1998).

N. J. Allen, C. M. Mann, and A. E. Mobius, J. Electroanal. Chem. 58, 18 (1975).

R. E. Kestner, P. G. Parsek, Ret... ...ahr, 1974.

J. Newman, in *Industrial and Engineering, No. 2, American Chem.*, Washington, 1974.

...

21

The Role of Water in the Surface Properties of Lipid Bilayers and Its Influence on Permeability

E. ANIBAL DISALVO   Laboratory of Physical Chemistry of Lipid
Membranes, University of Buenos Aires, Buenos Aires, Argentina

Abstract

The purpose of this work is to show that changes in the interface of lipid
membranes are relevant to the mechanism of permeation of water and
nonelectrolytes. The permeation of polar solutes and water is analyzed
as a function of the changes occurring at the membrane interface by the
presence of polar permeants and of the osmotic stress imposed by the
difference in permeant concentration at both sides of the membrane. It is
demonstrated that these variables affect the surface potential of the
membrane and that both are linked to changes in the amount and/or
organization of the interfacial water molecules. In consequence, the permeation process appears to be concomitant with changes in the polarity
of the interface, mainly the dipole potential. The variation of the dipole
potential, incorporated into a more general description of permeability
can explain the differences in the energy of activation observed for
polyols in isotonic and hypertonic conditions.

I. INTRODUCTION: WATER IN LIPID MEMBRANES, ELECTRICAL SURFACE PROPERTIES AND PERMEABILITY

A.   The Role of the Lipid Bilayer in Cell Membranes

The backbone structure of cell membranes is the lipid bilayer. This organization is a consequence of the amphiphilic character of the molecular constituents, i.e., the phospholipids, that spontaneously stabilize in water in a lamellar
form (Fig. 1). This structure consists of lipid bilayers separated by water.

The biological membranes contain a great variety of lipids. In the pure
form, some of them, such as phosphatidylcholines (PC), phosphatidylserines
(PS), phosphatidylglycerol (PG) and diglycosyl-diacylglycerol, stabilize in a
bilayer when hydrated in water. Other lipids, for example phosphatidylethanolamines (PE), monoglycosyldiacylglycerol and, in some conditions,
cardiolipins do not stabilize as a bilayer in the isolated form [1–4].

The bilayer is the principal permeability barrier of cells. Therefore, its stability is crucial for their compartmentalization. For this reason, the mixtures in
natural systems are a delicate balance between bilayer and nonbilayer forming
lipids [5]. Theoretical proposals have explained that the bilayers are formed
because, when hydrated in an excess of water, the lipid molecules keep a cylin-

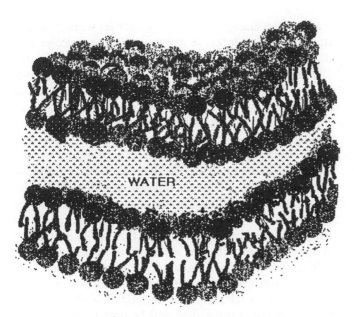

FIG. 1 The lipid membrane: the phospholipid molecules and its stabilization in lamellar structure. The area of the head group (dark circles) includes the hydration water molecules. This area is similar to that corresponding to the fatty acid chains. Thus, the cylindrical shape of the phosphatidylcholines promotes the formation of lamellar conformation. Water is located between the bilayers (shadow area) around the polar head groups and along the fatty acid chains (white points).

drical form due to balance between the area of the polar head groups and the area occupied by the acyl chains [6,7]. In this context, water bound to the phospholipid head groups plays a relevant role. The total area of the lipid head groups accounts for their hydration spheres. Thus, changes in the hydration level may alter the area relationship and result in destabilization of the lamellar phase by forming nonbilayer structures such as hexagonal, cubic or micellar phases [8].

Lamellar to hexagonal phase transitions are mainly found in processes in which the bilayer is subjected to desiccation or freezing. Examples of these transitions have been found in plant cells and bacteria and corroborated in model membrane systems composed by phosphatidylethanolamines [9]. The bilayer can also be destroyed by the action of surface active agents, such as Triton X-100, bile salts or lysophospholipids. In these cases, the lamellar structure is broken into mixed micelles resulting in a release of cellular material or of solutes encapsulated in vesicles [10,11]. There are, however, less drastic processes in which the bilayer can change its barrier properties without affecting the lamellar conformation. For instance, as shown in Fig. 2a, vesicles subjected to swelling leak gradually its content. A schematic picture of the swelling process and the leakage in a unilamellar vesicle, while the bilayer structure is maintained, is shown in Fig. 2b. It will be one of the purposes of this work to show that these changes in the barrier properties are related to the amount of water confined at the lipid interface composed by the polar head groups, and that the properties that this water organization imposes to the interface are relevant in determining the mechanism of permeation. In this context, the physical properties of water at the interface, such as its polarization and its behavior as a solvent for permeant molecules will be of importance. The first property is related to the dipole potential of the bilayer and the second in the definition of the bilayer as a heterogeneous solubility phase. This picture also should account for the dynamical response that the bilayer structure may have by exchanging water with the surrounding solutions in the process of permeation. Thus, this chapter will analyze the permeation of polar solutes in the light of the transient changes occurring at the membrane interface during permeation that appears related to the organization of water. For this reason, the interfacial properties during time will be determined by measuring the spectroscopical properties of a dye partitioning at the membrane interface that are correlated with the dipole potential.

B. Lipid Bilayers in the Context of Membrane Phenomena

A membrane is defined as a phase interposed between two compartments consisting of water solutions that may have extremely different compositions. For example, a unilamellar vesicle as that described in Fig. 2b is able to encapsulate a 0.1 M KCl solution in its internal volume and be stable in isosmotic conditions.

The physicochemical properties of this barrier control the rate of mass transfer between the two aqueous solutions. At least two steps in the process of mass transfer can be distinguished: the transference from the aqueous solution to the membrane phase and the diffusion of the substances across the membrane. The overall kinetics of transference is determined by the relative rates of these two processes. In lipid bilayers, the magnitude of the interfaces is relevant in relation to the total membrane thickness. Moreover, the lipid bilayer consists of a hydrocarbon slab sandwiched between two polar regions (see Fig. 1). In this sense, a bilayer composed by a single lipid, let us say dipalmitoylphosphatidylcholine (DPPC), is homogeneous in terms of chemical composition. However, it constitutes a heterogeneous structure when the different properties of the hydrocarbon core and the polar head groups regions are considered. Thus, the transference of solutes across the bilayer involves the mass transfer from the bulk aqueous solution to the polar region and the mass

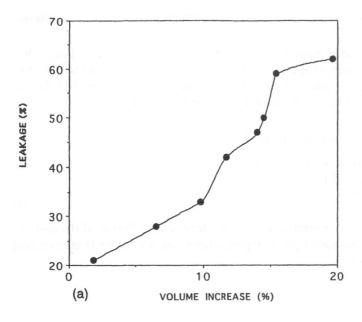

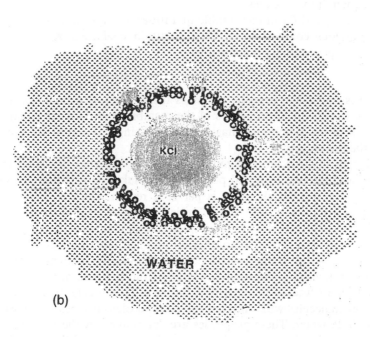

FIG. 2 Leakage of vesicle content in vesicles subjected to swelling. (a) Vesicles containing a solution of KCl leak their content when swollen in hypotonic solutions. The entrance of water is much faster than the KCl. Thus, the leakage is produced when a given volume has been attained. (b) Schematic representation of the vesicle swelling and leakage of the vesicle content. Gray areas indicates KCl solution and pointed areas water.

transfer from the polar region to the hydrocarbon core. The lipid bilayer has permeability properties that make it selective to ions and polar solutes in comparison to any other material in nature. Many of these properties are linked to the biological function that the lipid membrane play in cells.

C. The Basic Analysis of Permeability

The starting point in permeation studies is focused on the integrated form of the first Fick's law [12,13]

$$J = -D \, dC/dx \tag{1}$$

where J is the flux of substance, and D the diffusion coefficient of the molecular species in a continuous phase. Upon integration, assuming D independent of C, Eq. [1] results in

$$J = \frac{D}{\delta} (C'_2 - C'_1) \tag{2}$$

where δ is the membrane thickness.

To transform C'_2 and C'_1 in measurable quantities (i.e., the concentration in the bulk of aqueous compartments, C) a partition coefficient $K = C'/C$ is introduced. Thus, permeability is defined by

$$P = DK/\delta \tag{3}$$

This equation is applied to describe the mass transfer across a homogeneous phase. That is, the chemical properties of the membrane surface are equal to that of the bulk of the membrane phase and thus a single D and K are necessary to describe the process.

The differences in structure and physicochemical properties of the central nonpolar slab and the two hydrated polar regions make the partition process more complex. The interfacial region is per se a region which is chemically heterogeneous. Groups with different affinities to water, spatial orientation and H-bonding capabilities are confined in a complex network between the hydrocarbon chains and the bulk water solution. The most outstanding features of this region is that it may have a polarity drastically different from the hydrocarbon slab (dielectric constant $\varepsilon = 2$) and from the bulk aqueous solution ($\varepsilon = 78$). It constitutes a bidimensional lattice of H-bonds formed between lipids and water molecules with different solvent and dielectric properties with respect to the bulk water. These properties are determined by the polarizability of the water molecules around the chemical subgroups of the phospholipids. This water organization is decisive in several relevant biophysical phenomena such as: adhesion of membranes, fusion of vesicles, adsorption and penetration of peptides and proteins, insertion of chemical drugs, permeation of polar solutes, ion selectivity and mechanical behavior. In the context of this chapter, it will be important to determine the localization of water in the membrane. Its contributions to the barrier of permeation for water and nonelectrolytes will be related to its participation in the binding and adsorption of molecules from the aqueous bulk solution.

D. Localization of Water in the Bilayer Interface

The influence of the interfacial region on the permeability of a lipid membrane requires the understanding of how water is localized in the structure of a lipid membrane. From this basic standpoint, the dynamical properties and the response to penetrant or nonpenetrant molecules that may alter this water distribution will be analyzed.

The image that we have from a bilayer hydrated in the fluid state is the average spatial distribution of the submolecular groups projected onto the line normal to the plane of the membrane (Fig. 3). This bilayer profile provides a picture of the transbilayer distribution of water at the submolecular groups, necessary for understanding the permeability of membranes.

The first point is to establish the boundary between the hydrocarbon slab and the polar head groups, and its respective thickness. The thickness of the slab of the bilayer material has been calculated by using several methods. A resume of them is provided by White and Wiener [14]. The edge of the hydrocarbon slab comprises of the acyl chains beginning with the C_2 carbons [14,15]. Assuming the volumes of the methylenes, double bonds and methyls to be 27, 43 and 54 $Å^3$ the hydrocarbon slab thickness is 16.3 Å.

The comparison of the different methods makes a distinction between the transbilayer separation of the choline and glycerol groups, respectively. The mean between these two distances corresponds, according to White and Wiener [14], to the bilayer separation of the phosphate groups. The equivalent hydrocarbon slab is framed by the position of the carbonyl groups (Fig. 3).

The fine structure of this region is completed with the localization of water. Water seems to be distributed around the glycerol with a small but significant penetration into double bond regions. The volume of water associated to the lipids constitutes an excluded volume for solute solubilization. This amount of water associated to the membrane has been detected by calorimetry and has been shown to contribute to the barrier properties for nonelectrolytes [16]. Based on this observation, this chapter will analyze the permeability in a membrane described as a composite element consisting of the lipid leaflet and the water layers associated with the head groups. The mean thickness of water layers is about 6 Å in planar bilayers that may increase to 10 Å with the increase in curvature. This constitutes two-thirds of the total bilayer thickness.

The bilayer thickness is important for the description of the transport process according to Eq. (3). In this regard, the total thickness of the bilayer should be considered (water plus lipids) in order to calculate the concentration

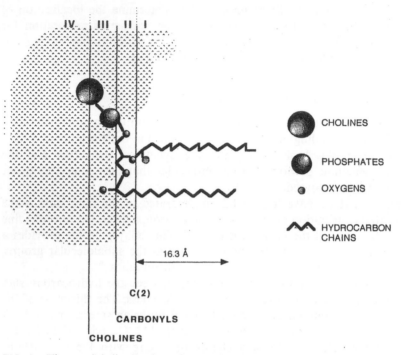

FIG. 3 The spatial distribution of submolecular groups in a lipid membrane and the localization of the water at the membrane interface. Region I comprises the hydrocarbon core, region II the glycerol backbone, region III the carbonyls of the sn_2 chain and region IV corresponds to the outer plane of the interface. The plane containing the carbonyls determines the limits of the hydrocarbon slab. The phosphates are in a different plane than the cholines. The shadow area denote the regions were water can be located. Note that water can be located around the glycerol backbone and the first methylene groups. In region III, water dipole would have an average orientation normal to the membrane plane. In region IV, water has no preferential orientation. For simplicity only half of the bilayer is drawn.

differences between the two bulk water solutions. More important, the magnitude and the type of the molecular interactions in the complex regions positioned between the hydrocarbon bulk and the water bulk (regions II, III and IV in Fig. 3) is a matter of general interest in the process of penetration of molecules. The structural properties of these regions will determine the processes of adsorption and binding of different types of compounds that may or may not permeate the membrane. In these processes the participation of the water at the interface will be reflected by its organization as a polarized layer of dipoles [63]. We will show later how this contributes to the permeability.

E.   The Role of Water in the Determination of the Electrical Properties of the Interface

The boundary between the hydrocarbon slab and the polar head group region, establishes the localization and orientation of the chemical groups that may affect the transference of solutes from the aqueous to the membrane phase.

The polar head groups of the phospholipid molecules are oriented at the water membrane interface as described in the Fig. 3. Carbonyls, phosphate groups and the positively (choline or ethanolamine) charged groups are the main points of hydration in a phospholipid membrane. The orientation of these groups and the organization of the water dipoles in its respective hydration spheres determine the polarity of the interface.

The polarity of the interface is defined by the contribution of the dipolar groups of the phospholipids and water dipoles to the surface potential (dipole potential) which is positive with respect to the water solution. This potential can be determined as the drop of potential across a monolayer spread in an air–water interface. McDonald and Simon [17] have shown that the dipole potential measured in this way decreases abruptly at a temperature corresponding closely to the bilayer phase transition. From this, they concluded that the organization of molecules in liposomes corresponds closely to that in monolayers in equilibrium with those liposomes. The dipole potential of dipalmitoylphosphatidylcholine (DPPC) in the gel phase is 466 ± 15 mV decreasing to 410 ± 20 mV in the fluid phase. The drastic decrease of the dipole potential at the phase transition, denotes a reorganization of the dipoles and hence a less polarized interface at the fluid in comparison to the gel state. The changes in the dipole potential can also be measured using an optical dye adsorbed to the membrane interface. In Fig. 4, the phase transition of dipalmitoylphosphatidylcholine (DPPC) measured with merocyanine 540, an optical probe partitioning at the glycerol backbone region of the lipid bilayer (region II in Fig. 3) is shown [18,19]. Merocyanine is a singly charged molecule that incorporates as a monomer when the bilayer is in the fluid state and as a dimer in the gel state. In the first case, an absorbance peak at 570 nm predominates, and in the second the highest absorbance is observed at 530 nm.

The drastic increase in the absorbance of merocyanine at 570 nm corresponds to the decrease in the dipole potential observed in monolayers.

[1]H nuclear magnetic resonance [^{1}H-NMR] or phospholipids deuterated in the polar head groups has shown that the phosphocholine group is oriented parallel to the bilayer plane contributing in a negligible form to the dipole potential [20,60]. In addition, ether linked instead of ester linked phospholipids show a potential of several hundred millivolts. Although not conclusive, it seems that water orientation contributes in a great extent to the dipole potential [21]. Simulation of the effect of a membrane composed by COO— groups on the water structure results in a layering of water molecules extending 7–8 Å into the liquid. The average density of the oxygen is between 2 and

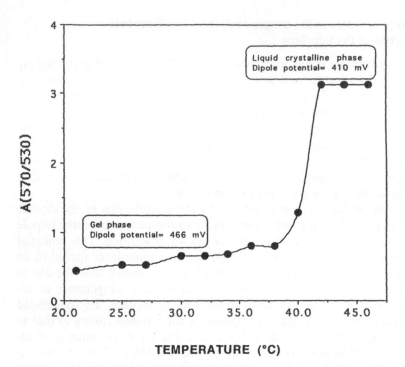

FIG. 4 Phase transition of DPPC measured by the changes in the absorbance at 570 nm corresponding to the monomer of merocyanine 540 incorporated in the membrane. The data of dipole potential measured in monolayers in the gels and the liquid crystalline state are included for comparison.

3.1 Å and those of the hydrogens at 2 Å. The shift between the oxygen and hydrogen peaks is an indication of the average orientation of the water molecules with respect to the surface normal of the membrane [22]. A second region between 4.5 and 6 Å is located for the oxygens but the location of hydrogens is washed out. This indicates that at 6 Å, the thickness of the aqueous excluded volume in planar bilayers, as described [16], constitutes a second water layer with no preferential orientation (see Fig. 3).

Thus, the optical probe can be used to detect changes at the interface concomitant with the changes in the dipole potential, assuming that this is completely determined by the orientation of water molecules at the interface. We will use this method to measure the changes occurring in the interface of bilayers during the permeation process.

F. Influence of the Surface Electric Fields on the Transference Processes

Electrostatic fields are associated to the membrane interface. Simple processes such as the permeation of organic ions are strongly influenced by membrane electrostatics, mentioned here in its wider meaning: the contribution of net charges and the dipoles. It is accepted that the permeation rates of hydrophobic ions such as tetraphenylborate and tetraphenyphosphonium is determined by the fact that the bilayer interior is positive resulting from the orientation of the water and hydrated chemical dipoles of the lipid molecules [23].

The distribution of ions and charges determines the properties of the electrical double layer and to transfer a solute from the aqueous phase to the membrane interior a potential barrier built by the charges (ϕ) and by the dipoles (χ) oriented in the surface must be surmounted (Bockris–Reddy [24]). With reference to Fig. 3, solute should be transferred across regions III and IV. Vice versa, in a structure like a lipid bilayer, that constitutes a bidimensional liquid crystal, polar molecules from the aqueous solution can also influence the charges and dipole distributions in those regions [25].

Nonionic permeants, such as water and polyalcohols, should not be influenced by the electrical charges at the interface. However, the water polarization at the interface constitute a region of different solvent properties in comparison to bulk water. Dipole–dipole and hydrogen bond interactions may affect the transference across the membrane interface, since the solute may adsorb to polarized groups and water dipoles. Dispersion forces, hydrogen bonds, dipole–dipole interactions, dipole-induced dipole interactions, donor acceptor bonds and electrostatic interactions may contribute to the surface tension. In the absence of net charges the interaction by dispersion forces and dipole–dipole cannot be neglected when, at least one dipole moment is greater than about 1.5 debye [26]. The water dipole is 1.84 debye and that of the $P - N +$ vector of the zwitterionic head group 22 debye and its orientation can be related to the hydration and presence of hydrogen-bonding compounds such as polyols.

This implies that variations in the dipole organization can change permeability. The purpose is to demonstrate that the changes in the surface properties, linked to changes in the amount and/or organization of water molecules, may change the permeability to polar permeants. Therefore, the changes in the polarity of the interface occurring during the permeation process should be measured concomitantly with the mass transfer. As a strategy to tackle this problem, the changes in the optical properties of merocyanine in relation to the dipole potential described above will be a useful tool.

The variations in the interfacial properties will then be incorporated into a general description of permeability redefining of the permeability coefficient given by Eq. (3).

II. THE LIPID BILAYER AS A HETEROGENEOUS SOLVENT. DYNAMIC AND STATIC PROPERTIES RELATED TO PERMEATION

The purpose of this section will be to demonstrate that the lipid membrane behaves as a heterogeneous barrier of solubility having dynamical properties depending on its water content.

A. Solubility of Permeants in Different Regions of the Bilayer

Equation (3) describes the permeability coefficient by including a partition coefficient K accounting for the relative solubility of the solute in the membrane phase and in the aqueous phase. The introduction of a solute in the membrane phase implies the formation of a hole with the size in which the solute can fit. This process requires energy, the larger is the solute the larger is the energy required. The solute, on the other hand, needs energy to abandon the aqueous phase by breaking the hydrogen bonds. The solvation energy of the solute in the membrane phase compensates the energy expended in the previous stages. Thus, the solubility of the solute into the membrane would be more favorable when the solvation energy of the solute in the membrane phase is higher (more negative).

As the solvent–solute interactions, both in the aqueous phase and the membrane phase, depend on the size of the molecule, the selectivity of the membrane is determined by a combination of size and chemical affinity. If the membrane is homogeneous its behavior as a solubility barrier for all solutes would be directly proportional to the solubility in the membrane phase. In other words, if the membrane is considered as a nonpolar phase only nonpolar solutes would be transferred; if the membrane is hydrophilic only polar solutes would be transferred. However, experimental data of different laboratories in the most varying conditions indicate that polar solutes such as water, urea, ethanol or propanol, having different hydrophilic–hydrophibic characters, can permeate lipid membranes to a significant extent.

The solubility of water and hydrogen-bonding molecules in the membrane decreases with the diminishing possibilities to make hydrogen bonds and the decreasing dielectrical constant of the surrounding media. In consequence, polar solutes such as glycerol would dissolve in the interface rather than in the hydrocarbon bulk. With the same argument, the diffusion coefficient will differ at the polar head group region and in the bulk nonpolar region. Thus, the mechanism of solubility and of diffusion will differ considerable in those parts of the bilayer normal. In consequence, the permeability coefficient described by Eq. (3) will be a combination of these alternatives.

To elucidate the question whether the bilayer behaves, in stationary conditions, as a homogeneous or a heterogeneous phase, the enthalpic and entropic contributions to the solubility phenomena will be analyzed. A plot of the entropy vs. the enthalpy of dissolution of different solutes in a bilayer is given in Fig. 5. We have drawn the data for families of solutes with similar structural characteristics. It is clear that each type of solutes fall into different straight lines with different slopes, except compounds 5, 6 and 9 corresponding to lineal monoalcohols.

One family corresponds to molecules in which a HCOH group is added (compounds 2–4 in Fig. 5). That is, the hydrophilic–hydrophobic balance is maintained but the total number of OH is increased. A second family is composed by compounds in which a methyl group is added maintaining the same number of OH groups in a tetrahedrical molecule (compounds 6–8). In this case, the size and the ability to form hydrogen bonds is maintained while the hydrophobic character increases [27,28]. A large enthalpy involves a large entropy in all cases. However, this enthalpic–entropic compensation is not equal for all the compounds assayed.

A slope is obtained for solutes with different size and increasing number of hydrogen bond groups and another for solutes with similar size and hydrogen bonding with increasing hydrophobicity.

The family composed by methanol, ethanol and *n*-butanol constitutes an

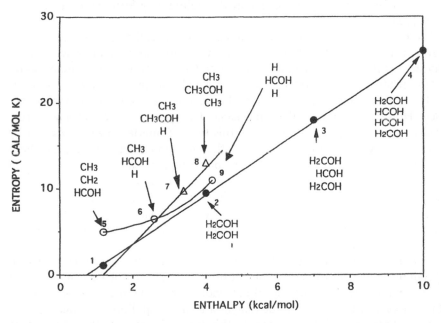

FIG. 5 Entropy vs. enthalpy compensation of the transference of different types of solutes from the aqueous solution into the membrane phase. (1) urea, (2) ethyleneglycol, (3) glycerol, (4) erythritol, (5) *n*-propanol, (6) ethanol, (7) iso-propanol, (8) *t*-butanol and (9) methanol. *Source*: data adapted from Refs. 27 and 59.

interesting case. It is observed that the values for this family do not fall in a straight line. Moreover, ethanol can be included in the family of compounds 7 and 8, and methanol is close to the line of family of compounds 1–4. This suggests that ethanol and methanol are partitioning into different regions of the bilayers. Which are the regions in which they are partitioning according to the four region model described in Fig. 3 has been the subject of recent works using molecular dynamic simulations [29,30].

For the purpose of this monograph we will focus on the behavior of glycerol. As shown in Fig. 5, glycerol has a high enthalpy in comparison to other compounds. This can be interpreted as a consequence of a stronger interaction of glycerol with the lipid phase than with the aqueous phase. In addition, a high entropy means a disordering of the system. The adsorption of glycerol to the membrane by hydrogen bonds would correspond to a decrease in entropy since the molecular degrees of freedom are restricted to a bidimensional region. Therefore, the increase in entropy can be ascribed to water molecules displaced from the interface to the bulk aqueous phase as a consequence of the glycerol–lipid interaction. This interpretation is supported by experimental results in which it was shown that glycerol may substitute for water in the membrane phase [31] and that the activation energy for permeation is related to the number of hydrogen bonds that this solute may form with the aqueous phase [32].

These results indicate that the usual comparison of the partition coefficients of solutes in saturated lecithin liposomes with those in octanol–water systems may be a coincidence but not provide useful information. The octanol–water system behaves as an isotropic solvent in which the amount of water saturating the organic phase is, in principle, the same as all the hydrocarbon methylenes. However, evidence that interfacial transport is rate limiting during passive membrane permeation across this type of interface has been given by Miller [33]. Due to the presence of the phosphocholine group, the limit between the hydrophobic and the hydrophilic regions can be very different in the bilayer in comparison to the octanol–water interface. Therefore, it seems reasonably to think that such a complex region can contribute to the permeation process. Thus, there would be no reason to assume that a hydrocarbon-like interior is the rate-limiting step of permeation of water-soluble compounds [34].

It is important to note that this conclusion is valid for a membrane system in equilibrium, i.e., in which the solvent properties of each phase is not affected by the penetration of solutes (ideal behavior) nor by the penetration of water. In principle, at each region of the bilayer a ternary equilibrium system formed by water, lipid and solutes is found. In this case, it is assumed that the amount of water in the membrane system remains constant when permeant solubilizes. This is not the case when permeation is measured driven by a macroscopic concentration gradient of permeant across the membrane. Tiny changes in the fine structure on the bilayer could be induced either by osmosis or by the permeant solutes. Thus, a further analysis should be done on the distribution of water in the membrane phase.

Considering the bilayer as a heterogeneous phase as described by the four region model, the partition coefficient of the permeant should vary with distance within the membrane. This is a consequence of the fact that the standard chemical potential of solute may be different at each region. The two main regions in which the standard chemical potential of solute may differ drastically are the hydrophilic region between the bulk aqueous solution and the carbonyl groups plane (regions II and III in Fig. 3) and the hydrophobic region from the carbonyl plane into the bilayer core (Region I). The standard chemical potential can vary with thickness within each of these regions. In region I, the standard chemical potential may depend on distance due to the different chemical environment in each plane of the hydrocarbon core or through the dependence of the standard chemical potential with water in the membrane phase. The first possibility would be possible if we can distinguish the solubilities at regions as thin as two or three methylenes. This could be accomplished by dynamical simulation but no significant differences in the potential energy wells have been observed. The second possibility can be considered negligible if coupling is not considered, since most of the water in the membrane is located at the interface, i.e., the region between bulk water and the carbonyl groups based on X-ray diffraction (see Fig. 3 and corresponding text).

At the interphase (regions I and II), the standard chemical potential of the solute can change due to changes in the amount and organization of water as a function of distance. Thus, as these properties are related with the polarization of the water dipoles giving place to the dipole potential the variation with distance will be a function of this potential.

To consider these properties in the permeability process of nonelectrolytes we have to face two problems. One of them is to identify a measurable property of the interface connected with water organization. The second is to adopt an experimental method providing information of those changes at the interface during the process of permeation. In this context, the contribution of water to the dipole potential and how this can be measured in a kinetic assay by means of the optical properties of merocyanine must be taken into account.

B. The Dynamical Structure of a Lipid Membrane in Relation to Stationary and Nonstationary Water

The static view given above is more complicated if one considers the dynamical properties as a consequence of the thermal motions of the molecules with respect to themselves and of each of their molecular portions. Several experimental studies of NMR and crystallographic measurements indicate that the glycerol backbone, which is the boundary of the hydrocarbon and water regions, is the less mobile part of the membrane (Fig. 6). It must be recalled that water is distributed around it (Fig. 3).

The relative mobilities of the different parts of the molecules is greater at the level of the methyl terminal groups of the acyl chains and in the extreme of the polar head groups. Because of the thermal motion a probability exists that polar molecules such as water or small nonelectrolytes may penetrate, at least transiently, into the deeper regions of the bilayer [35–37]. This means that nonstationary water can be found inside the hydrocarbon region, in addition to the stationary water bound to the polar submolecular groups. The distinction of these two types of water is crucial for the understanding of the mechanisms of permeability [34,38,39].

Water is known to permeate a bilayer with relative ease, much more than that expected from its solubility in hydrocarbon solvents. Moreover, solutes such as urea, glycerol, and ethyleneglycol, having a negligible partition in lipid bilayers, permeate at a considerable rate. Solubility of water increases dramatically with the presence of double bonds, suggesting that it may "catalyze" the transference of water. These "water clusters" may account for transient carriers of polar solutes.

As a guideline, stationary water is considered fixed to the polar head groups, and nonstationary water is travelling in clusters across the membrane coupled to solutes or diffusing along the lipid matrix. However, these two types of water may be exchanged. For instance, as in the case of glycerol given above, the solute may bind to the membrane groups displacing water from the hydration sphere of the phospholipid. Thus, stationary water at the interface will decrease at expense of an increase in the nonstationary one. The ability of the solute to exchange for water at the lipid interface will be related to its number of OH groups. We will return to this point when discussing the interpretation of the activation energy for solute permeation and the effects of glycerol and trehalose on the lipid membrane.

C. The Influence of the Aqueous Interface on the Permeability of Water and Solutes

The results shown in Fig. 5 and the interpretation of the glycerol penetration suggest that the interaction of solutes crossing the bilayer by passive transport are governed by a balance of water at the different regions of the membrane structure and its dynamics and not simply by the hydrophobicity of the solutes [34]. These conclusions are similar to those derived from molecular dynamics simulations [29].

The water transference is rather high in lipid bilayers in comparison to ions and large polar nonelectrolytes [40,41,64]. This semipermeability property accounts for the selective permeation that a membrane may have. By this, it is

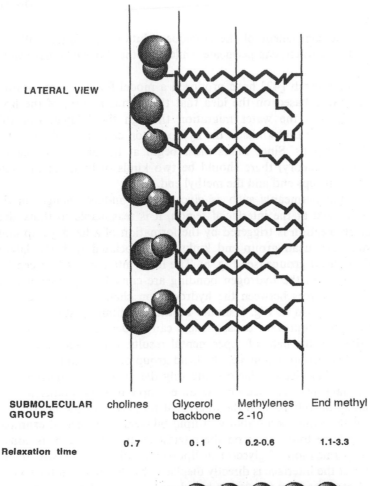

LATERAL VIEW

SUBMOLECULAR GROUPS	cholines	Glycerol backbone	Methylenes 2 -10	End methyl
Relaxation time	0.7	0.1	0.2-0.6	1.1-3.3

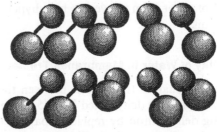

FIG. 6 Mobility of the different submolecular groups of a phospholipid molecule in a lipid bilayer. The degree of mobility of the different portions of the lipids molecules in a bilayer at 50°C as measured by ^{13}C NMR [20]. Lateral and front views of a bilayer show the possible orientations of the phosphocholine groups. The phosphocholine group can rotate in a plane parallel to the membrane surface or displace slightly the phosphates from the plane of the cholines. Because of these movements, the water boundary drawn in Fig. 3 can fluctuate.

understood that a component of the aqueous solution in contact with the membrane, let us say water, can permeate while the other (ions or polar solute) cannot.

Haines and Liebovitch [42] have proposed a model for water permeation into lipid membranes based on the idea that the lateral motion of the lipid molecules is linked to the water migration through the bilayer. For this purpose, they postulate that kinks in the hydrocarbon chains travel along the full length of the chains. Since kinks must begin at the end of the chains (according to Flory theory) there should be two kinds of kinks in the lipid bilayers: the head groups end and the methyl end.

In the light that permeants such as glycerol may induce changes in the stationary water fixed at the interfacial region, it is reasonable to think that the process of permeation is triggered by the formation of a head group kink at the interface. The head group end kinks are associated with the lateral movement of the head groups (see Fig. 6). The ionic interactions between the polar head groups and the hydrogen bonding are considerably greater than the van der Waals forces between the hydrocarbon chains. Hence, the head group movements shown in Fig. 6 should be the rate-limiting step for water transport. Thus, two important consequences can be derived and will be the subject of analysis in the light of experimental results. First, factors affecting the membrane head group region, i.e., the head group organization, may affect the water permeability. Second, factors affecting the membrane interface may change the mechanism of permeation. As an example of these points we will describe the effect of trehalose on the interfacial properties of the bilayer and its influence on the water permeability of lipid bilayers. In a second example, the effect of the hypertonic stress on the interfacial properties and its consequence on the permeation of glycerol in liposomes will be discussed. In the first case, water at the interface is directly displaced by the sugar. In the second case, extrusion of water from the vesicle by a hypertonic shock is done prior to solute permeation.

D.   Permeability of Water in Membranes Treated with Trehalose

Trehalose is a disaccharide that inserts between the polar head groups replacing water when lipids are dehydrated [43–45]. It incorporates into the bilayer structure during dehydration by replacing part of the water of the hydration sphere of the phospholipids [61]. This interaction affects the head groups through the formation of hydrogen bonds between the OH groups and the phosphate groups (see Fig. 3) as shown by the change in the PO_2 antisymmetric stretching mode [46]. When water is restored, the activation energy of water permeation induced by an osmotic gradient is lower for trehalose/DPPC mixtures (15.4 kcal/mol) than that corresponding to the gel state of lipids without trehalose (Table 1). This value is comparable to that obtained

TABLE 1 Activation Energies for Water Permeation in Multilamellar Liposomes in the Gel and the Fluid State and After Rehydration in Trehalose

Lipid	Activation energy for water permeation (kcal/mol)
DPPC gel	27.4
DPPC liquid crystalline	6.0
DPPC gel + trehalose	15.4
DPPC fluid + trehalose	6.3
DPPC gel + 4% DPPG	14.1

with DPPC multilamellar liposomes containing 4% dipalmitoylphosphatidylglycerol (DPPG) (14.1 kcal/mol) at the same temperature [45].

The importance of these results is that they reflect the fact that changes at the interface, maintaining the bilayer at the gel state, affects the energy of activation of water. This is a strong evidence that permeability is at least in part determined by the interfacial properties of the bilayer, since trehalose may substitute for water at the polar head group region.

E. Permeability of Glycerol in Membranes Under Osmotic Stress

There are two ways by which permeability induced by macroscopic permeant gradients can be determined [32,39,47,48].

One method consists of dispersing liposomes or lipid vesicles in a hypertonic solution of the permeant. When a vesicle is dispersed in a hypertonic solution of an impermeant an efflux of water is produced decreasing the volume particle to a constant minimum value. However, if this process is made with a permeant molecule, after reaching the minimum volume the permeant will enter as a consequence of the concentration difference. This permeant influx will drag water into the vesicle interior to produce an increase in the volume of the particle. Thus, a minimum volume is achieved corresponding to the condition in which the osmotic water outflux equals the diffusional water–solute influx (Fig. 7a).

In the isosmotic method, a permeant gradient across the bilayer is created without promoting osmotic perturbations at time zero of the experiment. In this case, the liposomes filled with a solution of an impermeant solute, such as sucrose, are dispersed in an osmotically equivalent solution of a permeant. At time zero, the chemical potential of water is equal inside and outside the liposome and hence no changes in volume are observed. However, solute will dissolve and diffuse across the membrane as a consequence of its macroscopic

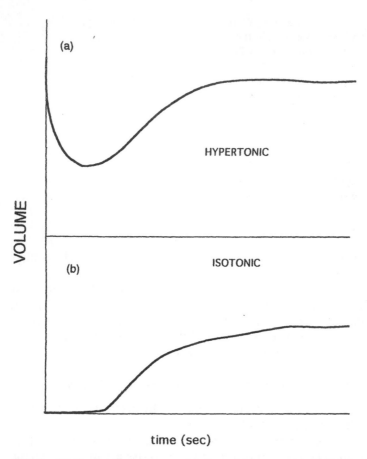

FIG. 7 Methods of inducing permeation of solutes across lipid bilayers. (a) Hypertonic method: vesicles filled with glucose 0.1 M and dispersed at time zero in a solution of 0.5 M glycerol or erythritol; (b) Isotonic method: vesicles filled with 0.1 M glucose are dispersed at time zero in an isotonic solution of glycerol or erythritol. It is observed in this last case that no volume change is produced at the initial time.

gradient. The osmotic imbalance produced by the entrance of permeant molecules into the liposome provokes swelling by an influx of water (Fig. 7b).

The ascending portions of curves a and b correspond to the solute influx from which the permeation rate at different temperatures can be calculated. The activation energy for glycerol and erythritol permeation is lower when it is measured by the hypertonic in comparison to the isotonic one (Table 2). Thus, it is clear that solute permeation is different whether the vesicles have been shrunken or not before permeant diffuses in.

A partial conclusion can be derived from the results of water permeation

TABLE 2 Activation Energies for the Permeation of Non-electrolytes Across Multilamellar Bilayers in the Fluid State Under Isotonic and Hypertonic Conditions

Permeant	Hypertonic method	Isotonic method	Number of hydrogen bonds in bulk water
Erythritol	16.1	21	8
Glycerol	11.0	18	6
Urea	9.3	—	5
Water	8.6	—	4

Source: Data adapted from Refs. 32 and 47.

obtained with trehalose-treated liposomes and the differences in glycerol and erythritol permeation in the hypertonic and isotonic methods. The changes in the water–membrane interface induced either by water displacement or by osmotic dehydration affects the permeation of water and non electrolytes. To consider how the extent of shrinkage effects the interface and its relationship to permeability analysis, the membrane properties achieved at each extent of shrinkage will be characterized.

F. The State of the Interface in Bilayers Treated with Trehalose or in Vesicles Subject to Hypertonic Stress

It is important now to describe how those factors affecting the activation energy for permeation may change the interfacial properties and how these variations can be measured to link them to the permeation process. The model of Haines [42] proposes that the highest barrier for permeation is the formation of a kink at the surface. Thus, the lipid head group and water must reorganize in order that this barrier be diminished.

This should bring changes in a measurable property related to the interface. As described in Fig. 4 the changes in the dipole potential can be followed by the changes in the absorbance at 570 nm of merocyanine. We will use this method, to show that trehalose and the osmotic shrinkage affects the interfacial properties in correlation to the changes in the dipole potential. These surface changes will be related with the changes in the activation energy for permeation shown in Tables 1 and 2.

1. Surface Changes Induced by Trehalose

An increase of the absorbance at 570 nm is observed in bilayers treated with trehalose (Table 3). These increase in the 570:530 ratio corresponds to a decrease in the activation energy of the water permeability membranes (Table

TABLE 3 Physical Changes in DPPC Bilayers in the Presence of 0.1 M Trehalose

Condition	$T(°C)$	A570/530
DPPC in the gel state without trehalose	25	0
DPPC gel state with 0.1 M trehalose	25	1.32
DPPC in the fluid state without trehalose	50	2.3

Source: Data adapted from Ref. 45.

1) and to a decrease in the dipole potential as shown in Fig. 4. Thus, the decrease in dipole potential is related to the increase in water permeability.

As shown in Fig. 4, an increase in the incorporation of the monomer of MC occurs when temperature is increased through the phase transition. The lowering of the activation energy shown in Table 1, achieved when the membrane in the gel state is treated with trehalose, corresponds to the increase in the incorporation of the dye probe.

A correspondence between absorbance at 570 nm and the decrease in dipole potential is observed when different types of sugars are in contact with the bilayer (Fig. 8). The 570 nm absorbance peak increases with the OH groups of the sugar with a parallel decrease in the dipole potential measured in monolayers. Thus, the replacement of water by trehalose decreases the activation energy for water permeation in membranes in the gel state, by a net decrease in the polarization of the interface.

This example illustrates that water replacement at the bilayer interface affects the dipole potential and that this change can be followed by means of the changes in the absorbance of the dye. This method will be useful to correlate the surface changes occurring simultaneously to the permeation process. A step in this direction is to show the changes in the interface when the hypertonic method for solute permeation is analyzed.

2. Surface Changes Induced by the Osmotic Stress

We will discuss now the correlation of the effect of shrinkage on membrane surface properties and the activation energy for solute permeation shown in Table 2.

We may name at least two possibilities about the effect of the hypertonic solution on the activation energy. One is that the high concentration of solute in contact with the bilayer may produce a change at the regions IV or III of Fig. 3, and therefore affecting the barrier properties for the same solute or for other solutes as shown in Fig. 2. Permeants, such as glycerol, can substitute for water at the bilayer interface affecting the packing, the area per lipid and the thickness [31]. At lower concentrations, a decrease of the surface potential by glycerol has been reported [49].

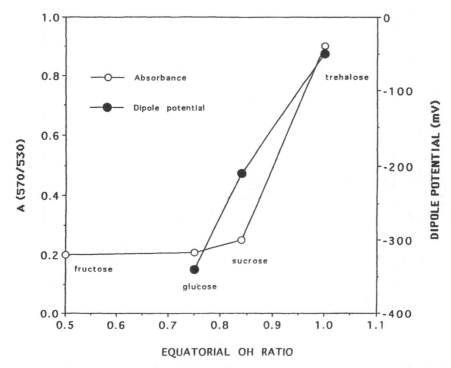

FIG. 8 Relation of the monomer absorption and the dipole potential. Relative incorporation of merocyanine monomer to bilayers and the dipole potential of monolayers as a function of the number of equatorial OH of different mono and disaccharides in contact with the interface.

The second possibility is related to the osmotic gradient imposed to induce permeation. In conditions in which the vesicles reach the minimum volume, as shown in the hypertonic method (Fig. 7a), water is extruded from the different bilayer regions causing additional packing [50]. Experimental evidences with the surface probe merocyanine have shown that these effects of water extrusion from the membrane by osmosis affect the interface [51].

Therefore, the effect of osmosis can be ascribed mainly to water extrusion from the bilayer interface. It will be the purpose to quantify such changes in terms of measurable properties that can be followed during the permeation process.

As shown in Fig. 9, dimyristoylphoshatidylcholine (DMPC) liposomes in the fluid state, (30°C) show a decrease in the peak at 570 nm of the monomer of merocyanine with the increase of osmotic pressure (Fig. 9). In the same figure, the effect of hypertonic stress on bilayers in the gel state shows an

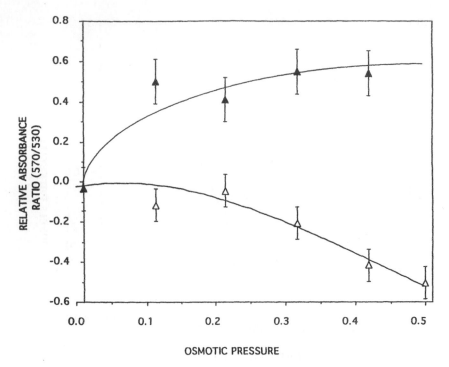

OSMOTIC PRESSURE

FIG. 9 Effect of the hypertonic stress on the surface properties of fluid ($\triangle$) and gel bilayers ($\blacktriangle$), measured by the penetration of MC 540 monomers.

opposite trend. Thus, the changes produced by the osmotic stress on the interface can be followed by measuring the binding of merocyanine to shrunken and nonshrunken liposomes.

The amount of merocyanine monomer adsorbed to the surface, given by the absorbance at 570 nm (ΔA), is related to the dye concentration in the aqueous solution (c_b) by the Langmuir adsorption isotherm:

$$\Delta A = NK_m c_i / [1 + K_m c_i]$$

where N is the maximum number of binding sites for the dye and K_m the association constant of the dye to the membrane.

Merocyanine [52] is sensitive to the state of the membrane reflecting changes in the area per phospholipid and water polarization in neutral phospholipid membranes. As shown in Fig. 4, the gel and fluid states of the membranes having different dipole potentials have markedly different absorbances at 570 nm. Thus, the distribution of the dye between the interface (c_i) surface and the solution (c_b) will depend on the dipole potential (χ) described by

$$c_i = c_b \exp[F\chi/(RT)]$$

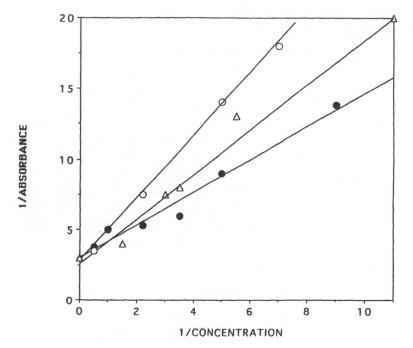

FIG. 10 Affinity of merocyanine monomer by bilayers subjected to hypotonic and hypertonic stress. The double reciprocal plots of monomer absorbance and merocyanine concentration for liposomes in isotonic ($\triangle$), hypertonic ($\bigcirc$) and hypotonic ($\bullet$) solutions were obtained by titrating liposomes in different osmotic states with merocyanine.

Thus,

$$\Delta A = N(K_m c_b \exp(F\chi/RT)/[1 + K_m c_b \exp(F\chi/RT)] \tag{4}$$

The double reciprocal plots corresponding to isosmotic and hypertonic conditions plotted in Fig. 10 according to Eq. (4), denotes that the surface properties of the external bilayer of shrunken liposomes have a different affinity for merocyanine 540 in comparison to that in isotonic conditions. The dissociation constants obtained from double reciprocal plots of a Langmuir type adsorption isotherm are 7.5×10^{-5} M and 14.0×10^{-5} M for the isotonic and the hypertonic conditions, respectively [53].

The value of the slope for the hypertonic conditions is displaced from that corresponding to the isotonic one by a $\Delta\chi = 6.6$ mV. This is in agreement with the behavior with temperature shown by the dipole potential and merocyanine in Fig. 4, indicating that bilayer dipole potential increases with packing when going from the fluid to the gel state. Thus, fluid bilayers of vesicles shrunken in hypertonic media show a higher dipole potential.

III.   DISCUSSION: INTERFACIAL CONTRIBUTIONS
TO THE ACTIVATION ENERGY

A.   Surface Potential Contributions to Permeability

There are several pieces of evidence indicating that the surface electrical properties of the bilayer affect the permeation rate of noncharged solutes. Permeability of water and nonelectrolytes are affected by the electrical charges present in the membrane surface. The water permeability of liposomes in the fluid state increases with the zeta potential of the negatively charged liposomes subjected to hypertonic stress [54]. In coincidence with these results, bilayers made with phosphatidylcholine and phosphatidylserine show an increase in the osmotic water permeability with pH [41]. Thus, the barrier for permeation of a noncharged molecule is influenced by the charges in the surface. These facts are not new, but has been ignored in the context of interpreting permeability in heterogeneous structures such as lipid interfaces [55].

In another line of investigation, our results show that the hypertonic stress affects the activation energy for permeation of nonelectrolytes across neutral phospholipid bilayers in parallel to changes in the surface properties related to water polarization.

The measurement of the dipole potential by means of the merocyanine absorbance allow to show that the surface changes occur within times comparable to those in which permeation occurs. The simultaneous determination of the volume changes with the changes at the interface are shown in Fig. 11. It is observed that the increase of shrinkage promotes a decrease of the absorbance at 570 nm corresponding to the merocyanine monomer. The decrease of the partition of the dye into the membrane with the osmotic stress denotes an increase in the packing of the membrane interface.

Thus, the changes in the surface properties as measured with merocyanine should be related to the changes in the activation energy.

As shown in Table 2, the activation energy for erythritol permeation decreases from 21 to 16.1 kcal/mol and from 18 to 11 kcal/mol for glycerol when the bilayer is subjected to a hypertonic stress. The difference between the activation energies in the isotonic and the hypertonic state requires to redefine the process of activation. For this purpose, the changes in the surface properties should be considered. As shown in Fig. 12, the logarithm of permeability for water is linear with the surface potential of liposomes subjected to hypertonic stress [54]. From this correlation it is immediate to deduce that permeability is a function of the surface potential according to

$$P = P^\circ \, e^{\alpha F \Delta V / RT} \tag{5}$$

where P° is the permeability of solutes in the absence of surface potential. The decrease of the activation energies for water permeation in membranes in the gel state when trehalose is intercalated (Table 1) suggests that the polar head

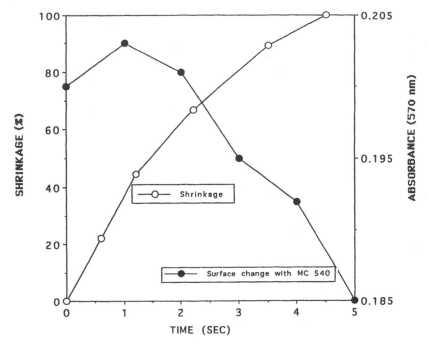

FIG. 11 Changes in vesicles volume and in surface properties. Vesicles were dispersed in hypertonic solution and shrinkage followed by light scattering at 600 nm. Simultaneously the absorbance at 570 nm for merocyanine was registered.

group region is involved, at least in part, in the control of water permeation. The factor α affecting the dipole potential in the argument of the exponential accounts for the symmetry of the water exchange at the interface and the possible orientation states of the dipoles.

This approach to interpret the permeability of water can be generalized for other polar permeants such glycerol and erythritol. Although these permeants are noncharged, it seems that the osmotic shock affects the barrier of activation energy. In this case, the surface properties of neutral phospholipid bilayers seem to be affected by the osmotic stress. According to the changes in the surface observed with merocyanine 540, they can be related with the polarization of the interface. The organization of water dipoles in the surface can be an additional physical barrier to the solute penetration. The jump of the permeant solute from the water to the membrane phase needs, as shown in Sec. 2.A, energy to break the hydrogen bonds with the surrounding molecules and to displace (or reorganize) water molecules. The possibility of the solute to form hydrogen bonds with the membrane interface and to eliminate water

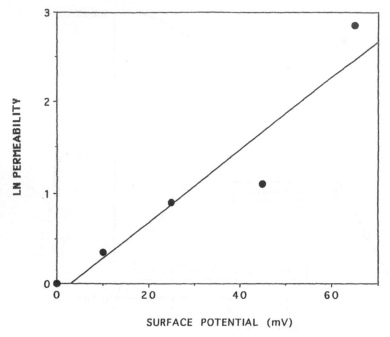

FIG. 12 Permeability of water as a function of the electrokinetic potential of MLVs (multilayer vesicles).

molecules from the interface would be favored by the osmotic shrinkage.

The experimental results shown above strongly suggest that the permeability coefficient cannot longer be interpreted unless the changes at the interface induced by osmosis are considered. The fine structure seems to be related to the reorganization of water at the interface. This water polarized at the interface determines the dipole potential [21]. In addition, the initiation step in the kink formation in the model formulated by Haines and Liebowitz [42] is considered to be a reaccomodation in the polar head groups. Thus, the osmotic extrusion of water from the membrane interface may alter the adsorption of the permeant in the first stage of permeation.

To redefine the permeability coefficient in the light of these results we must recall Eq. (2) in Sec. I.C.

$$J = D/\delta(C_2' - C_1')$$

As discussed, the partition of a nonelectrolyte cannot be described neglecting the interfacial properties. Thus, the concentration of solute in the bulk hydrocarbon phase (C') and in the head group region (C_i) is given by $K = C'/C_i$. The concentration in the head group region can be related to that in the bulk aqueous phase by considering that the water organized at the interphase affects the solubility in this region. This can be treated in a similar way as occurring in a surface in which the interface promotes a polarization by concentration. Thus, to surmount the interface and to reach the hydrocarbon region the solute must overcome an additional activation barrier. As we have measured changes in the activation barrier in parallel to changes in the dipole potential the permeability can be expressed as in Eq. (5) introducing an exponential factor in which the surface potential is included. The distribution of permeant between the bulk water phase and the interface can be expressed as affected by the water dipole arranged at the interface which has been experimentally determined as the dipole potential $(\Delta\chi)$:

$$C_i = C \exp[\alpha F\chi/(RT)]$$

where C_i and C are the permeant concentration at the water phase near the interface and in the bulk solution, respectively. The factor α now accounts for the symmetry factor of the water-permeant competition at the interface and the different orientations of water and permeant dipoles at the interface.

Thus, the partition coefficient of the permeant between the membrane phase and the water adjacent to the bilayer is given by

$$K = C'/C_i = C'/C \exp[\alpha F\chi/(RT)]$$

from where C' can be obtained and introduced in Eq. (2) giving

$$J = (D/\delta)K \exp[\alpha F\chi/(RT)]\Delta C$$

Thus the redefined permeability coefficient is

$$P^* = P \exp[\alpha F \Delta\chi/(RT)]$$

where P is the permeability coefficient defined in Eq. (3) for $\Delta\chi = 0$. This equation is analogous to Eq. (5).

The permeability expressed as an activated process becomes

$$P^* = A \, e^{-Ea/RT} \, e^{\alpha F\chi/RT} \tag{6}$$

where A is the preexponential factor of the Arrhenius equation.

From this equation, the difference between the activation energies for glycerol and erythritol in isotonic and hypertonic conditions gives a value of 491 mV for the surface potential. This value is displaced to positive values when compared to that for dipalmitoylphosphatidylcholine in the fluid state as shown in Fig. 4. Thus, the same conclusion as that deduced from the experiments with the surface dye probe merocyanine can be obtained from the analysis of permeability. The osmotic shrinkage produces a change of the dipole potential to positive values. This displacement in the interfacial properties decreases the barrier of activation for solute permeation.

IV. SUMMARY AND CONCLUSIONS

Water is an essential component of living cells. Many processes by which cells are dehydrated, such as liophylization, freeze-thaw and dessication, affect cellular structures in general and plasma membranes in particular [62]. Water is essential to maintain the semipermeable characteristics and structural integrity of the plasma membrane as requisite to survival.

In addition, water exchange in a living cell provides the adequate homeostatic equilibrium for cellular functions. In this regard, water is transfered across cell membranes in three different ways: (1) through diffusion across the lipid bilayer; (2) through transport proteins, and (3) through specialized water channel proteins [42,56–58].

In this chapter, the first mechanism of transference has been analyzed in relation to the more general process of nonelectrolyte permeation. Although the rate of transport in lipid bilayers is much more slow than through the water channels, its importance resides on its relation with the permeation of polar molecules with a very low partition in the lipid phase. These compounds, such glycerol, erythritol and ethylenglycol are known to be effective cryoprotectants, the mechanism of its action appearing to be the water replacement at the lipid structure.

A considerable amount of information allows us to conclude that water, localized at the head groups, is exchanged when solute adsorption or an osmotic extrusion are produced. In this chapter, we have shown that both factors affect the dipole potential, mainly established by the polarization of water molecules.

In general, it can be considered that the permeation process in a lipid bilayer is due to local perturbations involving the rearrangements of the hydrogen bond lattice. This way of seeing permeability denotes that the permeation phenomenon affects, at least in part, the bilayer stability, understanding for this the preservation of the barrier properties.

The permeability of water and non electrolytes is affected by the changes in the surface potential of the bilayer interface. The effect seems to be related to the organization of the water at the polar head group regions since surface potential varies accordingly to factors that alter the hydration of the bilayer. Among these, the effect of trehalose and the osmotic shrinkage has been tested. In consequence, a model explaining permeation as depending on the interfacial properties is described by including a term for the dipole potential in the permeability coefficient.

In the light of this analysis, the lipid bilayer cannot be considered as a single static slab separating two compartments. The osmotic stress and the interaction of solutes with the membrane interface appear to induce an exchange between stationary and nonstationary water modifying the solubility properties of the bilayers for solutes in a dynamical way. This dynamical response of the bilayer is a more complex process than that described by a passive solubility–diffusion mechanism. According to recent analysis of molecular dynamics simulation [30], the lipid bilayer is better described as a complex polymer matrix rather than a continuous hydrocarbon phase. The results presented in this chapter are congruent with that viewpoint. Shrinkage and water exchange affect the surface free energy of the material changing its sorption properties to water and other penetrant molecules. This is a well known property of polymeric structures.

The complete understanding of the physicochemical response of a bilayer deserves more detailed theoretical and experimental studies.

REFERENCES

1. H. Goldfine, N. C. Johnston, J. Mattai, and G. G. Shipley, Biochemistry 26:2814 (1987).
2. H. Hauser, I. Pascher, R. H. Pearson, and S. Sundell, Biochim. Biophys. Acta 650:21 (1981).
3. P. Cullis and M. J. Hope, in Biochemistry of Lipids and Membranes (D. E. Vance and J. E. Vance, eds), Benjamin/Cummings, Menlo Park, California, 1985, pp. 25–72.
4. M. W. Tate, E. F. Eikenberry, D. C. Turner, E. Shyamsunder, and S. M. Gruner, Chem. Phys. Lipids 57:147 (1991).
5. L. Rilfors, G. Lindbrom, A. Wieslander, and A. Christiansson, Biomembranes 12:205 (1984).
6. P. R. Cullis and B. de Kruijff, Biochem. Biophys. Acta 513:31 (1978).
7. J. N. Israelachvili, S. Marcelja, and R. G. Horn, Q. Rev. Biophys. 13:121 (1980).
8. D. P. Siegel, Biophys. J. 49:1155 (1986).
9. P. Steponkus, M. Uemura, and M. S. Webb, in Permeability and Stability of Lipid Bilayers, (E. A. Disalvo and S. A. Simon, eds.), CRC Press, Florida, 1995, pp. 77–104.
10. E. A. Disalvo, A. M. Campos, E. Abuin, and E. A. Lissi, Chem. Phys. Lipids 84:35 (1996).
11. E. A. Disalvo, L. I. Viera, L. S. Bakas, and G. A. Senisterra, J. Colloid Interface Sci. 178:417 (1996).
12. J. Crank, The Mathematics of Diffusion, Clarendon Press, Oxford, 1975.
13. N. A. Peppas and D. L. Meadows, J. Membrane Sci. 16:361 (1983).
14. S. H. White and M. C. Wiener, in Permeability and Stability of Lipid Bilayers, (E. A. Disalvo and S. A. Simon, eds.), CRC Press, Florida, 1995, pp. 1–20.
15. M. C. Wiener, R. M. Suter, and J. F. Nagle, Biophys. J. 55:315 (1989).
16. E. A. Disalvo and J. de Gier, Chem. Phys. Lipids 32:39 (1983).
17. R. C. McDonald and S. A. Simon, Proc. Natl. Acad. Sci. USA 84:4089 (1987).
18. P. Lelkes and I. R. Miller, J. Membrane Biol. 52:1 (1980).
19. J. C. Smith, Biochim. Biophys. Acta 1016:1 (1990).
20. J. Seelig, Biochim. Biophys. Acta 515:105 (1978).
21. K. Gawrisch, D. Ruston, J. Zimmerberg, V. A. Parsegian, R. P. Rand, and N. Fuller, Biophysical J. 61:1213 (1992).

22. K. Nicklas, J. Bocker, M. Schlenkrich, J. Brickman, and P. Bopp, Biophys. J. *60*:261 (1991).
23. R. F. Flewelling and W. L. Hubbel, Biophys. J. *49*:541 (1986).
24. J. O'M. Bockris and A. K. N. Reddy, *Modern Electrochemistry*, 2nd Ed., Plenum Press, New York, 1997.
25. A. Nayeem, S. B. Rananavare, V. S. S. Sastry, and J. H. Freed, J. Chem. Phys. *96*:3912 (1992).
26. M. J. Jaycock and M. Parfitt, *Chemistry of Interfaces*, Ellis Horwood Series in Physical Chemistry, Ellis Horwood Ltd, Chichester, UK, 1981.
27. W. R. Lieb and W. D. Stein, Nature *224*:240 (1969).
28. Y. Katz and J. M. Diamond, J. Membrane Biol. *17*:101 (1974).
29. T. R. Stouch and D. Bassolino, in *Biological Membranes* (K. Merz and B. Roux, eds.), Burkhauser, Boston, 1996, pp. 255–278.
30. S. J. Marrink, R. M. Sok, and H. J. C. Berendsen, J. Chem. Phys. *104*:9090 (1996).
31. R. V. McDaniel, T. J. McIntosh, and S. A. Simon, Biochim. Biophys. Acta *731*:97 (1983).
32. J. de Gier, J. G. Mandersloot, J. V. Hupkes, R. N. M. Mc Elhaney, and N. P. van Beek, Biochim. Biophys. Acta *223*:610 (1971).
33. D. M. Miller, Biochim. Biophys. Acta *1065*:75 (1991).
34. E. A. Disalvo, Adv. Colloid Interface Sci. *29*:141 (1988).
35. E. A. Lissi, E. Abuin, M. Saez, A. Zanucco and E. A. Disalvo, Langmuir *8*:348 (1992).
36. U. Essman, L. Perera, and M. Berkowitz, Langmuir *11*:4519 (1995).
37. S. J. Marrinck and M. Berkowitz, in *Permeability and Stability of Lipid Bilayers* (E. A. Disalvo and S. A. Simon, eds.), CRC Press, Florida, 1995, Chapter 2, pp. 21–48.
38. P. Meares, Phil. Trans. R. Soc. London *B278*:113 (1977).
39. E. A. Disalvo, Chem. Phys. Lipids *37*:385 (1985).
40. R. Lawaczeck, J. Membrane Biol. *51*:229 (1979).
41. J. P. Reeves and R. M. Dowben, J. Membrane Biol. *3*:123 (1970).
42. T. H. Haines and L. S. Liebowitz, in *Permeability and Stability of Lipid Bilayers* (E. A. Disalvo and S. A. Simon, eds.), CRC Press, Florida, 1995, pp. 123–136.
43. A. S. Rudolph and J. H. Crowe, Cryobiology *22*:367 (1985).
44. S. Alonso-Romanowski, A. C. Biondi, and E. A. Disalvo, J. Membrane Biol. *108*:1 (1989).
45. L. I. Viera, S. Alonso-Romanowski, V. Borovyagin, M. R. Feliz, and E. A. Disalvo, Biochim. Biophys. Acta *1145*:157 (1993).
46. J. H. Crowe, L. M. Crowe, and D. Chapman, Science *223*:701 (1984).
47. B. E. Cohen, J. Membrane Biol. *20*:205 (1975).
48. M. C. Blok, L. L. M. van Deenen, and J. de Gier, Biochim. Biophys. Acta *433*:1 (1976).
49. A. C. Biondi and E. A. Disalvo, Biochim. Biophys. Acta *1028*:43 (1990).
50. J. Y. A. Lehtonen and P. K. J. Kinnunen, Biophys. J. *60*:1981 (1994).
51. J. Arroyo, A. C. Biondi de Lopez, D. L. Bernik, and E. A. Disalvo, J. Colloid Interface Sci. *203*:106 (1998).
52. T. Aiuchi and Y. Kobatake, J. Membrane Biol. *45*:233 (1979).

53. A. C. Biondi, M. R. Feliz, and E. A. Disalvo, Biochim. Biophys. Acta *1069*:5 (1991).
54. A. D. Bangham, J. de Gier, and G. G. Greville, Chem. Phys. Lipids *1*:225 (1967).
55. D. E. Graham and E. J. Lea, Biochim. Biophys. Acta *274*:286 (1972).
56. A. S. Verkman, *Water Channels*, R. G. Landes Co., New York, 1993.
57. J. Fischbarg, K. Y. Kuang, and J. C. Vera et al., Proc. Natl. Acad. Sci. USA. *87*:3244 (1990).
58. E. A. Disalvo, E. A. Siddiqi, and T. H. Tien, in *Water Transport in Biological Membranes*, (G. Benga, ed.) CRC Press, Boca Raton, Florida, 1989, Vol. 1, Chapter 3.
59. J. M. Diamond and Y. Katz, J. Membrane Biol. *17*:121 (1974).
60. G. Beschiaschvili and J. Seelig, Biochemistry *31*:10044 (1992).
61. J. H. Crowe and L. M. Crowe, Cryobiology *19*:317 (1982).
62. W. J. Gordon-Kamn and P. L. Steponkus, Protoplasm *123*:83 (1984).
63. S. A. Simon and T. J. McIntosh, Proc. Natl. Acad. Sci. USA *86*:9263 (1989).
64. J. C. Walter and J. Gutknecht, J. Membrane Biol. *90*:207 (1986).

22

Surface Electrostatics of Biological Membranes and Ion Binding

SUREN A. TATULIAN Department of Molecular Physiology and Biological Physics, University of Virginia Health Sciences Center, Charlottesville, Virginia

Abstract

Electrostatic properties of biological membranes and ion adsorption at their surfaces play regulatory roles in many cellular processes, such as cell adhesion, binding of ligands, ion transport and excitability and others. Therefore, the theory of surface electrostatics and concepts of ion binding to membranes can be used to interpret a wide variety of phenomena at the molecular or cellular levels. Here the theory of surface electrostatics is presented in a comprehensive manner, with a specific tribute to the quantitative description of ion–membrane interactions. The thermotropic effects on membrane electrostatics and ion binding are briefly discussed. The roles of surface electrostatics and ion binding in some physiological processes in nerve, muscle and red blood cells are demonstrated. The available quantitative data on ion binding to artificial lipid bilayers and to biological membranes are summarized in several tables.

I. INTRODUCTION

Consideration of membrane electrostatics is important because the fixed surface charges at the membrane surface create extremely strong electrostatic fields which not only lead to considerable deviations from normal of such fundamental parameters as pH, ion concentrations, viscosity, dielectric constant, but also are able to induce conformational changes and reorientation of membrane-associating proteins and other molecules. The negative surface charge of biological membranes plays a catalytic role in the membrane binding of biologically active cationic species, such as anesthetics, ion channel antagonists, phospholipases, kinases and their substrates [1–11]. The difference in charge density or ion concentration at both sides of a membrane alters the potential drop inside the membrane thus affecting the translocation of charged species, nerve and muscle excitation, and probably the structure of integral membrane proteins. Proteins at a charged membrane surface are simultaneously exposed to a strong negative electrostatic field and are in a locally acidic environment, which in some cases leads to the formation of the molten globule conformation [12–14]. Changes in the cell surface components, such as glycosaminoglycans, proteoglycans, sialic acids and others during neoplastic transformations, inflammation or other pathological conditions lead to the alterations in cell surface charge density. This often significantly affects the "social behaviour" of the cells, i.e., their interactions with extracellular matrix components and with surrounding tissues, including the metastatic potential of malignant cells [15–17]. The surface charge of artificial and biological membranes also ensures the colloidal stability of cells and vesicles [18,19]. Even in the absence of fixed or adsorbed charges at the membrane surface, the membrane–solution interface represents a unique environment where the properties of matter considerably deviate from those in the bulk [20]. The physiological environment of biomembranes is an electrolyte solution of complex ionic composition, and ions in general adsorb to membranes and thus alter their surface charge. Therefore ion binding to membranes is a coherent part of membrane electrostatics and it is very useful to consider these two themes together. Ion binding to biological and artificial membranes affects not only their surface charge density, but also membrane structure, hydration, fluidity, phase transitions, conductivity, adhesion, aggregation and fusion capabilities and many others [21–41].

Negative electrostatic potential at membrane surface is essential for membrane binding and activation of cationic enzymes, such as secretory phospholipase A_2 (PLA_2) [2,4,9,10]. Addition of acidic lipids or detergents to zwitterionic lipid membranes substantially increases the binding and activity of secretory PLA_2s [2,10], and mutations of one or more Lys residues of the enzyme suppressed its membrane binding and activity [9,42]. These results strongly imply that the electrostatic interactions between the basic residues of secretory PLA_2s and the acidic lipids of the membrane play key roles in both membrane binding and activity of the enzyme.

Some enzymes involved in transmembrane signaling and other cellular processes, such as protein kinase C (PKC), phospholipase C, cytosolic PLA_2, mammalian lipoxygenases, are transiently bound to intracellular membranes and activated at elevated concentrations of Ca^{2+} during cell stimulation; Ca^{2+} serves as an ionic bridge between the enzymes and acidic lipids of the membrane [11,43–49]. At elevated intracellular Ca^{2+} concentrations during cell stimulation the cytosolic PLA_2 partitions to the intracellular membranes which results in a ~ 10-fold increase in the PLA_2 activity [43,50–55]. It was demonstrated that membrane binding of cytosolic PLA_2 was mediated by the N-terminal regulatory "Ca^{2+}-dependent lipid-binding" (CaLB) domain of the enzyme, which was independent of the C-terminal Ca^{2+} independent catalytic domain [44,56]. The CaLB domain of cytosolic PLA_2 exhibits up to 50% sequence homology with the membrane binding C_2 domains of other proteins, such as conventional PKC (i.e., the α, βI, βII and γ isozymes), phospholipase C-γ, synaptotagmin and some others [43,57]. Interestingly, upon activation of rat macrophages with a Ca^{2+} ionophore both cytosolic PLA_2 and the 5-lipoxygenase were shown to redistribute from the cytosol to the nuclear envelope [50]. In A23187-activated human neutrophils, the cytosolic PLA_2, 5-lipoxygenase and 5-lipoxygenase-activating protein were found colocalized in the nuclear membrane [58]. These findings demonstrate that Ca^{2+}-mediated membrane binding of these enzymes is essential for their efficient and coordinated functioning. There is strong evidence that the conventional PKCs are activated by Ca^{2+}-mediated binding to membranes containing phosphatidylserine (PS) and diacylglycerol (DAG) or phorbol ester [45,46,59,60]. The conserved C_2 (CaLB) domain of these enzymes is believed to interact with

PS via a Ca^{2+}-bridging mechanism and thus facilitate enzyme activation [11,45,46,61,62]. Replacement of two aspartic acid residues by arginines in the C_2 domain of PKC βII did not affect its ability to bind to bilayers containing PS in the absence of Ca^{2+}, but dramatically decreased both membrane binding of the enzyme and its catalytic activity in the presence of Ca^{2+}, providing further evidence for the Ca^{2+}-bridging mechanism of membrane binding of these proteins [11]. Clearly, the mechanisms of Ca^{2+}-dependent, interfacially activated enzymes cannot be fully understood before interaction of Ca^{2+} with membrane lipids is comprehensively examined, including the binding constants, binding stoichiometries, chemical groups directly involved in coordination, and accompanying electrostatic, (de)hydration and other effects.

As a fascinating example of the physiological importance of membrane electrostatics and ion binding, the mechanisms of membrane binding of secretory and cytosolic PLA_2s can be compared, keeping in mind that binding to membranes is a prerequisite for the activation of these enzymes. Secretory PLA_2s are cationic, and their binding to membranes is facilitated by direct interactions between basic residues of the enzyme and acidic lipids in the membrane [4,9]. The cytosolic enzymes interact with membranes using their CaLB domain, which carries excess negative charge [43,44,52]; Ca^{2+} ions bridge between the carboxyl oxygens of the side chains of Asp or Glu residues in the CaLB domain and the acidic lipids in the membrane. In spite of different mechanisms of membrane binding of the two types of enzyme, electrostatic effects at the membrane surface play crucial roles in both cases.

The aim of this review is to present the theory of membrane electrostatics and ion–membrane interactions with derivation of the most important relationships in a hope that this may help the others to interpret various membrane surface-related phenomena. Special attention is paid to the mechanism of Ca^{2+} binding to PS membranes in view of its potential physiological importance. A number of examples of the importance of cell surface electrostatics and ion binding in various physiological processes are presented.

II. THEORY

A. The Poisson–Boltzmann Theory

The Poisson–Boltzmann (PB) theory (for recent reviews see Refs. 20, 63, 64) is based on two fundamental laws, i.e., that the spatial variation of the electrostatic field strength ($\mathbf{E}$) at point r is proportional to the charge density at that point (ρ), and that the electrochemical potential of any species i (μ_i) is spatially invariable. In the SI system, these can be written as:

$$\text{div } \mathbf{E} = \rho(r)/\varepsilon\varepsilon_0, \tag{1}$$

and

$$\mu_i(r) = z_i e\psi(r) + kT \ln \chi_i(r) = \text{const} \tag{2}$$

Equation (2) is written using a system of reference where the standard chemical potential is zero. In Eqs. (1) and (2) div (short form of divergence) is $\partial/\partial x + \partial/\partial y + \partial/\partial z$, ε is the dielectric constant, ε_0 the permittivity of free space, ψ the mean-field electrostatic potential, z_i the valence number of charged species i, including sign, e the elementary charge, χ_i the mole fraction if the species i, k the Boltzmann constant, T the absolute temperature, and r the coordinate. The dielectric constant is supposed to be coordinate-independent in Eq. (1). Considering that $\mathbf{E} = -\text{grad } \psi$, Eq. (1) can be re-written as:

$$\text{div } (-\text{grad } \psi) = \rho(r)/\varepsilon\varepsilon_0 \tag{3}$$

Replacement of div grad in Eq. (3) by the Laplace operator, $\Delta = \partial^2/\partial x^2 + \partial^2/\partial y^2 + \partial^2/\partial z^2$ gives the Poisson equation:

$$\Delta\psi(r) = -\rho(r)/\varepsilon\varepsilon_0 \tag{4}$$

If there is excess charge at point r, it creates an electrostatic potential $\psi(r)$, which dissipates at infinity: $\psi(\infty) = 0$. With this boundary condition, Eq. (2) can be written in the form:

$$z_i e\psi(r) + kT \ln \chi_i(r) = kT \ln \chi_i(\infty). \tag{5}$$

Rearranging Eq. (5) using the approximation $n_i(r)/n_i(\infty) = \chi_i(r)/\chi_i(\infty)$, where n_i is the number concentration of the species i, we obtain the Boltzmann formula for the distribution of ions in an electrostatic field:

$$n_i(r) = n_i(\infty)\exp\left[-\frac{z_i e\psi(r)}{kT}\right] \tag{6}$$

or, in terms of charge density:

$$\rho_i(r) = z_i en_i(\infty)\exp\left[-\frac{z_i e\psi(r)}{kT}\right] \tag{7}$$

It is seen from Eqs. (6) and (7) that the concentration of coions [$\text{sgn}(z_i) = \text{sgn}(\psi)$] decreases and that of counterions [$\text{sgn}(z_i) = -\text{sgn}(\psi)$] increases near a charged surface adjacent to an electrolyte solution. Interpretation of the Boltzmann relation depends on the meaning of the potential in the exponent. Here the ions are supposed to be involved only in coulombic interactions, hence their distribution is determined by the electrostatic potential $\psi(r)$. In reality, higher order interactions of electrostatic character (ion–dipole, ion–induced dipole, dipole–dipole ...), as well as electrodynamic (such as the dispersion component of the van der Waals interactions) and indirect (i.e., through-solvent) interactions are equally effective. In general, the potential should include all types of force fields.

For a flat interface, described by the yz plane, Eq. (7) becomes one-dimensional. The total charge density at distance x from the charged wall is:

$$\rho(x) = \sum z_i\, en_i(\infty)\exp\left[-\frac{z_i\, e\psi(x)}{kT}\right] \tag{8}$$

Equation (8) and the one-dimensional version of Eq. (4):

$$\frac{d^2\psi(x)}{dx^2} = -\frac{\rho(x)}{\varepsilon\varepsilon_0} \tag{9}$$

yield the one-dimensional PB equation:

$$\frac{d^2\psi(x)}{dx^2} = -\frac{1}{\varepsilon\varepsilon_0}\sum z_i\, en_i(\infty)\exp\left[-\frac{z_i\, e\psi(x)}{kT}\right] \tag{10}$$

where summation is over all charged species.

The PB theory relies on somewhat oversimplified assumptions. The charge is assumed to be uniformly smeared over the surface, so the effects due to discreteness of charge are neglected. The ions in the aqueous phase are treated as point charges, implying that all interactions besides the long-range coulombic forces are neglected. This leads to infinite interaction energies at contact and unreasonably high counterion concentrations near charged surfaces. The "image charge" effects are ignored. The solvent is treated as a structureless dielectric continuum, and no dielectric saturation effects are considered. The ion correlation effects are neglected as well. Consequently, the primitive PB theory is based on inaccurate assumptions and therefore should not be able to adequately describe the real systems, especially the complex biological membranes. However, the unmodified PB theory, as well as the derived Gouy–Chapman (GC) theory, describe the electrostatic behavior of biological and artificial membranes surprisingly well [20,65,66]. This is because various corrections outweigh each other and therefore the modifications do not affect the final result considerably.

B. The Gouy–Chapman Theory

The GC theory [67,68] (for review see Refs. 20, 64–66) relates the surface charge density to the surface potential and other parameters of the system. Multiplying Eq. (10) by $d\psi$ and integrating from ∞ to 0 taking into account that at $x = \infty$ $\psi = 0$ and $d\psi/dx = 0$, we obtain:

$$\left[\frac{d\psi(x)}{dx}\right]^2_{x=0} = \frac{2kT}{\varepsilon\varepsilon_0}\sum n_i(\infty)\left[\exp\left(\frac{-z_i\, e\psi_0}{kT}\right) - 1\right] \tag{11}$$

where ψ_0 is the electrostatic potential at the interface.

According to the principle of electroneutrality, the fixed charge of the interface (σ_0) should be compensated by the mobile charges in the solution:

$$\sigma_0 = -\int_0^\infty \rho(x)\, dx \tag{12}$$

Substituting $\rho(x)$ from Eq. (9) and executing integration using the boundary condition $[d\psi(x)/dx]_{x=\infty} = 0$, we obtain

$$\left[\frac{d\psi(x)}{dx}\right]_{x=0} = -\frac{\sigma_0}{\varepsilon\varepsilon_0} \tag{13}$$

Equations (11) and (13) yield*.

$$\sigma_0 = \sqrt{2\varepsilon\varepsilon_0 kT \sum n_i(\infty)\left[\exp\left(\frac{-z_i e\psi_0}{kT}\right) - 1\right]} \tag{14}$$

In the case when the aqueous phase contains only "symmetric" electrolytes, i.e., when all cations have the same valency, z_+, and all anions the valency $z_- = -z_+ \equiv Z$, Eq. (14) is simplified to:

$$\sigma_0 = 2\sqrt{2\varepsilon\varepsilon_0 kTn(\infty)} \sinh \frac{Ze\psi_0}{2kT} \tag{15}$$

where $n(\infty)$ is the total concentration of the electrolyte.

The dependence between the surface charge density and the surface potential is depicted in Fig. 1 for 1:1, 2:2, 1:2 and 2:1 electrolytes. For a given charge density, increasing the valence number of a symmetric electrolyte by a factor of n results in an n-fold decrease in the surface potential. Since the counterions prevail at the charged surface, their effect on ψ_0 is much stronger than that of the coions. The effect of coions further decreases with increasing charge of counterions.

At very small potentials, when $\phi_0 \equiv e\psi_0/kT \ll 1$, the series expansion of the exponent in Eq. (14) up to the quadratic term yields:

$$\sigma_0 = \sqrt{2\varepsilon\varepsilon_0 kT \sum n_i(\infty)(-z_i \phi_0 + 0.5z_i^2\phi_0^2)} \tag{16}$$

Taking into account that, according to the principle of electroneutrality in the bulk phase, $\sum z_i n_i(\infty) = 0$, and that $0.5 \sum z_i^2 n_i(\infty)$ is the ionic strength (I), Eq. (16) becomes:

$$\sigma_0 = \phi_0 \sqrt{2\varepsilon\varepsilon_0 kTI} \tag{17}$$

C. Spatial Profile of the Potential

The distribution of the electrostatic potential in the electrolyte solution along the normal to the flat interface can be obtained by integration of the PB equation. This is easy to do for a symmetric electrolyte [69,70], in which case the

---

* Equation (14) was first published by Hans Müller [69]. However, this equation is repeatedly and erroneously attributed to David Grahame, who presented this equation in a review [70], giving the reference to the original paper by Müller [69].

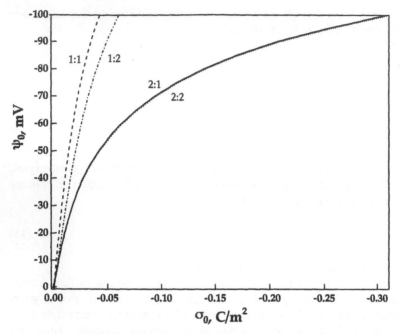

FIG. 1 Relationship between membrane surface charge density, σ_0 and surface potential ψ_0, calculated by Eq. (14). In all cases 10 mM electrolyte is present, $T = 20°C$. The valence type of electrolytes is indicated as $i:j$, where i is the valence (or charge) number of the counterion and j is that of the coion.

PB equation reads:

$$\frac{d^2\psi(x)}{dx^2} = -\frac{Zen(\infty)}{\varepsilon\varepsilon_0}\left[\exp\left(-\frac{Ze\psi(x)}{kT}\right) - \exp\left(\frac{Ze\psi(x)}{kT}\right)\right]$$

$$= \frac{2Zen(\infty)}{\varepsilon\varepsilon_0}\sinh\frac{Ze\psi(x)}{kT} \tag{18}$$

Multiplying Eq. (18) by $2d\psi(x)/dx$ and substituting $[2d\psi(x)/dx][d^2\psi(x)/dx^2]$ by $(d/dx)[d\psi(x)/dx]^2$, we obtain:

$$\frac{d}{dx}\left[\frac{d\psi(x)}{dx}\right]^2 = \frac{4Zen(\infty)}{\varepsilon\varepsilon_0}\sinh\frac{Ze\psi(x)}{kT}\frac{d\psi(x)}{dx} \tag{19}$$

Multiplying Eq. (19) by dx and integrating from 0 to $\psi(x)$ we then obtain:

$$\left[\frac{d\psi(x)}{dx}\right]^2 = \frac{4kTn(\infty)}{\varepsilon\varepsilon_0}\left[\cosh\frac{Ze\psi(x)}{kT} - 1\right] \tag{20}$$

or, using the identity $\cosh x \equiv 2(\sinh x/2)^2 + 1$,

$$\frac{d\psi(x)}{dx} = -\sqrt{\frac{8kTn(\infty)}{\varepsilon\varepsilon_0}} \sinh \frac{Ze\psi(x)}{2kT} \tag{21}$$

In Eq. (21) the negative sign is chosen to ensure that $d\psi(x)/dx$ and $\psi(x)$ have opposite signs, i.e., the absolute value of the potential decreases with distance from the charged wall. Using the identity $\sinh x \equiv 2 \sinh x/2 \cosh x/2$ and introducing $\phi(x) \equiv e\psi(x)/kT$, Eq. (21) acquires the form:

$$\frac{dZ\phi(x)/4}{\sinh Z\phi(x)/4 \cosh Z\phi(x)/4} = -Ze\sqrt{\frac{2n(\infty)}{\varepsilon\varepsilon_0 kT}} dx \tag{22}$$

Taking into account that $dx/\sinh x \cosh x = d \tanh x/\tanh x$, Eq. (22) becomes:

$$\frac{d \tanh[Z\phi(x)/4]}{\tanh[Z\phi(x)/4]} = -\kappa \, dx \tag{23}$$

where $\kappa = 1/\lambda$, and

$$\lambda = \sqrt{\frac{\varepsilon\varepsilon_0 kT}{e^2 \sum z_i^2 n_i(\infty)}} \tag{24}$$

is the Debye screening length. Integration of Eq. (23) from 0 to x yields:

$$\tanh[Z\phi(x)/4] = \tanh[Z\phi_0/4]\exp(-\kappa x), \tag{25}$$

where ϕ_0 is the dimensionless surface potential.

Using the approximation $\tanh x \approx x$ for $x \ll 1$, we find the potential distribution for low surface potentials:

$$\phi(x) = \phi_0 \exp(-\kappa x) \tag{26}$$

For very high surface potentials, $\tanh[Z\phi_0/4] \approx 1$. Since far from the surface the potentials are low irrespective of the surface potential, $\tanh[Z\phi(x)/4] \approx Z\phi(x)/4$. Therefore the potential distribution far from highly charged surfaces does not depend on the actual surface potential:

$$\phi(x) = \frac{4}{Z} \exp(-\kappa x) \tag{27}$$

The exact solution of PB equation is also available for some cases of asymmetric electrolytes. Thus, for 1:2 and 2:1 (i.e., monovalent counterion, divalent coion and divalent counterion, monovalent coion) electrolytes [71]:

$$\tanh\{v[\phi(x)]/4\} = \tanh[v(\phi_0)/4]\exp(-\kappa x) \tag{28}$$

where $v = \pm \ln\{[2 \exp(\pm\phi) + 1]/3\}$, and the plus and minus signs apply to 1:2 and 2:1 electrolytes, respectively. Potential distributions in the presence of electrolytes of more complex valence type have been treated elsewhere [72,73].

Figure 2 presents the distribution of surface potential along the normal to the charged wall calculated using the approximation (26) and the precise equations (25) and (28). For symmetric electrolytes, the potential decays with distance from the charged wall steeper than predicted by the simple exponential function. The situation is different for asymmetric electrolytes. In this case, the potential drop is much steeper for $|z_j| > |z_i|$ and less steeper for $|z_j| < |z_i|$ as compared to the approximation (26) (the subscripts i and j refer to the counterion and the coion, respectively).

Having determined the potential distribution along the normal to the interface, $\psi(x)$, the distribution of the counterions and coions can easily be calculated by the Boltzmann relationship [Eq. (6)]. The distributions of ions of different valence type in a 10 Mm salt solution adjacent to a flat charged surface with $\sigma_0 = -0.1e/nm^2$ are presented in Fig. 3. The concentration of the counterions (cations, in this case) increases and that of the coions (anions) decreases towards the charged surface. In the case of symmetric electrolytes

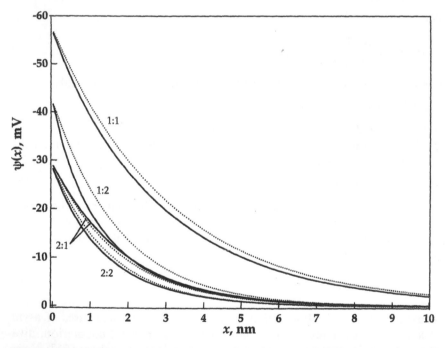

FIG. 2 The profile of electrostatic potential along the normal to a surface with a charge density $\sigma_0 = -0.1 \ e/nm^2$ ($= -0.016022 \ C/m^2$). In all cases 10 mM electrolyte is present, $T = 20°C$. The valence type of the electrolyte is indicated near each pair of curves. The dotted lines are calculated using the exponential approximation [Eq. (26)]. The solid lines for $1:1$ and $2:2$ electrolytes are calculated by Eq. (25), and the solid lines for the asymmetric electrolytes are calculated by Eq. (28).

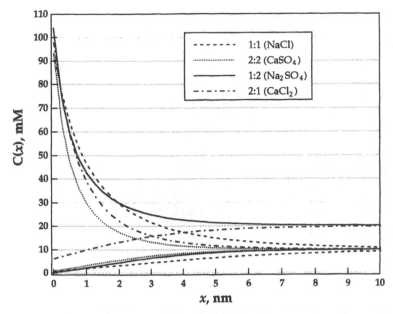

FIG. 3 The profiles of ion concentrations along the normal to the membrane surface, simulated according to the Boltzmann relation [Eq. (6)] using the surface potentials calculated by Eqs. (25) and (28). A negatively charged membrane with $\sigma_0 = -0.1 \; e/nm^2$ $(= -0.016022 \; C/m^2)$ is considered. The electrolyte concentration in the bulk solution is 10 mM. Note that the concentrations of the cations increase and those of the anions decrease towards the membrane surface.

(e.g. NaCl or $CaSO_4$), the interfacial concentrations of ions with like charges are similar independent of the valency because the increase in valency is compensated by the decrease in the surface potential so that the electrostatic energy of the ion at the interface, $z_i e \psi_0$, is constant. Also, the concentration gradient is steeper for a higher valency electrolyte because of a shorter Debye screening length [Eq. (24)].

D. The Gouy–Chapman–Stern Theory of Ion Binding

The ions in the electrolyte solution in contact with a dielectric with or without fixed surface charges interact with the (charged) surface not only by means of long-range coulombic forces. They can specifically bind to the chemical groups of the surface by means of short-range interactions, as well. Stern [74] introduced the compact layer, i.e., the layer between the (charged) wall ($x = 0$) and the plane of closest approach of dehydrated counterions ($x = b$) that specifically interact with the surface (Fig. 4). The plane $x = b$ is also known as the Stern layer, or the inner Helmholtz plane, while the plane $x = d$, i.e., that of

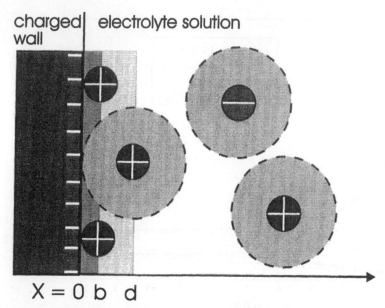

charged wall | electrolyte solution

X = 0 b d

FIG. 4 Schematic representation of a solid–fluid interface between a wall, carrying fixed negative charge at its surface (such as a lipid bilayer), and an electrolyte solution. The dashed circles indicate the hydration sphere of the ions. Two dehydrated cations are bound to the charged wall; they are supposed to form inner-sphere complexes with the chemical groups of the wall. One hydrated cation is adsorbed to the wall, forming an outer-sphere complex. The coordinate of the wall surface is $x = 0$, that of the plane of closest approach of dehydrated ions (the Stern or inner Helmhotz plane) is $x = b$, and that of the closest approach of hydrated ions (the outer Helmholtz plane) is $x = d$.

the closest approach of hydrated ions, which do not specifically interact with the surface, is referred to as the outer Helmholtz plane. The fixed charge at the surface and the adsorbed charges in the compact layer arise according to similar mechanisms. While the fixed surface charges owe to chemical binding (dissociation) of protons to (from) the chemical groups of the surface (*chemisorption*), the bound charge in the compact layer is thought to be created by physically adsorbed counterions (*physisorption*). In should be emphasized, however, that the ions in the Stern layer are involved in inner sphere complexes with the chemical groups of the surface. Therefore the binding of ions in the Stern layer may be accompanied with some overlap of outer shell electron orbitals and hence may have some covalent character. This does not apply to the ions in the outer Helmholtz plane, which are involved in outer sphere complexes. Following the logic of Langmuir adsorption model, we assume there is a finite number of binding sites per unit area of the wall. Then the process of ion binding to the wall can be described based on the mass action law:

$$S_f + I_f \rightarrow IS \tag{29}$$

where S_f, I_f, and IS stand for free site, free ion, and complex between the ion and the binding site, respectively. The association constant is defined as:

$$K = \frac{[IS]}{[S_f][I_f]} \tag{30}$$

where the square brackets indicate corresponding concentrations. Performing the following substitutions: $[IS] \equiv n_b$, $[I_f] \approx [I_{total}] \equiv n_i$, $[S_f] = [S_{total}] - [IS]$, and $[S_{total}] \equiv N$, and recalling that ions near the charged wall are distributed according to the Boltzmann law [Eq. (6)], Eq. (30) becomes:

$$n_b = \frac{NKn_i \exp\left(-\dfrac{z_i e\psi_b}{kT}\right)}{1 + Kn_i \exp\left(-\dfrac{z_i e\psi_b}{kT}\right)} \tag{31}$$

which represents the surface density of bound ions at the compact layer $(x = b)$. For the surface density of adsorbed charges we have:

$$\sigma_b = z_i e n_b = \frac{z_i eNKn_i \exp\left(-\dfrac{z_i e\psi_b}{kT}\right)}{1 + Kn_i \exp\left(-\dfrac{z_i e\psi_b}{kT}\right)} \tag{32}$$

It should be noted at this point that Eqs. (31) and (32) are derived assuming that the fraction of bound ions is negligible compared to the total ion concentration, which is true in most, but not all cases. In general, more than one ionic species may have affinity for the same binding sites; these ions are supposed to compete for binding. For two ionic species, i and k, the ion i can bind only to those sites which are not occupied by the species k:

$$n_{b,i} = \frac{(N - n_{b,k})K_i n_i \exp\left(-\dfrac{z_i e\psi_b}{kT}\right)}{1 + K_i n_i \exp\left(-\dfrac{z_i e\psi_b}{kT}\right)} \tag{33}$$

The proportion of bound species i and k will be determined by their binding constants and concentrations near the surface:

$$\frac{n_{b,i}}{n_{b,k}} = \frac{K_i n_i \exp\left(-\dfrac{z_i e\psi_b}{kT}\right)}{K_k n_k \exp\left(-\dfrac{z_k e\psi_b}{kT}\right)} \tag{34}$$

Substituting $n_{b,k}$ from Eq. (34) into Eq. (33) and solving the latter for $n_{b,i}$, we arrive at:

$$n_{b,i} = \frac{NK_i n_i \exp\left(-\dfrac{z_i e \psi_b}{kT}\right)}{1 + K_i n_i \exp\left(-\dfrac{z_i e \psi_b}{kT}\right) + K_k n_k \exp\left(-\dfrac{z_k e \psi_b}{kT}\right)} \tag{35}$$

In a more general case of competitive binding, when m ions are able to bind to the common sites, the density of total adsorbed charge is:

$$\sigma_b = \frac{Ne \displaystyle\sum_{j=1}^{m} z_j K_j n_j \exp\left(-\dfrac{z_j e \psi_b}{kT}\right)}{1 + \displaystyle\sum_{j=1}^{m} K_j n_j \exp\left(-\dfrac{z_j e \psi_b}{kT}\right)} \tag{36}$$

In many cases both cations and anions adsorb simultaneously to the same surface. If l different anions competitively bind to anion binding sites of density $N^{(-)}$ and m cations competitively bind to cation binding sites of density $N^{(+)}$, then:

$$\sigma_b = \frac{N^{(-)}e \displaystyle\sum_{j=1}^{l} z_j K_j n_j e^{-z_j \phi_b}}{1 + \displaystyle\sum_{j=1}^{l} K_j n_j e^{-z_j \phi_b}} + \frac{N^{(+)}e \displaystyle\sum_{i=1}^{m} z_i K_i n_i e^{-z_i \phi_b}}{1 + \displaystyle\sum_{i=1}^{m} K_i n_i e^{-z_i \phi_b}} \tag{37}$$

Now, the surface charge density is composed of the intrinsic charge, σ_0, and the adsorbed charge, σ_b. Using the sum of these in Eq. (14), we obtain the Gouy–Chapman–Stern (GCS) equation:

$$\frac{N^{(-)}e \displaystyle\sum_{j=1}^{l} z_j K_j n_j e^{-z_j \phi_b}}{1 + \displaystyle\sum_{j=1}^{l} K_j n_j e^{-z_j \phi_b}} + \frac{N^{(+)}e \displaystyle\sum_{i=1}^{m} z_i K_i n_i e^{-z_i \phi_b}}{1 + \displaystyle\sum_{i=1}^{m} K_i n_i e^{-z_i \phi_b}} + \sigma_0$$

$$= \mathrm{sgn}(\phi_b)\sqrt{2\varepsilon\varepsilon_0\, kT \sum n_k (e^{-z_k \phi_b} - 1)} \tag{38}$$

Thus, ions can not only shield the surface charge and decrease the surface potential by the GC mechanism. According to the GCS model, they can also affect the surface charge density by means of adsorption to the surface.

E. Dependence of Surface Potential on Ion Concentration

The parameters of ion binding, such as the binding constant and binding site density, can be determined based on the dependence of ψ_b on ion concentration. Therefore, description of the concentration dependence of ψ_b deserves a separate section. In the absence of ion binding, the surface potential monotonically decreases (in the absolute value) with increasing electrolyte concentration (Figs. 5 and 6, curve 1). Ion binding may lead to a variety of situations, including charge reversal and extrema in the dependence of the surface potential on ion concentration, as illustrated in Figs. 5–7. The charge reversal and the number of extrema depend on whether the signs of the intrinsic charge density, σ_0, and the charge number of the adsorbate, z_i, are similar or opposite. In the case of counterion binding, i.e. $\sigma_0/z_i < 0$, the dependence of ψ_b on log C_i (C_i is the molar concentration of the ion i) may exhibit no extremum if $|z_i eN| \leq |\sigma_0|$, or one extremum, if $|z_i eN| > |\sigma_0|$. In the first case, the surface potential decreases to zero more rapidly with increasing ion concentration than in the absence of ion binding (Figs. 5 and 6, curve 2). In the second case, the surface potential changes sign, passes through a maximum and then

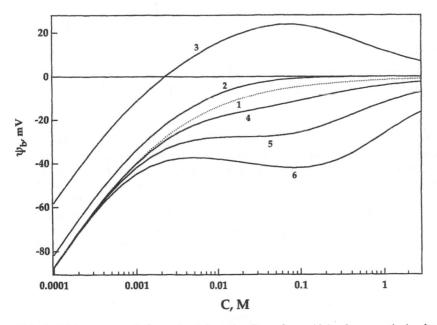

FIG. 5 Dependence of the potential at the Stern layer (ψ_b) of a negatively charged membrane ($\sigma_0 = -0.02$ $e/nm^2 = -3.2044$ mC/m^2) on the molar concentration of a 1:1 electrolyte at 20°C, calculated by Eq. (38). Curve 1: Gouy–Chapman screening without ion binding (no charge reversal, no extrema); curve 2: $K_i = 50$ M^{-1}, $K_j = 0$, $z_i eN = -\sigma_0$ (no charge reversal, no extrema); curve 3: $K_i = 50$ M^{-1}, $K_j = 0$, $z_i eN = -10\sigma_0$ (charge reversal and one extremum at $\psi_b > 0$); curve 4: $K_i = 0$, $K_j = 50$ M^{-1}, $z_j eN = 2\sigma_0$ (no charge reversal, no extrema); curve 5: $K_i = 0$, $K_j = 50$ M^{-1}, $z_i eN = 8\sigma_0$ (no charge reversal, no extrema, an inflection point with $d\psi_b/d$ log $C = 0$); curve 6: $K_i = 0$, $K_j = 50$ M^{-1}, $z_i eN = 20\sigma_0$ (no charge reversal, two extrema at $\psi_b < 0$). The subscripts i and j correspond to the cation and the anion, respectively.

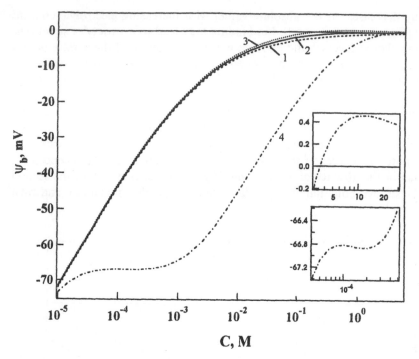

FIG. 6 Dependence of the potential at the Stern layer (ψ_b) of a negatively charged membrane ($\sigma_0 = -0.02\ e/\text{nm}^2 = -3.2044\ \text{mC/m}^2$) on the molar concentration of a 2:1 electrolyte (e.g. $CaCl_2$) at 20°C, calculated by Eq. (38). Curve 1: Gouy–Chapman screening without ion binding (no charge reversal, no extrema); curve 2: $K_i = 5\ M^{-1}$, $K_j = 0$, $z_i eN = -\sigma_0$ (no charge reversal, no extrema); curve 3: $K_i = 5\ M^{-1}$, $K_j = 0$, $z_i eN = -2\sigma_0$ (charge reversal and one extremum at $\psi_b > 0$); curve 4: $K_i = 2\ M^{-1}$, $K_j = 10^4\ M^{-1}$, $z_i eN = -24\sigma_0$, $z_j eN = 20\sigma_0$ (a charge reversal and three extrema, two at $\psi_b < 0$ and one at $\psi_b > 0$, as shown in two insets). The subscripts i and j correspond to the cation and the anion, respectively.

decreases to zero (Figs. 5 and 6, curve 3). In the case of coion binding, i.e., $\sigma_0/z_i > 0$, there may be either two extrema, provided $|z_i eN| > 8|\sigma_0|$, or none, when $|z_i eN| < 8|\sigma_0|$, as demonstrated in Fig. 5 [75]. When, $|z_i eN| = 8|\sigma_0|$, the surface potential passes through an inflection point where $d\psi_b/d \log C_i = 0$ (Fig. 5, curve 5). In the event of binding of both cations and anions, from zero to three extrema may occur, depending on the intrinsic surface charge density of the membrane and ion binding parameters. An example of a surface potential vs. ion concentration curve with three extrema is presented in Fig. 6 (curve 4). The two extrema at lower salt concentration and negative ψ_b and one at high salt concentrations and positive ψ_b are shown in two insets. It should be emphasized that nonmonotonic features of the $\psi_b(\log C_i)$ dependence take

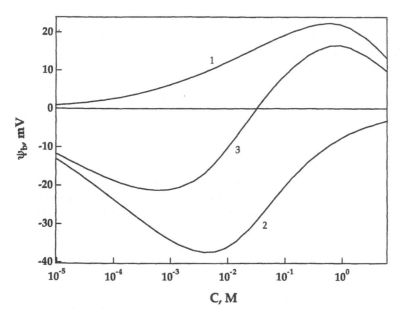

FIG. 7 Dependence of the potential at the Stern layer (ψ_b) of a neutral membrane on the molar concentration of a 2:1 electrolyte (e.g. $CaCl_2$) at 20°C, calculated by Eq. (38). Curve 1: $K_i = 10$ M^{-1}, $K_j = 0$, $z_i eN = 0.8$ $e/nm^2 = 0.128176$ C/m^2, i.e. one divalent cation binding site per 2.5 nm^2 (no charge reversal, one extremum at $\psi_b > 0$); curve 2: $K_i = 0$, $K_j = 500$ M^{-1}, $z_j eN = -0.2$ $e/nm^2 = -0.032044$ C/m^2, i.e., one binding site for the monovalent anion per 5 nm^2 (no charge reversal, one extremum at $\psi_b < 0$); curve 3: simultaneous adsorption of the divalent cation and the monovalent anion with the above parameters (a charge reversals and two extrema, one at $\psi_0 < 0$ and one at $\psi_b > 0$). The subscripts i and j correspond to the cation and the anion, respectively.

place provided the ionic strength of the electrolyte solution changes in parallel with the adsorbing ion concentration, i.e., when the ionic strength is not kept constant by indifferent electrolytes. In this case, the slope of the $\psi_b(\log C_i)$ curve is determined by ion binding and by GC screening. The ion binding may increase or decrease the surface potential, depending on the sign of σ_0/z_i, whereas the screening always suppresses the surface potential. Combination of these two factors may, under certain conditions, lead to nonmonotonic behavior of the $\psi_b(\log C_i)$ curve. For example, consider anion binding to a negatively charged membrane. At ion concentrations much lower than the reciprocal binding constant, $C_i \ll 1/K_i$, there is little binding and the predominant effect of increasing ion concentration is a decrease in ψ_b due to screening (Fig. 5, curves 4, 5, 6). In the concentration range $C_i \approx 1/K_i$, the coion binding leads to remarkable deviations of the $\psi_b(\log C_i)$ curve from the "screening only" pattern. At sufficiently high coion binding site density ($|z_i eN| > 8|\sigma_0|$), the ion binding effect overwhelms, resulting in the change of the slope of $\psi_b(\log C_i)$ curve (Fig. 5, curve 6). At higher concentrations, when ion binding is close to saturation, the screening effect again dominates and the potential eventually drops to zero, thus creating two extrema in the $\psi_b(\log C_i)$ curve.

For a net-neutral membrane, $\sigma_0 = 0$, any ion binding at varied ionic strength will result in an extremum in the $\psi_b(\log C_i)$ curve, except for a specific case when the adsorbed charges due to the cations and anions compensate each other. As illustrated in Fig. 7, binding of cations (curve 1) or anions (curve 2) produces positive or negative surface potential, respectively. The surface potential increases, passes through a maximum (in the absolute value), and decreases to zero at high ion concentrations. When both the cation and the anion bind to the membrane surface, two extrema may occur, one at $\psi_b < 0$, due to anion binding, and another at $\psi_b > 0$, due to cation binding (Fig. 7, curve 3). Clearly, these two extrema may only happen if there is a charge reversal, i.e., if the maximum bound charge density ($z_i eN$) of the ion with lower binding constant is higher than that of the ion with higher binding constant.

These peculiarities of the $\psi_b(\log C_i)$ dependence, i.e., the extrema and charge reversal, are of high practical interest because they provide information which can be used to determine ion binding parameters, such as the binding constant, binding site density, and ion–lipid binding stoichiometries. In a general case of binding of the ionic species i to a membrane with charge density σ_0, in the presence of indifferent electrolytes of arbitrary valence type, the binding constant and the binding site density of the ion i can be determined based on the surface potential at the extremum, $\phi_{ex} (= e\psi_{ex}/kT)$ and corresponding concentration, C_{ex} [75]:

$$K_i = \frac{2\sigma_{ex}(\sigma_{ex} - \sigma_0) - \xi}{\xi C_{i,ex} e^{-z_i \phi_{ex}}} \tag{39}$$

and

$$N = \frac{\sigma_{ex}(\sigma_{ex} - \sigma_0)^2}{z_i e[\sigma_{ex}(\sigma_{ex} - \sigma_0) - \xi/2]} \tag{40}$$

where

$$\xi = \sigma_{ex}^2 - 2\varepsilon\varepsilon_0 RT \sum_{k \neq i,j} C_k(e^{-z_k \phi_{ex}} - 1)$$

and σ_{ex} is the membrane surface charge density at the extremum. The advantage of this method of determination of ion binding parameters is that both K_i and N are determined simultaneously based on experimentally measured quantities. In the absence of extrema, the binding constant and the binding site density are evaluated by describing the surface potential vs. ion concentration curve using a combination of K_i and N yielding a good fit between the theory and experiment. The reliability of this latter approach is often questionable because none of the two parameters is determined independent of the other.

In the case when no extrema of the $\psi_b(\log C_i)$ curve are detected in the experimentally studied concentration range but there is a charge reversal, which occurs for instance when polyvalent cations bind to acidic membranes, the parameters K_i and N can be determined based on the ion concentration and the slope $d\psi_b/d \log C_i$ at $\psi_b = 0$ [76]. Let us consider competitive adsorption of a monovalent and a divalent cations to a membrane composed of a singly charged acidic lipid under conditions when the divalent cation concentration varies and that of the monovalent cation is constant. The total surface charge of the membrane, σ, is the sum of the intrinsic charge σ_0, and the adsorbed charge:

$$\sigma = \sigma_0 + \frac{eN(z_i K_i C_i e^{-z_i\phi} + z_n K_n C_n e^{-z_n\phi})}{1 + K_i C_i e^{-z_i\phi} + K_n C_n e^{-z_n\phi}} \tag{41}$$

where the subscripts i and n apply to the divalent and monovalent cations, ($z_i = 2$ and $z_n = 1$). At the charge reversal point, where $\phi = 0$ and $\sigma = 0$, Eq. (41) becomes:

$$eN = \frac{-\sigma_0(1 + K_i C_{i0} + K_n C_n)}{z_i K_i C_{i0} + z_n K_n C_n} \tag{42}$$

where C_{i0} is the divalent cation concentration corresponding to the charge reversal point. If the divalent cation binds with a 1:1 stoichiometry, then $eN = -\sigma_0$. Inserting this into Eq. (42) we immediately find the 1:1 binding constant of the divalent cation:

$$K_i = \frac{1}{C_{i0}} \tag{43}$$

This binding constant is only correct provided the binding of the divalent cation is governed exclusively by a 1:1 stoichiometry. If the interaction of an n-valent cation with a membrane containing singly charged acidic lipids was governed by pure coulombic forces, then ion binding would lead to electroneutrality at the membrane surface at saturation of adsorption, corresponding to a n:1 lipid-to-cation binding stoichiometry. In this case, which is referred to as *equivalent* adsorption, $\sigma_0 = -\sigma_b$. However, electrophoresis experiments demonstrate charge reversal of bilayers composed of such lipids as PS, phosphatidylglycerol (PG) or phosphatidylinositol (PI) upon increasing divalent cation concentration [77–81], providing evidence for at least partial 1:1 divalent cation binding stoichiometry. This *superequivalent* adsorption mechanism implies that apart from coulombic forces the cations experience specific, chemical affinity for acidic phospholipids. Since different physicochemical factors are involved in equivalent (2:1) and superequivalent (1:1) lipid to divalent cation interactions, it is very important to be able to distinguish between these two mechanisms of ion adsorption. It has been shown that this problem can be solved by determining the average density of binding sites from Eq. (42) and using it to evaluate the fraction of acidic lipid molecules involved in 2:1 binding at saturation [76]:

$$\Theta = 2\left(1 - \frac{eN}{|\sigma_0|}\right) \tag{44}$$

It should be noted that in the presence of a competitively adsorbing monovalent cation the parameters of the divalent cation binding can only be determined if those of the monovalent cation are known. The monomer–dimer problem of the adsorption of divalent cations to acidic membranes has been addressed by Cohen and Cohen [82,83] and Graham et al. [84]. Their approach has further been developed and analytic expressions for the 1:1 and 2:1 binding constants of the divalent cation and for the fractions of corresponding complexes have been provided [76]. Cohen and Cohen [82,83] showed that the adsorption of a divalent cation to a negatively charged membrane according to both 1:1 and 2:1 lipid-to-ion mechanisms, with corresponding binding constants K_{21} and K_{22}, which is accompanied by a competitive 1:1 adsorption of a monovalent cation with a binding constant K_{11}, can be described by:

$$\sigma_0(1 - \Theta)(1 - K_{21}C_2 e^{-2\phi}) = \sigma(1 + K_{11}C_1 e^{-\phi} + K_{21}C_2 e^{-2\phi}), \tag{45}$$

where

$$\Theta = \frac{f[1 + 2fb - \sqrt{1 + 4(f - 1)b}]}{2(1 + f^2 b)} \tag{46}$$

$$b = \frac{K_{22}C_2 e^{-2\phi}}{(1 + K_{11}C_1 e^{-\phi} + K_{21}C_2 e^{-2\phi})^2} \tag{47}$$

In Eqs. (45)–(47) C_1 is the (fixed) concentration of the monovalent cation and C_2 the (variable) concentration of the divalent cation, Θ is the fraction of lipid molecules involved in 2:1 lipid-to-divalent-cation complexes at a given ion concentration, and f is the coordination number characterizing the lipid lattice. At the charge reversal point ($\phi = 0$, $\sigma = 0$) Eq. (45) becomes:

$$\sigma_0(1 - \Theta_0)(1 - K_{21}C_{20}) = 0 \tag{48}$$

where Θ_0 and C_{20} are Θ and C_2 at $\phi = 0$. At $\sigma_0 \neq 0$ and $\Theta_0 \neq 1$ we obtain from Eq. (48):

$$K_{21} = \frac{1}{C_{20}} \tag{49}$$

which is the same as Eq. (43), although obtained in a quite different manner. Furthermore, Eq. (45) is differentiated with respect to log C_2 and written at $\phi = 0$, taking into account the relationship (49) as:

$$\Theta_0 = 1 - \frac{\Delta_0(2 + K_{11}C_1)\sqrt{2\varepsilon\varepsilon_0 RTI_0}}{\sigma_0(2\Delta_0 - \ln 10)} \tag{50}$$

where I_0 is the ionic strength at $\phi = 0$ and $\Delta_0 \equiv d\phi/d \log C_2$ at $\phi = 0$. Equation (50) is used to determine the fraction of lipids involved in 2:1 complexes at the charge reversal point, provided K_{11} is known.

Next, b_0 is determined from Eq. (46) as:

$$b_0 = -p \pm \sqrt{p^2 - q} \tag{51}$$

where

$$p = \frac{1 + \Theta_0(2\Theta_0 - f - 2)}{2f^2(1 - \Theta_0)^2}$$

$$q = \frac{\Theta_0(\Theta_0/f - 1)}{f^3(1 - \Theta_0)^2}$$

Generally, Eq. (51) yields a positive and a negative value for b_0, from which the positive value should be used to evaluate K_{22} as:

$$K_{22} = \frac{b_0(2 + K_{11}C_1)}{C_{20}} \tag{52}$$

Thus, the 1:1 and 2:1 binding constants and the fractions of the complexes of both types can be determined just using the divalent cation concentration corresponding to the charge reversal point and the slope of $\psi_b(\log C_2)$ dependence at $\psi_b = 0$.

III. ION BINDING TO LIPID BILAYERS

A. Neutral Lipids

It is well known that most biological membranes are composed of zwitterionic and acidic lipids and therefore are negatively charged. However, neutral lipids, such as mono- and diglycerides, even though constituting only a minor fraction of biomembranes, may play critical parts in various physiological processes. For example, one of phospholipase C products, DAG is essential for PKC activation, and hence is a key second messenger involved in transmembrane signaling in various cells. Monoacylglycerides are also of considerable interest because structurally they resemble physiologically important DAGs and phorbol esters. Cell stimulation gives rise to a transient increase in the intracellular free calcium concentration, another important second messenger which is required for activation of a wide variety of cytosolic enzymes and translocation of some of them to intracellular membranes. It is therefore important to have comprehensive information on the affinities of calcium ions for different membrane components, including neutral, zwitterionic and acidic lipids.

Data on the binding of Ca^{2+} cations and two anions (Cl^- and Br^-) to glycerolmonooleate (GMO) liposomes are presented in Fig. 8. Quantitative description of the binding of anions, such as Cl^-, is important because the binding of Ca^{2+} can only be accurately determined taking into account the accompanying anion effects. Figure 8 demonstrates that GMO liposomes carry excess negative charge at their surface; the surface charge density was estimated as $\sigma_0 = -2$ mC/m^2, or one negative charge per 80 nm.^{2} This is equivalent to the presence of $\sim 0.5\%$ free fatty acid in GMO samples. As follows from the panel a of Fig. 8, the dependence of the surface potential of

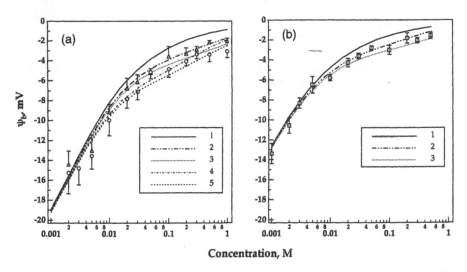

FIG. 8 Dependence of the surface potential of GMO liposomes on the concentration of (a) KCl (triangles) and KBr (circles) and (b) CaCl$_2$ at 22°C. The pH is adjusted to 7.2 with 1 mM tris-HCl. The Stern potentials are calculated by Eq. (26) based on measured ζ-potentials, using $\delta = 0.2$ nm for the thickness of the shear layer. The theoretical curves are calculated by Eq. (38) based on the following assumptions. Panel A: curve 1: Gouy–Chapman screening without ion binding; curve 2: $K_{Cl} = 5$ M^{-1}, $eN^{(-)} = 4$ mC/m^2, $K_K = 2$ M^{-1}, $eN^{(+)} = 2$ mC/m^2; curve 3: same parameters for Cl$^-$ binding but no cation binding; curve 4: $K_{Br} = 12$ M^{-1}, $eN^{(-)} = 4$ mC/m^2, $K_K = 2$ M^{-1}, $eN^{(+)} = 2$ mC/m^2; curve 5: same parameters for Br$^-$ binding but no cation binding; and panel b: curve 1: Gouy–Chapman screening without ion binding; curve 2: $K_{Cl} = 5$ M^{-1}, $eN^{(-)} = 4$ mC/m^2, $K_{Ca} = 2$ M^{-1}, $eN^{(+)} = 2$ mC/m^2; curve 3: same parameters for Cl$^-$ binding but no cation binding.

GMO liposomes on concentrations of KCl and KBr cannot be described by GC screening alone (curve 1). The deviation of the surface potential to more negative values at higher salt concentrations is most likely due to adsorption of corresponding anions to the surface of liposomes. The experimental curve corresponding to KCl can be satisfactorily described by theoretical curves 2 and 3, suggesting that Cl^- anions are able to bind to GMO membranes with parameters $K_{Cl} = 5$ M^{-1} and $eN^{(-)} = 4$ mC/m^2, while the binding of K^+ is weaker, $K_K = 0$ to 2 M^{-1} and $eN^{(+)} = 0$ to 2 mC/m^2. Binding of halide anions to GMO membranes is further supported by the dependence of the surface potential on KBr concentration. In this case, a stronger shift of the surface potential to more negative values is detected, implying that Br^- binds to GMO more strongly than Cl^-. The binding parameters of Br^- are determined as follows (curves 4 and 5): $K_{Br} = 12$ M^{-1}, $eN^{(-)} = 4$ mC/m^2. The binding of halides to mono- and diglyceride membranes is likely to involve OH ... halide hydrogen bonding between the hydroxyl groups of the lipid and the anions. Stronger binding of Br^- as compared to Cl^- may be due to either stronger hydrogen bonding capabilities of Br^- or by weaker image charge repulsion for Br^- due to its smaller charge density. The data obtained for KCl and KBr are intrinsically consistent because (a) the same density for anion binding sites are obtained for Cl^- and Br^- and (b) the binding of both Cl^- and Br^- is described using binding parameters for K^+ varying in the same range.

The dependence of the surface potential of GMO liposomes on $CaCl_2$ concentration is presented in panel b of Fig. 8. The surface potential is again shifted with respect to the pure screening curve to more negative values. When the binding of Cl^- is taken into account, with the parameters deduced from the data of the panel a, the fit between the experiment and theory becomes satisfactory (curve 3). Good fits may also be obtained allowing Ca^{2+} to adsorb with parameters $K_{Ca} = 2$ M^{-1}, $eN^{(+)} = 2$ mC/m^2 (curve 2). In conclusion, inorganic cations such as K^+ or Ca^{2+} have negligible affinity of glycerides. This result is not surprising because the only chemical group in GMO (or in diglycerides) that could potentially attract cations is the carbonyl oxygen, which is obviously not capable of creating a strong enough anionic field to dehydrate and coordinate cations. The quantitative results of ion binding to GMO membranes are summarized in Table 1.

B. Zwitterionic Lipids

Zwitterionic lipids, such as phosphatidylcholines and phosphatidylethanolamines, are the most abundant components of biological membranes, and there is vast literature on the interaction of ions with these lipids, especially PCs. Most of the literature on this topic published by 1992 has been reviewed earlier [85] and the reader is referred to that paper for more detailed

TABLE 1 Intrinsic Binding
Constants (K) and Lipid-to-
Ion Binding Stoichiometries
(n) Describing the Adsorption
of Some Inorganic Ions to
Glycerolmonooleate   Mem-
branes as Determined by Elec-
trophoresis at 22°C, pH 7.2

Ion	K (M^{-1})	n
Cl$^-$	5	~ 100
Br$^-$	12	~ 100
K$^+$	0–2	~ 200
Ca^{2+}	0–2	~ 200

information. Here only the most interesting aspects and some recent findings
are outlined.

1. Binding of Inorganic Anions to Zwitterionic Membranes

Studies on anion binding to artificial lipid membranes are basically restricted
to PC vesicles. The parameters of anion binding were determined by applying
the GCS theory to the experimental data, mostly obtained by NMR or electrophoresis techniques. As we discussed in the Theory section, the binding
constants and densities of binding sites can be accurately determined based on
the extrema of the membrane surface potential as a function of salt concentration, provided such extrema are experimentally detected. Nonmonotonic
$\psi_b(\log C_i)$ dependencies have first been observed by electrophoresis and were
used to determine the parameters K_i and N_i [75,85–88]. Maxima in the ζ-
potential of PC vesicles as a function of ion concentration have also been
observed by others [81,89–91].

Figure 9 represents electrophoresis data on the binding of NO$_3^-$, Br$^-$ and
SCN$^-$ anions to DMPC liposomes [75]. The measured ζ-potentials and the
ψ_b potentials, calculated using $\delta = 0.2$ nm for the separation of the shear plane
from the membrane surface [92], are presented in panels a and b, respectively.
In all cases, well-defined extrema in the values of the potential are present; the
curves corresponding to KBr and KNO$_3$ display two extrema, which is pre-
dicted for $|z_i e N_i| > 8|\sigma_0|$ (see the Theory section). The presence of two
extrema allows the parameters K_i and N_i to be determined using two pairs of
$C_{i,\,ex}$ and $\psi_{b,\,ex}$ (or ζ_{ex} at $\delta = 0$). The extrema at higher concentrations correspond to $C_{NO_3,ex} = 0.4 \pm 0.1$ M, $\zeta_{ex} = -4 \pm 0.4$ mV and $C_{Br,\,ex} = 0.2 \pm 0.1$ M,
$\zeta_{ex} = -7 \pm 0.7$ mV. For KSCN, $C_{SCN,\,ex} = 0.125 \pm 0.05$ M and $\zeta_{ex} = -16.5$
± 1.5 mV. Using these values, along with $\sigma_0 = -0.57$ mC/m^2 (in the presence

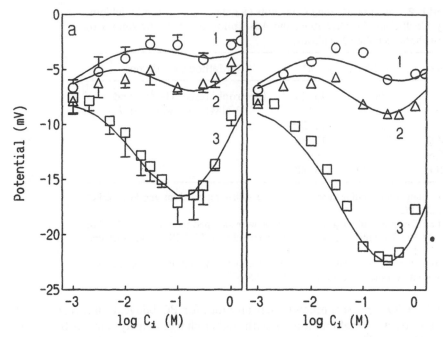

FIG. 9 Dependence of the ζ- (a) and Stern (b) potentials of DMPC liposomes on the concentration of KNO_3 (1), KBr (2) and KSCN (3) at 30°C. The pH is adjusted to 7.2 with 1 mM Tris-HCl. The Stern potentials are calculated by Eq. (26) based on measured ζ-potentials, using $\delta = 0.2$ nm for the thickness of the shear layer. The theoretical curves are calculated by the Gouy–Chapman–Stern equation. Panel a: $K = 2.3$ M^{-1}, $N = 0.072$ nm^{-2} for NO_3^-, $K = 5.5$ M^{-1}, $N = 0.087$ nm^{-2} for Br^-, $K = 14$ M^{-1}, $N = 0.165$ nm^{-2} for SCN^-; and panel b: $K = 2.2$ M^{-1}, $N = 0.119$ nm^{-2} for NO_3^-, $K = 4.2$ M^{-1}, $N = 0.138$ nm^{-2} for Br^-, $K = 7.6$ M^{-1}, $N = 0.355$ nm^{-2} for SCN^-. Reproduced from Tatulian [75].

of 3 mM KCl and 2 mM Tris-HCl (pH 7.2) the ζ-potential was -3.6 mV), we find the parameters K_i and N_i from Eqs. (39) and (40). It has been shown that the binding parameters are more reliably determined based on higher concentration extrema [75], so whenever more than one extremum is observed, that corresponding to higher salt concentration should be used to estimate the K_i and N_i.

The quantitative data on inorganic anion binding to PC bilayers are summarized in Table 2. A general trend has been observed indicating that the affinities of anions for PC bilayers increase in an order which is identical or similar to the Hofmeister series of anions: $SO_4^{2-} \approx Cl^- < NO_3^- < Br^- < SCN^- < I^- < ClO_4^-$ [86,87,93,94]. The more chaotropic (water-structure-breaking) anions with larger dimensions and lower charge density, such as I^-,

TABLE 2 Intrinsic Binding Constants (K) and Lipid-to-Ion Stoichiometry Coefficients (n) Describing the Adsorption of Inorganic Anions to Phosphatidylcholine Membranes[a]

Ion	K (M^{-1})	n^{b}	Methods, conditions
Cl^-	0.06–1.7	15–20[c]	Electrophoresis, ^{1}H-, ^{2}H- and
Br^-	2–5	9–17[c]	^{31}P-NMR, 25–30°C, pH 7.2–7.4
I^-	30–40	12–24[c]	
NO_3^-	2–8	13–36[c]	
SCN^-	10–80	4–9[c]	
ClO_4^-	70–230	23–48[c]	

[a] The ranges for binding constants include values reported for egg PC, POPC, and DMPC.
[b] The PC-to-anion binding stoichiometries were assumed to be 1:1 [91,93,95] or 2:1 [96,97]. The binding of SCN^- was described by a 7.5:1 PC/anion stoichiometry [98].
[c] Anion binding site densities increase by a factor of ~ 2 at the gel-to-liquid-crystal phase transition of the lipid [30, 75, 85–87].

SCN^-, ClO_4^-, possess much higher affinities for PC bilayers than cosmotropic (water-structure-making) anions with higher charge density, such as SO_4^{2-} and Cl^-. Higher affinities of chaotropic anions may be accounted for by various effects, such as lower image charge repulsion from bilayers, higher polarizabilities, stronger abilities to break the hydration shell of the lipid headgroups and probably others. Further details regarding anion binding to lipid bilayers may be found in Table 2 and in earlier reviews (e.g., Ref. 85).

2. Binding of Inorganic Cations to Zwitterionic Membranes

Interactions of cations with phospholipid bilayers are governed by two major types of forces, the long-range coulombic forces, in cases of charged membranes, and the short-range local atomic fields. The image charge effects and the ion–dipole interactions between the ions and the effective dipole potential of the interfacial region should be added to these factors to complete the picture. There is overwhelming evidence that the phosphate group of phospholipids plays a key role in cation–bilayer interactions. This is confirmed in particular by binding of multivalent cations to small phosphate-containing molecules in solution, which are used as fragments of phospholipid headgroups. For example, Pr^{3+} forms two types of complexes with dimethylphosphate (DMP) in aqueous solutions, $Pr(DMP)^{2+}$ and $Pr(DMP)_2^+$ with association constants 81 and 348 M^{-1}, respectively [99], and Ce^{3+} associates with glycerophosphocholine in methanol with $K = 2500$ M^{-1} [100]. The importance of the phosphate group in cation binding to lipid bilayers is also demonstrated by comparison between Ca^{2+} binding to a monoglyceride and to membranes of phosphatidic acid (PA), which differs from the glyceride in that the hydroxyl group at the glycerol sn-3 position is substituted by a phosphate group; the binding of Ca^{2+} to GMO membranes is negligible (Fig. 8b), whereas Ca^{2+} binds to PA bilayers with binding constants up to 200 M^{-1} [101–103]. Magnetic resonance, infrared spectroscopy, neutron diffraction and particle electrophoresis data also strongly implied that inorganic cations predominantly interact with the phosphodiester groups of phospholipid headgroups [23,27–29,81,97,104–111].

The binding of monovalent inorganic cations to zwitterionic membranes is very weak. Typically, binding constants ranging from 0 to 1 M^{-1} are reported and the binding stoichiometry is believed to be 1:1 (Table 3, for references see [85]).

The binding of alkaline-earth metal cations and several anions to egg PC, DMPC and DPPC membranes has been studied by particle electrophoresis [87]. Increasing concentrations of divalent cations induce positive ζ-potential of egg PC vesicles which increases, passes through a maximum and decreases at higher salt concentrations (Fig. 10, curves 1–6). These maxima were used to evaluate the binding constants and densities of binding sites characterizing the binding of the four divalent cations to PC membranes, using Eqs. (39) and (40). To demonstrate the effect of anions on the dependence of the surface potential on salt concentration, along with the chlorides of Mg^{2+}, Ca^{2+}, Sr^{2+} and Ba^{2+}, the bromide, nitrate, and perchlorate of Ba^{2+} were also tested. The ζ-potentials of vesicles in the presence of $BaBr_2$, $Ba(NO_3)_2$ and $Ba(ClO_4)_2$ is more negative than in $BaCl_2$ solutions, which is most likely caused by selective adsorption of anions at the vesicle membranes. The curves 4 and 7 of Fig. 10 allow the binding parameters (K_i and N_i) for Ba^{2+}, Cl^- and ClO_4^- to be determined based on the extrema in the positive (curve 4) and negative (curve 7) values of the ζ-potential. Having determined the parameters for Ba^{2+}, it is easy to find K_i and N_i values for Br^- and NO_3^- from the best fit between the theoretical curves 5 and 6 and the corresponding experimental results. Furthermore, the binding of Mg^{2+}, Ca^{2+} and Sr^{2+} are quantitatively characterized based on the ζ-potentials and ion concentrations at the extrema of corresponding curves, using a consistent pair of K and N for the Cl^- ion. The parameters of the binding of inorganic cations to zwitterionic lipid bilayers are summarized in Table 3. The surface densities of binding sites are converted into lipid-to-ion stoichiometry coefficients, n, using 0.6–0.7 nm^2 for cross-sectional areas of lipid molecules.

In general it is likely that for an efficient coordination of di- or trivalent cations by phospholipids, more than one phosphate group is involved in the complex formation, i.e., the lipid-to-ion stoichiometry is expected to be higher than 1:1. Determination of the binding stoichiometry is important because the binding constants can only be correctly interpreted if the stoichiometry is known. Combined electrophoresis and ^{31}P-NMR studies showed that Co^{2+} was interacting with egg PC bilayers with both 1:1 and 2:1 lipid-to-cation

TABLE 3 Intrinsic Binding Constants (K) and Lipid-to-Ion Stoichiometry Coefficients (n) Describing the Adsorption of Inorganic Cations to Zwitterionic Lipid Membranes[a]

Lipid	Ion	K (M^{-1})	n[b]	Methods, conditions[c]
PC	Li$^+$, Na$^+$, K$^+$, Bb$^+$, Cs$^+$	0.0–0.3	(1)	EP, 20°C
	Be^{2+}	400	(1)	EP, IFC, 22°C, diphytanoyl-PC
	Mg^{2+}	1–20	(1)	EP, X-ray, surface force, 5–25°C
		30	15	EP, 25°C, egg PC
	Ca^{2+}	1–5	(1–2)	EP, EPR, NMR, 25°C
		20	(1)	NMR (59°C), X-ray (5°C)
		190–256	13–15	EP, DMPC, DPPC, $T > T_m$
		392–440	14–16	EP, DMPC, DPPC, $T < T_m$
	Sr^{2+}	16	17	EP, egg PC, 25°C
	Ba^{2+}	10	18	EP, egg PC, 25°C
	Mn^{2+}	3.3	1–2	EP, egg PC, 25°C
		8–18	(1)	EPR, $T > T_m$
	Co^{2+}, Ni^{2+}	0.83	1–2	EP, egg PC, 25°C
	Fe^{3+}	7.5–110	300	EP, stronger binding at lower pH
	La^{3+}	4×10^3	24	POPC, titration calorimetry
	Ce^{3+}	2.5×10^3	(1)	gel filtration
	Pr^{3+}	435	(7)	NMR, DPPC, 52°C
	Eu^{3+}	700–2500	(1)	NMR, EP, centrifugation, 20°C
	Tb^{3+}	500–2×10^5	(2–3)	NMR, equilibrium dialysis
PE	Mg^{2+}	4	(1)	surface force, 22°C
	Ca^{2+}	2–12	(1)	EP, surface force, 25°C

[a] These data are collected from the references given in Tatulian [85] and a few papers which were either published later: Lehrmann and Seelig [112], Satoh [91], or not available at that time: Ermakov et al. [81]. See also Minami et al. [36], Bartucci and Sportelli [94].
[b] The n values in parentheses have been assumed arbitrarily and used in the GCS theory in combination with corresponding binding constants to fit the binding data. Therefore these parameters should be considered cautiously.
[c] EP = electrophoresis, IFC = internal field compensation, T_m is the main phase transition temperature of the lipid.

stoichiometries, with corresponding binding constants 0.33 and 1 M^{-1} [113] and Ca^{2+} was shown to be coordinated by phosphodiester groups of PC headgroups in a monodentate manner [111]. NMR results of Chrzeszczyk et al. [99] suggested that in the absence of trivalent cations, low affinity (2 M^{-1}) 1:1 binding sites were present at the surface of DPPC bilayers, whereas addi-

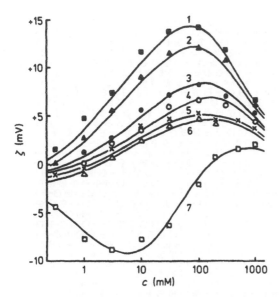

FIG. 10 Dependence of the ζ-potential of egg PC liposomes on the concentrations of $CaCl_2$, $MgCl_2$, $SrCl_2$, $BaCl_2$, $BaBr_2$, $Ba(NO_3)_2$ and $Ba(ClO_4)_2$ (curves 1 to 7, respectively) at 25°C and pH 7.4 (5 mM Tris-HCl). The theoretical curves were calculated by the Gouy–Chapman–Stern equation [Eq. (38)] using the parameters: $K = 42$, 30, 16, 10, 0.2, 2.0, 2.8 and 70 M^{-1} and $N = 0.0936$, 0.0874, 0.0749, 0.0749, 0.0749, 0.0749, 0.0749 and 0.0936 nm^{-2} for Ca^{2+}, Mg^{2+}, Sr^{2+} Ba^{2+}, Cl^-, Br^-, NO_3^- and ClO_4^-, respectively. Values for σ_0 used in Eq. (38) range from -0.2 to -0.36 mC/m^2. Reproduced from Tatulian [87].

tion of Pr^{3+} triggered appearance of high affinity (3000 M^{-1}) 2:1 binding sites, leading to an apparent cooperativity in Pr^{3+} binding. The GCS treatment of their results led to an effective binding constant of 435 M^{-1} and a DPPC:Pr^{3+} stoichiometry of $n = 7$. In other studies, n values between 8 and 33 were determined for Eu^{3+}, Nd^{3+} and UO_2^{2+} binding to PC bilayers [114–117]. Our electrophoresis results indicate that at the saturation of adsorption, about 13–17 lipid molecules correspond to one bound ion (Fig. 10 and Table 3). To rationalize these results, it was suggested that the inorganic ions bind at the point defects in the plane of the zwitterionic lipid lattice [87]. The lipid molecules were assumed to form closely packed domains so that the positive and negative poles of the headgroups were located at the points of a hexagonal lattice (Fig. 11). The domains were further assumed to be separated by local structural defects, namely point vacancies in the lattice. As shown in Fig. 11, these vacant points are surrounded by six charges creating a total charge hich can acquire values of -6, -4, -2, 0, 2, 4 or 6 elementary charges. Obviously, in the former three situations the defects may serve as good

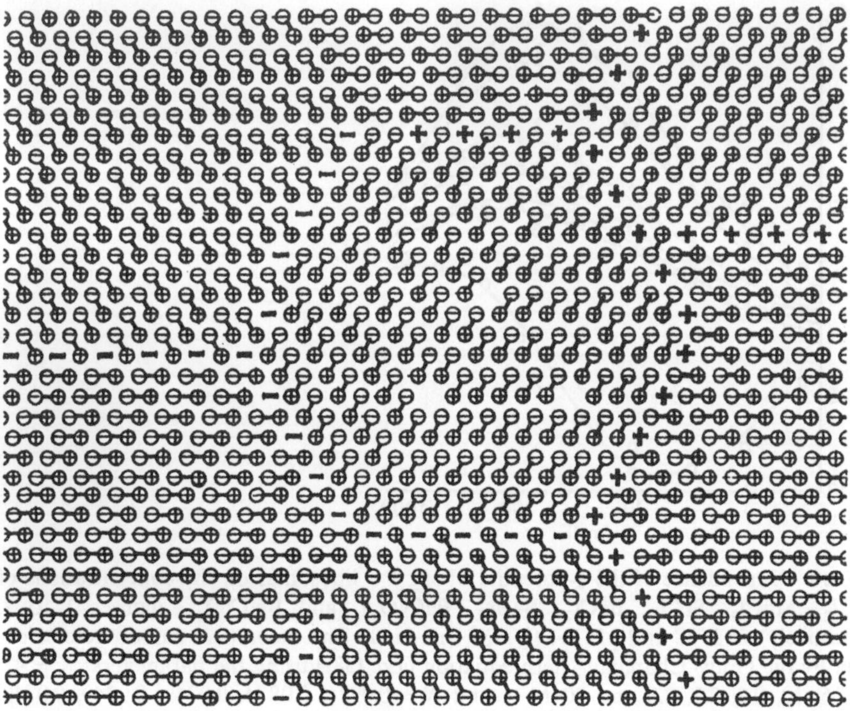

FIG. 11 A schematic model for the binding of ions at the point defects in the hexagonal lattice of a zwitterionic lipid. Each pair of connected circles with a plus and a minus inside represents a lipid polar headgroup. The lipid molecules are supposed to be packed in domains characterized, among other things, by headgroup orientational order. The vacant points between the domains serve as ion binding sites. The adsorbed cations and anions are indicated by bold-face pluses and minuses. Reproduced from Tatulian [87].

binding sites for cations, and in the latter three cases for anions. This model suggests that for a given membrane equal surface densities of binding sites are expected for cations and anions. Data from Tables 2 and 3 indicate that the effective lipid-to-ion binding ratios, which were determined experimentally, are approximately 10–20 for both anions and cations, providing evidence in favor of this model.

C. Acidic Lipids

Binding of inorganic ions, especially di- or trivalent cations, to membranes containing acidic lipids exerts profound effects on their structure, aggregation, fusion, hydration and other properties [23,24,27–29,32–35,38,39,118–122].

Infrared and NMR studies showed that inorganic cations primarily interact with the phosphate group of acidic phospholipids and cause its dehydration [23,27–29,121–123]. The carboxyl group of PS is not markedly dehydrated upon binding of divalent cations but is involved in cation coordination [27–29,122,124], and the amine group facilitates cation binding in the deprotonated state and inhibits cation binding in the protonated state.

The quantitative data describing inorganic cation binding to acidic lipid membranes are summarized in Table 4. Comparison of the data of Tables 3 and 4 indicate that the intrinsic binding constants of cations for acidic lipids are comparable to those for zwitterionic membranes. Nonetheless, under given conditions much more cations bind to membranes composed of acidic lipids than to zwitterionic lipid membranes for two reasons. First, since each acidic lipid possesses an excess negative charge, it may serve as an independent cation binding site providing a 1:1 lipid-to-ion binding stoichiometry. If the ion binding proceeds according to an equivalent mechanism, then for mono-, di- or trivalent cations the stoichiometry may be 1:1, 2:1 and 3:1, respectively. The ion binding site densities for zwitterionic lipids are much lower because otherwise ion binding would be thermodynamically unfavorable due to high electrostatic free energy of the membrane surface at high occupancies. Second, the local cation concentrations near membrane surfaces are much higher for acidic (negatively charged) membranes than for zwitterionic (positively charged due to cation binding) membranes. Thus, high local cation concentrations and high surface densities of binding sites provide more extensive cation binding to membranes containing acidic lipids.

As follows from Tables 3 and 4, in most cases the parameters of ion binding to lipid bilayers have been deduced from particle electrophoresis experiments. These experiments demonstrated reversal of the membrane surface charge at ~ 0.1 M divalent cation concentrations, providing some evidence in favor of a 1:1 binding of divalent cations to singly charged acidic lipids [77–80]. The 1:1 binding constants then were determined based on the cation concentration at the charge reversal point [see Eqs. (43) and (49)]. However, the question still remained whether the divalent cation binding was governed exclusively by a 1:1 stoichiometry or a combination of 1:1, 2:1 and possibly lower lipid-to-ion stoichiometry coefficients. This problem was addressed by processing the electrophoresis data of McLaughlin et al. [78] on the binding of Mg^{2+}, Ca^{2+}, Sr^{2+} and Ba^{2+} to PS vesicles using a newly developed theory which makes it possible to determine the 1:1 and 2:1 binding constants and the fractions of corresponding complexes [76]. Two different theoretical approaches have been tested, one based on the GCS formalism and the other on the Cohen–Cohen model [82,83]. Figure 12 represents the results of the application of these theories to the experimental data on Ca^{2+} binding to PS vesicles. In the case of ζ-potentials (Fig. 12, panel a), the Cohen–Cohen approach works better than the GCS model, whereas in the case of the Stern

TABLE 4 Intrinsic Binding Constants (K) and Lipid-to-Ion Stoichiometry Coefficients (n) Describing the Adsorption of Inorganic Cations to Acidic Lipid Membranes[a]

Lipid	Ion	K (M^{-1})	n	Methods, conditions
Singly charged phospholipids (PA[b], PG, PI, PS)	Li$^+$, Na$^+$, K$^+$, Bb$^+$, Cs$^+$	0.1–2.0[c]	(1)	EP, monolayer, NMR, EPR
	NH$_4^+$	0.17	(1)	EP, 25°C
	Be^{2+}	~ 100	(1)	EP, IFC, 22°C
	Mg^{2+}	2–10	(1–5)	EP, Equil. dial, AAS, monol.
	Ca^{2+}	3–100	(1–5)	EP, Eq. dial., AAS, surf. force
	Sr^{2+}	5–44	(1–2)	EP, light scattering (PG, PS)
	Ba^{2+}	6–36	(1–2)	EP, light scattering (PG, PS)
	Mn^{2+}	7–100	(1–2)	EP, EPR, AAS, Equilibr. dial.
	Ni^{2+}	14–40	(1–2)	EP, NMR, 20–25°C
	UO$_2^{2+}$	$(1-3) \times 10^3$	(1)	EP, 25°C
	VO$_2^{2+}$	$(2-10) \times 10^3$	(1–2)	EPR
	La^{3+}	$(4-100) \times 10^3$	(1–2)	EP, pH 4.5–7.4[d] (PS)
		2.5×10^4	~ 16	EP, pH 6.6 (PI)
PIP$_2$	Mg^{2+}	100	(1)	EP, 25°C
	Ca^{2+}	500	(1)	EP, 25°C
CL	Na$^+$	3.3	(1)	EP, 22°C
	Ca^{2+}	15.5	(1)	NMR
Gangliosides[e]	Mg^{2+}, Ca^{2+}	500	(1)	IFC, conductance
	Ca^{2+}	< 100	(1)	EP, conductance
SGC[f]	Na$^+$, K$^+$	~ 2.5	1	Monolayer
	Ca^{2+}	~ 12	2	Monolayer

[a] The majority of these data are collected from the references given in Tatulian [85]. See also Quinn and Sherman [125], McDaniel and McLaughlin [126], Reboiras and Jones [127], Graham et al. [84], Minami et al. [35], Tatulian [76]. The meaning of n values in parenthesis is the same as for Table 3. AAS = atomic absorption spectroscopy, SGC = sulfogalactosylceramide.
[b] At high pH, when PA acquired the second negative charge, cation binding was increased by a factor of ~ 2 [128].
[c] Binding of alkali metal cations to DLPG monolayers at low surface density (0.75 nm^2/molecule) was described by a lattice model using $K \approx 0.005$ M^{-1} [84].
[d] La^{3+} binding constant to PS increases from 4×10^3 at pH 4.5 to 10^5 M^{-1} at pH 7.4 [129].
[e] Similar binding constants of Ca^{2+} were obtained for mono-, di- and trisialogangliosides [89, 126].
[f] These intrinsic binding constants have been calculated using the apparent binding constants and the Stern potentials reported in the original paper [125].

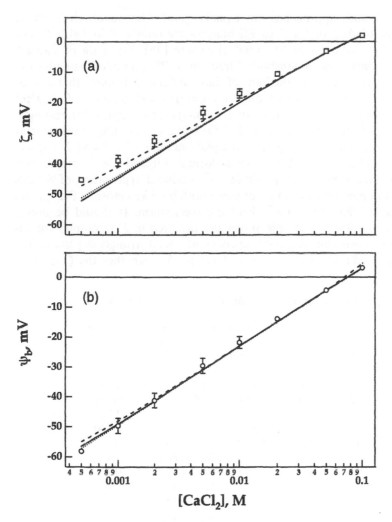

FIG. 12 Dependence of the ζ-potential (panel a) and surface potential (panel b) of PS vesicles on $CaCl_2$ concentration at 25°C and pH 7.4 (1 mM MOPS). The solid and dotted lines were calculated by Eq. (41), which is based on the GCS formalism, with and without consideration of the competitive binding of Na^+ ions with $K = 0.8\ M^{-1}$, respectively. The dashed lines were calculated by Eq. (45), which is based on the Cohen–Cohen approach, for a hexagonal lipid lattice; the calculations for a tetragonal lattice yield similar results. The experimental data points have been taken from McLaughlin et al. [78] and the theory was originally developed by Tatulian. Reproduced from Tatulian [76].

potentials, ψ_b, both approaches are equally good. The quantitative results describing the binding of Ca^{2+} to PS bilayers are tabulated in Table 5. The results for other cations can be found elsewhere [76]. The data of Table 5 immediately indicate that a substantial fraction of PS molecules is involved in 2:1 PS–Ca^{2+} association. In the light of these findings, it is likely that a combination of 1:1 and 2:1 stoichiometries governs the binding of divalent cations to membranes composed of singly charged acidic lipids. Interestingly, in an infrared spectroscopic study a 3:2 DPPS:Ca^{2+} binding stoichiometry was found [121], which corresponds to equal amounts of 1:1 and 2:1 lipid–ion complexes. The ability of Ca^{2+} ions to form 2:1 ligand–Ca^{2+} complexes is important because it plays a key role in Ca^{2+}-induced aggregation of vesicles and cells and in membrane binding of some proteins, like cytosolic PLA_2s and certain types of PKC, by a Ca^{2+}-bridging mechanism. It should be noted, however, that the fraction of lipid molecules involved in 2:1 complex formation (θ) and the corresponding binding constants (K_{22}) strongly depend on the choice of the thickness of the shearing layer (δ), i.e., whether the ζ or Stern

TABLE 5 Parameters Describing the Binding of Ca^{2+} Ions to PS Vesicles[a]

Model	δ (nm)	Δ_0	θ	K (M^{-1})	A (nm^2)
$GCS_{noncomp.}$	0	0.737	0.850	88.8	1.218
	0.2	0.965	0.391	21.9	0.870
$GCS_{comp.}$	0	0.737	0.854	94.3	1.222
	0.2	0.965	0.410	23.0	0.880
CC ($f = 6$)	0	0.737	0.730	$K_{21} = 13.3$	0.7
				$K_{22} = 84.0$	1.4
	0.2	0.965	0.213	$K_{21} = 13.4$	0.7
				$K_{22} = 3.2$	1.4
CC ($f = 4$)	0	0.737	0.730	$K_{21} = 13.3$	0.7
				$K_{22} = 117.2$	1.4
	0.2	0.965	0.213	$K_{21} = 13.4$	0.7
				$K_{22} = 4.7$	1.4

[a] These results are obtained by the application of the theory described by Tatulian [76] to the experimental data of McLaughlin et al. [78]. $GCS_{noncomp.}$ and $GCS_{comp.}$ mean that the extended Gouy–Chapman–Stern approach was used without and with competitive adsorption of Na^+ ions and CC indicates that the Cohen–Cohen approach was used. Δ_0 is the slope of $\phi(\log C_i)$ curve at the charge reversal point, θ is the fraction of PS molecules involved in 2:1 PS–calcium complexes at the saturation of adsorption (for GCS approach) and at the charge reversal point (for CC approach), K is the intrinsic binding constant (for GCS model, K is the "effective" binding constant), K_{21} and K_{22} are the intrinsic binding constants for the 1:1 and 2:1 PS–calcium complexes, A is the area per binding site.

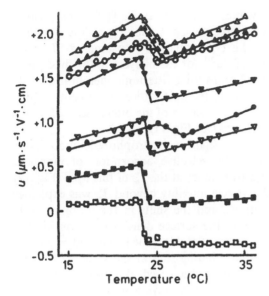

FIG. 13 Temperature-dependence of the electrophoretic mobility of DMPC liposomes at pH 7.2 (2 mM Tris-HCl) in the presence of $CaCl_2$ at concentrations (mM): 0.1 ($\square$), 0.3 ($\blacksquare$), 1.0 ($\triangledown$), 4.0 ($\blacktriangledown$), 20 ($\triangle$), 50 ($\blacktriangle$), 100 (O) and 500 ($\bullet$). Reproduced from Tatulian [87].

potentials are used. This means that these parameters can only be reliably evaluated provided the real Stern potentials have been determined.

D. Effects of Lipid Phase Transition

Lipids typically undergo a thermotropic phase transition from a "gel" to a "liquid crystalline" state, also referred to as a chain melting phase transition. These phase transitions have tremendous effects on almost all physicochemical properties of lipids, including their ionization state and ion binding properties. For example, upon the gel-to-liquid-crystal phase transition of PA membranes the lipid becomes partially deprotonated and the apparent pK decreases by ~ 0.8 units [130,131]. A decrease in the pK at the main transition temperature (T_m) was also detected for DPPS bilayers [132]. These pK shifts are explained by a decrease in the affinity of lipid molecules for protons above T_m because of decreased packing density of the lipid, and hence lower negative charge density of the membrane, and partially by a decrease in the intrinsic pK value (reviewed by Hauser [32]). The binding of divalent cations to phospholipid bilayers also significantly decreases above T_m [30,75,87,130,133–135].

Changes in ion binding parameters at T_m also occur for zwitterionic membranes, and these effects are difficult to interpret in simple electrostatic terms. Figure 13 demonstrates deviations of the electrophoretic mobility of DMPC liposomes toward more negative values occurring at T_m [87]. The positive mobility of zwitterionic liposomes is due to Ca^{2+} binding at the liposome surface. Shifts in the mobility, or the ζ-potential, of liposomes at T_m were described in terms of lower affinities of Ca^{2+} for PC bilayers in the fluid phase (Table 4). A decrease in the cation affinities for zwitterionic membranes at T_m may be explained by a lateral expansion of the lipid lattice at the gel-to-liquid-crystal phase transition resulting in the weakening of the interactions of bound cations with in the lipid polar headgroups (see Fig. 11).

It has been demonstrated that the negative electrophoretic mobility of DMPC vesicles, which was induced by selective adsorption of inorganic anions, strongly shifted to more negative values at the T_m of this lipid (Fig. 14). The temperature-dependence of the vesicle mobility beyond T_m was explained by changes in the viscosity of solutions, and the shifts in the mobility at T_m was attributed to an abrupt increase in the surface density of anion binding sites above T_m [86]. Interestingly, earlier Träuble [136] detected a 2.6-fold increase in the density of organic anion binding sites at the surface of DPPC at the gel-to-liquid-crystal phase transition. Increased affinities of anions to bilayers of zwitterionic lipids in the fluid phase have also been reported by Smejtek and Wong [137].

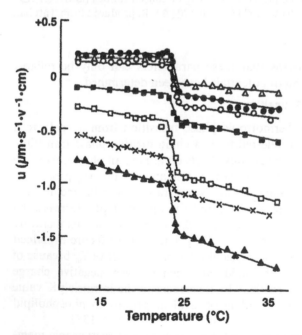

FIG. 14 Temperature-dependence of the electrophoretic mobility of DMPC liposomes in 10 mM solutions of K_2SO_4 (Δ), KCl (●), KNO_3 (O), KBr (■), KSCN (□), KI (×) and $KClO_4$ (▲) at pH 7.4 (5 mM Tris-HCl). Reproduced from Tatulian [86].

IV. BIOLOGICAL MEMBRANES

The negative surface charge of biological membranes first of all creates an overall negative electrostatic potential at the membrane surface which is important in such phenomena as cell adhesion and spreading, chemotaxix, endo- and exocytosis, hemostasis and others. On the other hand, negatively charged lipids produce local potentials which control ion concentrations near ion-conducting channels and hence regulate the channel conductance, as well as facilitate specific membrane binding of the basic residues of membrane-associating enzymes, their substrates, local anesthetics and other molecules. In many types of cell the charged lipids are distributed asymmetrically across the plasma membrane. The difference in the potentials at both surfaces of the membrane contributes to the potential drop inside the membrane (intramembrane potential, V_{IM}) and thus plays a significant role in voltage-dependent phenomena, like ion transport. Here I briefly review electrostatic phenomena and ion adsorption at the membrane surfaces of some specific types of cell, namely, nerve, muscle and red blood cells.

A. Nerve Cell Membranes

A common property of nerve cells is the abundance of ion channels in their membranes, such as Na^+-, K^+- and Ca^{2+}-channels, which provide a molecular machinery for the creation and transmittance of the action potential along the axon. This indicates how important the electrostatic surface potentials of these membranes are because the surface potentials determine the local ion concentrations at the channel orifice and also contribute to the V_{IM} felt by the channel molecule. In the 1960s and 1970s a number of studies demonstrated that variations of ion concentrations outside or inside perfused nerve cells affect the excitability thresholds and shift the current–voltage (I–V) curves along the voltage axis. These phenomena were attributed to GC screening of the fixed charges at the outer or inner surfaces of axon membranes and corresponding changes in the surface potential [138–141]. As schematically illustrated in Fig. 15, changes in the surface potential at the outer side of the membrane affects V_{IM} but not the transmembrane potential, V_{TM}. The difference between V_{IM} and V_{TM} is due to unequal potentials at both surfaces of the membrane: $V_{TM} = V_{IM} - \Delta\psi_0$, where $\Delta\psi_0$ is the difference in surface potentials (all potential differences are defined as potential inside minus potential outside). An increase in the ion concentration in bathing solution decreases the potential at the outer surface from ψ_{01} to ψ_{02} by screening or cation binding mechanisms, resulting in an enhancement in the V_{IM} by the difference between ψ_{01} and ψ_{02}. These variations in V_{IM} or in the surface potential cannot be measured by electrodes in the bulk solutions. However, since the steady-state ion conductance is sensitive to the ion concentration at the membrane surface near the ion channel, and to the V_{IM}, changes in the membrane surface potential can be estimated by measuring I–V characteristics of membranes under

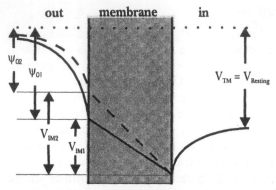

(a) No applied voltage

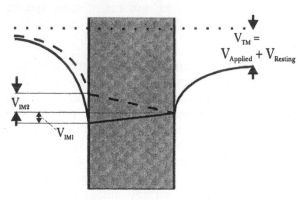

(b) With applied voltage

FIG. 15 Schematic representation of the distribution of the electrostatic potential across a cell plasma membrane. In panel a, there is no externally applied voltage. The transmembrane potential (V_{TM}) is determined by the distribution of charged species inside and outside the cell. The intramembrane potential, V_{IM}, is created by the sum of V_{TM} and the difference of the surface potentials at both surfaces of the membrane, $V_{IM} = V_{TM} + \Delta\psi_0$. In panel b, an external depolarizing potential is applied, which may cause, e.g., an excitation of nerve cells. The dashed line represents a situation when the external surface potential is reduced, e.g., by an increased ionic strength or cation binding. This may result in dramatic alterations in V_{IM}, including a change in its polarity, as shown in panel b.

varying ionic conditions. Information on the electrostatic properties of the ion selective filters inside the ion channels can be obtained in a similar manner based on pH- or cation-titration of the voltage dependence of instantaneous currents. These approaches were used in many studies to demonstrate that the surface and internal charges of ion channels in neuronal membranes are regulated not only by GC screening but by pH-titration of the ionizable groups and by binding of divalent cations as well [140,142–149]. Differential effects of divalent cations and protons on the voltage dependence of the peak Na^+ and steady-state K^+ conductances revealed acidic groups near both Na^+- and K^+-channels of frog nerve fibers with different pK values [142]. The density of acidic groups at the outer surface of a squid axon that bind Ca^{2+} ions with $K = 0.1$ M^{-1} were estimated by this method as $(3.5–8.3) \times 10^{17}/m^2$ [141]. Begenisich [150] found similar negative charge densities for a marine worm giant axon and suggested that the acidic groups, capable of binding Ca^{2+} with $K = 0.2$ M^{-1}, were located closer to the gating machinery rather than to the outer membrane surface. The dependence of steady-state conductance–voltage curves of K^+-channels in nodal membranes of frog axons on external pH and divalent cation concentrations were used to calculate membrane surface potentials [143]. Application of the GCS theory allowed these authors to establish the presence at the outer membrane surface of acidic groups with a surface density of $5.2 \times 10^{17}/m^2$ and pK = 4.5 as well as basic groups with a density of $2.8 \times 10^{17}/m^2$ and pK = 9.25. About 63% of the acidic (probably carboxyl) groups were able to bind Mg^{2+}, Ca^{2+}, Co^{2+} and Ni^{2+} ions with intrinsic binding constants, 3, 5, 8, and 10 M^{-1}, respectively. Cation binding to the rest of the acidic groups was much weaker because of nearby positive charges. Somewhat higher binding constants for alkaline-earth metal cations to the somatic membranes of mollusc neurons were determined by Kostyuk et al. [145]; the binding of divalent cations in the vicinity of Na^+-channels were characterized by $K_{Ca} = 90$, $K_{Sr} = 60$, $K_{Ba} = 25$ and $K_{Mg} = 16$ M^{-1} and the binding constants near the Ca^{2+}-channels were $K_{Ca} = 67$, $K_{Sr} = 20$ and $K_{Ba} = 18$ M^{-1}. Mildly acidic groups with pK = 6.2 were identified near both types of channels with a density of $(1.7–2.3) \times 10^{17}/m^2$. Based on the suppression of the Na^+ current through Ca^{2+}-channels in snail neurons by alkaline-earth metal cations in the external solution, these authors further suggested the presence of two types of ion-selective filters in Ca^{2+}-channels, one at the outer membrane surface possessing a strong anionic field, composed of several carboxyl groups and able to bind Ca^{2+}, Sr^{2+}, Ba^{2+} and Mg^{2+} with $K = 3.98 \times 10^6$, 3.16×10^5, 6.31×10^4 and 1.58×10^4, M^{-1}, respectively, and another inside the ion-conducting pore involving a single carboxyl group with high specificity and low affinity for the cations [146]. Different effects of divalent cations on the gating and permeation mechanisms of Ca^{2+}-channels in snail or frog neurons have been interpreted suggesting that cation-induced alterations in the surface charge affect the gating system stronger than the local ion concentrations near the channel entrance, probably due to lower charge density at the membrane surface than at the voltage sensor [148,149]. The quantitative data describing cation binding to nerve cell membranes are summarized in Table 6.

TABLE 6 Characterization of Ionizable Groups at the Surface of Biological Membranes. The Surface Density of Sites (N), their Location on the Membrane Surface, pK Values, and Intrinsic Binding Constants for Different Ions Are Presented[a]

Membrane	Location[b]	$N(m^{-2})$	pK	(Ion) $K(M^{-1})$
Nerve cells				
Squid axon	Outer surface	$(3.5-8.3) \times 10^{17}$	acidic	(Ca^{2+}) 0.1
Marine worm axon	Na^+-gating	8.3×10^{17}	acidic	$(Ca^{2+}) \leq 0.2$
Marine worm axon	K^+-gating	3.3×10^{17}	acidic	$(Ca^{2+}) \leq 0.2$
Frog axon	Ranvier node	3.3×10^{17}	4.5	(Ca^{2+}) 5
				(Mg^{2+}) 3
				(Co^{2+}) 8
				(Ni^{2+}) 10
		2.8×10^{17}	4.5[c]	0.0
		1.9×10^{17}	9.25	0.0
Mollusc neurons	Na^+-channels	1.7×10^{17}	6.2	(Ca^{2+}) 90
				(Mg^{2+}) 16
				(Sr^{2+}) 60
				(Ba^{2+}) 25
	Ca^{2+}-channels	2.3×10^{17}	6.2	(Ca^{2+}) 67
				(Ba^{2+}) 8
				(Sr^{2+}) 20
Mollusc neurons	Outer surface	?	carboxyl	(Ca^{2+}) 3.9×10^6
				(Mg^{2+}) 1.6×10^4
				(Sr^{2+}) 3.2×10^5
				(Ba^{2+}) 6.3×10^4
Mollusc neurons	Outer surface	11×10^{17}	acidic	(Ca^{2+}) 10[d]
				$(Ba^{2+}, Sr^{2+}, Mg^{2+})$ 2
Frog neurons	Ca^{2+}-channels	0.66×10^{17}	acidic	(Ba^{2+}) 15
Muscle cells				
G. pig smooth mus.	Ca^{2+}-channels	5×10^{17}	acidic	(Ca^{2+}) 833
				(Ba^{2+}) 104
				(Sr^{2+}) 556
Frog skelet. muscle	Ca^{2+}-channels	2×10^{17}	acidic	(Ca^{2+}) 45
Canine Purkinje	Outer surface	7.2×10^{17}	acidic	(La^{3+}) 33
				(Zn^{2+}) 4
				$(Ca^{2+}, Ni^{2+}, Ca^{2+})$ 0.8
				(Mn^{2+}) 0.7
				(Co^{2+}) 0.6
				(Ba^{2+}) 0.4
				(Mg^{2+}) 0.0
Purkinje, ventricles	Ca^{2+}-channels	4×10^{17}	acidic	(Ca^{2+}) 1

TABLE 6 *Continued*

Membrane	Location[b]	$N(m^{-2})$	pK	(Ion) $K(M^{-1})$
Erythrocytes				
Human erythrocytes	Outer surface	1.26×10^{17}	8.55[e]	(Li^+) 350
				(Na^+, K^+, NH_4^+) 180
				(Ca^{2+}) 630
				(Mg^{2+}) 436
				(Sr^{2+}) 600
				(Ba^{2+}) 400
		3.4×10^{16}	basic	(HPO_4^{2-}) 0.39
				(Cl^-) 0.50
				(Br^-) 28
				$(H_2PO_4^-)$ 85
				(SCN^-) 128
				(I^-) 216
				(salicylate) 216
				(ClO_4^-) 1220
				(IO_4^-) 4240

[a] The data on nerve cells are taken from Gilbert and Ehrenstein [141], Begenisich [150], Mozhayeva and Naumov [143], Kostyuk et al. [145,146], Zhou and Jones [149], Wilson et al. [147]. The data on muscle cells are from Gantikevich et al. [151], Hanck and Sheets [152], Kass and Krafte [153], Cota and Stefani [154]. The results on erythrocytes are taken from Tatulian et al. [155].

[b] Ion channels indicated in this column mean that the corresponding ionizable groups have been found in the vicinity of these channels.

[c] These groups, which were probably carboxyl groups, did not bind cations because of nearby basic groups [143].

[d] It was possible to describe the results without involving cation binding and using lower surface charge densities [147].

[e] Cation binding constant to the sites with pK = 8.55 were evaluated taking into account their competition with protons [155].

Much less data are available on the effects of anions on the excitability and conductivity of nerve cells, evidently because these effects are small and less important. Tasaki et al. [156] showed that the efficiency of anions in maintaining the excitability of axons decreased according to the sequence: $F^- > HPO_4^{2-} > Glu^- > Asp^- > SO_4^{2-} > Acetate^- > Cl^-$. The membranes were shown to leak in the absence of F^- [144,157].

The results presented in this section indicate that the ion transport in the nerve system is regulated by highly specific arrangement of ionizable groups in and around the ion-conducting channels. Any alterations in the arrangement, ionization state or the excess charge of these groups may have dramatic effects on both the excitability and conductivity of the channels, with corresponding physiological consequences. As illustrated in Fig. 15, a decrease in the outer surface potential of the membrane, e.g., by an increase in the outer ionic strength or by binding of divalent cations, may lead to a change in the polarity of the V_{IM} at a given applied voltage, and thus may crucially affect both the gating machinery and the steady-state conductivity. For example, upon an increase in the plasma Ca^{2+} levels, Ca^{2+} ions adsorb at the outer surface of nerve cells, leading to hyperpolarization of their membranes, increasing the excitation threshold and hence rendering the nerve system less responsive to external stimuli.

B. Muscle Cell Membranes

Like the nerve cells, muscle cells are excitable and are rich in different types of ion channels. Electrophysiological studies of muscle cells, similar to those described in the preceding section, revealed the importance of fixed charges near and inside the ion channels in the excitability and conductivity of the channels. The effects of Ca^{2+} and Ba^{2+} ions on the excitability threshold and the steady-state conductance of frog twitch skeletal muscle cells were described in the frame of the GCS theory, yielding a surface charge density of acidic groups near Ca^{2+}-channels of $2 \times 10^{17}/m^2$ which bind Ca^{2+} ions with $K = 45$ M^{-1} [154]. Shifts in excitatory Na^+ and Ca^{2+} currents in avian ventricular muscle upon elevation of extracellular Ca^{2+} concentrations were explained suggesting that Ca^{2+} ions reduce the negative charge near these channels [158]. Saturation of the current through Ca^{2+}-channels of guinea pig smooth muscle with increasing divalent cation concentrations was described by GCS theory, assuming a fixed negative charge near the Ca^{2+}-channels with a density of $5 \times 10^{17}/m^2$ and using binding constants $K = 833, 556$ and 104 M^{-1} for Ca^{2+}, Sr^{2+} and Ba^{2+} ions, respectively [151]. More data on ion binding to muscle cell membranes are presented in Table 6.

In respect of ion channel functioning cardiac cells are especially interesting because they themselves generate action potential and provide its transmittance and muscle contraction, thus resulting in the excitation–contraction (EC) coupling. These complex processes require the presence of different types of ion channels throughout the heart tissue, such as the L-type (i.e. long lasting) and T-type (i.e. transient) Ca^{2+}-channels. The effects of extracellular divalent and trivalent cations on the Na^+ and L-type Ca^{2+}-channels in mammalian ventricles and Purkinje fibers were described by the GCS theory [152,153,159]. A negative surface charge density of $4 \times 10^{17}/m^2$ near the voltage sensor of the L-type Ca^{2+}-channels was found to be responsible for the divalent cation-induced shifts of the inactivation curves [153]. Calcium ions were able to bind to these charges with $K \approx 1$ M^{-1}, but Ba^{2+} and Sr^{2+} did not bind at all. These authors suggested that surface potential-induced shifts in channel gating can account for the antagonism between divalent cations and 1,4-dihydropiridines. The allosteric coupling between the Ca^{2+}-binding and dihydropiridine-binding domains of L-type Ca^{2+}-channels was demonstrated by site-directed mutagenesis experiments [160]. Electrophysiological data on the Na^+-channels in canine Purkinje cells revealed a very high density of negative charge at the external surface of the membranes, $\sigma = 7.2 \times 10^{17}/m^2$ [152].

These acidic groups were able to bind di- and trivalent cations, which were arranged in the following sequence according to their binding constants (in M^{-1}, shown in parentheses): La^{3+} (33) > Zn^{2+} (4) > Ni^{2+} (0.8) ≈ Cd^{2+} ≈ Ca^{2+} > Mn^{2+} (0.7) > Co^{2+} (0.6) > Ba^{2+} (0.4). It was suggested that Mg^{2+}, which exerted the smallest effect, screened but did not bind to the surface charges.

Using a potentiometric dye in the voltage-clamped transverse tubule membranes of frog twitch skeletal muscle fibers, Heiny and Jong [161] and Jong et al. [162] detected a sharp increase in the membrane surface potential at a threshold of the applied potential of ~ −60 mV, leading to additional depolarization. This result was interpreted in terms of a voltage-dependent conformational change in the dihydropyridine binding domain of the L-type Ca^{2+}-channel, resulting in a ~1 nm displacement of the intramembrane charged residue(s) of the protein thus providing a gating mechanism for the EC coupling. Interestingly, perchlorate anions, which potentiate EC coupling in the skeletal muscle, were shown to shift the voltage-dependence of this process by 13–14 mV to more negative potentials. Other chaotropic anions, such as Br^-, I^- and NO_3^- exert similar effects on skeletal muscle membranes, probably due to the adsorption of these anions at the membrane surface [163]. This is in good agreement with high affinities of perchlorate and other chaotropic anions for PC bilayers, as described in Sec. III.B.1.

Ion channels reconstituted in artificial lipid bilayers have been used to study the effects of membrane surface charge on the channel conductance [164–166]. Laver and Curtis [166] reconstituted the skeletal and cardiac muscle ryanodine receptor Ca^{2+} release channels in planar bilayers and used a rapid solution exchange apparatus to measure the response of channels to rapid changes in Ca^{2+} concentration (Ca^{2+}-dependent gating). Their estimates of the shifts in the bilayer surface potential caused by changes in the ion concentration were in good agreement with the predictions of the GC theory. Coronado and Affolter [165] showed that Ba^{2+} currents through Ca^{2+}-channels of rat skeletal muscle transverse tubules reconstituted in planar bilayers were insensitive to the negative charge of membranes, and Na^+ currents were only 2 times higher in PS than PE bilayers. To rationalize these results, which did not agree very well with the experiments of Apell et al. [164] on gramicidin reconstituted in planar bilayers, these authors suggested that the channel entrance was located in the aqueous phase ~2 nm away from the membrane surface, where the membrane surface potential was shielded by Ba^{2+} ions more strongly than by Na^+ ions.

C. Erythrocytes

Erythrocytes, as other types of cell, carry excess negative charge at their surface [155,167–174] which is necessary to prevent the aggregation of these cells and their adhesion to the blood vessel wall. Treatment of erythrocytes with neuraminidase reduced their electrophoretic mobility, which correlated with the amount of sialic acid released from the cell surface [175–179]. These and other results indicated that the carboxyl groups of the sialic acid attached to the cell surface glycoproteins and glycolipids account for 60–65% of the total negative surface charge of erythrocytes [180–186], whereas other researchers reported that up to 100% of erythrocyte surface sialic acid could be removed by neuraminidase, decreasing the cell electrophoretic mobility to zero [178,179,187]. These results indicate that the negative charge at the red blood cell surface results mainly from carboxyl groups of sialic acid.

Particle electrophoresis has been extensively employed to study the surface electrostatics of erythrocytes and ion binding to their membranes (see Refs. 155 and 173 and references therein). In most cases the electrophoretic mobility was converted to the ζ-potential using the Helmholtz–Smoluchowski equation: $\zeta = \eta u/\varepsilon\varepsilon_0$, where u is the electrophoretic mobility, η and ε are the dynamic viscosity and the dielectric constant of the medium, ε_0 is the permittivity of free space. This approach considers the cell surface as a two-dimensional charged interface and hence all the results of the GCS theory are applicable. The cell surface has also been treated as a three-dimensional interface with a given thickness and charge distribution, which seems more realistic taking into account that the glycocalyx is 5–10 nm thick [173,174,188–191]. The parameters used in the latter approach are the glycocalyx thickness, the mean glycoprotein segment radius, and the volume charge density. Both approaches face certain difficulties in describing the dependence of the cell ζ-potential on salt concentration. A disagreement between the experimental and theoretical curves occurs at low ionic strengths, typically below 50–75 mM salt. This has been explained in terms of glycocalyx swelling due to reduced charge screening at low ionic strengths [171,191].

A number of studies demonstrated selective interactions of inorganic ions with erythrocyte membranes [192–198]. Ion binding to red cell membranes has a number of physiological consequences, such as suppression of their surface potential, divalent cation-induced cell aggregation and anion-induced inhibition of anion transport [169,194,195]. Strongly divergent data on ion binding to erythrocyte membranes have been reported. Seaman et al. [199] found a Ca^{2+} binding constant of 11.4 M^{-1}, whereas others established three types of Ca^{2+}-binding sites at the outer surface of human red cells with binding constants $(3–25) \times 10^4$, $(3–14) \times 10^3$ and $(1–6) \times 10^2$ M^{-1} [197,198, 200]. The binding site characterized by $K_{Ca} = 100–1000$ M^{-1} was attributed to sialic acid residues. Involvement of sialic acids in the binding of Ca^{2+} ions was demonstrated by abolition of the ability of Ca^{2+} to reduce erythrocyte negative surface potential after removal of the cell surface sialic acids by neuraminidase [186].

Anions were reported to increase the cation (Na^+, K^+) permeability and suppress the anion (Cl^-, SO_4^{2-}) permeability of erythrocyte membranes, the efficiency of anions decreasing in the sequence: salicylate $>$ SCN^- $>$ I^- $>$ NO_3^- $>$ Br^- $>$ Cl^- [194,195]. These results were interpreted in terms of selective adsorption of the anions to the cationic groups of cell membranes. In a detailed analysis of the influence of a number of anions and cations on the electrostatic properties of human erythrocytes, basic, anion binding sites and two types of acidic, cation binding sites on the external cell surface were identified [155]. Upon a decrease in the ambient ionic strength from 145 to 18 mM, the density of low-affinity cation binding sites was increased and that of the high-affinity cation binding sited decreased, paralleled with a decrease in the density of acidic groups. This resulted in a decrease in the total negative surface charge density of erythrocytes at low ionic strengths. These effects have been interpreted in terms of ionic strength dependent structural rearrangement in the glycocalyx. The dependence of the ζ-potential of erythrocytes on concentrations of various ions were used to determine the ion binding constants and the binding site densities, as summarized in Table 6. The anion binding constants are arranged in a sequence which is in good agreement with the data of Wieth [194,195] on the influence of anions on ion transport in red blood cell membranes. These results again demonstrate that physiologically important processes taking place in cell membranes may be explained by the influence of ion adsorption on the electrostatic properties of membranes.

V. CONCLUSIONS

Electrostatic potentials and ion adsorption at membrane surfaces exert profound effects on their properties, including membrane structure, phase transitions, adhesion, aggregation and fusion, binding of biologically active molecules to membranes, ion transport and others. Here the theory of membrane electrostatics is presented with an emphasis on the peculiarities of ion binding to membranes. Inorganic ions do bind to lipid bilayers with appreciable binding constants. Cations interact with the phosphate groups of phospholipids, and cation binding constants increase with their charge. The mechanism of anion binding seems to be quite different because their binding constants decrease with increasing anion charge density. The stoichiometries of ion binding to zwitterionic membranes correspond to 10–20 lipid molecules per bound ion, indicating the existence of specific structural elements, presumably point defects, in the lipid lattice which serve as ion binding sites. In the case of acidic lipids, the cation binding stoichiometry is a combination of a 1:1 and 2:1, and probably other, lipid-to-ion ratios. This allows the cations to completely compensate the negative surface charge of the membranes, according to the *equivalent* binding mechanism, and further cause a charge reversal and induce some excess positive charge, according to the *superequivalent* adsorption mechanism. The gel-to-liquid-crystal phase transitions of lipids result in a shift of membrane surface potential to more negative values, probably caused by additional adsorption of anions or desorption of cations, or perhaps both. A novel theoretical approach is presented which allows one to simultaneously determine the ion binding constants and binding site densities based on the observed peculiarities of the dependence of membrane surface potential on ion concentration.

The role of the surface electrostatics of biological membranes is discussed, specifically focusing on three types of cell, the nerve cells, muscle cells and erythrocytes. In the case of excitable cells, such as neurons and muscle cells, the electrostatic surface charge influences the excitability properties of the membranes and ion binding to the charges in the vicinity of ion channels affects the ion transport characteristics. For erythrocytes, as for other blood cells, the surface potential is important to ensure the colloidal stability of the cells and to maintain the hemostasis. Binding of ions to the surface of these cells exerts considerable effects on the ion transport through their plasma membranes, and divalent cations cause cell aggregation and blood flocculation.

LIST OF ABBREVIATIONS

AAS, atomic absorption spectroscopy; CaLB, Ca^{2+}-dependent lipid binding; CL, cardiolipin; DAG, diacylglycerol; DLPG, dilauroylphosphatidylglycerol; DMP, dimethylphosphate; DMPC, dimyristoylphosphatidylcholine; DPPC, dipalmitoylphosphatidylcholine; EC, excitation–contraction; EP, electrophoresis; GC, Gouy–Chapman; GCS, Gouy–Chapman–Stern; GMO, glycerolmonooleate; IFC, internal field compensation; PA, phosphatidic acid; PB, Poisson–Boltzmann; PC, phosphatidylcholine; PE, phosphatidylethanolamine; PG, phosphatidylglycerol; PI, phosphatidylinositol; PIP_2, phosphatidylinositolbisphosphate; PKC, protein kinase C; PLA_2, phospholipase A_2; POPC, 1-palmitoyl-2-oleoylphosphatidylcholine; PS, phosphatidylserine; SGC, sulfogalactosylceramide.

REFERENCES

1. L. Wojtczak, K. S. Famulski, M. J. Nalecz, and J. Zborowski, FEBS Lett. 139:221 (1982).
2. J. J. Volwerk, P. C. Jost, G. H. de Haas, and O. H. Griffith, Biochemistry 25:1726 (1986).
3. H-D. Bäuerle, and J. Seelig, Biochemistry 30:7203 (1991).
4. D. L. Scott, A. M. Mandel, P. B. Sigler, and B. Honig, Biophys. J. 67:493 (1994).
5. S. Duinhoven, R. Poort, G. Van der Voet, W. G. M. Agterof, W. Norde, and J. Lyklema, J. Colloid Interface Sci. 170:340 (1995).
6. S. Duinhoven, R. Poort, G., Van der Voet, W. G. M. Agterof, W. Norde, and J. Lyklema, J. Colloid Interface Sci. 170:351 (1995).

7. S. McLaughlin, and A. Aderem,, Trends Biochem. Sci. *20*: 272 (1995).

8. P. Garcia, R. Gupta, S. Shah, A. J. Morris, S. A. Rudge, S. Scarlata, V. Petrova, S. McLaughlin, and M. J. Rebecchi, Biochemistry *34*: 16228 (1995).

9. R. Dua, S.-K. Wu, and W. Cho, J. Biol. Chem. *270*: 263 (1995).

10. S. K. Han, E. T. Yoon, D. L. Scott, P. B. Sigler, and W. Cho J. Biol. Chem. *272*: 3573 (1997).

11. A. S. Edwards and A. C. Newton, Biochemistry *36*: 15615 (1997).

12. F. G. Van de Goot, J. M. Gonzáles-Mañas, J. H. Lakey, and F. Pattus, Nature *354*: 408 (1991).

13. V. E. Bychkova, A. E. Dujsekina, S. I. Klenin, E. I. Tiktopulo, V. N. Uversky, and O. B. Ptitsyn, Biochemistry *35*: 6058 (1996).

14. S. D. Zakharov, J. B. Heymann, Y.-L. Zhang, and W. A. Cramer, Biophys. J. *70*: 2774 (1996).

15. N. J. Klein, G. I. Shennan, R. S. Heyderman, and M. Levin, J. Cell Sci. *102*: 821 (1992).

16. K. Makino, T. Taki, M. Ogura, S. Handa, M. Nakajima, T. Kondo, and H. Ohshima, Biophys. Chem. *47*: 261 (1993).

17. V. G. Prieto, J. A. Reed, N. S. McNutt, J. K. Bogdany, J. Lugo, and C. R. Shea, Am. J. Dermatol. *17*: 447 (1995).

18. T. Bohler, O. Linderkamp, A. Leo, A. M. Wingen, and K. Scharer, Clin. Nephr. *38*: 119 (1992).

19. F. J. Carrión, A. De la Maza, and J. L. Parra, J. Colloid Interface Sci. *164*: 78 (1994).

20. G. Cevc, Biochim. Biophys. Acta *1031*: 311 (1990).

21. Y. Inoko, T. Yamaguchi, K. Furuya, and T. Mitsui, Biochim. Biophys. Acta *413*: 24 (1975).

22. L. J. Lis, V. A. Parsegian, and R. P. Rand, Biochemistry *20*: 1761 (1981).

23. R. A. Dluhy, D. G. Cameron, H. H. Mantsch, and R. Mendelsohn, Biochemistry *22*: 6318 (1983).

24. S. Ohki, J. Membrane Biol. *77*: 265 (1984).

25. S. Ohki, and H. Ohshima, Biochim. Biophys. Acta *812*: 147 (1985).

26. J. Marra and J. Israelachvili, Biochemistry *24*: 4608 (1985).

27. H. L. Casal, H. H. Mantsch, and H. Hauser, Biochemistry *26*: 4408 (1987).

28. H. L. Casal, A. Martin, H. H. Mantsch, F. Paltauf, and H. Hauser, Biochemistry *26*: 7395 (1987).

29. H. L. Casal, H. H. Mantsch, F. Paltauf, and H. Hauser, Biochim. Biophys. Acta *919*: 275 (1987).

30. S. A. Tatulian, Biochim. Biophys. Acta *901*: 161 (1987).

31. S. A. Tatulian, V. I. Gordeliy, A. E. Sokolova, and A. G. Syrykh, Biochim. Biophys. Acta *1070*: 143 (1991).

32. H. Hauser, Chem. Phys. Lipids *57*: 309 (1991).

33. S. Ohki and O. Zschörnig, Chem. Phys. Lipids *65*: 193 (1993).

34. H. Minami, T. Inoue, and R. Shimozawa, J. Colloid Interface Sci. *158*: 460 (1993).

35. H. Minami, T. Inoue, and R. Shimozawa, J. Colloid Interface Sci. *164*: 9 (1994).

36. H. Minami, T. Inoue, and R. Shimozawa, Langmuir *12*: 3574 (1996).

37. J. R. Coorssen, and R. P. Rand, Biophys. J. *68*: 1009 (1995).

38. S. A. Summers, B. A. Guebert, and M. F. Shanahan, Biophys. J. *71*: 3199 (1996).

39. L. A. Flanagan, C. C. Cunningham, J. Chen, G. D. Prestwich, K. S. Kosik, and P. A. Janmey, Biophys. J. *73*:1440 (1997).
40. R. Koynova, J. Brankov, and B. Tenchov, Eur. Biophys. J. *25*:261 (1997).
41. K. D. Collins, Biophys. J. *72*:65 (1997).
42. L. Chang, K. Kuo, S. Lin, and C. Chang, J. Protein Chem. *13*:641 (1994).
43. J. D. Clark, A. R. Schievella, E. A. Nalefski, and L.-L. Lin, J. Lipid Mediators Cell Signaling *12*:83 (1995).
44. E. A. Nalefski, L. A. Sultzman, D. M. Martin, R. W. Kriz, P. S. Towler, J. L. Knopf, and J. D. Clark, J. Biol. Chem. *269*:18239 (1994).
45. A. C. Newton, Annu. Rev. Biophys. Biomol. Struct. *22*:1 (1993).
46. Y. Nishizuka, Science *258*:607 (1992).
47. A. Baba, S. Sakuma, H. Okatomo, T. Inoue, and H. Iwata, J. Biol. Chem. *264*:15790 (1989).
48. A. Watson and F. J. Doherty, Biochem. J. *298*:377 (1994).
49. R. Malaviya, R. Malaviya, and B. A. Jakschik, J. Biol. Chem. *268*:4939 (1993).
50. M. Peters-Golden and R. W. McNish, Biochem. Biophys. Res. Commun. *196*:147 (1993).
51. M. Durstin, S. Durstin, T. P. F. Molski, E. L. Becker, and R. I. Sha'afi, Proc. Natl. Acad. Sci. USA *91*:3142 (1994).
52. J. D. Clark, L.-L. Lin, R. W. Kriz, C. S. Ramesha, L. A. Sultzman, A. Y. Lin, N. Milona, and J. L. Knopf, Cell *65*:1043 (1991).
53. S. Glover, T. Bayburt, M. Jones, E. Chi, and M. H. Gelb, J. Biol. Chem. *270*:15359 (1995).
54. A. R. Schievella, M. K. Regiers, W. L. Smith, and L.-L. Lin, J. Biol. Chem. *270*:30749 (1995).
55. R. M. Kramer and J. D. Sharp, FEBS Lett. *410*:49 (1997).
56. J. Wijkander, and R. Sundler, Biochem. Biophys. Res. Commun. *184*:118 (1992).
57. E. A. Nalefski and J. J. Falke, Protein Sci. *5*:2375 (1996).
58. M. Pouliot, P. P. McDonald, E. Krump, J. A. Mancini, S. McColl, P. K. Weech, and P. Borgeat, Eur. J. Biochem. *238*:250 (1996).
59. A. C. Newton and L. M. Keranen, Biochemistry *33*:6651 (1994).
60. S. Jaken, Current Opin. Cell Biol. *8*:168 (1996).
61. J. W. Orr and A. C. Newton, Biochemistry *31*:4661 (1992).
62. J. W. Orr and A. C. Newton, Biochemistry *31*:4667 (1992).
63. R. J. Hunter, *Foundations of Colloid Science*, Vol. 1, Clarendon Press, Oxford, 1987.
64. D. Andelman, in *Structure and Dynamics of Membranes*, Vol. 1B, *Generic and Specific interactions* (R. Lipowsky and E. Sackmann, eds.) Elsevier, Amsterdam, 1995, pp. 603–642.
65. S. McLaughlin, Curr. Topics Membranes Transport *9*:71 (1977).
66. S. McLaughlin, Annu. Rev. Biophys. Biophys. Chem. *18*:113 (1989).
67. G-L. Gouy, J. Phys. (Paris) *9*:457 (1910).
68. D. L. Chapman, Phil. Mag. *25*:475 (1913).
69. H. Müller, Cold Spring Harbor Symp. Quant. Biol. *1*:1 (1933).
70. D. C. Grahame, Chem. Rev. *41*:441 (1947).
71. B. V. Derjaguin, N. V. Churaev, and V. M. Muller, in *Surface Forces*, (J. A. Kitchener, ed.) Plenum, New York, 1987.
72. J. Bentz, J. Colloid Interface Sci. *90*:164 (1982).

73. J.-P. Hsu and Y.-C Kuo, J. Colloid Interface Sci. *166*: 208 (1994).
74. O. Stern, Z. Elektrochem. *30*: 508 (1924).
75. S. A. Tatulian, J. Phys. Chem. *98*: 4963 (1994).
76. S. A. Tatulian, J. Colloid Interface Sci. *175*: 131 (1995).
77. A. Lau, A. McLaughlin, and S. McLaughlin, Biochim. Biophys. Acta *645*: 279 (1981).
78. S. McLaughlin, N. Mulrine, T. Gresalfi, G. Vaio, and A. McLaughlin, J. Gen. Physiol. *77*: 445 (1981).
79. S. A. Tatulian, in *Water and Ions in Biological Systems* (P. Läuger, L. Packer, and V. Vasilescu, eds.) Birkhäuser Verlag, Berlin, 1988, pp. 99–110.
80. M. Toner, G. Vaio, A. McLaughlin, and S. McLaughlin, Biochemistry *27*: 7435 (1988).
81. Yu. A. Ermakov, V. V. Cherny, and V. S. Sokolov, Biol. Mem. *9*: 201 (1992).
82. J. A. Cohen and M. Cohen, Biophys. J. *36*: 623 (1981).
83. J. A. Cohen and M. Cohen, Biophys. J. *46*: 487 (1984).
84. I. S. Graham, J. A. Cohen, and M. J. Zuckermann, J. Colloid Interface Sci. *135*: 335 (1990).
85. S. A. Tatulian, in *Phospholipids Handbook* (G. Cevc, ed.), Marcel Dekker, New York, 1993, Chapter 14, pp. 511–552.
86. S. A. Tatulian, Biochim. Biophys. Acta *736*: 189 (1983).
87. S. A. Tatulian, Eur. J. Biochem. *170*: 413 (1987).
88. S. A. Tatulian, Yu. A. Ermakov, V. I. Gordeliy, A. E. Sokolova, and A. G. Syrykh, Biol Mem. *9*: 741 (1992).
89. N. S. Matinyan, G. B. Melikyan, V. B. Arakelyan, S. L. Kocharov, N. V. Prokazova, and Ts. M. Avakian, Biochim. Biophys. Acta *984*: 313 (1989).
90. Yu. A. Ermakov, S. S. Mahmudova, E. V. Shevchenko, and V. I. Lobyshev, Biol. Mem. *10*: 212 (1993).
91. K. Satoh, Biochim. Biophys. Acta *1239*: 239 (1995).
92. M. Eisenberg, T. Gresalfi, T. Riccio, and S. McLaughlin, Biochemistry *18*: 5213 (1979).
93. J. R. Rydall and P. M. Macdonald, Biochemistry *31*: 1092 (1992).
94. R. Bartucci and L. Sportelli, Biochim. Biophys. Acta *1195*: 229 (1994).
95. L. I. Barsukov, V. I. Volkova, Yu. E. Shapiro, A. V. Viktorov, V. F. Bystrov, and L. D. Bergelson, Bioorg. Khimiia *3*: 1355 (1977).
96. H. Grasdalen, L. E. G. Eriksson, J. Westman, and A. Ehrenberg, Biochim. Biophys. Acta *469*: 151 (1977).
97. J. Westman and L. E. G. Eriksson, Biochim. Biophys. Acta *557*: 62 (1979).
98. P. M. Macdonald and J. Seelig, Biochemistry *27*: 6769 (1988).
99. A. Chrzeszczyk, A. Wishnia, and C. S. Springer, Jr., Biochim. Biophys. Acta *648*: 28 (1981).
100. R. L. Misiorowski and M. A. Wells, Biochemistry *12*: 967 (1973).
101. D. H. Haynes, J. Membrane Biol. *17*: 341 (1974).
102. S. A. Sundberg and W. L. Hubbell, Biophys. J. *49*: 553 (1986).
103. F. Bellemare and R. Lesage, J. Colloid Interface Sci. *147*: 462 (1991).
104. P. W. Nolden and T. Ackermann, Biophys. Chem. *4*: 297 (1976).
105. H. Hauser, C. C. Hinckley, J. Krebs, B. A. Levine, M. C. Phillips, and R. J. P. Williams, Biochim. Biophys. Acta *468*: 364 (1977).

106. H. Hauser, M. C. Phillips, B. A. Levine, and R. J. P. Williams, Eur. J. Biochem. 58:133 (1975).
107. A. McLaughlin, Biochemistry 21:4879 (1982).
108. L. Herbette, C. Napolitano, and R. V. McDaniel, Biophys. J. 46:677 (1984).
109. M. Bozsik, C. Helm, L. Laxhuber, and H. Möhwald, J. Colloid Interface Sci. 107:514 (1985).
110. M. Petersheim and J. Sun, Biophys. J. 55:631 (1989).
111. M. Petersheim, H. N. Halladay, and J. Blodnieks, Biophys. J. 56:551 (1989).
112. R. Lehrmann and J. Seelig, Biochim. Biophys. Acta 1189:89 (1994).
113. A. McLaughlin, C. Grathwohl, and S. McLaughlin, Biochim. Biophys. Acta 513:338 (1978).
114. Y. K. Levine, A. G. Lee, N. J. M. Birdsall, J. C. Metcalfe, and J. D. Robinson, Biochim. Biophys. Acta 291:592 (1973).
115. C.-H. Huang, J. P. Sipe, S. T. Chow, and R. B. Martin, Proc. Natl. Acad. Sci. USA 71:359 (1974).
116. B. Sears, W. C. Hutton, and T. E. Thompson, Biochemistry 15:1635 (1976).
117. L. Pasquale, A. Winiski, C. Oliva, G. Vaio, and S. McLaughlin, J. Gen. Physiol. 88:697 (1986).
118. C. Newton, W. Pangborn, S. Nir, and D. Papahadjopoulos, Biochim. Biophys. Acta 506:281 (1978).
119. S. Tupper, P. T. T. Wong, and N. Tanphaichitr, Biochemistry 31:11902 (1992).
120. S. Tupper, P. T. T. Wong, M. Kates, and N. Tanphaichitr, Biochemistry 33:13250 (1994).
121. F. López-García, V. Micol, J. Villalaín, and J. C. Gómez-Fernandez, Biochim. Biophys. Acta 1169:264 (1993).
122. F. López-García, J. Villalaín, and J. C. Gómez-Fernandez, Biochim. Biophys. Acta 1236:279 (1995).
123. W. Hübner, H. H. Mantsch, F. Paltauf, and H. Hauser, Biochemistry 33:320 (1994).
124. D. L. Holwerda, P. D. Ellis, and R. E. Wuthier, Biochemistry 20:418 (1981).
125. P. J. Quinn and W. R. Sherman, Biochim. Biophys. Acta 233:734 (1971).
126. R. McDaniel and S. McLaughlin, Biochim. Biophys. Acta 819:153 (1985).
127. M. D. Reboiras and M. N. Jones, Colloids Surf. 15:239 (1985).
128. H.-J. Galla and E. Sackmann, Biochim. Biophys. Acta 401:509 (1975).
129. J. Bentz, D. Alford, J. Cohen, and N. Düzgünes, Biophys. J. 53:593 (1988).
130. H. Träuble, in Structure of Biological Membranes (S. Abrahamsson and I. Pascher, eds.), Plenum Press, New York, 1977, pp. 509–550.
131. A. Blume and J. Tuchtenhagen, Biochemistry 31:4636 (1992).
132. R. C. MacDonald, S. A. Simon, and E. Baer, Biochemistry 15:885 (1976).
133. M. Papánková and D. Horvát, Biochim. Biophys. Acta 778:17 (1984).
134. J. S. Puskin and T. Martin, Biochim. Biophys. Acta 552:53 (1979).
135. B. A. Cunningham, E. Gelerinter, and L. J. Lis, Chem. Phys. Lipids 46:205 (1988).
136. H. Träuble, Naturwissenschaften 58:277 (1971).
137. P. Smejtek and S. Wong, Biophys. J. 58:1285 (1990).
138. P. F. Baker, A. L. Hodgkin, and H. Meves, J. Physiol. 170:541 (1964).
139. W. K. Chandler, A. L. Hodgkin, and H. Meves, J. Physiol. 180:821 (1965).

140. M. P. Blaustein and D. E. Goldman, J. Gen. Physiol. *51*:279 (1968).
141. D. L. Gilbert and G. Ehrenstein, Biophys. J. *9*:447 (1969).
142. B. Hille, J. Gen. Physiol. *51*:221 (1968).
143. G. N. Mozhayeva and A. P. Naumov, Nature *228*:164 (1970).
144. T. Begenisich and C. Lynch, J. Gen. Physiol. *63*:675 (1974).
145. P. G. Kostyuk, S. L. Mironov, P. A. Doroshenko, and V. N. Ponomarev, J. Membrane Biol. *70*:171 (1982).
146. P. G. Kostyuk, S. L. Mironov, and Ya. M. Shuba, J. Membrane Biol. *76*:83 (1983).
147. D. L. Wilson, K. Morimoto, Y. Tsada, and A. M. Brown, J. Membrane Biol. *72*:117 (1983).
148. L. Byerly, P. B. Chase, and J. R. Stimers, J. Gen. Physiol. *85*:491 (1985).
149. W. Zhou and S. W. Jones, J. Gen. Physiol. *105*:441 (1995).
150. T. Begenisich, J. Gen. Physiol. *66*:47 (1975).
151. V. Ya. Gantikevich, M. F. Shuba, and S. V. Smirnov, J. Physiol. *399*:419 (1988).
152. D. A. Hanck and M. F. Sheets, J. Physiol. *454*:267 (1992).
153. R. S. Kass and D. S. Krafte, J. Gen. Physiol. *89*:629 (1987).
154. G. Cota and E. Stefani, J. Physiol. *351*:135 (1984).
155. S. A. Tatulian, A. N. Tulupov, and E. V. Polishchuk, Gen. Physiol. Biophys. 7:613 (1988).
156. I. Tasaki, I. Singer, and T. Takanaka, J. Gen. Physiol. *48*:1095 (1965).
157. W. J. Adelman, Jr., F. Dyro, and J. P. Senft, Science *151*:1392 (1966).
158. D. Inoue and A. J. Pappano, Circ. Res. *52*:625 (1983).
159. M. F. Sheets and D. A. Hanck, J. Physiol. *454*:299 (1992).
160. B. Z. Peterson and W. A. Catterall, J. Biol. Chem. *270*:18201 (1995).
161. J. A. Heiny, and D. Jong, J. Gen. Physiol. *95*:147 (1990).
162. D. Jong, K. Stroffekova, and J. A. Heiny, J. Physiol. *499*:787 (1997).
163. W. G. Nayler and J. M. Price, Am. J. Physiol. *213*:1459 (1967).
164. H. J. Apell, E. Bamberg, and P. Läuger, Biochim. Biophys. Acta *522*:369 (1979).
165. R. Coronado and H. Affolter, J. Gen. Physiol. *87*:933 (1986).
166. D. R. Laver and B. A. Curtis, Biophys. J. *71*:722 (1996).
167. G. V. F. Scaman and D. H. Heard, J. Gen. Physiol. *44*:251 (1960).
168. K. Jan and S. Chien, J. Gen. Physiol. *61*:638 (1973).
169. K. Jan and S. Chien, J. Gen. Physiol. *61*:655 (1973).
170. G. V. F. Seaman, Ann. N. Y. Acad. Sci. *416*:176 (1983).
171. P. Snabre and P. Mills, Colloid Polym. Sci. *263*:494 (1985).
172. P. Snabre, P. Mills, and A. B. Thiam, Colloid Polym. Sci. *264*:103 (1986).
173. M. Nakamura, H. Ohshima, and T. Kondo, Colloids Surf. B: Biointerfaces *2*:445 (1994).
174. Y. Nakano, K. Makino, H. Ohshima, and T. Kondo, Biophys. Chem. *50*:249 (1994).
175. D. H. Heard, and G. V. F. Seaman, J. Gen. Physiol. *43*:635 (1960).
176. E. H. Eylar, M. A. Madoff, O. V. Brody, and J. L. Oncley, J. Biol. Chem. *237*:1992 (1962).
177. G. V. F. Seaman and G. M. W. Cook, in *Cell Electrophoresis* (E. J. Ambrose, ed.), J. and A. Churchill Ltd., London, 1965, pp. 48–65.
178. F. J. Nordt, R. J. Knox, and G. V. F. Seaman, J. Gen. Physiol. *97*:209 (1978).

179. H. Walter, C. H. Tamblyn, E. J. Krob, and G. V. F. Seaman, Biochim. Biophys. Acta *734*: 368 (1983).
180. G. M. W. Cook, D. H. Heard, and G. V. F. Seaman, Nature *191*: 44 (1961).
181. G. M. W. Cook, Nature *195*: 159 (1962).
182. D. A. Haydon, and G. V. F. Seaman, Arch. Biochem. Biophys. *122*: 126 (1967).
183. J. N. Mehrishi, Prog. Biophys. Mol. Biol. *25*: 1 (1972).
184. G. V. F. Seaman, J. Supramol. Struct. *1*: 437 (1973).
185. J. Viitala and J. Järnefelt, Trends Biochem. Sci. *10*: 392 (1985).
186. J. Mészáros, L. Villanova, and A. J. Pappano, J. Mol. Cell Cardiol. *20*: 481 (1988).
187. E. Donath and D. Lerche, Bioelectrochem. Bioenerg. *7*: 41 (1980).
188. V. Pastushenko and E. Donath, Stud. Biophys. *56*: 7 (1976).
189. E. Donath and V. Pastushenko, J. Electroanal. Chem. *104*: 543 (1979).
190. E. Donath and V. Pastushenko, Bioelectrochem. Bioenerg. *7*: 31 (1980).
191. S. Levine, M. Levine, K. A. Sharp, and D. E. Brooks, Biophys. J. *42*: 127 (1983).
192. W. L. G. Gent, J. R. Trounce, and M. Walser, Arch. Biochem. Biophys. *105*: 582 (1964).
193. G. V. F. Seaman and B. A. Pethica, Biochem. J. *90*: 573 (1964).
194. J. O. Wieth, J. Physiol. *207*: 563 (1970).
195. J. O. Wieth, J. Physiol. *207*: 581 (1970).
196. R. B. Mikkelsen and D. F. H. Wallach, Biochim. Biophys. Acta *363*: 211 (1974).
197. C. Long and B. Mouat, Biochem. J. *123*: 829 (1971).
198. C. M. Cohen and A. K. Solomon, J. Membrane Biol. *29*: 345 (1976).
199. G. V. F. Seaman, P. S. Vassar, and M. J. Kendall, Arch. Biochem. Biophys. *135*: 356 (1969).
200. R. B. Moore, E. E. Dryden, D. I. Kells, and J. F. Manery, Can. J. Biochem. Mol. Biol. *62*: 398 (1984).

23

Ion Transport Across a Membrane with Soft Polar Interfaces

VICTOR LEVADNY The Scientific Council for Cybernetics, Russian Academy of Sciences, Moscow, Russia

VICENTE AGUILELLA Departament de Ciències Experimentals, Universitat "Jaume I," de Castelló, Castelló, Spain

MARINA BELAYA Institute of Plant Physiology, Russian Academy of Sciences, Moscow, Russia

Abstract

The ion transport across membranes with extended soft permeable interfaces (polar zones), placed in an aqueous solution, is considered. These membranes have three layers: an inner hydrophobic layer and two polar zones which usually contain fixed charges and dipoles. Nernst–Planck's and Poisson's equation are used for analyzing ion transport under general conditions and in two limit cases: (a) when the internal hydrophobic layer is the rate-controlling barrier; and (b) when the polar zones are the rate-controlling barrier. The influence of the electrolyte concentration, the surface dipole density and the thickness of the polar zone on the total ion flux and permselectivity is studied.

I. INTRODUCTION

Soft interfaces are a distinctive feature of a large group of membranes in which the most representative group is formed by some biological structures such as proteins, cells and lipid membranes [1–6]. In these membrane systems the hydrophobic groups form, in some sense, a core which is shielded from the aqueous medium by the hydrophilic groups. The latter extend into the water region and create a polar zone whose boundaries are far from being sharp. Actually, the polar zone thickness L is a phenomenological parameter that describes the extent of water and ion penetration into this region of the membrane.

Such interfaces have been called *soft*, because they are filled with water molecules and ions from the solution in addition to the membrane surface molecular structures. Besides, their thickness is large enough in comparison with the characteristic size of the total membrane system. In the case of lipid membranes, the interfaces are the zones of lipid polar heads, whereas in the case of biological membranes they are defined by the cytoskeleton, spectrin layer, glycocalyx and/or other surface structures [2–4]. The presence of charged groups, either compensated (e.g., in phosphatidylcholine bilayers) or uncompensated (e.g., in phosphatidylserine bilayers) contributes to the existence of a dipole moment distribution in the polar zones, together with the dipole moment of the interfacial water molecules. However, the origin of the so-called *dipole potential* is not so simple and is still under discussion. Here we analyze a general system without reference to any particular membrane.

Usually, L is much greater than the characteristic spatial extent of the electric charges and dipoles and can vary from $5 - 10$ Å for lipid membranes [1,3, 32–34,58] to 40–70 Å for some cells [36]. The same membrane can exhibit different polar zone thickness according to its phase state and external conditions [1,26]. For example, it is known that Ca^{2+} and prolepherin [31] push out the water molecules from the lipid polar zones and thereby decrease its thickness. In addition, NMR and ESR data suggest that the presence of ions increases the mobility of the lipid head groups [34] and hence, makes L bigger. All this evidence suggest analyzing the influence of the polar zone thickness on ion transport.

Usually, the membrane fixed charges and dipoles are located inside this boundary zone. Besides, due to the specific structure of soft interfaces, the

electric fields created by them differ from the fields that appear in the electrolyte near the common membranes. It is well known that the electric field of an
infinitely large layer of a constant distribution of dipoles is identically zero.
But in this kind of membranes with soft interfaces, the surface dipoles are able
to create a significant electric field in the solution [8,9] which depends on the
thickness of the soft interface. Due to the effect of dipoles, for instance, a
positively charged surface can give rise to an apparent negative "surface"
potential (and vice versa), the electric field can change from negative far from
the membrane to positive near the interface [9], and changing the ion concentration or the polar zone thickness can cause the surface potential to change
its sign [10]. As mentioned above, surface dipoles play an unusual role in the
considered systems, so they deserve a special attention. Apart from creating an
electric barrier for ions, in the case of nonzero polar zone thickness they have
some effect on the electric field distribution in solution.

Another reason for a detailed study of the ion transport across membranes
with soft polar interfaces can be illustrated with a particular experimental fact.
Different lipid membranes may have similar inner hydrophobic parts, which
consist of short CH_2-chains, while at the same time their polar zones are
remarkably different [1,26]. For hydrophilic ions, such as Ca^{2+}, Na^+, K^+ the
inner hydrophobic layer of the membrane is the main barrier and hence, the
permeability of any hydrophilic ion should be expected to be the same in any
lipid membrane. However, there is evidence that this is not true (see for
example [27]). It means that the polar zones of such membranes exert some
influence on the ionic transport. In addition, it has been also demonstrated in
other cases that the polar zones determine the transport properties of the
membrane system [28,29]. Apart from this, the interaction between ions and
fixed charges in the polar region of a phospholipid bilayer have been shown to
be important in determining ionic permeability [25].

We will consider here how polar zone parameters influence on the steady-
state ionic transport through such a membrane. Particularly, the way the
polar zone thickness L, and the surface density of charges σ and dipoles v have
some effect on the permeability, permselectivity and conductance of the membrane.

The transport of ions through the system under consideration includes a
few steps: (a) passage of ions across the unstirred layers; (b) passage of ions
across the polar zones (that actually includes passage of ions across dipole
interfaces and ion diffusion and migration in the polar zones itself); and (c)
transport thorough the hydrophobic layer. For the sake of simplicity, it is
worth to consider the two main limit cases, namely, (i) the inner hydrophobic
layer as the rate-determining barrier; and (ii) the polar zones (together with
the dipole interfaces) as the rate-determining barrier. The steady state transport of ions is described by the combination of Nernst–Planck's and Poisson's
equations. The first one describes electrodiffusion migration of ions in any
medium [11–14] and the second one relates the electric potential distribution

$\psi(x)$ with the sources of the electric field. Thus, to analyze the ion transport across a membrane with soft interfaces, it is necessary to determine first the potential profile $\psi(x)$ in the whole system.

The real translocation of ions across membranes is of course a complicated process, too complex to model in a simple way. Nevertheless, it seems appropriate firstly to get the main qualitative result on the basis of a relatively simple model and secondly to exhaust the possibilities of a simple model before introducing additional complications. After analyzing the electric potential profiles near the membrane in absence of ion fluxes, we study the nonequilibrium case when electric current is small enough. Then, after a general description of ion transport, we explore in detail the two limit cases of transport controlled by the hydrophobic layer and transport controlled by the polar zones.

II. THE ELECTRIC POTENTIAL PROFILE NEAR A MEMBRANE UNDER QUASI-EQUILIBRIUM CONDITIONS

Let us consider a planar, charged inhomogeneous membrane separating two aqueous solution of a binary electrolyte with concentrations C_1 and C_2 on the left and right side, respectively of the membrane. The membrane consists of three layers: a central hydrophobic one and two hydrophilic zones. The geometry of the system is illustrated in Fig. 1, where the Cartesian spatial

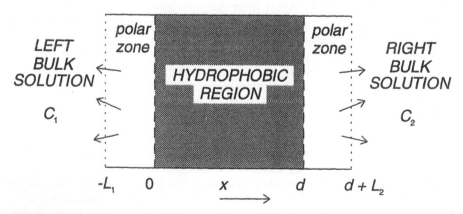

FIG. 1 Schematic cross-section of the membrane system. The hydrophobic region is shown cross-hatched and the charges and dipoles are assumed to be on the planes at $x = -L_1$ and $x = d + L_2$. The aqueous solution region extends from $x = -\infty$ to $x = 0$ and from $x = d$ to $x = d + \infty$. The hydrophilic zones extend from $x = -L_1$ to $x = 0$ and from $x = d$ to $x = d + L_2$ [40].

coordinate system has been chosen in such a manner that the y and z axes lie in the membrane plane and the x-axis is perpendicular to it. We are interested here in charged membranes. Moreover, inside the hydrophilic polar zones of the membrane there are fixed charges and dipoles that are strongly bound to the hydrophobic core [1,2,25]. It is well known that near such kind of membranes bathed in electrolyte solution there is a region typically 10–1000 Å thick where a Double Electric Layer (DEL) arises, with considerable departure from electroneutrality [1,11,15]. Generally the distribution of the electric potential $\phi(x)$ (unit V) in any system is determined by Poisson's equation:

$$\frac{d}{dx}\left[\varepsilon(x)\frac{d\phi(x)}{dx}\right] = -\frac{\rho(x)}{\varepsilon_0} \tag{1}$$

(where ε_0 is the permittivity of vacuum). To apply this general equation to the system considering here it is necessary to take into account all sources of electric field that contribute to the volume charge density $\rho(x)$ (unit $e/\text{Å}^3$). Remember that the system consists of a central hydrophobic layer; two hydrophilic polar zones and two outside solutions. Let us discuss shortly $\rho(x)$ for each part of the system.

As for hydrophobic zone, it is necessary to take into account that we are considering here only inorganic ions transport (Na^+, K^+, Cl^-, etc.), whose partition coefficients are usually very small for real membranes (e.g. of the order 10^{-30} for nonmodified lipid membranes [1,14]). So $\rho(x) = 0$ everywhere inside the hydrophobic zone.

In the region outside the hydrophobic layer $\rho(x)$ includes both mobile free ions of solution and fixed sources of electric field of the membrane. The latter consists of the mentioned above fixed charges and dipoles. It is important to underline that apart from this, in hydrophilic zones there are a number of water molecules and ions from the bathing solution. (Although these zones are denoted as *polar zones*, strictly speaking, only a few membranes, e.g., lipid membranes, have their polar groups only in these regions. So the hydrophilic zone thickness L is a phenomenological parameter that describes the extent of water and ion penetration into this loose region of the membrane). In reality the space distributions of fixed charges and dipoles inside the polar zones can be complicated enough. Their specific distributions influence on the electric potential profile $\phi(x)$ significantly, but there are some characteristics that are common for all specific distributions. To clarify just these characteristics it is worth analyzing an idealized, simplified charge and dipole distribution. First of all we assume that the membrane fixed charge and dipole densities depend only upon x and neither upon z nor upon y. Besides, we shall consider here only the effect of the normal x-component of the dipoles. This is because the lateral component contributes much less than the x-component of the electric dipole to the electric field [37].

Then we also assume that the electric dipoles and membrane surface charges in each polar zone are located on one plane that is placed on the external boundary of the polar zone, i.e., the total effective fixed charge density $\rho_{i,\,\text{fix}}$ of each polar zone (unit $e/\text{Å}^3$) can be mathematically represented as

$$\rho_{i,\,\text{fix}}(x) = \sigma_i \delta[\bar{x} - (-1)^i L_i] - v_i \delta'[\bar{x} - (-1)^i L_i]\,; \tag{2}$$

$$\bar{x} = \begin{cases} x & i = 1 \\ x - d & i = 2 \end{cases}$$

where σ_i is the surface charge density (unit $e/\text{Å}^2$); v_i is the surface dipole density of the normal dipole component (unit $e/\text{Å}$); $\delta(x - L)$ is Dirac's delta function and $\delta'(x - L)$ is its derivative; e is the elementary charge. Here and everywhere subscript 1 denotes the left side of the membrane and subscript 2 denotes the right side.

The distribution (2) represents the simplified idealized model of the real distribution. However there are two reasons to use just Eq. (2). Firstly, as we shall see below, this distribution really contains the main common characteristics of a DEL near a membrane with soft interfaces, namely the influence of the surface dipoles v and polar zone thickness L on the electric potential profile $\phi(x)$. Secondly, generalization for any distribution of fixed charges and dipoles can be easily obtained by summation or integration of the solution obtained on the basis of Eq. (2) (see [10,40]).

Summarizing these speculations we can represent the charge density $\rho(x)$ in the system considered here in the following manner:

$$\rho_i(x) = \begin{cases} 0 & 0 < x < d \\ \rho_{i,\,\text{fix}} + e(z^+ C_i^+ + z^- C_i^-) & 0 \le (-1)^i \bar{x} < \infty \end{cases} \tag{3}$$

Here $C_i^\pm(x)$ (unit ion/cm³) and $z^\pm$ denote the local ion concentration and valence of positive and negative ions of the ith solution. The expression for $\rho_{i,\,\text{fix}}(x)$ is found in Eq. (2). As for ion concentration profiles $C_i^\pm(x)$ in Eq. (3), under zero flux conditions the DEL is in thermodynamic equilibrium and hence the ion concentration profiles can be described by Boltzmann's equation. Strictly speaking, the electric current perturbs the DEL and transforms it into a nonequilibrium Double Electric Layer (NDEL) (see [52–56] and references therein). However, usually, for the sake of simplicity, the influence of the ion fluxes on the electric potential profiles is neglected, i.e., it is assumed that the electric current is small enough. To clarify the main characteristics of the DEL near a charged membrane with a soft interfaces, we shall also use this assumption.

The dielectric permittivity profile $\varepsilon(x)$ is the last that we have to determine to apply eq. (1) to the membrane system considered. As the latter consists of a central hydrophobic layer; two hydrophilic polar zones and two outside solutions then $\varepsilon(x)$ can be represented by three dielectric constants: the dielectric constant of aqueous solution $\varepsilon = 78$ for $-\infty < x < -L_1$ and $d + L_2 < x < +\infty$; the dielectric constant of the polar zone $\varepsilon_p = 10\text{--}40$ (see [35] for $-L_1 < x < 0$ and $d < x < d + L_2$; and the dielectric constant of the hydrophobic layer $\varepsilon_h = 2\text{--}3$ (see [1,2]) for $0 < x < d$. If Eq. (1) is combined with the usual boundary conditions $\phi(-\infty) = 0$ and $\phi(+\infty) = -\phi_{ext}$ (where ϕ_{ext} is the externally applied electric potential), then an electric potential distribution $\phi(x)$ in the considered membrane system can be obtained [10,40] which allows analysis of any membrane. However to clarify the main properties of the membrane system we will concentrate on the symmetrical membrane system and neglect the differences between the polar zone dielectric constant ε_p and the one in the aqueous solution ε, i.e.,

$$L_1 = L_2 \equiv L$$
$$\sigma_1 = \sigma_2 \equiv \sigma$$
$$v_1 = -v_2 \equiv -v$$
$$\varepsilon_p = \varepsilon = 78$$

To simplify, it is worth considering the case of small potentials to ensure the validity of Debye–Hückel's approximation. Then, introducing the dimensionless electric potential $\psi(x)$, we can represent the Eqs. (1)–(3) as the following Poisson–Boltzmann's equation:

$$\frac{d^2\psi}{dx^2} = \begin{cases} 0; & 0 < x < d \\ k_i^2\psi(x) - \alpha\rho_{i,\,\text{fix}}(x); & 0 \le (-1)^i\bar{x} \le L \\ k_i^2\psi(x); & L < (-1)^i\bar{x} < \infty \end{cases} \qquad (4)$$

with boundary conditions:

$$\psi(-\infty) = 0; \qquad \psi(\infty) = -\psi_{ext} \qquad (5)$$

where: $\alpha = \beta/\varepsilon\varepsilon_0$ and k_i is the inverse Debye length of the solution in i-semispace, which for a binary symmetrical electrolyte ($|z^+| = |z^-| = z$) reads:

$$k_i^2 = \frac{2C_i e^2 z^2}{\varepsilon\varepsilon_0 k_B T} = \frac{2C_i ez^2\beta}{\varepsilon\varepsilon_0} \qquad (i = 1, 2)$$

C_i is the bulk concentration in ith solution. The dimensionless electric potential $\psi(x)$ is connected with the real electric potential $\phi(x)$ in the usual way $\psi(x) = \beta\phi(x)$, $\beta = e/k_B T$ (for room temperature $\beta^{-1} = 25.7$ mV); k_B is Boltzmann's constant.

Equations (4) and (5) determine the electric potential profile $\psi(x)$ in the membrane system. There are a few methods for solution of Eqs. (4) and (5). The simplest one is the following: let us "cut" the total electric profile $\psi(x)$ into five parts. Each of them is valid only in corresponding part of the considered membrane system, i.e., $\psi_i(x)$ for outside solutions; $\psi_{pi}(x)$ for polar zones; $\psi_h(x)$ for the hydrophobic layer. To get the solution it is necessary to take into account that they must satisfy the following matching conditions:

at the polar zone boundaries:

$$\psi_2(d + L + 0) - \psi_{p2}(d + L - 0) = \alpha v \tag{6}$$

$$\frac{d\psi_2}{dx}(d + L + 0) - \frac{d\psi_{p2}}{dx}(d + L - 0) = \alpha\sigma \tag{7}$$

$$\psi_{p1}(-L + 0) - \psi_1(-L - 0) = -\alpha v \tag{8}$$

$$\frac{d\psi_{p1}}{dx}(-L + 0) - \frac{d\psi_1}{dx}(-L - 0) = \alpha\sigma \tag{9}$$

at the boundaries between the hydrophobic layer and the polar zones:

$$\psi_{p2}(d + 0) = \psi_h(d - 0) \tag{10}$$

$$\varepsilon\frac{d\psi_{p2}}{dx}(d + 0) = \varepsilon_h\frac{d\psi_h}{dx}(d - 0) \tag{11}$$

$$\psi_h(+0) = \psi_{p1}(-0) \tag{12}$$

$$\varepsilon_h\frac{d\psi_h}{dx}(+0) = \varepsilon\frac{d\psi_{p1}}{dx}(-0) \tag{13}$$

The solution of Eqs. (4)–(13) is (for details see [33]):

(a) for outside solutions $(-\infty < x < -L$ and $d + L < x < +\infty)$

$$\psi_i(x) = \alpha\left\{\left[\frac{\sigma\cosh(k_i L)}{k_i} + (-1)^i v \sinh(k_i L)\right]\exp[-(-1)^i k_i \bar{x}] - \psi_{ext}\delta_2^i\right\} \tag{14}$$

(b) for polar zones $(-L < x < 0$ and $d < x < d + L)$

$$\psi_{pi}(x) = \alpha\left[\left(\frac{\sigma}{k_i} - v\right)\exp(k_i L)\cosh(k_i \bar{x}) - \psi_{ext}\delta_2^i\right] \tag{15}$$

(c) for the hydrophobic layer $(0 < x < d)$

$$\psi_h(x) = \alpha\left\{[\psi_{p2}(d) - \psi_{p1}(0)]\frac{x}{d} + \psi_{p1}(0)\right\} \tag{16}$$

Kronecker's symbol δ_2^i allows the introduction of ψ_{ext} only in the right solution. These equations describe the electric potential distribution in the system upon neglecting the influence of the electric current on the DEL. [In Eqs. (14)–(16) we have omitted the terms that take into account the influence of the electric field inside the hydrophobic layer on the electric potential profiles in

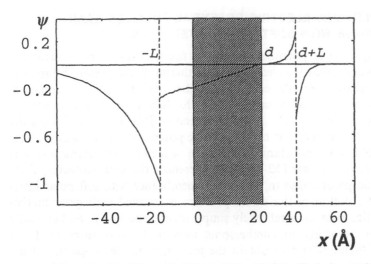

FIG. 2   An example of the typical electric potential profile in a membrane system with negative surface charge density ($\sigma_1 = \sigma_2 = -10^{-4}$ $e/\text{Å}^2$) and dipole density of opposite sign on each polar zone ($v_2 = -v_1 = -8.5 \times 10^{-3}$ $e/\text{Å}$) [40].

outside solutions. These terms are negligibly small because the influence is proportional to the parameter [59] $\gamma = \varepsilon_h/\varepsilon k d$ and usually $\gamma \sim 1/200$].

Figure 2 displays the typical electric profile in such system. Note that apart from other features, Eq. (14) shows an important peculiarity of the membranes with soft interfaces. As it follows from this equation, the electric field in the surrounding solution is determined by both surface charges and surface dipoles, i.e., a significant electric field exists near a dipole neutral surface in an electrolytic solution. Systems which involve both surface charges and surface dipoles display a more complicated behavior. As can be seen from Eq. (14); both the sign and the magnitude of surface potential $\psi(\bar{x} = 0)$ are determined by the surface charge density, σ, and the surface dipole density, v. If, for example, both σ and v have the same sign, then they increase their effects, while if they have opposite signs their competition leads to new qualitative effects. For example, charged lipid phosphatidyl-cholines or -serines membranes usually have $\sigma < 0$ and $v > 0$ [1]. One consequence of this is that the sign of $\psi(\bar{x} = 0)$ can be opposite to the sign of σ. In particular, the apparent surface potential will be positive, if $\sigma > -vk \tanh(kL)$.

Here we give a simple description of the problem of the electric field in an aqueous solution near a membrane with soft interfaces. Readers more interested in this problem can get more information from the original papers [9,10, 40]. Moreover, the influence of the spatial variation of the permittivity of the solvent near the interface on the electric field has been considered in Ref. 62.

III. NONEQUILIBRIUM ELECTRIC POTENTIAL PROFILES NEAR A MEMBRANE WITH SOFT POLAR INTERFACES

When analyzing electric potential profiles in the previous part we used the common assumption that the electrolyte is in thermodynamic equilibrium and the ion concentration profile can be described by Boltzmann's equation. However, in reality the electric current perturbs these profiles and transforms them into nonequilibrium ones. In this connection, it is worth to discuss the influence of the electric current on the electric potential profiles near a membrane. This problem is important for any type of membrane systems and was investigated extensively (see [52–56] and references therein). However, there are some specific peculiarities in the case of membranes with soft polar interfaces. An exact solution of the whole problem is entailed with great mathematical difficulties even for a relatively simple membrane system and can only be obtained by resorting to cumbersome numerical calculations [56]. To bypass these difficulties and to obtain the main qualitative properties of the system considered, it is worth to use a perturbation theory [53,57] and analyze only the cases of small ion fluxes.

Generally the steady-state ion distribution $C^{\pm}(x)$ (unit ion/cm^3) in any medium, in particular inside liquid solutions, in presence of ion fluxes $J^{\pm}$ (unit ion/s cm^2) is determined by the combination of Nernst–Planck's electrodiffusion equations (see Eq. (23) below) and Poisson's equation (1) and can be represented as [18,57]

$$c^{\pm}(x) = \left\{ 1 - j^{\pm}k \int_0^x \exp[z^{\pm}\psi(\tau)\,d\tau \right\}\exp[-z^{\pm}\psi(x)] \tag{17}$$

Here we introduced the dimensionless variables $c^{\pm}$ and $j^{\pm}$ that are connected with the dimensional ones $C^{\pm}$ and $J^{\pm}$ in the following manner: $c^{\pm} = C^{\pm}/C_1$; $j^{\pm} = J^{\pm}/D_s^{\pm}C_1k$; where $D_s^{\pm}$ denote the aqueous solution diffusion coefficients; k is inverse Debye's length of solution.

Let us consider only the case when both ion fluxes $j^{\pm}$ and total dimensionless current density $j_t = j^+ - j^-$ are small*, i.e., $j^{\pm} \approx \Delta$ and $j_t \approx \Delta$. Then, let Δ be small enough so that the real nonequilibrium electric potential profile $\psi(x)$ can be represented as a perturbed equilibrium electric potential $\psi_e(x)$

$$\psi(x) = \psi_e(x) + j_t a(x) + j_t^2 b(x) + \cdots \tag{18}$$

where $a(x)$ and $b(x)$ are unknown functions. By inserting Eq. (18) into Eq. (17) and holding only first-order terms, we obtain

$$c^{\pm}(x) = \exp[-z^{\pm}\psi(x)] - j^{\pm}\exp[-z^{\pm}\psi_e(x)] \int_0^x \exp[z^{\pm}\psi_e(\tau)]\,d\tau + o(\Delta^2) \tag{19}$$

---

* Generally, $j_t = z^+j^+ + z^-j^-$. For simplicity we are considering here the case of a symmetrical binary 1:1 solution.

The essential difference between Eqs. (17) and (19) is that the integral part of the expression is determined now only by the equilibrium electric potential $\psi_e(x)$. The latter is relatively easy to obtain for any membrane system. Expression (19) allows analyzing the nonequilibrium Double Electric Layer in any membrane system provided that ion fluxes are small and $\psi_e(x)$ is known. Generally, the integral in Eq. (19) must be computed numerically, but in the case of small equilibrium potentials we can get an analytical expression for $c^{\pm}(x)$. By taking $|\psi_e(x)| \approx \Delta$ and holding only first-order terms, Eq. (19) becomes

$$c^{\pm}(x) = \exp[-z^{\pm}\psi(x)] - j^{\pm}xk + o(\Delta^2) \tag{20}$$

Finally from Eqs. (1), (2) and (20) the first-order approximation of the nonequilibrium electric potential profile can be obtained [57]. Here we will discuss only the solution for the right part of our membrane system:

for polar zone: $0 \leq \bar{x} \leq L$

$$\psi_{p2}(x) \approx \alpha\left[\left(\frac{\sigma}{k} - v\right)\exp(-kL) + \frac{\varepsilon_h}{\varepsilon k}E_h\right]\cosh(k\bar{x}) - \frac{j_t}{2}[k\bar{x} + \exp(-k\bar{x})] \tag{21}$$

for outside solution: $L < \bar{x}$ (but within the diffusion layer and far from its boundary)

$$\psi_2(x) \approx \alpha\left[\frac{\sigma_0}{k} + \frac{\varepsilon_h}{\varepsilon k}E_h\right]\exp(-k\bar{x}) - \frac{j_t}{2}[k\bar{x} + \exp(-k\bar{x})] \tag{22}$$

where E_h and ε_h are the electric field and the dielectric constant, respectively, in the hydrophobic region ($x < d$) and $\sigma_0 = \sigma\cosh(kL) + vk\sinh(kL)$.

To solve the problem we use the common electrostatic boundary and matching conditions that take into account the discontinuity of the electric field and the electric potential at $x = L$ due to the surface charges and surface dipoles, respectively. So, as it follows from Eqs. (21) and (22) the nonequilibrium electric potential (and hence the ion concentration profiles, see Eq. (20)) in the considered system, within the first-order approximation, is the sum of the equilibrium potential profile and a simple linear function. Moreover, $\psi(x)$ in the outside solutions can be in general nonmonotonic [see Eq. (22)]. If $k|\sigma_0| < |j_t/2|$ then $\psi(x)$ reaches a maximum or a minimum value at the point $x^* \approx d - \ln[1 + 2\sigma_0/(j_tk - 2\sigma_0)]$ depending on the specific values of σ, v and j_t. Note that the space-charge $\rho = (\varepsilon k/8\pi\beta)(j_tk - 2\sigma_0)\exp(-k\bar{x})$ changes monotonically. It means, firstly, that the space–charge distribution has neither maximum nor minimum. However, in contrast with ρ, the concentration distribution of each ionic species $c^{\pm}(x)$ has an extreme value at the point $x^{**} \approx \ln[(j_tk - 2j^{\pm})/(j_tk - 2z^{\pm}\sigma_0)] + d$.

Figure 3 shows the influence of the flux on $\psi(x)$ in the right solution for the

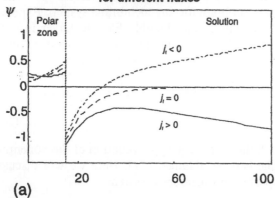

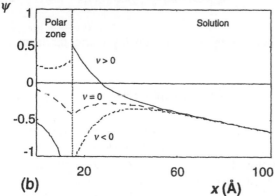

FIG. 3 Dimensionless electric potential profile in the right NDEL: (a) as a function of the distance from the hydrophobic region, for different values of total ionic flux in the case when the voltage drop across the membrane is created by the concentration difference on both sides of the membrane (i.e., $C_1 \neq C_2$). $k_2^{-1} = 10$ Å; $k_1^{-1} = 17$ Å; $L = 15$ Å; $\sigma = -8 \times 10^{-4}$ $e/Å^2$, $v = -1.6 \times 10^{-2}$ $e/Å$; and $|j_t| = 0.5$; (b) as a function of the distance from the hydrophobic region, for different values of the dipole density v. $k_2^{-1} = 10$ Å; $k_1^{-1} = 17$ Å; $L = 15$ Å; $\sigma = -8 \times 10^{-4}$ $e/Å^2$; $j_t = -0.5$ and $|v| = 1.6 \times 10^{-2}$ $e/Å$ [57].

case when the voltage drop on the membrane is created by a concentration difference on both sides of the membrane (i.e., $C_1 \neq C_2$, and hence $E_h \neq 0$ also). The polarization effects in the NDEL become apparent in a region of 3–4 debye lengths. Outside this region the potential profile varies linearly and is determined mainly by the total flux. As it seems from Fig. 3a, $\psi(x)$ is monotonic for $j_t < 0$, but it has a maximum at the point x^* for $j_t > 0$.

The surface dipoles turn out to change dramatically the electric potential profile $\psi(x)$ in the NDEL (see Fig. 3b). However their influences becomes apparent only on a region 3–4 k^{-1} thick; further away it is essentially zero. Moreover, $\psi(x)$ is monotonic for $v > 0$, but for $v < 0$ it has maximum at the point x^*.

The existence of a maximum for $\psi(x)$ is an important feature of the considered systems, because it creates an additional barrier for one kind of ions and facilitates the transport of others. It means that surface dipoles can significantly change the apparent permselectivity of the membrane system.

IV. ION TRANSPORT ACROSS A MEMBRANE WITH SOFT INTERFACES: GENERAL DESCRIPTION

The steady-state transport of ions across a medium, in particular inside liquid solutions, is described by the combination of the Nernst–Planck's electrodiffusion equations [11–14]

$$j^{\pm} = -\frac{D^{\pm}(x)}{k}\left[\frac{dc^{\pm}(x)}{dx} + z^{\pm}c^{\pm}(x)\frac{d\psi(x)}{dx}\right] \tag{23}$$

and Poisson's equation (1). Here $D^{\pm}(x)$ denote the dimensionless diffusion coefficients (i.e., expressed in $D_s^{\pm}$ units, where $D_s^{\pm}$ are the dimensional diffusion coefficients in aqueous solution). Generally, when ions pass through any complex inhomogeneous medium, diffusion coefficients and dielectric constants are spatial variables. First of all let us discuss Eq. (23). With the help of the integration factor $\exp(z^{\pm}\psi)$, this equation can be rewritten as [1,14,30,33]

$$j^{\pm} = z^{\pm}P^{\pm}\{c^{\pm}(x_1)\exp[z^{\pm}\psi(x_1)] - c^{\pm}(x_2)\exp[z^{\pm}\psi(x_2)]\} \tag{24}$$

where $x = x_1$ and $x = x_2$ are the boundaries of the medium under consideration, and the dimensionless parameter $P^{\pm}$ is determined by the expression:

$$P^{\pm} = \left[k\int_{x_1}^{x_2}\frac{\exp[z^{\pm}\psi(x)]}{D^{\pm}(x)}dx\right]^{-1} \tag{25}$$

It is worth stressing that Eqs. (24) and (25) do not solve the ion transport problem. They are only another form of Nernst–Planck's equations. However, in certain cases it is more convenient to use them instead of the original equation. As already mentioned, we will analyse this system under short circuit conditions, which means that the membrane separates two solutions with different concentration but with the same electric potential, namely $\psi(x_1) = \psi(x_2) = 0$. In this case Eq. (24) becomes:

$$j^\pm = z^\pm P^\pm [c^\pm(x_1) - c^\pm(x_2)] \equiv z^\pm P^\pm \Delta c^\pm \tag{26}$$

Now the parameter $P^\pm$ is an effective permeability of the system for each ionic species. It is rather convenient because, on one hand, all transport properties of the system are summarized in $P^\pm$. On the other hand, this parameter can be measured by experiment. If the membrane can be represented as a set of homogeneous layers, then Eq. (25) is valid for each part of it and can be written as

$$P_m^\pm = D_m^\pm \bigg/ \left\{ k \int_{b_1}^{b_2} \exp[z^\pm \psi_m(x)] \, dx \right\} \tag{27}$$

where b_1 and b_2 are the limits of the m-part of the membrane system according to the following notation:

m = h   hydrophobic layer

m = p_1, p_2 polar zones

m = d_1, d_2 dipole interfaces

In addition, D_m^+ and $\psi_m^\pm(x)$ are the dimensionless ionic diffusion coefficients and the electric potential, respectively, in part m. Thus, according to Eq. (27), the permeability $P^\pm$ of the whole system is connected with permeabilities of all parts in this way:

$$\frac{1}{P^\pm} = \sum_m \frac{1}{P_m^\pm} \tag{28}$$

It is worth making a few general comments on the mathematical side of the problem. Strictly speaking, the problem cannot be solved with only Eqs. (1) and (23), because five unknown functions have to be found: $j^+, j^-, c^+(x), c^-(x), \psi(x)$. Therefore, in order to obtain j^+ and j^-, the system of Eqs. (1) and (23) has to be supplemented with two equations and/or with the equations that can determine the connection between $c^\pm(x)$ and $\psi(x)$. Generally, there are two ways to do it. The first way (direct and general one) is to consider the corresponding time-dependent transport problem instead of using the steady-state equations (see Ref. 30 and references therein) and analysing if for $t \to \infty$. But in this case, the Poisson (1) and Nernst–Planck (23) equations have to be supplemented by two continuity equations. Then, the dependence of the concentration on the potential in the steady state can be obtained as a result of the solution of the whole system of equations.

This approach seems not suitable usually because the numerical solution of the time-dependent equations in our system is rather complicated [30]. The difficulties involved in obtaining a numerical solution could hide the main objective of analyzing the influence of the structure of the polar zone on ion transport. Besides, this approach also demands some a priori assumptions about boundary conditions that can influence significantly the final result. So another approach is more convenient in many cases. It consists in introducing a priori some determined dependence between $c^{\pm}(x)$ and $\psi(x)$. It is impossible to get this dependence generally. For each specific system, this dependence can be found from the preliminary analysis of its physicochemical characteristics. For example, this approach is used to Goldman's and Planck's approximation [11,12], and also when the Double Electrical Layer near the membrane is assumed to be in thermodynamic equilibrium (even with a nonzero ion flux across it [15–18]).

In the case considered here the problem can also be simplified if we introduce some additional assumptions that help us to find the connection between the ion concentration and electric potential profiles. Such assumptions have to be introduced for each separate part of the membrane system, i.e., for the hydrophobic layer, the polar zones and bulk electrolyte solutions. As regards the latter they are regarded to be always in thermodynamic equilibrium so that the dimensionless concentration profiles $c_i^{\pm}(x)$ are determined by Boltzmann's equation.

$$c_i^{\pm}(x) = c_i \exp[-z^{\pm}\psi_i(x)]; \qquad (i = 1, 2) \tag{29}$$

As above, here subscript 1 denotes also the left side of the membrane and subscript 2 denotes the right side. Here c_i denotes the dimensionless bulk concentration in ith solution, that is connected with the dimensional one C_i and $c_i = C_i/C_1$.

As for the hydrophobic layer, due to its small dielectric constant ($\varepsilon_h = 2$–3 [1,2,31]), Debye's length there is usually much bigger than its thickness [32, 33] ($d \approx 30$ Å^3), so Goldman's approximation [50] is valid here and hence the concentration profile is determined by the following expression [14]

$$c_h^{\pm}(x) = c_1 \exp(z^{\pm}\Delta\psi x/d) + \frac{j^{\pm}kd}{(z^{\pm})^2 D_h^{\pm}\Delta\psi} [1 - \exp(z^{\pm}\Delta\psi x/d)] \tag{30}$$

where $\Delta\psi = \psi(d) - \psi(0)$.

Unlike the hydrophobic layer, a similar general hypothesis cannot be made for the polar zones. The reason is that their thickness is of the same order as Debye's length. However, in the following limit cases a realistic assumption can be made to determine the concentration profiles in the polar zones: (1) the inner hydrophobic layer is the rate-determining barrier; and (ii) the polar zones are the rate-determining barrier. It is obvious that concentration profiles will be different for each one of these cases.

V. ION TRANSPORT WHEN THE INNER HYDROPHOBIC LAYER IS THE RATE-DETERMINING BARRIER

The statement "hydrophobic layer is the rate-determining barrier" means that the permeabilities of all parts of the membrane except the hydrophobic layer are assumed to be large enough. This can happen if $D_h^\pm \ll D_{pi}^\pm$ and $D_h^\pm \ll D_{di}^\pm$. For polar zones it means that very small deviations from thermodynamic equilibrium inside them will be enough to give a finite value for the ion flux. Hence, the ion flux has to be finite despite the fact that its diffusion coefficient tends to infinity $D_{pi}^\pm \to \infty$. This can occur only if the expression in brackets within Eqs. (23) or (24) is equal to zero for polar zones and hence concentration profiles inside them are determined by Boltzmann's law

$$c_{pi}^\pm(x) = c_{pi} \exp[-z^\pm(\psi_{pi}(x) - \psi_{pi}^*)] \tag{31}$$

where $\psi_{pi}(x)$ is the electric potential profile, ψ_{pi}^* is an "additional" potential ($\psi_{pi}^* = $ constant), and c_{pi} is the bulk electrolyte concentration in i-polar zone. Generally, $c_{pi} \neq c_i$ and $\psi_{pi}^* \neq 0$, which means that the electrolyte inside the polar zones can be charged, i.e., the electroneutrality condition is not valid here as a rule. The values for ψ_{pi}^* and c_{pi} can be obtained from the condition that the dipole interfaces themselves are not the rate controlling barrier either in this limit case. Then, by repeating for dipole interfaces the above speculations made for the polar zones, the following expression for the left dipole interface (i.e., at $x = -L$) follows from Eq. (24).

$$c_1^\pm(-L - 0)\exp[z^\pm\psi_1(-L - 0)] = c_{p1}^\pm(-L + 0)\exp[z^\pm\psi_{p1}(-L + 0)] \tag{32}$$

and from Eqs. (31) and (32) we finally get $c_1 = c_{p1} \exp(z^\pm\psi_{p1}^*)$. Similar expressions can be also obtained for the right dipole interface. As these expressions are valid both for cations ($z^+ = 1$) and anions ($z^- = -1$), it means that in the considered case for both polar zones $\psi_{pi}^* = 0$ and $c_i = c_{pi}$.

So, these equations, together with Eq. (29), allow us to solve the ion transport problem when the inner hydrophobic layer is the rate controlling barrier and to determine the main parameters of the ion transport across the membrane, namely ion fluxes $j^\pm$, permeabilities $P^\pm$, and permselectivity η. As it follows from Eqs. (24) and (29) the steady-state ion flux is

$$j^\pm = z^+ P_h^\pm(c_1 - c_2) = z^\pm P_h^\pm \, \Delta c \tag{33}$$

Then, by using the common Goldman's assumption that the electric field inside the hydrophobic layer is constant, the following expression for the permeability can be obtained

$$P_h^\pm = z^\pm \frac{D_h^\pm}{kd} [\psi_{p1}(0) - \psi_{p2}(d)]/\{\exp[z^\pm\psi_{p1}(0)] - \exp[z^\pm\psi_{p2}(d)]\} \tag{34}$$

These expressions (32)–(34) determine the separate ion fluxes $j^{\pm}$ and the total flux $j_t = j^+ - j^-$.

$$j_t = (P_h^+ - P_h^-)\,\Delta c$$
$$= \frac{1}{kd}\,\frac{[\psi_{p1}(0) - \psi_{p2}(d)][D_h^+ - D_h^-\,\exp(\psi_{p1}(0) + \psi_{p2}(d))]}{\exp[\psi_{p1}(0)] - \exp[\psi_{p2}(d)]}\,\Delta c \qquad (35)$$

The total flux j_t (or electric current) is the main characteristics of the membrane system that is usually measured in experiments. The characteristic difference in membrane permèability for cations and anions can be described by the permselectivity [10] η defined as

$$\eta = \frac{j^+}{j^-} = \frac{P_h^+}{P_h^-} = \frac{D_h^+}{D_h^-}\bigg/ \exp[\psi_{p1}(0) + \psi_{p2}(d)] \qquad (36)$$

Now we have all expressions to analyze the ion transport problem in the considered system when the inner hydrophobic layer is the rate-controlling barrier. We start by analyzing the influence of the surface dipoles on the ion transport across the membranes. Note that the widespread hypothesis is that the negative surface dipoles cause the anion selectivity of the lipid membrane (see for example [45,46]). In particular, it has been suggested that the Born-image energy, the hydrophobic energy and the dipole electric energy [47] determine the ion permeability of these membranes. Moreover, the positive dipole potential (i.e. $v_2 = v < 0$ in our notation) of the ester groups of lipid carbonyls is believed to be the main contribution to the dipole electric energy. It results in a low energy barrier for anions as compared to cations and anion selectivity of lipid membranes. This theory has been corroborated by an experimental investigation of organic ions permeation across lipid bilayers [36]. However, the generalization of this theory to other membrane systems is not supported by the experimental results. In particular, planar lipid bilayers formed from thylakoid lipids showed a selective permeability to K^+ over Cl^- (see [27] and references there) but their membrane dipole potential is known to be positive inside ($v < 0$ in our notation) [48]. So it appears that the dipole theory of membrane permselectivity is in contradiction with the observed cation selectivity (see discussion in Ref. 27). However, the approach developed above shows that the sign of the surface dipole by itself is not enough to explain cation or anion permselectivity of the membrane system. To demonstrate this, let us consider the ion flux calculated according to equations (33)–(35). To avoid overcomplicating the expression we shall omit now the subscript "h". Consider as an example that the concentration at the left side solution c_1 is fixed and c_2 is variable.

The dipoles usually play a two-fold role, firstly they charge the interior of the membrane [45–47]; secondly, they influence on the outside double electric layer [8,9]. Therefore, to rule out the second effect from the beginning let us

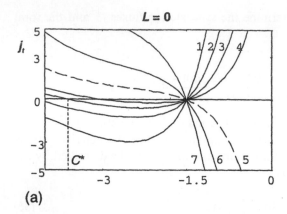

(a)

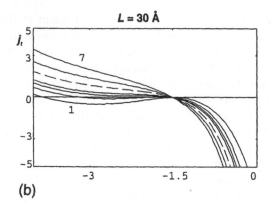

(b)

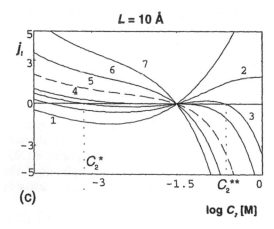

(c)

log C_2 [M]

consider the limit cases when the polar zones are very small ($L \approx 0$). As it seems from Fig. 4, the surface dipoles have a great influence on the total ion flux and the permselectivity. Moreover, this influence is connected only with the charging of the membrane interior because the polar zone thickness is assumed to be zero and hence the dipoles have not effect on the outside solution [9,10]. However, the total permselectivity (Fig. 5) is determined not only by the sign of v but also by electrolyte concentration c_1 and c_2, by the surface charge density σ and by the ratio D_s^+/D_s^-. Furthermore, in some cases the membrane is anion-selective for some concentration range and cation-selective for another (see curves 3 and 4 in Fig. 5). Generally, for $L \cong 0$ the membrane is cation selective if

$$v > \frac{1}{2}\left[\sigma\left(\frac{1}{k_1} + \frac{1}{k_2}\right) - \frac{1}{\alpha}\ln\frac{D_s^+}{D_s^-}\right] \tag{37}$$

and hence for certain conditions in experiments with constant c_1 and variable c_2 the *blocking concentration* c^* (see curve 3 on Fig. 4a) can be obtained [40] when total flux is zero (and so is the electric current).

The results for the other limit case of very large polar zone ($L \gg k_1^{-1}$) are shown in Fig. 4b. As it follows from comparison of this figure with Fig. 4a the difference between these cases lies in the fact that permselectivity of the membranes with large polar zones for concentrated solutions ($c_2 > c_1$) does not depend on the sign of the surface dipoles and is determined only by the diffusion coefficients of cations D_s^+ and anions D_s^-. The functional dependence $j_t(c_2)$ becomes more complicated for the intermediate cases of moderate polar zones (see Fig. 4c). In particular, for certain conditions, there is a second *blocking concentration* c^{**} in the range of large concentrations (curves 2 and 3). In this connection it is worth to note that the existence of these *blocking concentrations* is a general characteristic of the membrane systems under consideration. In addition, these blocking concentrations may serve as a test of the theory because they can be obtained experimentally [40].

These results demonstrate two important peculiarities of the membranes systems with polar zones. First, the permselectivity of such systems is not only

---

FIG. 4 The total flux j_t through the hydrophobic layer in dimensionless units ($D_s^+ C_1/d$) as a function of right solution concentration C_2 for a symmetrical membrane $\sigma_1 = \sigma_2 = \sigma = -10^{-4}$ $e/\text{Å}^2$; $v_1 = -v_2$ in the case $C_1 = 10^{-1.5}$ M, for different dipole densities: (1) $v_2 = -2.5 \times 10^{-2}$ $e/\text{Å}$; (2) $v_2 = -1.7 \times 10^{-2}$ $e/\text{Å}$; (3) $v_2 = -1.17 \times 10^{-2}$ $e/\text{Å}$; (4) $v_2 = -8.5 \times 10^{-3}$ $e/\text{Å}$; (5) $v_2 = 0$; (6) $v_2 = 8.5 \times 10^{-3}$ $e/\text{Å}$; (7) $v_2 = 1.7 \times 10^{-2}$ $e/\text{Å}$. The thickness of the hydrophobic layer is $d = 30$ Å and the diffusion coefficients are related through $D_s^+/D_s^- = 2$. The thickness of the polar zone is (a) $L = 0$; (b) $L = 30$ Å; (c) $L = 10$ Å [40].

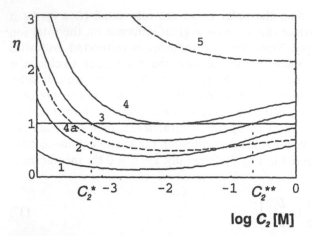

FIG. 5 The permselectivity η as a function of right solution concentration C_2 for different values of the surface dipole density v: (1) $v_2 = -2.5 \times 10^{-2}\ e/\text{Å}$; (2) $v_2 = -1.7 \times 10^{-2}\ e/\text{Å}$; (3) $v_2 = -1.17 \times 10^{-2}\ e/\text{Å}$; (4) $v_2 = -8.5 \times 10^{-3}\ e/\text{Å}$; (5) $v_2 = 0$; The polar zone thickness is $L = 10\ \text{Å}$. All other parameters are the same as in Fig. 4 except for the dashed line (curve 4a), which reproduces curve 4 for the case of $D_s^+/D_s^- = 1$ [40].

determined by the surface dipoles but also by the surface charges and by the thickness of the polar zone. From equations (36) and (15) it follows that, generally speaking, a membrane is cation selective ($\eta > 1$) if $v > b_1\sigma - b_2$, where

$$b_1 = \frac{k_1\exp(k_1 L) + k_2\exp(k_2 L)}{k_1 k_2[\exp(k_1 L) + \exp(k_2 L)]} \quad \text{and} \quad b_2 = \frac{\ln(D_s^+/D_s^-)}{\alpha[\exp(-k_1 L) + \exp(-k_2 L)]}$$

The second peculiarity is that, for this kind of membrane systems, permselectivity is no longer a constant parameter but depends on the electrolyte concentration. Figure 6 shows that the permselectivity of the system is determined not only by v but also by σ and c_2. It is seen that permselectivity changes with c_2. Moreover, in certain cases this dependence is nonmonotonic and the membrane can be cation selective in one region (e.g. curve 3 in Fig. 6 for $c_2 > c_2^{**}$ and $c_2 < c_2^*$) and anion selective in another one (e.g. curve 3 for $c^* < c_2 < c^{**}$). It should be stressed that the variation of the permselectivity in this approach is connected with the redistribution of the electric field in the system. The selectivity determined by diffusion coefficients—described here by the ratio D_s^+/D_s^-—remains unchanged. What determines this behavior of the permselectivity $\eta(c_2)$? To clarify this problem let us consider in detail a particular membrane system, e.g., that represented by curve 3 in Fig. 6. The dependence of permselectivity, flux, cation and anion permeability upon right bulk

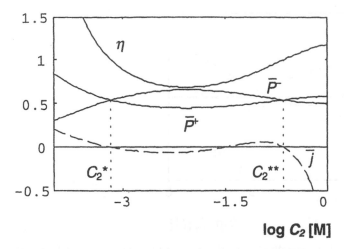

FIG. 6 The dependence of the main transport parameters on the right solution concentration C_2 for the same membrane system represented by curve 3 on Fig. 4c. The permselectivity $\eta(C_2)$, the normalized total flux $\bar{j} = j_t(C_2)/j_t(C_2 = 10^{-4})$, and the normalized cation and anion permeability $\bar{P}^\pm = P^\pm(C_2)/P^+(C_2 = C_1)$ for this membrane system [40].

concentration is shown in Fig. 7 for this membrane system. As it is seen, both cation and anion permeability change with the concentration c_2. Moreover, in the region where $c^* < c_2 < c^{**}$ the former is bigger than the latter ($P^+ > P^-$) but for the regions where $c_2 > c_2^{**}$ and $c_2 < c_2^*$ the opposite happens ($P^+ < P^-$). The variation of $P^\pm$ is determined mainly by the change of $\Delta\psi$. Note that in this case $P^\pm \approx P_h^\pm$. For a negatively charged membrane ($\sigma < 0$) any decrease in the right electrolyte concentration leads to a decrease in the potential $\psi_{p2}(d)$. Generally, it has two sequences: (i) *transhydrophobic* potential increases $\Delta\psi$; and (ii) cation concentration increases and anion concentration decreases at $x = d$. As for cation permeability P^+, the first effect accelerates the cation flux, and hence increases the cation permeability of the hydrophobic zone. The second one decreases the difference of concentrations at the hydrophobic zone boundary and hence decreases the cation permeability [12]. However for our membrane system the second effect, connected with the variations $\Delta c^\pm$, is negligible. Actually, as it is seen in Fig. 7b, the concentration difference Δc^+ in the region $C_2 < 10^{-2}$ M is changing weakly but P^+ is growing. As it follows from Eq. (15) $\Delta\psi$ consists of two terms, namely, the surface charge term and the dipole one; the first one is decreasing but the second one is increasing with increased concentration. The balance between these terms determine the potential difference $\Delta\psi$ and hence the permeability $P^\pm$ of the membrane system.

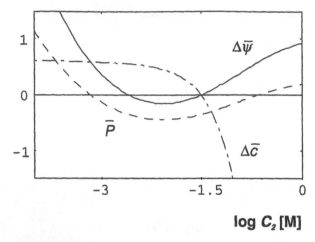

FIG. 7 Transhydrophobic normalized potential $\Delta\bar{\psi} = \Delta\psi/\psi_{p1}(0)$ (——); total normalized permeability $\bar{P} = P/P^{+}(C_2 = C_1)$ (– – –) and normalized cation concentration difference $\Delta\bar{c} = \Delta c/c_1$ (– · – · –) [40].

Another important question is the influence of the polar zone thickness L on the ionic transport because it is well known that lipid membranes of similar chemical composition can have the same inner hydrophobic layer, but quite different structure and size of their polar zones, as it happens, e.g., in phosphatidylcholine and phosphatidylethanolamine bilayers [1,21]. In Fig. 8 the dependence of permselectivity η and total ion flux j_t on L are shown. From this figure it is seen that the membrane permselectivity η in the region of the small L is determined mainly by the sign of the surface dipoles and the ratio between D_s^{+} and D_s^{-}. The permselectivity changes with the increasing of the polar zone thickness. Moreover, as the polar zone thickness is growing, an anion selective membrane (in the region of small L; see, e.g., curve 1 on Fig. 8) can become cation selective in the region of large L (provided that $D_s^{+} > D_s^{-}$). The permselectivity η and total ion flux j_t of membranes with large polar zones $(L \gg k_1^{-1})$ do not depend neither on dipole density nor on charge density and are determined only by anion and cation diffusion coefficients. It should be underlined that the total ion flux will be the highest if the polar zone thickness is

$$L^{**} \cong \frac{1}{k_1 - k_2} \ln\left(\frac{vk_2 - \sigma}{\sigma - vk_1}\right).$$

Summarizing the above considerations we can say that in the case of negative surface dipole densities $v < 0$, membranes with bigger polar zones should exhibit higher cation selectivity (curve 1 on Fig. 8) and hence higher cation permeability.

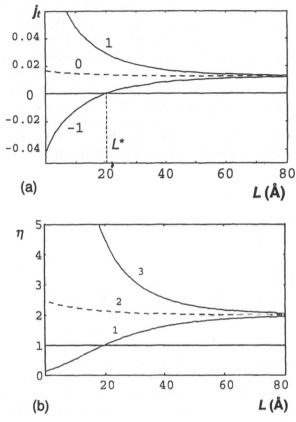

FIG. 8 The influence of the polar zone thickness L on the main transport parameters of the membrane system in the case $C_1 = 0.1$ M, $C_2 = 0.225$ M, $\sigma_1 = \sigma_2 = \sigma = -10^{-4}$ $e/\text{Å}^2$; for different dipole densities ($v_1 = -v_2$): (1) $v_2 = -1.7 \times 10^{-2}$ $e/\text{Å}$; (2) $v_2 = 0$; (3) $v_2 = 1.7 \times 10^{-2}$ $e/\text{Å}$. The thickness of the hydrophobic layer is $d = 30$ Å and $D_s^+/D_s^- = 2$; (a) the total flux j_t through the hydrophobic layer in dimensionless units $(D_s^+ C_1/d)$ as a function of L; (b) the permselectivity η as a function of L [40].

How can the approach developed here help in a correct interpretation of measurements? For example, it can explain the experimental fact that thylakoid membranes are more cation permeable that phospholipid membranes [27] because the polar zone thickness of the former is $L = 3$–8 Å [1,2,26] while for the latter L is 11–15 Å [3].

Another example is the following. It is known that the addition of some small molecules to the solution changes the bilayer permeability, e.g., salicilamide and phloretin. Phloretin has been reported to increase dramatically the cation flux and decrease the anion flux across artificial and natural membranes

[29,31,49,50]. These experimental data were earlier interpreted as a result of conformational changes of the lipid head in such a manner that the surface density of the normal component of the dipoles changes [31,49,51], but this is not enough to account for the observed changes. If we take into account that these NMR studies have shown that phloretin also pushes out the boundary water from the polar zone regions, this means in our approach that the effective thickness of the polar zone L is decreased. Hence Phloretin has a double effect on the bilayer: (1) it changes the normal component of surface dipoles; and (2) it changes the effective thickness of the polar zones. Taking into account both of these effects enables one to find a better interpretation of the experimental results.

VI. ION TRANSPORT WHEN THE POLAR ZONE IS THE RATE-DETERMINING BARRIER

It is known that the polar zones of some membranes, e.g. phospholipid ones, are important in determining ionic permeability [25]. And more, in certain cases just these interfacial regions are the rate-determining barriers [60]. The latter means that the permeability of the polar zones $P_{pi}^{\pm}$ ($i = 1, 2$) is sufficiently smaller than the permeability of the inner hydrophobic layer, i.e. $P_{pi}^{\pm} \ll P_{h}^{\pm}$. To describe this limit case in the framework of the approach developed above, it is necessary to determine electric potential $\psi(x)$ and concentration $c^{\pm}(x)$ profiles for each part of the considered membrane system, namely, for the outside solution $\psi_i(x)$ and $c_i^{\pm}(x)$; for polar zones $\psi_{pi}(x)$ and $c_{pi}^{\pm}(x)$; and for hydrophobic layer $\psi_h(x)$ and $c_h^{\pm}(x)$. As regards the first it is worth to consider them as before to be always in thermodynamic equilibrium so that concentration profiles $c_h^{\pm}(x)$ to be determined by Boltzmann's equation (29). At the same time $\psi_i(x)$ is determined by Eq. (14).

Let us consider now the potential profiles $\psi_{pi}(x)$ and concentration profiles $c_{pi}^{\pm}(x)$ in the polar zones. Remember that the polar zone is regarded here as composed of two parts: polar zone itself and outer boundary plane covered by membrane fixed charges and dipoles. Generally the dielectric constant and the viscosity of the electrolyte inside the polar zone can differ from those in the bulk solution. But to understand the main ion transport characteristics of the considered membrane system, at the beginning this fact can be ignored, i.e., we will consider $D_{pi}^{+} = 1$ and $D_{pi}^{-} = 1$. Note that $D_{pi}^{\pm}$ are dimensionless. Then the permeability of the electrolyte inside the polar zone is the same as outside and actually the outer boundary plane covered by dipoles becomes the rate-determining step. So in this case electrolyte solutions everywhere, including the polar zone, are in thermodynamic equilibrium, i.e. Eq. (31) continues to be valid. But now the condition of electroneutrality inside the polar zone is not valid any more. Some additional space charge can be accumulated in polar zones in such a way to keep the equality of ion fluxes through the right and left polar zones, i.e., in contrast to the limit case considered above now $\psi_{pi}^* \neq 0$ and $c_i \neq c_{pi}$. Then, by making use of Eq. (24) for the hydrophobic layer and taking into account that now this layer is not the rate-controlling step, i.e., $P_h^\pm \to \infty$, we obtain

$$c_{p1}^\pm(0)\exp[z^\pm\psi_{p1}(0)] = c_{p2}^\pm(d)\exp[z^\pm\psi_{p2}(d)] \tag{38}$$

Then, from Eqs. (31) and (38) it follows

$$c_{p1} \exp[z^\pm\psi_{p1}^*] = c_{p2} \exp[z^\pm\psi_{p2}^*] \tag{39}$$

As these expressions are valid both for cations ($z^+ = 1$) and anions ($z^- = -1$), it means that for both polar zones $\psi_{p1}^* = \psi_{p2}^* = \psi_p^* \neq 0$ and $c_{p1} = c_{p2} = c_p$. So to solve our problem now we have to obtain ψ_p^* and c_p. But before it is necessary to determine the permeability of the dipole layer $P_{di}^\pm$ in the general case. The latter can be done in the following manner. Any dipole layer can be represented as a layer of small but finite thickness Δ, its boundaries being covered by charges of opposite signs. As Δ is small, the electric field inside the layer can be regarded constant. Then, by taking into account that Δ is formally connected with the dipole surface density as $v = e\Delta/A$ (where A is the surface area per molecule on the membrane), the permeability of the dipole layer $P_{di}^\pm$ is obtained from Eq. (27):

$$P_{d1}^\pm = \gamma z^\pm D^\pm \frac{\exp[-z^\pm\psi_1(-L)]}{|1 - \exp(-\alpha z^\pm v)|} \tag{40}$$

$$P_{d2}^\pm = \gamma z^\pm D^\pm \frac{\exp[-z^\pm\psi_2(d + L)]}{|1 - \exp(\alpha z^\pm v)|} \tag{41}$$

where $\gamma = \beta e/\varepsilon_0\varepsilon A$. The last step to solve our ion transport problem is to obtain ψ_p^* and c_p, which can be done on the basis of the steady-state condition, i.e., assuming that ion fluxes through the left dipole interface and the right one are the same in the steady state: $j_{d1}^\pm = j_{d2}^\pm$. These fluxes can be obtained from Eq. (24), by taking into account, e.g., that for the left dipole plane, $c^\pm(x_1) = c_1^\pm(-L)$; $c^\pm(x_2) = c_{p1}^\pm(-L)$; $\psi(x_1) = \psi_1(-L)$ and $\psi(x_2) = \psi_{p1}(-L)$ (for the right side similar expressions hold):

$$j_{di}^\pm = (-1)^i P_{di}^\pm[c_p \exp(z^\pm\psi_p^*) - c_i] \tag{42}$$

Finally, from $j_{d1}^\pm = j_{d2}^\pm$ we obtain the two unknown parameters ψ_p^* and c_p

$$c_p = \frac{\{[c_1 + c_2 \exp(\Delta\psi)][c_2 + c_1 \exp(\Delta\psi)]\}^{1/2}}{1 + c_2 \exp(\Delta\psi)}$$

$$\approx \frac{c_1 + c_2}{2}\left[1 + \frac{1}{2}\left(\frac{c_1 - c_2}{c_1 + c_2}\frac{\Delta\psi}{2}\right)^2\right]^{1/2} \tag{43}$$

$$\psi_p^* = \frac{1}{2} \ln \frac{c_2 + c_1 \exp(\Delta\psi)}{c_1 + c_2 \exp(\Delta\psi)} \approx \frac{\Delta\psi}{2} \frac{c_1 - c_2}{c_1 + c_2} \tag{44}$$

Now we have everything to analyze the ion transport if the rate-determining barriers are the polar zones. First of all it is worth comparing the behavior of the main transport parameters in this and the above limit case. Figure 9 shows the total dimensionless ion flux $j_t(c_2)$ for different values of the surface dipole density and the same parameter values as in Fig. 4. As it can be seen from Fig. 9, the way the total flux changes with concentration c_2 strongly depends on the sign of surface dipoles. With the growth of concentration c_2 the total flux j_t decreases for negative dipoles $v_2 < 0$ (positive surface dipole density, $v_2 > 0$, means dipoles "point" outwards, and $v_2 < 0$ means dipoles "point" inwards), achieves a minimum value and then increases rapidly. The dependence of $j_t(c_2)$ in the case when the inner hydrophobic zone is the rate determining barrier is similar, as shown in Fig. 4c. But now the *blocking* concentration C_2^* is much closer to $C_1 = 10^{-1.5}$. So the difference between the two cases is only quantitative for negative dipoles v_2. Another behavior is expected in membranes with positive v_2 (Fig. 9, curves 4 and 5). From the comparison of these curves with the corresponding ones in Fig. 4c it is seen that for $v_2 > 0$ the behavior of $j_t(c_2)$ is different. Particularly, when polar zones are the rate-determining step, the dependence $j_t(c_2)$ is nonmonotonous, achieving a maximum value at certain concentration (curves 4 and 5 in Fig. 9). While

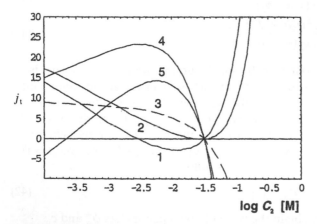

FIG. 9 The total ion flux j_t in dimensionless units $(D_s^+ C_1/L)$ as a function of the right solution concentration C_2 in the case when the polar zones are the rate-determining step. Parameter values are the same as in Fig. 4 and dipole densities take different values: (1) $v_2 = -1.7 \times 10^{-2}$ $e/\text{Å}$; (2) $v_2 = -8.5 \times 10^{-3}$ $e/\text{Å}$; (3) $v_2 \approx 0$; (4) $v_2 = 8.5 \times 10^{-3}$ $e/\text{Å}$; (5) $v_2 = 1.7 \times 10^{-2}$ $e/\text{Å}$. The thickness of the polar zone is $L = 10$ Å and diffusion coefficients are related through $D_s^+/D_s^- = 2$.

in the case of the hydrophobic zone being the rate-determining step, the dependence $j_t(c_2)$ is monotonous (curves 4–7 in Fig. 4c).

The behavior of another important parameter, i.e., the permselectivity $\eta(c_2)$ (see Fig. 10) differs now significantly from that in the case when the rate-determining barrier is the hydrophobic layer (Fig. 5) as for positive the surface dipoles $v_2 > 0$ (i.e., dipoles "point" outwards) as for negative ones $v_2 < 0$ (i.e., dipoles "point" inwards). For $v_2 > 0$ the membrane is always a cation selective one and its permselectivity exceeds considerably the original selectivity of the system (i.e., $\eta = D_s^+/D_s^- = 2$). Moreover, as concentration c_2 decreases the permselectivity is also lowered (curves 5–7 in Fig. 10). But for $v_2 < 0$ the membrane is always anion selective and as concentration c_2 decreases the permselectivity increases (curves 1–3 in Fig. 10). Note that in these examples we have assumed different values of the diffusion coefficients for cations and anions. $D_s^+ = 2D_s^-$, i.e., the original selectivity of the system is assumed to be cationic. The fact that in this case, of polar zones as the rate-determining barrier, the solutions inside these zones are not electroneutral can give the physical explanation of such unusual behavior of the permselectivity $\eta(c_2)$. Since the concentration in the left and right solutions are different, then initially the ion fluxes across the left $j_{d1}^{\pm}$ and right $j_{d2}^{\pm}$ dipole interfaces are different. Let us assume that $j_{d1}^{\pm} > j_{d2}^{\pm}$, then at the initial moment the number of ions that enter the left polar zone is greater than the number of ions that leave the right one. Consequently, there will be an accumulation of ions inside the polar

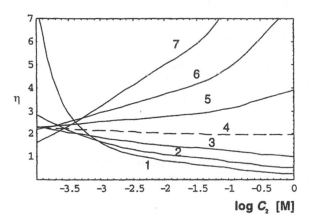

FIG. 10 The permselectivity η as a function of right solution concentration C_2 in the case when the polar zones are the rate-determining step, for the same value of the parameters as in Fig. 4 and different values of the surface dipole density v: (1) $v_2 = -1.25 \times 10^{-2}$ $e/\text{Å}$; (2) $v_2 = -8.5 \times 10^{-3}$ $e/\text{Å}$; (3) $v_2 = -4.25 \times 10^{-3}$ $e/\text{Å}$; (4) $v_2 \approx 0$; (5) $v_2 = 4.25 \times 10^{-3}$ $e/\text{Å}$; (6) $v_2 = 8.5 \times 10^{-3}$ $e/\text{Å}$; (7) $v_2 = 1.25 \times 10^{-2}$ $e/\text{Å}$.

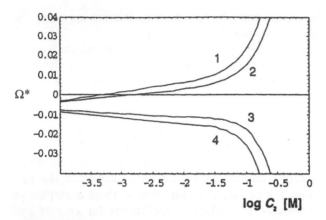

FIG. 11 The additional net space charge Ω^* in the polar zones as a function of right solution concentration C_2 for the same value of the parameters as in Fig. 10 and different values of the surface dipole density v: (1) $v_2 = -8.5 \times 10^{-3}$ $e/\text{Å}$; (2) $v_2 = -1.25 \times 10^{-3}$ $e/\text{Å}$; (3) $v_2 = 1.25 \times 10^{-3}$ $e/\text{Å}$; (4) $v_2 = 8.5 \times 10^{-3}$ $e/\text{Å}$. See explanation in the text.

zones. Generally $P_{di}^+ \neq P_{di}^-$ and $j_{di}^+ \neq j_{di}^-$, hence, some space charge density Ω^* (see Fig. 11) will appear inside the polar zones [61]

$$\Omega^* = \int_{-L}^{0} \rho(x) \, dx = \frac{\varepsilon \varepsilon_0}{\beta} \left[\frac{d\psi_{p1}}{dx}(-L) - \frac{d\psi_{p1}}{dx}(0) \right]$$

$$= -\frac{1}{2}(\sigma - vk_1)[1 - \exp(-2k_1 L)] \tag{45}$$

This additional space charge will decrease $j_{d1}^{\pm}$ and increase $j_{d2}^{\pm}$. The process of accumulation of additional space charge will continue till steady state condition $j_{d1}^{\pm} = j_{d2}^{\pm}$ will be met. It is obvious that the final state depends on the electrolyte concentrations, hence the final value of the additional space charges Ω^* will be different for different values of c_2. As it seems from Fig. 11, for negative surface dipoles $v_2 < 0$ the sign of Ω^* is positive (curve 1 and 2) which makes the membrane anion selective. In case of positive dipoles $v_2 > 0$ the sign of Ω^* is negative (curve 3 and 4), which increases cation selectivity of the membrane.

VII. CONCLUSION

Let us summarize the main results above described. First of all, it should be underlined once more that such parameters of the polar zones as its thickness and surface dipole density have considerable influence on ion transport across a membrane with soft interfaces. Moreover their influence will change depending on the conditions. It means that a membrane could be anion selective or cation selective, depending on the value of bulk concentrations. So, if such peculiarities of these membranes are not taken into account the experimental results could be misinterpreted.

As can be seen in the reference list the studies about membranes with soft interfaces are abundant, but most of them deal with the interaction between these membranes. However, the study of the ion transport phenomena in such kind of systems is only starting. A few words about some problems that we haven't discussed here. For instance, we have used a simple model of the membrane–solution interfaces. In reality, charges and dipoles are spread throughout the whole polar zone and its distribution can be rather complex. It is reasonable to think that the specific details of this distribution will influence on the ion transport.

Another important question not mentioned here is that of the influence of the membrane system dielectric characteristics on ion transport. As it is known the dielectric constant of bound water and polar zones differ significantly from that in the bulk (see [2,5,52] and references therein). It is obvious that these effects will influence significantly on the ion fluxes and membrane permselectivity in the system.

And last but not least, the problem of the surface dipoles orientation. As we have seen, the normal component of the surface dipoles influences very much on the transport properties of the membrane. But we assumed their value to be constant. In real membrane systems this is not correct. Firstly, there is a thermal orientation oscillation of the dipoles, secondly, the electric current has generally some influence on the dipole orientation. So, there is a very important question of mutual influence between surface dipoles and electric current across the membrane. All these questions await their solutions.

LIST OF SYMBOLS

Superscripts indicate the type of ion ("$+$" and "$-$" indicate cations and anions, respectively; "$\pm$" indicates both possibilities) and subscripts indicate the part of the membrane system. All the values with subscript "1" deal with the left part and those with subscript "2" with the right one. Subscript d indicates dipole layers, subscript p indicates polar zones and subscript h indicates hydrophobic layer. Generally, upper case letters are used for dimensional variables and lower case letters for dimensionless variables. α, β, γ, Ω^*, σ_0, b_1, b_2, ψ_e, are auxiliary parameters defined in the text. In particular, $\beta = e/k_B T$ and $\alpha = \beta/\varepsilon\varepsilon_0$.

C_i, c_i bulk solution concentration (dimensional and dimensionless, respectively),

$C_m^\pm(x), c_m^\pm(x)$ cation and anion concentration profiles in m-part (dimensional and dimensionless, respectively),

d thickness of the hydrophobic layer of the membrane,

$D_m^\pm$ dimensionless diffusion coefficient in the m-part of the membrane system,

$J_m^\pm, j_m^\pm$ ionic flux in the m-part (dimensional and dimensionless, respectively),

j_t total ionic flux (dimensionless),

k_i inverse Debye length of the i-solution,

k_B Boltzmann's constant,

L_i thickness of i-polar zone,

$P_m^\pm$ cation and anion permeability of the m-part of the membrane system (dimensionless),

T absolute temperature,

$x, \bar{x}$ spatial coordinates ($\bar{x} = x$ for $i = 1$; $\bar{x} = x - d$ for $i = 2$),

$z^\pm$ valence of the cation and anion, respectively,

ε_0 vacuum permittivity,

$\varepsilon, \varepsilon_m$ dielectric constants of the aqueous solution and of the m part, respectively,

η permselectivity,

$\phi(x), \phi_{ext}$ electric potential profile, and externally applied potential, respectively,

$\psi_m(x)$ dimensionless electric potential profile in the m part,

$\rho(x)$ volume charge density,

$\rho_{i, fix}(x)$ effective fixed charge density in i-polar zone,

σ_i surface charge density in i-polar zone; (for a symmetrical system $\sigma_1 = \sigma_2 = \sigma$),

ν_i surface dipole density in i-polar zone, (for a symmetrical system ($\nu_1 = -\nu_2 = \nu$),

E_h electric field in the hydrophobic region.

REFERENCES

1. G. Cevc and D. Marsh, *Phospholipid Bilayers*, J. Wiley & Sons, New York, 1987.
2. J.-F. Tocanne and J. Teissie, Biochim. Biophys. Acta. *1031*: 111 (1990).
3. S. W. Thorne and J. T. Duniec, Quart. Rev. Biophys. *16*: 197 (1983).
4. R. Heinrich, M. Gaestel, and R. Glaser, J. Theor. Biol. *96*: 211 (1982).
5. H. Ohshima and T. Kondo, J. Theor. Biol. *128*: 187 (1987); J. Colloid. Interface Sci. *157*: 504 (1993).
6. W.-C. Hsu, J.-P. Hsu, and Y.-I. Chang, J. Colloid. Interface Sci. *155*: 1 (1993).
7. E. Dickinson, in *Interactions of Surfactants with Polymers and Proteins.* (E. D. Goddard and K. P. Anunthapadmanabhan, eds.), CRC Press, Boca Raton, 1992, p. 295.
8. G. M. Bell and P. L. Levine, J. Colloid. Interface Sci. *74*: 530 (1980).

9. M. Belaya, M. Feigelman, and V. Levadny, Langmuir *3*:648 (1987).
10. M. Belaya, V. Levadny, and D. Pink, Langmuir *10*:2010 (1994).
11. N. Lakshminarayanaiah, *Transport Phenomena in Membranes*, Academic Press, New York, 1969; *Equations of Membrane Biophysics*, Academic Press, New York, 1984.
12. F. Helfferich, *Ion Exchange*, McGraw-Hill, New York, 1962.
13. A. V. Anderson, in *Membrane Transport in Biology* (G. Giebisch, D. C. Tostesson, and H. H. Ussing, eds.), Springer, New York, 1978, Vol. 1, p. 349.
14. V. S. Markin and Yu. A. Chizmadzev, *Induced Ionic Transport*, Nauka, Moscow, 1974.
15. A. Pullman, Chem. Rev. *91*:793 (1991).
16. B. Neumcke and P. Läuger, Biophys. J. *9*:1160 (1969).
17. A. H. Hainsworth and S. B. Hladky, Biophys. J. *51*:27 (1987).
18. D. Levitt, Ann. Rev. Biophys. Biophys. Chem. *15*:29 (1986); Biophys. J. *2*:209 (1978).
19. B. Neumcke, D. Waltz, and P. Läuger, Biophys. J. *10*:172 (1970).
20. W. H. Green and O. S. Andersen, Ann. Rev. Physiol. *53*:341 (1991).
21. E. Donath and V. Pastushenko, J. Electroanal. Chem. *104*:543 (1979); Stud. Biophys. *56*:7 (1976).
22. E. Donath and A. Voigt, Biophys. J. *49*:493 (1986).
23. I. S. Jones, J. Colloid Interface Sci. *68*:451 (1979).
24. M. Vorotyntsev, Yu. Ermakov, V. Markin, and A. Rubashkin, Elektrokhimiya *29*:596 (1992).
25. L. A. Meijer, F. A. M. Leermakers, and A. Nelson, Langmuir *10*:1199 (1994).
26. V. G. Ivkov and G. N. Berestovskii, *Dynamical Structure of the Lipid Bilayers*, Nauka, Moscow, 1981.
27. B. Fucks and F. Homble, Biophys. J. *66*:1404 (1994).
28. T. R. Stouch, D. Bassolino, and H. Alpper, Biophys. J. *66*:A16 (1995).
29. Y. Antonenko and A. A. Bulychev, Biochim. Biophys. Acta *1070*:474 (1991).
30. J. A. Manzanares, W. D. Murphy, S. Mafe, and H. Reiss, J. Phys. Chem. *97*:8524 (1993).
31. B. Bechinger and J. Seelig, Biochemistry, *30*:3923 (1991).
32. V. I. Gordeliy and M. A. Kiselev, Biophys. J. *69*:424 (1995).
33. R. G. Ashcroft, H. G. L. Coster, and J. R. Smith, Biochim. Biophys. Acta *643*:191 (1981).
34. H. Hauser and M. C. J. Phillips, Progr. Surf. Membr Sci. *13*:297 (1979).
35. G. B. Melikyan, N. S. Matinyan, and V. B. Arakelian, Biochim. Biophys. Acta *1030*:11 (1990).
36. G. Poste and L. W. Greenham, Cytobios. *2*:243 (1970).
37. P. G. Dzavakhidze, A. A. Kornyshev, and V. G. Levadny, Nuovo Cimento *10*:627 (1988).
38. A. V. Sokirko, J. A. Manzanares, and J. Pellicer, J. Colloid Interface Sci. *168*:32 (1994).
39. R. Petihig, in *Dielectric and Related Molecular Processes*, Special Periodical Report Chemical Society, London, 1977, vol. 3, p. 219.
40. V. M. Aguilella, M. Belaya, and V. Levadny, Langmuir *12*:4817 (1996).
41. V. M. Aguilella, M. Belaya, and V. Levadny, Thin Solid Films *272*:10 (1996).

42. C. A. Barlow, in *Physical Chemistry: IXA, Electrochemistry.* (H. Eyring, ed.), Academic Press, New York, 1970, p. 167.
43. A. Raudino and D. Mauzerall, Biophys. J. *50*:441 (1986).
44. H. G. L. Coster and J. R. Smith, Biochim. Biophys. Acta *373*:151 (1974).
45. E. Gross, R. S. Bedlack, and L. M. Loew, Biophys. J. *67*:208 (1994).
46. J. C. Franklin and D. S. Cafiso, Biophys. J. *65*:289 (1993).
47. R. F. Flewelling and W. L. Hubbell, Biophys. J. *49*:541 (1986).
48. D. Oldani, H. Hanser, B. W. Nichols, and M. C. Phillips, Biochim. Biophys. Acta *382*:1 (1975).
49. C. Zheng and G. Vanderkooi, Biophys. J. *63*:95 (1992).
50. O. S. Andersen, A. Finkelstein, I. Katz, and A. Cass, J. Gen Physiol. *67*:749 (1976).
51. E. Melnik, R. Latorre, J. E. Hall, and D. C. Tosteson, J. Gen Physiol. *69*:243 (1977).
52. L. Bass, Trans. Farad. Soc. *60*:1656 (1964).
53. J. Newman, Trans. Farad. Soc. *61*:2229 (1965).
54. V. V. Nikonenko, V. I. Zabolotskii, and N. P. Gnusin, Elektrokhimiya *25*:301 (1989).
55. L. Listovnicii, Elektrokhimiya *27*:316 (1990).
56. J. A. Manzanares, W. D. Murphy, S. Mafé, and H. Reiss, J. Phys. Chem. *97*:8524 (1993).
57. V. M. Aguilella, M. Belaya and V. Levadny, J. Colloid Interface Sci. *186*:212 (1997).
58. N. K. Rogers, in *Prediction of Protein Structure and the Principles of Protein Conformation* (G. D. Fasman, ed.), Plenum Press, New York, 1987, p. 359.
59. S. Aytian and M. Belaya, Electrochemistry (USSR) *16*:691 (1980).
60. C. Selvey and H. Reiss, J. Membrane Sci. *30*:75 (1987).
61. V. Levadny, V. M. Aguilella, M. Belaya, and M. Yamazaki, Langmuir *14*:4630 (1998).
62. M. Belaya, V. Levadny, and D. Pink, Langmuir *10*:2015 (1995).

24

Nonlinear Instability of Biological Membrane Surfaces with Application to Bioadhesion

DOMINIQUE GALLEZ Service de Chimie Physique,
Université Libre de Bruxelles, Brussels, Belgium

Abstract

One of the important problems which can be treated in a nonlinear thermodynamics perspective is the relation between structure and function of membranes (biological membranes or reconstituted lipid membranes). In this paper, we will address the process of bioadhesion (adhesion of two cells/vesicles or adhesion of a cell/vesicle to a substratum). The structure of the membrane affects the ability of the membrane to deform and to be fixed to some other cell or to some substratum. This structure is highly heterogeneous, composed usually of a fluid lipidic bilayer where proteins are inserted. The possibility of the appearance of organized behavior (dissipative structures) in such systems has recently received attention. Indeed, in the thin aqueous layer (100–1000 Å) between the cells or between cell and substratum, long-range molecular forces due to van der Waals attraction usually compete with the presence of repulsive forces of different origins (electrical, hydration or steric) and lead to the formation of a new stable stationary state (spatially periodic pattern). These patterns are observed in cell/cell or cell/solid support interactions (periodic contacts of the order of 1 μm), or also in lipid vesicles of different composition adhering to a solid. The appearance of those patterns can be explained by an interfacial instability theory. Based on the asymptotic procedure of reduction of the full set of governing (Navier–Stokes) equations and boundary conditions, the dynamics of the aqueous layer is well described by a set of nonlinear evolution equations (NEE). Specific interactions (present for instance in bioadhesion by lock-and-key molecules) can also be included in the dynamical formalism by considering a chemical reaction between receptors (on the membrane) and sites (on a solid substratum). The method proposed here is composed of three different steps: a linear stability analysis to identify thresholds for constraints, a bifurcation calculus to predict the onset of new patterns near critical points, and numerical simulations to describe the full nonlinear dynamics. At each step, comparison with experimental data confirms the validity of the nonlinear thermodynamics approach to analyze the appearance and the dynamics of bioadhesion in a number of different situations.

I. INTRODUCTION

Several important biophysical problems related to membrane surface have already found an explanation in the general framework of nonlinear thermodynamics, as examples of dissipatives structures formed far from equilibrium [1]. Amongst these problems let us cite the problem of ion transport through membranes [2,3], the formation of structures in morphogenesis [4,5] or the onset and control of biological rhythms [6,7]. One of the best examples of a nonlinear approach in biophysics is the use of reaction–diffusion equations in models for pulse propagation along a nerve membrane [2]. In this case, the active medium is the membrane itself, which uses chemical energy to create a nonequilibrium distribution of the various ions, and sustains voltage pulses that serve to transmit information in the nervous system. In this paper, we will address a problem treated recently with the nonequilibrium approach, i.e., the bioadhesion of cells and vesicles. This subject which has many technological implications has benefited recently from the nonlinear thermodynamics perspective [8,9].

Plasma membranes, which have a very complex structure including a bilayer and a glycocalyx, regulate the onset and the characteristics of bioadhesion. The molecular composition of a cell outer membrane has been best established for the human erythrocyte. This characterization and the ready availability of the cell has led to a concentration of effort of elucidating the physical properties of this membrane [10]. However the ubiquitous occurrence of adhesion phenomena requires that the properties of other cell surfaces also be considered. Some important physicochemical properties of mammalian cell membranes are summarized in Table 1. The plasma membrane may be viewed as a three-section interfacial region which separates the cell suspending phase from the cytoplasm. Starting from the extracellular phase these sections are the glycocalyx, the bilayer and the cytoplasmic-face membrane skeleton complex which is essentially tangential to the bilayer (see Fig. 1).

Lipid vesicles are model cells, where the reconstituted membrane can mimic real biological membranes. In this chapter, we will also consider these model membranes, since they become more and more important in order to under-

TABLE 1 Physicochemical Properties of Mammalian Cell Membranes [9]

Property	Value	Cell
Charge density of cell surface	-5×10^6 C/m^3	average
Surface charge	-1.6×10^{-2} C/m^2	average
Hamaker constant A	10^{-22}–10^{-19} Joules	average
Debye length (ionic strength ≈ 0.1 M)	≈ 1 nm	average
Thickness of:		
lipid bilayer	4–6 nm	RBC
glycocalyx	5.5 nm	RBC
spectrin layer	3.5 nm	RBC
Surface diffusion coefficient D_s (for proteins)	4×10^{-15} m^2/s	RBC
Membrane tension σ_0	10^{-3}–1 mN/m	RBC
Bending elastic modulus B	1.8×10^{-16} mN/m	RBC
Inner surface potential ϕ_i	60 mV	RBC
Outer surface potential ϕ_o	0–15 mV	RBC
Number of receptors per cell N	10^5	lymphocyte
Spring constant K_s (for ligand–receptor bond)	10^{-16} Nm	lymphocyte
Compressibility coefficient (for glycocalyx)	10^{-11} N	lymphocyte
Bond length L_R	5–30 nm	lymphocyte

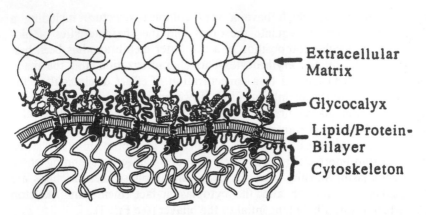

FIG. 1 Schematic diagram of the fine structure of plasma membrane as a three section interfacial region: the extracellular phase with the glycocalyx extending in the solution, the lipid–protein bilayer and the cytoplasmic-face membrane skeleton complex [12].

stand the specific and universal forces in biological membrane surfaces. Let us cite for instance recent experiments on supported membranes [11] where lipopolymers are incorporated in lipid vesicles as artificial glycocalyx in order to mimic lock-and-key forces present in bioadhesion.

When a living cell or a vesicle approaches another cell or a solid substratum, adhesion can take place due to physicochemical forces. Bioadhesion regulates many aspects of cellular physiology, including growth, differentiation, motility or cell activation in immune networks. A set of nonspecific interactions (electrical, hydration, steric ...) or specific interactions (as for lock-and-key molecules) are involved in the process of bioadhesion. As concern long-range interactions, van der Waals forces are attractive while electrostatic forces due to electric double layers in the intercellular media are repulsive. Then, the system can reach an equilibrium state corresponding to a free energy minimum (secondary minimum h^* in Fig. 2). As concerns short-range forces, they can be attractive or repulsive and a new energy minimum corresponding to a primary minimum L_R appears, related to a repulsive length L_R due to the surface molecules.

Many theoretical approaches have been proposed to understand adhesion phenomena (for a review see [12]). However recently, cell-to-cell and cell-to-substratum interactions have motivated a nonequilibrium approach by considering the formation of periodic patterns in the thin interstitial aqueous layer (contact zone). Due to the relevance of dynamic processes in phenomena involved in thin liquid films dynamics, an electrohydrodynamical theory was formulated [13,14] for the membrane case. Cellular adhesion was viewed as an interfacial instability generated in the fluid film due to external constraints.

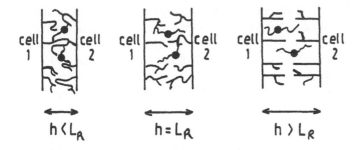

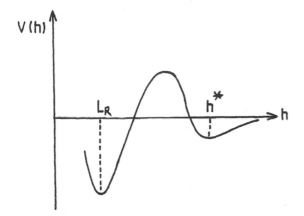

FIG. 2 Three positions of interacting cells in the presence of polycations (above). L_R is related to the combined thickness of the glycocalyx of the two cells. Sketch of the total interaction energy as a function of separation distance h (below). The primary minimum at $h \approx L_R$ is due to attractive cross-bridging and repulsive interactions, while the secondary minimum at $h \approx h^*$ is due to attractive van der Waals and repulsive (electrostatic or steric) interactions.

Several aspects were considered: the role of surfactants [15], the role of a chemical reaction between receptors and sites [16] and the role of electrical constraints [17].

The method proposed is composed of three different steps:

1. A linear stability analysis based on the appropriate nonlinear evolution equation (NEE) established in the different cases the existence of a critical value of the control parameter at which the system switches from asymptotic stability to instability [8].
2. Numerical solutions of the NEE provided a description of finite-amplitude

deformation [15–17]. The solutions describe different regimes (stability, rupture or pattern formation): this last phenomenon cannot be predicted by a linear theory.

3. A weakly nonlinear analysis in the vicinity of the bifurcation point for the uniform solution can be performed. From the amplitude equation, conditions for a subcritical unstable bifurcation and a supercritical stable bifurcation are predicted [18,19].

Experimental evidence is provided with aggregation of erythrocytes with polymers (polylysine, dextran) or lectins. Patterns are observed in cell–cell [8,9,21] or cell–solid support [20] interactions (periodic contacts of the order of 1 μm). In lipid vesicles of different composition adhering to a solid, blisters are formed in response to a change in pH [22], or to insertion of lipopolymers as artificial glycocalixes [11].

II. INTERFACIAL INSTABILITY APPROACH TO BIOADHESION

A.   Adhesion of Two Cells or Two Vesicles (Case A)

1. Hydrodynamic Model and Linear Stability Analysis

Let us first consider cell–cell interactions or vesicle–vesicle interactions, where the thin aqueous film between the cells or vesicles has two free surfaces (see Fig. 3). We will refer to this situation as case A. More precisely, region I is the cytoplasmic intracellular medium (or intravesicular medium), region II is the liquid between the two cell (vesicle) surfaces. The surface I–II is the membrane itself, composed of a fluid lipidic matrix where proteins can be embedded. As a

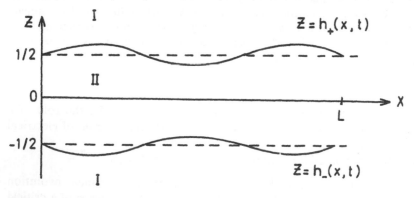

FIG. 3 Sketch of a free film with fluctuating surfaces. The dashed lines indicate the mean position of the surfaces at $h = \pm 1/2$. For the case of cell–cell adhesion, region I is the cytoplasmic intracellular medium, region II is the liquid between the two cell surfaces. The surface I–II is the membrane itself.

first approach, this membrane will be considered as a 2D fluid (the lipidic matrix), with surface molecules (the proteins) moving laterally with a diffusion coefficient of about 10^{-10}–10^{-8} cm^2/s (see Table 1). A nonlinear description of the membrane itself considered as a 3D lipidic fluid, has been given elsewhere [23].

The model considered is a thin liquid layer bounded by two surfaces. The longitudinal direction is denoted by x while z corresponds to the transverse direction. The film is bounded by two free surfaces located at $z = h_{\pm}(x, t)$ separating the liquid from the gas. There are two modes of vibration for a free liquid film: a bending mode, where the two surfaces move in phase, and the squeezing mode where the two surfaces are 180° out-of-phase (see Fig. 4). The analysis will be based on the squeezing mode, which is symmetric along the x axis, since it leads to film rupture or formation of contact points and is the most unstable.

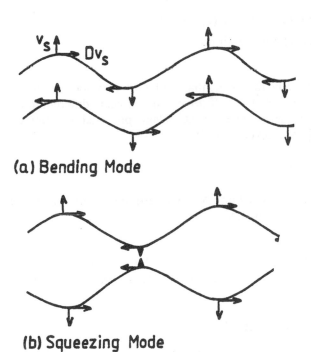

(a) Bending Mode

(b) Squeezing Mode

FIG. 4 The two modes of fluctuations for a free film: (a) for the bending mode (BE), the two interfaces move transversely in phase leading to the deformation of the thin film. The arrows indicate the orientation of normal v_s and tangential Dv_s velocities at the surfaces. (b) for the squeezing mode (SQ), the two interfaces move 180° out-of-phase leading to thickness variation of the thin film and eventually rupture or periodic pattern formation.

The liquid layer is assumed to be thin enough so that van der Waals forces are effective and yet thick enough so that a continuum theory of the liquid is applicable. The film is supposed to be of finite extent, its length L far exceeding its thickness h_0. The free surfaces possess surface properties like surface tension and surface coverage. Consequently, if the surfactants are free to diffuse along the surface, the surface tension will vary in accordance with surface concentration (Marangoni effect). The liquid film is described as a Newtonian viscous fluid having viscosity μ, density ρ and kinematic viscosity v. Dimensionless variables are introduced using the following scales: length h_0, time h_0^2/v, velocity v/h_0 and pressure $\rho v^2/h_0^2$. In addition, we use the equilibrium value Γ_0 as a unit measure for the concentration of the surfactants. The two-dimensional motion of the liquid in the film phase is given by the dimensionless Navier–Stokes equations [9]:

$$(u_t + uu_x + vu_z) = -(p + W_V + W_R)_x + (u_{xx} + u_{zz}) \tag{1a}$$

$$(v_t + uv_x + vv_z) = -(p + W_V + W_R)_z + (v_{xx} + v_{zz}) \tag{1b}$$

together with the incompressibility condition

$$u_x + v_z = 0 \tag{1c}$$

where u and v are respectively the tangential and normal velocities in the Cartesian coordinate system (x,z). The suffices x and z indicate differentiation while p is the mechanical pressure. The van der Waals potential at a point $\mathbf{r}$ due to other points $\mathbf{r}'$ in space is given by [8]:

$$W_V(\mathbf{r}) = \int \Lambda_0/(|\mathbf{r} - \mathbf{r}'|)^6 \rho(\mathbf{r}')\, d\mathbf{r}' \tag{2a}$$

with the dimensionless London constant Λ_0. The attractive van der Waals potential W_V depends on the film thickness h as:

$$W_V = A(h_+ - h_-)^{-3} \tag{2b}$$

where the dimensionless Hamaker constant A can be linked to the dimensional constant A_H as $A = A_H/(h_0^2 \rho v^2)$. The repulsive potential has the following form [8]:

$$W_R(r) = \int P \exp(-(|\mathbf{r} - \mathbf{r}'|)/L_R)\rho(\mathbf{r}')\, d\mathbf{r}' \tag{3}$$

where P is the amplitude of the repulsion and L_R the decay length depending of the type of molecules considered (glycocalyx, free polymer, receptor ...).

At the free interfaces $h_\pm(x,t)$, we have the following boundary conditions:

a normal momentum balance, in which the *capillary force* (involving the surface tension T) is balanced by the normal stress exerted on either sides of the surface;

a tangential momentum balance, in which the *Marangoni force* (involving the gradient of surface tension) is balanced by the tangential stress exerted by the adjacent bulk phases;

electrostatic boundary conditions if the surfaces are charged (continuity of surface potential and discontinuity of electric field);

kinematic boundary conditions

$$v = h_{\pm t} + h_{\pm x} u \tag{4}$$

where v and u are respectively the normal and tangential velocity;

a surface mass balance, if the surface bears surfactants molecules. We will give explicitly this condition, since it will be used in the following:

$$\Gamma_t = -(\Gamma u)_x + (D_s/v)\Gamma_{xx} + F(\Gamma) \tag{5}$$

The r.h.s. of this equation involves surface convection, surface diffusion and reaction terms, respectively, for the surfactants. D_s is the surface diffusion coefficient of surfactants.

Last, the perturbations at the two surfaces are symmetric for the squeezing mode in which

$$h_+(x, t) = -h_-(x, t)$$

The conditions for the SQ mode at the center of the film $z = 0$ are then:

$$u_z = v = 0 \tag{6}$$

A long wavelength approximation is used in a nonlinear theory to obtain successive approximations to the solutions of the equations of motion (1). The solutions derived for each component of the velocity field will then be substituted in the kinematic equation (4) and in the conservation equation (5). We formalize the long wavelength theory by rescaling the variables with a small parameter ε inversely proportional to the wavelength of the disturbance which is supposed to be much larger than the film thickness. We define thus new dimensionless rescaled variables as follows:

$$
\begin{aligned}
X &= \varepsilon x & Z &= z \\
U &= u/\varepsilon & V &= v/\varepsilon^2 \\
t &= \varepsilon^2 t & P &= p/\varepsilon^2 & H &= h
\end{aligned}
\tag{7}
$$

The rescaled variables and derivatives with respect to the upper case variables are all of unit order as $\varepsilon \to 0$. Approximate solutions of this new system of equations can be obtained by introducing the following regular perturbation expansion for U, V and P into Eqs. (1)–(6)

$$(U, V, P) = (U_0, V_0, P_0) + \varepsilon^2(U_1, V_1, P_1) + \cdots \tag{8}$$

At lower orders of ε, we obtain a simple model describing the evolution of free films with insoluble surfactants thanks to three coupled NEE for the thickness h of the film, the concentration Γ of the surfactants and the tangential velocity u of the fluid in the film, i.e.

$$h_t = -(uh)_x \tag{9a}$$

$$\Gamma_t = \Gamma_{xx}/Sc - (\Gamma u)_x \tag{9b}$$

$$(u_t + uu_x - Th_{xxx} + (A/h^3)_x - (P\exp(-(h-d)/L_R))_x)h = (-M\Gamma + 4hu_x) \tag{9c}$$

with the Schmidt number $Sc = D_s/v$ and d is a cut-off distance depending on the repulsive interaction. The dimensionless parameters used are the Marangoni number M, the tension T, the Hamaker constant A and the repulsive parameters P and L_R.

Linear stability analysis, which is restricted to situations where the vertical displacement of the thin film surface is small compared to the thickness of the film which again must be small compared to the wavelength of the disturbance, is applied below because of the guidance provided by its analytical solutions. A complete linear stability analysis of Eqs. (9) can be found in [15]. Numerical solutions will be described afterwards for the high amplitude nonlinear dynamic behavior of an unstable aqueous film between two membranes [14,15].

In the linear analysis below, we concentrate on the stability of Eq. (9a). The development, with time t, of a single-frequency vertical disturbance (of initial amplitude delta) of the surface is described by $h = 1/2 + delta.\exp(\omega t + ikx)$ where w (the sum of the real and virtual angular frequencies) is the complex angular frequency of the perturbation and k is its wavenumber. If w_R, the real part of w, is negative the disturbance will die out with time and the system is stable, if w_R is positive the displacement will grow exponentially and the interface is unstable. Dimitrov [24], as part of an analysis of squeezing mode stability for a thin film where the resistance to deformation was effected by bending elasticity B and membrane tension T constructed an equation for the component of the hydrodynamic pressure due to wave motion of amplitude z in the film. Ruckenstein and Jain [25] and Prevost and Gallez [13] isolated conditions for bending and squeezing mode development for a charged aqueous film with tangentially immobile surfaces. Gallez and Coakley [8] generalized these results for the case of a nonthinning aqueous layer between two interacting cells (for $M = 0$) to give the following expression for w (in dimensional form) [Eq. (10) is derived from a general viscoelastic approach, taking into account the intrinsic bending elasticity of the membrane considered as a complex two-dimensional surface.]:

$$\omega = (h^3k^2/24\mu)(2\,dP_T/dh - k^2\sigma_T - k^4B) \tag{10}$$

where h is the thickness of the undisturbed film, $k = 2\pi/\lambda$ with λ as the disturbance wavelength, μ is the film viscosity and B is the membrane bending modulus. The total surface tension $\sigma_T = 2\sigma_S + \sigma_R + \sigma_A$ with σ_S as the pure surface tension and σ_R and σ_A as the contributions of repulsive and attractive interactions to surface tension. The total or net disjoining pressure P_T is the sum of the different normal membrane–membrane interaction pressures due, for instance, to the van der Waals (P_W), electrostatic (P_E), hydration (P_H), glycocalyx stereo-repulsion (P_R) and dissolved-macromolecule induced attraction (P_A). The criterion for a positive growth rate w and thus for growth of a squeezing mode instability is that the second bracketed term of Eq. (10) should be positive. Therefore the squeezing mode stability criterion is given by:

$$k^2\sigma_T + k^4 B - 2\, dP_T/dh > 0 \tag{11a}$$

It can be seen from criterion (11a) that an aqueous intermembrane film is more likely to be stable when bounded by membranes of high surface tension and/or high bending elasticity. The stabilizing contributions of these parameters is reduced when k is small, i.e., at long wavelength ($k = 2\pi/\lambda$). The dependence on intercellular water layer thickness h of a number of the contributions $P(h)$ to the net normal interaction pressure P_T can be described, excluding the case of van der Waals attraction, by terms of the form

$$P(h) = P_0 \cdot \exp(-h/L_0) \tag{11b}$$

where P_0 is a constant and L_0 is a characteristic length for the interaction. When the pressure is repulsive (P_0 positive) the contribution of the first derivative of $P(h)$ terms as in Eq. (11a) (or indeed for any function where repulsion increases with decreasing separation) to Criterion (11a) is positive and therefore stabilizing. When the pressure is attractive the contribution is destabilizing. The derivative dP_T/dh of disjoining pressure is the second derivative of the net interaction potential so that a high positive curvature of the interaction potential profile will be destabilizing.

The wavelength which will dominate disturbance growth in an unstable film is obtained by differentiating w [Eq. (10)] with respect to k and setting $d\omega/dk = 0$ to give

$$\lambda = 2\pi[\sigma_T/dP_T/dh]^{0.5} \tag{12a}$$

when B in criterion (11) can be ignored compared with σ_T and

$$\lambda = 2\pi[B/dP_T/dh]^{0.25} \tag{12b}$$

when σ_T can be ignored compared with B. When a squeezing wave of wavelength λ grows exponentially on the intercellular water, it follows that the membrane will make localized contact at points separated by the distance λ along the membrane. If the formation of localized membrane contacts is to be described as an interfacial instability phenomenon then the experimentally determined intercontact distances should be a measure of λ. It follows also from Eq. (12) that, where it is possible to quantify the dP_T/dh at the onset of growth of the dominant instability, a log–log plot of λ against dP_T/dh should

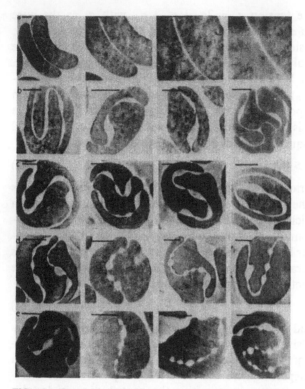

FIG. 5 Transmission electron micrographs of the contact seams of erythrocytes adhered in suspension in 2% w/v 450 kD dextran following pretreatment with 0.5 mg/ml pronase for different times: Row (a): control cells (no pronase pretreatment) showing, at different magnifications, the continuous parallel membrane seam between adhering cells. Rows (b) 0.5 min–1.0 min pronase pretreatment (charge removal (CR = 27%); (c) 5 min pretreatment (CR = 46%); (d) 25 min (CR = 53%) and (e) 2*h* (CR = 56%). Bars represent 1 μm (row a) and 2 μm (rows b–e) [27].

have a slope of -0.5 or -0.25 when membrane reunion σ_T or bending modulus B, respectively, to determine the outcome of the membrane interaction. The relative importance of stretching and bending resistance is of general interest in the understanding of membrane interactions and will be discussed in more detail hereafter.

2. Comparison with Experiments on Red Blood Cells

An estimation of some dynamical parameters is already possible, in order to check the relevance of the interfacial instability approach to bioadhesion. We will perform it using experiments on aggregation of red blood cells in the presence of polymers [8,9].

(a) *Topology of Adhesive Contact Seam.*   Two types of seam geometry have been identified in molecular-induced adhesion of erythrocytes. In one type the membranes of adhered cells are parallel with each other along the seam of contact. In the second case contact occurs at spatially periodic local points which are separated by regions where the membranes are not in close contact. The seam topology and its dependence on experimental conditions is given below for different macromolecules:

Cells in dextran.   The cell–cell contact seams formed on suspending normal human erythrocytes in dextran solutions is usually made up of parallel membranes, an example of which is shown in Fig. 5 (row a) for cells exposed to 2% w/v 450 kD dextran. However when the cell surface is treated with pronase before exposure to dextran, spatial periodicity of contact regions is observed as shown in Fig. 5 (rows b–e). The effect on contact separation of dextran concentration and molecular weight and of pronase concentration and duration of enzyme pretreatment of the cells has been examined in detail [26, 27]. The principal results were that: (i) plane parallel contacts occurred when control cells were exposed to dextran concentrations of 4% w/v and lower; and (ii) spatially periodic contact patterns were a feature of almost all cases where pronase pretreated cells were exposed to dextran (Table 2). Experimental procedures that increased attractive interactions (e.g., increase in dextran concentration or pretreatment time) led to a transition from parallel membrane contact through a long (> 1.8 μm) to a medium and finally short limiting separation distance of about 0.7 μm.

Cells in polylysine.   Spatially periodic contact occurs in all cases when normal erythrocytes are exposed to polylysine [28] or polyarginine, above the adhesion threshold. Figure 6a shows a regular pattern of contact in a flat cell-doublet. Figure 6b shows that the pattern occurs in cells in partial contact only in the region of cell overlap. Regular spacing of contact regions between cells in a polylysine induced clump are shown in the transmission electron microcopy shows (Fig. 6c). The wavy profile is confined to areas where cell surfaces oppose each other, i.e., the erythrocyte membrane on the outside of the clump shows no undulation. The scanning electron micrograph of fixed cell clumps which were sheared to expose the contact surface (Fig. 6d) confirm, with Fig. 6c, that the pattern is confined to opposite discrete regions of the cell surface. While control erythrocytes adhered in polylysine always gave spatially periodic contact it was found that the separation distance increased and the extent of adhesion decreased following mild decrease in sialic acid (polylysine interaction site) on the surface of neuraminidase pretreated cells (Table 2).

The lateral separation distance of polylysine contacts is sensitive to polylysine concentration only when close to the threshold concentration for adhesion. The separation rapidly reaches a limiting lower value of about 0.8 μm as polycation concentration increases.

TABLE 2 Lateral Separation of Contact Regions for Erythrocytes which Have Been Adhered by Different Macromolecules

Macromolecule mass (kD), conc. (% w/v)	Enzyme pretreatment	Constraint	Effect on net attraction (P_T)	Separation distance (μm)
Dextran				
450, 2%–8%	P	Extent of pronase pretreatment	Increase	3.4–0.8
20, 3%–8%	P	Increased dextran concentration	Increase	1.4–0.8
72, 6%	P	Decreased ionic strength	Decrease	$1.0 \rightarrow 1.5$
Polylysine				
228, $10^{-4} \rightarrow$	C	Increased polylysine concentration	Increase	1.5–0.8
20, 10^{-3}	N	Depleted polylysine binding sites	Decrease	0.8–1.6
Lectins				
WGA, 10^{-4}	C	N.A.[a]	N.A.[a]	0.84
con A, 10^{-2}	P	N,A.[a]	N.A.[a]	0.66
con A, 10^{-2}	N	N.A.[a]	N.A.[a]	0.5

The cell glycocalyx was, in some cases, subjected to enzyme pretreatment. Where a range of lateral separations is given the controlling variable is identified, together with its effect of the net intermembrane attraction. The enzyme notation P, N, C is for Pronase, Neuraminidase, Control [9].
[a] Not applicable in the absence of published studies of contact separation as a function of an interaction variable.

Cells in lectin solutions. Darmani and her colleagues investigated the seam of contact formed during agglutination by the lectins (WGA) and (con A) [29]. In contrast to the rapid (< 1.0 s) completion of erythrocyte adhesion in polymer solutions, the area of contact of erythrocytes agglutinating in solutions of the lectins wheat germ agglutinin and concanavalin A spread slowly over times of the order of 2 h [29]. The contact spreading proceeded by the formation of spatially periodic contacts.

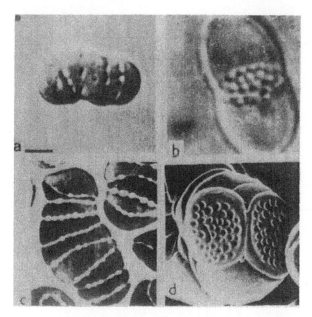

FIG. 6 Light micrographs showing spatial periodicity of contacts in erythrocytes (a) treated with 5 mg/ml 275 kD polylysine [98], (b) partially overlapping following exposure to 20 mg/ml 14 kD polylysine, (c) transmission electron micrograph of cells treated as in (b), (d) scanning electron micrographs of cell contact surfaces exposed by shearing of glutaraldehyde fixed cell clumps (b–d, [28]).

For those three cases, the first parameter to estimate is the order of magnitude of the dominant wavelength. Using Eq. (12a) with a total interfacial tension of the order of 10^{-1} mN/m (Table 1), and an estimate of dP_T/dh at the onset of the instability (equality sign in Eq. (11)), we obtain a dominant wavelength $\lambda \approx 0.63$ μm, which is of the same order of magnitude as the average spacing between contact regions of periodic patterns (≈ 0.8 μm) produced by polycation adhesion of erythrocytes [8,9]. It is also comparable to the order of magnitude of the damped surface waves observed during flickering of red blood cells ≈ 0.59 μm [30]. The same estimation is obtained using Eq. (12b) with a bending modulus of the order of 1.8×10^{-16} mN/m (Table 1).

(b) Dependence of Lateral Contact Separation Distance on Polymer Concentration. The lateral contact separations which were detected had an upper limit of about 3.5 μm, set by the 7–8 μm diameter of the discoid erythrocyte, and a lower limit of about 0.7 μm. The lateral contact separation dependence on polymer concentration is shown in Fig. 7 for pronase pretreated cells in dextrans of a number of different molecular weights. The slope of the log–log plot was -0.62 and was independent of dextran molecular mass. Different pronase

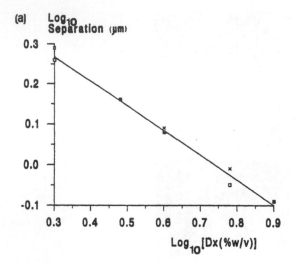

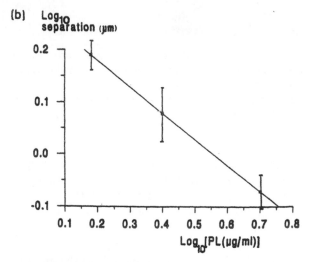

FIG. 7 The polymer concentration dependence of the average intercontact distance on the adhesion seam of erythrocytes exposed to polymers: (a) cells pretreated with 0.5 mg/ml pronase for 60, 20 or 15 min and exposed to ($\times$) 20 kD, ($\blacksquare$) 72 kD or ($\square$) 450 kD dextran, respectively. (The 72 kD data are from [21], the remaining data are from [26]). (b) Normal erythrocytes exposed to 228 kD polylysine. The error bars are 95% confidence limits on wavelength determinations from a single suspension [21].

pretreatments were carried out to modify the cell surface interactions for the molecular masses shown in Fig. 7 so that the contact separations would fall within the above 3.5–0.7 μm limits for each molecular mass. The similar slopes observed for the different dextran molecular masses in Fig. 7 then did not imply that the change in interaction itself was independent of molecular mass. The slope of the log–log plot of the dependence of lateral separation of contact regions on polylysine concentration for normal erythrocytes was -0.50 [9].

Figure 7 then gives the relationships between dominant wavelength and dextran [DX] and polylysine [PL] concentrations respectively as

$$\lambda = C^{DX} \cdot [DX]^{-0.62} \tag{13a}$$

and

$$\lambda = C^{PL} \cdot [PL]^{-0.50} \tag{13b}$$

Changes in polymer concentration, the only constraint varied in obtaining the intercontact spacings for each subset of data in Fig. 7, can be expected to modify the coefficient P_0 rather than the characteristic length L_0 in Eq. (11b). The dominant wavelength would then, for a fixed value of h, change with the coefficient of P_A, through the contribution of the latter to P_T in dP_T/dh.

(c) *Electrostatic Effects on Lateral Separation of Dextran-Induced Contacts in Erythrocyte–Erythrocyte Adhesion.* The contact seam topology in erythrocyte–erythrocyte adhesion changes from plane parallel to localized spatially periodic contact regions when the cells are pretreated with neuraminidase or with pronase. The contact separation distance decreases with increasing pronase pretreatment. For a given surface charge removal by enzymic pretreatment the lateral contact separation was less for pronase than for neuramidinase pretreated cells. This result was in agreement with a much earlier conclusion that, in addition to modifying cell–cell interaction by reducing electrostatic repulsion, pronase pretreatment also reduced repulsion by removing steric hinderances to adhesion. While the above contact separation results were in agreement with the general conclusion (Table 2) that a net increase in attractive interactions led to a decrease in λ it was not possible to quantitatively separate the electrostatic and stereorepulsion consequences of the two enzyme pretreatments. An approach was adopted in which cells were pretreated with a fixed pronase regime (so that stereo-repulsion or other non-electrostatic effects of pronase pretreatment remained (constant) and the consequences of changing ionic strength on contact separation were examined.

The lateral separation of contact regions increased as ionic strength was decreased from 0.150 to 0.95. Ionic strength dependent changes in the stability criterion (11a) were taken as arising from changes in (i) the electrostatic repulsive contribution P_E of the remaining surface charge to the net interaction P_T and (ii) the negative contribution of the electrical free energy of formation of the double layer to the membrane tension. Calculations for cells in 145 mM saline showed [21] that the free energy of formation of the double layer makes the net electrostatic contribution to the stability criterion destabilizing for values of $h > 10$ nm and that electrostatic repulsion dominates to give a net stabilizing contribution of values of $h < 10$ nm. The dependence of lateral contact separation (λ) on change $D(EI)$ in the ionic strength contribution to the stability criterion was taken to be of a form

$$\lambda = 2\pi(S)^M(D(EI))^{-M} \tag{14}$$

where S becomes s_T or B and M becomes 0.5 or 0.25 for membrane bending or tension controlled mechanisms, respectively. A restricted set of allowed combinations of M and S were obtained from linear regressions of $\log(\lambda)$ against $\log(D(EI))$ for values (in the range 13–2 nm) of the normal separation distances h at which the dominant instability began to grow. The set included S values close to published values for membrane bending or membrane tension when $M = 0.25$ or 0.50, respectively [21]. It was concluded that, for ionic strength dependent effects, within the limits of linear theory and the assumption of a fixed film thickness for the growth of instability, experimental results were consistent with an instability mechanism but did not resolve in favour of membrane bending or tension control.

The second parameter which allows a test of the validity of the interfacial hypothesis is the maximum rate of growth of the instability. The rate of development of the fluctuations will be given by the fastest rate of growth (for which $dw/dk = 0$). Equation (10) shows immediately that this rate of growth will be inversely proportional to the viscosity of the intercellular layer. For an aqueous intercellular layer, the viscosity of pure water ($\mu = 10^{-2}$ poises (i.e., g/cm.s)) will lead to a fastest rate of growth of 3×10^3/s. This is certainly an overestimation, since the viscosity of the intercellular layer is enhanced by the presence of the glycocalyx. A higher viscosity $\mu = 1$ poise would lead to a fastest rate of growth of the order of 10/s (see Fig. 8). In this case, the time of the development of the instability, which is the inverse of the rate of growth, will be of the order of 0.1 s. This estimate is in good agreement with experimental observations for the development of periodic patterns between erythrocytes [8,9].

B. Cell–Substratum or Vesicle–Substratum Adhesion (Case B)

1. Hydrodynamic Model and Linear Stability Analysis

Let us now consider cell–substratum or vesicle–substratum interactions, where the thin aqueous film has a free surface and a rigid surface on the solid substratum (see Fig. 9). We will refer to this case as case B. More precisely, region I is again the intracellular (or intravesicular) fluid, region II is the thin liquid film between the cell (vesicle) and the substratum, and region III is the solid support.

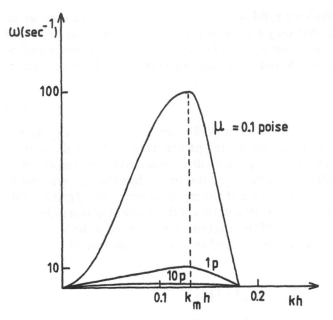

FIG. 8 Rate of growth of the SQ mode as a function of the dimensionless wavenumber kh, for several values of the viscosity of the intercellular layer [8].

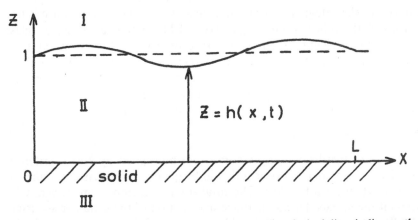

FIG. 9 Sketch of a film on a solid substrate. The dashed line indicates the mean position of the free surface. For the case of cell–substrate adhesion, region I is the intracellular fluid, II is the thin liquid film between the cell and the substrate, and region III is the solid support.

For the case of a film on a solid substratum, Eqs. (1)–(6) are the same as for the case of a free film but only for the upper free surface $h_+(x, t)$. It is now more natural to take the lower rigid surface at $z = 0$. Since the lower surface $h(x, t)$ is rigid, Eq. (6) is replaced by a no-slip condition at the lower surface $z = 0$:

$$u = v = 0 \tag{15}$$

This change in the boundary conditions profoundly affects the velocity field in the film. The choice of the scaling for the parameter $A = O(1)$ is dictated by the new condition (15) which allows one to determine directly the velocity field at zero order. This different scaling is justified by the fact that the gradient of pressure, the van der Waals forces and the repulsive forces are playing a role at leading order allowing a complete solution of the problem at this order.

We end thus with a set of 2 NEE governing the position of the free surface and the surfactants concentration, instead of 3 NEE in the case of a free film [15]:

$$h_t = [M\Gamma_x h^2/2 - \phi_x h^3/3 - Th_{xxx} h^3/3]_x \tag{16a}$$

$$\Gamma_t = \Gamma_{xx}/Sc + [M\Gamma_x \Gamma h - \Gamma\phi_x h^2/2 - \Gamma Th_{xxx} h^2/2]_x \tag{16b}$$

with

$$\phi(x, t) = -A/h^3 + P \exp(-(h - d)/L_R) \tag{16c}$$

For this case, a complete linear and nonlinear analysis was performed [15]. The nonlinear aspects will be described in more details in the following. This case enters into the category of asymmetrical systems, where one surface is free to deform and the other is more rigid like red blood cells adhering on glass [20]. Other systems sharing this common property are host–prey contacts during phagocytosis, erythrocyte–yeast interaction in the presence of polylysine or amoebae interacting with cells [8]. This case will also describe the adhesion of lipid vesicles on supported membranes [22].

The linear stability analysis gives the following criterion:

$$k^2\sigma_T + k^4 B - dP_T/dh > 0 \tag{17}$$

The derivative of the disjoining pressure is not multiplied by 2 as is criterion (11a), so that the dominant wavelength will be greater in the case of a film on solid support than for a free film. The total surface tension σ_T must here take into account the surface tension (surface free energy) of the solid surface itself, so that different stability regimes should be obtained for different types of solid support. For low surface energies of the support, the linear analysis will lead to a dominant wavelength of the same order of magnitude as for cell–cell interactions.

2. Comparison with Red Blood Cell Adhesion to Glass

For cells exposed to polylysine and then allowed to settle on glass, scanning electron microscopy has revealed patterns with a typical periodicity of 1 μm [20]. The periodic distance decreases with polycation concentration, demonstrating also a decrease in lateral separation of contact points with increasing net attraction.

In these experiments the cells were weakly attached to the glass by polylysine of a low molecular mass (1.5 kD) selected so that undulations of the cell dimple were not inhibited, as was the case with higher molecular mass polylysine. It has been shown by light microscopy that the edge-of-cell contacts formed when erythrocytes interact with glass in the presence of polylysine are regularly spaced. The underside of the attached erythrocytes was also examined by scanning electron microscopy. In this technique erythrocytes on glass coverslips were fixed, dehydrated and dried in preparation for electron microscopy. The dried coverslips were etched with a diamond. The diagonal etched line stopped at the edges of the small area covered by red blood cells so that the cells were not disturbed by the diamond. The coverslips were then snapped along the centre exposing the erythrocyte–glass contact regions. This technique showed that the undersurfaces of control red blood cells which had settled on glass were relatively smooth with some evidence of slight rippling but no suggestions of spatially periodic patterns. In contrast erythrocytes in suspension in 1.0 or 5.0 mg/ml 193 or 205 kD polylysine made contact seams with the glass which were interrupted by patterns of concavities on the erythrocyte underside (Fig. 10). The mean lateral separations of the concavities were 1.5 and 0.98 μm for cells in 1.0 and 5.0 mg/ml polylysine, respectively. The mean spacing for cells in 5.0 mg/ml was similar to that measured for spacing on the contact seam of erythrocytes in cell agglutinates at the same polycation concentration [28]. The result that lateral separation distance decreased with increasing polycation concentration for erythrocyte–glass interaction is consistent with the result for the concentration dependence of contact separation in erythrocyte–erythrocyte adhesion.

Further experiments have still to be performed, for the case of erythrocyte adhesion to glass, especially by varying the adhesiveness of the solid support. However, we may already advance the fact that the interfacial stability theory provides also here a coherent explanation of the localized contacts points between the cells and the substrate (case B).

Agglutination of a yeast with a human erythrocyte in the presence of polylysine shows also periodic patterns of wavelength ≈ 0.9 μm in the interaction zone [9].

3. Lipid Vesicle Adhesion to Supported Membranes

The behavior of unilamellar vesicle systems interacting with carefully designed substrata has recently been examined microscopically [22], in relation to

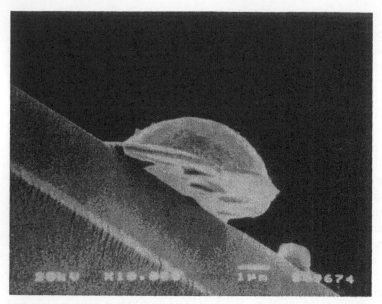

FIG. 10 Scanning electron micrographs of the undersides of erythrocytes which were exposed by cracking the glass substratum following settling of cells on the glass. The saline contains 5.0 mg/ml 193 kD polylysine [courtesy of W. T. Coakley].

membrane adhesion. A model system was established consisting of partially charged giant lipid vesicles and an oppositely charged supported membrane. The adhesion is controlled by charging the supported membrane through pH changes. It has been shown by interferometry that adhesion induced segregation of charged lipids in one of the membrane in the contact zone. This leads to patches of tight contact and blisters. There is a pH threshold for blister formation. Work is now in progress to describe these blisters as patterns in the thin liquid film forming the contact zone. The change in the membrane–membrane pressure is due here to a change in the electrostatic disjoining pressure P_E. Preliminary results are in agreement with the previous conclusions of the interfacial stability theory that a decreased repulsion leads to a transition from parallel membrane contact to a spatially periodic contact.

On the other hand, previous results on liposome fusion [31] show also patterned indentations just before fusion. Indeed, during proton-induced fusion (pH 5.3) of oleic acid PA oligolamellar giant vesicles, quick-freezing freeze-fracture electron micrographs shows a range of intermediate forms with patterns of 100 nm scale circular indentation.

As close membrane–membrane contact is a prerequisite to membrane fusion, these results together with results on lipid vesicle adhesion, suggest that oligolamellar and multilamellar liposomes provide new applicable models to test instability theory.

C. Role of a Specific Chemical Reaction (Case C)

When the adhesion is mediated by specific membrane molecules (proteins) reacting with binding sites on the substratum, it becomes important to describe explicitly the dynamics of receptor–ligand interactions. We will refer to this case as case C. However, here the dynamical approach clarifies the time development of the adhesion processes, and the dynamics of the receptors. The role of a surface chemical reaction between receptors on the membrane and binding sites on the substrate [16] was also treated recently in a nonlinear analysis.

Let us summarize this latter case, which is the most relevant for bio-adhesion: A reversible surface chemical reaction is considered between the insoluble surfactant molecules ("receptors") on the free surface and homogeneously distributed binding sites ("ligands") on the substratum (see Fig. 11).

For simple binding kinetics, we can adopt the following reversible scheme:

$$R + S \underset{k_2}{\overset{k_1}{\longleftrightarrow}} C \tag{18}$$

where R is the concentration of free receptor molecules, S the concentration of binding sites and C the concentration of complexes. k_1 and k_2 are the associ-

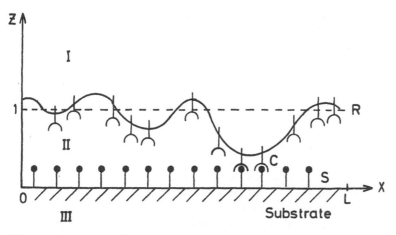

FIG. 11 Sketch of a film on solid substrate with some receptors molecules present on the free surface (membrane). These receptor molecules R can diffuse along the membrane and bind to substrate molecules S to form complexes C.

ation and dissociation kinetic constants, respectively. The following assumptions are taken into account:

1. The free receptor molecules R are surface active, i.e., their local concentration will modify the local gradient of surface tension.
2. The free receptors R are laterally mobile with a surface diffusion coefficient D_s.
3. The complexes C are more or less firmly bound to the fixed substrate molecules of density S_0 so that their diffusion coefficient is set to zero.
4. There is no recruitment of receptor molecules at the boundaries of the contact zone which is of length L.
5. The receptors and sites are uncharged, a provisional simplifying assumption.

After a longwave analysis [16], the following set of dimensionless evolution equations is obtained for the film thickness $h(x, t) = h/h_0$, the receptor concentration $r(x, t) = R/R_0$, and the complex concentration $c(x, t) = C/R_0$ (h_0 and R_0 are the dimensional equilibrium values of the film thickness and receptor concentration):

$$h_t = [Mr_x h^2/2 - \phi_x h^3/3 - Th_{xxx} h^3/3]_x \tag{19a}$$
$$r_t = (D_s/v)r_{xx} + [Mr_x rh - r\phi_x h^2/2 - rTh_{xxx} h^2/2]_x + F(r, c) \tag{19b}$$
$$c_t = -F(r, c) \tag{19c}$$

where the potential term ϕ is given by Eq. (16c). The source term $F(r,c)$ depends on the specific chemical reaction and will be discussed later.

Let us consider the cases where k_1/k_2, the affinity of the binding/dissociation reaction, is a function of the thickness of the film h. The binding step is then favored when the receptors r are close to the substrate s. For nonlinear reaction kinetics, the source term $F(r, c)$ reads:

$$F(r, c) = -k_1(h)r(s_0 - c) + k_2 c \tag{20}$$

with

$$k_1(h) = k_1 \exp(-K(h - h_0))$$

The dimensionless density of fixed binding sites $s_0 = S_0/R_0$.

For $0 \leq h \leq h_0$, the binding kinetics will be favored as the thickness of the film decreases from the equilibrium thickness h_0, with a *binding factor* K. For $h > h_0$, the association kinetics are highly unfavorable at large film thickness. The kinetic constant of dissociation k_2 remains independent of h.

Three roots are obtained in a linear stability analysis: a hydrodynamic root, similar to case B, and two "chemical roots", which control the dynamics of the film, especially for nonlinear chemical reactions (oscillatory solutions) [16] (see Fig. 12).

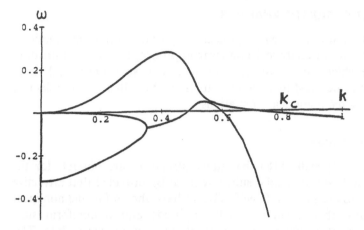

FIG. 12 Real parts of the roots obtained in a linear stability analysis for case C. Three roots appear: a positive real root for $k < k_c$ (the hydrodynamic root), and two complex conjugate roots (the chemical roots), the real part of which can become positive [16].

The following dynamical features have been qualitatively identified, in the case of a cell adhering to a solid substrate bearing fixed sites [16]:

1. The cell may develop a nonuniform morphology in the contact zone for an unstable hydrodynamical mode.
2. The cell will make contact faster at the boundary of the contact zone, so that a tip can be formed at the ring of the adhering cell.
3. A clustering of the receptors can be predicted at the local points of contact.
4. The relative time scales of the hydrodynamical processes and the receptor–ligand kinetics or receptor diffusion will influence the final morphology.

A complete nonlinear analysis of this case, including different nonlinear chemical schema (like autocatalysis), and repulsive forces is still to be done.

The role of specific forces for the adhesion of giant cells on solid supported membranes has been studied recently [11]. Lipopolymers (phospholipids with specific headgroups) were incorporated in the vesicles as artificial glycocalyxes and lock-and-key forces were mimicked by incorporating biotinylated lipids in both membranes mediating strong coupling by streptavidin. It has been shown that adhesion is accompanied by lateral phase separation leading to the formation of domains of tight adhesion (adhesion plaques) separated by area of weak adhesion showing pronounced flickering. A detailed comparison with those experiments remains to be done, but the formation of these adhesion plaques could be explained by the clustering of receptors described in case C.

III. NONLINEAR STABILITY ANALYSIS

Let us now show what a nonlinear approach can provide as new informations. We will first develop an analytical nonlinear approach, based on bifurcation calculus [18,19], which will prove the existence of new spatio-temporal structures (dissipative structures) in a simple situation. We will then complement this approach by some numerical simulations.

A. Bifurcation Calculus

We have shown analytically [18] that stable structures are possible for the case of a thin liquid film on a solid substrate (case B), provided that attractive and repulsive forces are present. Specifically, we have shown for one nonlinear evolution equation that a stable, small amplitude and nonuniform state appears as a result of a change in stability of the uniform basic state. This bifurcation transition is the simplest scenario leading to new patterns in thin liquid films. Those patterns have been observed recently in thin liquid films [32]. The calculus is briefly recalled here. An extension to a bifurcation calculus for the complete system of 2 NEE given by Eq. (14), showing the role of surfactants, was performed afterwards [19].

The evolution equation for the interface $h(x, t)$ without surfactants reads [Eq. (14a) with $M = 0$]:

$$h_t = -1/3[T(h^3 h_{xxx})_x + (h^3 \phi_x)_x] \qquad (21)$$

with

$$\phi(h) = -A/h^3 + P \exp(-(h - d)/L_R)$$

The solution is of the form $h = 1 + u(x, t)$ in the interval $0 < x < L$ with periodic boundary conditions.

The linear problem admits normal modes $u = \exp(ikx + wt)$ with $k = n\pi/L(n = 1, 2, \ldots)$. The condition $w = 0$ evaluated at $n = 1$ gives the bifurcation point $A = A_c$

$$A_c = 1/3[P/L_R \exp(-(1 - d)/L_R) + T\pi^2/L^2] \qquad (22)$$

For $A = A_c + \eta^2 a$ $(a = \pm 1)$ a stationary solution is constructed of the form [33]:

$$u(x, \eta) = \eta u_1(x) + \eta^2 u_2(x) + \cdots \qquad (23)$$

This solution is replaced in the Eq. (20) at the successive orders. At order 1, we obtain $u_1(x) = \alpha \exp(ikx) + \text{c.c.}$ At order 2 we obtain $u_2(x) = (\beta \exp(ikx) + \text{c.c.}) + (\alpha^2 p \exp(2ikx) + \text{c.c.})$, with $p = \phi''/6T(\pi^2/L^2)$. Using the Fredholm alternative [33] at order 3, the amplitude equation for α is found to be:

$$1/6\alpha^2\alpha[\phi''^2/3T + \phi'''\pi^2] + a\pi^2/L^2]\alpha = 0 \qquad (24)$$

The sign of the coefficient of the nonlinear term in Eq. (24) determines the direction of the bifurcation. We define the coefficient C as

$$C = -6(\pi^2/L^2)/(\phi''^2/3T + \phi'''\pi^2) \tag{25}$$

where ϕ'' and ϕ''' are evaluated at $h = 1$.

The leading expression for the solution reads:

$$h = 1 + 2[(A - A_c)C]^{1/2}\sin(\pi x/L) + O(|A - A_c|) \tag{26}$$

Because of the square-root in Eq. (26), the solution only exists for $A \geq A_c$ if $C > 0$ (only exists for $A \leq A_c$ if $C < 0$). Following standard bifurcation theory and since we know that the basic state is unstable as $A > A_c$, the bifurcation leads to a new stable solution if $C > 0$ (*supercritical bifurcation*, i.e., above the critical point), or to an unstable solution if $C < 0$ (*subcritical bifurcation*, i.e., below the critical point). Figure 13 illustrates the two possibilities. Comparison with some numerical simulations will be described hereafter.

This scenario has been applied to spatio-temporal instabilities in thin liquid films (dewetting experiments where small droplets or nanodrops are formed on the solid substrate). The parameters used to check the scenario were relevant for aqueous films without surfactants [18]. An extension of the bifurcation calculus for the complete case of two variables, given by the 2 NEE (14) was recently performed [19]: preliminary results indicate that the bifurcating point A_c is the same, so that the formation of patterns for the variable $h(x, t)$ will be similar. The dynamics of the second variable $\Gamma(x, t)$ is more complex, as will be verified by the numerical simulations.

We are presently applying the complete formalism of 2 NEE for the formation of blisters in vesicles adhering to supported membranes [22], and to red blood cells adhering to glass in the presence of polylysine [20]. In these biological examples, the attractive forces are provided by the usual van der Waals attraction, but attractive and repulsive forces are provided by electrostatic interactions between the two biological surfaces in contact.

B. Numerical Simulations for Nonlinear Evolution Equations

1. Case A

We have solved numerically the set of Eqn (9) using finite difference methods [34]. We will present here the results for a particular case relevant for experiments on erythrocytes adhering in dextran suspension following pronase pretreatment (see Fig. 5). We suppose that the surfaces are tangential immobiles (no diffusion of surfactants), and repulsive electrical forces arise, due to the remaining surface charges at ionic strength of about 0.1 M NaCl. The set of NEE (9) reduces to one nonlinear evolution equation for the thickness h of the aqueous layer between the two cells (SQ mode instability [17]):

$$h_t = -(1/4)(\phi_x h^3 + T h_{xxx} h^2)_x \tag{27a}$$

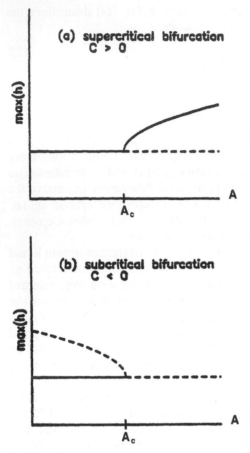

FIG. 13 Bifurcation diagrams. (a) and (b) illustrate the cases of a supercritical and subcritical bifurcation, respectively. Full and broken lines correspond to stable and unstable solutions, respectively [18]. The bifurcation point $A = A_c$ is given by Eq. (22).

with

$$\phi = \phi_E + \phi_N \tag{27b}$$

The electrical part ϕ_E of the disjoining pressure is given by [17]

$$\phi_E = P_E \exp(-h/\lambda_D) \tag{28a}$$

(with P_E proportional to the square of the outer surface potential ϕ_0 and λ_D the dimensionless Debye length) while the nonelectrical part ϕ_N includes the disjoining pressure due to van der Waals forces, steric forces and cross-linking in the presence of dextran [17]:

$$\phi_N = -P_N \exp(-h/\lambda_N) \tag{28b}$$

The results for the simulation are shown in Fig. 14. Periodic boundary conditions are used, while initial conditions are at random. The dimensional parameters values are from Table 1: membrane tension of about 10^- mN/m, outer surface potential $\phi_0 \approx 6$ mV, Debye length ≈ 1 nm. The dimensionless parameter values used in the simulation are $T = 0.03$, $P_E = 0.011$, $P_N = 0.0016$, $\lambda_D = 0.1$ and $\lambda_N = 0.45$. The temporal evolution of the minimum of h is represented on Fig. 14a. After a short time, the evolution of the minimum thickness goes to a stationary value, which represents the nodes of the SQ mode. Figure 14b shows the finals pattern after the dimensionless evolution time $t_F \approx 10^7$. The corresponding dimensional time is of the order of 1 m s, for a viscosity of the aqueous film in the contact zone of about 10^{-2} poises. If we consider as before that the viscosity of the intercellular layer is enhanced by the presence of the glycocalyx, this would lead to a time of about 0.1 s for the development of the pattern, which is a lower bound compared with the predictions of the linear analysis (nonlinearity always accelerate the dynamic processes) and with th experimental observations. In Fig. 14b, we observe about 12 wavelengths for the periodic pattern, for a dimensionless length of the contact zone $L = 150$. This is in agreement with the number of wavelengths observed in the experiments with dextran (Fig. 5, row e). A detailed analysis of the dependence of the wavelength on the ionic strength will be published elsewhere, together with a discussion on the role of the bending [17].

2. Case B

We have solved numerically the set of Eqs. (16), using the same explicit finite difference methods [14,15]. Periodic boundary conditions will be considered here. We select her two different regimes corresponding to the two different situations predicted by the bifurcation calculus.

First, let us take a choice of parameters where the coefficient C defined in (25) is negative. The bifurcating solution will then be subcritical and unstable. We choose the following dimensionless parameters: $A = 5$, $T = 1$, $M = 0.1$, $S_c = 30$, $P = 100$, $d = 0.2$ and $L_R = 0.15$. Using Eq. (22), this corresponds to a critical value of $A_c = 1.23$. For $A > A_c$, the basic situation will be unstable and small perturbations will grow. We choose an initial condition of the form $(h_{in}, \Gamma_{in}) = (\cos(6\pi/L), 1)$. The temporal evolution of the minimum value of h and Γ is represented in Fig. 15a. It is clearly seen that after a short time, the thickness of the film and the concentration will suddenly go to zero (rupture). The spatio-temporal evolution respectively of the height $h(x, t)$ of the film and of the concentration $\Gamma(x, t)$ is represented in Figs. 15b and 15c. The plotted curves show successive spatial situations separated by an interval $\Delta t = 0.036$.

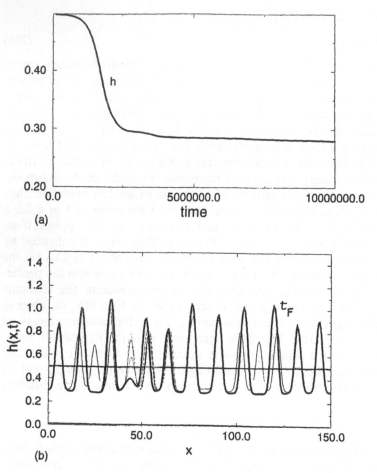

FIG. 14 Numerical simulations for pattern formation between two red blood cells adhering in the presence of dextran. The parameters are chosen to represent data of Fig. 5, row e. The dimensionless parameters are $T = 0.03$, $P_E = 0.011$, $P_N = 0.0016$, $\lambda_D = 0.1$ and $\lambda_N = 0.45$. (a) Temporal evolution of the minimum value of h. (b) Stationary pattern after evolution time t_F. Only one interface is represented. By symmetry, the periodic pattern is similar to the SQ mode predicted by the theory [17].

The dimensionless length of the film is taken to be 18, so that the asymptotic expansion in long wavelengths is justified. The initial perturbation of h is amplified leading to rupture when h reaches zero, keeping the same wavelength (which was an unstable wavelength close to the most unstable one). The concentration of surfactants will also be zero at the points of rupture. The surfactants will thus flow away from the rupture points.

Second, if we take a choice of parameters where the coefficient C is positive,

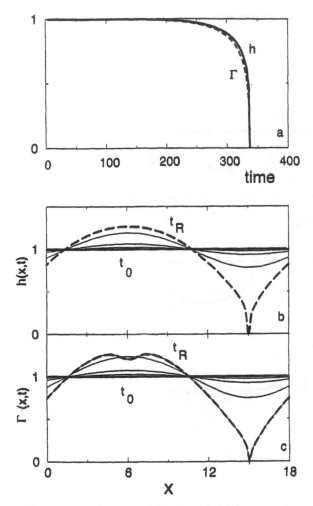

FIG. 15 Rupture of a film on a solid substrate with periodic boundary conditions. The parameters are $A = 5$, $T = 1$, $M = 0.1$, $S_c = 30$, $P = 100$, $d = 0.2$ and $L_R = 0.15$. (a) Temporal evolution of the minimum value of h and Γ. (b) Spatio-temporal evolution of the thickness $h(x, t)$. The curves plotted show successive spatial situations. Periodic initial conditions are imposed at time t_0. The film ruptures at time t_R at the minimum adjacent to the edge. (c) Spatio-temporal evolution of the concentration $\Gamma(x, t)$. At time t_R, the surfactants flow away from the rupture point [19].

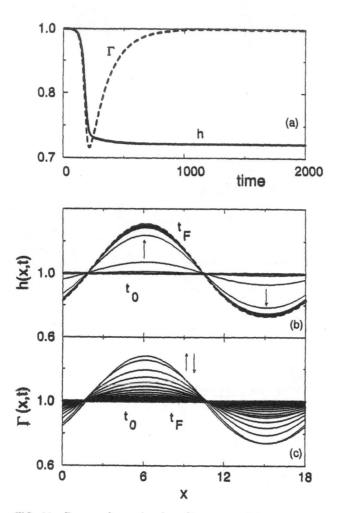

FIG. 16 Pattern formation in a film on a solid substrate with periodic boundary conditions. The parameters are $A = 3.8$, $T = 1$, $M = 0.1$, $S_c = 30$, $P = 280$, $d = 0.2$ and $L_R = 0.15$. (a) Temporal evolution of the minimum value of h and Γ. The minimum value of h saturates to a stationary value different from zero and related to the repulsive forces. The minimum value of Γ goes back to an homogeneous concentration after a transient behavior. (b) Spatio-temporal evolution for the thickness $h(x, t)$. Random initial conditions are imposed (thermal fluctuations). As time evolves, the pattern becomes stationary at time t_F with a final wavelength. (c) Spatio-temporal evolution for the concentration $\Gamma(x, t)$. Starting from an initial homogeneous concentration, the concentrations follows the formation of the pattern, and returns finally to the homogeneous state, due to the diffusion of the surfactants along the surface [19].

we expect that the bifurcating solution for $A > A_c$ will be supercritical and stable. This is confirmed by the numerical simulations. We choose the following parameters: $A = 3.8$, $T = 1$, $M = 0.1$, $S_c = 30$, $P = 280$, $d = 0.2$ and $L_R = 0.15$, so that $A_c = 3.37$. The temporal evolution of the minimum value of h and Γ is represented in Fig. 16a and is completely different from the case of rupture. The dynamics of $h(x, t)$ shows a slow evolution to a stationary state, which will correspond to a stable pattern of the thin film. The dynamics of $\Gamma(x, t)$ shows a complex evolution, characterized by two transient peaks, followed by a slow evolution back to the initial state. The spatio-temporal evolution of the height $h(x, t)$ is represented in Fig. 16b for four different times. The initial condition is a small random perturbation. At time $t = 75$, the film develops two patterns, followed at time $t = 225$ by a selection of wavelengths leading to a single pattern which persists for $t \gg 225$. The change of wavelength is seen in Fig. 16a as a small kink in the time evolution of the minimum of h. The spatio-temporal evolution of the concentration $\Gamma(x, t)$ is represented for four different times in Fig. 16c. For $t = 0$, the concentration was homogeneous. For $t = 75$, two patterns appear, followed by a change of wavelength but the final situation at $t = 1900$ is again homogeneous. The physicochemical explanation is the following: at the onset of the pattern formation, the surfactants will "follow" the dynamics of the film, and will flow away from the regions of minimum thickness. After a certain time, controlled by the time of diffusion of the surfactants along the surface, the concentration will become again homogeneous due to the diffusion. It was shown [19], that if the diffusion of the surfactants is suppressed (diffusion coefficient D_s going to zero), the pattern for the concentration $\Gamma(x, t)$ will remain as the pattern for the height $h(x, t)$.

3. Case C: Oscillatory Solution and Clustering of Receptors

The set of equations (19) have been solved numerically [16] and different situations (stable or unstable) have been simulated. In Fig. 17, we select a simulation where the system is unstable according to the linear stability analysis: the same hydrodynamical root as already identified in thin films (see Fig. 12) is recovered, but coupled now to new chemical roots. Fixed boundary conditions are applied at the boundaries of the contact zone ($x = 0$ and $x = L$). The choosen dimensionless parameters influencing the hydrodynamical mode are $A = 5$, $T = 30$, $M = 1$, and $P_0 = 0$. The choosen dimensionless parameters influencing the chemical mode are the binding factor $K = 30$, the kinetic constants $k_1 = 0.1$ and $k_2 = 0.675$, and the density of binding sites $s_0 = 2.5$. Each numerical simulation starts from the initial condition $(h_{in}, r_{in}, c_{in}) = (h_s \cos(6\pi/L), r_s, c_s)$.

 The spatio-temporal evolution respectively of the height h of the film, the normalized concentration r of receptors and c of the complexes is represented in (Figs. 17b–d). The plotted curves show successive spatial situations separat-

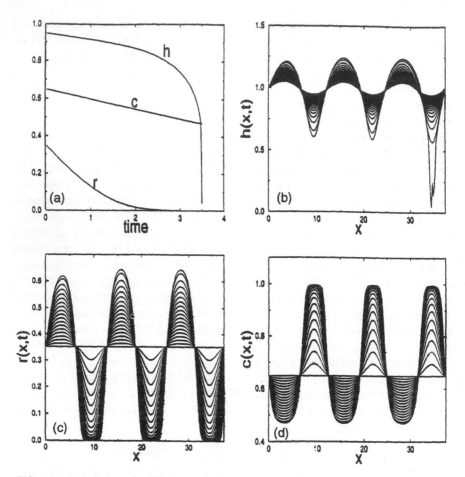

FIG. 17 Dynamics of a film on which the receptors undergo a binding/unbinding reaction with the substrates. (a) Minimum of each of the variables h, r and c on the domain $[0, L]$ as a function of time. (b), (c) and (d) Spatio-temporal evolution respectively of the thickness h of the film, the concentration r of receptors and the concentrations c of complexes between the receptors and the substrates. The curves plotted show successive spatial situations. The initial small perturbation of h is amplified leading to periodic pattern formation for r and c. A clustering of the complexes c is observed at the contact points [16].

ed in time by an interval $\Delta t = 0.2$. The initial perturbation of h is amplified leading to rupture when h reaches zero (no repulsive forces in this simulation). It is to be noted that the film height reaches zero faster close to a boundary ($x = L$ on this simulation) than in the remaining of the contact zone, so that a "tip" is formed at the end of the contact zone. Starting from a homogeneous distribution, the receptors and the complexes evolve at 90° out-of-phase. Complexes accumulate at the location of the minima of h well before the film thickness goes to zero (local contact points). We interpret this dynamics as an aggregation phenomena, where a *clustering of fixed receptors* occurs at locations regularly separated by a distance $\lambda = 2\pi/k$ where k is given by the linear analysis. In this simulation, the timescale of the formation of the complexes is shorter than the timescale of the film rupture (hydrodynamic time). We define the nonlinear rupture time t_{NL} as the time where h goes suddenly to zero (see Fig. 17a). Other timescales are possible (hydrodynamic time is much faster than receptor–ligand kinetics or receptor diffusion), especially when the repulsive interactions are taken into account, so that stationary periodic patterns will emerge from the simulations instead of the rupture of the film [18,19]. The spatial extent of the molecules will then prevent the system reaching the state $h = 0$.

While a complete parametric study remains to be done, the following dynamical features have been qualitatively identified, in the case of a cell adhering to a solid substrate bearing fixed sites:

1. The cell may develop a nonuniform morphology in the contact zone for an unstable hydrodynamical mode.
2. The cell will make contact faster at the boundary of the contact zone, so that a tip can be formed at the ring of the adhering cell.
3. A clustering of the receptors can be predicted at the local points of contact.
4. The relative timescales of the hydrodynamical processes and the receptor–ligand kinetics or receptor diffusion will influence the final morphology.

It is to be noted that the numerical simulations presented in case B and C have been performed using parameters for aqueous films with insoluble surfactants. The simulations for biological systems were only performed for case A (red blood cells adhering with polymers with no diffusion–reaction). The role of proteins in biological membranes and the study of artificial lipid systems (electrostatic adhesion of lipid vesicles on supported membranes, adhesion of lipid vesicles possessing relevant lock-and-key molecules) are in progress.

IV. CONCLUSIONS

This review has concentrated on nonlinear aspects of biomembranes, related to bioadhesion. Some concluding remarks are in order now.

It appears that the biological membrane at the macroscopic level, has intrinsic nonlinear devices, allowing extremely diversified and complex behavior, as well in ionic transport or in bioadhesion. These behaviors seem to be different from the traditional equilibrium approach.

In fact, what can be gained by the localized close contact approach of bio-adhesion developed here? Beyond the exact details of the interfacial instability approach, we have realized that two approaching cells or a cell approaching a solid surface will adapt to the external physicochemical constraints imposed: in some cases, the intercellular layer gives some advantage in adopting a non-uniform morphology, allowing strong cross-bridging of the macromolecules involved. In other cases, when receptors are present, the dynamics of the surface molecules can allow a clustering of the complexes at the local points of contacts. This provides a possible mechanism for the local reorganization of the composite membrane in specific conditions. Experimental studies of adhesion of erythrocytes provide reasonable tests of some predictions of the model, such as the observed wavelength of the patterns or the time of development of the instability. Work is still in progress to refine the analysis, for instance in selecting between a bending or a tension induced mechanism, or in assessing the role of the substrate.

Finally, this review could provide some original ground to pursue future research topics related to other functions of biological membranes, especially at the molecular level. Much work is still to be devoted to these open questions.

ACKNOWLEDGMENTS

The financial support of the Belgian Government (Pôle d'Attraction Inter-universitaire "Phénomènes Nonlinéaires et Processus Irréversibles") is grate-fully acknowledged. The author wishes to thank A. De Wit, M. Kaufman, T. Erneux, E. Ramos de Souza for their collaboration to this work at the ULB and for numerous and useful discussions. She acknowledges also the very fruit-ful collaboration with W. T. Coakley and his team in Cardiff, who performed the experiments on red blood cells described in the paper. The author is grate-ful to E. Sackmann and J. Nardi, from TUM, Garching for introducing her to blistering during adhesion of lipid vesicles.

REFERENCES

1. G. Nicolis and I. Prigogine, *Self-organization in Nonequilibrium Systems*, J. Wiley, New York, 1977.
2. J. D. Murray, *Mathematical Biology*, Springer, Berlin, 1993.
3. R. Larter, Chem. Rev. *90*:355 (1990).
4. J. D. Murray, J. Theor. Biol. *88*:161 (1981).
5. M. Cross and P. C. Hohenberg, Rev. of Modern Physics. *65*:851 (1993).
6. A. Goldbeter, *Biochemical Oscillations and Cellular Rhythms*, Cambridge University Press, 1990.
7. D. Gallez and A. Babloyantz, Biol. Cybern. *64*:381 (1991).
8. D. Gallez and W. T. Coakley, Prog. Biophys. Molec. Biol. *48*:155 (1986).

9. D. Gallez and W. T. Coakley, Heterogeneous Chem. Rev. *3*: 443 (1997).
10. J. Viitala and J. Jarnefelt, Trends Biochem. Sci. *10*: 392 (1985).
11. L. E. Sackmann, Science *271*: 43 (1996).
12. R. Lipowsky and E. Sackmann, Handbook of Biological Physics, Volumes I and II, Elsevier, Amsterdam, 1995.
13. M. Prevost and D. Gallez, J. Chem. Soc. Far. Trans. II. *80*: 517 (1984).
14. M. Prevost and D. Gallez, J. Chem. Phys. *84*: 4043 (1986).
15. A. De Wit, D. Gallez, and C. I. Christov, Physics of Fluids *6*: 3256 (1994).
16. D. Gallez, A. De Wit, and M. Kaufman. J. Colloid Interface Sci. *180*: 524 (1996).
17. W. T. Coakley, D. Gallez, E. Ramos de Souza, and E. Gaucci, Biophys. J., submitted.
18. T. Erneux and D. Gallez, Physics of Fluids *9*: 1194 (1997).
19. E. Ramos de Souza and D. Gallez, Physics of Fluids, *10*: 1804 (1998).
20. N. E. Thomas, W. T. Coakley, and C. Winters, Colloids and Surfaces B: Biointerfaces *6*: 139 (1995).
21. N. E. Thomas and W. T. Coakley, Biophys. J. *69*: 1387 (1995).
22. J. Nardi, T. Feder, R. Bruinsma, and E. Sackmann, Europhys Lett. *37*: 371 (1997).
23. E. Ramos de Souza, C. Anteneodo, N. M. Costa-Pinto, and P. M. Bisch, J. Colloid Interface Sci. *187*: 313 (1997).
24. D. S. Dimitrov, Colloid Polym. Sci. *260*: 1137 (1982).
25. E. Ruckenstein and R. Jain, J. Chem. Soc. Far. Trans. II *70*: 132 (1974).
26. A. J. Baker, W. T. Coakley, and D. Gallez, Eur. Biophys. J. *22*: 53 (1993).
27. W. T. Coakley, L. A. Hewison, and D. Tilley, Eur. Biophys. J. *13*: 123 (1985).
28. H. Darmani and W. T. Coakley, Biochim. Biophys. Acta *1021*: 182 (1990).
29. H. Darmani and W. T. Coakley, Cell Biophys. *18*: 1 (1991).
30. F. Brochard and J. F. Lennon, J. Phys. (Paris) *36*: 134 (1975).
31. N. Duzgunes, R. M. Straubinger, P. A. Baldwin, D. S. Friends, and D. Papahadjopoulos, Biochemistry *24*: 3091 (1985).
32. A. Sharma and A. T. Jameel, J. Colloid Interface Sci. *161*: 190 (1993).
33. G. Nicolis, *Introduction to Nonlinear Science*, Cambridge University Press, Cambridge, 1995.
34. W. H. Press, B. P. Flannery, S. A. Teukolsky, and W. T. Vetterling, *Numerical Recipes*, Cambridge University Press, Cambridge, 1989.

Index